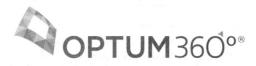

General Surgery/ Gastroenterology

A comprehensive illustrated guide
to coding and reimbursement

2022   optum360coding.com

Publisher's Notice

Coding Companion for General Surgery/Gastroenterology is designed to be an authoritative source of information about coding and reimbursement issues affecting general surgery and gastroenterology procedures. Every effort has been made to verify accuracy and all information is believed reliable at the time of publication. Absolute accuracy cannot be guaranteed, however. This publication is made available with the understanding that the publisher is not engaged in rendering legal or other services that require a professional license.

American Medical Association Notice

Our Commitment to Accuracy

Optum360 is committed to producing accurate and reliable materials.

To report corrections, please email accuracy@optum.com. You can also reach customer service by calling 1.800.464.3649, option 1.

Copyright

Acknowledgments

Marianne Randall, CPC, *Product Manager*
Stacy Perry, *Manager, Desktop Publishing*
Jacqueline Petersen, BS, RHIA, CHDA, CPC, *Subject Matter Expert*
Nichole VanHorn, CPC, CCS-P, *Subject Matter Expert*
Tracy Betzler, *Senior Desktop Publishing Specialist*
Hope M. Dunn, *Senior Desktop Publishing Specialist*
Katie Russell, *Desktop Publishing Specialist*
Kimberli Turner, *Editor*

Technical Editors

Jacqueline Petersen, BS, RHIA, CHDA, CPC

Ms. Petersen has more than 25 years of experience in the health care profession. She has served as Senior Clinical Product Research Analyst with Optum360 developing business requirements for edits to support correct coding and reimbursement for claims processing applications. Her experience includes development of data-driven and system rules for both professional and facility claims and in-depth analysis of claims data inclusive of ICD-10-CM, CPT, HCPCS, and modifiers. Her background also includes consulting work for Optum, serving as a SME, providing coding and reimbursement education to internal and external clients. Ms. Petersen is a member of the American Academy of Professional Coders (AAPC), and the American Health Information Management Association (AHIMA).

Nichole VanHorn, CPC, CCS-P

Ms. VanHorn has more than 20 years of experience in the health care profession. Her areas of expertise include CPT and ICD-10-CM coding in multiple specialties, auditing, and education. Most recently she served as Clinical Auditor for a multi-specialty group. Ms. VanHorn was responsible for the oversight of the physician coding and education section of the Corporate Compliance Program. She has been an active member of her local American Academy of Professional Coders (AAPC) chapter for several years and has also served as an officer.

At our core, we're about coding.

Essential medical code sets are just that — essential to your revenue cycle. In our ICD-10-CM/PCS, CPT®, HCPCS and DRG coding tools, we apply our collective coding expertise to present these code set resources in a way that is comprehensive, plus easy to use and apply. Print books are budget-friendly and easily referenced, created with intuitive features and formats, such as visual alerts, color-coding and symbols to identify important coding notes and instructions — plus, great coding tips.

Find the same content, tips and features of our code books in a variety of formats. Choose from print products, online coding tools, data files or web services.

Your coding, billing and reimbursement product team,

Ryan Nichole Greg LaJuana
       Ken
Jacqui Marianne Denise Leanne
        Anita Debbie Elizabeth Nann
                      Karen

Put Optum360 medical coding, billing and reimbursement content at your fingertips today. Choose what works for you.

📖 Print books

🛠 Online coding tools

📁 Data files

🖥 Web services

Visit us at **optum360coding.com** to browse our products, or call us at **1-800-464-3649, option 1,** for more information.

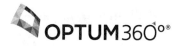

What if you could go back in time?

How much time do you think you spend researching elusive codes? Too much, probably. Time you would like to have back. We can't give time back, but we can help you save it. Our all-in-one coding solutions consolidate specialty coding processes so you can find information more easily and quickly. Each specialty-specific procedure code includes its official and lay descriptions, coding tips, cross-coding to common ICD-10-CM codes, relative value units, Medicare edit guidance, *CPT Assistant®* references, CCI edits and, when relevant, specific reimbursement and documentation tips.

With tools available for 30 specialties, we're sure you'll find the right resource to meet your organization's unique needs, even if those needs are allergy, anesthesia/pain management, behavioral health, cardiology, cardiothoracic surgery, dental, dermatology, emergency medicine, ENT, gastroenterology, general surgery, hematology, laboratory/pathology, nephrology, neurology, neurosurgery, OB/GYN, OMS, oncology, ophthalmology, orthopaedics, pediatrics, physical therapy, plastics, podiatry, primary care, pulmonology, radiology, urology or vascular surgery.

Say good-bye to time wasted digging for those elusive codes.

Your coding, billing and reimbursement product team,

Ryan Nichole Greg LaJuana
Ken Denise Leanne
Jacqui Marianne Elizabeth Nann
Anita Debbie Karen

Put Optum360 medical coding, billing and reimbursement content at your fingertips today. Choose what works for you.

Print books

Online coding tools

Data files

Web services

Visit us at **optum360coding.com** to browse our products, or call us at **1-800-464-3649, option 1,** for more information.

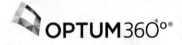

Contents

Getting Started with Coding Companion

Coding Companion for General Surgery/Gastroenterology is designed to be a guide to the specialty procedures classified in the CPT® book. It is structured to help coders understand procedures and translate physician narrative into correct CPT codes by combining many clinical resources into one, easy-to-use source book.

The book also allows coders to validate the intended code selection by providing an easy-to-understand explanation of the procedure and associated conditions or indications for performing the various procedures. As a result, data quality and reimbursement will be improved by providing code-specific clinical information and helpful tips regarding the coding of procedures.

CPT Codes

For ease of use, evaluation and management codes related to General Surgery/Gastroenterology are listed first in the *Coding Companion*. All other CPT codes in *Coding Companion* are listed in ascending numeric order. Included in the code set are all surgery, radiology, laboratory, and medicine codes pertinent to the specialty. Each CPT code is followed by its official CPT code description.

Resequencing of CPT Codes

The American Medical Association (AMA) employs a resequenced numbering methodology. According to the AMA, there are instances where a new code is needed within an existing grouping of codes, but an unused code number is not available to keep the range sequential. In the instance where the existing codes were not changed or had only minimal changes, the AMA assigned a code out of numeric sequence with the other related codes being grouped together. The resequenced codes and their descriptions have been placed with their related codes, out of numeric sequence.

CPT codes within the Optum360 *Coding Companion* series display in their resequenced order. Resequenced codes are enclosed in brackets for easy identification.

ICD-10-CM

Overall, in the 10th revision of the ICD-10-CM codes, conditions are grouped with general epidemiological purposes and the evaluation of health care in mind. Features include icons to identify newborn, pediatric, adult, male only, female only, and laterality. Refer to the ICD-10-CM book for more ICD-10-CM coding information.

Detailed Code Information

One or more columns are dedicated to each procedure or service or to a series of similar procedures/services. Following the specific CPT code and its narrative, is a combination of features. A sample is shown on page ii. The black boxes with numbers in them correspond to the information on the pages following the sample.

Appendix Codes and Descriptions

Some CPT codes are presented in a less comprehensive format in the appendix. The CPT codes appropriate to the specialty are included in the appendix with the official CPT code description. The codes are presented in numeric order, and each code is followed by an easy-to-understand lay description of the procedure.

The codes in the appendix are presented in the following order:

- E/M Services
- Surgery
- Radiology
- Pathology and Laboratory
- Medicine Services
- Category III

Category II codes are not published in this book. Refer to the CPT book for code descriptions.

CCI Edits and Other Coding Updates

The *Coding Companion* includes the list of codes from the official Centers for Medicare and Medicaid Services' National Correct Coding Policy Manual for Part B Medicare Contractors that are considered to be an integral part of the comprehensive code or mutually exclusive of it and should not be reported separately. The codes in the Correct Coding Initiative (CCI) section are from version 27.3, the most current version available at press time. CCI edits are updated quarterly and will be posted on the product updates page listed below. The CCI edits are located in a section at the back of the book. As other CPT (including COVID-related vaccine and administration codes) and ICD-10-CM codes relevant to your specialty are released, updates will be posted to the Optum360 website. The website address is http://www.optum360coding.com/ProductUpdates/. The 2022 edition password is: **CODING22**. Log in frequently to ensure you receive the most current updates.

Index

A comprehensive index is provided for easy access to the codes. The index entries have several axes. A code can be looked up by its procedural name or by the diagnoses commonly associated with it. Codes are also indexed anatomically. For example:

47600   Cholecystectomy;

could be found in the index under the following main terms:

Cholecystectomy
  Open Approach, 47600-47620
OR
Excision
  Gallbladder
    Open, 47600-47620
OR
Gallbladder
  Cholecystectomy, 47600

General Providers

The AMA advises coders that while a particular service or procedure may be assigned to a specific section, it is not limited to use only by that specialty group (see paragraphs two and three under "Instructions for Use of the CPT Codebook" on page xiv of the CPT Book). Additionally, the procedures and services listed throughout the book are for use by any qualified physician or other qualified health care professional or entity (e.g., hospitals, laboratories, or home health agencies). Keep in mind that there may be other policies or guidance that can affect who may report a specific service.

Supplies

Some payers may allow physicians to separately report drugs and other supplies when reporting the place of service as office or other nonfacility setting. Drugs and supplies are to be reported by the facility only when performed in a facility setting.

Professional and Technical Component

Radiology and some pathology codes often have a technical and a professional component. When physicians do not own their own equipment and send their patients to outside testing facilities, they should append modifier 26 to the procedural code to indicate they performed only the professional component.

44705

44705 Preparation of fecal microbiota for instillation, including assessment of donor specimen

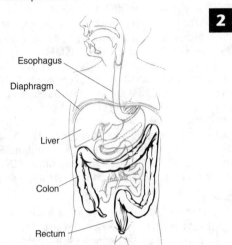

Microbiota is instilled in the digestive tract

Explanation

Fecal microbiota transplantation (FMT) is the process of instilling fecal matter from a donor to a patient to treat a Clostridium difficile (C. diff) infection, most commonly. The donor stool is thinned using a normal saline solution and filtered for use in a nasogastric tube or an enema application. This code includes the screening protocol of the donor specimen for C. diff and other enteric bacterial pathogens and any ova or parasites.

Coding Tips

Do not report 44705 with 74283. For fecal instillation via enema or oro- or nasogastric tube, see 44799. Medicare and some other payers may require G0455 be reported for this service.

ICD-10-CM Diagnostic Codes

A04.71	Enterocolitis due to Clostridium difficile, recurrent
A04.72	Enterocolitis due to Clostridium difficile, not specified as recurrent
K50.011	Crohn's disease of small intestine with rectal bleeding
K50.012	Crohn's disease of small intestine with intestinal obstruction
K50.013	Crohn's disease of small intestine with fistula
K50.014	Crohn's disease of small intestine with abscess
K50.018	Crohn's disease of small intestine with other complication
K50.111	Crohn's disease of large intestine with rectal bleeding
K50.112	Crohn's disease of large intestine with intestinal obstruction
K50.113	Crohn's disease of large intestine with fistula
K50.114	Crohn's disease of large intestine with abscess
K50.118	Crohn's disease of large intestine with other complication
K51.00	Ulcerative (chronic) pancolitis without complications
K51.011	Ulcerative (chronic) pancolitis with rectal bleeding
K51.012	Ulcerative (chronic) pancolitis with intestinal obstruction
K51.013	Ulcerative (chronic) pancolitis with fistula
K51.014	Ulcerative (chronic) pancolitis with abscess
K51.018	Ulcerative (chronic) pancolitis with other complication
K51.80	Other ulcerative colitis without complications
K51.811	Other ulcerative colitis with rectal bleeding
K51.812	Other ulcerative colitis with intestinal obstruction
K51.813	Other ulcerative colitis with fistula
K51.814	Other ulcerative colitis with abscess
K51.818	Other ulcerative colitis with other complication
K55.021	Focal (segmental) acute infarction of small intestine
K55.022	Diffuse acute infarction of small intestine
K55.031	Focal (segmental) acute (reversible) ischemia of large intestine
K55.032	Diffuse acute (reversible) ischemia of large intestine
K55.041	Focal (segmental) acute infarction of large intestine
K55.042	Diffuse acute infarction of large intestine
K58.0	Irritable bowel syndrome with diarrhea
K58.1	Irritable bowel syndrome with constipation
K58.2	Mixed irritable bowel syndrome
K58.8	Other irritable bowel syndrome
K59.01	Slow transit constipation
K59.02	Outlet dysfunction constipation
K59.03	Drug induced constipation
K59.04	Chronic idiopathic constipation
K59.09	Other constipation

Associated HCPCS Codes

G0455	Preparation with instillation of fecal microbiota by any method, including assessment of donor specimen

AMA: 44705 2018,Jan,8; 2017,Jan,8; 2016,Jan,13; 2015,Jan,16

Relative Value Units/Medicare Edits

Non-Facility RVU	Work	PE	MP	Total
44705	1.42	1.72	0.13	3.27
Facility RVU	Work	PE	MP	Total
44705	1.42	0.55	0.13	2.1

	FUD	Status	MUE	Modifiers				IOM Reference
44705	N/A	I	1(3)	N/A	N/A	N/A	N/A	None

* with documentation

Terms To Know

colitis. Inflammation of the colon, caused by an infection or external influences such as laxatives, radiation, or antibiotics.

instillation. Administering a liquid slowly over time, drop by drop.

nasogastric tube. Long, hollow, cylindrical catheter made of soft rubber or plastic that is inserted through the nose down into the stomach, and is used for feeding, instilling medication, or withdrawing gastric contents.

1. CPT Codes and Descriptions

This edition of *Coding Companion* is updated with CPT codes for year 2022.

The following icons are used in *Coding Companion*:

● This CPT code is new for 2022.

▲ This CPT code description is revised for 2022.

✛ This CPT code is an add-on code.

Add-on codes are not subject to bilateral or multiple procedure rules, reimbursement reduction, or appending modifier 50 or 51. Add-on codes describe additional intraservice work associated with the primary procedure performed by the same physician on the same date of service and are not reported as stand-alone procedures. Add-on codes for procedures performed on bilateral structures are reported by listing the add-on code twice.

★ This CPT code is identified by CPT as appropriate for telemedicine services.

The Centers for Medicare and Medicaid Services (CMS) have identified additional services that may be performed via telehealth. Due to the COVID-19 public health emergency (PHE), some services have been designated as temporarily appropriate for telehealth. These CMS approved services are identified in the coding tips where appropriate. Payers may require telehealth/telemedicine to be reported with place of service 02 Telehealth Provided Other than the Patient's Home or 10 Telehealth Provided in Patient's Home and modifier 95 appended. If specialized equipment is used at the originating site, HCPCS Level II code Q3014 may be reported. Individual payers should be contacted for additional or different guidelines regarding telehealth/telemedicine services. Documentation should include the type of technology used for the treatment in addition to the patient evaluation, treatment, and consents.

[ ] CPT codes enclosed in brackets are resequenced and may not appear in numerical order.

2. Illustrations

The illustrations that accompany the *Coding Companion* series provide coders a better understanding of the medical procedures referenced by the codes and data. The graphics offer coders a visual link between the technical language of the operative report and the cryptic descriptions accompanying the codes. Although most pages will have an illustration, there will be some pages that do not.

3. Explanation

Every CPT code or series of similar codes is presented with its official CPT code description. However, sometimes these descriptions do not provide the coder with sufficient information to make a proper code selection. In *Coding Companion*, an easy-to-understand step-by-step clinical description of the procedure is provided. Technical language that might be used by the physician is included and defined. *Coding Companion* describes the most common method of performing each procedure.

4. Coding Tips

Coding tips provide information on how the code should be used, provides related CPT codes, and offers help concerning common billing errors, modifier usage, and anesthesia. This information comes from consultants and subject matter experts at Optum360 and from the coding guidelines provided in the CPT book and by the Centers for Medicare and Medicaid Services (CMS).

5. ICD-10-CM Diagnostic Codes

ICD-10-CM diagnostic codes listed are common diagnoses or reasons the procedure may be necessary. This list in most cases is inclusive to the specialty. Some ICD-10-CM codes are further identified with the following icons:

N Newborn: 0

P Pediatric: 0-17

M Maternity: 9-64

A Adult: 15-124

♂ Male only

♀ Female Only

☑ Laterality

Please note that in some instances the ICD-10-CM codes for only one side of the body (right) have been listed with the CPT code. The associated ICD-10-CM codes for the other side and/or bilateral may also be appropriate. Codes that refer to the right or left are identified with the ☑ icon to alert the user to check for laterality. In some cases, not every possible code is listed and the ICD-10-CM book should be referenced for other valid codes.

6. Associated HCPCS Codes

Medicare and some other payers require the use of HCPCS Level II codes and not CPT codes when reporting certain services. The HCPCS codes and their description are displayed in this field. If there is not a HCPCS code for this service, this field will not be displayed.

7. AMA References

The AMA references for *CPT Assistant* are listed by CPT code, with the most recent reference listed first. Generally only the last six years of references are listed.

8. Relative Value Units/Medicare Edits

Medicare edits are provided for most codes. These Medicare edits were current as of November 2021.

The 2022 Medicare edits were not available at the time this book went to press. Updated 2022 values will be posted at https://www.optum360coding.com/ProductUpdates/. The 2022 edition password is **CODING22**.

Relative Value Units

In a resource based relative value scale (RBRVS), services are ranked based on the relative costs of the resources required to provide those services as opposed to the average fee for the service, or average prevailing Medicare charge. The Medicare RBRVS defines three distinct components affecting the value of each service or procedure:

- Physician work component, reflecting the physician's time and skill

- Practice expense (PE) component, reflecting the physician's rent, staff, supplies, equipment, and other overhead

- Malpractice (MP) component, reflecting the relative risk or liability associated with the service

- Total RVUs are a sum of the work, PE, and MP RVUs

There are two groups of RVUs listed for each CPT code. The first RVU group is for facilities (Facility RVU), which includes provider services performed in hospitals, ambulatory surgical centers, or skilled nursing facilities. The second RVU group is for nonfacilities (Non-Facility RVU), which represents provider services performed in physician offices, patient's homes, or other nonhospital settings. The appendix includes RVU components for facility and non-facility. Because no values have been established by CMS for the Category III codes, no relative value unit/grids are identified. Refer to the RBRVS tool or guide for the RVUs when the technical (modifier TC) or professional (modifier26) component of a procedure is provided.

Medicare Follow-Up Days (FUD)

Information on the Medicare global period is provided here. The global period is the time following a surgery during which routine care by the physician is considered postoperative and included in the surgical fee. Office visits or other routine care related to the original surgery cannot be separately reported if they occur during the global period.

Status

The Medicare status indicates if the service is separately payable by Medicare. The Medicare RBRVS includes:

A   Active code—separate payment may be made

B   Bundled code—payment is bundled into other service

C   Carrier priced—individual carrier will price the code

I   Not valid—Medicare uses another code for this service

N   Non-covered—service is not covered by Medicare

R   Restricted—special coverage instructions apply

T   Paid as only service—These codes are paid only if there are no other services payable under the PFS billed on the same date by the same practitioner. If any other services payable under the PFS are billed on the same date by the same practitioner, these services are bundled into the service(s) for which payment is made.

X   Statutory exclusion—no RVUs or payment

Medically Unlikely Edits

This column provides the maximum number of units allowed by Medicare. However, it is also important to note that not every code has a Medically Unlikely Edit (MUE) available. Medicare has assigned some MUE values that are not publicly available. If there is no information in the MUE column for a particular code, this doesn't mean that there is no MUE. It may simply mean that CMS has not released information on that MUE. Watch the remittance advice for possible details on MUE denials related to those codes. If there is not a published MUE, a dash will display in the field.

An additional component of the MUE edit is the MUE Adjudication Indicator (MAI). This edit is the result of an audit by the Office of the Inspector General (OIG) that identified inappropriate billing practices that bypassed the MUE edits. These included inappropriate reporting of bilateral services and split billing.

There are three MUE Adjudication Indicators.

- 1 Line Edit
- 2 Date of Service Edit: Policy
- 3 Date of Service Edit: Clinical

The MUE will be listed following the MAI value. For example code 11446 has a MUE value of 2 and a MAI value of 3. This will display in the MUE field as "2(3)."

Modifiers

Medicare identifies some modifiers that are required or appropriate to report with the CPT code. When the modifiers are not appropriate, it will be indicated with N/A. Four modifiers are included.

51   Multiple Procedure
Medicare and other payers reduce the reimbursement of second and subsequent procedures performed at the same session to 50 percent of the allowable. For endoscopic procedures, the reimbursement is reduced by the value of the endoscopic base code.

50   Bilateral Procedures
This modifier is used to identify when the same procedure is performed bilaterally. Medicare requires one line with modifier 50 and the reimbursement is 50 percent of the allowable. Other payers may require two lines and will reduce the second procedure.

62*   Two Surgeons
Medicare identifies procedures that may be performed by co-surgeons. The reimbursement is split between both providers. Both surgeons must report the same code when using this modifier.

80*   Assistant Surgeon
An assistant surgeon is allowed if modifier 80 is listed. Reimbursement is usually 20 percent of the allowable. For Medicare it is 16 percent to account for the patient's co-pay amount.

* with documentation

Modifiers 62 and 80 may require supporting documentation to justify the co- or assistant surgeon.

Medicare Official Regulatory Information

Medicare official regulatory information provides official regulatory guidelines. Also known as the CMS Online Manual System, the Internet-only Manuals (IOM) contain official CMS information pertaining to program issuances, instructions, policies, and procedures based on statutes, regulations, guidelines, models, and directives. Optum360 has provided the reference for the surgery codes. The full text of guidelines can be found online at http://www.cms.gov/Regulations-and-Guidance/Guidance/Manuals/.

9.   Terms to Know

Some codes are accompanied by general information pertinent to the procedure, labeled "Terms to Know." This information is not critical to code selection, but is a useful supplement to coders hoping to expand their knowledge of the specialty.

99202-99205

★**99202** Office or other outpatient visit for the evaluation and management of a new patient, which requires a medically appropriate history and/or examination and straightforward medical decision making. When using time for code selection, 15-29 minutes of total time is spent on the date of the encounter.

★**99203** Office or other outpatient visit for the evaluation and management of a new patient, which requires a medically appropriate history and/or examination and low level of medical decision making. When using time for code selection, 30-44 minutes of total time is spent on the date of the encounter.

★**99204** Office or other outpatient visit for the evaluation and management of a new patient, which requires a medically appropriate history and/or examination and moderate level of medical decision making. When using time for code selection, 45-59 minutes of total time is spent on the date of the encounter.

★**99205** Office or other outpatient visit for the evaluation and management of a new patient, which requires a medically appropriate history and/or examination and high level of medical decision making. When using time for code selection, 60-74 minutes of total time is spent on the date of the encounter.

Explanation

Providers report these codes for new patients being seen in the doctor's office, a multispecialty group clinic, or other outpatient environment. All require a medically appropriate history and/or examination. Code selection is based on the level of medical decision making (MDM) or total time personally spent by the physician and/or other qualified health care professional(s) on the date of the encounter. Factors to be considered in MDM include the number/complexity of problems addressed during the encounter, amount and complexity of data requiring review and analysis, and the risk of complications and/or morbidity or mortality associated with patient management. The most basic service is represented by 99202, which entails straightforward MDM. If time is used for code selection, 15 to 29 minutes of total time is spent on the day of encounter. Report 99203 for a visit requiring a low level of MDM or 30 to 44 minutes of total time; 99204 for a visit requiring a moderate level of MDM or 45 to 59 minutes of total time; and 99205 for a visit requiring a high level of MDM or 60 to 74 minutes of total time.

Coding Tips

These codes are used to report office or other outpatient services for a new patient. A medically appropriate history and physical examination, as determined by the treating provider, should be documented. The level of history and physical examination are no longer used when determining the level of service. Codes should be selected based upon the current CPT Medical Decision Making table. Alternately, time alone may be used to select the appropriate level of service. Total time for reporting these services includes face-to-face and non-face-to-face time personally spent by the physician or other qualified health care professional on the date of the encounter. For office or other outpatient services for an established patient, see 99211-99215. For observation care services, see 99217-99226. For patients admitted and discharged from observation or inpatient status on the same date, see 99234-99236. Telemedicine services may be reported by the performing provider by adding modifier 95 to these procedure codes and using the appropriate place of service. Services at the origination site are reported with HCPCS Level II code Q3014.

ICD-10-CM Diagnostic Codes

The application of this code is too broad to adequately present ICD-10-CM diagnostic code links here. Refer to your ICD-10-CM book.

AMA: **99202** 2020,Sep,14; 2020,Sep,3; 2020,Oct,14; 2020,Nov,3; 2020,May,3; 2020,Jun,3; 2020,Jan,3; 2020,Feb,3; 2020,Dec,11; 2019,Oct,10; 2019,Jan,3; 2019,Feb,3; 2018,Sep,14; 2018,Mar,7; 2018,Jan,8; 2018,Apr,9; 2018,Apr,10; 2017,Jun,6; 2017,Jan,8; 2017,Aug,3; 2016,Sep,6; 2016,Mar,10; 2016,Jan,7; 2016,Jan,13; 2016,Dec,11; 2015,Oct,3; 2015,Jan,12; 2015,Jan,16; 2015,Dec,3 **99203** 2020,Sep,3; 2020,Sep,14; 2020,Oct,14; 2020,Nov,3; 2020,May,3; 2020,Jun,3; 2020,Jan,3; 2020,Feb,3; 2019,Oct,10; 2019,Jan,3; 2019,Feb,3; 2018,Sep,14; 2018,Mar,7; 2018,Jan,8; 2018,Apr,10; 2018,Apr,9; 2017,Jun,6; 2017,Jan,8; 2017,Aug,3; 2016,Sep,6; 2016,Mar,10; 2016,Jan,7; 2016,Jan,13; 2016,Dec,11; 2015,Oct,3; 2015,Jan,12; 2015,Jan,16; 2015,Dec,3 **99204** 2020,Sep,14; 2020,Sep,3; 2020,Oct,14; 2020,Nov,12; 2020,Nov,3; 2020,May,3; 2020,Jun,3; 2020,Jan,3; 2020,Feb,3; 2019,Oct,10; 2019,Jan,3; 2019,Feb,3; 2018,Sep,14; 2018,Mar,7; 2018,Jan,8; 2018,Apr,9; 2018,Apr,10; 2017,Jun,6; 2017,Jan,8; 2017,Aug,3; 2016,Sep,6; 2016,Mar,10; 2016,Jan,7; 2016,Jan,13; 2016,Dec,11; 2015,Oct,3; 2015,Jan,16; 2015,Jan,12; 2015,Dec,3 **99205** 2020,Sep,14; 2020,Sep,3; 2020,Oct,14; 2020,Nov,12; 2020,Nov,3; 2020,May,3; 2020,Jun,3; 2020,Jan,3; 2020,Feb,3; 2019,Oct,10; 2019,Jan,3; 2019,Feb,3; 2018,Sep,14; 2018,Mar,7; 2018,Jan,8; 2018,Apr,9; 2018,Apr,10; 2017,Jun,6; 2017,Jan,8; 2017,Aug,3; 2016,Sep,6; 2016,Mar,10; 2016,Jan,7; 2016,Jan,13; 2016,Dec,11; 2015,Oct,3; 2015,Jan,12; 2015,Jan,16; 2015,Dec,3

Relative Value Units/Medicare Edits

Non-Facility RVU	Work	PE	MP	Total
99202	0.93	1.1	0.09	2.12
99203	1.6	1.51	0.15	3.26
99204	2.6	2.04	0.23	4.87
99205	3.5	2.62	0.31	6.43
Facility RVU	Work	PE	MP	Total
99202	0.93	0.41	0.09	1.43
99203	1.6	0.67	0.15	2.42
99204	2.6	1.11	0.23	3.94
99205	3.5	1.54	0.31	5.35

	FUD	Status	MUE	Modifiers				IOM Reference
99202	N/A	A	1(2)	N/A	N/A	N/A	80*	None
99203	N/A	A	1(2)	N/A	N/A	N/A	80*	
99204	N/A	A	1(2)	N/A	N/A	N/A	80*	
99205	N/A	A	1(2)	N/A	N/A	N/A	80*	

* with documentation

99211-99215

▲★**99211** Office or other outpatient visit for the evaluation and management of an established patient that may not require the presence of a physician or other qualified health care professional

★**99212** Office or other outpatient visit for the evaluation and management of an established patient, which requires a medically appropriate history and/or examination and straightforward medical decision making. When using time for code selection, 10-19 minutes of total time is spent on the date of the encounter.

★**99213** Office or other outpatient visit for the evaluation and management of an established patient, which requires a medically appropriate history and/or examination and low level of medical decision making. When using time for code selection, 20-29 minutes of total time is spent on the date of the encounter.

★**99214** Office or other outpatient visit for the evaluation and management of an established patient, which requires a medically appropriate history and/or examination and moderate level of medical decision making. When using time for code selection, 30-39 minutes of total time is spent on the date of the encounter.

★**99215** Office or other outpatient visit for the evaluation and management of an established patient, which requires a medically appropriate history and/or examination and high level of medical decision making. When using time for code selection, 40-54 minutes of total time is spent on the date of the encounter.

Explanation

Providers report these codes for established patients being seen in the doctor's office, a multispecialty group clinic, or other outpatient environment. All require a medically appropriate history and/or examination excluding the most basic service represented by 99211 that describes an encounter that may not require the presence of a physician or other qualified health care professional. For the remainder of codes within this range, code selection is based on the level of medical decision making (MDM) or total time personally spent by the physician and/or other qualified health care professional(s) on the date of the encounter. Factors to be considered in MDM include the number/complexity of problems addressed during the encounter, amount and complexity of data requiring review and analysis, and the risk of complications and/or morbidity or mortality associated with patient management. Report 99212 for a visit that entails straightforward MDM. If time is used for code selection, 10 to 19 minutes of total time is spent on the day of encounter. Report 99213 for a visit requiring a low level of MDM or 20 to 29 minutes of total time; 99214 for a moderate level of MDM or 30 to 39 minutes of total time; and 99215 for a high level of MDM or 40 to 54 minutes of total time.

Coding Tips

These codes are used to report office or other outpatient services for an established patient. A medically appropriate history and physical examination, as determined by the treating provider, should be documented. The level of history and physical examination are no longer used when determining the level of service. Codes should be selected based upon the current CPT Medical Decision Making table. Alternately, time alone may be used to select the appropriate level of service. Total time for reporting these services includes face-to-face and non-face-to-face time personally spent by the physician or other qualified health care professional on the date of the encounter. Code

99211 does not require the presence of a physician or other qualified health care professional. For office or other outpatient services for a new patient, see 99202-99205. For observation care services, see 99217-99226. For patients admitted and discharged from observation or inpatient status on the same date, see 99234-99236. Telemedicine services may be reported by the performing provider by adding modifier 95 to these procedure codes and using the appropriate place of service. Services at the origination site are reported with HCPCS Level II code Q3014.

ICD-10-CM Diagnostic Codes

The application of this code is too broad to adequately present ICD-10-CM diagnostic code links here. Refer to your ICD-10-CM book.

AMA: 99211 2020,Sep,14; 2020,Sep,3; 2020,Oct,14; 2020,Nov,3; 2020,Nov,12; 2020,May,3; 2020,Jun,3; 2020,Jan,3; 2020,Feb,3; 2019,Oct,10; 2019,Jan,3; 2019,Feb,3; 2018,Sep,14; 2018,Mar,7; 2018,Jan,8; 2018,Apr,10; 2018,Apr,9; 2017,Mar,10; 2017,Jun,6; 2017,Jan,8; 2017,Aug,3; 2016,Sep,6; 2016,Mar,10; 2016,Jan,7; 2016,Jan,13; 2016,Dec,11; 2015,Oct,3; 2015,Jan,12; 2015,Jan,16; 2015,Dec,3 **99212** 2020,Sep,14; 2020,Sep,3; 2020,Oct,14; 2020,Nov,3; 2020,May,3; 2020,Jun,3; 2020,Jan,3; 2020,Feb,3; 2019,Oct,10; 2019,Jan,3; 2019,Feb,3; 2018,Sep,14; 2018,Mar,7; 2018,Jan,8; 2018,Apr,9; 2018,Apr,10; 2017,Oct,5; 2017,Jun,6; 2017,Jan,8; 2017,Aug,3; 2016,Sep,6; 2016,Mar,10; 2016,Jan,13; 2016,Jan,7; 2016,Dec,11; 2015,Oct,3; 2015,Jan,12; 2015,Jan,16; 2015,Dec,3 **99213** 2020,Sep,14; 2020,Sep,3; 2020,Oct,14; 2020,Nov,3; 2020,May,3; 2020,Jun,3; 2020,Jan,3; 2020,Feb,3; 2019,Oct,10; 2019,Jan,3; 2019,Feb,3; 2018,Sep,14; 2018,Mar,7; 2018,Jan,8; 2018,Apr,10; 2018,Apr,9; 2017,Jun,6; 2017,Jan,8; 2017,Aug,3; 2016,Sep,6; 2016,Mar,10; 2016,Jan,7; 2016,Jan,13; 2016,Dec,11; 2015,Oct,3; 2015,Jan,12; 2015,Jan,16; 2015,Dec,3 **99214** 2020,Sep,14; 2020,Sep,3; 2020,Oct,14; 2020,Nov,3; 2020,Nov,12; 2020,May,3; 2020,Jun,3; 2020,Jan,3; 2020,Feb,3; 2019,Oct,10; 2019,Jan,3; 2019,Feb,3; 2018,Sep,14; 2018,Mar,7; 2018,Jan,8; 2018,Apr,10; 2018,Apr,9; 2017,Jun,6; 2017,Jan,8; 2017,Aug,3; 2016,Sep,6; 2016,Mar,10; 2016,Jan,7; 2016,Jan,13; 2016,Dec,11; 2015,Oct,3; 2015,Jan,16; 2015,Jan,12; 2015,Dec,3 **99215** 2020,Sep,3; 2020,Sep,14; 2020,Oct,14; 2020,Nov,3; 2020,Nov,12; 2020,May,3; 2020,Jun,3; 2020,Jan,3; 2020,Feb,3; 2019,Oct,10; 2019,Jan,3; 2019,Feb,3; 2018,Sep,14; 2018,Mar,7; 2018,Jan,8; 2018,Apr,9; 2018,Apr,10; 2017,Jun,6; 2017,Jan,8; 2017,Aug,3; 2016,Sep,6; 2016,Mar,10; 2016,Jan,7; 2016,Jan,13; 2016,Dec,11; 2015,Oct,3; 2015,Jan,12; 2015,Jan,16; 2015,Dec,3

Relative Value Units/Medicare Edits

Non-Facility RVU	Work	PE	MP	Total
99211	0.18	0.47	0.01	0.66
99212	0.7	0.88	0.05	1.63
99213	1.3	1.25	0.1	2.65
99214	1.92	1.7	0.14	3.76
99215	2.8	2.24	0.21	5.25
Facility RVU	Work	PE	MP	Total
99211	0.18	0.07	0.01	0.26
99212	0.7	0.29	0.05	1.04
99213	1.3	0.55	0.1	1.95
99214	1.92	0.82	0.14	2.88
99215	2.8	1.23	0.21	4.24

	FUD	Status	MUE	Modifiers				IOM Reference
99211	N/A	A	1(3)	N/A	N/A	N/A	80*	None
99212	N/A	A	2(3)	N/A	N/A	N/A	80*	
99213	N/A	A	2(3)	N/A	N/A	N/A	80*	
99214	N/A	A	2(3)	N/A	N/A	N/A	80*	
99215	N/A	A	1(3)	N/A	N/A	N/A	80*	

* with documentation

Terms To Know

established patient. Patient who has received professional services in a face-to-face setting within the last three years from the same physician/qualified health care professional or another physician/qualified health care professional of the exact same specialty and subspecialty who belongs to the same group practice. If the patient is seen by a physician/qualified health care professional who is covering for another physician/qualified health care professional, the patient will be considered the same as if seen by the physician/qualified health care professional who is unavailable.

medical decision making. Consideration of the differential diagnoses, the amount and/or complexity of data reviewed and considered (medical records, test results, correspondence from previous treating physicians, etc.), current diagnostic studies ordered, and treatment or management options and risk (complications of the patient's condition, the potential for complications, continued morbidity, risk of mortality, any comorbidities associated with the patient's disease process).

99217

99217 Observation care discharge day management (This code is to be utilized to report all services provided to a patient on discharge from outpatient hospital "observation status" if the discharge is on other than the initial date of "observation status." To report services to a patient designated as "observation status" or "inpatient status" and discharged on the same date, use the codes for Observation or Inpatient Care Services [including Admission and Discharge Services, 99234-99236 as appropriate.])

Explanation

This code describes the final processes associated with discharging a patient from outpatient hospital observation status and includes a patient exam, a discussion about the hospital stay, instructions for ongoing care, as well as preparing the medical discharge records. Report this code only when the patient has been discharged from observation services on a date other than the initial date of observation care. There are no key components or time estimates associated with this service.

Coding Tips

This code is used to report hospital outpatient observation discharge services. This code includes patient examination, discharge and follow-up care instructions, and preparation of all medical records. Time is not a factor when selecting this E/M service. For patients admitted and discharged from observation or inpatient status on the same date, see 99234-99236; for hospital inpatient discharge services, see 99238-99239. Medicare has provisionally identified this code as a telehealth/telemedicine service. Current Medicare coverage guidelines should be reviewed. Commercial payers should be contacted regarding their coverage guidelines. Telemedicine services may be reported by the performing provider by adding modifier 95 to this procedure code and using the appropriate place of service. Services at the origination site are reported with HCPCS Level II code Q3014.

ICD-10-CM Diagnostic Codes

The application of this code is too broad to adequately present ICD-10-CM diagnostic code links here. Refer to your ICD-10-CM book.

AMA: 99217 2019,Jul,10; 2018,Jan,8; 2017,Jun,6; 2017,Jan,8; 2017,Aug,3; 2016,Jan,13; 2016,Jan,7; 2016,Dec,11; 2015,Jan,16; 2015,Dec,3

Relative Value Units/Medicare Edits

Non-Facility RVU	Work	PE	MP	Total
99217	1.28	0.7	0.09	2.07
Facility RVU	Work	PE	MP	Total
99217	1.28	0.7	0.09	2.07

	FUD	Status	MUE	Modifiers				IOM Reference
99217	N/A	A	1(2)	N/A	N/A	N/A	80*	100-04,11,40.1.3; 100-04,12,30.6.4; 100-04,12,30.6.8; 100-04,12,100; 100-04,32,130.1

* with documentation

99218-99220

99218 Initial observation care, per day, for the evaluation and management of a patient which requires these 3 key components: A detailed or comprehensive history; A detailed or comprehensive examination; and Medical decision making that is straightforward or of low complexity. Counseling and/or coordination of care with other physicians, other qualified health care professionals, or agencies are provided consistent with the nature of the problem(s) and the patient's and/or family's needs. Usually, the problem(s) requiring admission to outpatient hospital "observation status" are of low severity. Typically, 30 minutes are spent at the bedside and on the patient's hospital floor or unit.

99219 Initial observation care, per day, for the evaluation and management of a patient, which requires these 3 key components: A comprehensive history; A comprehensive examination; and Medical decision making of moderate complexity. Counseling and/or coordination of care with other physicians, other qualified health care professionals, or agencies are provided consistent with the nature of the problem(s) and the patient's and/or family's needs. Usually, the problem(s) requiring admission to outpatient hospital "observation status" are of moderate severity. Typically, 50 minutes are spent at the bedside and on the patient's hospital floor or unit.

99220 Initial observation care, per day, for the evaluation and management of a patient, which requires these 3 key components: A comprehensive history; A comprehensive examination; and Medical decision making of high complexity. Counseling and/or coordination of care with other physicians, other qualified health care professionals, or agencies are provided consistent with the nature of the problem(s) and the patient's and/or family's needs. Usually, the problem(s) requiring admission to outpatient hospital "observation status" are of high severity. Typically, 70 minutes are spent at the bedside and on the patient's hospital floor or unit.

Explanation

Initial hospital observation service codes describe the first visit of the patient's admission for hospital outpatient observation care by the supervising qualified clinician. Hospital outpatient observation status includes the supervision of the care plan for observation as well as periodic reassessments. The patient is not required to be physically located in a designated observation area within a hospital; however, if such an area is utilized, these codes should be reported. When a patient is admitted to observation status during the course of another encounter from a different site of service, such as the physician's office, a nursing home, or the emergency department, all of the E/M services rendered by the supervising clinician as part of the observation status are considered part of the initial observation care services when they are performed on the same day; the level of initial observation code reported by the clinician should incorporate the other services related to the hospital outpatient observation admission that were provided in any other sites of services as well as those provided in the actual observation setting. Codes are reported per day and do not differentiate between new or established patients. Under the initial observation care category, there are three levels represented by 99218, 99219, and 99220. These levels require all three key components to be documented. The lowest level of care within this category, 99218, requires a detailed or comprehensive history and exam as well as straightforward or low complexity medical decision making (MDM) with approximately 30 minutes time being spent at the patient's bedside and on the patient's floor or unit. For the mid-level and highest level observation care codes, a comprehensive history and examination are required. Medical decision making is the differentiating factor for these two levels. For moderate complexity, report 99219. For observation care requiring MDM of high complexity, report 99220. The clinician

typically spends 50 (99219) to 70 (99220) minutes at the patient's bedside or on the unit accordingly.

Coding Tips

These codes are used to report initial hospital outpatient observation services. All three key components (history, exam, and medical decision making) must be met or exceeded for the level of service selected. Time may be used to select the level of service when counseling and coordination of care are documented as at least half of the time spent face-to-face with the patient. All evaluation and management services provided by the clinician leading up to the initiation of the observation status are part of the patient's initial observation care when performed on the same date of service. The designation of "observation status" refers to the initiation of observation care and not to a specific area of the facility. CPT guidelines indicate these services are reported only by the admitting/supervising provider; all other providers should report 99224-99226 or 99241-99245. Medicare and some payers may allow providers of different specialties to report initial hospital services and require the admitting/supervising provider to append modifier AI. For observation discharge on a different date of service than the admission, see 99217. For patients admitted and discharged from observation or inpatient status on the same date, see 99234-99236. Medicare has provisionally identified these codes as telehealth/telemedicine services. Current Medicare coverage guidelines, including place of service, should be reviewed. Commercial payers should be contacted regarding their coverage guidelines. Telemedicine services may be reported by the performing provider by adding modifier 95 to these procedure codes and using the appropriate place of service. Services at the origination site are reported with HCPCS Level II code Q3014.

ICD-10-CM Diagnostic Codes

The application of this code is too broad to adequately present ICD-10-CM diagnostic code links here. Refer to your ICD-10-CM book.

AMA: 99218 2020,Sep,3; 2019,Jul,10; 2018,Jan,8; 2018,Dec,8; 2018,Dec,8; 2017,Jun,6; 2017,Jan,8; 2017,Aug,3; 2016,Jan,13; 2016,Jan,7; 2016,Dec,11; 2015,Mar,3; 2015,Jul,3; 2015,Jan,16; 2015,Dec,3 **99219** 2020,Sep,3; 2019,Jul,10; 2018,Jan,8; 2018,Dec,8; 2018,Dec,8; 2017,Jun,6; 2017,Jan,8; 2017,Aug,3; 2016,Jan,13; 2016,Jan,7; 2016,Dec,11; 2015,Jul,3; 2015,Jan,16; 2015,Dec,3 **99220** 2020,Sep,3; 2019,Jul,10; 2018,Jan,8; 2018,Dec,8; 2018,Dec,8; 2017,Jun,6; 2017,Jan,8; 2017,Aug,3; 2016,Jan,13; 2016,Jan,7; 2016,Dec,11; 2015,Jul,3; 2015,Jan,16; 2015,Dec,3

Relative Value Units/Medicare Edits

Non-Facility RVU	Work	PE	MP	Total
99218	1.92	0.74	0.16	2.82
99219	2.6	1.05	0.2	3.85
99220	3.56	1.4	0.25	5.21
Facility RVU	Work	PE	MP	Total
99218	1.92	0.74	0.16	2.82
99219	2.6	1.05	0.2	3.85
99220	3.56	1.4	0.25	5.21

	FUD	Status	MUE	Modifiers				IOM Reference
99218	N/A	A	1(2)	N/A	N/A	N/A	80*	100-04,12,100
99219	N/A	A	1(2)	N/A	N/A	N/A	80*	
99220	N/A	A	1(2)	N/A	N/A	N/A	80*	

* with documentation

[99224, 99225, 99226]

99224   Subsequent observation care, per day, for the evaluation and management of a patient, which requires at least 2 of these 3 key components: Problem focused interval history; Problem focused examination; Medical decision making that is straightforward or of low complexity. Counseling and/or coordination of care with other physicians, other qualified health care professionals, or agencies are provided consistent with the nature of the problem(s) and the patient's and/or family's needs. Usually, the patient is stable, recovering, or improving. Typically, 15 minutes are spent at the bedside and on the patient's hospital floor or unit.

99225   Subsequent observation care, per day, for the evaluation and management of a patient, which requires at least 2 of these 3 key components: An expanded problem focused interval history; An expanded problem focused examination; Medical decision making of moderate complexity. Counseling and/or coordination of care with other physicians, other qualified health care professionals, or agencies are provided consistent with the nature of the problem(s) and the patient's and/or family's needs. Usually, the patient is responding inadequately to therapy or has developed a minor complication. Typically, 25 minutes are spent at the bedside and on the patient's hospital floor or unit.

99226   Subsequent observation care, per day, for the evaluation and management of a patient, which requires at least 2 of these 3 key components: A detailed interval history; A detailed examination; Medical decision making of high complexity. Counseling and/or coordination of care with other physicians, other qualified health care professionals, or agencies are provided consistent with the nature of the problem(s) and the patient's and/or family's needs. Usually, the patient is unstable or has developed a significant complication or a significant new problem. Typically, 35 minutes are spent at the bedside and on the patient's hospital floor or unit.

Explanation

Subsequent hospital observation service codes describe visits that occur after the first encounter of the patient's admission for observation care by the supervising qualified clinician. Observation status includes supervision of the care plan for observation as well as periodic reassessments. The patient is not required to be physically located in a designated observation area within a hospital; however, if such an area is utilized, these codes are reported. Codes are reported per day and, as with the initial observation care codes, do not differentiate between new or established patients. Under the subsequent observation care category, there are three levels represented by resequenced codes 99224, 99225, and 99226. All three of these levels require at least two out of the three key components to be documented. The lowest level of care, 99224, describes a problem-focused interval history as well as a problem-focused examination with straightforward or low complexity medical decision making and involves approximately 15 minutes of time by the provider at the patient's bedside or on the unit. For mid-level observation care code 99225, an expanded problem-focused history and examination are required with moderate medical decision making. Time associated with this level usually involves 25 minutes at the bedside or on the patient's floor. The third and highest level of follow-up observation care, 99226, requires a detailed history and exam as well as medical decision making of high complexity; the provider typically spends around 35 minutes with the patient or on the unit. All three levels of subsequent observation care involve the clinician reviewing the patient's medical record, results from diagnostic studies, as well as any changes to the patient's status such as the condition, response to treatments, or changes in health history since the last assessment.

Coding Tips

These codes are used to report subsequent hospital outpatient observation services. Two of the three key components (history, exam, and medical decision making) must be met or exceeded for the level of service selected. Time may be used to select the level of service when counseling and coordination of care are documented as at least half of the time spent face-to-face with the patient. Subsequent hospital outpatient observation care services include review of the medical record, including all diagnostic studies, as well as changes noted in the patient's condition and response to treatment since the last evaluation. The designation of "observation status" refers to the initiation of observation care and not to a specific area of the facility. For initial observation care, see 99218-99220; for observation discharge on a different date of service than the admission, see 99217. For patients admitted and discharged from observation or inpatient status on the same date, see 99234-99236. Medicare has provisionally identified these codes as telehealth/telemedicine services. Current Medicare coverage guidelines, including place of service, should be reviewed. Commercial payers should be contacted regarding their coverage guidelines. Telemedicine services may be reported by the performing provider by adding modifier 95 to these procedure codes and using the appropriate place of service. Services at the origination site are reported with HCPCS Level II code Q3014.

ICD-10-CM Diagnostic Codes

The application of this code is too broad to adequately present ICD-10-CM diagnostic code links here. Refer to your ICD-10-CM book.

AMA: **99224** 2020,Sep,3; 2019,Jul,10; 2018,Jan,8; 2017,Jun,6; 2017,Jan,8; 2017,Aug,3; 2016,Jan,13; 2016,Jan,7; 2016,Dec,11; 2015,Jan,16; 2015,Dec,3 **99225** 2020,Sep,3; 2019,Jul,10; 2018,Jan,8; 2017,Jun,6; 2017,Jan,8; 2017,Aug,3; 2016,Jan,13; 2016,Jan,7; 2016,Dec,11; 2015,Jan,16; 2015,Dec,3 **99226** 2020,Sep,3; 2019,Jul,10; 2018,Jan,8; 2017,Jun,6; 2017,Jan,8; 2017,Aug,3; 2016,Jan,13; 2016,Jan,7; 2016,Dec,11; 2015,Jan,16; 2015,Dec,3

Relative Value Units/Medicare Edits

Non-Facility RVU	Work	PE	MP	Total
99224	0.76	0.3	0.05	1.11
99225	1.39	0.57	0.1	2.06
99226	2.0	0.82	0.14	2.96
Facility RVU	**Work**	**PE**	**MP**	**Total**
99224	0.76	0.3	0.05	1.11
99225	1.39	0.57	0.1	2.06
99226	2.0	0.82	0.14	2.96

	FUD	Status	MUE	Modifiers				IOM Reference
99224	N/A	A	1(2)	N/A	N/A	N/A	80*	None
99225	N/A	A	1(2)	N/A	N/A	N/A	80*	
99226	N/A	A	1(2)	N/A	N/A	N/A	80*	

* with documentation

99221-99223

99221 Initial hospital care, per day, for the evaluation and management of a patient, which requires these 3 key components: A detailed or comprehensive history; A detailed or comprehensive examination; and Medical decision making that is straightforward or of low complexity. Counseling and/or coordination of care with other physicians, other qualified health care professionals, or agencies are provided consistent with the nature of the problem(s) and the patient's and/or family's needs. Usually, the problem(s) requiring admission are of low severity. Typically, 30 minutes are spent at the bedside and on the patient's hospital floor or unit.

99222 Initial hospital care, per day, for the evaluation and management of a patient, which requires these 3 key components: A comprehensive history; A comprehensive examination; and Medical decision making of moderate complexity. Counseling and/or coordination of care with other physicians, other qualified health care professionals, or agencies are provided consistent with the nature of the problem(s) and the patient's and/or family's needs. Usually, the problem(s) requiring admission are of moderate severity. Typically, 50 minutes are spent at the bedside and on the patient's hospital floor or unit.

99223 Initial hospital care, per day, for the evaluation and management of a patient, which requires these 3 key components: A comprehensive history; A comprehensive examination; and Medical decision making of high complexity. Counseling and/or coordination of care with other physicians, other qualified health care professionals, or agencies are provided consistent with the nature of the problem(s) and the patient's and/or family's needs. Usually, the problem(s) requiring admission are of high severity. Typically, 70 minutes are spent at the bedside and on the patient's hospital floor or unit.

Explanation

Initial hospital inpatient service codes describe the first encounter with the patient by the admitting physician or qualified clinician. For initial encounters by a physician other than the admitting physician, see the initial inpatient consultation codes or subsequent inpatient care codes. When the patient is admitted to the hospital under inpatient status during the course of another encounter from a different site of service, such as the physician's office, a nursing home, or the emergency department, all of the E/M services rendered by the supervising clinician as part of the inpatient admission status are considered part of the initial inpatient care services when they are performed on the same day. The level of initial inpatient care reported by the clinician should incorporate the other services related to the hospital admission that were provided in any other sites of services as well as those provided in the actual inpatient setting. Codes are reported per day and do not differentiate between new or established patients. Under the initial inpatient care category, there are three levels represented by 99221, 99222, and 99223. All of these levels require all three key components, history, exam, and medical decision-making (MDM), to be documented. The lowest level of care within this category, 99221, requires a detailed or comprehensive history and exam as well as straightforward or low complexity medical decision-making with approximately 30 minutes time being spent at the patient's bedside and on the patient's floor or unit. For the mid-level and highest level initial inpatient care codes, a comprehensive history and examination are required. MDM is the differentiating factor for these two levels; for moderate complexity, report 99222 and for initial inpatient care requiring MDM of high complexity, report 99223. The clinician typically spends 50 (99222) to 70 (99223) minutes at the patient's bedside or on the unit accordingly. Note that these codes include services provided to patients in a "partial hospital" setting.

Coding Tips

These codes are used to report initial hospital inpatient services. All three key components (history, exam, and medical decision making) must be met or exceeded for the level of service selected. Time may be used to select the level of service when counseling and coordination of care are documented as at least half of the floor/unit time spent with the patient. Evaluation and management services provided by the clinician leading up to the initiation of observation status or inpatient admission are part of the patient's initial hospital care when performed on the same date of service. Codes may be selected based upon the 1995 or the 1997 Evaluation and Management Guidelines. CPT guidelines indicate these services are reported only by the admitting/supervising provider; all other providers should report 99231-99233 or 99251-99255. Medicare and some payers may allow providers of different specialties to report initial hospital services and require the admitting/supervising provider to append modifier AI. For subsequent inpatient care, see 99231-99233. For discharge from an inpatient stay on a different date of service than the admission, see 99238-99239. For patients admitted and discharged from observation or inpatient status on the same date, see 99234-99236. Medicare has provisionally identified these codes as telehealth/telemedicine services. Current Medicare coverage guidelines, including place of service, should be reviewed. Commercial payers should be contacted regarding their coverage guidelines. Telemedicine services may be reported by the performing provider by adding modifier 95 to these procedure codes and using the appropriate place of service. Services at the origination site are reported with HCPCS Level II code Q3014.

ICD-10-CM Diagnostic Codes

The application of this code is too broad to adequately present ICD-10-CM diagnostic code links here. Refer to your ICD-10-CM book.

AMA: 99221 2020,Sep,3; 2020,Oct,14; 2018,Jan,8; 2018,Dec,8; 2018,Dec,8; 2017,Jun,6; 2017,Jan,8; 2017,Aug,3; 2016,Mar,10; 2016,Jan,13; 2016,Jan,7; 2016,Dec,11; 2015,Jul,3; 2015,Jan,16; 2015,Dec,3; 2015,Dec,18 **99222** 2020,Sep,3; 2020,Oct,14; 2018,Jan,8; 2018,Dec,8; 2018,Dec,8; 2017,Jun,6; 2017,Jan,8; 2017,Aug,3; 2016,Mar,10; 2016,Jan,7; 2016,Jan,13; 2016,Dec,11; 2015,Mar,3; 2015,Jul,3; 2015,Jan,16; 2015,Dec,3; 2015,Dec,18 **99223** 2020,Sep,3; 2020,Oct,14; 2018,Jan,8; 2018,Dec,8; 2018,Dec,8; 2017,Jun,6; 2017,Jan,8; 2017,Aug,3; 2016,Mar,10; 2016,Jan,13; 2016,Jan,7; 2016,Dec,11; 2015,Jul,3; 2015,Jan,16; 2015,Dec,18; 2015,Dec,3

Relative Value Units/Medicare Edits

Non-Facility RVU	Work	PE	MP	Total
99221	1.92	0.78	0.2	2.9
99222	2.61	1.08	0.21	3.9
99223	3.86	1.6	0.28	5.74
Facility RVU	Work	PE	MP	Total
99221	1.92	0.78	0.2	2.9
99222	2.61	1.08	0.21	3.9
99223	3.86	1.6	0.28	5.74

	FUD	Status	MUE	Modifiers				IOM Reference
99221	N/A	A	1(3)	N/A	N/A	N/A	80*	100-04,12,30.6.4;
99222	N/A	A	1(3)	N/A	N/A	N/A	80*	100-04,12,30.6.9;
99223	N/A	A	1(3)	N/A	N/A	N/A	80*	100-04,12,30.6.9.1;
								100-04,12,30.6.15.1;
								100-04,12,100

* with documentation

99231-99233

★99231 Subsequent hospital care, per day, for the evaluation and management of a patient, which requires at least 2 of these 3 key components: A problem focused interval history; A problem focused examination; Medical decision making that is straightforward or of low complexity. Counseling and/or coordination of care with other physicians, other qualified health care professionals, or agencies are provided consistent with the nature of the problem(s) and the patient's and/or family's needs. Usually, the patient is stable, recovering or improving. Typically, 15 minutes are spent at the bedside and on the patient's hospital floor or unit.

★99232 Subsequent hospital care, per day, for the evaluation and management of a patient, which requires at least 2 of these 3 key components: An expanded problem focused interval history; An expanded problem focused examination; Medical decision making of moderate complexity. Counseling and/or coordination of care with other physicians, other qualified health care professionals, or agencies are provided consistent with the nature of the problem(s) and the patient's and/or family's needs. Usually, the patient is responding inadequately to therapy or has developed a minor complication. Typically, 25 minutes are spent at the bedside and on the patient's hospital floor or unit.

★99233 Subsequent hospital care, per day, for the evaluation and management of a patient, which requires at least 2 of these 3 key components: A detailed interval history; A detailed examination; Medical decision making of high complexity. Counseling and/or coordination of care with other physicians, other qualified health care professionals, or agencies are provided consistent with the nature of the problem(s) and the patient's and/or family's needs. Usually, the patient is unstable or has developed a significant complication or a significant new problem. Typically, 35 minutes are spent at the bedside and on the patient's hospital floor or unit.

Explanation

Subsequent hospital inpatient service codes describe visits that occur after the first encounter of the patient's inpatient hospital admission by the supervising physician or qualified clinician. Codes are reported per day and do not differentiate between new or established patients. Under the subsequent inpatient care category, there are three levels represented by 99231, 99232, and 99233. All of these levels require at least two out of the three key components—history, exam, and medical decision making—to be documented. The lowest level of care within this category, 99231, describes a problem-focused interval history as well as a problem-focused examination with straightforward or low complexity medical decision making and involves approximately 15 minutes of time by the provider at the patient's bedside or on the unit. For the mid-level subsequent inpatient care code, 99232, an expanded problem-focused history and examination are required with moderate medical decision making. Time associated with this level usually involves 25 minutes at the bedside or on the patient's floor. The third and highest level of subsequent inpatient care, 99233, requires a detailed history and exam as well as medical decision making of high complexity. For this level of care, the provider typically spends around 35 minutes with the patient or on the unit. All three levels of subsequent inpatient care involve the clinician reviewing the patient's medical record, results from diagnostic studies, as well as any changes to the patient's status such as physical condition, response to treatments, or changes in health history since the last assessment.

Coding Tips

These codes are used to report subsequent hospital inpatient services. Two of the three key components (history, exam, and medical decision making) must be met or exceeded for the level of service selected. Time may be used to select the level of service when counseling and coordination of care are documented as at least half of the floor/unit time spent with the patient. Codes may be selected based upon the 1995 or the 1997 Evaluation and Management Guidelines. Subsequent inpatient care services include review of the medical record, including all diagnostic studies, as well as changes noted in the patient's condition and response to treatment since the last evaluation. For initial inpatient care, see 99221-99223. For discharge from an inpatient stay on a different date of service than the admission, see 99238-99239. For patients admitted and discharged from observation or inpatient status on the same date, see 99234-99236. Telemedicine services may be reported by the performing provider by adding modifier 95 to these procedure codes and using the appropriate place of service. Services at the origination site are reported with HCPCS Level II code Q3014.

ICD-10-CM Diagnostic Codes

The application of this code is too broad to adequately present ICD-10-CM diagnostic code links here. Refer to your ICD-10-CM book.

AMA: **99231** 2020,Sep,3; 2018,Jan,8; 2018,Dec,8; 2018,Dec,8; 2017,Jun,6; 2017,Jan,8; 2017,Aug,3; 2016,Jan,7; 2016,Jan,13; 2016,Dec,11; 2015,Jul,3; 2015,Jan,16; 2015,Dec,3 **99232** 2020,Sep,3; 2018,Jan,8; 2018,Dec,8; 2018,Dec,8; 2017,Jun,6; 2017,Jan,8; 2017,Aug,3; 2016,Oct,8; 2016,Jan,7; 2016,Jan,13; 2016,Dec,11; 2015,Jul,3; 2015,Jan,16; 2015,Dec,3 **99233** 2020,Sep,3; 2018,Jan,8; 2018,Dec,8; 2018,Dec,8; 2017,Jun,6; 2017,Jan,8; 2017,Aug,3; 2016,Oct,8; 2016,Jan,13; 2016,Jan,7; 2016,Dec,11; 2015,Jul,3; 2015,Jan,16; 2015,Dec,3

Relative Value Units/Medicare Edits

Non-Facility RVU	Work	PE	MP	Total
99231	0.76	0.29	0.05	1.1
99232	1.39	0.57	0.1	2.06
99233	2.0	0.82	0.14	2.96
Facility RVU	Work	PE	MP	Total
99231	0.76	0.29	0.05	1.1
99232	1.39	0.57	0.1	2.06
99233	2.0	0.82	0.14	2.96

	FUD	Status	MUE	Modifiers				IOM Reference
99231	N/A	A	1(3)	N/A	N/A	N/A	80*	100-04,12,30.6.9.2; 100-04,12,100
99232	N/A	A	1(3)	N/A	N/A	N/A	80*	
99233	N/A	A	1(3)	N/A	N/A	N/A	80*	

* with documentation

99234-99236

99234 Observation or inpatient hospital care, for the evaluation and management of a patient including admission and discharge on the same date, which requires these 3 key components: A detailed or comprehensive history; A detailed or comprehensive examination; and Medical decision making that is straightforward or of low complexity. Counseling and/or coordination of care with other physicians, other qualified health care professionals, or agencies are provided consistent with the nature of the problem(s) and the patient's and/or family's needs. Usually the presenting problem(s) requiring admission are of low severity. Typically, 40 minutes are spent at the bedside and on the patient's hospital floor or unit.

99235 Observation or inpatient hospital care, for the evaluation and management of a patient including admission and discharge on the same date, which requires these 3 key components: A comprehensive history; A comprehensive examination; and Medical decision making of moderate complexity. Counseling and/or coordination of care with other physicians, other qualified health care professionals, or agencies are provided consistent with the nature of the problem(s) and the patient's and/or family's needs. Usually the presenting problem(s) requiring admission are of moderate severity. Typically, 50 minutes are spent at the bedside and on the patient's hospital floor or unit.

99236 Observation or inpatient hospital care, for the evaluation and management of a patient including admission and discharge on the same date, which requires these 3 key components: A comprehensive history; A comprehensive examination; and Medical decision making of high complexity. Counseling and/or coordination of care with other physicians, other qualified health care professionals, or agencies are provided consistent with the nature of the problem(s) and the patient's and/or family's needs. Usually the presenting problem(s) requiring admission are of high severity. Typically, 55 minutes are spent at the bedside and on the patient's hospital floor or unit.

Explanation

Hospital observation or inpatient care service in cases where the patient is admitted and discharged on the same date of service by the supervising or qualified clinician is reported with 99234-99236. Observation status includes the supervision of the care plan for observation, as well as the periodic reassessments. The patient is not required to be physically located in a designated observation area within a hospital; however, if such an area is utilized, these codes should be reported. When a patient is admitted to the hospital from observation status on the same date of service, the clinician should only report the appropriate level of initial hospital care code. The level of care reported should reflect all of the other services from the observation status services the clinician rendered to the patient on the same date of service, as well as those provided in the actual inpatient setting. Codes do not differentiate between new or established patients. Under this care category, there are three levels represented by 99234, 99235, and 99236. All of these levels require all three key components (history, exam, and medical decision-making [MDM]) to be documented. The lowest level of care within this category, 99234, requires a detailed or comprehensive history and exam, as well as straightforward medical decision-making or that of low complexity with approximately 40 minutes time being spent at the patient's bedside and on the patient's floor or unit. For the mid-level and highest level observation or inpatient care codes, a comprehensive history and examination are required. Medical decision-making is the differentiating factor for these two levels; for moderate complexity, report 99235 and for observation or inpatient care requiring MDM of high complexity, report 99236. The clinician typically spends 50 (99235) to 55 (99236) minutes at the patient's bedside or on the unit

accordingly. Note that these codes should be reported only when the patient has been admitted and discharged on the same date of service.

Coding Tips

These codes are used to report observation or initial hospital services for the patient admitted and discharged on the same date of service. All three key components (history, exam, and medical decision making) must be met or exceeded for the level of service selected. Evaluation and management services provided by the clinician leading up to the initiation of observation status or inpatient admission are part of the patient's initial hospital care when performed on the same date of service. The designation of "observation status" refers to the initiation of observation care and not to a specific area of the facility. For patients admitted to observation status, initial care, see 99218-99220; subsequent observation care, see 99224-99226; for observation discharge on a different date of service than the admission, see 99217. For initial inpatient care, see 99221-99223; subsequent inpatient care, see 99231-99233. For discharge from an inpatient stay on a different date of service than the admission, see 99238-99239. Medicare has provisionally identified these codes as telehealth/telemedicine services. Current Medicare coverage guidelines, including place of service, should be reviewed. Commercial payers should be contacted regarding their coverage guidelines. Telemedicine services may be reported by the performing provider by adding modifier 95 to these procedure codes and using the appropriate place of service. Services at the origination site are reported with HCPCS Level II code Q3014.

ICD-10-CM Diagnostic Codes

The application of this code is too broad to adequately present ICD-10-CM diagnostic code links here. Refer to your ICD-10-CM book.

AMA: 99234 2020,Sep,3; 2018,Jan,8; 2018,Dec,8; 2018,Dec,8; 2018,Apr,10; 2017,Jun,6; 2017,Jan,8; 2017,Aug,3; 2016,Jan,13; 2016,Dec,11; 2015,Jul,3; 2015,Jan,16 **99235** 2020,Sep,3; 2018,Jan,8; 2018,Dec,8; 2018,Dec,8; 2018,Apr,10; 2017,Jun,6; 2017,Jan,8; 2017,Aug,3; 2016,Jan,13; 2016,Dec,11; 2015,Jul,3; 2015,Jan,16 **99236** 2020,Sep,3; 2018,Jan,8; 2018,Dec,8; 2018,Dec,8; 2018,Apr,10; 2017,Jun,6; 2017,Jan,8; 2017,Aug,3; 2016,Jan,13; 2016,Dec,11; 2015,Jul,3; 2015,Jan,16

Relative Value Units/Medicare Edits

Non-Facility RVU	Work	PE	MP	Total
99234	2.56	1.0	0.21	3.77
99235	3.24	1.32	0.23	4.79
99236	4.2	1.65	0.3	6.15
Facility RVU	Work	PE	MP	Total
99234	2.56	1.0	0.21	3.77
99235	3.24	1.32	0.23	4.79
99236	4.2	1.65	0.3	6.15

	FUD	Status	MUE	Modifiers				IOM Reference
99234	N/A	A	1(3)	N/A	N/A	N/A	80*	100-04,12,30.6.4;
99235	N/A	A	1(3)	N/A	N/A	N/A	80*	100-04,12,30.6.9; 100-04,12,30.6.9.1;
99236	N/A	A	1(3)	N/A	N/A	N/A	80*	100-04,12,30.6.9.2; 100-04,12,100

* with documentation

99241-99245

★99241 Office consultation for a new or established patient, which requires these 3 key components: A problem focused history; A problem focused examination; and Straightforward medical decision making. Counseling and/or coordination of care with other physicians, other qualified health care professionals, or agencies are provided consistent with the nature of the problem(s) and the patient's and/or family's needs. Usually, the presenting problem(s) are self limited or minor. Typically, 15 minutes are spent face-to-face with the patient and/or family.

★99242 Office consultation for a new or established patient, which requires these 3 key components: An expanded problem focused history; An expanded problem focused examination; and Straightforward medical decision making. Counseling and/or coordination of care with other physicians, other qualified health care professionals, or agencies are provided consistent with the nature of the problem(s) and the patient's and/or family's needs. Usually, the presenting problem(s) are of low severity. Typically, 30 minutes are spent face-to-face with the patient and/or family.

★99243 Office consultation for a new or established patient, which requires these 3 key components: A detailed history; A detailed examination; and Medical decision making of low complexity. Counseling and/or coordination of care with other physicians, other qualified health care professionals, or agencies are provided consistent with the nature of the problem(s) and the patient's and/or family's needs. Usually, the presenting problem(s) are of moderate severity. Typically, 40 minutes are spent face-to-face with the patient and/or family.

★99244 Office consultation for a new or established patient, which requires these 3 key components: A comprehensive history; A comprehensive examination; and Medical decision making of moderate complexity. Counseling and/or coordination of care with other physicians, other qualified health care professionals, or agencies are provided consistent with the nature of the problem(s) and the patient's and/or family's needs. Usually, the presenting problem(s) are of moderate to high severity. Typically, 60 minutes are spent face-to-face with the patient and/or family.

★99245 Office consultation for a new or established patient, which requires these 3 key components: A comprehensive history; A comprehensive examination; and Medical decision making of high complexity. Counseling and/or coordination of care with other physicians, other qualified health care professionals, or agencies are provided consistent with the nature of the problem(s) and the patient's and/or family's needs. Usually, the presenting problem(s) are of moderate to high severity. Typically, 80 minutes are spent face-to-face with the patient and/or family.

Explanation

Office and other outpatient consultation service codes describe encounters where another qualified clinician's advice or opinion regarding diagnosis and treatment or determination to accept transfer of care of a patient is rendered at the request of the primary treating provider. Consultations may also be requested by another appropriate source; for example, a third-party payer may request a second opinion. The request for a consultation must be documented in the medical record, as well as a written report of the consultation findings. During the course of a consultation, the physician consultant can initiate diagnostic or therapeutic services at the same encounter or at a follow-up visit. Other separately reportable procedures or services performed in conjunction with the consultation may be reported separately. Codes do not differentiate between new or established patients. Services are reported based on meeting all three key components (history, exam, and medical decision-making [MDM]) within each level of service. The most basic service, 99241, describes a problem-focused history and exam with straightforward medical decision-making encompassing approximately 15 minutes of face-to-face time with the patient and/or family discussing a minor or self-limiting complaint. The mid-level services describe problems involving an expanded problem focused history and exam or a detailed history and exam as represented by 99242 and 99243, respectively. Medical decision-making for 99242 is the same as for a level one visit (straightforward) and is designated as low complexity for the level three service (99243). At these levels of service, the encounter can involve face-to-face time of 30 (99242) to 40 (99243) minutes involving minimal to low severity concerns. The last two levels of service in this category represent moderate to high-severity problems and both services involve comprehensive history and examination components. The differentiating factor between the two levels is the medical decision-making; code 99244 involves moderate complexity MDM and approximately 60 minutes of face-to-face time with the patient and/or family, while the highest level of service in this category, 99245, involves MDM of high complexity and approximately 80 minutes of face-to-face time.

Coding Tips

These codes are used to report consultations in the office or outpatient setting. All three key components (history, exam, and medical decision making) must be met or exceeded for the level of service selected. Time may be used to select the level of service when counseling and coordination of care are documented as at least half of the time spent face-to-face with the patient. Codes may be selected based upon the 1995 or the 1997 Evaluation and Management Guidelines. Consultation codes are not covered by Medicare and some payers. Report new or established outpatient E/M codes for consultation services. Consultation services should not be reported when the care and management of a problem or condition is assumed prior to the initial examination of the patient. In these situations, the appropriate initial or subsequent evaluation and management service should be reported. For office or other outpatient services for a new patient, see 99202-99205; for an established patient, see 99211-99215. For inpatient consultation services, see 99251-99255. Telemedicine services may be reported by the performing provider by adding modifier 95 to these procedure codes and using the appropriate place of service. Services at the origination site are reported with HCPCS Level II code Q3014.

ICD-10-CM Diagnostic Codes

The application of this code is too broad to adequately present ICD-10-CM diagnostic code links here. Refer to your ICD-10-CM book.

AMA: 99241 2020,Sep,3; 2020,Oct,14; 2020,Nov,3; 2018,Mar,7; 2018,Jan,8; 2018,Apr,10; 2018,Apr,9; 2017,Jun,6; 2017,Jan,8; 2017,Aug,3; 2016,Sep,6; 2016,Jan,13; 2016,Jan,7; 2016,Dec,11; 2015,Jan,16; 2015,Jan,12 **99242** 2020,Sep,3; 2020,Oct,14; 2020,Nov,3; 2018,Mar,7; 2018,Jan,8; 2018,Apr,9; 2018,Apr,10; 2017,Jun,8; 2017,Jun,6; 2017,Jan,8; 2017,Aug,3; 2016,Sep,6; 2016,Jan,13; 2016,Jan,7; 2016,Dec,11; 2015,Jan,12; 2015,Jan,16 **99243** 2020,Sep,3; 2020,Oct,14; 2020,Nov,3; 2018,Mar,7; 2018,Jan,8; 2018,Apr,9; 2018,Apr,10; 2017,Jun,6; 2017,Jan,8; 2017,Aug,3; 2016,Sep,6; 2016,Jan,7; 2016,Jan,13; 2016,Dec,11; 2015,Jan,16; 2015,Jan,12 **99244** 2020,Sep,3; 2020,Oct,14; 2020,Nov,3; 2018,Mar,7; 2018,Jan,8; 2018,Apr,9; 2018,Apr,10; 2017,Jun,6; 2017,Jan,8; 2017,Aug,3; 2016,Sep,6; 2016,Jan,13; 2016,Jan,7; 2016,Dec,11; 2015,Jan,12; 2015,Jan,16 **99245** 2020,Sep,3; 2020,Oct,14; 2020,Nov,3; 2018,Mar,7; 2018,Jan,8; 2018,Apr,10; 2018,Apr,9; 2017,Jun,6; 2017,Jan,8; 2017,Aug,3; 2016,Sep,6; 2016,Jan,7; 2016,Jan,13; 2016,Dec,11; 2015,Jan,16; 2015,Jan,12

Relative Value Units/Medicare Edits

Non-Facility RVU	Work	PE	MP	Total
99241	0.64	0.66	0.05	1.35
99242	1.34	1.1	0.11	2.55
99243	1.88	1.46	0.15	3.49
99244	3.02	1.96	0.25	5.23
99245	3.77	2.3	0.3	6.37
Facility RVU	**Work**	**PE**	**MP**	**Total**
99241	0.64	0.24	0.05	0.93
99242	1.34	0.51	0.11	1.96
99243	1.88	0.71	0.15	2.74
99244	3.02	1.14	0.25	4.41
99245	3.77	1.38	0.3	5.45

	FUD	Status	MUE	Modifiers				IOM Reference
99241	N/A	I	0(3)	N/A	N/A	N/A	N/A	100-04,4,160;
99242	N/A	I	0(3)	N/A	N/A	N/A	N/A	100-04,12,30.6.4;
99243	N/A	I	0(3)	N/A	N/A	N/A	N/A	100-04,12,30.6.10;
99244	N/A	I	0(3)	N/A	N/A	N/A	N/A	100-04,12,30.6.15.1;
99245	N/A	I	0(3)	N/A	N/A	N/A	N/A	100-04,12,100

* with documentation

Terms To Know

consultation. Advice or opinion regarding diagnosis and treatment or determination to accept transfer of care of a patient rendered by a medical professional at the request of the primary care provider.

Medicare. Federally funded program authorized as part of the Social Security Act that provides for health care services for people age 65 or older, people with disabilities, and people with end-stage renal disease (ESRD).

99251-99255

★**99251** Inpatient consultation for a new or established patient, which requires these 3 key components: A problem focused history; A problem focused examination; and Straightforward medical decision making. Counseling and/or coordination of care with other physicians, other qualified health care professionals, or agencies are provided consistent with the nature of the problem(s) and the patient's and/or family's needs. Usually, the presenting problem(s) are self limited or minor. Typically, 20 minutes are spent at the bedside and on the patient's hospital floor or unit.

★**99252** Inpatient consultation for a new or established patient, which requires these 3 key components: An expanded problem focused history; An expanded problem focused examination; and Straightforward medical decision making. Counseling and/or coordination of care with other physicians, other qualified health care professionals, or agencies are provided consistent with the nature of the problem(s) and the patient's and/or family's needs. Usually, the presenting problem(s) are of low severity. Typically, 40 minutes are spent at the bedside and on the patient's hospital floor or unit.

★**99253** Inpatient consultation for a new or established patient, which requires these 3 key components: A detailed history; A detailed examination; and Medical decision making of low complexity. Counseling and/or coordination of care with other physicians, other qualified health care professionals, or agencies are provided consistent with the nature of the problem(s) and the patient's and/or family's needs. Usually, the presenting problem(s) are of moderate severity. Typically, 55 minutes are spent at the bedside and on the patient's hospital floor or unit.

★**99254** Inpatient consultation for a new or established patient, which requires these 3 key components: A comprehensive history; A comprehensive examination; and Medical decision making of moderate complexity. Counseling and/or coordination of care with other physicians, other qualified health care professionals, or agencies are provided consistent with the nature of the problem(s) and the patient's and/or family's needs. Usually, the presenting problem(s) are of moderate to high severity. Typically, 80 minutes are spent at the bedside and on the patient's hospital floor or unit.

★**99255** Inpatient consultation for a new or established patient, which requires these 3 key components: A comprehensive history; A comprehensive examination; and Medical decision making of high complexity. Counseling and/or coordination of care with other physicians, other qualified health care professionals, or agencies are provided consistent with the nature of the problem(s) and the patient's and/or family's needs. Usually, the presenting problem(s) are of moderate to high severity. Typically, 110 minutes are spent at the bedside and on the patient's hospital floor or unit.

Explanation

Inpatient consultation service codes describe encounters with patients admitted to the hospital, residing in nursing facilities, or to patients in a partial hospital setting where another qualified clinician's advice or opinion regarding diagnosis and treatment or determination to accept transfer of care of a patient is rendered at the request of the primary treating provider. The request for a consultation must be documented in the patient's medical record, as well as a written report of the findings of the consultation to the primary treating physician. During the course of a consultation, the physician consultant can initiate diagnostic or therapeutic services at the same encounter or at a follow-up visit. Other procedures or services performed in conjunction with the consultation may be reported separately. Codes do not differentiate between new or established patients and only one inpatient consultation services code should be reported per admission. Services are reported based on meeting all three key components (history, exam, and medical decision-making [MDM]) within each level of service. The most basic service, as represented by 99251, describes a problem focused history and exam with straightforward medical decision-making for a minor or self-limiting complaint encompassing approximately 20 minutes of time at the patient's bedside or on the unit. The mid-level services describe problems involving an expanded problem focused history and exam or a detailed history and exam as represented by 99252 and 99253, respectively. Medical decision-making for 99252 is the same (straightforward) as for a level one visit (99251) and is designated as low complexity for the level three service (99253). At these levels of service, the encounter can involve time at the patient's bedside or on the unit of 40 (99252) to 55 (99253) minutes involving minimal to low severity concerns. The last two levels of service in this category represent moderate to high-severity problems and both services involve comprehensive history and examination components. The differentiating factor between the two levels is the medical decision-making. Code 99254 involves moderate complexity MDM and approximately 80 minutes of time at the patient's bedside or on the unit, while the highest level of service in this category, 99255, involves MDM of high complexity and approximately 110 minutes at the patient's bedside or on the unit.

Coding Tips

These codes are used to report consultations in the inpatient setting. All three key components (history, exam, and medical decision making) must be met or exceeded for the level of service selected. Time may be used to select the level of service when counseling and coordination of care are documented as at least half of the time spent face-to-face with the patient. Consultation codes are not covered by Medicare and some payers. Report new or established inpatient E/M codes for consultation services. Consultation services should not be reported when the care and management of a problem or condition is assumed prior to the initial examination of the patient. In these situations, the appropriate initial or subsequent evaluation and management service should be reported. Do not report an inpatient and outpatient consultation when both are related to the same inpatient admission. For initial hospital care services, see 99221-99223; for subsequent hospital care services, see 99231-99233. For office or other outpatient consultation services, see 99241-99245. Telemedicine services may be reported by the performing provider by adding modifier 95 to these procedure codes and using the appropriate place of service. Services at the origination site are reported with HCPCS Level II code Q3014.

ICD-10-CM Diagnostic Codes

The application of this code is too broad to adequately present ICD-10-CM diagnostic code links here. Refer to your ICD-10-CM book.

AMA: **99251** 2020,Sep,3; 2018,Jan,8; 2017,Jun,6; 2017,Jan,8; 2017,Aug,3; 2016,Jan,13; 2016,Jan,7; 2016,Dec,11; 2015,Jan,16 **99252** 2020,Sep,3; 2018,Jan,8; 2017,Jun,6; 2017,Jan,8; 2017,Aug,3; 2016,Jan,13; 2016,Jan,7; 2016,Dec,11; 2015,Jan,16 **99253** 2020,Sep,3; 2018,Jan,8; 2017,Jun,6; 2017,Jan,8; 2017,Aug,3; 2016,Jan,13; 2016,Jan,7; 2016,Dec,11; 2015,Jan,16 **99254** 2020,Sep,3; 2018,Jan,8; 2017,Jun,6; 2017,Jan,8; 2017,Aug,3; 2016,Jan,13; 2016,Jan,7; 2016,Dec,11; 2015,Jan,16 **99255** 2020,Sep,3; 2018,Jan,8; 2017,Jun,6; 2017,Jan,8; 2017,Aug,3; 2016,Jan,13; 2016,Jan,7; 2016,Dec,11; 2015,Jan,16

Relative Value Units/Medicare Edits

Non-Facility RVU	Work	PE	MP	Total
99251	1.0	0.32	0.09	1.41
99252	1.5	0.52	0.13	2.15
99253	2.27	0.84	0.19	3.3
99254	3.29	1.23	0.26	4.78
99255	4.0	1.44	0.32	5.76
Facility RVU	Work	PE	MP	Total
99251	1.0	0.32	0.09	1.41
99252	1.5	0.52	0.13	2.15
99253	2.27	0.84	0.19	3.3
99254	3.29	1.23	0.26	4.78
99255	4.0	1.44	0.32	5.76

	FUD	Status	MUE	Modifiers				IOM Reference
99251	N/A	I	0(3)	N/A	N/A	N/A	N/A	100-04,12,30.6.4;
99252	N/A	I	0(3)	N/A	N/A	N/A	N/A	100-04,12,30.6.10;
99253	N/A	I	0(3)	N/A	N/A	N/A	N/A	100-04,12,100
99254	N/A	I	0(3)	N/A	N/A	N/A	N/A	
99255	N/A	I	0(3)	N/A	N/A	N/A	N/A	

* with documentation

Terms To Know

consultation. Advice or opinion regarding diagnosis and treatment or determination to accept transfer of care of a patient rendered by a medical professional at the request of the primary care provider.

inpatient. Time period in which a patient is housed in a hospital or facility offering medical, surgical, and/or psychiatric services, usually without interruption.

medical decision making. Consideration of the differential diagnoses, the amount and/or complexity of data reviewed and considered (medical records, test results, correspondence from previous treating physicians, etc.), current diagnostic studies ordered, and treatment or management options and risk (complications of the patient's condition, the potential for complications, continued morbidity, risk of mortality, any comorbidities associated with the patient's disease process).

99291-99292

	99291	Critical care, evaluation and management of the critically ill or critically injured patient; first 30-74 minutes
+	**99292**	each additional 30 minutes (List separately in addition to code for primary service)

Explanation

Critical care services are reported by a physician or other qualified health care provider for critically ill or injured patients. Critical illnesses or injuries are defined as those with impairment to one or more vital organ systems with an increased risk of rapid or imminent health deterioration. Critical care services require direct patient/provider involvement with highly complex decision making in order to evaluate, control, and support vital systems functions to treat one or more vital organ system failures and/or to avoid further decline of the patient's condition. Vital organ system failure includes, but is not limited to, failure of the central nervous, circulatory, or respiratory systems; kidneys; liver; shock; and other metabolic processes. Generally, critical care services necessitate the interpretation of many physiologic parameters and/or other applications of advanced technology as available in a critical care unit, pediatric intensive care unit, respiratory care unit, in an emergency facility, patient room or other hospital department; however, in emergent situations, critical care may be provided where these elements are not available. Critical care may be provided so long as the patient's condition continues to warrant the level of care according to the criteria described. Care provided to patients residing in a critical care unit but not fitting the criteria for critical care is reported using other E/M codes, as appropriate. These codes are time based codes, meaning the total time spent must be documented and includes direct patient care bedside or time spent on the patient's floor or unit (reviewing laboratory results or imaging studies and discussing the patient's care with medical staff, time spent with family members, caregivers, or other surrogate decision makers to gather information on the patient's medical history, reviewing the patient's condition or prognosis, and discussing various treatment options or limitations of treatment), as long as the clinician is immediately available and not providing services to any other patient during the same time period. Time spent outside of the patient's unit or floor, including telephone calls, caregiver discussions, or time spent in actions that do not directly contribute to the patient's care rendered in the critical unit are not reported as critical care. Report these codes for attendance of the patient during transport for patients 24 months of age or older to or from a facility. Code 99291 represents the first 30 to 74 minutes of critical care and is reported once per day. Additional time beyond the first 74 minutes is reported in 30 minute increments with 99292.

Coding Tips

These codes are used to report critical care services. These are time-based services and the total time spent providing critical care must be documented in the medical record. All time spent providing critical care on the same date of service is added together and does not need to be contiguous. Time is reported for practitioner time spent in care of the critically ill or injured patient at the patient's bedside and on the floor/unit. Time spent off the patient unit, even if related to patient care, is not counted. Do not report critical care for patients who may be in the critical care unit but are not currently critically ill. The following services are considered inclusive to the critical care codes when reported by the clinician: interpretation of cardiac output measurements, chest x-rays, pulse oximetry, blood gases, collection and interpretation of physiologic data, computer data such as ECGs, gastric intubation, vascular access, and ventilation management. Code 99291 is reported once per day. Code 99292 is reported in addition to code 99291. Medicare and some other payers may allow 99292 to be reported alone when critical care is reported by another physician of the same group and specialty the same date as another provider reporting 99291. For care of the critically ill neonate, see 99468-99469;

for patients 29 days through 24 months, see 99471-99472; and for patients 2 through 5 years, see 99475-99476. Medicare has provisionally identified these codes as telehealth/telemedicine services. Current Medicare coverage guidelines, including place of service, should be reviewed. Commercial payers should be contacted regarding their coverage guidelines. Telemedicine services may be reported by the performing provider by adding modifier 95 to these procedure codes and using the appropriate place of service. Services at the origination site are reported with HCPCS Level II code Q3014.

ICD-10-CM Diagnostic Codes

The application of this code is too broad to adequately present ICD-10-CM diagnostic code links here. Refer to your ICD-10-CM book.

AMA: 99291 2020,Jan,12; 2020,Feb,7; 2019,Jul,10; 2019,Dec,14; 2019,Aug,8; 2018,Jun,9; 2018,Jan,8; 2018,Dec,8; 2018,Dec,8; 2017,Jun,6; 2017,Jan,8; 2017,Aug,3; 2016,Oct,8; 2016,May,3; 2016,Jan,13; 2016,Aug,9; 2015,Jul,3; 2015,Jan,16; 2015,Feb,10 **99292** 2020,Feb,7; 2019,Jul,10; 2019,Dec,14; 2019,Aug,8; 2018,Jun,9; 2018,Jan,8; 2018,Dec,8; 2018,Dec,8; 2017,Jun,6; 2017,Jan,8; 2017,Aug,3; 2016,May,3; 2016,Jan,13; 2016,Aug,9; 2015,Jul,3; 2015,Jan,16; 2015,Feb,10

Relative Value Units/Medicare Edits

Non-Facility RVU	Work	PE	MP	Total
99291	4.5	3.2	0.41	8.11
99292	2.25	1.09	0.21	3.55
Facility RVU	**Work**	**PE**	**MP**	**Total**
99291	4.5	1.42	0.41	6.33
99292	2.25	0.72	0.21	3.18

	FUD	Status	MUE	Modifiers				IOM Reference
99291	N/A	A	1(2)	N/A	N/A	N/A	80*	100-04,4,160;
99292	N/A	A	8(3)	N/A	N/A	N/A	80*	100-04,12,30.6.9; 100-04,12,100

* with documentation

Terms To Know

documentation. Physician's written or transcribed notations about a patient encounter, including a detailed operative report or written notes about a routine encounter. Source documentation must be the treating provider's own account of the encounter and may be transcribed from dictation, dictated by the physician into voice recognition software, or be hand- or typewritten. A signature or authentication accompanies each entry.

monitoring. Recording of events; keep track, regulate, or control patient activities and record findings.

99354-99359

+ ★**99354** Prolonged service(s) in the outpatient setting requiring direct patient contact beyond the time of the usual service; first hour (List separately in addition to code for outpatient Evaluation and Management or psychotherapy service, except with office or other outpatient services [99202, 99203, 99204, 99205, 99212, 99213, 99214, 99215])

+ ★**99355** each additional 30 minutes (List separately in addition to code for prolonged service)

+ ★**99356** Prolonged service in the inpatient or observation setting, requiring unit/floor time beyond the usual service; first hour (List separately in addition to code for inpatient or observation Evaluation and Management service)

+ ★**99357** each additional 30 minutes (List separately in addition to code for prolonged service)

99358 Prolonged evaluation and management service before and/or after direct patient care; first hour

+ **99359** each additional 30 minutes (List separately in addition to code for prolonged service)

Explanation

Prolonged services involve face-to-face patient contact or psychotherapy services beyond the typical service time and should only be reported once per day. Direct patient contact also includes additional non-face-to-face time, such as time spent on the patient's floor or unit in the hospital or nursing facility setting. For prolonged services rendered in the outpatient setting for the first hour, report 99354; for each additional 30 minutes, report 99355. For prolonged services rendered in the inpatient or observation setting for the first hour, report 99356; for each additional 30 minutes, report 99357. Codes should be reported using the total duration of face-to-face time spent by the clinician on the date of service even when the time spent is not continuous. Report prolonged service without direct patient contact with 99358-99359.

Coding Tips

These codes are used to report prolonged services, with direct patient contact (99354-99357) or without direct patient contact (99358-99359) beyond the usual service. These are time-based codes and time spent with the patient must be documented in the medical record. Codes 99354-99357 are only reported in addition to other time-based E/M services. Time spent on other separately reported services excluding the E/M service should not be counted toward the prolonged service time. Code selection is based on whether the service is provided in the outpatient setting or an inpatient or observation setting. For prolonged services provided by a physician or other qualified health care professional with or without direct patient contact in the office or other outpatient setting (i.e., 99205 or 99215), see 99417. For prolonged services provided by a physician or other qualified health care professional involving total time spent at the patient's bedside and on the floor/unit in the hospital or nursing facility, see 99356-99357. For prolonged services provided by a physician or other qualified health care professional without face-to-face contact or unit/floor time, see 99358-99359. Codes 99358-99359 may be reported on a different date of service than the primary service and do not require the primary service to have an established time. Prolonged service of less than 30 minutes should not be reported separately. Report 99354, 99356, and 99358 only once per day for the initial hour of prolonged service care; for each additional 30-minute block of time beyond the initial hour, see 99355, 99357, and 99359. For prolonged services provided by clinical staff, see 99415-99416. Do not report 99354-99355 with 99202-99205, 99212-99215, or 99415-99417. Report 99354 in addition to 90837, 90847, 99241-99245, 99324-99337, 99341-99350, and 99483. Report 99355 in addition to 99354. Report 99356 in addition to 90837, 90847, 99218-99220, 99221-99223,

99224-99226, 99231-99233, 99234-99236, 99251-99255, and 99304-99310. Report 99357 in addition to 99356. Do not report 99358-99359 on the same date of service as 99202-99205, 99212-99215, or 99417. Do not report 99358 or 99359 for time spent performing the following E/M or monitoring services: 93792-93793, 99339, 99340, 99366-99368, 99374-99380, 99421-99423, 99424, 99446-99449, 99451-99452, or 99491. Report 99359 in addition to 99358. Medicare has identified 99356 and 99357 as telehealth/telemedicine services. Commercial payers should be contacted regarding their coverage guidelines. Telemedicine services may be reported by the performing provider by adding modifier 95 to these procedure codes and using the appropriate place of service. Services at the origination site are reported with HCPCS Level II code Q3014.

ICD-10-CM Diagnostic Codes

The application of this code is too broad to adequately present ICD-10-CM diagnostic code links here. Refer to your ICD-10-CM book.

AMA: 99354 2020,Sep,3; 2020,Feb,3; 2020,Dec,11; 2019,Oct,10; 2019,Jun,7; 2018,Jan,8; 2017,Jan,8; 2016,Jan,13; 2016,Dec,11; 2015,Oct,9; 2015,Oct,3; 2015,Jan,16 **99355** 2020,Sep,3; 2020,Feb,3; 2020,Dec,11; 2019,Oct,10; 2019,Jun,7; 2018,Jan,8; 2017,Jan,8; 2016,Jan,13; 2016,Dec,11; 2015,Oct,9; 2015,Oct,3; 2015,Jan,16 **99356** 2020,Sep,3; 2020,Dec,11; 2019,Jun,7; 2018,Jan,8; 2017,Jan,8; 2016,Jan,13; 2016,Dec,11; 2015,Oct,9; 2015,Oct,3; 2015,Jan,16 **99357** 2020,Sep,3; 2020,Dec,11; 2019,Jun,7; 2018,Jan,8; 2017,Jan,8; 2016,Jan,13; 2016,Dec,11; 2015,Oct,9; 2015,Oct,3; 2015,Jan,16 **99358** 2020,Sep,3; 2020,Feb,3; 2019,Jun,7; 2019,Jan,13; 2018,Oct,9; 2018,Jan,8; 2017,Jan,8; 2016,Jan,13; 2015,Jan,16 **99359** 2020,Sep,3; 2020,Feb,3; 2019,Jun,7; 2019,Jan,13; 2018,Oct,9; 2018,Jan,8; 2017,Jan,8; 2016,Jan,13; 2015,Jan,16

Relative Value Units/Medicare Edits

Non-Facility RVU	Work	PE	MP	Total
99354	2.33	1.22	0.15	3.7
99355	1.77	0.88	0.11	2.76
99356	1.71	0.8	0.11	2.62
99357	1.71	0.81	0.11	2.63
99358	2.1	0.95	0.15	3.2
99359	1.0	0.47	0.06	1.53

Facility RVU	Work	PE	MP	Total
99354	2.33	0.98	0.15	3.46
99355	1.77	0.67	0.11	2.55
99356	1.71	0.8	0.11	2.62
99357	1.71	0.81	0.11	2.63
99358	2.1	0.95	0.15	3.2
99359	1.0	0.47	0.06	1.53

	FUD	Status	MUE	Modifiers				IOM Reference
99354	N/A	A	1(2)	N/A	N/A	N/A	80*	100-04,11,40.1.3;
99355	N/A	A	4(3)	N/A	N/A	N/A	80*	100-04,12,30.6.4;
99356	N/A	A	1(2)	N/A	N/A	N/A	80*	100-04,12,30.6.13;
99357	N/A	A	4(3)	N/A	N/A	N/A	80*	100-04,12,30.6.14;
99358	N/A	A	1(2)	N/A	N/A	N/A	80*	100-04,12,30.6.15.1;
99359	N/A	A	2(3)	N/A	N/A	N/A	80*	100-04,12,30.6.15.2; 100-04,12,100

* with documentation

[99415, 99416]

+ **99415** Prolonged clinical staff service (the service beyond the highest time in the range of total time of the service) during an evaluation and management service in the office or outpatient setting, direct patient contact with physician supervision; first hour (List separately in addition to code for outpatient Evaluation and Management service)

+ **99416** Prolonged clinical staff service (the service beyond the highest time in the range of total time of the service) during an evaluation and management service in the office or outpatient setting, direct patient contact with physician supervision; each additional 30 minutes (List separately in addition to code for prolonged service)

Explanation

Prolonged clinical staff services are reported with resequenced codes that were added to describe special situations in which the physician's staff provided assistance to a patient beyond the usual time associated with circumstances requiring observation of the patient, such as in cases where the patient was administered a new medication or inhaled drug requiring monitoring to ensure patient safety in the office or outpatient setting. Such cases do not necessitate the clinician being face-to-face with the patient throughout the entire time period; observation and monitoring of the patient can be performed by a member of the clinician's staff under the provider's supervision. Report these codes in conjunction with the designated E/M service code along with any other service provided at the same encounter. Codes in this category should report the total amount of face-to-face time spent with the patient by the clinical staff on the same date of service even if the time is not continuous; time spent rendering other separately reportable services other than the E/M service do not count toward the prolonged services time. The highest total time in the time ranges of the code descriptions is used in defining when prolonged services time should begin. Report the first hour of prolonged services on a given date with 99415; for each additional 30 minutes of prolonged services, report 99416.

Coding Tips

These codes are used to report prolonged face-to-face services beyond the highest total time indicated in the code description provided by the clinical staff in the office or outpatient setting. These are time-based codes and time spent with the patient must be documented in the medical record. Time spent on other separately reported services excluding the E/M service should not be counted toward the prolonged service time. These codes are reported in addition to the other E/M service provided on the same date of service. A provider must be available to provide direct supervision of the clinical staff. Report 99415 only once per day for the initial hour of prolonged service care; for each additional 30-minute block of time beyond the initial hour, see 99416. Prolonged service of less than 30 minutes should not be reported separately. For prolonged services with or without direct patient contact provided by the physician or other qualified health care provider in the office or other outpatient setting, see 99417. Do not report 99415-99416 with 99354, 99355, or 99417. Report 99415 in addition to 99202-99205 and 99212-99215. Report 99416 in addition to 99415.

ICD-10-CM Diagnostic Codes

The application of this code is too broad to adequately present ICD-10-CM diagnostic code links here. Refer to your ICD-10-CM book.

AMA: **99415** 2020,Sep,3; 2020,Nov,12; 2020,Feb,3; 2019,Oct,10; 2018,Jan,8; 2017,Jan,8; 2016,Mar,8; 2016,Jan,13; 2016,Feb,13; 2015,Oct,3 **99416** 2020,Sep,3; 2020,Nov,12; 2020,Feb,3; 2019,Oct,10; 2018,Jan,8; 2017,Jan,8; 2016,Mar,8; 2016,Jan,13; 2016,Feb,13; 2015,Oct,3

Relative Value Units/Medicare Edits

Non-Facility RVU	Work	PE	MP	Total
99415	0.0	0.28	0.01	0.29
99416	0.0	0.15	0.0	0.15
Facility RVU	Work	PE	MP	Total
99415	0.0	0.28	0.01	0.29
99416	0.0	0.15	0.0	0.15

	FUD	Status	MUE	Modifiers				IOM Reference
99415	N/A	A	1(2)	N/A	N/A	N/A	80*	None
99416	N/A	A	3(3)	N/A	N/A	N/A	80*	

* with documentation

Terms To Know

clinical staff. Someone who works for, or under, the direction of a physician or qualified health care professional and does not bill services separately. The person may be licensed or regulated to help the physician perform specific duties.

direct supervision. Situation in which the physician must be present in the office suite and immediately available to provide assistance and direction throughout a given procedure. The physician is not, however, required to be present in the room when the procedure is performed.

face to face. Interaction between two parties, usually provider and patient, that occurs in the physical presence of each other.

[99417]

+ ★99417 Prolonged office or other outpatient evaluation and management service(s) beyond the minimum required time of the primary procedure which has been selected using total time, requiring total time with or without direct patient contact beyond the usual service, on the date of the primary service, each 15 minutes of total time (List separately in addition to codes 99205, 99215 for office or other outpatient Evaluation and Management services)

Explanation

Code 99417 reports prolonged total time (time with and without direct patient contact combined) that is provided by the physician or other qualified health care professional on the date of an office visit or other outpatient service. This code is assigned only when the code for the primary E/M service has been selected based solely on total time, and only after exceeding by 15 minutes the minimum time that is required to report the highest-level service. For example, when reporting an established patient encounter (99215), code 99417 would not be reported until at least 15 minutes of time beyond 40 minutes has been accumulated (i.e., 55 minutes) on the day of the encounter.

Coding Tips

This code is used to report prolonged service time by the physician or other qualified health care professional provided on the same date as 99205 or 99215. The prolonged time may be with or without direct patient contact. This service is reported only when time was the criteria used to select code 99205 or 99215 and the time exceeds the minimum time required to report these levels of service by at least 15 minutes. Code 99417 may be reported once for each additional 15 minutes spent providing prolonged services. Time performing other reportable services is not counted as prolonged service. Prolonged services provided on a date other than the date of the face-to-face encounter may be reported with 99358-99359. Prolonged services provided by clinical staff are reported with 99415-99416. Do not report 99417 with 99354-99355, 99358-99359, or 99415-99416. Telemedicine services may be reported by the performing provider by adding modifier 95 to this procedure code and using the appropriate place of service. Services at the origination site are reported with HCPCS Level II code Q3014.

ICD-10-CM Diagnostic Codes

Relative Value Units/Medicare Edits

Non-Facility RVU	Work	PE	MP	Total
99417	0.61	0.3	0.05	0.96
Facility RVU	Work	PE	MP	Total
99417	0.61	0.27	0.05	0.93

	FUD	Status	MUE	Modifiers				IOM Reference
99417	N/A	I	4(3)	N/A	N/A	N/A	N/A	None

* with documentation

99360

99360 Standby service, requiring prolonged attendance, each 30 minutes (eg, operative standby, standby for frozen section, for cesarean/high risk delivery, for monitoring EEG)

Explanation

Standby services are those requested of a qualified clinician that involves prolonged attendance without face-to-face contact with the patient (e.g., operative or cesarean/high-risk delivery standby, EEG monitoring, or standby to obtain a frozen section specimen). The clinician on standby is not permitted to provide care or services to other patients during the standby period. This code should not be used to report time spent proctoring another individual nor should it be used if the standby period ends with the standby clinician performing a procedure that is subject to the surgical package. This code encompasses the total duration of time spent on standby on a given date; standby services of less than 30 minutes total duration are not reported separately. A second and subsequent period of standby, after the initial 30 minutes, may be reported contingent that each unit of standby service equates to a full 30 minutes.

Coding Tips

This code is used to report standby services requested by another clinician for prolonged attendance without face-to-face patient contact. This is a time-based code representing the total duration of time spent providing standby services and must be documented in the medical record. Standby services of less than 30 minutes should not be reported separately. Report each additional 30 minutes of time beyond the initial time only when a full 30-minute period is provided. Report this code in addition to 99460 or 99465, if applicable. Do not report 99360 with 99464.

ICD-10-CM Diagnostic Codes

The application of this code is too broad to adequately present ICD-10-CM diagnostic code links here. Refer to your ICD-10-CM book.

AMA: 99360 2018,Jan,8; 2017,Jan,8; 2016,Jan,13; 2015,Jan,16

Relative Value Units/Medicare Edits

Non-Facility RVU	Work	PE	MP	Total
99360	1.2	0.46	0.1	1.76
Facility RVU	Work	PE	MP	Total
99360	1.2	0.46	0.1	1.76

	FUD	Status	MUE	Modifiers				IOM Reference
99360	N/A	X	1(3)	N/A	N/A	N/A	N/A	100-04,12,30.6.4; 100-04,12,30.6.15.3

* with documentation

99366-99368

99366	Medical team conference with interdisciplinary team of health care professionals, face-to-face with patient and/or family, 30 minutes or more, participation by nonphysician qualified health care professional
99367	Medical team conference with interdisciplinary team of health care professionals, patient and/or family not present, 30 minutes or more; participation by physician
99368	participation by nonphysician qualified health care professional

Explanation

A medical team conference is defined as a service where at least three qualified health care professionals from different specialties or disciplines, each of whom provides direct care to the patient, actively engage in the evolution, revision, coordination, and implementation of health care services needed by the patient. The conferences may or may not involve the presence of the patient, family members, community agencies, surrogate decision makers/legal guardians, and/or caregivers. Medical team clinicians should report the time spent in a team conference with the patient and/or family present with the appropriate E/M code, using time as a key controlling factor for selecting a code when counseling and/or coordination of care dominates the service. The individual clinician must be directly involved with rendering face-to-face services outside of the conference visit with other clinicians or agencies. All medical professionals participating on the medical team must document their own individual participation in the team conference, in addition to their contributed information and follow-up treatment recommendations. However, only one individual from the same specialty may report a code from this category at the same encounter. No individuals may report a code from range 99366-99368 if participation in the medical team conference is a part of a facility or organizational service contractually provided by the facility or organization. Team conferences commence upon review of the individual patient case and conclude once the review has come to a conclusion. Record keeping and report generation time is not reportable. The clinician must report all time for which he or she was present. Reportable time is not limited to the time that the clinician is communicating with other team members, the patient, and/or the patient's family. Note that time spent in medical team conferences should not be used toward determining other E/M services such as care plan oversight services, home, domiciliary, or rest home care plan oversight, prolonged services, psychotherapy, or any other E/M service. Nonphysician qualified health care professionals may report 99366, medical team conference, direct (face-to-face) contact with patient and/or family, when the patient is present for any or all of the medical conference with a duration of at least 30 minutes. This includes such providers as speech-language pathologists, physical therapists, occupational therapists, social workers, and dieticians. Medical conferences of less than 30 minutes duration are not reported. Codes 99367-99368 describe team conferences without direct, face-to-face patient and/or family contact.

Coding Tips

These codes are used to report medical team conferences, with direct patient and/or family contact (99366) or without direct patient and/or family contact (99367-99368). For medical team participation by a nonphysician health care professional with direct patient and/or family contact, see 99366; without direct patient or family contact, see 99368. For medical team participation by the physician without direct patient and/or family contact, see 99367. Medical team meetings of less than 30 minutes should not be reported separately. For physician participation with face-to-face patient contact, report the appropriate E/M code. Do not report medical team conference codes in the same month as 99424-99427, 99437, 99439, 99487, or 99489-99491.

ICD-10-CM Diagnostic Codes

The application of this code is too broad to adequately present ICD-10-CM diagnostic code links here. Refer to your ICD-10-CM book.

AMA: **99366** 2018,Jan,8; 2018,Apr,9; 2017,Jan,8; 2016,Jan,13; 2015,Jan,16 **99367** 2019,Dec,14; 2018,Jan,8; 2018,Apr,9; 2017,Jan,8; 2016,Jan,13; 2015,Jan,16 **99368** 2018,Jan,8; 2018,Apr,9; 2017,Jan,8; 2016,Jan,13; 2015,Jan,16

Relative Value Units/Medicare Edits

Non-Facility RVU	Work	PE	MP	Total
99366	0.82	0.35	0.06	1.23
99367	1.1	0.43	0.09	1.62
99368	0.72	0.28	0.05	1.05
Facility RVU	Work	PE	MP	Total
99366	0.82	0.32	0.06	1.2
99367	1.1	0.43	0.09	1.62
99368	0.72	0.28	0.05	1.05

	FUD	Status	MUE	Modifiers				IOM Reference
99366	N/A	B	0(3)	N/A	N/A	N/A	N/A	100-02,15,230.4; 100-04,11,40.1.3
99367	N/A	B	0(3)	N/A	N/A	N/A	N/A	
99368	N/A	B	0(3)	N/A	N/A	N/A	N/A	

* with documentation

Terms To Know

interdisciplinary care. Two or more health care professions working in a collaborative manner for the benefit of the patient.

other qualified health care professional. Individual who is qualified by education, training, licensure/regulation, and facility privileging to perform a professional service within his or her scope of practice and independently (or as incident-to) report the professional service without requiring physician supervision. Payers may state exemptions in writing or state and local regulations may not follow this definition for performance of some services. Always refer to any relevant plan policies and federal and/or state laws to determine who may perform and report services.

99441-99443

99441 Telephone evaluation and management service by a physician or other qualified health care professional who may report evaluation and management services provided to an established patient, parent, or guardian not originating from a related E/M service provided within the previous 7 days nor leading to an E/M service or procedure within the next 24 hours or soonest available appointment; 5-10 minutes of medical discussion

99442 11-20 minutes of medical discussion

99443 21-30 minutes of medical discussion

Explanation

Telephone services are non-face-to-face encounters originating from the established patient for evaluation or management of a problem provided by a qualified clinician. The problem may not be related to an E/M encounter that occurred within the previous seven days nor can the problem lead to an E/M encounter or other service within the following 24 hours or next available in-office appointment opening. Report 99441 for services lasting five to 10 minutes; 99442 for services lasting 11 to 20 minutes; and 99443 for calls lasting 21 to 30 minutes.

Coding Tips

These codes are used to report non-face-to-face patient services initiated by an established patient via the telephone. These are time-based codes and time spent with the patient must be documented in the medical record. These codes should not be reported if the provider decides to see the patient within 24 hours or by the next available urgent visit appointment, or if the provider performed a related E/M service within the previous seven days or the call is initiated within a postoperative period. Medicare and other payers may not reimburse separately for these services. Check with the specific payer to determine coverage. Do not report 99441-99443 when the same provider has reported 99421-99423 for the same problem in the previous seven days. For nonphysician telephone medical services, see 98966-98968. Do not report these services when performed concurrently with other billable services, such as 99339-99340, 99374-99380, 99487-99489, or 99495-99496. Do not report these services for INR monitoring when reporting 93792 or 93793. Medicare has provisionally identified these codes as telehealth/telemedicine services. Current Medicare coverage guidelines should be reviewed. Commercial payers should be contacted regarding their coverage guidelines. Telemedicine services may be reported by the performing provider by adding modifier 95 to these procedure codes and using the appropriate place of service. Services at the origination site are reported with HCPCS Level II code Q3014.

ICD-10-CM Diagnostic Codes

The application of this code is too broad to adequately present ICD-10-CM diagnostic code links here. Refer to your ICD-10-CM book.

AMA: 99441 2020,Jul,1; 2019,Mar,8; 2018,Mar,7; 2018,Jan,8; 2017,Jan,8; 2016,Jan,13; 2015,Jan,16 **99442** 2020,Jul,1; 2019,Mar,8; 2018,Mar,7; 2018,Jan,8; 2017,Jan,8; 2016,Jan,13; 2015,Jan,16 **99443** 2020,Jul,1; 2019,Mar,8; 2018,Mar,7; 2018,Jan,8; 2017,Jan,8; 2016,Jan,13; 2015,Jan,16

Relative Value Units/Medicare Edits

Non-Facility RVU	Work	PE	MP	Total
99441	0.7	0.88	0.05	1.63
99442	1.3	1.25	0.11	2.66
99443	1.92	1.7	0.15	3.77
Facility RVU	**Work**	**PE**	**MP**	**Total**
99441	0.7	0.29	0.05	1.04
99442	1.3	0.55	0.11	1.96
99443	1.92	0.82	0.15	2.89

	FUD	Status	MUE	Modifiers				IOM Reference
99441	N/A	A	1(2)	N/A	N/A	N/A	80*	None
99442	N/A	A	1(2)	N/A	N/A	N/A	80*	
99443	N/A	A	1(2)	N/A	N/A	N/A	80*	

* with documentation

Terms To Know

established patient. Patient who has received professional services in a face-to-face setting within the last three years from the same physician/qualified health care professional or another physician/qualified health care professional of the exact same specialty and subspecialty who belongs to the same group practice. If the patient is seen by a physician/qualified health care professional who is covering for another physician/qualified health care professional, the patient will be considered the same as if seen by the physician/qualified health care professional who is unavailable.

other qualified health care professional. Individual who is qualified by education, training, licensure/regulation, and facility privileging to perform a professional service within his or her scope of practice and independently (or as incident-to) report the professional service without requiring physician supervision. Payers may state exemptions in writing or state and local regulations may not follow this definition for performance of some services. Always refer to any relevant plan policies and federal and/or state laws to determine who may perform and report services.

[99421, 99422, 99423]

99421 Online digital evaluation and management service, for an established patient, for up to 7 days, cumulative time during the 7 days; 5-10 minutes

99422 Online digital evaluation and management service, for an established patient, for up to 7 days, cumulative time during the 7 days; 11-20 minutes

99423 Online digital evaluation and management service, for an established patient, for up to 7 days, cumulative time during the 7 days; 21 or more minutes

Explanation

Online medical evaluation services are non-face-to-face encounters originating from the established patient to the physician or other qualified health care professional for evaluation or management of a problem utilizing internet resources. The service includes all communication, prescription, and laboratory orders with permanent storage in the patient's medical record. The service may include more than one provider responding to the same patient and is only reportable once during seven days for the same encounter. Do not report these codes if the online patient request is related to an E/M service that occurred within the previous seven days or within the global period following a procedure. Report 99421 if the cumulative time during the seven-day period is five to 10 minutes; 99422 for 11 to 20 minutes; and 99423 for 21 or more minutes.

Coding Tips

These codes are used to report non-face-to-face patient services initiated by an established patient via an on-line inquiry. Providers must provide a timely response to the inquiry and the encounter must be stored permanently to report this service. These services are reported once in a seven-day period and are reported for the cumulative time devoted to the service over the seven days. Cumulative time of less than five minutes should not be reported. A new/unrelated problem initiated within seven days of a previous E/M visit that addresses a different problem may be reported separately. Medicare and other payers may not reimburse separately for these services. Check with the specific payer to determine coverage. For nonphysician on-line medical services, see 98970, 98971, and 98972. Do not report these services when performed concurrently with other billable services, such as 99202-99205, 99212-99215, 99241-99245, or when using the following for the same communication: 99091, 99339-99340, 99374-99380, 99424-99427, 99437, 99487-99489, 99491, and 99495-99496. Do not report these services for INR monitoring when reporting 93792 or 93793.

ICD-10-CM Diagnostic Codes

The application of this code is too broad to adequately present ICD-10-CM diagnostic code links here. Refer to your ICD-10-CM book.

AMA: **99421** 2020,Jan,3 **99422** 2020,Jan,3 **99423** 2020,Jan,3

Relative Value Units/Medicare Edits

Non-Facility RVU	Work	PE	MP	Total
99421	0.25	0.16	0.02	0.43
99422	0.5	0.32	0.04	0.86
99423	0.8	0.51	0.05	1.36
Facility RVU	Work	PE	MP	Total
99421	0.25	0.1	0.02	0.37
99422	0.5	0.21	0.04	0.75
99423	0.8	0.33	0.05	1.18

	FUD	Status	MUE	Modifiers				IOM Reference
99421	N/A	A	1(2)	N/A	N/A	N/A	80*	None
99422	N/A	A	1(2)	N/A	N/A	N/A	80*	
99423	N/A	A	1(2)	N/A	N/A	N/A	80*	

* with documentation

Terms To Know

established patient. Patient who has received professional services in a face-to-face setting within the last three years from the same physician/qualified health care professional or another physician/qualified health care professional of the exact same specialty and subspecialty who belongs to the same group practice. If the patient is seen by a physician/qualified health care professional who is covering for another physician/qualified health care professional, the patient will be considered the same as if seen by the physician/qualified health care professional who is unavailable.

99446-99449 [99451, 99452]

99446 Interprofessional telephone/Internet/electronic health record assessment and management service provided by a consultative physician, including a verbal and written report to the patient's treating/requesting physician or other qualified health care professional; 5-10 minutes of medical consultative discussion and review

99447 11-20 minutes of medical consultative discussion and review

99448 21-30 minutes of medical consultative discussion and review

99449 31 minutes or more of medical consultative discussion and review

99451 Interprofessional telephone/Internet/electronic health record assessment and management service provided by a consultative physician, including a written report to the patient's treating/requesting physician or other qualified health care professional, 5 minutes or more of medical consultative time

99452 Interprofessional telephone/Internet/electronic health record referral service(s) provided by a treating/requesting physician or other qualified health care professional, 30 minutes

Explanation

Interprofessional telephone/internet/electronic health record consultation services are utilized when the attending qualified clinician requests the input of another provider with specific knowledge of the condition. This specialist may assist in diagnosis or treatment of the patient without seeing the patient and often occurs when the situation is urgent and/or complex in nature. The patient may be a new or established patient with a new problem or exacerbation of a current problem in the eyes of the consulting physician; however, the consultant may not have seen the patient within the previous 14 days. This code may not be reported for transfer of care or to schedule a face-to-face with the consultant within the next 14 days or next available appointment opening. This discussion includes appropriate review of medical records, laboratory and radiology results, medication review/tolerance, and pathology results. The consult should account for more than 50 percent of the time in discussion; if more than one discussion is necessary, the time is cumulative with the code reported one time. The patient's medical record should contain a request for consult with an explanation as to the medical necessity of the request and the consulting physician should provide a verbal and written report to the requesting/treating clinician. These codes are not reportable if the discussion requires less than five minutes of time. Report 99446 for encounters of five- to 10 minutes duration; 99447 for 11 to 20 minutes; 99448 for 21 to 30 minutes; and 99449 for encounters of more than 30 minutes duration. Report 99451 for encounters of five or more minutes that include a written report only from the consulting physician. The attending qualified clinician can report 99452 when 16 to 30 minutes of the clinician's time is spent preparing for or communicating with the consultant; 99452 can only be reported once during a 14-day period.

Coding Tips

These codes are used to report an assessment and management service requested by the patient's treating clinician for guidance from a specialist in treating the patient. These are time-based codes and time spent in medical consultation must be documented in the medical record. These codes do not differentiate between a new or established patient. Do not report these codes for the sole purpose of arranging a transfer of care or other face-to-face services. Report 99446-99449 for time spent in telephone/internet/electronic health record assessment and review with verbal and written report of findings. Report 99451 for written report of findings without a verbal report. Report

99452 for the time a provider spends, on a service day, preparing for or communicating with the consultant. Prolonged service codes 99354-99357 may be reported by the treating/requesting provider in addition to these services when the patient is present (on-site) and the telephone/internet/electronic health record discussion with the consultant exceeds 30 minutes. Prolonged service codes 99358-99359 may be reported by the treating/requesting provider in addition to these services when the patient is not present and the telephone/internet discussion with the consultant exceeds 30 minutes. For telephone services conducted by the physician directly with the patient, see 99441-99443. For on-line digital medical evaluation and management services provided by the physician directly with the patient, see 99421-99423. For nonphysician telephone or online medical services, see 98966-98968.

ICD-10-CM Diagnostic Codes

The application of this code is too broad to adequately present ICD-10-CM diagnostic code links here. Refer to your ICD-10-CM book.

AMA: 99446 2019,Jun,7; 2019,Jan,3; 2018,Jan,8; 2017,Jan,8; 2016,Jan,13; 2015,Jan,16 **99447** 2019,Jun,7; 2019,Jan,3; 2018,Jan,8; 2017,Jan,8; 2016,Jan,13; 2015,Jan,16 **99448** 2019,Jun,7; 2019,Jan,3; 2018,Jan,8; 2017,Jan,8; 2016,Jan,13; 2015,Jan,16 **99449** 2019,Jun,7; 2019,Jan,3; 2018,Jan,8; 2017,Jan,8; 2016,Jan,13; 2015,Jan,16 **99451** 2019,Jun,7; 2019,Jan,3 **99452** 2020,Jun,3; 2019,Jun,7; 2019,Jan,3

Relative Value Units/Medicare Edits

Non-Facility RVU	Work	PE	MP	Total
99446	0.35	0.15	0.04	0.54
99447	0.7	0.21	0.06	0.97
99448	1.05	0.4	0.09	1.54
99449	1.4	0.59	0.11	2.1
99451	0.7	0.29	0.05	1.04
99452	0.7	0.3	0.05	1.05

Facility RVU	Work	PE	MP	Total
99446	0.35	0.15	0.04	0.54
99447	0.7	0.21	0.06	0.97
99448	1.05	0.4	0.09	1.54
99449	1.4	0.59	0.11	2.1
99451	0.7	0.29	0.05	1.04
99452	0.7	0.3	0.05	1.05

	FUD	Status	MUE	Modifiers				IOM Reference
99446	N/A	A	1(2)	N/A	N/A	N/A	80*	None
99447	N/A	A	1(2)	N/A	N/A	N/A	80*	
99448	N/A	A	1(2)	N/A	N/A	N/A	80*	
99449	N/A	A	1(2)	N/A	N/A	N/A	80*	
99451	N/A	A	1(2)	N/A	N/A	N/A	80*	
99452	N/A	A	1(2)	N/A	N/A	N/A	80*	

* with documentation

[99437, 99439, 99490, 99491]

▲ **99490** Chronic care management services with the following required elements: multiple (two or more) chronic conditions expected to last at least 12 months, or until the death of the patient, chronic conditions that place the patient at significant risk of death, acute exacerbation/decompensation, or functional decline, comprehensive care plan established, implemented, revised, or monitored; first 20 minutes of clinical staff time directed by a physician or other qualified health care professional, per calendar month.

+▲ **99439** Chronic care management services with the following required elements: multiple (two or more) chronic conditions expected to last at least 12 months, or until the death of the patient, chronic conditions that place the patient at significant risk of death, acute exacerbation/decompensation, or functional decline, comprehensive care plan established, implemented, revised, or monitored; each additional 20 minutes of clinical staff time directed by a physician or other qualified health care professional, per calendar month (List separately in addition to code for primary procedure)

▲ **99491** Chronic care management services with the following required elements: multiple (two or more) chronic conditions expected to last at least 12 months, or until the death of the patient, chronic conditions that place the patient at significant risk of death, acute exacerbation/decompensation, or functional decline, comprehensive care plan established, implemented, revised, or monitored; first 30 minutes provided personally by a physician or other qualified health care professional, per calendar month.

+● **99437** Chronic care management services with the following required elements: multiple (two or more) chronic conditions expected to last at least 12 months, or until the death of the patient, chronic conditions that place the patient at significant risk of death, acute exacerbation/decompensation, or functional decline, comprehensive care plan established, implemented, revised, or monitored; each additional 30 minutes by a physician or other qualified health care professional, per calendar month (List separately in addition to code for primary procedure)

Explanation

Care management services are defined as those management and support services that are 1) rendered by clinical staff while under the direction of a clinician who may be a physician or other qualified health care professional (QHP) or 2) provided personally by a physician or other QHP to a patient who resides in a personal residence or in an assisted living facility, domiciliary, or rest home. Some components of care management services include the establishment, implementation, monitoring, or revision of the patient's individual care plan; coordination of the care provided by other agencies and professionals; and education afforded to the patient or their caregiver regarding the patient's care plan, condition, and prognosis. Intended to improve coordination of care and patient engagement while reducing hospitalizations and disjointed care, care management services also take into account the patient's other medical conditions, psychosocial needs, and normal activities of daily living (ADL). Chronic care management services are represented by resequenced codes 99490, 99439, 99491, and 99437. Typically, patients receiving this care have a minimum of two and possibly more chronic ongoing or episodic health conditions that are anticipated to last at least one year (or until the patient expires) and that put the patient at increased risk of death, exacerbation, or functional decline. Chronic care management services include the establishment, implementation, revision, or monitoring of a comprehensive care plan. Code 99490 should be reported once per calendar month for the first 20 minutes of clinical staff time when directed by a physician or other QHP; for each additional 20 minutes, report 99439. Code 99439 should not be reported more than twice per calendar month. Code 99491 is also reported once per calendar month and represents the first 30 minutes provided personally by the physician or other QHP involved with care management activities; report 99437 for each additional 30 minutes.

Coding Tips

These codes are used to report care management services provided by the clinical staff under the direction of a qualified health care professional or directly by a physician or other qualified health care professional to a patient residing at home or in an assisted living facility, domiciliary, or rest home. These are time-based codes and total time spent performing care management services during the calendar month should be documented in the patient record. Do not report these codes if all elements listed in the code description are not performed. If the physician provides face-to-face E/M visits in the same calendar month, these visits may be reported separately. Do not count clinical staff time for a particular day if the physician reports an E/M service on that day. Code 99490 and 99491 may only be reported once per calendar month by the provider that assumes the care management role for the patient. Do not report 99490 if less than 20 minutes of chronic care management is provided in the calendar month. Code 99439 should be reported in addition to 99490 for each additional 20 minutes of clinical staff time provided. Report 99491 when more than 30 minutes of chronic care management is provided by the physician or other qualified health care provider in the same calendar month. Code 99437 should be reported in addition to 99491 for each additional 30 minutes of physician time provided. Do not report 99439 or 99490 with 99437 or 99491 during the same calendar month; do not report any of these codes with 99487 or 99489. Do not report these codes with 90951-90970 for ESRD services or in the postoperative period of a reported surgery. Do not report these codes with 99339-99340, 99374-99380, 99424-99427, 99437, 99487, 99489, 99491, or 99605-99607 in the same calendar month. Do not report these codes for service time reported with 93792-93793, 98960-98962, 98966-98968, 98970-98972, 99071, 99078, 99080, 99091, 99358-99359, 99366-99368, 99421-99423, 99441-99443, 99495-99496, or 99605-99607.

ICD-10-CM Diagnostic Codes

AMA: 99490 2020,Feb,7; 2020,Apr,5; 2019,Jan,6; 2018,Oct,9; 2018,Mar,7; 2018,Mar,5; 2018,Jul,12; 2018,Jan,8; 2018,Feb,7; 2018,Apr,9; 2017,Jan,8; 2016,Jan,13; 2015,Jan,16; 2015,Feb,3 **99491** 2020,Apr,5

Relative Value Units/Medicare Edits

Non-Facility RVU	Work	PE	MP	Total
99490	0.61	0.53	0.04	1.18
99439	0.54	0.5	0.04	1.08
99491	1.45	0.82	0.09	2.36
99437				
Facility RVU	Work	PE	MP	Total
99490	0.61	0.26	0.04	0.91
99439	0.54	0.23	0.04	0.81
99491	1.45	0.82	0.09	2.36
99437				

	FUD	Status	MUE	Modifiers				IOM Reference
99490	N/A	A	1(2)	N/A	N/A	N/A	80*	None
99439	N/A	A	2(2)	N/A	N/A	N/A	80*	
99491	N/A	A	1(2)	N/A	N/A	N/A	80*	
99437	N/A		-	N/A	N/A	N/A	N/A	

* with documentation

Terms To Know

chronic. Persistent, continuing, or recurring.

clinical staff. Someone who works for, or under, the direction of a physician or qualified health care professional and does not bill services separately. The person may be licensed or regulated to help the physician perform specific duties.

medical decision making. Consideration of the differential diagnoses, the amount and/or complexity of data reviewed and considered (medical records, test results, correspondence from previous treating physicians, etc.), current diagnostic studies ordered, and treatment or management options and risk (complications of the patient's condition, the potential for complications, continued morbidity, risk of mortality, any comorbidities associated with the patient's disease process).

E/M Services

99487-99489

▲ **99487** Complex chronic care management services with the following required elements: multiple (two or more) chronic conditions expected to last at least 12 months, or until the death of the patient, chronic conditions that place the patient at significant risk of death, acute exacerbation/decompensation, or functional decline, comprehensive care plan established, implemented, revised, or monitored, moderate or high complexity medical decision making; first 60 minutes of clinical staff time directed by a physician or other qualified health care professional, per calendar month.

+▲ **99489** each additional 30 minutes of clinical staff time directed by a physician or other qualified health care professional, per calendar month (List separately in addition to code for primary procedure)

Explanation

Care management services are defined as those management and support services that are 1) rendered by clinical staff while under the direction of a clinician who may be a physician or other qualified health care professional (QHP) or 2) provided personally by a physician or other QHP to a patient who resides in a personal residence or in an assisted living facility, domiciliary, or rest home. Some components of care management services include the establishment, implementation, monitoring, or revision of the patient's individual care plan; coordination of the care provided by other agencies and professionals; and education afforded to the patient or their caregiver regarding the patient's care plan, condition, and prognosis. Intended to improve coordination of care and patient engagement while reducing hospitalizations and disjointed care, care management services also consider the patient's other medical conditions, psychosocial needs, and normal activities of daily living (ADL). Complex chronic care management services (99487, 99489) are provided to patients who typically have a minimum of two and possibly more chronic ongoing or episodic health conditions that are anticipated to last at least one year (or until the patient expires) and that put the patient at increased risk of death, exacerbation, or functional decline. Included is the establishment, implementation, revision, or monitoring of a comprehensive care plan that requires moderate or high complexity medical decision making. Code 99487 is reported once per calendar month for the first 60 minutes of clinical staff time when directed by a physician or other QHP; for each additional 30 minutes, report 99489. Code 99489 should not be reported more than twice per calendar month.

Coding Tips

These codes are used to report care management services provided by the clinical staff under the direction of a qualified health care professional to a patient residing at home or in an assisted living facility, domiciliary, or rest home. These are time-based codes and total time spent performing care management services during the calendar month should be documented in the patient record. Do not report these codes if all elements listed in the code description are not performed. If the physician provides face-to-face E/M visits in the same calendar month, these visits may be reported separately. Do not count clinical staff time for a particular day if the physician reports an E/M service on that day. Code 99487 may only be reported once per calendar month by the provider that assumes the care management role for the patient. Code 99489 should only be reported in addition to 99487. Do not report 99487 if less than 60 minutes of complex chronic care management is provided in a calendar month. Do not report 99489 if less than 30 minutes of additional time beyond the first 60 minutes of complex chronic care is provided. Do not report these codes in addition to 90951-90970 for ESRD services or in the postoperative period of a reported surgery. Do not report these codes in

addition to 99339-99340, 99374-99380, 99424-99427, 99437, 99439, or 99490-99491 in the same calendar month. Do not report 99487 or 99489 for service time reported with 93792-93793, 98960-98962, 98966-98968, 98970-98972, 99071, 99078, 99080, 99091, 99358-99359, 99366-99368, 99421-99423, 99441-99443, or 99605-99607.

ICD-10-CM Diagnostic Codes

The application of this code is too broad to adequately present ICD-10-CM diagnostic code links here. Refer to your ICD-10-CM book.

AMA: **99487** 2020,Feb,7; 2020,Apr,5; 2019,Jan,6; 2018,Oct,9; 2018,Mar,5; 2018,Mar,7; 2018,Jul,12; 2018,Jan,8; 2018,Feb,7; 2018,Apr,9; 2017,Jan,8; 2017,Apr,9; 2016,Jan,13; 2015,Jan,16 **99489** 2020,Feb,7; 2020,Apr,5; 2019,Jan,6; 2018,Oct,9; 2018,Mar,5; 2018,Mar,7; 2018,Jul,12; 2018,Jan,8; 2018,Feb,7; 2018,Apr,9; 2017,Jan,8; 2017,Apr,9; 2016,Jan,13; 2015,Jan,16

Relative Value Units/Medicare Edits

Non-Facility RVU	Work	PE	MP	Total
99487	1.0	1.58	0.05	2.63
99489	0.5	0.72	0.04	1.26
Facility RVU	Work	PE	MP	Total
99487	1.0	0.42	0.05	1.47
99489	0.5	0.2	0.04	0.74

	FUD	Status	MUE	Modifiers				IOM Reference
99487	N/A	A	1(2)	N/A	N/A	N/A	80*	None
99489	N/A	A	10(3)	N/A	N/A	N/A	80*	

* with documentation

Terms To Know

clinical staff. Someone who works for, or under, the direction of a physician or qualified health care professional and does not bill services separately. The person may be licensed or regulated to help the physician perform specific duties.

10010-10021 [10004, 10005, 10006, 10007, 10008, 10009]

	10021	Fine needle aspiration biopsy, without imaging guidance; first lesion
+	10004	Fine needle aspiration biopsy, without imaging guidance; each additional lesion (List separately in addition to code for primary procedure)
	10005	Fine needle aspiration biopsy, including ultrasound guidance; first lesion
+	10006	Fine needle aspiration biopsy, including ultrasound guidance; each additional lesion (List separately in addition to code for primary procedure)
	10007	Fine needle aspiration biopsy, including fluoroscopic guidance; first lesion
+	10008	Fine needle aspiration biopsy, including fluoroscopic guidance; each additional lesion (List separately in addition to code for primary procedure)
	10009	Fine needle aspiration biopsy, including CT guidance; first lesion
+	10010	Fine needle aspiration biopsy, including CT guidance; each additional lesion (List separately in addition to code for primary procedure)
	10011	Fine needle aspiration biopsy, including MR guidance; first lesion
+	10012	Fine needle aspiration biopsy, including MR guidance; each additional lesion (List separately in addition to code for primary procedure)

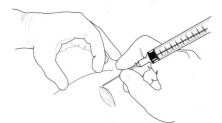

Fine needle aspiration biopsy with or without imaging guidance

Explanation

Fine needle aspiration (FNA) is a diagnostic percutaneous procedure that uses a fine gauge needle (often 22 or 25 gauge) and a syringe to sample fluid from a cyst or remove clusters of cells from a solid mass. The skin is cleansed. If a lump can be felt, the radiologist or surgeon guides a needle into the area by palpating the lump. If the lump is non-palpable, the FNA procedure is performed using ultrasound, fluoroscopy, computed tomography (CT), or MR imaging with the patient positioned according to the area of concern. Ultrasonography-guided aspiration biopsy involves inserting an aspiration catheter needle device through the accessory channel port of the echoendoscope; the needle is placed into the area to be sampled under endoscopic ultrasonographic guidance. After the needle is placed into the region of the lesion, a vacuum is created and multiple in and out needle motions are performed. Several needle insertions are usually required to ensure that an adequate tissue sample is taken. In fluoroscopic guidance, intermittent fluoroscopy guides the advancement of the needle. CT image guidance allows computer-assisted targeting of the area to be sampled. At the completion of the procedure, the needle is withdrawn and a small bandage is placed over

the area. MR image guidance involves the use of a magnetic field, radiowaves, and computer-assisted targeting to identify the area for biopsy without the use of ionizing radiation. Report 10021 for fine needle aspiration of the initial lesion performed without imaging guidance; for each subsequent lesion, report 10004. Report 10005 for FNA of the first lesion using ultrasound guidance; for each additional lesion, report 10006. Report 10007 for FNA of the first lesion using fluoroscopy; for each additional lesion, report 10008. Report 10009 for FNA of the first lesion utilizing CT imaging; for each subsequent lesion, report 10010. Report 10011 when MR imaging is used for the initial lesion; for each additional lesion, report 10012.

Coding Tips

When these codes are performed with another separately identifiable procedure, the highest dollar value code is listed as the primary procedure and subsequent procedures are appended with modifier 51. If multiple areas are aspirated, report 10004–10012 and 10021 for each site taken and append modifier 59 or an X{EPSU} modifier to the additional codes. For evaluation of fine needle aspirate, see 88172–88173. For percutaneous placement of a localization device during breast biopsy, see 19081–19086. For percutaneous needle biopsy, muscle, see 20206; lung or mediastinum and pleura, see 32408; salivary gland, see 42400; liver, see 47000; pancreas, see 48102; abdominal or retroperitoneal mass, see 49180; kidney, see 50200; and thyroid, see 60100. For percutaneous image-guided fluid collection drainage of soft tissue via catheter, see 10030.

ICD-10-CM Diagnostic Codes

C25.0	Malignant neoplasm of head of pancreas
C25.1	Malignant neoplasm of body of pancreas
C25.2	Malignant neoplasm of tail of pancreas
C25.3	Malignant neoplasm of pancreatic duct
C34.01	Malignant neoplasm of right main bronchus ☑
C34.02	Malignant neoplasm of left main bronchus ☑
C34.11	Malignant neoplasm of upper lobe, right bronchus or lung ☑
C34.12	Malignant neoplasm of upper lobe, left bronchus or lung ☑
C34.2	Malignant neoplasm of middle lobe, bronchus or lung
C34.31	Malignant neoplasm of lower lobe, right bronchus or lung ☑
C34.32	Malignant neoplasm of lower lobe, left bronchus or lung ☑
C34.81	Malignant neoplasm of overlapping sites of right bronchus and lung ☑
C34.82	Malignant neoplasm of overlapping sites of left bronchus and lung ☑
C50.011	Malignant neoplasm of nipple and areola, right female breast ♀ ☑
C50.021	Malignant neoplasm of nipple and areola, right male breast ♂ ☑
C50.111	Malignant neoplasm of central portion of right female breast ♀ ☑
C50.121	Malignant neoplasm of central portion of right male breast ♂ ☑
C50.211	Malignant neoplasm of upper-inner quadrant of right female breast ♀ ☑
C50.221	Malignant neoplasm of upper-inner quadrant of right male breast ♂ ☑
C50.311	Malignant neoplasm of lower-inner quadrant of right female breast ♀ ☑
C50.321	Malignant neoplasm of lower-inner quadrant of right male breast ♂ ☑
C50.411	Malignant neoplasm of upper-outer quadrant of right female breast ♀ ☑
C50.421	Malignant neoplasm of upper-outer quadrant of right male breast ♂ ☑

C50.511	Malignant neoplasm of lower-outer quadrant of right female breast ♀ ☑
C50.521	Malignant neoplasm of lower-outer quadrant of right male breast ♂ ☑
C50.611	Malignant neoplasm of axillary tail of right female breast ♀ ☑
C50.621	Malignant neoplasm of axillary tail of right male breast ♂ ☑
C76.2	Malignant neoplasm of abdomen
C76.41	Malignant neoplasm of right upper limb ☑
C76.51	Malignant neoplasm of right lower limb ☑
C7A.092	Malignant carcinoid tumor of the stomach
C81.25	Mixed cellularity Hodgkin lymphoma, lymph nodes of inguinal region and lower limb
D09.3	Carcinoma in situ of thyroid and other endocrine glands
D13.5	Benign neoplasm of extrahepatic bile ducts
D13.6	Benign neoplasm of pancreas
D13.7	Benign neoplasm of endocrine pancreas
D17.21	Benign lipomatous neoplasm of skin and subcutaneous tissue of right arm ☑
D17.23	Benign lipomatous neoplasm of skin and subcutaneous tissue of right leg ☑
D17.5	Benign lipomatous neoplasm of intra-abdominal organs
D24.1	Benign neoplasm of right breast ☑
D37.6	Neoplasm of uncertain behavior of liver, gallbladder and bile ducts
D37.8	Neoplasm of uncertain behavior of other specified digestive organs
D44.0	Neoplasm of uncertain behavior of thyroid gland
D48.3	Neoplasm of uncertain behavior of retroperitoneum
D48.4	Neoplasm of uncertain behavior of peritoneum
D48.61	Neoplasm of uncertain behavior of right breast ☑
E01.0	Iodine-deficiency related diffuse (endemic) goiter
E01.1	Iodine-deficiency related multinodular (endemic) goiter
E04.0	Nontoxic diffuse goiter
E04.1	Nontoxic single thyroid nodule
E04.2	Nontoxic multinodular goiter
K70.11	Alcoholic hepatitis with ascites 🅐
K70.2	Alcoholic fibrosis and sclerosis of liver 🅐
K70.31	Alcoholic cirrhosis of liver with ascites 🅐
K71.0	Toxic liver disease with cholestasis
K71.10	Toxic liver disease with hepatic necrosis, without coma
K71.3	Toxic liver disease with chronic persistent hepatitis
K71.51	Toxic liver disease with chronic active hepatitis with ascites
K74.3	Primary biliary cirrhosis
K75.0	Abscess of liver
K86.3	Pseudocyst of pancreas
L02.216	Cutaneous abscess of umbilicus
L03.311	Cellulitis of abdominal wall
L03.316	Cellulitis of umbilicus
N60.01	Solitary cyst of right breast ☑
N60.11	Diffuse cystic mastopathy of right breast 🅐 ☑
N60.21	Fibroadenosis of right breast ☑
N60.31	Fibrosclerosis of right breast ☑
R19.01	Right upper quadrant abdominal swelling, mass and lump
R19.03	Right lower quadrant abdominal swelling, mass and lump
R19.05	Periumbilic swelling, mass or lump
R19.06	Epigastric swelling, mass or lump
R22.31	Localized swelling, mass and lump, right upper limb ☑
R22.41	Localized swelling, mass and lump, right lower limb ☑

AMA: **10004** 2019,Feb,8; 2019,Apr,4 **10005** 2019,May,10; 2019,Feb,8; 2019,Apr,4 **10006** 2019,Feb,8; 2019,Apr,4 **10007** 2019,Feb,8; 2019,Apr,4 **10008** 2019,Feb,8; 2019,Apr,4 **10009** 2019,Feb,8; 2019,Apr,4 **10010** 2019,Feb,8; 2019,Apr,4 **10011** 2019,Feb,8; 2019,Apr,4 **10012** 2019,Feb,8; 2019,Apr,4 **10021** 2019,May,10; 2019,Feb,8; 2019,Apr,4; 2018,Jan,8; 2017,Jan,8; 2016,Jan,13; 2015,Jan,16

Relative Value Units/Medicare Edits

Non-Facility RVU	Work	PE	MP	Total
10021	1.03	1.85	0.14	3.02
10004	0.8	0.59	0.11	1.5
10005	1.46	2.38	0.15	3.99
10006	1.0	0.67	0.1	1.77
10007	1.81	7.06	0.19	9.06
10008	1.18	3.52	0.11	4.81
10009	2.26	11.44	0.21	13.91
10010	1.65	6.42	0.15	8.22
10011	0.0	0.0	0.0	0.0
10012	0.0	0.0	0.0	0.0
Facility RVU	**Work**	**PE**	**MP**	**Total**
10021	1.03	0.44	0.14	1.61
10004	0.8	0.34	0.11	1.25
10005	1.46	0.5	0.15	2.11
10006	1.0	0.37	0.1	1.47
10007	1.81	0.67	0.19	2.67
10008	1.18	0.41	0.11	1.7
10009	2.26	0.78	0.21	3.25
10010	1.65	0.56	0.15	2.36
10011	0.0	0.0	0.0	0.0
10012	0.0	0.0	0.0	0.0

	FUD	Status	MUE	Modifiers				IOM Reference
10021	N/A	A	1(2)	51	N/A	N/A	80*	100-04,13,80.1; 100-04,13,80.2
10004	N/A	A	3(3)	N/A	N/A	N/A	80*	
10005	N/A	A	1(2)	51	N/A	N/A	80*	
10006	N/A	A	3(3)	N/A	N/A	N/A	80*	
10007	N/A	A	1(2)	51	N/A	N/A	80*	
10008	N/A	A	2(3)	N/A	N/A	N/A	80*	
10009	N/A	A	1(2)	51	N/A	N/A	80*	
10010	N/A	A	3(3)	N/A	N/A	N/A	80*	
10011	N/A	C	1(2)	51	N/A	N/A	80*	
10012	N/A	C	3(3)	N/A	N/A	N/A	80*	

* with documentation

10030

10030 Image-guided fluid collection drainage by catheter (eg, abscess, hematoma, seroma, lymphocele, cyst), soft tissue (eg, extremity, abdominal wall, neck), percutaneous

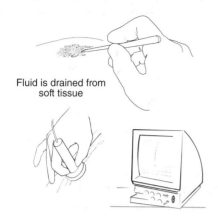

Fluid is drained from soft tissue

A transducer is passed over the site and the results are viewed on a monitor

Explanation

A fluid collection in the soft tissue, such as a hematoma, seroma, abscess, lymphocele, or cyst, is drained using a catheter. The area over the abnormal tissue is cleansed and local anesthesia is administered. Imaging is performed to assist in the insertion of a needle or guidewire into the fluid collection. Small tissue samples may be collected from the site for pathological examination. A catheter is inserted to drain and collect the fluid for analysis. More imaging may be performed to ensure hemostasis. In some cases, the catheter may be attached to a drainage system to allow for further drainage over the course of days. Once the fluid has completely drained, the catheter is removed. A bandage is applied. Report 10030 for each fluid collection drained using a separate catheter.

Coding Tips

Report 10030 once per individual collection drained with a separate catheter. Do not report 10030 with imaging codes 75989, 76942, 77002–77003, 77012, or 77021. For percutaneous or transvaginal/transrectal, image-guided fluid collection of the visceral, peritoneal, or retroperitoneal areas, see 49405–49407.

ICD-10-CM Diagnostic Codes

L02.11	Cutaneous abscess of neck
L02.211	Cutaneous abscess of abdominal wall
L02.212	Cutaneous abscess of back [any part, except buttock]
L02.213	Cutaneous abscess of chest wall
L02.214	Cutaneous abscess of groin
L02.215	Cutaneous abscess of perineum
L02.216	Cutaneous abscess of umbilicus
L02.31	Cutaneous abscess of buttock
L02.411	Cutaneous abscess of right axilla ☑
L02.412	Cutaneous abscess of left axilla ☑
L02.413	Cutaneous abscess of right upper limb ☑
L02.414	Cutaneous abscess of left upper limb ☑
L02.415	Cutaneous abscess of right lower limb ☑
L02.416	Cutaneous abscess of left lower limb ☑
L02.511	Cutaneous abscess of right hand ☑
L02.512	Cutaneous abscess of left hand ☑
L02.611	Cutaneous abscess of right foot ☑
L02.612	Cutaneous abscess of left foot ☑
L02.818	Cutaneous abscess of other sites
L76.21	Postprocedural hemorrhage of skin and subcutaneous tissue following a dermatologic procedure
L76.22	Postprocedural hemorrhage of skin and subcutaneous tissue following other procedure
L76.31	Postprocedural hematoma of skin and subcutaneous tissue following a dermatologic procedure
L76.32	Postprocedural hematoma of skin and subcutaneous tissue following other procedure
L76.33	Postprocedural seroma of skin and subcutaneous tissue following a dermatologic procedure
L76.34	Postprocedural seroma of skin and subcutaneous tissue following other procedure
M72.8	Other fibroblastic disorders
M79.81	Nontraumatic hematoma of soft tissue
M96.830	Postprocedural hemorrhage of a musculoskeletal structure following a musculoskeletal system procedure
M96.831	Postprocedural hemorrhage of a musculoskeletal structure following other procedure
N61.1	Abscess of the breast and nipple
N61.21	Granulomatous mastitis, right breast ☑
O91.02	Infection of nipple associated with the puerperium Ⓜ ♀
O91.12	Abscess of breast associated with the puerperium Ⓜ ♀
T79.2XXA	Traumatic secondary and recurrent hemorrhage and seroma, initial encounter
T81.42XA	Infection following a procedure, deep incisional surgical site, initial encounter
T87.89	Other complications of amputation stump

AMA: 10030 2019,Apr,4; 2018,Jan,8; 2017,Jan,8; 2017,Aug,9; 2016,Jan,13; 2015,Jan,16

Relative Value Units/Medicare Edits

Non-Facility RVU	Work	PE	MP	Total
10030	2.75	16.52	0.26	19.53
Facility RVU	**Work**	**PE**	**MP**	**Total**
10030	2.75	0.94	0.26	3.95

	FUD	Status	MUE	Modifiers				IOM Reference
10030	0	A	2(3)	51	N/A	N/A	80*	None

* with documentation

10035-10036

10035 Placement of soft tissue localization device(s) (eg, clip, metallic pellet, wire/needle, radioactive seeds), percutaneous, including imaging guidance; first lesion

+ **10036** each additional lesion (List separately in addition to code for primary procedure)

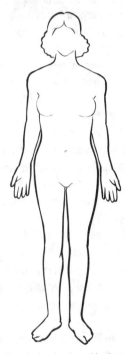

Localization device is placed in the soft tissue

Explanation

The physician places a soft tissue localization device prior to a biopsy. Using image guidance, the physician places a metallic clip, pellet, wire, needle, or radioactive seed adjacent to a soft tissue lesion to mark the site for an open soft tissue procedure or a percutaneous soft tissue biopsy to be performed during the same or a different encounter. Report 10035 for the first lesion and 10036 for each additional lesion, whether on the same or the contralateral side, marked using imaging guidance.

Coding Tips

Report 10036 in addition to 10035. These codes should be used for placement of a localization device identified only as soft tissue; if another more specific site is identified, use the appropriate site-specific code. Report these codes once per treatment site regardless of the number of markers used. Do not report 10035–10036 with 76942, 77002, 77012, or 77021. To report a second, subsequent procedure on the same or contralateral side, see 10036.

ICD-10-CM Diagnostic Codes

The application of this code is too broad to adequately present ICD-10-CM diagnostic code links here. Refer to your ICD-10-CM book.

AMA: 10035 2018,Jan,8; 2017,Jan,8; 2016,Jun,3 **10036** 2018,Jan,8; 2017,Jan,8; 2016,Jun,3

Relative Value Units/Medicare Edits

Non-Facility RVU	Work	PE	MP	Total
10035	1.7	10.72	0.15	12.57
10036	0.85	9.82	0.1	10.77
Facility RVU	**Work**	**PE**	**MP**	**Total**
10035	1.7	0.61	0.15	2.46
10036	0.85	0.3	0.1	1.25

	FUD	Status	MUE	Modifiers				IOM Reference
10035	0	A	1(2)	51	50	N/A	80*	None
10036	N/A	A	2(3)	N/A	N/A	N/A	80*	

* with documentation

Terms To Know

imaging. Radiologic means of producing pictures for clinical study of the internal structures and functions of the body, such as x-ray, ultrasound, magnetic resonance, or positron emission tomography.

lesion. Area of damaged tissue that has lost continuity or function, due to disease or trauma.

localization. Limitation to one area.

percutaneous. Through the skin.

soft tissue. Nonepithelial tissues outside of the skeleton that includes subcutaneous adipose tissue, fibrous tissue, fascia, muscles, blood and lymph vessels, and peripheral nervous system tissue.

10060 Incision and drainage of abscess (eg, carbuncle, suppurative hidradenitis, cutaneous or subcutaneous abscess, cyst, furuncle, or paronychia); simple or single

10061 complicated or multiple

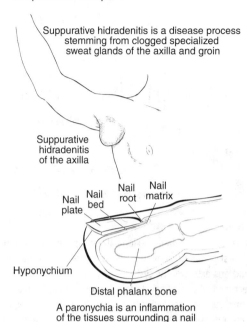

Suppurative hidradenitis is a disease process stemming from clogged specialized sweat glands of the axilla and groin

Suppurative hidradenitis of the axilla

A paronychia is an inflammation of the tissues surrounding a nail

Explanation

The physician makes a small incision through the skin overlying an abscess for incision and drainage (e.g., carbuncle, cyst, furuncle, paronychia, hidradenitis). The abscess or cyst is opened with a surgical instrument, allowing the contents to drain. The lesion may be curetted and irrigated. The physician leaves the surgical wound open to allow for continued drainage or the physician may place a Penrose latex drain or gauze strip packing to allow continued drainage. Report 10060 for incision and drainage of a simple or single abscess. Report 10061 for complex or multiple cysts. Complex or multiple cysts may require surgical closure at a later date.

Coding Tips

For puncture aspiration of an abscess, hematoma, bulla, or cyst, see 10160. For incision and drainage of a pilonidal cyst, simple, see 10080; complicated, see 10081. Local anesthesia is included in this service. Surgical trays, A4550, are not separately reimbursed by Medicare; however, other third-party payers may cover them. Check with the specific payer to determine coverage.

ICD-10-CM Diagnostic Codes

K12.2	Cellulitis and abscess of mouth
L02.01	Cutaneous abscess of face
L02.02	Furuncle of face
L02.03	Carbuncle of face
L02.11	Cutaneous abscess of neck
L02.12	Furuncle of neck
L02.13	Carbuncle of neck
L02.211	Cutaneous abscess of abdominal wall
L02.212	Cutaneous abscess of back [any part, except buttock]
L02.213	Cutaneous abscess of chest wall
L02.216	Cutaneous abscess of umbilicus
L02.221	Furuncle of abdominal wall
L02.222	Furuncle of back [any part, except buttock]
L02.223	Furuncle of chest wall
L02.226	Furuncle of umbilicus
L02.231	Carbuncle of abdominal wall
L02.232	Carbuncle of back [any part, except buttock]
L02.233	Carbuncle of chest wall
L02.236	Carbuncle of umbilicus
L02.31	Cutaneous abscess of buttock
L02.32	Furuncle of buttock
L02.33	Carbuncle of buttock
L02.411	Cutaneous abscess of right axilla ☑
L02.412	Cutaneous abscess of left axilla ☑
L02.413	Cutaneous abscess of right upper limb ☑
L02.414	Cutaneous abscess of left upper limb ☑
L02.415	Cutaneous abscess of right lower limb ☑
L02.416	Cutaneous abscess of left lower limb ☑
L02.421	Furuncle of right axilla ☑
L02.422	Furuncle of left axilla ☑
L02.423	Furuncle of right upper limb ☑
L02.424	Furuncle of left upper limb ☑
L02.425	Furuncle of right lower limb ☑
L02.426	Furuncle of left lower limb ☑
L02.431	Carbuncle of right axilla ☑
L02.432	Carbuncle of left axilla ☑
L02.433	Carbuncle of right upper limb ☑
L02.434	Carbuncle of left upper limb ☑
L02.435	Carbuncle of right lower limb ☑
L02.436	Carbuncle of left lower limb ☑
L02.511	Cutaneous abscess of right hand ☑
L02.512	Cutaneous abscess of left hand ☑
L02.521	Furuncle right hand ☑
L02.522	Furuncle left hand ☑
L02.531	Carbuncle of right hand ☑
L02.532	Carbuncle of left hand ☑
L02.611	Cutaneous abscess of right foot ☑
L02.612	Cutaneous abscess of left foot ☑
L02.621	Furuncle of right foot ☑
L02.622	Furuncle of left foot ☑
L02.631	Carbuncle of right foot ☑
L02.632	Carbuncle of left foot ☑
L02.811	Cutaneous abscess of head [any part, except face]
L03.011	Cellulitis of right finger ☑
L03.012	Cellulitis of left finger ☑
L03.031	Cellulitis of right toe ☑
L03.032	Cellulitis of left toe ☑
L03.111	Cellulitis of right axilla ☑
L03.112	Cellulitis of left axilla ☑
L03.113	Cellulitis of right upper limb ☑
L03.114	Cellulitis of left upper limb ☑
L03.115	Cellulitis of right lower limb ☑
L03.116	Cellulitis of left lower limb ☑
L03.211	Cellulitis of face

L03.221	Cellulitis of neck
L03.311	Cellulitis of abdominal wall
L03.312	Cellulitis of back [any part except buttock]
L03.313	Cellulitis of chest wall
L03.314	Cellulitis of groin
L03.316	Cellulitis of umbilicus
L03.317	Cellulitis of buttock
L73.2	Hidradenitis suppurativa
N61.21	Granulomatous mastitis, right breast ☑

AMA: **10060** 2018,Jan,8; 2017,Jan,8; 2016,Jan,13; 2015,Jan,16 **10061** 2018,Jan,8; 2017,Jan,8; 2016,Jan,13; 2015,Jan,16

Relative Value Units/Medicare Edits

Non-Facility RVU	Work	PE	MP	Total
10060	1.22	2.27	0.13	3.62
10061	2.45	3.45	0.31	6.21
Facility RVU	Work	PE	MP	Total
10060	1.22	1.66	0.13	3.01
10061	2.45	2.57	0.31	5.33

	FUD	Status	MUE	Modifiers				IOM Reference
10060	10	A	1(2)	51	N/A	N/A	N/A	None
10061	10	A	1(2)	51	N/A	N/A	N/A	

* with documentation

Terms To Know

carbuncle. Infection of the skin that arises from a collection of interconnected infected boils or furuncles, usually from hair follicles infected by staphylococcus. This condition can produce pus and form drainage cavities.

cellulitis. Infection of the skin and subcutaneous tissues, most often caused by Staphylococcus or Streptococcus bacteria secondary to a cutaneous lesion. Progression of the inflammation may lead to abscess and tissue death, or even systemic infection-like bacteremia.

furuncle. Inflamed, painful abscess, cyst, or nodule on the skin caused by bacteria, often Staphylococcus, entering along the hair follicle.

sebaceous cyst. Benign cyst of the skin or hair follicle filled with keratin and debris rich in lipids. Cysts of the integumentary system may be treated by incision and drainage or puncture aspiration.

10080-10081

10080 Incision and drainage of pilonidal cyst; simple
10081   complicated

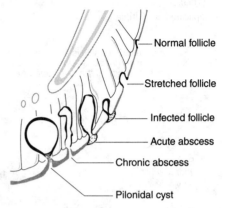

A pilonidal cyst is incised and drained

Explanation

The physician incises and drains a pilonidal cyst. A pilonidal cyst is an abnormal pocket in the skin and subcutaneous tissue that may contain hair follicles, skin debris, fluid, and exudate. The cyst is usually located in the sacrococcygeal region near the tailbone and cleft of the buttocks. An incision overlying the pocket is made to allow drainage of the contents. The wound may be left open and packed until the cyst heals. Report 10081 if the procedure is more complicated and requires marsupialization, approximation of the wound's edges, and/or primary closure.

Coding Tips

For excision of a pilonidal cyst, see 11770–11772. For incision and drainage of an abscess, other than a pilonidal cyst, simple or single, see 10060; complicated or multiple, see 10061. Surgical trays, A4550, are not separately reimbursed by Medicare; however, other third-party payers may cover them. Check with the specific payer to determine coverage.

ICD-10-CM Diagnostic Codes

L05.01	Pilonidal cyst with abscess
L05.02	Pilonidal sinus with abscess
L05.91	Pilonidal cyst without abscess
L05.92	Pilonidal sinus without abscess

AMA: **10080** 2018,Jan,8; 2017,Jan,8; 2016,Jan,13; 2015,Jan,16 **10081** 2018,Jan,8; 2017,Jan,8; 2016,Jan,13; 2015,Jan,16

Relative Value Units/Medicare Edits

Non-Facility RVU	Work	PE	MP	Total
10080	1.22	5.83	0.19	7.24
10081	2.5	7.09	0.41	10.0
Facility RVU	Work	PE	MP	Total
10080	1.22	1.65	0.19	3.06
10081	2.5	2.15	0.41	5.06

	FUD	Status	MUE	Modifiers				IOM Reference
10080	10	A	1(3)	51	N/A	N/A	N/A	None
10081	10	A	1(3)	51	N/A	N/A	N/A	

* with documentation

Terms To Know

abscess. Circumscribed collection of pus resulting from bacteria, frequently associated with swelling and other signs of inflammation.

curettage. Removal of tissue by scraping.

cyst. Elevated encapsulated mass containing fluid, semisolid, or solid material with a membranous lining.

drain. Device that creates a channel to allow fluid from a cavity, wound, or infected area to exit the body.

epithelial tissue. Cells arranged in sheets that cover internal and external body surfaces that can absorb, protect, and/or secrete and includes the protective covering for external surfaces (skin), absorptive linings for internal surfaces such as the intestine, and secreting structures such as salivary or sweat glands.

excision. Surgical removal of an organ or tissue.

exudate. Fluid or other material, such as debris from cells, that has escaped blood vessel circulation and is deposited in or on tissues and usually occurs due to inflammation.

hair follicle. Tube-like opening in the epidermis where the hair shaft develops.

incision. Act of cutting into tissue or an organ.

marsupialization. Creation of a pouch in surgical treatment of a cyst in which one wall is resected and the remaining cut edges are sutured to adjacent tissue creating an open pouch of the previously enclosed cyst.

pilonidal cyst. Sac or sinus cavity of trapped epithelial tissues in the sacrococcygeal region, usually associated with ingrown hair.

10120-10121

10120   Incision and removal of foreign body, subcutaneous tissues; simple
10121   complicated

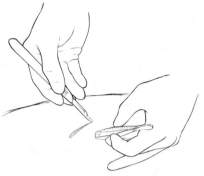

A foreign body is removed through an incision into subcutaneous tissues

Explanation

The physician removes a foreign body embedded in subcutaneous tissue. The physician makes a simple incision in the skin overlying the foreign body. The foreign body is retrieved using hemostats or forceps. The skin may be sutured or allowed to heal secondarily. Report 10121 if the procedure is more complicated, requiring dissection of underlying tissues.

Coding Tips

These codes may be used when foreign body removal is confined to the skin and/or subcutaneous tissues. To report debridement associated with an open fracture and/or dislocation, see 11010–11012. Surgical trays, A4550, are not separately reimbursed by Medicare; however, other third-party payers may cover them. Check with the specific payer to determine coverage.

ICD-10-CM Diagnostic Codes

L92.3	Foreign body granuloma of the skin and subcutaneous tissue
M79.5	Residual foreign body in soft tissue
S00.05XA	Superficial foreign body of scalp, initial encounter
S00.35XA	Superficial foreign body of nose, initial encounter
S00.452A	Superficial foreign body of left ear, initial encounter ☑
S00.551A	Superficial foreign body of lip, initial encounter
S00.552A	Superficial foreign body of oral cavity, initial encounter
S01.02XA	Laceration with foreign body of scalp, initial encounter
S01.422A	Laceration with foreign body of left cheek and temporomandibular area, initial encounter ☑
S01.442A	Puncture wound with foreign body of left cheek and temporomandibular area, initial encounter ☑
S01.82XA	Laceration with foreign body of other part of head, initial encounter
S01.84XA	Puncture wound with foreign body of other part of head, initial encounter
S20.152A	Superficial foreign body of breast, left breast, initial encounter ☑
S20.351A	Superficial foreign body of right front wall of thorax, initial encounter
S20.354A	Superficial foreign body of middle front wall of thorax, initial encounter
S20.452A	Superficial foreign body of left back wall of thorax, initial encounter

Skin

is in margin.

S21.122A	Laceration with foreign body of left front wall of thorax without penetration into thoracic cavity, initial encounter
S21.221A	Laceration with foreign body of right back wall of thorax without penetration into thoracic cavity, initial encounter
S21.241A	Puncture wound with foreign body of right back wall of thorax without penetration into thoracic cavity, initial encounter
S21.242A	Puncture wound with foreign body of left back wall of thorax without penetration into thoracic cavity, initial encounter
S30.851A	Superficial foreign body of abdominal wall, initial encounter
S30.852A	Superficial foreign body of penis, initial encounter ♂
S30.853A	Superficial foreign body of scrotum and testes, initial encounter ♂
S30.854A	Superficial foreign body of vagina and vulva, initial encounter ♀
S31.020A	Laceration with foreign body of lower back and pelvis without penetration into retroperitoneum, initial encounter
S31.040A	Puncture wound with foreign body of lower back and pelvis without penetration into retroperitoneum, initial encounter
S31.124A	Laceration of abdominal wall with foreign body, left lower quadrant without penetration into peritoneal cavity, initial encounter ☑
S31.144A	Puncture wound of abdominal wall with foreign body, left lower quadrant without penetration into peritoneal cavity, initial encounter ☑
S31.814A	Puncture wound with foreign body of right buttock, initial encounter ☑
S40.251A	Superficial foreign body of right shoulder, initial encounter ☑
S40.851A	Superficial foreign body of right upper arm, initial encounter ☑
S41.021A	Laceration with foreign body of right shoulder, initial encounter ☑
S50.352A	Superficial foreign body of left elbow, initial encounter ☑
S50.852A	Superficial foreign body of left forearm, initial encounter ☑
S51.022A	Laceration with foreign body of left elbow, initial encounter ☑
S51.821A	Laceration with foreign body of right forearm, initial encounter ☑
S51.842A	Puncture wound with foreign body of left forearm, initial encounter ☑
S60.351A	Superficial foreign body of right thumb, initial encounter ☑
S60.451A	Superficial foreign body of left index finger, initial encounter ☑
S60.452A	Superficial foreign body of right middle finger, initial encounter ☑
S60.551A	Superficial foreign body of right hand, initial encounter ☑
S60.851A	Superficial foreign body of right wrist, initial encounter ☑
S60.852A	Superficial foreign body of left wrist, initial encounter ☑
S61.041A	Puncture wound with foreign body of right thumb without damage to nail, initial encounter ☑
S61.122A	Laceration with foreign body of left thumb with damage to nail, initial encounter ☑
S61.220A	Laceration with foreign body of right index finger without damage to nail, initial encounter ☑
S61.223A	Laceration with foreign body of left middle finger without damage to nail, initial encounter ☑
S61.224A	Laceration with foreign body of right ring finger without damage to nail, initial encounter ☑
S61.241A	Puncture wound with foreign body of left index finger without damage to nail, initial encounter ☑
S61.242A	Puncture wound with foreign body of right middle finger without damage to nail, initial encounter ☑
S61.321A	Laceration with foreign body of left index finger with damage to nail, initial encounter ☑
S61.322A	Laceration with foreign body of right middle finger with damage to nail, initial encounter ☑
S61.342A	Puncture wound with foreign body of right middle finger with damage to nail, initial encounter ☑
S61.421A	Laceration with foreign body of right hand, initial encounter ☑
S61.442A	Puncture wound with foreign body of left hand, initial encounter ☑
S61.522A	Laceration with foreign body of left wrist, initial encounter ☑
S61.541A	Puncture wound with foreign body of right wrist, initial encounter ☑
S70.251A	Superficial foreign body, right hip, initial encounter ☑
S70.351A	Superficial foreign body, right thigh, initial encounter ☑
S71.022A	Laceration with foreign body, left hip, initial encounter ☑
S71.041A	Puncture wound with foreign body, right hip, initial encounter ☑
S71.042A	Puncture wound with foreign body, left hip, initial encounter ☑
S71.122A	Laceration with foreign body, left thigh, initial encounter ☑
S71.142A	Puncture wound with foreign body, left thigh, initial encounter ☑
S80.852A	Superficial foreign body, left lower leg, initial encounter ☑
S81.022A	Laceration with foreign body, left knee, initial encounter ☑
S81.042A	Puncture wound with foreign body, left knee, initial encounter ☑
S81.821A	Laceration with foreign body, right lower leg, initial encounter ☑
S90.451A	Superficial foreign body, right great toe, initial encounter ☑
S90.551A	Superficial foreign body, right ankle, initial encounter ☑
S90.851A	Superficial foreign body, right foot, initial encounter ☑
S91.021A	Laceration with foreign body, right ankle, initial encounter ☑
S91.041A	Puncture wound with foreign body, right ankle, initial encounter ☑
S91.042A	Puncture wound with foreign body, left ankle, initial encounter ☑

AMA: 10120 2018,Jan,8; 2017,Jan,8; 2016,Jan,13; 2015,Jan,16 10121 2018,Jan,8; 2017,Jan,8; 2016,Jan,13; 2015,Jan,16

Relative Value Units/Medicare Edits

Non-Facility RVU	Work	PE	MP	Total
10120	1.22	3.14	0.14	4.5
10121	2.74	4.85	0.39	7.98
Facility RVU	Work	PE	MP	Total
10120	1.22	1.68	0.14	3.04
10121	2.74	2.27	0.39	5.4

	FUD	Status	MUE	Modifiers				IOM Reference
10120	10	A	3(3)	51	N/A	N/A	N/A	None
10121	10	A	2(3)	51	N/A	N/A	N/A	

* with documentation

Terms To Know

foreign body. Any object or substance found in an organ and tissue that does not belong under normal circumstances.

subcutaneous tissue. Sheet or wide band of adipose (fat) and areolar connective tissue in two layers attached to the dermis.

© 2021 Optum360, LLC   N Newborn: 0   P Pediatric: 0-17   M Maternity: 9-64   A Adult: 15-124   ♂ Male Only   ♀ Female Only   CPT © 2021 American Medical Association. All Rights Reserved.

30   Coding Companion for General Surgery/Gastroenterology

10140

10140 Incision and drainage of hematoma, seroma or fluid collection

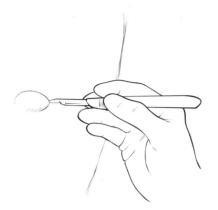

A hematoma, seroma, or fluid collection is incised and drained

Explanation

The physician makes an incision in the skin to decompress and drain a hematoma, seroma, or other collection of fluid. A hemostat bluntly penetrates the fluid pockets, allowing the fluid to evacuate. A latex drain or gauze packing may be placed into the incision site. This will allow the escape of any fluids that may continue to enter the pocket. A pressure dressing may be placed over the region. Any drain or packing is removed within 48 hours. The incision can be closed primarily or may be left to granulate without closure.

Coding Tips

Hematomas, seromas, or fluid collections can result from trauma or postoperative complications. These fluid-filled pockets can cause infections or lead to permanent erosion of bone and/or cartilage. Removal of a drain is not reported separately. If tissue is transported to an outside laboratory, report 99000 for handling and/or conveyance. Any local anesthesia is not reported separately. When image guidance is performed, report 10140 with 76942, 77012, or 77021, depending on modality. Surgical trays, A4550, are not separately reimbursed by Medicare; however, other third-party payers may cover them. Check with the specific payer to determine coverage.

ICD-10-CM Diagnostic Codes

K64.5	Perianal venous thrombosis
L76.02	Intraoperative hemorrhage and hematoma of skin and subcutaneous tissue complicating other procedure
L76.31	Postprocedural hematoma of skin and subcutaneous tissue following a dermatologic procedure
L76.32	Postprocedural hematoma of skin and subcutaneous tissue following other procedure
L76.33	Postprocedural seroma of skin and subcutaneous tissue following a dermatologic procedure
L76.34	Postprocedural seroma of skin and subcutaneous tissue following other procedure
S00.03XA	Contusion of scalp, initial encounter
S00.11XA	Contusion of right eyelid and periocular area, initial encounter ☑
S00.12XA	Contusion of left eyelid and periocular area, initial encounter ☑
S00.33XA	Contusion of nose, initial encounter
S00.431A	Contusion of right ear, initial encounter ☑
S00.432A	Contusion of left ear, initial encounter ☑
S00.531A	Contusion of lip, initial encounter
S00.83XA	Contusion of other part of head, initial encounter
S10.83XA	Contusion of other specified part of neck, initial encounter
S20.01XA	Contusion of right breast, initial encounter ☑
S20.02XA	Contusion of left breast, initial encounter ☑
S20.211A	Contusion of right front wall of thorax, initial encounter
S20.212A	Contusion of left front wall of thorax, initial encounter
S20.213A	Contusion of bilateral front wall of thorax, initial encounter
S20.214A	Contusion of middle front wall of thorax, initial encounter
S20.221A	Contusion of right back wall of thorax, initial encounter
S20.222A	Contusion of left back wall of thorax, initial encounter
S20.224A	Contusion of middle back wall of thorax, initial encounter
S30.0XXA	Contusion of lower back and pelvis, initial encounter
S30.1XXA	Contusion of abdominal wall, initial encounter
S30.21XA	Contusion of penis, initial encounter ♂
S30.22XA	Contusion of scrotum and testes, initial encounter ♂
S30.23XA	Contusion of vagina and vulva, initial encounter ♀
S30.3XXA	Contusion of anus, initial encounter
S40.011A	Contusion of right shoulder, initial encounter ☑
S40.012A	Contusion of left shoulder, initial encounter ☑
S40.021A	Contusion of right upper arm, initial encounter ☑
S40.022A	Contusion of left upper arm, initial encounter ☑
S50.01XA	Contusion of right elbow, initial encounter ☑
S50.02XA	Contusion of left elbow, initial encounter ☑
S50.11XA	Contusion of right forearm, initial encounter ☑
S50.12XA	Contusion of left forearm, initial encounter ☑
S60.011A	Contusion of right thumb without damage to nail, initial encounter ☑
S60.012A	Contusion of left thumb without damage to nail, initial encounter ☑
S60.021A	Contusion of right index finger without damage to nail, initial encounter ☑
S60.022A	Contusion of left index finger without damage to nail, initial encounter ☑
S60.031A	Contusion of right middle finger without damage to nail, initial encounter ☑
S60.041A	Contusion of right ring finger without damage to nail, initial encounter ☑
S60.042A	Contusion of left ring finger without damage to nail, initial encounter ☑
S60.052A	Contusion of left little finger without damage to nail, initial encounter ☑
S60.111A	Contusion of right thumb with damage to nail, initial encounter ☑
S60.112A	Contusion of left thumb with damage to nail, initial encounter ☑
S60.121A	Contusion of right index finger with damage to nail, initial encounter ☑
S60.131A	Contusion of right middle finger with damage to nail, initial encounter ☑
S60.151A	Contusion of right little finger with damage to nail, initial encounter ☑
S60.152A	Contusion of left little finger with damage to nail, initial encounter ☑
S60.211A	Contusion of right wrist, initial encounter ☑
S60.212A	Contusion of left wrist, initial encounter ☑
S60.221A	Contusion of right hand, initial encounter ☑

S60.222A	Contusion of left hand, initial encounter ☑	
S70.01XA	Contusion of right hip, initial encounter ☑	
S70.02XA	Contusion of left hip, initial encounter ☑	
S70.11XA	Contusion of right thigh, initial encounter ☑	
S70.12XA	Contusion of left thigh, initial encounter ☑	
S80.11XA	Contusion of right lower leg, initial encounter ☑	
S80.12XA	Contusion of left lower leg, initial encounter ☑	
S90.111A	Contusion of right great toe without damage to nail, initial encounter ☑	
S90.112A	Contusion of left great toe without damage to nail, initial encounter ☑	
S90.121A	Contusion of right lesser toe(s) without damage to nail, initial encounter ☑	
S90.122A	Contusion of left lesser toe(s) without damage to nail, initial encounter ☑	
S90.221A	Contusion of right lesser toe(s) with damage to nail, initial encounter ☑	
S90.222A	Contusion of left lesser toe(s) with damage to nail, initial encounter ☑	
T79.2XXA	Traumatic secondary and recurrent hemorrhage and seroma, initial encounter	
T87.89	Other complications of amputation stump	

AMA: 10140 2018,Jan,8; 2017,Jan,8; 2016,Jan,13; 2015,Jan,16

Relative Value Units/Medicare Edits

Non-Facility RVU	Work	PE	MP	Total
10140	1.58	3.26	0.21	5.05
Facility RVU	Work	PE	MP	Total
10140	1.58	1.67	0.21	3.46

	FUD	Status	MUE	Modifiers			IOM Reference
10140	10	A	2(3)	51	N/A	N/A	N/A	100-04,13,80.1; 100-04,13,80.2

* with documentation

Terms To Know

evacuation. Removal or purging of waste material.

granulation. Formation of small, bead-like masses of cytoplasm or granules on the surface of healing wounds of an organ, membrane, or tissue.

hematoma. Tumor-like collection of blood in some part of the body caused by a break in a blood vessel wall, usually as a result of trauma.

seroma. Swelling caused by the collection of serum, or clear fluid, in the tissues.

10160

10160 Puncture aspiration of abscess, hematoma, bulla, or cyst

A subcutaneous fluid pocket is aspirated

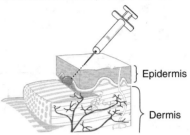

Schematic of layers of the skin

Explanation

The physician performs a puncture aspiration of an abscess, hematoma, bulla, or cyst. The palpable collection of fluid is located subcutaneously. The physician cleanses the overlying skin and introduces a large bore needle on a syringe into the fluid space. The fluid is aspirated into the syringe, decompressing the fluid space. A pressure dressing may be placed over the site.

Coding Tips

For incision and drainage of an abscess (e.g., carbuncle, suppurative hidradenitis, cutaneous or subcutaneous abscess, cyst, furuncle, or paronychia), simple or single, see 10060; complicated or multiple, see 10061. For incision and drainage of a pilonidal cyst, simple, see 10080; complicated, see 10081. For imaging guidance, see 76942, 77002, 77012, and 77021. Surgical trays, A4550, are not separately reimbursed by Medicare; however, other third-party payers may cover them. Check with the specific payer to determine coverage.

ICD-10-CM Diagnostic Codes

L02.01	Cutaneous abscess of face
L02.02	Furuncle of face
L02.03	Carbuncle of face
L02.11	Cutaneous abscess of neck
L02.211	Cutaneous abscess of abdominal wall
L02.212	Cutaneous abscess of back [any part, except buttock]
L02.214	Cutaneous abscess of groin
L02.31	Cutaneous abscess of buttock
L02.411	Cutaneous abscess of right axilla ☑
L02.412	Cutaneous abscess of left axilla ☑
L02.413	Cutaneous abscess of right upper limb ☑
L02.415	Cutaneous abscess of right lower limb ☑
L02.611	Cutaneous abscess of right foot ☑
L02.612	Cutaneous abscess of left foot ☑
L72.0	Epidermal cyst
L72.11	Pilar cyst
L72.12	Trichodermal cyst
L72.3	Sebaceous cyst
L72.8	Other follicular cysts of the skin and subcutaneous tissue
L76.32	Postprocedural hematoma of skin and subcutaneous tissue following other procedure
O90.2	Hematoma of obstetric wound Ⓜ ♀
S00.03XA	Contusion of scalp, initial encounter

S00.33XA	Contusion of nose, initial encounter
S00.431A	Contusion of right ear, initial encounter ☑
S00.432A	Contusion of left ear, initial encounter ☑
S00.531A	Contusion of lip, initial encounter
S20.01XA	Contusion of right breast, initial encounter ☑
S20.02XA	Contusion of left breast, initial encounter ☑
S20.211A	Contusion of right front wall of thorax, initial encounter
S20.214A	Contusion of middle front wall of thorax, initial encounter
S20.221A	Contusion of right back wall of thorax, initial encounter
S20.224A	Contusion of middle back wall of thorax, initial encounter
S30.0XXA	Contusion of lower back and pelvis, initial encounter
S30.1XXA	Contusion of abdominal wall, initial encounter
S30.3XXA	Contusion of anus, initial encounter
S40.011A	Contusion of right shoulder, initial encounter ☑
S40.012A	Contusion of left shoulder, initial encounter ☑
S40.021A	Contusion of right upper arm, initial encounter ☑
S50.01XA	Contusion of right elbow, initial encounter ☑
S50.02XA	Contusion of left elbow, initial encounter ☑
S50.11XA	Contusion of right forearm, initial encounter ☑
S60.012A	Contusion of left thumb without damage to nail, initial encounter ☑
S60.022A	Contusion of left index finger without damage to nail, initial encounter ☑
S60.031A	Contusion of right middle finger without damage to nail, initial encounter ☑
S60.041A	Contusion of right ring finger without damage to nail, initial encounter ☑
S60.042A	Contusion of left ring finger without damage to nail, initial encounter ☑
S60.051A	Contusion of right little finger without damage to nail, initial encounter ☑
S60.111A	Contusion of right thumb with damage to nail, initial encounter ☑
S60.122A	Contusion of left index finger with damage to nail, initial encounter ☑
S60.131A	Contusion of right middle finger with damage to nail, initial encounter ☑
S60.142A	Contusion of left ring finger with damage to nail, initial encounter ☑
S60.151A	Contusion of right little finger with damage to nail, initial encounter ☑
S60.152A	Contusion of left little finger with damage to nail, initial encounter ☑
S60.211A	Contusion of right wrist, initial encounter ☑
S60.212A	Contusion of left wrist, initial encounter ☑
S60.221A	Contusion of right hand, initial encounter ☑
S60.222A	Contusion of left hand, initial encounter ☑
S70.02XA	Contusion of left hip, initial encounter ☑
S70.11XA	Contusion of right thigh, initial encounter ☑
S70.12XA	Contusion of left thigh, initial encounter ☑
S80.01XA	Contusion of right knee, initial encounter ☑
S80.02XA	Contusion of left knee, initial encounter ☑
S80.11XA	Contusion of right lower leg, initial encounter ☑
S90.01XA	Contusion of right ankle, initial encounter ☑

S90.02XA	Contusion of left ankle, initial encounter ☑
S90.111A	Contusion of right great toe without damage to nail, initial encounter ☑
S90.112A	Contusion of left great toe without damage to nail, initial encounter ☑
S90.122A	Contusion of left lesser toe(s) without damage to nail, initial encounter ☑
S90.212A	Contusion of left great toe with damage to nail, initial encounter ☑
S90.221A	Contusion of right lesser toe(s) with damage to nail, initial encounter ☑
S90.222A	Contusion of left lesser toe(s) with damage to nail, initial encounter ☑
S90.31XA	Contusion of right foot, initial encounter ☑
S90.32XA	Contusion of left foot, initial encounter ☑

AMA: **10160** 2018,Jan,8; 2017,Jan,8; 2017,Aug,9; 2016,Jan,13; 2015,Jan,16

Relative Value Units/Medicare Edits

Non-Facility RVU	Work	PE	MP	Total
10160	1.25	2.43	0.15	3.83
Facility RVU	**Work**	**PE**	**MP**	**Total**
10160	1.25	1.37	0.15	2.77

	FUD	Status	MUE	Modifiers				IOM Reference
10160	10	A	3(3)	51	N/A	N/A	N/A	100-04,13,80.1; 100-04,13,80.2

* with documentation

Terms To Know

abscess. Circumscribed collection of pus resulting from bacteria, frequently associated with swelling and other signs of inflammation.

bulla. Large, elevated, membranous sac or blister on the skin containing serous or seropurulent fluid. Bullae are usually treated by incision and drainage or puncture aspiration.

cyst. Elevated encapsulated mass containing fluid, semisolid, or solid material with a membranous lining.

hematoma. Tumor-like collection of blood in some part of the body caused by a break in a blood vessel wall, usually as a result of trauma.

Skin

10180

10180   Incision and drainage, complex, postoperative wound infection

An operation site that has become infected
is incised and the wound is drained

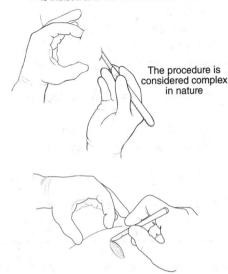

The procedure is
considered complex
in nature

Explanation

This procedure treats an infected postoperative wound. A more complex than usual incision and drainage procedure is necessary to remove the fluid and allow the surgical wound to heal. The physician first removes the surgical sutures or staples and/or makes additional incisions into the skin. The wound is drained of infected fluid. Any necrotic tissue is removed from the surgical site and the wound is irrigated. The wound may be sutured closed or packed open with gauze to allow additional drainage. If closed, the surgical site may have suction or latex drains placed into the wound. If packed open, the wound may be sutured again during a later procedure.

Coding Tips

Drain placement is included in the code and should not be reported separately. If drainage is of a hematoma, seroma, or fluid collection, see 10140. For simple secondary closure of a surgical wound, see 12020–12021. For extensive or complicated secondary closure of a surgical wound or dehiscence, see 13160. Supplies used when providing this procedure may be reported with the appropriate HCPCS level II code. Surgical trays, A4550, are not separately reimbursed by Medicare; however, other third-party payers may cover them. Check with the specific payer to determine coverage.

ICD-10-CM Diagnostic Codes

A48.52	Wound botulism
K68.11	Postprocedural retroperitoneal abscess
O86.02	Infection of obstetric surgical wound, deep incisional site Ⓜ ♀
O86.03	Infection of obstetric surgical wound, organ and space site Ⓜ ♀
O86.04	Sepsis following an obstetrical procedure Ⓜ ♀
T81.42XA	Infection following a procedure, deep incisional surgical site, initial encounter
T81.43XA	Infection following a procedure, organ and space surgical site, initial encounter
T81.44XA	Sepsis following a procedure, initial encounter

AMA: **10180** 2018,Jan,8; 2017,Jan,8; 2016,Jan,13; 2015,Jan,16

Relative Value Units/Medicare Edits

Non-Facility RVU	Work	PE	MP	Total
10180	2.3	4.99	0.48	7.77
Facility RVU	**Work**	**PE**	**MP**	**Total**
10180	2.3	2.44	0.48	5.22

	FUD	Status	MUE	Modifiers				IOM Reference
10180	10	A	2(3)	51	N/A	N/A	N/A	None

* with documentation

Terms To Know

drain. Device that creates a channel to allow fluid from a cavity, wound, or infected area to exit the body.

hematoma. Tumor-like collection of blood in some part of the body caused by a break in a blood vessel wall, usually as a result of trauma.

incision and drainage. Cutting open body tissue for the removal of tissue fluids or infected discharge from a wound or cavity.

infected postoperative seroma. Infection within a pocket of serum following surgery.

infection. Presence of microorganisms in body tissues that may result in cellular damage.

necrosis. Death of cells or tissue within a living organ or structure.

packing. Material placed into a cavity or wound, such as gels, gauze, pads, and sponges.

postpartum. Period of time following childbirth.

seroma. Swelling caused by the collection of serum, or clear fluid, in the tissues.

Skin

11004-11006

11004 Debridement of skin, subcutaneous tissue, muscle and fascia for necrotizing soft tissue infection; external genitalia and perineum
11005   abdominal wall, with or without fascial closure
11006   external genitalia, perineum and abdominal wall, with or without fascial closure

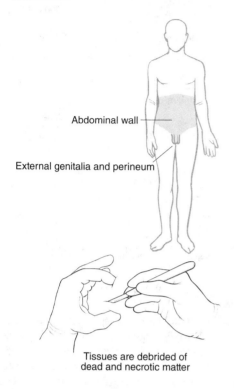

Abdominal wall

External genitalia and perineum

Tissues are debrided of dead and necrotic matter

Explanation

Debridement is carried out for a severe type of tissue infection that causes gangrenous changes, systemic disease, and tissue death. These types of infections are caused by virulent strains of bacteria, such as "flesh-eating" streptococcus, and affect the skin, subcutaneous fat, fascia, and muscle tissue. Surgery is performed immediately upon diagnosis to open and drain the infected area and excise the dead or necrotic tissue. Report 11004 for surgical debridement of necrotic soft tissue of the external genitalia and perineum; 11005 for the abdominal wall, with or without repair of the abdominal fascia; and 11006 for both areas, with or without repair of the abdominal fascia.

Coding Tips

This type of debridement is done on high-risk patients who have a life-threatening infection such as Fournier's gangrene. Necrosis is often caused by infection from a combination of dangerously virulent microorganisms. Fistulas, herniations, and organ destruction may occur, requiring an extensive level of repair involved with the debridement. Tissue flaps or skin grafting are reported separately when used for repair or closure. For removal of prosthetic material or mesh from the abdominal wall, see 11008. Report skin grafts or flaps separately when performed for closure at the same session as 11004–11006.

ICD-10-CM Diagnostic Codes

A48.0	Gas gangrene
A48.52	Wound botulism
A48.8	Other specified bacterial diseases

B95.0	Streptococcus, group A, as the cause of diseases classified elsewhere
B95.1	Streptococcus, group B, as the cause of diseases classified elsewhere
B95.2	Enterococcus as the cause of diseases classified elsewhere
B95.3	Streptococcus pneumoniae as the cause of diseases classified elsewhere
B95.4	Other streptococcus as the cause of diseases classified elsewhere
B95.61	Methicillin susceptible Staphylococcus aureus infection as the cause of diseases classified elsewhere
B95.62	Methicillin resistant Staphylococcus aureus infection as the cause of diseases classified elsewhere
B95.7	Other staphylococcus as the cause of diseases classified elsewhere
B96.1	Klebsiella pneumoniae [K. pneumoniae] as the cause of diseases classified elsewhere
B96.21	Shiga toxin-producing Escherichia coli [E. coli] [STEC] O157 as the cause of diseases classified elsewhere
B96.22	Other specified Shiga toxin-producing Escherichia coli [E. coli] [STEC] as the cause of diseases classified elsewhere
B96.29	Other Escherichia coli [E. coli] as the cause of diseases classified elsewhere
B96.4	Proteus (mirabilis) (morganii) as the cause of diseases classified elsewhere
B96.5	Pseudomonas (aeruginosa) (mallei) (pseudomallei) as the cause of diseases classified elsewhere
B96.6	Bacteroides fragilis [B. fragilis] as the cause of diseases classified elsewhere
B96.7	Clostridium perfringens [C. perfringens] as the cause of diseases classified elsewhere
B96.82	Vibrio vulnificus as the cause of diseases classified elsewhere
B96.89	Other specified bacterial agents as the cause of diseases classified elsewhere
I96	Gangrene, not elsewhere classified
M72.6	Necrotizing fasciitis
N49.3	Fournier gangrene ♂
T81.42XA	Infection following a procedure, deep incisional surgical site, initial encounter
T81.43XA	Infection following a procedure, organ and space surgical site, initial encounter
T81.44XA	Sepsis following a procedure, initial encounter
T81.49XA	Infection following a procedure, other surgical site, initial encounter

AMA: **11004** 2019,Nov,14; 2018,Jan,8; 2018,Feb,10; 2017,Jan,8; 2016,Jan,13; 2015,Jan,16 **11005** 2019,Nov,14; 2018,Jan,8; 2018,Feb,10; 2017,Jan,8; 2016,Jan,13; 2015,Jan,16 **11006** 2019,Nov,14; 2018,Jan,8; 2017,Jan,8; 2016,Jan,13; 2015,Jan,16

Skin

Relative Value Units/Medicare Edits

Non-Facility RVU	Work	PE	MP	Total
11004	10.8	3.95	1.98	16.73
11005	14.24	5.35	3.25	22.84
11006	13.1	4.89	2.6	20.59
Facility RVU	**Work**	**PE**	**MP**	**Total**
11004	10.8	3.95	1.98	16.73
11005	14.24	5.35	3.25	22.84
11006	13.1	4.89	2.6	20.59

	FUD	Status	MUE	Modifiers				IOM Reference
11004	0	A	1(2)	51	N/A	N/A	N/A	None
11005	0	A	1(2)	N/A	N/A	N/A	80*	
11006	0	A	1(2)	51	N/A	N/A	N/A	

* with documentation

Terms To Know

Escherichia coli. Gram negative, anaerobic of the family *Enterobacteriaceae* found in the large intestine of warm-blooded animals, generally as a nonpathologic entity aiding in digestion. They become pathogenic when an opportunity to grow somewhere outside this relationship presents itself, such as ingestion of fecal-contaminated food or water. The species coli is the principle organism found in the human intestine and has pathogenic and nonpathogenic strains. The enterotoxigenic form causes cholera-like illness while the enteroinvasive form causes dysentery by invading the epithelial cells of the human colon. Bloody stools are seen with the enterohemorrhagic strain. A relatively new strain of *E. coli* has been identified as *E. coli* O157:H7, found in undercooked beef and unpasteurized apple juice.

irrigation. To wash out or cleanse a body cavity, wound, or tissue with water or other fluid.

soft tissue. Nonepithelial tissues outside of the skeleton.

streptococcus group B colonization. Bacteria normally found in the vagina or lower intestine of many healthy adult women that may infect the fetus during childbirth, causing mental or physical handicaps or death. Women who test positive for *Streptococcus* group B during pregnancy are considered a "colonized" status and are treated with IV antibiotics at the time of delivery and may also be treated with oral antibiotics during the pregnancy.

11008

+ **11008** Removal of prosthetic material or mesh, abdominal wall for infection (eg, for chronic or recurrent mesh infection or necrotizing soft tissue infection) (List separately in addition to code for primary procedure)

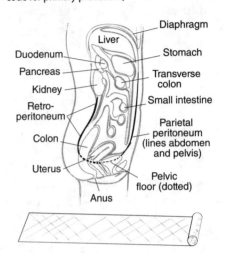

Synthetic mesh is often placed as a surgical wound of the abdominal wall is being closed. The mesh provides support and structure for the healing process

Explanation

The physician removes prosthetic material or mesh previously placed in the abdominal wall. This may be done due to the presence of a chronic infection, a necrotizing soft tissue infection, or a recurrent mesh infection. Surgery is performed immediately after diagnosis and usually under general anesthesia. The skin is incised and the tissue dissected exposing the prosthetic material. Debridement of the tissue adjacent to or incorporated in the mesh may be performed with instruments or irrigation. Unincorporated or infected areas of the mesh are excised and removed with any remaining areas of infection or necrotic tissue. Incorporated mesh that is not infected may be left in the wound. The area is irrigated and the wound is sutured. Note that 11008 is reported in addition to the code for the primary procedure of complex incision and drainage of a postoperative wound infection or debridement of a necrotizing soft tissue infection.

Coding Tips

Report 11008 in addition to 10180 or 11004–11006 as the necrotizing soft tissue infection must also be debrided at the same time as the previously placed prosthetic material is being removed. Skin grafts or flaps may be reported separately when performed for closure at the same session as 11008.

ICD-10-CM Diagnostic Codes

This/these CPT code(s) are add-on code(s). See the primary procedure code that this code is performed with for your ICD-10-CM code selections.

AMA: 11008 2019,Jan,14; 2018,Jan,8; 2017,Jan,8; 2016,Jan,13; 2015,Jan,16

Skin

Relative Value Units/Medicare Edits

Non-Facility RVU	Work	PE	MP	Total
11008	5.0	1.87	1.16	8.03
Facility RVU	Work	PE	MP	Total
11008	5.0	1.87	1.16	8.03

	FUD	Status	MUE	Modifiers				IOM Reference
11008	N/A	A	1(2)	N/A	N/A	N/A	80*	None

* with documentation

Terms To Know

acute. Sudden, severe.

debridement. Removal of dead or contaminated tissue and foreign matter from a wound.

fascia. Fibrous sheet or band of tissue that envelops organs, muscles, and groupings of muscles.

gangrene. Death of tissue, usually resulting from a loss of vascular supply, followed by a bacterial attack or onset of disease.

mesh. Synthetic fabric used as a prosthetic patch in hernia repair.

necrosis. Death of cells or tissue within a living organ or structure.

11042 [11045]

11042 Debridement, subcutaneous tissue (includes epidermis and dermis, if performed); first 20 sq cm or less

+ **11045** Debridement, subcutaneous tissue (includes epidermis and dermis, if performed); each additional 20 sq cm, or part thereof (List separately in addition to code for primary procedure)

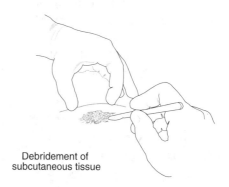

Debridement of
subcutaneous tissue

Explanation

The physician surgically removes foreign matter and contaminated or devitalized subcutaneous tissue (including epidermis and dermis, if performed) caused by injury, infection, wounds (excluding burn wounds), or chronic ulcers. Using a scalpel or dermatome, the physician excises the affected subcutaneous tissue until viable, bleeding tissue is encountered. A topical antibiotic is placed on the wound. A gauze dressing or an occlusive dressing may be placed over the surgical site. Report 11042 for the first 20 sq cm or less and 11045 for each additional 20 sq cm or part thereof.

Coding Tips

Report 11045 in addition to 11042. When reporting debridement of a single wound, the deepest level of tissue removed determines the correct code. The debridement of multiple wounds at the same tissue level may be added together to determine the appropriate code. Different tissue depths should not be added together for code selection. According to the AMA, the debridement of skin (epidermis/dermis) is reported with the codes describing active wound care management (97597 or 97598). Surgical trays, A4550, are not separately reimbursed by Medicare; however, other third-party payers may cover them. Check with the specific payer to determine coverage.

ICD-10-CM Diagnostic Codes

E09.621	Drug or chemical induced diabetes mellitus with foot ulcer
E09.622	Drug or chemical induced diabetes mellitus with other skin ulcer
E13.621	Other specified diabetes mellitus with foot ulcer
E13.622	Other specified diabetes mellitus with other skin ulcer
I70.231	Atherosclerosis of native arteries of right leg with ulceration of thigh 🅰 ☑
I70.235	Atherosclerosis of native arteries of right leg with ulceration of other part of foot 🅰 ☑
I70.238	Atherosclerosis of native arteries of right leg with ulceration of other part of lower leg 🅰 ☑
I70.241	Atherosclerosis of native arteries of left leg with ulceration of thigh 🅰 ☑
I70.245	Atherosclerosis of native arteries of left leg with ulceration of other part of foot 🅰 ☑
I70.448	Atherosclerosis of autologous vein bypass graft(s) of the left leg with ulceration of other part of lower leg 🅰 ☑

I70.533	Atherosclerosis of nonautologous biological bypass graft(s) of the right leg with ulceration of ankle 🅰 ☑	
I70.542	Atherosclerosis of nonautologous biological bypass graft(s) of the left leg with ulceration of calf 🅰 ☑	
I70.734	Atherosclerosis of other type of bypass graft(s) of the right leg with ulceration of heel and midfoot 🅰 ☑	
I83.012	Varicose veins of right lower extremity with ulcer of calf 🅰 ☑	
I83.013	Varicose veins of right lower extremity with ulcer of ankle 🅰 ☑	
I83.018	Varicose veins of right lower extremity with ulcer other part of lower leg 🅰 ☑	
I87.2	Venous insufficiency (chronic) (peripheral)	
I87.312	Chronic venous hypertension (idiopathic) with ulcer of left lower extremity ☑	
I87.333	Chronic venous hypertension (idiopathic) with ulcer and inflammation of bilateral lower extremity ☑	
L89.011	Pressure ulcer of right elbow, stage 1 ☑	
L89.012	Pressure ulcer of right elbow, stage 2 ☑	
L89.013	Pressure ulcer of right elbow, stage 3 ☑	
L89.021	Pressure ulcer of left elbow, stage 1 ☑	
L89.022	Pressure ulcer of left elbow, stage 2 ☑	
L89.023	Pressure ulcer of left elbow, stage 3 ☑	
L89.111	Pressure ulcer of right upper back, stage 1 ☑	
L89.113	Pressure ulcer of right upper back, stage 3 ☑	
L89.121	Pressure ulcer of left upper back, stage 1 ☑	
L89.122	Pressure ulcer of left upper back, stage 2 ☑	
L89.131	Pressure ulcer of right lower back, stage 1 ☑	
L89.132	Pressure ulcer of right lower back, stage 2 ☑	
L89.133	Pressure ulcer of right lower back, stage 3 ☑	
L89.141	Pressure ulcer of left lower back, stage 1 ☑	
L89.142	Pressure ulcer of left lower back, stage 2 ☑	
L89.143	Pressure ulcer of left lower back, stage 3 ☑	
L89.151	Pressure ulcer of sacral region, stage 1	
L89.152	Pressure ulcer of sacral region, stage 2	
L89.153	Pressure ulcer of sacral region, stage 3	
L89.212	Pressure ulcer of right hip, stage 2 ☑	
L89.213	Pressure ulcer of right hip, stage 3 ☑	
L89.221	Pressure ulcer of left hip, stage 1 ☑	
L89.223	Pressure ulcer of left hip, stage 3 ☑	
L89.311	Pressure ulcer of right buttock, stage 1 ☑	
L89.313	Pressure ulcer of right buttock, stage 3 ☑	
L89.321	Pressure ulcer of left buttock, stage 1 ☑	
L89.322	Pressure ulcer of left buttock, stage 2 ☑	
L89.323	Pressure ulcer of left buttock, stage 3 ☑	
L89.41	Pressure ulcer of contiguous site of back, buttock and hip, stage 1	
L89.42	Pressure ulcer of contiguous site of back, buttock and hip, stage 2	
L89.43	Pressure ulcer of contiguous site of back, buttock and hip, stage 3	
L89.511	Pressure ulcer of right ankle, stage 1 ☑	
L89.512	Pressure ulcer of right ankle, stage 2 ☑	
L89.521	Pressure ulcer of left ankle, stage 1 ☑	
L89.522	Pressure ulcer of left ankle, stage 2 ☑	
L89.523	Pressure ulcer of left ankle, stage 3 ☑	

L89.612	Pressure ulcer of right heel, stage 2 ☑
L89.613	Pressure ulcer of right heel, stage 3 ☑
L89.621	Pressure ulcer of left heel, stage 1 ☑
L89.623	Pressure ulcer of left heel, stage 3 ☑
L89.891	Pressure ulcer of other site, stage 1
L89.892	Pressure ulcer of other site, stage 2
L89.893	Pressure ulcer of other site, stage 3
L97.111	Non-pressure chronic ulcer of right thigh limited to breakdown of skin ☑
L97.121	Non-pressure chronic ulcer of left thigh limited to breakdown of skin ☑
L97.211	Non-pressure chronic ulcer of right calf limited to breakdown of skin ☑
L97.221	Non-pressure chronic ulcer of left calf limited to breakdown of skin ☑
L97.311	Non-pressure chronic ulcer of right ankle limited to breakdown of skin ☑
L97.321	Non-pressure chronic ulcer of left ankle limited to breakdown of skin ☑
L97.421	Non-pressure chronic ulcer of left heel and midfoot limited to breakdown of skin ☑
L97.821	Non-pressure chronic ulcer of other part of left lower leg limited to breakdown of skin ☑
L98.411	Non-pressure chronic ulcer of buttock limited to breakdown of skin
L98.421	Non-pressure chronic ulcer of back limited to breakdown of skin
T33.012A	Superficial frostbite of left ear, initial encounter ☑
T33.02XA	Superficial frostbite of nose, initial encounter
T33.42XA	Superficial frostbite of left arm, initial encounter ☑
T33.531A	Superficial frostbite of right finger(s), initial encounter ☑
T33.71XA	Superficial frostbite of right knee and lower leg, initial encounter ☑
T33.812A	Superficial frostbite of left ankle, initial encounter ☑
T33.832A	Superficial frostbite of left toe(s), initial encounter ☑

AMA: **11042** 2018,Jan,8; 2017,Jan,8; 2016,Oct,3; 2016,Jan,13; 2016,Feb,13; 2016,Aug,9; 2015,Jan,16 **11045** 2018,Jan,8; 2017,Jan,8; 2016,Oct,3; 2016,Jan,13; 2016,Aug,9; 2015,Jan,16

Relative Value Units/Medicare Edits

Non-Facility RVU	Work	PE	MP	Total
11042	1.01	2.68	0.13	3.82
11045	0.5	0.62	0.09	1.21
Facility RVU	Work	PE	MP	Total
11042	1.01	0.62	0.13	1.76
11045	0.5	0.18	0.09	0.77

	FUD	Status	MUE	Modifiers				IOM Reference
11042	0	A	1(2)	51	N/A	N/A	N/A	None
11045	N/A	A	12(3)	N/A	N/A	N/A	80*	

* with documentation

11043 [11046]

11043 Debridement, muscle and/or fascia (includes epidermis, dermis, and subcutaneous tissue, if performed); first 20 sq cm or less

+   11046 Debridement, muscle and/or fascia (includes epidermis, dermis, and subcutaneous tissue, if performed); each additional 20 sq cm, or part thereof (List separately in addition to code for primary procedure)

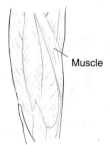

Muscle

A debridement into the muscle

Explanation

The physician surgically removes necrotic muscle and/or fascia, including epidermis, dermis, and subcutaneous tissue, if performed. The physician uses the appropriate surgical instrument (i.e., scalpel) to excise the affected tissue into the muscle layer. The dissection is continued until viable, bleeding tissue is encountered. Depending on wound size, closure may be immediate or delayed. The wound may be packed open with gauze and require immediate or delayed reconstruction. Report 11043 for the first 20 sq cm or less and 11046 for each additional 20 sq cm or part thereof.

Coding Tips

Report 11046 in addition to 11043. When reporting debridement of a single wound, the deepest level of tissue removed determines the correct code. The debridement of multiple wounds at the same tissue level may be added together to determine the appropriate code. Different tissue depths should not be added together for code selection. According to the AMA, the debridement of skin (epidermis/dermis) is reported with the codes describing active wound care management (97597 or 97598).

ICD-10-CM Diagnostic Codes

E09.52	Drug or chemical induced diabetes mellitus with diabetic peripheral angiopathy with gangrene
E09.621	Drug or chemical induced diabetes mellitus with foot ulcer
E09.622	Drug or chemical induced diabetes mellitus with other skin ulcer
H95.31	Accidental puncture and laceration of the ear and mastoid process during a procedure on the ear and mastoid process
H95.32	Accidental puncture and laceration of the ear and mastoid process during other procedure
I73.01	Raynaud's syndrome with gangrene
I87.011	Postthrombotic syndrome with ulcer of right lower extremity ☑
I87.013	Postthrombotic syndrome with ulcer of bilateral lower extremity ☑
I87.031	Postthrombotic syndrome with ulcer and inflammation of right lower extremity ☑
I87.033	Postthrombotic syndrome with ulcer and inflammation of bilateral lower extremity ☑
I96	Gangrene, not elsewhere classified

L89.010	Pressure ulcer of right elbow, unstageable ☑
L89.014	Pressure ulcer of right elbow, stage 4 ☑
L89.020	Pressure ulcer of left elbow, unstageable ☑
L89.024	Pressure ulcer of left elbow, stage 4 ☑
L89.114	Pressure ulcer of right upper back, stage 4 ☑
L89.120	Pressure ulcer of left upper back, unstageable ☑
L89.134	Pressure ulcer of right lower back, stage 4 ☑
L89.136	Pressure-induced deep tissue damage of right lower back ☑
L89.150	Pressure ulcer of sacral region, unstageable
L89.154	Pressure ulcer of sacral region, stage 4
L89.156	Pressure-induced deep tissue damage of sacral region
L89.214	Pressure ulcer of right hip, stage 4 ☑
L89.216	Pressure-induced deep tissue damage of right hip ☑
L89.220	Pressure ulcer of left hip, unstageable ☑
L89.310	Pressure ulcer of right buttock, unstageable ☑
L89.314	Pressure ulcer of right buttock, stage 4 ☑
L89.514	Pressure ulcer of right ankle, stage 4 ☑
L89.610	Pressure ulcer of right heel, unstageable ☑
L89.614	Pressure ulcer of right heel, stage 4 ☑
L89.616	Pressure-induced deep tissue damage of right heel ☑
L89.624	Pressure ulcer of left heel, stage 4 ☑
L97.113	Non-pressure chronic ulcer of right thigh with necrosis of muscle ☑
L97.115	Non-pressure chronic ulcer of right thigh with muscle involvement without evidence of necrosis ☑
L97.212	Non-pressure chronic ulcer of right calf with fat layer exposed ☑
L97.214	Non-pressure chronic ulcer of right calf with necrosis of bone ☑
L97.215	Non-pressure chronic ulcer of right calf with muscle involvement without evidence of necrosis ☑
L97.222	Non-pressure chronic ulcer of left calf with fat layer exposed ☑
L97.224	Non-pressure chronic ulcer of left calf with necrosis of bone ☑
L97.313	Non-pressure chronic ulcer of right ankle with necrosis of muscle ☑
L97.314	Non-pressure chronic ulcer of right ankle with necrosis of bone ☑
L97.315	Non-pressure chronic ulcer of right ankle with muscle involvement without evidence of necrosis ☑
L97.415	Non-pressure chronic ulcer of right heel and midfoot with muscle involvement without evidence of necrosis ☑
L97.513	Non-pressure chronic ulcer of other part of right foot with necrosis of muscle ☑
L97.515	Non-pressure chronic ulcer of other part of right foot with muscle involvement without evidence of necrosis ☑
L97.524	Non-pressure chronic ulcer of other part of left foot with necrosis of bone ☑
L97.814	Non-pressure chronic ulcer of other part of right lower leg with necrosis of bone ☑
L98.412	Non-pressure chronic ulcer of buttock with fat layer exposed
L98.413	Non-pressure chronic ulcer of buttock with necrosis of muscle
L98.415	Non-pressure chronic ulcer of buttock with muscle involvement without evidence of necrosis
L98.423	Non-pressure chronic ulcer of back with necrosis of muscle
L98.425	Non-pressure chronic ulcer of back with muscle involvement without evidence of necrosis
M60.011	Infective myositis, right shoulder ☑

M60.022	Infective myositis, left upper arm ☑
M60.041	Infective myositis, right hand ☑
M60.045	Infective myositis, left finger(s) ☑
M60.052	Infective myositis, left thigh ☑
M60.076	Infective myositis, right toe(s) ☑
M60.077	Infective myositis, left toe(s) ☑
M60.09	Infective myositis, multiple sites
M96.820	Accidental puncture and laceration of a musculoskeletal structure during a musculoskeletal system procedure
M96.821	Accidental puncture and laceration of a musculoskeletal structure during other procedure
S07.0XXA	Crushing injury of face, initial encounter
S47.1XXA	Crushing injury of right shoulder and upper arm, initial encounter ☑
S57.02XA	Crushing injury of left elbow, initial encounter ☑
S57.82XA	Crushing injury of left forearm, initial encounter ☑
S67.02XA	Crushing injury of left thumb, initial encounter ☑
S67.190A	Crushing injury of right index finger, initial encounter ☑
S67.192A	Crushing injury of right middle finger, initial encounter ☑
S67.197A	Crushing injury of left little finger, initial encounter ☑
S67.22XA	Crushing injury of left hand, initial encounter ☑
S67.31XA	Crushing injury of right wrist, initial encounter ☑
S77.01XA	Crushing injury of right hip, initial encounter ☑
S77.12XA	Crushing injury of left thigh, initial encounter ☑
S77.22XA	Crushing injury of left hip with thigh, initial encounter ☑
S87.81XA	Crushing injury of right lower leg, initial encounter ☑
S97.01XA	Crushing injury of right ankle, initial encounter ☑
S97.02XA	Crushing injury of left ankle, initial encounter ☑
S97.111A	Crushing injury of right great toe, initial encounter ☑
S97.121A	Crushing injury of right lesser toe(s), initial encounter ☑
S97.81XA	Crushing injury of right foot, initial encounter ☑
S97.82XA	Crushing injury of left foot, initial encounter ☑

AMA: **11043** 2020,Apr,8; 2018,Jan,8; 2017,Jan,8; 2016,Oct,3; 2016,Jan,13; 2016,Aug,9; 2015,Jan,16 **11046** 2018,Jan,8; 2017,Jan,8; 2016,Oct,3; 2016,Jan,13; 2016,Aug,9; 2015,Jan,16

Relative Value Units/Medicare Edits

Non-Facility RVU	Work	PE	MP	Total
11043	2.7	3.78	0.42	6.9
11046	1.03	0.94	0.2	2.17
Facility RVU	**Work**	**PE**	**MP**	**Total**
11043	2.7	1.4	0.42	4.52
11046	1.03	0.4	0.2	1.63

	FUD	Status	MUE	Modifiers				IOM Reference
11043	0	A	1(2)	51	N/A	N/A	N/A	None
11046	N/A	A	10(3)	N/A	N/A	N/A	80*	

* with documentation

11044, 11047

	11044	Debridement, bone (includes epidermis, dermis, subcutaneous tissue, muscle and/or fascia, if performed); first 20 sq cm or less
+	11047	each additional 20 sq cm, or part thereof (List separately in addition to code for primary procedure)

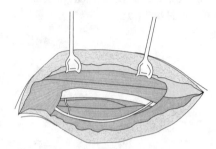

Debridement into the bone

Explanation

The physician surgically removes foreign matter and contaminated or devitalized bone (including epidermis, dermis, subcutaneous tissue, muscle, and/or fascia, if performed) caused by injury, infection, wounds (excluding burn wounds), or chronic ulcers. The physician uses a scalpel to excise the affected tissues into the bone. Depending on wound size, closure may be immediate or delayed. The wound may be packed open with gauze and require immediate or delayed reconstruction. Report 11044 for the first 20 sq cm or less and 11047 for each additional 20 sq cm or part thereof.

Coding Tips

Report 11047 in addition to 11044. These codes report debridement of contaminated devitalized skin, subcutaneous tissue, muscle, and bone not associated with open fractures or dislocations. To report debridement with open fractures/dislocations, see 11010–11012. When reporting debridement of a single wound, the deepest level of tissue removed determines the correct code. Debridement of multiple wounds at the same tissue level may be added together to determine the appropriate code. Different tissue depths should not be added together for code selection. According to the AMA, the debridement of skin (epidermis/dermis) is reported with the codes describing active wound care management (97597 or 97598).

ICD-10-CM Diagnostic Codes

E09.52	Drug or chemical induced diabetes mellitus with diabetic peripheral angiopathy with gangrene
I70.231	Atherosclerosis of native arteries of right leg with ulceration of thigh △ ☑
I70.232	Atherosclerosis of native arteries of right leg with ulceration of calf △ ☑
I70.233	Atherosclerosis of native arteries of right leg with ulceration of ankle △ ☑
I70.234	Atherosclerosis of native arteries of right leg with ulceration of heel and midfoot △ ☑
I70.261	Atherosclerosis of native arteries of extremities with gangrene, right leg △ ☑
I70.439	Atherosclerosis of autologous vein bypass graft(s) of the right leg with ulceration of unspecified site △ ☑
I70.534	Atherosclerosis of nonautologous biological bypass graft(s) of the right leg with ulceration of heel and midfoot △ ☑
I73.01	Raynaud's syndrome with gangrene

I87.011	Postthrombotic syndrome with ulcer of right lower extremity ☑
I87.031	Postthrombotic syndrome with ulcer and inflammation of right lower extremity ☑
I96	Gangrene, not elsewhere classified
L89.016	Pressure-induced deep tissue damage of right elbow ☑
L89.110	Pressure ulcer of right upper back, unstageable ☑
L89.114	Pressure ulcer of right upper back, stage 4 ☑
L89.130	Pressure ulcer of right lower back, unstageable ☑
L89.134	Pressure ulcer of right lower back, stage 4 ☑
L89.154	Pressure ulcer of sacral region, stage 4
L89.210	Pressure ulcer of right hip, unstageable ☑
L89.214	Pressure ulcer of right hip, stage 4 ☑
L89.216	Pressure-induced deep tissue damage of right hip ☑
L89.220	Pressure ulcer of left hip, unstageable ☑
L89.224	Pressure ulcer of left hip, stage 4 ☑
L89.314	Pressure ulcer of right buttock, stage 4 ☑
L89.324	Pressure ulcer of left buttock, stage 4 ☑
L89.44	Pressure ulcer of contiguous site of back, buttock and hip, stage 4
L89.514	Pressure ulcer of right ankle, stage 4 ☑
L89.516	Pressure-induced deep tissue damage of right ankle ☑
L89.520	Pressure ulcer of left ankle, unstageable ☑
L89.524	Pressure ulcer of left ankle, stage 4 ☑
L89.610	Pressure ulcer of right heel, unstageable ☑
L89.614	Pressure ulcer of right heel, stage 4 ☑
L89.624	Pressure ulcer of left heel, stage 4 ☑
L89.894	Pressure ulcer of other site, stage 4
L97.114	Non-pressure chronic ulcer of right thigh with necrosis of bone ☑
L97.116	Non-pressure chronic ulcer of right thigh with bone involvement without evidence of necrosis ☑
L97.124	Non-pressure chronic ulcer of left thigh with necrosis of bone ☑
L97.214	Non-pressure chronic ulcer of right calf with necrosis of bone ☑
L97.216	Non-pressure chronic ulcer of right calf with bone involvement without evidence of necrosis ☑
L97.314	Non-pressure chronic ulcer of right ankle with necrosis of bone ☑
L97.316	Non-pressure chronic ulcer of right ankle with bone involvement without evidence of necrosis ☑
L97.414	Non-pressure chronic ulcer of right heel and midfoot with necrosis of bone ☑
L97.416	Non-pressure chronic ulcer of right heel and midfoot with bone involvement without evidence of necrosis ☑
L97.424	Non-pressure chronic ulcer of left heel and midfoot with necrosis of bone ☑
L97.516	Non-pressure chronic ulcer of other part of right foot with bone involvement without evidence of necrosis ☑
L97.524	Non-pressure chronic ulcer of other part of left foot with necrosis of bone ☑
L97.814	Non-pressure chronic ulcer of other part of right lower leg with necrosis of bone ☑
L97.816	Non-pressure chronic ulcer of other part of right lower leg with bone involvement without evidence of necrosis ☑
L98.414	Non-pressure chronic ulcer of buttock with necrosis of bone
L98.416	Non-pressure chronic ulcer of buttock with bone involvement without evidence of necrosis
L98.424	Non-pressure chronic ulcer of back with necrosis of bone
L98.426	Non-pressure chronic ulcer of back with bone involvement without evidence of necrosis
L98.494	Non-pressure chronic ulcer of skin of other sites with necrosis of bone
S07.0XXA	Crushing injury of face, initial encounter
S47.1XXA	Crushing injury of right shoulder and upper arm, initial encounter ☑
S47.2XXA	Crushing injury of left shoulder and upper arm, initial encounter ☑
S57.01XA	Crushing injury of right elbow, initial encounter ☑
S57.02XA	Crushing injury of left elbow, initial encounter ☑
S57.81XA	Crushing injury of right forearm, initial encounter ☑
S57.82XA	Crushing injury of left forearm, initial encounter ☑
S67.01XA	Crushing injury of right thumb, initial encounter ☑
S67.02XA	Crushing injury of left thumb, initial encounter ☑
S67.190A	Crushing injury of right index finger, initial encounter ☑
S67.191A	Crushing injury of left index finger, initial encounter ☑
S67.194A	Crushing injury of right ring finger, initial encounter ☑
S67.195A	Crushing injury of left ring finger, initial encounter ☑
S67.196A	Crushing injury of right little finger, initial encounter ☑
S67.197A	Crushing injury of left little finger, initial encounter ☑
S67.198A	Crushing injury of other finger, initial encounter
S67.21XA	Crushing injury of right hand, initial encounter ☑
S67.31XA	Crushing injury of right wrist, initial encounter ☑
S67.32XA	Crushing injury of left wrist, initial encounter ☑
S68.011A	Complete traumatic metacarpophalangeal amputation of right thumb, initial encounter ☑
S68.012A	Complete traumatic metacarpophalangeal amputation of left thumb, initial encounter ☑
S68.021A	Partial traumatic metacarpophalangeal amputation of right thumb, initial encounter ☑
S68.511A	Complete traumatic transphalangeal amputation of right thumb, initial encounter ☑
S68.512A	Complete traumatic transphalangeal amputation of left thumb, initial encounter ☑
S68.521A	Partial traumatic transphalangeal amputation of right thumb, initial encounter ☑
S87.01XA	Crushing injury of right knee, initial encounter ☑
S87.02XA	Crushing injury of left knee, initial encounter ☑
S87.81XA	Crushing injury of right lower leg, initial encounter ☑
S87.82XA	Crushing injury of left lower leg, initial encounter ☑
S88.112A	Complete traumatic amputation at level between knee and ankle, left lower leg, initial encounter ☑
S88.121A	Partial traumatic amputation at level between knee and ankle, right lower leg, initial encounter ☑
S88.122A	Partial traumatic amputation at level between knee and ankle, left lower leg, initial encounter ☑
S97.01XA	Crushing injury of right ankle, initial encounter ☑
S97.02XA	Crushing injury of left ankle, initial encounter ☑
S97.111A	Crushing injury of right great toe, initial encounter ☑
S97.122A	Crushing injury of left lesser toe(s), initial encounter ☑
S97.81XA	Crushing injury of right foot, initial encounter ☑
S97.82XA	Crushing injury of left foot, initial encounter ☑
S98.011A	Complete traumatic amputation of right foot at ankle level, initial encounter ☑

Skin

S98.012A	Complete traumatic amputation of left foot at ankle level, initial encounter ☑
S98.022A	Partial traumatic amputation of left foot at ankle level, initial encounter ☑
S98.111A	Complete traumatic amputation of right great toe, initial encounter ☑
S98.132A	Complete traumatic amputation of one left lesser toe, initial encounter ☑
S98.221A	Partial traumatic amputation of two or more right lesser toes, initial encounter ☑
S98.311A	Complete traumatic amputation of right midfoot, initial encounter ☑
T79.8XXA	Other early complications of trauma, initial encounter
T81.33XA	Disruption of traumatic injury wound repair, initial encounter
T87.41	Infection of amputation stump, right upper extremity ☑
T87.43	Infection of amputation stump, right lower extremity ☑

AMA: 11044 2018,Jan,8; 2017,Jan,8; 2016,Oct,3; 2016,Jan,13; 2016,Aug,9; 2015,Jan,16 **11047** 2018,Jan,8; 2017,Jan,8; 2016,Oct,3; 2016,Jan,13; 2016,Aug,9; 2015,Jan,16

Relative Value Units/Medicare Edits

Non-Facility RVU	Work	PE	MP	Total
11044	4.1	4.42	0.64	9.16
11047	1.8	1.44	0.34	3.58
Facility RVU	**Work**	**PE**	**MP**	**Total**
11044	4.1	1.83	0.64	6.57
11047	1.8	0.71	0.34	2.85

	FUD	Status	MUE	Modifiers				IOM Reference
11044	0	A	1(2)	51	N/A	N/A	N/A	None
11047	N/A	A	10(3)	N/A	N/A	N/A	80*	

* with documentation

Terms To Know

debridement. Removal of dead or contaminated tissue and foreign matter from a wound.

devitalized. Deprivation of vital necessities or of life itself.

fascia. Fibrous sheet or band of tissue that envelops organs, muscles, and groupings of muscles.

packing. Material placed into a cavity or wound, such as gels, gauze, pads, and sponges.

11102-11107

	11102	Tangential biopsy of skin (eg, shave, scoop, saucerize, curette); single lesion
+	11103	each separate/additional lesion (List separately in addition to code for primary procedure)
	11104	Punch biopsy of skin (including simple closure, when performed); single lesion
+	11105	each separate/additional lesion (List separately in addition to code for primary procedure)
	11106	Incisional biopsy of skin (eg, wedge) (including simple closure, when performed); single lesion
+	11107	each separate/additional lesion (List separately in addition to code for primary procedure)

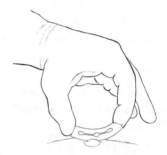

Tangential biopsy by shaving or saucerization

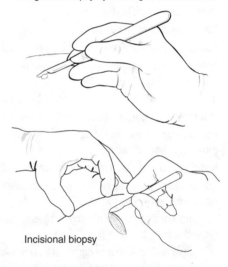

Incisional biopsy

Explanation

The physician removes a biopsy sample of skin or subcutaneous tissue for the purpose of performing a diagnostic histopathologic study under a microscope. Skin biopsies are reported based on one of three techniques used: tangential, punch, or incisional. Tangential technique describes a biopsy performed via a sharp blade to obtain a superficial, epidermal tissue specimen that may or may not include sections of underlying dermis and does not involve a full-thickness biopsy. Punch technique involves the use of a specific punch tool to obtain a full-thickness, barrel-shaped, or columnar-shaped specimen. Simple closure, including any manipulation of the biopsy defect, is included in the performance of a punch biopsy. The incisional biopsy technique describes a biopsy utilizing a sharp blade (no punch tool) to obtain a full-thickness specimen via a wedge or vertical incision. This technique type may involve specimens of subcutaneous fat. Closure of an incisional biopsy, other than simple closure, is reported separately. Report 11102 for a tangential biopsy, initial lesion; each additional lesion, report 11103. Report 11104 for a punch biopsy, initial lesion; each additional lesion, report 11105. Report 11106 for an incisional biopsy, initial lesion; each additional lesion, report 11107.

Coding Tips

These biopsy codes may be reported when the procedure is performed for the specific purpose of obtaining tissue samples for diagnostic examination. Report 11103, 11105, or 11107 in addition to 11102, 11104, and 11106 according to type of biopsy techniques. Any local anesthesia is not reported separately. If tissue is transported to an outside laboratory, report 99000 for handling and/or conveyance. For excision of a lesion, see 11440–11446 or 11640–11646.

ICD-10-CM Diagnostic Codes

C43.39	Malignant melanoma of other parts of face
C43.4	Malignant melanoma of scalp and neck
C43.51	Malignant melanoma of anal skin
C43.52	Malignant melanoma of skin of breast
C43.59	Malignant melanoma of other part of trunk
C44.311	Basal cell carcinoma of skin of nose
C44.319	Basal cell carcinoma of skin of other parts of face
C44.321	Squamous cell carcinoma of skin of nose
C44.329	Squamous cell carcinoma of skin of other parts of face
C44.391	Other specified malignant neoplasm of skin of nose
C44.399	Other specified malignant neoplasm of skin of other parts of face
C44.41	Basal cell carcinoma of skin of scalp and neck
C44.42	Squamous cell carcinoma of skin of scalp and neck
C44.510	Basal cell carcinoma of anal skin
C44.511	Basal cell carcinoma of skin of breast
C44.521	Squamous cell carcinoma of skin of breast
C44.529	Squamous cell carcinoma of skin of other part of trunk
C44.590	Other specified malignant neoplasm of anal skin
C44.712	Basal cell carcinoma of skin of right lower limb, including hip ☑
C44.722	Squamous cell carcinoma of skin of right lower limb, including hip ☑
C46.0	Kaposi's sarcoma of skin
C49.0	Malignant neoplasm of connective and soft tissue of head, face and neck
C76.0	Malignant neoplasm of head, face and neck
C79.2	Secondary malignant neoplasm of skin
D03.39	Melanoma in situ of other parts of face
D03.51	Melanoma in situ of anal skin
D03.52	Melanoma in situ of breast (skin) (soft tissue)
D04.39	Carcinoma in situ of skin of other parts of face
D04.4	Carcinoma in situ of skin of scalp and neck
D17.23	Benign lipomatous neoplasm of skin and subcutaneous tissue of right leg ☑
D18.01	Hemangioma of skin and subcutaneous tissue
D22.39	Melanocytic nevi of other parts of face
D22.4	Melanocytic nevi of scalp and neck
D23.39	Other benign neoplasm of skin of other parts of face
D23.4	Other benign neoplasm of skin of scalp and neck
D23.71	Other benign neoplasm of skin of right lower limb, including hip ☑
I78.1	Nevus, non-neoplastic
L02.212	Cutaneous abscess of back [any part, except buttock]
L02.413	Cutaneous abscess of right upper limb ☑
L03.211	Cellulitis of face
L03.212	Acute lymphangitis of face
L03.221	Cellulitis of neck
L03.222	Acute lymphangitis of neck
L03.313	Cellulitis of chest wall
L10.0	Pemphigus vulgaris
L10.1	Pemphigus vegetans
L10.2	Pemphigus foliaceous
L10.3	Brazilian pemphigus [fogo selvagem]
L10.4	Pemphigus erythematosus
L10.5	Drug-induced pemphigus
L10.81	Paraneoplastic pemphigus
L11.1	Transient acantholytic dermatosis [Grover]
L40.0	Psoriasis vulgaris
L57.5	Actinic granuloma
L72.0	Epidermal cyst
L72.3	Sebaceous cyst
L82.0	Inflamed seborrheic keratosis
L82.1	Other seborrheic keratosis
Q82.5	Congenital non-neoplastic nevus

AMA: **11102** 2020,May,13; 2019,Jan,9; 2019,Dec,9 **11103** 2020,May,13; 2019,Jan,9; 2019,Dec,9 **11104** 2019,Jan,9; 2019,Dec,9 **11105** 2019,Jan,9; 2019,Dec,9 **11106** 2019,Jan,9; 2019,Dec,9 **11107** 2019,Jan,9; 2019,Dec,9

Relative Value Units/Medicare Edits

Non-Facility RVU	Work	PE	MP	Total
11102	0.66	2.34	0.05	3.05
11103	0.38	1.13	0.04	1.55
11104	0.83	2.9	0.09	3.82
11105	0.45	1.29	0.05	1.79
11106	1.01	3.55	0.11	4.67
11107	0.54	1.55	0.05	2.14

Facility RVU	Work	PE	MP	Total
11102	0.66	0.38	0.05	1.09
11103	0.38	0.22	0.04	0.64
11104	0.83	0.46	0.09	1.38
11105	0.45	0.25	0.05	0.75
11106	1.01	0.56	0.11	1.68
11107	0.54	0.31	0.05	0.9

	FUD	Status	MUE	Modifiers				IOM Reference
11102	0	A	1(2)	51	N/A	N/A	N/A	None
11103	N/A	A	6(3)	N/A	N/A	N/A	N/A	
11104	0	A	1(2)	51	N/A	N/A	N/A	
11105	N/A	A	3(3)	N/A	N/A	N/A	N/A	
11106	0	A	1(2)	51	N/A	N/A	N/A	
11107	N/A	A	2(3)	N/A	N/A	N/A	N/A	

* with documentation

11400-11406

11400 Excision, benign lesion including margins, except skin tag (unless listed elsewhere), trunk, arms or legs; excised diameter 0.5 cm or less
11401   excised diameter 0.6 to 1.0 cm
11402   excised diameter 1.1 to 2.0 cm
11403   excised diameter 2.1 to 3.0 cm
11404   excised diameter 3.1 to 4.0 cm
11406   excised diameter over 4.0 cm

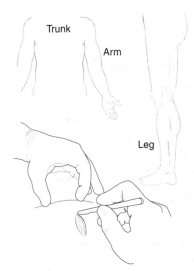

Trunk

Arm

Leg

Excision of benign lesion, trunk, arms, legs

Explanation

The physician removes a benign skin lesion located on the trunk, arms, or legs. After administering a local anesthetic, the physician makes a full thickness incision through the dermis with a scalpel, usually in an elliptical shape around and under the lesion. The lesion and a margin of normal tissue are removed. The wound is repaired using a single layer of sutures, chemical or electrocauterization. Complex or layered closure is reported separately, if required. Each lesion removed is reported separately. Report 11400 for an excised diameter 0.5 cm or less; 11401 for 0.6 cm to 1 cm; 11402 for 1.1 cm to 2 cm; 11403 for 2.1 cm to 3 cm; 11404 for 3.1 cm to 4 cm; and 11406 if the excised diameter is greater than 4 cm.

Coding Tips

These procedures include simple (nonlayered) closure. If intermediate (layered) or complex closure is necessary, see 12031–12037 or 13100–13122. If significant additional time and effort is documented, append modifier 22 and submit a cover letter and operative report. When these codes are performed with another separately identifiable procedure, the highest dollar value code is listed as the primary procedure and subsequent procedures are appended with modifier 51. When a specimen is transported to an outside laboratory, report 99000 for handling or conveyance. For excision of a malignant lesion, trunk, arms, or legs, see 11600–11606. For destruction of premalignant lesions, by any method, including laser, see 17000–17004; benign, see 17106–17111. Destruction of extensive (50 to 100) cutaneous neurofibroma lesions is reported with 0419T–0420T. For removal of skin tags, see 11200–11201. Surgical trays, A4550, are not separately reimbursed by Medicare; however, other third-party payers may cover them. Check with the specific payer to determine coverage.

ICD-10-CM Diagnostic Codes

B07.8	Other viral warts
D17.1	Benign lipomatous neoplasm of skin and subcutaneous tissue of trunk
D17.21	Benign lipomatous neoplasm of skin and subcutaneous tissue of right arm ☑
D17.22	Benign lipomatous neoplasm of skin and subcutaneous tissue of left arm ☑
D17.23	Benign lipomatous neoplasm of skin and subcutaneous tissue of right leg ☑
D17.24	Benign lipomatous neoplasm of skin and subcutaneous tissue of left leg ☑
D17.39	Benign lipomatous neoplasm of skin and subcutaneous tissue of other sites
D18.01	Hemangioma of skin and subcutaneous tissue
D22.5	Melanocytic nevi of trunk
D22.61	Melanocytic nevi of right upper limb, including shoulder ☑
D22.62	Melanocytic nevi of left upper limb, including shoulder ☑
D22.71	Melanocytic nevi of right lower limb, including hip ☑
D22.72	Melanocytic nevi of left lower limb, including hip ☑
D23.5	Other benign neoplasm of skin of trunk
D23.61	Other benign neoplasm of skin of right upper limb, including shoulder ☑
D23.62	Other benign neoplasm of skin of left upper limb, including shoulder ☑
D23.71	Other benign neoplasm of skin of right lower limb, including hip ☑
D23.72	Other benign neoplasm of skin of left lower limb, including hip ☑
D48.5	Neoplasm of uncertain behavior of skin
D49.2	Neoplasm of unspecified behavior of bone, soft tissue, and skin
I78.1	Nevus, non-neoplastic
L72.0	Epidermal cyst
L72.11	Pilar cyst
L72.12	Trichodermal cyst
L72.2	Steatocystoma multiplex
L72.3	Sebaceous cyst
L72.8	Other follicular cysts of the skin and subcutaneous tissue
L82.0	Inflamed seborrheic keratosis
L82.1	Other seborrheic keratosis
L90.5	Scar conditions and fibrosis of skin
L91.0	Hypertrophic scar
L92.3	Foreign body granuloma of the skin and subcutaneous tissue
L92.8	Other granulomatous disorders of the skin and subcutaneous tissue
Q82.5	Congenital non-neoplastic nevus

AMA: **11400** 2019,Nov,3; 2018,Sep,7; 2018,Jan,8; 2018,Feb,10; 2017,Jan,8; 2016,Jan,13; 2016,Apr,3; 2015,Jan,16 **11401** 2019,Nov,3; 2018,Sep,7; 2018,Jan,8; 2018,Feb,10; 2017,Jan,8; 2016,Jan,13; 2016,Apr,3; 2015,Jan,16 **11402** 2019,Nov,3; 2018,Sep,7; 2018,Jan,8; 2018,Feb,10; 2017,Jan,8; 2016,Jan,13; 2016,Apr,3; 2015,Jan,16 **11403** 2019,Nov,3; 2018,Sep,7; 2018,Jan,8; 2018,Feb,10; 2017,Jan,8; 2016,Jan,13; 2016,Apr,3; 2015,Jan,16 **11404** 2019,Nov,3; 2018,Sep,7; 2018,Jan,8; 2018,Feb,10; 2017,Jan,8; 2016,Jan,13; 2016,Apr,3; 2015,Jan,16 **11406** 2019,Nov,3; 2018,Sep,7; 2018,Jan,8; 2018,Feb,10; 2017,Jan,8; 2016,Jan,13; 2016,Apr,3; 2015,Jan,16

Skin

Relative Value Units/Medicare Edits

Non-Facility RVU	Work	PE	MP	Total
11400	0.9	2.78	0.11	3.79
11401	1.28	3.18	0.15	4.61
11402	1.45	3.45	0.19	5.09
11403	1.84	3.75	0.26	5.85
11404	2.11	4.21	0.34	6.66
11406	3.52	5.27	0.65	9.44
Facility RVU	**Work**	**PE**	**MP**	**Total**
11400	0.9	1.41	0.11	2.42
11401	1.28	1.62	0.15	3.05
11402	1.45	1.72	0.19	3.36
11403	1.84	2.21	0.26	4.31
11404	2.11	2.31	0.34	4.76
11406	3.52	3.07	0.65	7.24

	FUD	Status	MUE	Modifiers				IOM Reference
11400	10	A	3(3)	51	N/A	N/A	N/A	None
11401	10	A	3(3)	51	N/A	N/A	N/A	
11402	10	A	3(3)	51	N/A	N/A	N/A	
11403	10	A	2(3)	51	N/A	N/A	N/A	
11404	10	A	2(3)	51	N/A	N/A	N/A	
11406	10	A	2(3)	51	N/A	N/A	N/A	

* with documentation

Terms To Know

benign. Mild or nonmalignant in nature.

diameter. Straight line connecting two opposite points on the surface of a lesion, spheric, or cylindric body.

hemangioma. Benign neoplasm arising from vascular tissue or malformations of vascular structures. It is most commonly seen in children and infants as a tumor of newly formed blood vessels due to malformed fetal angioblastic tissues.

keloid. Progressive overgrowth of cutaneous scar tissue that is raised and irregular in shape, caused by excessive formation of collagen during connective tissue repair.

lesion. Area of damaged tissue that has lost continuity or function, due to disease or trauma.

pilar cyst. Cyst of the skin containing sebum and keratin and occurring more commonly in the scalp.

sebaceous cyst. Benign cyst of the skin or hair follicle filled with keratin and debris rich in lipids. Cysts of the integumentary system may be treated by incision and drainage or puncture aspiration.

11420-11426

11420 Excision, benign lesion including margins, except skin tag (unless listed elsewhere), scalp, neck, hands, feet, genitalia; excised diameter 0.5 cm or less

11421 excised diameter 0.6 to 1.0 cm

11422 excised diameter 1.1 to 2.0 cm

11423 excised diameter 2.1 to 3.0 cm

11424 excised diameter 3.1 to 4.0 cm

11426 excised diameter over 4.0 cm

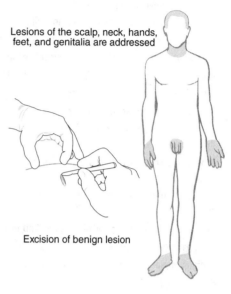

Lesions of the scalp, neck, hands, feet, and genitalia are addressed

Excision of benign lesion

Explanation

The physician removes a benign skin lesion located on the scalp, neck, hands, feet, or genitalia. After administering a local anesthetic, the physician makes a full thickness incision through the dermis with a scalpel, usually in an elliptical shape around and under the lesion. The lesion and a margin of normal tissue are removed. The wound is repaired using a single layer of sutures, chemical or electrocauterization. Complex or layered closure is reported separately, if required. Each lesion removed is reported separately. Report 11420 for an excised diameter 0.5 cm or less; 11421 for 0.6 cm to 1 cm; 11422 for 1.1 cm to 2 cm; 11423 for 2.1 cm to 3 cm; 11424 for 3.1 cm to 4 cm; and 11426 if the excised diameter is greater than 4 cm.

Coding Tips

These procedures include simple (nonlayered) closure. If intermediate (layered) or complex closure is necessary, see 12031–12047 or 13120–13133. If significant additional time and effort is documented, append modifier 22 and submit a cover letter and operative report. If the specimen is transported to an outside laboratory, report 99000 for handling or conveyance. For excision of a malignant lesion of the scalp, neck, hands, feet, or genitalia, see 11620–11626. For destruction of premalignant lesions, by any method, including laser, see 17000–17004; benign, see 17106–17111. For removal of skin tags, see 11200–11201. Surgical trays, A4550, are not separately reimbursed by Medicare; however, other third-party payers may cover them. Check with the specific payer to determine coverage.

ICD-10-CM Diagnostic Codes

D17.0	Benign lipomatous neoplasm of skin and subcutaneous tissue of head, face and neck
D17.21	Benign lipomatous neoplasm of skin and subcutaneous tissue of right arm ☑

D17.22	Benign lipomatous neoplasm of skin and subcutaneous tissue of left arm ☑
D17.23	Benign lipomatous neoplasm of skin and subcutaneous tissue of right leg ☑
D17.24	Benign lipomatous neoplasm of skin and subcutaneous tissue of left leg ☑
D17.39	Benign lipomatous neoplasm of skin and subcutaneous tissue of other sites
D17.72	Benign lipomatous neoplasm of other genitourinary organ
D18.01	Hemangioma of skin and subcutaneous tissue
D22.4	Melanocytic nevi of scalp and neck
D22.61	Melanocytic nevi of right upper limb, including shoulder ☑
D22.62	Melanocytic nevi of left upper limb, including shoulder ☑
D22.71	Melanocytic nevi of right lower limb, including hip ☑
D22.72	Melanocytic nevi of left lower limb, including hip ☑
D23.4	Other benign neoplasm of skin of scalp and neck
D23.5	Other benign neoplasm of skin of trunk
D23.61	Other benign neoplasm of skin of right upper limb, including shoulder ☑
D23.62	Other benign neoplasm of skin of left upper limb, including shoulder ☑
D23.71	Other benign neoplasm of skin of right lower limb, including hip ☑
D23.72	Other benign neoplasm of skin of left lower limb, including hip ☑
D28.0	Benign neoplasm of vulva ♀
D28.7	Benign neoplasm of other specified female genital organs ♀
D29.0	Benign neoplasm of penis ♂
D29.4	Benign neoplasm of scrotum ♂
D40.8	Neoplasm of uncertain behavior of other specified male genital organs ♂
D48.5	Neoplasm of uncertain behavior of skin
D49.2	Neoplasm of unspecified behavior of bone, soft tissue, and skin
I78.1	Nevus, non-neoplastic
L72.0	Epidermal cyst
L72.11	Pilar cyst
L72.12	Trichodermal cyst
L72.2	Steatocystoma multiplex
L72.3	Sebaceous cyst
L72.8	Other follicular cysts of the skin and subcutaneous tissue
L82.0	Inflamed seborrheic keratosis
L82.1	Other seborrheic keratosis
L91.0	Hypertrophic scar
L91.8	Other hypertrophic disorders of the skin
L92.2	Granuloma faciale [eosinophilic granuloma of skin]
L92.3	Foreign body granuloma of the skin and subcutaneous tissue
L92.8	Other granulomatous disorders of the skin and subcutaneous tissue
Q82.5	Congenital non-neoplastic nevus

AMA: **11420** 2019,Nov,3; 2018,Sep,7; 2018,Jan,8; 2018,Feb,10; 2017,Jan,8; 2016,Jan,13; 2016,Apr,3; 2015,Jan,16 **11421** 2019,Nov,3; 2018,Sep,7; 2018,Jan,8; 2018,Feb,10; 2017,Jan,8; 2016,Jan,13; 2016,Apr,3; 2015,Jan,16 **11422** 2019,Nov,3; 2018,Sep,7; 2018,Jan,8; 2018,Feb,10; 2017,Jan,8; 2016,Jan,13; 2016,Apr,3; 2015,Jan,16 **11423** 2019,Nov,3; 2018,Sep,7; 2018,Jan,8; 2018,Feb,10; 2017,Jan,8; 2016,Jan,13; 2016,Apr,3; 2015,Jan,16 **11424** 2019,Nov,3; 2018,Sep,7; 2018,Jan,8; 2018,Feb,10; 2017,Jan,8; 2016,Jan,13; 2016,Apr,3; 2015,Jan,16 **11426** 2019,Nov,3; 2018,Sep,7; 2018,Jan,8; 2018,Feb,10; 2017,Jan,8; 2016,Jan,13; 2016,Apr,3; 2015,Jan,16

Relative Value Units/Medicare Edits

Non-Facility RVU	Work	PE	MP	Total
11420	1.03	2.66	0.11	3.8
11421	1.47	3.1	0.16	4.73
11422	1.68	3.44	0.21	5.33
11423	2.06	3.73	0.27	6.06
11424	2.48	4.11	0.36	6.95
11426	4.09	5.19	0.66	9.94
Facility RVU	**Work**	**PE**	**MP**	**Total**
11420	1.03	1.25	0.11	2.39
11421	1.47	1.54	0.16	3.17
11422	1.68	2.04	0.21	3.93
11423	2.06	2.19	0.27	4.52
11424	2.48	2.32	0.36	5.16
11426	4.09	3.25	0.66	8.0

	FUD	Status	MUE	Modifiers				IOM Reference
11420	10	A	3(3)	51	N/A	N/A	N/A	None
11421	10	A	3(3)	51	N/A	N/A	N/A	
11422	10	A	3(3)	51	N/A	N/A	N/A	
11423	10	A	2(3)	51	N/A	N/A	N/A	
11424	10	A	2(3)	51	N/A	N/A	N/A	
11426	10	A	2(3)	51	N/A	N/A	N/A	

* with documentation

Terms To Know

benign. Mild or nonmalignant in nature.

dermis. Skin layer found under the epidermis that contains a papillary upper layer and the deep reticular layer of collagen, vascular bed, and nerves.

diameter. Straight line connecting two opposite points on the surface of a lesion, spheric, or cylindric body.

excision. Surgical removal of an organ or tissue.

full thickness. Consisting of skin and subcutaneous tissue.

incision. Act of cutting into tissue or an organ.

lesion. Area of damaged tissue that has lost continuity or function, due to disease or trauma.

11440-11446

11440 Excision, other benign lesion including margins, except skin tag (unless listed elsewhere), face, ears, eyelids, nose, lips, mucous membrane; excised diameter 0.5 cm or less
11441 excised diameter 0.6 to 1.0 cm
11442 excised diameter 1.1 to 2.0 cm
11443 excised diameter 2.1 to 3.0 cm
11444 excised diameter 3.1 to 4.0 cm
11446 excised diameter over 4.0 cm

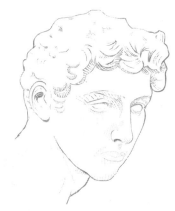

Benign lesions of the face, ears, eyelids, nose,
lips, or mucous membranes are excised

Explanation

The physician removes a benign skin lesion located on the face, ears, eyelids, nose, lips, or mucous membranes. After administering a local anesthetic, the physician makes a full thickness incision through the dermis with a scalpel, usually in an elliptical shape around and under the lesion. The lesion and a margin of normal tissue are removed. The wound is repaired using a single layer of sutures, chemical or electrocauterization. Complex or layered closure is reported separately, if required. Each lesion removed is reported separately. Report 11440 for an excised diameter 0.5 cm or less; 11441 for 0.6 cm to 1 cm; 11442 for 1.1 cm to 2 cm; 11443 for 2.1 cm to 3 cm; 11444 for 3.1 cm to 4 cm; and 11446 if the excised diameter is greater than 4 cm.

Coding Tips

These procedures include simple (nonlayered) closure. If intermediate (layered) or complex closure is necessary, see 12051–12057 or 13131–13153. If significant additional time and effort is documented, append modifier 22 and submit a cover letter and operative report. When these codes are performed with another separately identifiable procedure, the highest dollar value code is listed as the primary procedure and subsequent procedures are appended with modifier 51. When a specimen is transported to an outside laboratory, report 99000 for handling or conveyance. For excision of a malignant lesion, face, ears, eyelid, nose, or lips, see 11640–11646. For destruction of premalignant lesions, by any method, including laser, see 17000–17004; benign, see 17106–17111. Surgical trays, A4550, are not separately reimbursed by Medicare; however, other third-party payers may cover them. Check with the specific payer to determine coverage.

ICD-10-CM Diagnostic Codes

D10.0	Benign neoplasm of lip
D17.0	Benign lipomatous neoplasm of skin and subcutaneous tissue of head, face and neck
D18.01	Hemangioma of skin and subcutaneous tissue
D21.0	Benign neoplasm of connective and other soft tissue of head, face and neck
D22.0	Melanocytic nevi of lip
D22.111	Melanocytic nevi of right upper eyelid, including canthus ☑
D22.112	Melanocytic nevi of right lower eyelid, including canthus ☑
D22.21	Melanocytic nevi of right ear and external auricular canal ☑
D22.22	Melanocytic nevi of left ear and external auricular canal ☑
D22.39	Melanocytic nevi of other parts of face
D23.0	Other benign neoplasm of skin of lip
D23.111	Other benign neoplasm of skin of right upper eyelid, including canthus ☑
D23.112	Other benign neoplasm of skin of right lower eyelid, including canthus ☑
D23.21	Other benign neoplasm of skin of right ear and external auricular canal ☑
D23.22	Other benign neoplasm of skin of left ear and external auricular canal ☑
D23.39	Other benign neoplasm of skin of other parts of face
D48.1	Neoplasm of uncertain behavior of connective and other soft tissue
D48.5	Neoplasm of uncertain behavior of skin
D49.2	Neoplasm of unspecified behavior of bone, soft tissue, and skin
I78.1	Nevus, non-neoplastic
K13.29	Other disturbances of oral epithelium, including tongue
L57.0	Actinic keratosis
L72.0	Epidermal cyst
L72.11	Pilar cyst
L72.12	Trichodermal cyst
L72.2	Steatocystoma multiplex
L72.3	Sebaceous cyst
L72.8	Other follicular cysts of the skin and subcutaneous tissue
L82.0	Inflamed seborrheic keratosis
L82.1	Other seborrheic keratosis
L85.8	Other specified epidermal thickening
L91.0	Hypertrophic scar
L91.8	Other hypertrophic disorders of the skin
L92.2	Granuloma faciale [eosinophilic granuloma of skin]
L92.3	Foreign body granuloma of the skin and subcutaneous tissue
L92.8	Other granulomatous disorders of the skin and subcutaneous tissue
Q82.5	Congenital non-neoplastic nevus

AMA: 11440 2019,Nov,3; 2019,Jan,14; 2018,Sep,7; 2018,Jan,8; 2018,Feb,10; 2017,Jan,8; 2016,Jan,13; 2016,Apr,3; 2015,Jan,16 **11441** 2019,Nov,3; 2019,Jan,14; 2018,Sep,7; 2018,Jan,8; 2018,Feb,10; 2017,Jan,8; 2016,Jan,13; 2016,Apr,3; 2015,Jan,16 **11442** 2019,Nov,3; 2019,Jan,14; 2018,Sep,7; 2018,Jan,8; 2018,Feb,10; 2017,Jan,8; 2016,Jan,13; 2016,Apr,3; 2015,Jan,16 **11443** 2019,Nov,3; 2019,Jan,14; 2018,Sep,7; 2018,Jan,8; 2018,Feb,10; 2017,Jan,8; 2016,Jan,13; 2016,Apr,3; 2015,Jan,16 **11444** 2019,Nov,3; 2019,Jan,14; 2018,Sep,7; 2018,Jan,8; 2018,Feb,10; 2017,Jan,8; 2016,Jan,13; 2016,Apr,3; 2015,Jan,16 **11446** 2019,Nov,3; 2019,Jan,14; 2018,Sep,7; 2018,Jan,8; 2018,Feb,10; 2017,Jan,8; 2016,Jan,13; 2016,Apr,3; 2015,Jan,16

Skin

Relative Value Units/Medicare Edits

Non-Facility RVU	Work	PE	MP	Total
11440	1.05	3.08	0.11	4.24
11441	1.53	3.42	0.19	5.14
11442	1.77	3.7	0.23	5.7
11443	2.34	4.09	0.32	6.75
11444	3.19	4.77	0.45	8.41
11446	4.8	6.0	0.66	11.46
Facility RVU	Work	PE	MP	Total
11440	1.05	1.87	0.11	3.03
11441	1.53	2.1	0.19	3.82
11442	1.77	2.22	0.23	4.22
11443	2.34	2.52	0.32	5.18
11444	3.19	2.94	0.45	6.58
11446	4.8	3.91	0.66	9.37

	FUD	Status	MUE	Modifiers				IOM Reference
11440	10	A	4(3)	51	N/A	N/A	N/A	None
11441	10	A	3(3)	51	N/A	N/A	N/A	
11442	10	A	3(3)	51	N/A	N/A	N/A	
11443	10	A	2(3)	51	N/A	N/A	N/A	
11444	10	A	2(3)	51	N/A	N/A	N/A	
11446	10	A	2(3)	51	N/A	N/A	N/A	

* with documentation

Terms To Know

benign. Mild or nonmalignant in nature.

dermis. Skin layer found under the epidermis that contains a papillary upper layer and the deep reticular layer of collagen, vascular bed, and nerves.

full thickness. Consisting of skin and subcutaneous tissue.

hemangioma. Benign neoplasm arising from vascular tissue or malformations of vascular structures. It is most commonly seen in children and infants as a tumor of newly formed blood vessels due to malformed fetal angioblastic tissues.

lesion. Area of damaged tissue that has lost continuity or function, due to disease or trauma.

nevus. Benign, pigmented skin lesion that includes congenital lesions of the skin such as birthmarks, telangiectasias (permanent dilations of small blood vessels), vascular spider veins, hemangiomas, and moles.

11450-11451

11450   Excision of skin and subcutaneous tissue for hidradenitis, axillary; with simple or intermediate repair

11451   with complex repair

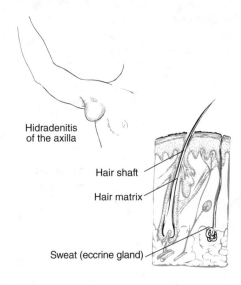

Hidradenitis of the axilla

Hair shaft

Hair matrix

Sweat (eccrine gland)

Explanation

Hidradenitis is a chronic, relapsing disease that occurs in tissue where apocrine glands are found. Localized nodules develop from occlusion of the apocrine ducts. Recurrence of the lesions may produce superimposed infections, recurrent abscesses with or without sinus formation, and scarring. The physician performs an excision of the affected skin and subcutaneous tissue of the axilla including margins. Intraoperative mapping of any existing sinus tracts may be performed to ensure complete removal. In 11450, the wound is left open to heal by granulation or is repaired using single or multiple layers of sutures. Report 11451 if more than layered closure (complex repair) is required.

Coding Tips

These are unilateral procedures. If performed bilaterally, some payers require that the service be reported twice with modifier 50 appended to the second code while others require identification of the service only once with modifier 50 appended. Check with individual payers. Modifier 50 identifies a procedure performed identically on the opposite side of the body (mirror image). If reconstructive closure is required, see 15002–15261 or 15570–15770. Surgical trays, A4550, are not separately reimbursed by Medicare; however, other third-party payers may cover them. Check with the specific payer to determine coverage.

ICD-10-CM Diagnostic Codes

L73.2   Hidradenitis suppurativa

AMA: 11450 2019,Nov,3; 2018,Sep,7; 2018,Jan,8; 2018,Feb,10; 2017,Jan,8; 2016,Jan,13; 2016,Aug,9; 2015,Jan,16 **11451** 2019,Nov,3; 2018,Sep,7; 2018,Jan,8; 2018,Feb,10; 2017,Jan,8; 2016,Jan,13; 2016,Aug,9; 2015,Jan,16

Skin

Relative Value Units/Medicare Edits

Non-Facility RVU	Work	PE	MP	Total
11450	3.22	8.85	0.71	12.78
11451	4.43	10.33	0.93	15.69
Facility RVU	Work	PE	MP	Total
11450	3.22	3.67	0.71	7.6
11451	4.43	4.3	0.93	9.66

	FUD	Status	MUE	Modifiers				IOM Reference
11450	90	A	1(2)	51	50	N/A	N/A	None
11451	90	A	1(2)	51	50	N/A	80*	

* with documentation

Terms To Know

abscess. Circumscribed collection of pus resulting from bacteria, frequently associated with swelling and other signs of inflammation.

axillary. Area under the arm.

epidermis. Outermost, nonvascular layer of skin that contains four to five differentiated layers depending on its body location: stratum corneum, lucidum, granulosum, spinosum, and basale.

excision. Surgical removal of an organ or tissue.

graft. Tissue implant from another part of the body or another person.

granulation. Formation of small, bead-like masses of cytoplasm or granules on the surface of healing wounds of an organ, membrane, or tissue.

hidradenitis. Infection or inflammation of a sweat gland, usually treated by incision and drainage.

lesion. Area of damaged tissue that has lost continuity or function, due to disease or trauma.

pedicle flap. Full-thickness skin and subcutaneous tissue for grafting that remains partially attached to the donor site by a pedicle or stem in which the blood vessels supplying the flap remain intact.

subcutaneous tissue. Sheet or wide band of adipose (fat) and areolar connective tissue in two layers attached to the dermis.

suppurative. Forming pus.

unilateral. Located on or affecting one side.

wound repair. Surgical closure of a wound is divided into three categories: simple, intermediate, and complex. *simple repair:* Surgical closure of a superficial wound, requiring single layer suturing of the skin epidermis, dermis, or subcutaneous tissue. *intermediate repair:* Surgical closure of a wound requiring closure of one or more of the deeper subcutaneous tissue and non-muscle fascia layers in addition to suturing the skin; contaminated wounds with single layer closure that need extensive cleaning or foreign body removal. *complex repair:* Repair of wounds requiring more than layered closure (debridement, scar revision, stents, retention sutures).

11462-11463

11462   Excision of skin and subcutaneous tissue for hidradenitis, inguinal; with simple or intermediate repair

11463   with complex repair

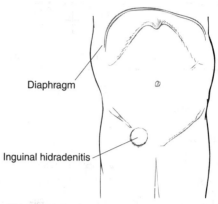

Diaphragm

Inguinal hidradenitis

Hidradenitis is often seen among obese patients

Explanation

Hidradenitis is a chronic, relapsing disease that occurs in tissue where apocrine glands are found. Localized nodules develop from occlusion of the apocrine ducts. Recurrence of the lesions may produce superimposed infections, recurrent abscesses with or without sinus formation, and scarring. The physician performs a wide excision of the affected skin and subcutaneous tissue of the groin (inguinal) region including margins. Intraoperative mapping of any existing sinus tracts may be performed to ensure complete removal. In 11462, the wound is left open to heal by granulation or is repaired using single or multiple layers of sutures. Report 11463 if more than layered closure (complex repair) is required.

Coding Tips

These are unilateral procedures. If performed bilaterally, some payers require that the service be reported twice with modifier 50 appended to the second code while others require identification of the service only once with modifier 50 appended. Check with individual payers. Modifier 50 identifies a procedure performed identically on the opposite side of the body (mirror image). If reconstructive closure is required, see 15002–15261 or 15570–15770. Surgical trays, A4550, are not separately reimbursed by Medicare; however, other third-party payers may cover them. Check with the specific payer to determine coverage.

ICD-10-CM Diagnostic Codes

L73.2   Hidradenitis suppurativa

AMA: 11462 2019,Nov,3; 2018,Sep,7; 2018,Jan,8; 2018,Feb,10; 2017,Jan,8; 2016,Jan,13; 2016,Aug,9; 2015,Jan,16 **11463** 2019,Nov,3; 2018,Sep,7; 2018,Jan,8; 2018,Feb,10; 2017,Jan,8; 2016,Jan,13; 2016,Aug,9; 2015,Jan,16

Relative Value Units/Medicare Edits

Non-Facility RVU	Work	PE	MP	Total
11462	3.0	8.72	0.64	12.36
11463	4.43	10.5	0.91	15.84
Facility RVU	Work	PE	MP	Total
11462	3.0	3.57	0.64	7.21
11463	4.43	4.36	0.91	9.7

	FUD	Status	MUE	Modifiers				IOM Reference
11462	90	A	1(2)	51	50	N/A	80*	None
11463	90	A	1(2)	51	50	N/A	80*	

* with documentation

Terms To Know

abscess. Circumscribed collection of pus resulting from bacteria, frequently associated with swelling and other signs of inflammation.

dermis. Skin layer found under the epidermis that contains a papillary upper layer and the deep reticular layer of collagen, vascular bed, and nerves.

epidermis. Outermost, nonvascular layer of skin that contains four to five differentiated layers depending on its body location: stratum corneum, lucidum, granulosum, spinosum, and basale.

excision. Surgical removal of an organ or tissue.

graft. Tissue implant from another part of the body or another person.

granulation. Formation of small, bead-like masses of cytoplasm or granules on the surface of healing wounds of an organ, membrane, or tissue.

hidradenitis. Infection or inflammation of a sweat gland, usually treated by incision and drainage.

lesion. Area of damaged tissue that has lost continuity or function, due to disease or trauma.

pedicle flap. Full-thickness skin and subcutaneous tissue for grafting that remains partially attached to the donor site by a pedicle or stem in which the blood vessels supplying the flap remain intact.

subcutaneous tissue. Sheet or wide band of adipose (fat) and areolar connective tissue in two layers attached to the dermis.

suppurative. Forming pus.

wound repair. Surgical closure of a wound is divided into three categories: simple, intermediate, and complex. *simple repair:* Surgical closure of a superficial wound, requiring single layer suturing of the skin epidermis, dermis, or subcutaneous tissue. *intermediate repair:* Surgical closure of a wound requiring closure of one or more of the deeper subcutaneous tissue and non-muscle fascia layers in addition to suturing the skin; contaminated wounds with single layer closure that need extensive cleaning or foreign body removal. *complex repair:* Repair of wounds requiring more than layered closure (debridement, scar revision, stents, retention sutures).

11470-11471

11470 Excision of skin and subcutaneous tissue for hidradenitis, perianal, perineal, or umbilical; with simple or intermediate repair

11471 with complex repair

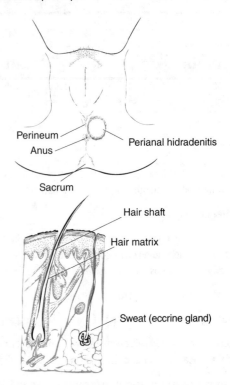

Perineum

Anus

Perianal hidradenitis

Sacrum

Hair shaft

Hair matrix

Sweat (eccrine gland)

Explanation

Hidradenitis is a chronic, relapsing disease that occurs in tissue where apocrine glands are found. Localized nodules develop from occlusion of the apocrine ducts. Recurrence of the lesions may produce superimposed infections, recurrent abscesses with or without sinus formation, and scarring. The physician performs a wide excision of the affected skin and subcutaneous tissue of the perianal, perineal, or umbilical region including margins. Intraoperative mapping of any existing sinus tracts may be performed to ensure complete removal. In 11470, the wound is left open to heal by granulation or is repaired using single or multiple layers of sutures. Report 11471 if more than layered closure (complex repair) is required.

Coding Tips

These are unilateral procedures. If performed bilaterally, some payers require that the service be reported twice with modifier 50 appended to the second code while others require identification of the service only once with modifier 50 appended. Check with individual payers. Modifier 50 identifies a procedure performed identically on the opposite side of the body (mirror image). Report skin grafts or flaps separately when performed for closure at the same session as 11470–11471. Surgical trays, A4550, are not separately reimbursed by Medicare; however, other third-party payers may cover them. Check with the specific payer to determine coverage.

ICD-10-CM Diagnostic Codes

L73.2 Hidradenitis suppurativa

AMA: 11470 2019,Nov,3; 2018,Sep,7; 2018,Jan,8; 2018,Feb,10; 2017,Jan,8; 2016,Jan,13; 2016,Aug,9; 2015,Jan,16 **11471** 2019,Nov,3; 2018,Sep,7; 2018,Jan,8; 2018,Feb,10; 2017,Jan,8; 2016,Jan,13; 2016,Aug,9; 2015,Jan,16

Relative Value Units/Medicare Edits

Non-Facility RVU	Work	PE	MP	Total
11470	3.74	8.96	0.74	13.44
11471	4.89	10.38	0.94	16.21
Facility RVU	**Work**	**PE**	**MP**	**Total**
11470	3.74	3.84	0.74	8.32
11471	4.89	4.42	0.94	10.25

	FUD	Status	MUE	Modifiers				IOM Reference
11470	90	A	3(2)	51	N/A	N/A	N/A	None
11471	90	A	2(3)	51	N/A	N/A	80*	

* with documentation

Terms To Know

abscess. Circumscribed collection of pus resulting from bacteria, frequently associated with swelling and other signs of inflammation.

dermis. Skin layer found under the epidermis that contains a papillary upper layer and the deep reticular layer of collagen, vascular bed, and nerves.

excision. Surgical removal of an organ or tissue.

graft. Tissue implant from another part of the body or another person.

granulation. Formation of small, bead-like masses of cytoplasm or granules on the surface of healing wounds of an organ, membrane, or tissue.

hidradenitis. Infection or inflammation of a sweat gland, usually treated by incision and drainage.

lesion. Area of damaged tissue that has lost continuity or function, due to disease or trauma.

pedicle flap. Full-thickness skin and subcutaneous tissue for grafting that remains partially attached to the donor site by a pedicle or stem in which the blood vessels supplying the flap remain intact.

perineal. Pertaining to the pelvic floor area between the thighs; the diamond-shaped area bordered by the pubic symphysis in front, the ischial tuberosities on the sides, and the coccyx in back.

subcutaneous tissue. Sheet or wide band of adipose (fat) and areolar connective tissue in two layers attached to the dermis.

suppurative. Forming pus.

wound repair. Surgical closure of a wound is divided into three categories: simple, intermediate, and complex. *simple repair:* Surgical closure of a superficial wound, requiring single layer suturing of the skin epidermis, dermis, or subcutaneous tissue. *intermediate repair:* Surgical closure of a wound requiring closure of one or more of the deeper subcutaneous tissue and non-muscle fascia layers in addition to suturing the skin; contaminated wounds with single layer closure that need extensive cleaning or foreign body removal. *complex repair:* Repair of wounds requiring more than layered closure (debridement, scar revision, stents, retention sutures).

11600-11606

11600 Excision, malignant lesion including margins, trunk, arms, or legs; excised diameter 0.5 cm or less
11601 excised diameter 0.6 to 1.0 cm
11602 excised diameter 1.1 to 2.0 cm
11603 excised diameter 2.1 to 3.0 cm
11604 excised diameter 3.1 to 4.0 cm
11606 excised diameter over 4.0 cm

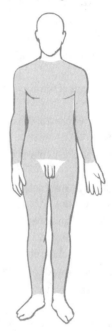

Malignant lesion, including margins, trunk, arms, or legs are excised

Explanation

The physician removes a malignant lesion located on the trunk, arms, or legs. After administering a local anesthetic, the physician makes a full-thickness incision through the dermis, usually in an elliptical shape around and under the lesion. The lesion and a margin of normal tissue are removed. The wound is repaired using a single layer of sutures, chemical or electrocauterization. Complex, layered, or reconstructive (excluding adjacent tissue transfer) wound repair is reported separately, if required. Each lesion removed is reported separately. Report 11600 for an excised diameter 0.5 cm or less; 11601 for 0.6 cm to 1 cm; 11602 for 1.1 cm to 2 cm; 11603 for 2.1 cm to 3 cm; 11604 for 3.1 cm to 4 cm; and 11606 if the excised diameter is greater than 4 cm.

Coding Tips

When these procedures are performed with another separately identifiable procedure, the highest dollar value code is listed as the primary procedure and subsequent procedures are appended with modifier 51. If significant additional time and effort is documented, append modifier 22 and submit a cover letter and operative report. When a specimen is transported to an outside laboratory, report 99000 for handling or conveyance. If intermediate (layered) or complex closure is necessary, see 12031–12037 or 13100–13122. For closure requiring skin grafts, see 15050–15261, by anatomical location. For excision of a benign lesion, trunk, arms, or legs, see 11400–11406. For destruction of premalignant lesions, by any method, including laser, see 17000–17004; benign, see 17110–17111; malignant, see 17260–17266. Surgical trays, A4550, are not separately reimbursed by Medicare; however, other third-party payers may cover them. Check with the specific payer to determine coverage.

Skin

ICD-10-CM Diagnostic Codes

C43.52	Malignant melanoma of skin of breast
C43.59	Malignant melanoma of other part of trunk
C43.61	Malignant melanoma of right upper limb, including shoulder ☑
C43.62	Malignant melanoma of left upper limb, including shoulder ☑
C43.71	Malignant melanoma of right lower limb, including hip ☑
C43.72	Malignant melanoma of left lower limb, including hip ☑
C43.8	Malignant melanoma of overlapping sites of skin
C44.511	Basal cell carcinoma of skin of breast
C44.519	Basal cell carcinoma of skin of other part of trunk
C44.521	Squamous cell carcinoma of skin of breast
C44.529	Squamous cell carcinoma of skin of other part of trunk
C44.591	Other specified malignant neoplasm of skin of breast
C44.612	Basal cell carcinoma of skin of right upper limb, including shoulder ☑
C44.619	Basal cell carcinoma of skin of left upper limb, including shoulder ☑
C44.622	Squamous cell carcinoma of skin of right upper limb, including shoulder ☑
C44.629	Squamous cell carcinoma of skin of left upper limb, including shoulder ☑
C44.692	Other specified malignant neoplasm of skin of right upper limb, including shoulder ☑
C44.699	Other specified malignant neoplasm of skin of left upper limb, including shoulder ☑
C44.712	Basal cell carcinoma of skin of right lower limb, including hip ☑
C44.719	Basal cell carcinoma of skin of left lower limb, including hip ☑
C44.722	Squamous cell carcinoma of skin of right lower limb, including hip ☑
C44.729	Squamous cell carcinoma of skin of left lower limb, including hip ☑
C44.792	Other specified malignant neoplasm of skin of right lower limb, including hip ☑
C44.799	Other specified malignant neoplasm of skin of left lower limb, including hip ☑
C44.81	Basal cell carcinoma of overlapping sites of skin
C44.82	Squamous cell carcinoma of overlapping sites of skin
C44.89	Other specified malignant neoplasm of overlapping sites of skin
C46.0	Kaposi's sarcoma of skin
C4A.52	Merkel cell carcinoma of skin of breast
C4A.59	Merkel cell carcinoma of other part of trunk
C4A.61	Merkel cell carcinoma of right upper limb, including shoulder ☑
C4A.71	Merkel cell carcinoma of right lower limb, including hip ☑
C76.41	Malignant neoplasm of right upper limb ☑
C76.42	Malignant neoplasm of left upper limb ☑
C79.2	Secondary malignant neoplasm of skin
C7B.1	Secondary Merkel cell carcinoma
D03.52	Melanoma in situ of breast (skin) (soft tissue)
D03.59	Melanoma in situ of other part of trunk
D03.61	Melanoma in situ of right upper limb, including shoulder ☑
D03.62	Melanoma in situ of left upper limb, including shoulder ☑
D03.71	Melanoma in situ of right lower limb, including hip ☑
D03.72	Melanoma in situ of left lower limb, including hip ☑
D03.8	Melanoma in situ of other sites
D04.5	Carcinoma in situ of skin of trunk
D04.61	Carcinoma in situ of skin of right upper limb, including shoulder ☑
D04.62	Carcinoma in situ of skin of left upper limb, including shoulder ☑
D04.71	Carcinoma in situ of skin of right lower limb, including hip ☑
D04.72	Carcinoma in situ of skin of left lower limb, including hip ☑
D48.5	Neoplasm of uncertain behavior of skin

AMA: 11600 2019,Nov,3; 2018,Sep,7; 2018,Jan,8; 2017,Jan,8; 2016,Jan,13; 2015,Jan,16 **11601** 2019,Nov,3; 2018,Sep,7; 2018,Jan,8; 2017,Jan,8; 2016,Jan,13; 2015,Jan,16 **11602** 2019,Nov,3; 2018,Sep,7; 2018,Jan,8; 2017,Jan,8; 2016,Jan,13; 2015,Jan,16 **11603** 2019,Nov,3; 2018,Sep,7; 2018,Jan,8; 2017,Jan,8; 2016,Jan,13; 2015,Jan,16 **11604** 2019,Nov,3; 2018,Sep,7; 2018,Jan,8; 2017,Jan,8; 2016,Jan,13; 2015,Jan,16 **11606** 2019,Nov,3; 2018,Sep,7; 2018,Jan,8; 2017,Jan,8; 2016,Jan,13; 2015,Jan,16

Relative Value Units/Medicare Edits

Non-Facility RVU	Work	PE	MP	Total
11600	1.63	4.08	0.21	5.92
11601	2.07	4.49	0.25	6.81
11602	2.27	4.75	0.25	7.27
11603	2.82	5.12	0.32	8.26
11604	3.17	5.63	0.42	9.22
11606	5.02	7.39	0.78	13.19

Facility RVU	Work	PE	MP	Total
11600	1.63	1.72	0.21	3.56
11601	2.07	1.99	0.25	4.31
11602	2.27	2.16	0.25	4.68
11603	2.82	2.45	0.32	5.59
11604	3.17	2.6	0.42	6.19
11606	5.02	3.43	0.78	9.23

	FUD	Status	MUE	Modifiers			IOM Reference
11600	10	A	2(3)	51	N/A	N/A	N/A	None
11601	10	A	2(3)	51	N/A	N/A	N/A	
11602	10	A	3(3)	51	N/A	N/A	N/A	
11603	10	A	2(3)	51	N/A	N/A	N/A	
11604	10	A	2(3)	51	N/A	N/A	N/A	
11606	10	A	2(3)	51	N/A	N/A	N/A	

* with documentation

Terms To Know

carcinoma in situ. Malignancy that arises from the cells of the vessel, gland, or organ of origin that remains confined to that site or has not invaded neighboring tissue.

diameter. Straight line connecting two opposite points on the surface of a lesion, spheric, or cylindric body.

malignant. Any condition tending to progress toward death, specifically an invasive tumor with a loss of cellular differentiation that has the ability to spread or metastasize to other body areas.

Skin

11620-11626

11620 Excision, malignant lesion including margins, scalp, neck, hands, feet, genitalia; excised diameter 0.5 cm or less
11621   excised diameter 0.6 to 1.0 cm
11622   excised diameter 1.1 to 2.0 cm
11623   excised diameter 2.1 to 3.0 cm
11624   excised diameter 3.1 to 4.0 cm
11626   excised diameter over 4.0 cm

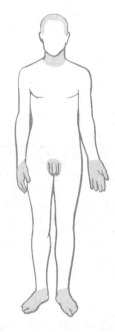

Malignant lesions, including margins, scalp, neck, hands, feet, or genitalia are excised

Explanation

The physician removes a malignant lesion located on the scalp, neck, hands, feet, or genitalia. After administering a local anesthetic, the physician makes a full-thickness incision through the dermis, usually in an elliptical shape around and under the lesion. The lesion and a margin of normal tissue are removed. The wound is repaired using a single layer of sutures, chemical or electrocauterization. Complex, layered, or reconstructive (excluding adjacent tissue transfer) wound repair is reported separately, if required. Each lesion removed is reported separately. Report 11620 for an excised diameter 0.5 cm or less; 11621 for 0.6 cm to 1 cm; 11622 for 1.1 cm to 2 cm; 11623 for 2.1 cm to 3 cm; 11624 for 3.1 cm to 4 cm; and 11626 if the excised diameter is greater than 4 cm.

Coding Tips

These procedures often require a larger excision than a similarly sized benign lesion; excision of a malignant lesion requires a full thickness incision and removal of the lesion and a rim of normal tissue margins. Local anesthesia is included in these services. However, these procedures may be performed under general anesthesia, depending on the age and/or condition of the patient. These procedures include simple (nonlayered) repair of the skin and/or subcutaneous tissues. If intermediate repair involving layered closure of deeper subcutaneous or non-muscle fascia is required, it is reported separately. For destruction of premalignant lesions, by any method, including laser, see 17000–17004; benign, see 17110–17111; malignant, see 17270–17276. Surgical trays, A4550, are not separately reimbursed by Medicare; however, other third-party payers may cover them. Check with the specific payer to determine coverage.

ICD-10-CM Diagnostic Codes

C43.4	Malignant melanoma of scalp and neck
C43.61	Malignant melanoma of right upper limb, including shoulder ☑
C43.62	Malignant melanoma of left upper limb, including shoulder ☑
C43.71	Malignant melanoma of right lower limb, including hip ☑
C43.72	Malignant melanoma of left lower limb, including hip ☑
C43.8	Malignant melanoma of overlapping sites of skin
C44.41	Basal cell carcinoma of skin of scalp and neck
C44.42	Squamous cell carcinoma of skin of scalp and neck
C44.49	Other specified malignant neoplasm of skin of scalp and neck
C44.612	Basal cell carcinoma of skin of right upper limb, including shoulder ☑
C44.619	Basal cell carcinoma of skin of left upper limb, including shoulder ☑
C44.622	Squamous cell carcinoma of skin of right upper limb, including shoulder ☑
C44.629	Squamous cell carcinoma of skin of left upper limb, including shoulder ☑
C44.692	Other specified malignant neoplasm of skin of right upper limb, including shoulder ☑
C44.699	Other specified malignant neoplasm of skin of left upper limb, including shoulder ☑
C44.712	Basal cell carcinoma of skin of right lower limb, including hip ☑
C44.719	Basal cell carcinoma of skin of left lower limb, including hip ☑
C44.722	Squamous cell carcinoma of skin of right lower limb, including hip ☑
C44.729	Squamous cell carcinoma of skin of left lower limb, including hip ☑
C44.792	Other specified malignant neoplasm of skin of right lower limb, including hip ☑
C44.799	Other specified malignant neoplasm of skin of left lower limb, including hip ☑
C4A.4	Merkel cell carcinoma of scalp and neck
C4A.61	Merkel cell carcinoma of right upper limb, including shoulder ☑
C4A.62	Merkel cell carcinoma of left upper limb, including shoulder ☑
C4A.71	Merkel cell carcinoma of right lower limb, including hip ☑
C4A.72	Merkel cell carcinoma of left lower limb, including hip ☑
C4A.8	Merkel cell carcinoma of overlapping sites
C51.0	Malignant neoplasm of labium majus ♀
C51.1	Malignant neoplasm of labium minus ♀
C51.2	Malignant neoplasm of clitoris ♀
C51.8	Malignant neoplasm of overlapping sites of vulva ♀
C57.8	Malignant neoplasm of overlapping sites of female genital organs ♀
C60.0	Malignant neoplasm of prepuce ♂
C60.1	Malignant neoplasm of glans penis ♂
C60.2	Malignant neoplasm of body of penis ♂
C60.8	Malignant neoplasm of overlapping sites of penis ♂
C63.2	Malignant neoplasm of scrotum ♂
C63.8	Malignant neoplasm of overlapping sites of male genital organs ♂
C76.41	Malignant neoplasm of right upper limb ☑

Skin

Skin

C76.42	Malignant neoplasm of left upper limb ☑
C76.51	Malignant neoplasm of right lower limb ☑
C76.52	Malignant neoplasm of left lower limb ☑
C79.2	Secondary malignant neoplasm of skin
C79.82	Secondary malignant neoplasm of genital organs
C7B.1	Secondary Merkel cell carcinoma
D03.4	Melanoma in situ of scalp and neck
D03.61	Melanoma in situ of right upper limb, including shoulder ☑
D03.62	Melanoma in situ of left upper limb, including shoulder ☑
D03.71	Melanoma in situ of right lower limb, including hip ☑
D03.72	Melanoma in situ of left lower limb, including hip ☑
D03.8	Melanoma in situ of other sites
D04.4	Carcinoma in situ of skin of scalp and neck
D04.61	Carcinoma in situ of skin of right upper limb, including shoulder ☑
D04.62	Carcinoma in situ of skin of left upper limb, including shoulder ☑
D04.71	Carcinoma in situ of skin of right lower limb, including hip ☑
D04.72	Carcinoma in situ of skin of left lower limb, including hip ☑
D07.1	Carcinoma in situ of vulva ♀
D07.4	Carcinoma in situ of penis ♂
D07.60	Carcinoma in situ of unspecified male genital organs ♂
D07.61	Carcinoma in situ of scrotum ♂
D39.8	Neoplasm of uncertain behavior of other specified female genital organs ♀
D40.8	Neoplasm of uncertain behavior of other specified male genital organs ♂

AMA: 11620 2019,Nov,3; 2018,Sep,7; 2018,Jan,8; 2017,Jan,8; 2016,Jan,13; 2015,Jan,16 **11621** 2019,Nov,3; 2018,Sep,7; 2018,Jan,8; 2017,Jan,8; 2016,Jan,13; 2015,Jan,16 **11622** 2019,Nov,3; 2018,Sep,7; 2018,Jan,8; 2017,Jan,8; 2016,Jan,13; 2015,Jan,16 **11623** 2019,Nov,3; 2018,Sep,7; 2018,Jan,8; 2017,Jan,8; 2016,Jan,13; 2015,Jan,16 **11624** 2019,Nov,3; 2018,Sep,7; 2018,Jan,8; 2017,Jan,8; 2016,Jan,13; 2015,Jan,16 **11626** 2019,Nov,3; 2018,Sep,7; 2018,Jan,8; 2017,Jan,8; 2016,Jan,13; 2015,Jan,16

Relative Value Units/Medicare Edits

Non-Facility RVU	Work	PE	MP	Total
11620	1.64	4.09	0.21	5.94
11621	2.08	4.5	0.25	6.83
11622	2.41	4.83	0.26	7.5
11623	3.11	5.28	0.38	8.77
11624	3.62	5.86	0.48	9.96
11626	4.61	6.69	0.74	12.04
Facility RVU	**Work**	**PE**	**MP**	**Total**
11620	1.64	1.73	0.21	3.58
11621	2.08	1.99	0.25	4.32
11622	2.41	2.22	0.26	4.89
11623	3.11	2.59	0.38	6.08
11624	3.62	2.8	0.48	6.9
11626	4.61	3.17	0.74	8.52

	FUD	Status	MUE	Modifiers				IOM Reference
11620	10	A	2(3)	51	N/A	N/A	N/A	None
11621	10	A	2(3)	51	N/A	N/A	N/A	
11622	10	A	2(3)	51	N/A	N/A	N/A	
11623	10	A	2(3)	51	N/A	N/A	N/A	
11624	10	A	2(3)	51	N/A	N/A	N/A	
11626	10	A	2(3)	51	N/A	N/A	N/A	

* with documentation

Terms To Know

carcinoma. Malignant growth of epithelial cells in the coverings and linings of organs and tissues. The cells tend to spread to other locations via the bloodstream or lymphatic channels.

melanoma. Highly metastatic malignant neoplasm composed of melanocytes that occur most often on the skin from a preexisting mole or nevus but may also occur in the mouth, esophagus, anal canal, or vagina.

11640-11646

11640 Excision, malignant lesion including margins, face, ears, eyelids, nose, lips; excised diameter 0.5 cm or less
11641 excised diameter 0.6 to 1.0 cm
11642 excised diameter 1.1 to 2.0 cm
11643 excised diameter 2.1 to 3.0 cm
11644 excised diameter 3.1 to 4.0 cm
11646 excised diameter over 4.0 cm

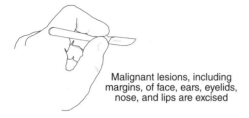

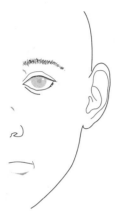

Malignant lesions, including margins, of face, ears, eyelids, nose, and lips are excised

Explanation

The physician removes a malignant lesion located on the face, ears, eyelids, nose, or lips. After administering a local anesthetic, the physician makes a full-thickness incision through the dermis, usually in an elliptical shape around and under the lesion. The lesion and a margin of normal tissue are removed. The wound is repaired using a single layer of sutures, chemical or electrocauterization. Complex, layered, or reconstructive (excluding adjacent tissue transfer) wound repair is reported separately, if required. Each lesion removed is reported separately. Report 11640 for an excised diameter 0.5 cm or less; 11641 for 0.6 cm to 1 cm; 11642 for 1.1 cm to 2 cm; 11643 for 2.1 cm to 3 cm; 11644 for 3.1 cm to 4 cm; and 11646 if the excised diameter is greater than 4 cm.

Coding Tips

These procedures often require a larger excision than a similarly sized benign lesion; excision of a malignant lesion requires a full thickness incision and removal of the lesion and a rim of normal tissue margins. Local anesthesia is included in these services. However, these procedures may be performed under general anesthesia, depending on the age and/or condition of the patient. These procedures include simple (nonlayered) repair of the skin and/or subcutaneous tissues. If intermediate repair involving layered closure of deeper subcutaneous or non-muscle fascia is required, it is reported separately. For destruction of premalignant lesions, by any method, including laser, see 17000–17004; benign, see 17110–17111; malignant, see 17280–17286. Surgical trays, A4550, are not separately reimbursed by Medicare; however, other third-party payers may cover them. Check with the specific payer to determine coverage.

ICD-10-CM Diagnostic Codes

C00.0	Malignant neoplasm of external upper lip
C00.1	Malignant neoplasm of external lower lip
C00.8	Malignant neoplasm of overlapping sites of lip
C43.0	Malignant melanoma of lip
C43.111	Malignant melanoma of right upper eyelid, including canthus ☑
C43.112	Malignant melanoma of right lower eyelid, including canthus ☑
C43.21	Malignant melanoma of right ear and external auricular canal ☑
C43.22	Malignant melanoma of left ear and external auricular canal ☑
C43.31	Malignant melanoma of nose
C43.39	Malignant melanoma of other parts of face
C44.01	Basal cell carcinoma of skin of lip
C44.02	Squamous cell carcinoma of skin of lip
C44.09	Other specified malignant neoplasm of skin of lip
C44.1121	Basal cell carcinoma of skin of right upper eyelid, including canthus ☑
C44.1122	Basal cell carcinoma of skin of right lower eyelid, including canthus ☑
C44.1221	Squamous cell carcinoma of skin of right upper eyelid, including canthus ☑
C44.1222	Squamous cell carcinoma of skin of right lower eyelid, including canthus ☑
C44.1921	Other specified malignant neoplasm of skin of right upper eyelid, including canthus ☑
C44.1922	Other specified malignant neoplasm of skin of right lower eyelid, including canthus ☑
C44.212	Basal cell carcinoma of skin of right ear and external auricular canal ☑
C44.219	Basal cell carcinoma of skin of left ear and external auricular canal ☑
C44.222	Squamous cell carcinoma of skin of right ear and external auricular canal ☑
C44.229	Squamous cell carcinoma of skin of left ear and external auricular canal ☑
C44.292	Other specified malignant neoplasm of skin of right ear and external auricular canal ☑
C44.299	Other specified malignant neoplasm of skin of left ear and external auricular canal ☑
C44.311	Basal cell carcinoma of skin of nose
C44.319	Basal cell carcinoma of skin of other parts of face
C44.321	Squamous cell carcinoma of skin of nose
C44.329	Squamous cell carcinoma of skin of other parts of face
C44.391	Other specified malignant neoplasm of skin of nose
C44.399	Other specified malignant neoplasm of skin of other parts of face
C4A.0	Merkel cell carcinoma of lip
C4A.111	Merkel cell carcinoma of right upper eyelid, including canthus ☑
C4A.112	Merkel cell carcinoma of right lower eyelid, including canthus ☑
C4A.21	Merkel cell carcinoma of right ear and external auricular canal ☑
C4A.22	Merkel cell carcinoma of left ear and external auricular canal ☑
C4A.31	Merkel cell carcinoma of nose
C4A.39	Merkel cell carcinoma of other parts of face
C4A.8	Merkel cell carcinoma of overlapping sites
C76.0	Malignant neoplasm of head, face and neck
C79.2	Secondary malignant neoplasm of skin

Skin

C7B.1	Secondary Merkel cell carcinoma	
D00.01	Carcinoma in situ of labial mucosa and vermilion border	
D03.0	Melanoma in situ of lip	
D03.111	Melanoma in situ of right upper eyelid, including canthus	☑
D03.112	Melanoma in situ of right lower eyelid, including canthus	☑
D03.21	Melanoma in situ of right ear and external auricular canal	☑
D03.22	Melanoma in situ of left ear and external auricular canal	☑
D03.39	Melanoma in situ of other parts of face	
D04.0	Carcinoma in situ of skin of lip	
D04.111	Carcinoma in situ of skin of right upper eyelid, including canthus	☑
D04.112	Carcinoma in situ of skin of right lower eyelid, including canthus	☑
D04.21	Carcinoma in situ of skin of right ear and external auricular canal	☑
D04.22	Carcinoma in situ of skin of left ear and external auricular canal	☑
D04.39	Carcinoma in situ of skin of other parts of face	
D37.01	Neoplasm of uncertain behavior of lip	
D48.5	Neoplasm of uncertain behavior of skin	

AMA: **11640** 2019,Nov,3; 2018,Sep,7; 2018,Jan,8; 2017,Jan,8; 2016,Jan,13; 2015,Jan,16 **11641** 2019,Nov,3; 2018,Sep,7; 2018,Jan,8; 2017,Jan,8; 2016,Jan,13; 2015,Jan,16 **11642** 2019,Nov,3; 2018,Sep,7; 2018,Jan,8; 2017,Jan,8; 2016,Jan,13; 2015,Jan,16 **11643** 2019,Nov,3; 2018,Sep,7; 2018,Jan,8; 2017,Jan,8; 2016,Jan,13; 2015,Jan,16 **11644** 2019,Nov,3; 2018,Sep,7; 2018,Jan,8; 2017,Jan,8; 2016,Jan,13; 2015,Jan,16 **11646** 2019,Nov,3; 2018,Sep,7; 2018,Jan,8; 2017,Jan,8; 2016,Jan,13; 2015,Jan,16

Relative Value Units/Medicare Edits

Non-Facility RVU	Work	PE	MP	Total
11640	1.67	4.19	0.21	6.07
11641	2.17	4.62	0.26	7.05
11642	2.62	5.02	0.31	7.95
11643	3.42	5.48	0.44	9.34
11644	4.34	6.56	0.61	11.51
11646	6.26	7.76	0.93	14.95

Facility RVU	Work	PE	MP	Total
11640	1.67	1.79	0.21	3.67
11641	2.17	2.07	0.26	4.5
11642	2.62	2.34	0.31	5.27
11643	3.42	2.75	0.44	6.61
11644	4.34	3.27	0.61	8.22
11646	6.26	4.21	0.93	11.4

	FUD	Status	MUE	Modifiers				IOM Reference
11640	10	A	2(3)	51	N/A	N/A	N/A	None
11641	10	A	2(3)	51	N/A	N/A	N/A	
11642	10	A	3(3)	51	N/A	N/A	N/A	
11643	10	A	2(3)	51	N/A	N/A	N/A	
11644	10	A	2(3)	51	N/A	N/A	N/A	
11646	10	A	2(3)	51	N/A	N/A	N/A	

* with documentation

11770-11772

11770 Excision of pilonidal cyst or sinus; simple
11771 extensive
11772 complicated

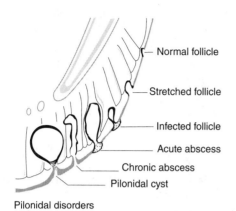

Pilonidal disorders

A pilonidal cyst is excised

Explanation

A pilonidal cyst or sinus is entrapped epithelial tissue located in the sacrococcygeal region above the buttocks. These lesions are usually associated with ingrown hair. A sinus cavity is present and may have a fluid-producing cystic lining. With a small or simple sinus in 11770, the physician uses a scalpel to completely excise the involved tissue. The wound is sutured in a single layer. In 11771, an extensive sinus is present superficial to the fascia overlying the sacrum but with subcutaneous extensions. The physician uses a scalpel to completely excise the cystic tissue. The wound may be sutured in several layers. In 11772, the sinus involves many subcutaneous extensions superficial to the fascia overlying the sacrum. The physician uses a scalpel to completely excise the cystic tissue. Local soft tissue flaps (i.e., Z-plasty, Y-V plasty, myofasciocutaneous flap) may be required for closure of a large defect or the wound may be left open to heal by granulation.

Coding Tips

Closure of the defect is included in this code and should not be reported separately. For incision and drainage of a pilonidal cyst, simple, see 10080; complicated, see 10081. Surgical trays, A4550, are not separately reimbursed by Medicare; however, other third-party payers may cover them. Check with the specific payer to determine coverage.

ICD-10-CM Diagnostic Codes

L05.01	Pilonidal cyst with abscess
L05.02	Pilonidal sinus with abscess
L05.91	Pilonidal cyst without abscess
L05.92	Pilonidal sinus without abscess

AMA: 11772 2018,Jan,8; 2017,Jan,8; 2016,Jan,13; 2015,Sep,12

Relative Value Units/Medicare Edits

Non-Facility RVU	Work	PE	MP	Total
11770	2.66	7.1	0.59	10.35
11771	6.09	11.13	1.37	18.59
11772	7.35	13.96	1.62	22.93
Facility RVU	**Work**	**PE**	**MP**	**Total**
11770	2.66	2.24	0.59	5.49
11771	6.09	5.66	1.37	13.12
11772	7.35	8.32	1.62	17.29

	FUD	Status	MUE	Modifiers				IOM Reference
11770	10	A	1(3)	51	N/A	N/A	N/A	None
11771	90	A	1(3)	51	N/A	N/A	N/A	
11772	90	A	1(3)	51	N/A	N/A	N/A	

* with documentation

Terms To Know

abscess. Circumscribed collection of pus resulting from bacteria, frequently associated with swelling and other signs of inflammation.

epithelial tissue. Cells arranged in sheets that cover internal and external body surfaces that can absorb, protect, and/or secrete and includes the protective covering for external surfaces (skin), absorptive linings for internal surfaces such as the intestine, and secreting structures such as salivary or sweat glands.

fascia. Fibrous sheet or band of tissue that envelops organs, muscles, and groupings of muscles.

lesion. Area of damaged tissue that has lost continuity or function, due to disease or trauma.

pilonidal cyst. Sac or sinus cavity of trapped epithelial tissues in the sacrococcygeal region, usually associated with ingrown hair.

pilonidal sinus. Fistula, tract, or channel that extends from an infected area of ingrown hair to another site within the skin or out to the skin surface.

subcutaneous tissue. Sheet or wide band of adipose (fat) and areolar connective tissue in two layers attached to the dermis.

wound repair. Surgical closure of a wound is divided into three categories: simple, intermediate, and complex. *simple repair:* Surgical closure of a superficial wound, requiring single layer suturing of the skin epidermis, dermis, or subcutaneous tissue. *intermediate repair:* Surgical closure of a wound requiring closure of one or more of the deeper subcutaneous tissue and non-muscle fascia layers in addition to suturing the skin; contaminated wounds with single layer closure that need extensive cleaning or foreign body removal. *complex repair:* Repair of wounds requiring more than layered closure (debridement, scar revision, stents, retention sutures).

z-plasty. Plastic surgery technique used primarily to release tension or elongate contracted scar tissue in which a Z-shaped incision is made with the middle line of the Z crossing the area of greatest tension. The triangular flaps are then rotated so that they cross the incision line in the opposite direction, creating a reversed Z.

11960

11960 Insertion of tissue expander(s) for other than breast, including subsequent expansion

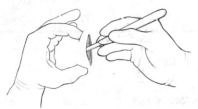

The skin is incised and separated from subcutaneous layers

A balloon-like tissue expander is inserted

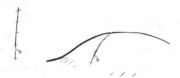

Later, the insert is inflated. The skin expands and stretches in preparation for reconstruction

Explanation

The physician uses a tissue expander to stretch skin and soft tissue prior to definitive reconstruction of tissue other than breast. These expanders are balloon-type devices that stretch the skin and enhance epithelial and collagen expansion and reduce or eliminate the need for skin grafts during reconstruction. The physician makes an incision into the skin. The subcutaneous layer is identified. Blunt dissection is used to separate the skin and subcutaneous layers. The tissue expander is placed into the prepared site. The wound is sutured. The expander is inflated. During the postoperative visits, greater volume is placed into the expander stretching the skin. The expander remains in place until the final reconstruction is performed.

Coding Tips

When 11960 is performed with another separately identifiable procedure, the highest dollar value code is listed as the primary procedure and subsequent procedures are appended with modifier 51. For replacement of a tissue expander with a permanent implant, other than breast, see 11970; for removal of a tissue expander without insertion of an implant, see 11971. For breast reconstruction with tissue expander, see 19357. Do not report 11960 with 11971, 13160, 29848, or 64702-64726. Surgical trays, A4550, are not separately reimbursed by Medicare; however, other third-party payers may cover them. Check with the specific payer to determine coverage.

ICD-10-CM Diagnostic Codes

L90.5	Scar conditions and fibrosis of skin
S21.311D	Laceration without foreign body of right front wall of thorax with penetration into thoracic cavity, subsequent encounter
S21.321D	Laceration with foreign body of right front wall of thorax with penetration into thoracic cavity, subsequent encounter
S21.331D	Puncture wound without foreign body of right front wall of thorax with penetration into thoracic cavity, subsequent encounter
S21.341D	Puncture wound with foreign body of right front wall of thorax with penetration into thoracic cavity, subsequent encounter
S21.351D	Open bite of right front wall of thorax with penetration into thoracic cavity, subsequent encounter
S21.411D	Laceration without foreign body of right back wall of thorax with penetration into thoracic cavity, subsequent encounter
S21.421D	Laceration with foreign body of right back wall of thorax with penetration into thoracic cavity, subsequent encounter
S21.431D	Puncture wound without foreign body of right back wall of thorax with penetration into thoracic cavity, subsequent encounter
S21.441D	Puncture wound with foreign body of right back wall of thorax with penetration into thoracic cavity, subsequent encounter
S21.451D	Open bite of right back wall of thorax with penetration into thoracic cavity, subsequent encounter
S28.1XXD	Traumatic amputation (partial) of part of thorax, except breast, subsequent encounter
S28.211D	Complete traumatic amputation of right breast, subsequent encounter ☑
S28.221D	Partial traumatic amputation of right breast, subsequent encounter ☑
S31.020D	Laceration with foreign body of lower back and pelvis without penetration into retroperitoneum, subsequent encounter
S31.021D	Laceration with foreign body of lower back and pelvis with penetration into retroperitoneum, subsequent encounter
S31.041D	Puncture wound with foreign body of lower back and pelvis with penetration into retroperitoneum, subsequent encounter
S31.120D	Laceration of abdominal wall with foreign body, right upper quadrant without penetration into peritoneal cavity, subsequent encounter ☑
S31.122D	Laceration of abdominal wall with foreign body, epigastric region without penetration into peritoneal cavity, subsequent encounter
S31.123D	Laceration of abdominal wall with foreign body, right lower quadrant without penetration into peritoneal cavity, subsequent encounter ☑
S31.610D	Laceration without foreign body of abdominal wall, right upper quadrant with penetration into peritoneal cavity, subsequent encounter ☑
S31.612D	Laceration without foreign body of abdominal wall, epigastric region with penetration into peritoneal cavity, subsequent encounter
S31.613D	Laceration without foreign body of abdominal wall, right lower quadrant with penetration into peritoneal cavity, subsequent encounter ☑
S31.620D	Laceration with foreign body of abdominal wall, right upper quadrant with penetration into peritoneal cavity, subsequent encounter ☑
S31.640D	Puncture wound with foreign body of abdominal wall, right upper quadrant with penetration into peritoneal cavity, subsequent encounter ☑
S31.642D	Puncture wound with foreign body of abdominal wall, epigastric region with penetration into peritoneal cavity, subsequent encounter
S31.643D	Puncture wound with foreign body of abdominal wall, right lower quadrant with penetration into peritoneal cavity, subsequent encounter ☑
S31.645D	Puncture wound with foreign body of abdominal wall, periumbilic region with penetration into peritoneal cavity, subsequent encounter
S31.650D	Open bite of abdominal wall, right upper quadrant with penetration into peritoneal cavity, subsequent encounter ☑

S31.652D	Open bite of abdominal wall, epigastric region with penetration into peritoneal cavity, subsequent encounter
S31.812D	Laceration with foreign body of right buttock, subsequent encounter ☑
S31.813D	Puncture wound without foreign body of right buttock, subsequent encounter ☑
S31.832D	Laceration with foreign body of anus, subsequent encounter
T21.32XD	Burn of third degree of abdominal wall, subsequent encounter
T21.33XD	Burn of third degree of upper back, subsequent encounter
T21.34XD	Burn of third degree of lower back, subsequent encounter
T21.35XD	Burn of third degree of buttock, subsequent encounter
T21.72XD	Corrosion of third degree of abdominal wall, subsequent encounter
T21.73XD	Corrosion of third degree of upper back, subsequent encounter
T21.74XD	Corrosion of third degree of lower back, subsequent encounter
T21.75XD	Corrosion of third degree of buttock, subsequent encounter
T22.311D	Burn of third degree of right forearm, subsequent encounter ☑
T22.321D	Burn of third degree of right elbow, subsequent encounter ☑
T22.331D	Burn of third degree of right upper arm, subsequent encounter ☑
T22.341D	Burn of third degree of right axilla, subsequent encounter ☑
T22.351D	Burn of third degree of right shoulder, subsequent encounter ☑
T22.361D	Burn of third degree of right scapular region, subsequent encounter ☑
T22.711D	Corrosion of third degree of right forearm, subsequent encounter ☑
T22.721D	Corrosion of third degree of right elbow, subsequent encounter ☑
T22.741D	Corrosion of third degree of right axilla, subsequent encounter ☑
T23.311D	Burn of third degree of right thumb (nail), subsequent encounter ☑
T23.321D	Burn of third degree of single right finger (nail) except thumb, subsequent encounter ☑
T23.331D	Burn of third degree of multiple right fingers (nail), not including thumb, subsequent encounter ☑
T23.341D	Burn of third degree of multiple right fingers (nail), including thumb, subsequent encounter ☑
T23.351D	Burn of third degree of right palm, subsequent encounter ☑
T23.361D	Burn of third degree of back of right hand, subsequent encounter ☑
T23.371D	Burn of third degree of right wrist, subsequent encounter ☑
T23.391D	Burn of third degree of multiple sites of right wrist and hand, subsequent encounter ☑
T23.721D	Corrosion of third degree of single right finger (nail) except thumb, subsequent encounter ☑
T23.731D	Corrosion of third degree of multiple right fingers (nail), not including thumb, subsequent encounter ☑
T23.741D	Corrosion of third degree of multiple right fingers (nail), including thumb, subsequent encounter ☑
T23.751D	Corrosion of third degree of right palm, subsequent encounter ☑
T23.761D	Corrosion of third degree of back of right hand, subsequent encounter ☑
T23.771D	Corrosion of third degree of right wrist, subsequent encounter ☑
T23.791D	Corrosion of third degree of multiple sites of right wrist and hand, subsequent encounter ☑
T24.311D	Burn of third degree of right thigh, subsequent encounter ☑
T24.321D	Burn of third degree of right knee, subsequent encounter ☑
T24.331D	Burn of third degree of right lower leg, subsequent encounter ☑
T24.391D	Burn of third degree of multiple sites of right lower limb, except ankle and foot, subsequent encounter ☑
T24.711D	Corrosion of third degree of right thigh, subsequent encounter ☑
T24.721D	Corrosion of third degree of right knee, subsequent encounter ☑
T24.731D	Corrosion of third degree of right lower leg, subsequent encounter ☑
T24.791D	Corrosion of third degree of multiple sites of right lower limb, except ankle and foot, subsequent encounter ☑
T25.311D	Burn of third degree of right ankle, subsequent encounter ☑
T25.321D	Burn of third degree of right foot, subsequent encounter ☑
T25.331D	Burn of third degree of right toe(s) (nail), subsequent encounter ☑
T25.391D	Burn of third degree of multiple sites of right ankle and foot, subsequent encounter ☑
T25.711D	Corrosion of third degree of right ankle, subsequent encounter ☑
T25.721D	Corrosion of third degree of right foot, subsequent encounter ☑
T25.731D	Corrosion of third degree of right toe(s) (nail), subsequent encounter ☑
T25.791D	Corrosion of third degree of multiple sites of right ankle and foot, subsequent encounter ☑

AMA: 11960 1991,Win,1

Relative Value Units/Medicare Edits

Non-Facility RVU	Work	PE	MP	Total
11960	11.49	16.42	2.04	29.95
Facility RVU	Work	PE	MP	Total
11960	11.49	16.42	2.04	29.95

	FUD	Status	MUE	Modifiers				IOM Reference
11960	90	A	2(3)	51	N/A	N/A	N/A	None

* with documentation

Terms To Know

collagen. Protein based substance of strength and flexibility that is the major component of connective tissue, found in cartilage, bone, tendons, and skin.

epithelial tissue. Cells arranged in sheets that cover internal and external body surfaces that can absorb, protect, and/or secrete and includes the protective covering for external surfaces (skin), absorptive linings for internal surfaces such as the intestine, and secreting structures such as salivary or sweat glands.

prosthesis. Man-made substitute for a missing body part.

reconstruction. Recreating, restoring, or rebuilding a body part or organ.

subcutaneous tissue. Sheet or wide band of adipose (fat) and areolar connective tissue in two layers attached to the dermis.

11970

11970 Replacement of tissue expander with permanent implant

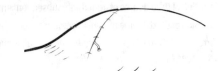

A balloon-like tissue expander is removed

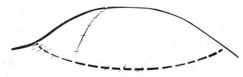

A permanent implant is inserted

Explanation

The physician removes a subcutaneous tissue expander and places a permanent implant for final reconstruction. The tissue expander is deflated. The physician uses a scalpel to make an incision. Blunt dissection is used to remove the tissue expander. The permanent implant is placed into the recipient bed. The implant may be an autologous graft or a commercially prepared synthetic material. The graft implant may require stabilization with sutures, wires, or screws. The incision is closed with sutures.

Coding Tips

When 11970 is performed with another separately identifiable procedure, the highest dollar value code is listed as the primary procedure and subsequent procedures are appended with modifier 51. For insertion of a tissue expander, other than breast, see 11960; for removal of a tissue expander without insertion of an implant, see 11971. For breast reconstruction with a tissue expander, see 19357. Surgical trays, A4550, are not separately reimbursed by Medicare; however, other third-party payers may cover them. Check with the specific payer to determine coverage.

ICD-10-CM Diagnostic Codes

L90.5	Scar conditions and fibrosis of skin
S21.011D	Laceration without foreign body of right breast, subsequent encounter ☑
S21.021D	Laceration with foreign body of right breast, subsequent encounter ☑
S21.031D	Puncture wound without foreign body of right breast, subsequent encounter ☑
S21.041D	Puncture wound with foreign body of right breast, subsequent encounter ☑
S21.051D	Open bite of right breast, subsequent encounter ☑
S21.311D	Laceration without foreign body of right front wall of thorax with penetration into thoracic cavity, subsequent encounter
S21.321D	Laceration with foreign body of right front wall of thorax with penetration into thoracic cavity, subsequent encounter
S21.331D	Puncture wound without foreign body of right front wall of thorax with penetration into thoracic cavity, subsequent encounter
S21.341D	Puncture wound with foreign body of right front wall of thorax with penetration into thoracic cavity, subsequent encounter
S21.351D	Open bite of right front wall of thorax with penetration into thoracic cavity, subsequent encounter
S21.411D	Laceration without foreign body of right back wall of thorax with penetration into thoracic cavity, subsequent encounter
S21.421D	Laceration with foreign body of right back wall of thorax with penetration into thoracic cavity, subsequent encounter
S21.431D	Puncture wound without foreign body of right back wall of thorax with penetration into thoracic cavity, subsequent encounter
S21.441D	Puncture wound with foreign body of right back wall of thorax with penetration into thoracic cavity, subsequent encounter
S21.451D	Open bite of right back wall of thorax with penetration into thoracic cavity, subsequent encounter
S28.1XXD	Traumatic amputation (partial) of part of thorax, except breast, subsequent encounter
S28.211D	Complete traumatic amputation of right breast, subsequent encounter ☑
S28.221D	Partial traumatic amputation of right breast, subsequent encounter ☑
S31.020D	Laceration with foreign body of lower back and pelvis without penetration into retroperitoneum, subsequent encounter
S31.021D	Laceration with foreign body of lower back and pelvis with penetration into retroperitoneum, subsequent encounter
S31.041D	Puncture wound with foreign body of lower back and pelvis with penetration into retroperitoneum, subsequent encounter
S31.120D	Laceration of abdominal wall with foreign body, right upper quadrant without penetration into peritoneal cavity, subsequent encounter ☑
S31.123D	Laceration of abdominal wall with foreign body, right lower quadrant without penetration into peritoneal cavity, subsequent encounter ☑
S31.610D	Laceration without foreign body of abdominal wall, right upper quadrant with penetration into peritoneal cavity, subsequent encounter ☑
S31.612D	Laceration without foreign body of abdominal wall, epigastric region with penetration into peritoneal cavity, subsequent encounter
S31.613D	Laceration without foreign body of abdominal wall, right lower quadrant with penetration into peritoneal cavity, subsequent encounter ☑
S31.620D	Laceration with foreign body of abdominal wall, right upper quadrant with penetration into peritoneal cavity, subsequent encounter ☑
S31.640D	Puncture wound with foreign body of abdominal wall, right upper quadrant with penetration into peritoneal cavity, subsequent encounter ☑
S31.642D	Puncture wound with foreign body of abdominal wall, epigastric region with penetration into peritoneal cavity, subsequent encounter
S31.643D	Puncture wound with foreign body of abdominal wall, right lower quadrant with penetration into peritoneal cavity, subsequent encounter ☑
S31.645D	Puncture wound with foreign body of abdominal wall, periumbilic region with penetration into peritoneal cavity, subsequent encounter
S31.650D	Open bite of abdominal wall, right upper quadrant with penetration into peritoneal cavity, subsequent encounter ☑
S31.652D	Open bite of abdominal wall, epigastric region with penetration into peritoneal cavity, subsequent encounter

Introduction

S31.812D Laceration with foreign body of right buttock, subsequent encounter ☑

S31.813D Puncture wound without foreign body of right buttock, subsequent encounter ☑

S31.832D Laceration with foreign body of anus, subsequent encounter

T21.32XD Burn of third degree of abdominal wall, subsequent encounter

T21.33XD Burn of third degree of upper back, subsequent encounter

T21.34XD Burn of third degree of lower back, subsequent encounter

T21.35XD Burn of third degree of buttock, subsequent encounter

T21.72XD Corrosion of third degree of abdominal wall, subsequent encounter

T21.73XD Corrosion of third degree of upper back, subsequent encounter

T21.74XD Corrosion of third degree of lower back, subsequent encounter

T21.75XD Corrosion of third degree of buttock, subsequent encounter

T22.311D Burn of third degree of right forearm, subsequent encounter ☑

T22.321D Burn of third degree of right elbow, subsequent encounter ☑

T22.331D Burn of third degree of right upper arm, subsequent encounter ☑

T22.341D Burn of third degree of right axilla, subsequent encounter ☑

T22.351D Burn of third degree of right shoulder, subsequent encounter ☑

T22.361D Burn of third degree of right scapular region, subsequent encounter ☑

T22.711D Corrosion of third degree of right forearm, subsequent encounter ☑

T22.721D Corrosion of third degree of right elbow, subsequent encounter ☑

T22.741D Corrosion of third degree of right axilla, subsequent encounter ☑

T22.751D Corrosion of third degree of right shoulder, subsequent encounter ☑

T23.311D Burn of third degree of right thumb (nail), subsequent encounter ☑

T23.321D Burn of third degree of single right finger (nail) except thumb, subsequent encounter ☑

T23.331D Burn of third degree of multiple right fingers (nail), not including thumb, subsequent encounter ☑

T23.341D Burn of third degree of multiple right fingers (nail), including thumb, subsequent encounter ☑

T23.351D Burn of third degree of right palm, subsequent encounter ☑

T23.361D Burn of third degree of back of right hand, subsequent encounter ☑

T23.371D Burn of third degree of right wrist, subsequent encounter ☑

T23.391D Burn of third degree of multiple sites of right wrist and hand, subsequent encounter ☑

T23.721D Corrosion of third degree of single right finger (nail) except thumb, subsequent encounter ☑

T23.731D Corrosion of third degree of multiple right fingers (nail), not including thumb, subsequent encounter ☑

T23.741D Corrosion of third degree of multiple right fingers (nail), including thumb, subsequent encounter ☑

T23.751D Corrosion of third degree of right palm, subsequent encounter ☑

T23.761D Corrosion of third degree of back of right hand, subsequent encounter ☑

T23.771D Corrosion of third degree of right wrist, subsequent encounter ☑

T23.791D Corrosion of third degree of multiple sites of right wrist and hand, subsequent encounter ☑

T24.311D Burn of third degree of right thigh, subsequent encounter ☑

T24.321D Burn of third degree of right knee, subsequent encounter ☑

T24.331D Burn of third degree of right lower leg, subsequent encounter ☑

T24.391D Burn of third degree of multiple sites of right lower limb, except ankle and foot, subsequent encounter ☑

T24.711D Corrosion of third degree of right thigh, subsequent encounter ☑

T24.721D Corrosion of third degree of right knee, subsequent encounter ☑

T24.731D Corrosion of third degree of right lower leg, subsequent encounter ☑

T24.791D Corrosion of third degree of multiple sites of right lower limb, except ankle and foot, subsequent encounter ☑

T25.311D Burn of third degree of right ankle, subsequent encounter ☑

T25.321D Burn of third degree of right foot, subsequent encounter ☑

T25.331D Burn of third degree of right toe(s) (nail), subsequent encounter ☑

T25.391D Burn of third degree of multiple sites of right ankle and foot, subsequent encounter ☑

T25.711D Corrosion of third degree of right ankle, subsequent encounter ☑

T25.721D Corrosion of third degree of right foot, subsequent encounter ☑

T25.731D Corrosion of third degree of right toe(s) (nail), subsequent encounter ☑

T25.791D Corrosion of third degree of multiple sites of right ankle and foot, subsequent encounter ☑

AMA: **11970** 2018,Jan,8; 2017,Jan,8; 2016,Jan,13; 2015,Jan,16

Relative Value Units/Medicare Edits

Non-Facility RVU	Work	PE	MP	Total
11970	7.49	7.66	1.34	16.49
Facility RVU	**Work**	**PE**	**MP**	**Total**
11970	7.49	7.66	1.34	16.49

	FUD	Status	MUE	Modifiers				IOM Reference
11970	90	A	2(3)	51	50	N/A	N/A	None

* with documentation

Terms To Know

autologous. Tissue, cells, or structure obtained from the same individual.

blunt dissection. Surgical technique used to expose an underlying area by separating along natural cleavage lines of tissue, without cutting.

prosthesis. Man-made substitute for a missing body part.

subcutaneous tissue. Sheet or wide band of adipose (fat) and areolar connective tissue in two layers attached to the dermis.

Introduction

11971

11971 Removal of tissue expander without insertion of implant

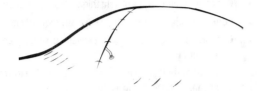

A balloon-like tissue expander is removed
without placing a permanent implant

Explanation

The physician removes a subcutaneous tissue expander without placing an
implant or performing final reconstruction. Initially, the tissue expander is
deflated. The physician uses a scalpel to make an incision. Blunt dissection is
used to remove the tissue expander. A surgical drain may be placed in the
wound. The incision is closed with sutures.

Coding Tips

When 11971 is performed with another separately identifiable procedure, the
highest dollar value code is listed as the primary procedure and subsequent
procedures are appended with modifier 51. For insertion of a tissue expander,
other than for breast, see 11960. For replacement of a tissue expander with a
permanent implant, other than breast, see 11970. For breast reconstruction
with tissue expander, see 19357. Do not report 11971 with 11960 or 11970.
Surgical trays, A4550, are not separately reimbursed by Medicare; however,
other third-party payers may cover them. Check with the specific payer to
determine coverage.

ICD-10-CM Diagnostic Codes

T81.31XA	Disruption of external operation (surgical) wound, not elsewhere classified, initial encounter
T81.32XA	Disruption of internal operation (surgical) wound, not elsewhere classified, initial encounter
T81.42XA	Infection following a procedure, deep incisional surgical site, initial encounter
T81.43XA	Infection following a procedure, organ and space surgical site, initial encounter
T81.44XA	Sepsis following a procedure, initial encounter
T85.618A	Breakdown (mechanical) of other specified internal prosthetic devices, implants and grafts, initial encounter
T85.628A	Displacement of other specified internal prosthetic devices, implants and grafts, initial encounter
T85.638A	Leakage of other specified internal prosthetic devices, implants and grafts, initial encounter
T85.698A	Other mechanical complication of other specified internal prosthetic devices, implants and grafts, initial encounter
T85.79XA	Infection and inflammatory reaction due to other internal prosthetic devices, implants and grafts, initial encounter
T85.818A	Embolism due to other internal prosthetic devices, implants and grafts, initial encounter
T85.828A	Fibrosis due to other internal prosthetic devices, implants and grafts, initial encounter
T85.838A	Hemorrhage due to other internal prosthetic devices, implants and grafts, initial encounter
T85.848A	Pain due to other internal prosthetic devices, implants and grafts, initial encounter
T85.858A	Stenosis due to other internal prosthetic devices, implants and grafts, initial encounter
T85.868A	Thrombosis due to other internal prosthetic devices, implants and grafts, initial encounter
T85.898A	Other specified complication of other internal prosthetic devices, implants and grafts, initial encounter
Z41.1	Encounter for cosmetic surgery
Z42.8	Encounter for other plastic and reconstructive surgery following medical procedure or healed injury

AMA: 11971 2018,Jan,8; 2017,Jan,8; 2016,Jan,13; 2015,Jan,16

Relative Value Units/Medicare Edits

Non-Facility RVU	Work	PE	MP	Total
11971	7.02	7.8	1.25	16.07
Facility RVU	**Work**	**PE**	**MP**	**Total**
11971	7.02	7.8	1.25	16.07

	FUD	Status	MUE	Modifiers				IOM Reference
11971	90	A	2(3)	51	50	N/A	80*	None

* with documentation

Terms To Know

blunt dissection. Surgical technique used to expose an underlying area by
separating along natural cleavage lines of tissue, without cutting.

drain. Device that creates a channel to allow fluid from a cavity, wound, or
infected area to exit the body.

prosthesis. Man-made substitute for a missing body part.

11981-11983

▲ **11981** Insertion, drug-delivery implant (ie, bioresorbable, biodegradable, non-biodegradable)
11982 Removal, non-biodegradable drug delivery implant
11983 Removal with reinsertion, non-biodegradable drug delivery implant

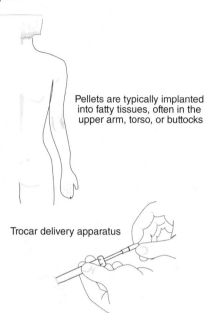

Pellets are typically implanted into fatty tissues, often in the upper arm, torso, or buttocks

Trocar delivery apparatus

Explanation

A drug delivery implant, which may be nonbiodegradable or biodegradable/bioresorbable, is inserted to deliver a therapeutic dose of a drug continuously at a predetermined rate of release. One such system works via a semipermeable membrane at one end of the subcutaneous cylinder that permits the entrance of fluid; the drug is delivered from a port at the other end of the cylinder at a controlled rate appropriate to the specific therapeutic agent. The physician injects local anesthesia and makes a small incision in the skin with a scalpel to insert the miniature drug-containing cylinder, which is held in place with sutures tied by a knot or secured by a single running stitch. Various types of medications for different indications may be administered via drug delivery implants. In 11982, the physician removes a previously placed nonbiodegradable drug delivery implant, such as a miniature drug-containing titanium cylinder, through a small incision. In 11983, the physician removes and then reinserts the previously placed nonbiodegradable implant through a small incision. The wounds are sutured closed.

Coding Tips

For subcutaneous implantation of hormone pellets, see 11980. For removal of implantable contraceptive capsules, see 11976; for removal with reinsertion, see 11976 and 11981. For removal of biodegradable or bioresorbable implant, see 17999. Surgical trays, A4550, are not separately reimbursed by Medicare; however, other third-party payers may cover them. Check with the specific payer to determine coverage. Medicare and some payers may require HCPCS Level II codes G0516-G0518 be reported for four or more implants. Do not report 11981 with 20700, 20702, or 20704. Do not report 11982 with 20701, 20703, or 20705. For subfascial, intramedullary, or intra-articular drug delivery devices, which include manual preparation and insertion, see 20700, 20702, and 20704; for removal, see 20701, 20703, and 20705.

ICD-10-CM Diagnostic Codes

C50.011	Malignant neoplasm of nipple and areola, right female breast ♀ ☑
C50.021	Malignant neoplasm of nipple and areola, right male breast ♂ ☑
C50.111	Malignant neoplasm of central portion of right female breast ♀ ☑
C50.121	Malignant neoplasm of central portion of right male breast ♂ ☑
C50.211	Malignant neoplasm of upper-inner quadrant of right female breast ♀ ☑
C50.221	Malignant neoplasm of upper-inner quadrant of right male breast ♂ ☑
C50.311	Malignant neoplasm of lower-inner quadrant of right female breast ♀ ☑
C50.321	Malignant neoplasm of lower-inner quadrant of right male breast ♂ ☑
C50.411	Malignant neoplasm of upper-outer quadrant of right female breast ♀ ☑
C50.421	Malignant neoplasm of upper-outer quadrant of right male breast ♂ ☑
C50.511	Malignant neoplasm of lower-outer quadrant of right female breast ♀ ☑
C50.621	Malignant neoplasm of axillary tail of right male breast ♂ ☑
C61	Malignant neoplasm of prostate ♂
D25.0	Submucous leiomyoma of uterus ♀
D25.1	Intramural leiomyoma of uterus ♀
D25.2	Subserosal leiomyoma of uterus ♀
E08.3211	Diabetes mellitus due to underlying condition with mild nonproliferative diabetic retinopathy with macular edema, right eye ☑
E08.3311	Diabetes mellitus due to underlying condition with moderate nonproliferative diabetic retinopathy with macular edema, right eye ☑
E08.37X1	Diabetes mellitus due to underlying condition with diabetic macular edema, resolved following treatment, right eye ☑
E10.311	Type 1 diabetes mellitus with unspecified diabetic retinopathy with macular edema
E10.3311	Type 1 diabetes mellitus with moderate nonproliferative diabetic retinopathy with macular edema, right eye ☑
E10.65	Type 1 diabetes mellitus with hyperglycemia
E11.3211	Type 2 diabetes mellitus with mild nonproliferative diabetic retinopathy with macular edema, right eye ☑
E11.3311	Type 2 diabetes mellitus with moderate nonproliferative diabetic retinopathy with macular edema, right eye ☑
E11.3411	Type 2 diabetes mellitus with severe nonproliferative diabetic retinopathy with macular edema, right eye ☑
E11.3511	Type 2 diabetes mellitus with proliferative diabetic retinopathy with macular edema, right eye ☑
E11.37X1	Type 2 diabetes mellitus with diabetic macular edema, resolved following treatment, right eye ☑
E11.65	Type 2 diabetes mellitus with hyperglycemia
F11.21	Opioid dependence, in remission
F11.220	Opioid dependence with intoxication, uncomplicated
F11.221	Opioid dependence with intoxication delirium
F11.222	Opioid dependence with intoxication with perceptual disturbance
F11.250	Opioid dependence with opioid-induced psychotic disorder with delusions

Introduction

F11.251	Opioid dependence with opioid-induced psychotic disorder with hallucinations	
F11.281	Opioid dependence with opioid-induced sexual dysfunction	
F11.282	Opioid dependence with opioid-induced sleep disorder	
F11.288	Opioid dependence with other opioid-induced disorder	
G20	Parkinson's disease	
G89.21	Chronic pain due to trauma	
G89.22	Chronic post-thoracotomy pain	
G89.3	Neoplasm related pain (acute) (chronic)	
G89.4	Chronic pain syndrome	
H34.8110	Central retinal vein occlusion, right eye, with macular edema ☑	
H35.81	Retinal edema	
T85.618A	Breakdown (mechanical) of other specified internal prosthetic devices, implants and grafts, initial encounter	
T85.628A	Displacement of other specified internal prosthetic devices, implants and grafts, initial encounter	
T85.698A	Other mechanical complication of other specified internal prosthetic devices, implants and grafts, initial encounter	
T85.79XA	Infection and inflammatory reaction due to other internal prosthetic devices, implants and grafts, initial encounter	
T85.848A	Pain due to other internal prosthetic devices, implants and grafts, initial encounter	
T85.898A	Other specified complication of other internal prosthetic devices, implants and grafts, initial encounter	
T88.7XXA	Unspecified adverse effect of drug or medicament, initial encounter	
Z30.017	Encounter for initial prescription of implantable subdermal contraceptive	

AMA: 11981 2018,Jan,8; 2017,Jan,8; 2016,Jan,13; 2015,Jan,16

Relative Value Units/Medicare Edits

Non-Facility RVU	Work	PE	MP	Total
11981	1.14	1.7	0.21	3.05
11982	1.34	1.85	0.25	3.44
11983	1.91	2.03	0.32	4.26
Facility RVU	Work	PE	MP	Total
11981	1.14	0.52	0.21	1.87
11982	1.34	0.61	0.25	2.2
11983	1.91	0.81	0.32	3.04

	FUD	Status	MUE	Modifiers				IOM Reference
11981	0	A	1(3)	51	N/A	N/A	80*	None
11982	0	A	1(3)	51	N/A	N/A	80*	
11983	0	A	1(3)	51	N/A	N/A	80*	

* with documentation

Terms To Know

hormone. Chemical substance produced by the body that has a regulatory effect on the function of its specific target organ(s).

implant. Material or device inserted or placed within the body for therapeutic, reconstructive, or diagnostic purposes.

subcutaneous tissue. Sheet or wide band of adipose (fat) and areolar connective tissue in two layers attached to the dermis.

12001-12007

12001	Simple repair of superficial wounds of scalp, neck, axillae, external genitalia, trunk and/or extremities (including hands and feet); 2.5 cm or less
12002	2.6 cm to 7.5 cm
12004	7.6 cm to 12.5 cm
12005	12.6 cm to 20.0 cm
12006	20.1 cm to 30.0 cm
12007	over 30.0 cm

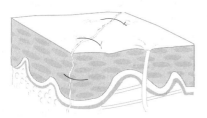

Example of a simple closure involving
only one skin layer, the epidermis

Explanation

The physician performs wound closure of superficial lacerations of the scalp, neck, axillae, external genitalia, trunk, or extremities using sutures, staples, tissue adhesives, or a combination of these materials. A local anesthetic is injected around the wound and it is cleansed, explored, and often irrigated with a saline solution. The physician performs a simple, one-layer repair of the epidermis, dermis, or subcutaneous tissues. For multiple wounds of the same complexity and in the same anatomical area, the length of all wounds sutured is summed and reported as one total length. Report 12001 for a total length of 2.5 cm or less; 12002 for 2.6 cm to 7.5 cm; 12004 for 7.6 cm to 12.5 cm; 12005 for 12.6 cm to 20 cm; 12006 for 20.1 cm to 30 cm; and 12007 if the total length is greater than 30 cm.

Coding Tips

Wounds treated with tissue glue or staples qualify as a simple repair even if they are not closed with sutures. When chemical cauterization, electrocauterization, or adhesive strips are the only material used for wound closure, the service is included in the appropriate E/M code. Anesthesia (local or topical) and hemostasis are not reported separately. Intermediate repair is used when layered closure of one or more of the deeper layers of subcutaneous tissue and superficial fascia are required in addition to limited undermining. Single-layer closure of a wound requiring extensive cleaning or removal of contaminated foreign matter or damaged tissue is classified as an intermediate repair. For extensive debridement of soft tissue and/or bone, not associated with open fractures and/or dislocations, resulting from penetrating and/or blunt trauma, see 11042–11047. For wound care closure by tissue adhesive(s) only, see HCPCS Level II code G0168. Surgical trays, A4550, are not separately reimbursed by Medicare; however, other third-party payers may cover them. Check with the specific payer to determine coverage.

ICD-10-CM Diagnostic Codes

S01.01XA	Laceration without foreign body of scalp, initial encounter
S01.03XA	Puncture wound without foreign body of scalp, initial encounter
S01.05XA	Open bite of scalp, initial encounter
S21.011A	Laceration without foreign body of right breast, initial encounter ☑
S21.032A	Puncture wound without foreign body of left breast, initial encounter ☑
S21.051A	Open bite of right breast, initial encounter ☑
S21.052A	Open bite of left breast, initial encounter ☑
S31.010A	Laceration without foreign body of lower back and pelvis without penetration into retroperitoneum, initial encounter
S31.030A	Puncture wound without foreign body of lower back and pelvis without penetration into retroperitoneum, initial encounter
S31.110A	Laceration without foreign body of abdominal wall, right upper quadrant without penetration into peritoneal cavity, initial encounter ☑
S31.114A	Laceration without foreign body of abdominal wall, left lower quadrant without penetration into peritoneal cavity, initial encounter ☑
S31.115A	Laceration without foreign body of abdominal wall, periumbilic region without penetration into peritoneal cavity, initial encounter
S31.130A	Puncture wound of abdominal wall without foreign body, right upper quadrant without penetration into peritoneal cavity, initial encounter ☑
S31.132A	Puncture wound of abdominal wall without foreign body, epigastric region without penetration into peritoneal cavity, initial encounter
S31.152A	Open bite of abdominal wall, epigastric region without penetration into peritoneal cavity, initial encounter
S31.153A	Open bite of abdominal wall, right lower quadrant without penetration into peritoneal cavity, initial encounter ☑
S31.155A	Open bite of abdominal wall, periumbilic region without penetration into peritoneal cavity, initial encounter
S31.21XA	Laceration without foreign body of penis, initial encounter ♂
S31.35XA	Open bite of scrotum and testes, initial encounter ♂
S31.43XA	Puncture wound without foreign body of vagina and vulva, initial encounter ♀
S31.831A	Laceration without foreign body of anus, initial encounter
S41.012A	Laceration without foreign body of left shoulder, initial encounter ☑
S41.031A	Puncture wound without foreign body of right shoulder, initial encounter ☑
S41.051A	Open bite of right shoulder, initial encounter ☑
S41.132A	Puncture wound without foreign body of left upper arm, initial encounter ☑
S41.151A	Open bite of right upper arm, initial encounter ☑
S51.011A	Laceration without foreign body of right elbow, initial encounter ☑
S51.032A	Puncture wound without foreign body of left elbow, initial encounter ☑
S51.052A	Open bite, left elbow, initial encounter ☑
S51.812A	Laceration without foreign body of left forearm, initial encounter ☑
S51.831A	Puncture wound without foreign body of right forearm, initial encounter ☑
S51.852A	Open bite of left forearm, initial encounter ☑
S61.032A	Puncture wound without foreign body of left thumb without damage to nail, initial encounter ☑
S61.052A	Open bite of left thumb without damage to nail, initial encounter ☑
S61.151A	Open bite of right thumb with damage to nail, initial encounter ☑

Repair

S61.214A	Laceration without foreign body of right ring finger without damage to nail, initial encounter ☑	
S61.231A	Puncture wound without foreign body of left index finger without damage to nail, initial encounter ☑	
S61.251A	Open bite of left index finger without damage to nail, initial encounter ☑	
S61.254A	Open bite of right ring finger without damage to nail, initial encounter ☑	
S61.257A	Open bite of left little finger without damage to nail, initial encounter ☑	
S61.316A	Laceration without foreign body of right little finger with damage to nail, initial encounter ☑	
S61.330A	Puncture wound without foreign body of right index finger with damage to nail, initial encounter ☑	
S61.350A	Open bite of right index finger with damage to nail, initial encounter ☑	
S61.353A	Open bite of left middle finger with damage to nail, initial encounter ☑	
S61.356A	Open bite of right little finger with damage to nail, initial encounter ☑	
S61.412A	Laceration without foreign body of left hand, initial encounter ☑	
S61.512A	Laceration without foreign body of left wrist, initial encounter ☑	
S61.531A	Puncture wound without foreign body of right wrist, initial encounter ☑	
S61.551A	Open bite of right wrist, initial encounter ☑	
S61.552A	Open bite of left wrist, initial encounter ☑	
S65.211A	Laceration of superficial palmar arch of right hand, initial encounter ☑	
S65.312A	Laceration of deep palmar arch of left hand, initial encounter ☑	
S71.031A	Puncture wound without foreign body, right hip, initial encounter ☑	
S71.051A	Open bite, right hip, initial encounter ☑	
S71.132A	Puncture wound without foreign body, left thigh, initial encounter ☑	
S71.151A	Open bite, right thigh, initial encounter ☑	
S81.031A	Puncture wound without foreign body, right knee, initial encounter ☑	
S81.051A	Open bite, right knee, initial encounter ☑	
S81.811A	Laceration without foreign body, right lower leg, initial encounter ☑	
S81.831A	Puncture wound without foreign body, right lower leg, initial encounter ☑	
S81.852A	Open bite, left lower leg, initial encounter ☑	
S91.011A	Laceration without foreign body, right ankle, initial encounter ☑	
S91.012A	Laceration without foreign body, left ankle, initial encounter ☑	
S91.032A	Puncture wound without foreign body, left ankle, initial encounter ☑	
S91.051A	Open bite, right ankle, initial encounter ☑	
S91.131A	Puncture wound without foreign body of right great toe without damage to nail, initial encounter ☑	
S91.134A	Puncture wound without foreign body of right lesser toe(s) without damage to nail, initial encounter ☑	
S91.135A	Puncture wound without foreign body of left lesser toe(s) without damage to nail, initial encounter ☑	
S91.152A	Open bite of left great toe without damage to nail, initial encounter ☑	
S91.154A	Open bite of right lesser toe(s) without damage to nail, initial encounter ☑	
S91.214A	Laceration without foreign body of right lesser toe(s) with damage to nail, initial encounter ☑	
S91.231A	Puncture wound without foreign body of right great toe with damage to nail, initial encounter ☑	
S91.235A	Puncture wound without foreign body of left lesser toe(s) with damage to nail, initial encounter ☑	
S91.251A	Open bite of right great toe with damage to nail, initial encounter ☑	
S91.255A	Open bite of left lesser toe(s) with damage to nail, initial encounter ☑	
S91.311A	Laceration without foreign body, right foot, initial encounter ☑	

Associated HCPCS Codes

G0168	Wound closure utilizing tissue adhesive(s) only

AMA: **12001** 2018,Sep,7; 2018,Jan,8; 2017,Jan,8; 2017,Dec,14; 2016,Jan,13; 2015,Jan,16 **12002** 2018,Sep,7; 2018,Jan,8; 2017,Jan,8; 2016,Jan,13; 2015,Jan,16 **12004** 2018,Sep,7; 2018,Jan,8; 2017,Jan,8; 2016,Jan,13; 2015,Jan,16 **12005** 2018,Sep,7; 2018,Jan,8; 2017,Jan,8; 2016,Jan,13; 2015,Jan,16 **12006** 2018,Sep,7; 2018,Jan,8; 2017,Jan,8; 2016,Jan,13; 2015,Jan,16 **12007** 2018,Sep,7; 2018,Jan,8; 2017,Jan,8; 2016,Jan,13; 2015,Jan,16

Relative Value Units/Medicare Edits

Non-Facility RVU	Work	PE	MP	Total
12001	0.84	1.77	0.15	2.76
12002	1.14	1.99	0.21	3.34
12004	1.44	2.18	0.26	3.88
12005	1.97	2.84	0.38	5.19
12006	2.39	3.22	0.45	6.06
12007	2.9	3.42	0.58	6.9
Facility RVU	Work	PE	MP	Total
12001	0.84	0.31	0.15	1.3
12002	1.14	0.37	0.21	1.72
12004	1.44	0.44	0.26	2.14
12005	1.97	0.46	0.38	2.81
12006	2.39	0.59	0.45	3.43
12007	2.9	0.81	0.58	4.29

	FUD	Status	MUE	Modifiers				IOM Reference
12001	0	A	1(2)	51	N/A	N/A	N/A	None
12002	0	A	1(2)	51	N/A	N/A	N/A	
12004	0	A	1(2)	51	N/A	N/A	N/A	
12005	0	A	1(2)	51	N/A	N/A	N/A	
12006	0	A	1(2)	51	N/A	N/A	N/A	
12007	0	A	1(2)	51	N/A	62*	N/A	

* with documentation

Terms To Know

simple repair. Surgical closure of a superficial wound requiring single layer suturing of the skin (epidermis, dermis, or subcutaneous tissue).

superficial. On the skin surface or near the surface of any involved structure or field of interest.

wound. Injury to living tissue often involving a cut or break in the skin.

Repair

12011-12018

12011	Simple repair of superficial wounds of face, ears, eyelids, nose, lips and/or mucous membranes; 2.5 cm or less
12013	2.6 cm to 5.0 cm
12014	5.1 cm to 7.5 cm
12015	7.6 cm to 12.5 cm
12016	12.6 cm to 20.0 cm
12017	20.1 cm to 30.0 cm
12018	over 30.0 cm

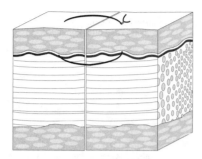

Simple (single layer) repair

Explanation

Superficial wounds located on the face, ears, eyelids, nose, lips, and/or mucous membranes are repaired. A local anesthetic is injected around the laceration and the wound is cleansed, explored, and often irrigated with a saline solution. The physician performs a simple, one-layer repair of the epidermis, dermis, or subcutaneous tissue with sutures. With multiple wounds of the same complexity and in the same anatomical area, the length of all wounds sutured is summed and reported as one total length. Report 12011 for a total length of 2.5 cm or less; 12013 for 2.6 cm to 5 cm; 12014 for 5.1 cm to 7.5 cm; 12015 for 7.6 cm to 12.5 cm; 12016 for 12.6 cm to 20 cm; 12017 for 20.1 cm to 30 cm; and 12018 if the total length is greater than 30 cm.

Coding Tips

Wounds treated with tissue glue or staples qualify as a simple repair even if they are not closed with sutures. When chemical cauterization, electrocauterization, or adhesive strips are the only material used for wound closure, the service is included in the appropriate E/M code. Anesthesia (local or topical) and hemostasis are not reported separately. Suture removal is included in these procedures. Intermediate repair is used when layered closure of one or more of the deeper layers of subcutaneous tissue and superficial fascia are required in addition to limited undermining. Single-layer closure of a wound requiring extensive cleaning or removal of contaminated foreign matter or damaged tissue is classified as an intermediate repair. For extensive debridement of soft tissue and/or bone, not associated with open fractures and/or dislocations, resulting from penetrating and/or blunt trauma, see 11042–11047. For wound closure by tissue adhesive(s) only, see HCPCS Level II code G0168. Surgical trays, A4550, are not separately reimbursed by Medicare; however, other third-party payers may cover them. Check with the specific payer to determine coverage.

ICD-10-CM Diagnostic Codes

S00.471A	Other superficial bite of right ear, initial encounter ☑
S00.472A	Other superficial bite of left ear, initial encounter ☑
S00.511A	Abrasion of lip, initial encounter
S00.512A	Abrasion of oral cavity, initial encounter
S00.571A	Other superficial bite of lip, initial encounter
S00.572A	Other superficial bite of oral cavity, initial encounter
S01.111A	Laceration without foreign body of right eyelid and periocular area, initial encounter ☑
S01.112A	Laceration without foreign body of left eyelid and periocular area, initial encounter ☑
S01.121A	Laceration with foreign body of right eyelid and periocular area, initial encounter ☑
S01.122A	Laceration with foreign body of left eyelid and periocular area, initial encounter ☑
S01.131A	Puncture wound without foreign body of right eyelid and periocular area, initial encounter ☑
S01.132A	Puncture wound without foreign body of left eyelid and periocular area, initial encounter ☑
S01.141A	Puncture wound with foreign body of right eyelid and periocular area, initial encounter ☑
S01.142A	Puncture wound with foreign body of left eyelid and periocular area, initial encounter ☑
S01.151A	Open bite of right eyelid and periocular area, initial encounter ☑
S01.152A	Open bite of left eyelid and periocular area, initial encounter ☑
S01.21XA	Laceration without foreign body of nose, initial encounter
S01.23XA	Puncture wound without foreign body of nose, initial encounter
S01.25XA	Open bite of nose, initial encounter
S01.311A	Laceration without foreign body of right ear, initial encounter ☑
S01.312A	Laceration without foreign body of left ear, initial encounter ☑
S01.331A	Puncture wound without foreign body of right ear, initial encounter ☑
S01.332A	Puncture wound without foreign body of left ear, initial encounter ☑
S01.351A	Open bite of right ear, initial encounter ☑
S01.352A	Open bite of left ear, initial encounter ☑
S01.411A	Laceration without foreign body of right cheek and temporomandibular area, initial encounter ☑
S01.412A	Laceration without foreign body of left cheek and temporomandibular area, initial encounter ☑
S01.431A	Puncture wound without foreign body of right cheek and temporomandibular area, initial encounter ☑
S01.432A	Puncture wound without foreign body of left cheek and temporomandibular area, initial encounter ☑
S01.451A	Open bite of right cheek and temporomandibular area, initial encounter ☑
S01.452A	Open bite of left cheek and temporomandibular area, initial encounter ☑
S01.511A	Laceration without foreign body of lip, initial encounter
S01.512A	Laceration without foreign body of oral cavity, initial encounter
S01.531A	Puncture wound without foreign body of lip, initial encounter
S01.532A	Puncture wound without foreign body of oral cavity, initial encounter
S01.551A	Open bite of lip, initial encounter
S01.552A	Open bite of oral cavity, initial encounter
S05.8X1A	Other injuries of right eye and orbit, initial encounter ☑
S05.8X2A	Other injuries of left eye and orbit, initial encounter ☑

Associated HCPCS Codes

G0168	Wound closure utilizing tissue adhesive(s) only

Repair

AMA: **12011** 2018,Sep,7; 2018,Jan,8; 2017,Jan,8; 2016,Nov,7; 2016,Jan,13; 2015,Jan,16 **12013** 2018,Sep,7; 2018,Jan,8; 2017,Jan,8; 2016,Jan,13; 2015,Jan,16 **12014** 2018,Sep,7; 2018,Jan,8; 2017,Jan,8; 2016,Jan,13; 2015,Jan,16 **12015** 2018,Sep,7; 2018,Jan,8; 2017,Jan,8; 2016,Jan,13; 2015,Jan,16 **12016** 2018,Sep,7; 2018,Jan,8; 2017,Jan,8; 2016,Jan,13; 2015,Jan,16 **12017** 2018,Sep,7; 2018,Jan,8; 2017,Jan,8; 2016,Jan,13; 2015,Jan,16 **12018** 2018,Sep,7; 2018,Jan,8; 2017,Jan,8; 2016,Jan,13; 2015,Jan,16

Relative Value Units/Medicare Edits

Non-Facility RVU	Work	PE	MP	Total
12011	1.07	2.06	0.21	3.34
12013	1.22	2.02	0.23	3.47
12014	1.57	2.37	0.3	4.24
12015	1.98	2.74	0.38	5.1
12016	2.68	3.3	0.51	6.49
12017	3.18	0.67	0.64	4.49
12018	3.61	0.74	0.74	5.09
Facility RVU	**Work**	**PE**	**MP**	**Total**
12011	1.07	0.35	0.21	1.63
12013	1.22	0.26	0.23	1.71
12014	1.57	0.33	0.3	2.2
12015	1.98	0.42	0.38	2.78
12016	2.68	0.59	0.51	3.78
12017	3.18	0.67	0.64	4.49
12018	3.61	0.74	0.74	5.09

	FUD	Status	MUE	Modifiers				IOM Reference
12011	0	A	1(2)	51	N/A	N/A	N/A	None
12013	0	A	1(2)	51	N/A	N/A	N/A	
12014	0	A	1(2)	51	N/A	N/A	N/A	
12015	0	A	1(2)	51	N/A	N/A	N/A	
12016	0	A	1(2)	51	N/A	N/A	N/A	
12017	0	A	1(2)	51	N/A	N/A	80*	
12018	0	A	1(2)	51	N/A	N/A	80	

* with documentation

Terms To Know

dermis. Skin layer found under the epidermis that contains a papillary upper layer and the deep reticular layer of collagen, vascular bed, and nerves.

epidermis. Outermost, nonvascular layer of skin that contains four to five differentiated layers depending on its body location: stratum corneum, lucidum, granulosum, spinosum, and basale.

repair. Surgical closure of a wound. The wound may be a result of injury/trauma or it may be a surgically created defect. Repairs are divided into three categories: simple, intermediate, and complex.

subcutaneous. Below the skin.

superficial. On the skin surface or near the surface of any involved structure or field of interest.

wound. Injury to living tissue often involving a cut or break in the skin.

12020-12021

12020	Treatment of superficial wound dehiscence; simple closure
12021	with packing

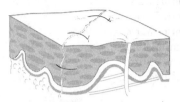

Example of a simple closure involving only one skin layer

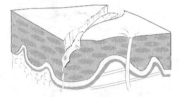

Example of a wound left open with packing due to infection

Explanation

There has been a breakdown of the healing skin either before or after suture removal. The skin margins have opened. The physician cleanses the wound with irrigation and antimicrobial solutions. The skin margins may be trimmed to initiate bleeding surfaces. Report 12020 if the wound is sutured in a single layer. Report 12021 if the wound is left open and packed with gauze strips due to the presence of infection. This allows infection to drain from the wound and the skin closure will be delayed until the infection is resolved.

Coding Tips

When chemical cauterization, electrocauterization, or adhesive strips are the only material used for wound closure, the service is included in the appropriate E/M code. For extensive or complicated secondary wound closure, see 13160. For wound closure by tissue adhesive(s) only, see HCPCS Level II code G0168. For extensive debridement of soft tissue and/or bone, not associated with open fractures and/or dislocations, resulting from penetrating and/or blunt trauma, see 11042–11047. Surgical trays, A4550, are not separately reimbursed by Medicare; however, other third-party payers may cover them. Check with the specific payer to determine coverage.

ICD-10-CM Diagnostic Codes

T81.31XA	Disruption of external operation (surgical) wound, not elsewhere classified, initial encounter
T81.32XA	Disruption of internal operation (surgical) wound, not elsewhere classified, initial encounter
T81.33XA	Disruption of traumatic injury wound repair, initial encounter

AMA: **12020** 2019,Nov,3; 2018,Jan,8; 2017,Jan,8; 2016,Jan,13; 2015,Jan,16 **12021** 2019,Nov,3; 2018,Jan,8; 2017,Jan,8; 2016,Jan,13; 2015,Jan,16

Repair

Relative Value Units/Medicare Edits

Non-Facility RVU	Work	PE	MP	Total
12020	2.67	5.82	0.43	8.92
12021	1.89	2.97	0.3	5.16
Facility RVU	Work	PE	MP	Total
12020	2.67	2.43	0.43	5.53
12021	1.89	1.91	0.3	4.1

	FUD	Status	MUE	Modifiers				IOM Reference
12020	10	A	2(3)	51	N/A	N/A	N/A	None
12021	10	A	3(3)	51	N/A	N/A	N/A	

* with documentation

Terms To Know

closure. Repairing an incision or wound by suture or other means.

dehiscence. Complication of healing in which the surgical wound ruptures or bursts open, superficially or through multiple layers.

infection. Presence of microorganisms in body tissues that may result in cellular damage.

irrigation. To wash out or cleanse a body cavity, wound, or tissue with water or other fluid.

packing. Material placed into a cavity or wound, such as gels, gauze, pads, and sponges.

simple repair. Surgical closure of a superficial wound requiring single layer suturing of the skin (epidermis, dermis, or subcutaneous tissue).

skin. Outer protective covering of the body composed of the epidermis and dermis, situated above the subcutaneous tissues.

subcutaneous tissue. Sheet or wide band of adipose (fat) and areolar connective tissue in two layers attached to the dermis.

superficial. On the skin surface or near the surface of any involved structure or field of interest.

12031-12037

12031	Repair, intermediate, wounds of scalp, axillae, trunk and/or extremities (excluding hands and feet); 2.5 cm or less
12032	2.6 cm to 7.5 cm
12034	7.6 cm to 12.5 cm
12035	12.6 cm to 20.0 cm
12036	20.1 cm to 30.0 cm
12037	over 30.0 cm

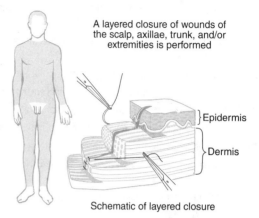

A layered closure of wounds of the scalp, axillae, trunk, and/or extremities is performed

Epidermis

Dermis

Schematic of layered closure

Explanation

The physician performs a repair of a wound of the scalp, axillae, trunk, and/or extremities (except hands and feet) using sutures, staples, tissue adhesives, or a combination of these materials to perform a layered closure. Due to deeper or more complex lacerations, deep subcutaneous or layered repair techniques are required. A local anesthetic is injected around the laceration, and the wound is cleansed, explored, and often irrigated with a saline solution. Extensive cleaning or removal of foreign matter from a heavily contaminated wound that is closed with a single layer may also be reported as an intermediate repair. For multiple wounds of the same complexity and in the same anatomical area, the length of all wounds repaired is summed and reported as one total length. Report 12031 for a total length of 2.5 cm or less; 12032 for 2.6 cm to 7.5 cm; 12034 for 7.6 cm to 12.5 cm; 12035 for 12.6 cm to 20 cm; 12036 for 20.1 cm to 30 cm; and 12037 if the total length is greater than 30 cm.

Coding Tips

Intermediate repair includes the repair of wounds that require layered closure of one or more of the deeper layers of subcutaneous tissue and superficial fascia in addition to limited undermining. Single-layer closure of a wound requiring extensive cleaning or removal of contaminated foreign matter or damaged tissue is classified as an intermediate repair. For simple (nonlayered) closure of the scalp, axillae, trunk, and/or extremities, see 12001–12007. For complex repairs, see 13100–13133. For wound closure by tissue adhesive(s) only, see HCPCS Level II code G0168.

ICD-10-CM Diagnostic Codes

C43.4	Malignant melanoma of scalp and neck
C43.52	Malignant melanoma of skin of breast
C43.61	Malignant melanoma of right upper limb, including shoulder ☑
C43.72	Malignant melanoma of left lower limb, including hip ☑
C44.42	Squamous cell carcinoma of skin of scalp and neck
C44.511	Basal cell carcinoma of skin of breast
C44.521	Squamous cell carcinoma of skin of breast

Repair

C44.612	Basal cell carcinoma of skin of right upper limb, including shoulder ☑
C44.719	Basal cell carcinoma of skin of left lower limb, including hip ☑
C4A.59	Merkel cell carcinoma of other part of trunk
C4A.61	Merkel cell carcinoma of right upper limb, including shoulder ☑
C4A.72	Merkel cell carcinoma of left lower limb, including hip ☑
C4A.8	Merkel cell carcinoma of overlapping sites
D17.22	Benign lipomatous neoplasm of skin and subcutaneous tissue of left arm ☑
D17.23	Benign lipomatous neoplasm of skin and subcutaneous tissue of right leg ☑
D17.24	Benign lipomatous neoplasm of skin and subcutaneous tissue of left leg ☑
S01.01XA	Laceration without foreign body of scalp, initial encounter
S01.02XA	Laceration with foreign body of scalp, initial encounter
S01.03XA	Puncture wound without foreign body of scalp, initial encounter
S01.04XA	Puncture wound with foreign body of scalp, initial encounter
S01.05XA	Open bite of scalp, initial encounter
S21.011A	Laceration without foreign body of right breast, initial encounter ☑
S21.012A	Laceration without foreign body of left breast, initial encounter ☑
S21.031A	Puncture wound without foreign body of right breast, initial encounter ☑
S21.032A	Puncture wound without foreign body of left breast, initial encounter ☑
S21.051A	Open bite of right breast, initial encounter ☑
S21.112A	Laceration without foreign body of left front wall of thorax without penetration into thoracic cavity, initial encounter
S21.132A	Puncture wound without foreign body of left front wall of thorax without penetration into thoracic cavity, initial encounter
S21.151A	Open bite of right front wall of thorax without penetration into thoracic cavity, initial encounter
S21.212A	Laceration without foreign body of left back wall of thorax without penetration into thoracic cavity, initial encounter
S21.231A	Puncture wound without foreign body of right back wall of thorax without penetration into thoracic cavity, initial encounter
S21.252A	Open bite of left back wall of thorax without penetration into thoracic cavity, initial encounter
S31.010A	Laceration without foreign body of lower back and pelvis without penetration into retroperitoneum, initial encounter
S31.030A	Puncture wound without foreign body of lower back and pelvis without penetration into retroperitoneum, initial encounter
S31.050A	Open bite of lower back and pelvis without penetration into retroperitoneum, initial encounter
S31.112A	Laceration without foreign body of abdominal wall, epigastric region without penetration into peritoneal cavity, initial encounter
S31.113A	Laceration without foreign body of abdominal wall, right lower quadrant without penetration into peritoneal cavity, initial encounter ☑
S31.115A	Laceration without foreign body of abdominal wall, periumbilic region without penetration into peritoneal cavity, initial encounter

S31.130A	Puncture wound of abdominal wall without foreign body, right upper quadrant without penetration into peritoneal cavity, initial encounter ☑
S31.134A	Puncture wound of abdominal wall without foreign body, left lower quadrant without penetration into peritoneal cavity, initial encounter ☑
S31.151A	Open bite of abdominal wall, left upper quadrant without penetration into peritoneal cavity, initial encounter ☑
S31.155A	Open bite of abdominal wall, periumbilic region without penetration into peritoneal cavity, initial encounter
S31.811A	Laceration without foreign body of right buttock, initial encounter ☑
S31.813A	Puncture wound without foreign body of right buttock, initial encounter ☑
S31.815A	Open bite of right buttock, initial encounter ☑
S31.823A	Puncture wound without foreign body of left buttock, initial encounter ☑
S31.825A	Open bite of left buttock, initial encounter ☑
S41.011A	Laceration without foreign body of right shoulder, initial encounter ☑
S41.012A	Laceration without foreign body of left shoulder, initial encounter ☑
S41.032A	Puncture wound without foreign body of left shoulder, initial encounter ☑
S41.051A	Open bite of right shoulder, initial encounter ☑
S41.112A	Laceration without foreign body of left upper arm, initial encounter ☑
S41.131A	Puncture wound without foreign body of right upper arm, initial encounter ☑
S41.132A	Puncture wound without foreign body of left upper arm, initial encounter ☑
S41.151A	Open bite of right upper arm, initial encounter ☑
S41.152A	Open bite of left upper arm, initial encounter ☑
S51.011A	Laceration without foreign body of right elbow, initial encounter ☑
S51.012A	Laceration without foreign body of left elbow, initial encounter ☑
S51.032A	Puncture wound without foreign body of left elbow, initial encounter ☑
S51.811A	Laceration without foreign body of right forearm, initial encounter ☑
S51.831A	Puncture wound without foreign body of right forearm, initial encounter ☑
S51.832A	Puncture wound without foreign body of left forearm, initial encounter ☑
S51.851A	Open bite of right forearm, initial encounter ☑
S61.511A	Laceration without foreign body of right wrist, initial encounter ☑
S61.532A	Puncture wound without foreign body of left wrist, initial encounter ☑
S61.551A	Open bite of right wrist, initial encounter ☑
S61.552A	Open bite of left wrist, initial encounter ☑
S71.012A	Laceration without foreign body, left hip, initial encounter ☑
S71.032A	Puncture wound without foreign body, left hip, initial encounter ☑
S71.051A	Open bite, right hip, initial encounter ☑
S71.111A	Laceration without foreign body, right thigh, initial encounter ☑

Repair

S71.132A	Puncture wound without foreign body, left thigh, initial encounter ☑	
S71.151A	Open bite, right thigh, initial encounter ☑	
S81.011A	Laceration without foreign body, right knee, initial encounter ☑	
S81.032A	Puncture wound without foreign body, left knee, initial encounter ☑	
S81.052A	Open bite, left knee, initial encounter ☑	
S81.812A	Laceration without foreign body, left lower leg, initial encounter ☑	
S81.831A	Puncture wound without foreign body, right lower leg, initial encounter ☑	
S81.852A	Open bite, left lower leg, initial encounter ☑	
S91.011A	Laceration without foreign body, right ankle, initial encounter ☑	
S91.012A	Laceration without foreign body, left ankle, initial encounter ☑	
S91.031A	Puncture wound without foreign body, right ankle, initial encounter ☑	
S91.052A	Open bite, left ankle, initial encounter ☑	

AMA: **12031** 2019,Nov,3; 2018,Sep,7; 2018,Jan,8; 2017,Jan,8; 2016,Jan,13; 2015,Jan,16 **12032** 2019,Nov,3; 2018,Sep,7; 2018,Jan,8; 2017,Jan,8; 2016,Jan,13; 2015,Jan,16 **12034** 2019,Nov,3; 2018,Sep,7; 2018,Jan,8; 2017,Jan,8; 2016,Jan,13; 2015,Jan,16 **12035** 2019,Nov,3; 2018,Sep,7; 2018,Jan,8; 2017,Jan,8; 2016,Jan,13; 2015,Jan,16 **12036** 2019,Nov,3; 2018,Sep,7; 2018,Jan,8; 2017,Jan,8; 2016,Jan,13; 2015,Jan,16 **12037** 2019,Nov,3; 2018,Sep,7; 2018,Jan,8; 2017,Jan,8; 2016,Jan,13; 2015,Jan,16

Relative Value Units/Medicare Edits

Non-Facility RVU	Work	PE	MP	Total
12031	2.0	5.54	0.25	7.79
12032	2.52	6.28	0.26	9.06
12034	2.97	6.53	0.41	9.91
12035	3.5	7.58	0.64	11.72
12036	4.23	7.86	0.84	12.93
12037	5.0	8.45	1.02	14.47
Facility RVU	**Work**	**PE**	**MP**	**Total**
12031	2.0	2.15	0.25	4.4
12032	2.52	2.71	0.26	5.49
12034	2.97	2.6	0.41	5.98
12035	3.5	2.92	0.64	7.06
12036	4.23	3.22	0.84	8.29
12037	5.0	3.61	1.02	9.63

	FUD	Status	MUE	Modifiers				IOM Reference
12031	10	A	1(2)	51	N/A	N/A	N/A	None
12032	10	A	1(2)	51	N/A	N/A	N/A	
12034	10	A	1(2)	51	N/A	N/A	N/A	
12035	10	A	1(2)	51	N/A	N/A	N/A	
12036	10	A	1(2)	51	N/A	N/A	N/A	
12037	10	A	1(2)	51	N/A	62*	80*	

* with documentation

Terms To Know

closure. Repairing an incision or wound by suture or other means.

12041-12047

12041	Repair, intermediate, wounds of neck, hands, feet and/or external genitalia; 2.5 cm or less
12042	2.6 cm to 7.5 cm
12044	7.6 cm to 12.5 cm
12045	12.6 cm to 20.0 cm
12046	20.1 cm to 30.0 cm
12047	over 30.0 cm

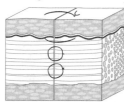

Layered suturing

The physician repairs intermediate lacerations. The lacerations are deep and require layered closure

Explanation

The physician performs a repair of a wound located on the neck, hands, feet, and/or external genitalia. A local anesthetic is injected around the laceration, and the wound is cleansed, explored, and often irrigated with a saline solution. Due to deeper or more complex lacerations, deep subcutaneous or layered suturing techniques are required. The physician closes tissue layers under the skin with dissolvable sutures before suturing the skin. Extensive cleaning or removal of foreign matter from a heavily contaminated wound that is closed with a single layer may also be reported as an intermediate repair. With multiple wounds of the same complexity and in the same anatomical area, the length of all wounds sutured is summed and reported as one total length. Report 12041 for a total length of 2.5 cm or less; 12042 for 2.6 cm to 7.5 cm; 12044 for 7.6 cm to 12.5 cm; 12045 for 12.6 cm to 20 cm; 12046 for 20.1 cm to 30 cm; and 12047 if the total length is greater than 30 cm.

Coding Tips

Intermediate repair includes the repair of wounds that require layered closure of one or more of the deeper layers of subcutaneous tissue and superficial fascia in addition to limited undermining. Single-layer closure of a wound requiring extensive cleaning or removal of contaminated foreign matter or damaged tissue is classified as an intermediate repair. For simple (nonlayered) closure of the neck, hands, feet, and/or external genitalia, see 12001–12007. For complex repairs, see 13131–13133. For wound closure by tissue adhesive(s) only, see HCPCS Level II code G0168.

ICD-10-CM Diagnostic Codes

C43.4	Malignant melanoma of scalp and neck	
C43.61	Malignant melanoma of right upper limb, including shoulder ☑	
C43.71	Malignant melanoma of right lower limb, including hip ☑	
C44.41	Basal cell carcinoma of skin of scalp and neck	
C44.42	Squamous cell carcinoma of skin of scalp and neck	
C44.612	Basal cell carcinoma of skin of right upper limb, including shoulder ☑	
C44.622	Squamous cell carcinoma of skin of right upper limb, including shoulder ☑	
C44.712	Basal cell carcinoma of skin of right lower limb, including hip ☑	
C44.722	Squamous cell carcinoma of skin of right lower limb, including hip ☑	

Repair

C44.792	Other specified malignant neoplasm of skin of right lower limb, including hip ☑
C4A.4	Merkel cell carcinoma of scalp and neck
C4A.61	Merkel cell carcinoma of right upper limb, including shoulder ☑
C4A.71	Merkel cell carcinoma of right lower limb, including hip ☑
C63.2	Malignant neoplasm of scrotum ♂
D03.4	Melanoma in situ of scalp and neck
D04.4	Carcinoma in situ of skin of scalp and neck
D04.61	Carcinoma in situ of skin of right upper limb, including shoulder ☑
D07.2	Carcinoma in situ of vagina ♀
D07.4	Carcinoma in situ of penis ♂
D07.61	Carcinoma in situ of scrotum ♂
D17.21	Benign lipomatous neoplasm of skin and subcutaneous tissue of right arm ☑
D17.23	Benign lipomatous neoplasm of skin and subcutaneous tissue of right leg ☑
D22.4	Melanocytic nevi of scalp and neck
D22.61	Melanocytic nevi of right upper limb, including shoulder ☑
D22.71	Melanocytic nevi of right lower limb, including hip ☑
D29.0	Benign neoplasm of penis ♂
D29.4	Benign neoplasm of scrotum ♂
S31.21XA	Laceration without foreign body of penis, initial encounter ♂
S31.25XA	Open bite of penis, initial encounter ♂
S31.32XA	Laceration with foreign body of scrotum and testes, initial encounter ♂
S31.34XA	Puncture wound with foreign body of scrotum and testes, initial encounter ♂
S31.35XA	Open bite of scrotum and testes, initial encounter ♂
S31.41XA	Laceration without foreign body of vagina and vulva, initial encounter ♀
S31.42XA	Laceration with foreign body of vagina and vulva, initial encounter ♀
S31.44XA	Puncture wound with foreign body of vagina and vulva, initial encounter ♀

AMA: **12041** 2019,Nov,3; 2018,Sep,7; 2018,Jan,8; 2017,Jan,8; 2016,Jan,13; 2015,Jan,16 **12042** 2019,Nov,3; 2018,Sep,7; 2018,Jan,8; 2017,Jan,8; 2016,Jan,13; 2015,Jan,16 **12044** 2019,Nov,3; 2018,Sep,7; 2018,Jan,8; 2017,Jan,8; 2016,Jan,13; 2015,Jan,16 **12045** 2019,Nov,3; 2018,Sep,7; 2018,Jan,8; 2017,Jan,8; 2016,Jan,13; 2015,Jan,16 **12046** 2019,Nov,3; 2018,Sep,7; 2018,Jan,8; 2017,Jan,8; 2016,Jan,13; 2015,Jan,16 **12047** 2019,Nov,3; 2018,Sep,7; 2018,Jan,8; 2017,Jan,8; 2016,Jan,13; 2015,Jan,16

Relative Value Units/Medicare Edits

Non-Facility RVU	Work	PE	MP	Total
12041	2.1	5.46	0.26	7.82
12042	2.79	6.05	0.31	9.15
12044	3.19	7.68	0.45	11.32
12045	3.75	7.69	0.64	12.08
12046	4.3	9.67	1.04	15.01
12047	4.95	10.26	1.21	16.42
Facility RVU	Work	PE	MP	Total
12041	2.1	1.86	0.26	4.22
12042	2.79	2.58	0.31	5.68
12044	3.19	2.57	0.45	6.21
12045	3.75	3.48	0.64	7.87
12046	4.3	3.99	1.04	9.33
12047	4.95	4.23	1.21	10.39

	FUD	Status	MUE	Modifiers				IOM Reference
12041	10	A	1(2)	51	N/A	N/A	N/A	None
12042	10	A	1(2)	51	N/A	N/A	N/A	
12044	10	A	1(2)	51	N/A	N/A	N/A	
12045	10	A	1(2)	51	N/A	N/A	N/A	
12046	10	A	1(2)	51	N/A	N/A	80*	
12047	10	A	1(2)	51	N/A	62*	80	

* with documentation

Terms To Know

foreign body. Any object or substance found in an organ and tissue that does not belong under normal circumstances.

laceration. Tearing injury; a torn, ragged-edged wound.

puncture. Creating a hole.

wound. Injury to living tissue often involving a cut or break in the skin.

12051-12057

12051 Repair, intermediate, wounds of face, ears, eyelids, nose, lips and/or mucous membranes; 2.5 cm or less
12052   2.6 cm to 5.0 cm
12053   5.1 cm to 7.5 cm
12054   7.6 cm to 12.5 cm
12055   12.6 cm to 20.0 cm
12056   20.1 cm to 30.0 cm
12057   over 30.0 cm

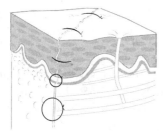

Layered suturing

Explanation

The physician performs a repair of a wound located on the face, ears, eyelids, nose, lips, and/or mucous membranes. A local anesthetic is injected around the laceration, and the wound is cleansed, explored, and often irrigated with a saline solution. Due to deeper or more complex lacerations, deep layered suturing techniques are required. The physician closes tissue layers under the skin with dissolvable sutures before suturing the skin. Extensive cleaning or removal of foreign matter from a heavily contaminated wound that is closed with a single layer may also be reported as an intermediate repair. With multiple wounds of the same complexity and in the same anatomical area, the length of all wounds sutured is summed and reported as one total length. Report 12051 for a total length of 2.5 cm or less; 12052 for 2.6 cm to 5 cm; 12053 for 5.1 cm to 7.5 cm; 12054 for 7.6 cm to 12.5 cm; 12055 for 12.6 cm to 20 cm; 12056 for 20.1 cm to 30 cm; and 12057 if the total length is greater than 30 cm.

Coding Tips

Intermediate repair includes the repair of wounds that require layered closure of one or more of the deeper layers of subcutaneous tissue and superficial fascia in addition to limited undermining. Single-layer closure of a wound requiring extensive cleaning or removal of contaminated foreign matter or damaged tissue is classified as an intermediate repair. For simple (nonlayered) closure of the face, ears, eyelids, nose, lips, and/or mucous membranes, see 12011–12018. For complex repairs, see 13131–13153. Surgical trays, A4550, are not separately reimbursed by Medicare; however, other third-party payers may cover them. Check with the specific payer to determine coverage.

ICD-10-CM Diagnostic Codes

C00.0	Malignant neoplasm of external upper lip
C00.1	Malignant neoplasm of external lower lip
C00.3	Malignant neoplasm of upper lip, inner aspect
C00.4	Malignant neoplasm of lower lip, inner aspect
C43.0	Malignant melanoma of lip
C43.111	Malignant melanoma of right upper eyelid, including canthus ☑
C43.112	Malignant melanoma of right lower eyelid, including canthus ☑
C43.21	Malignant melanoma of right ear and external auricular canal ☑
C43.22	Malignant melanoma of left ear and external auricular canal ☑
C43.31	Malignant melanoma of nose
C43.39	Malignant melanoma of other parts of face
C44.01	Basal cell carcinoma of skin of lip
C44.02	Squamous cell carcinoma of skin of lip
C44.09	Other specified malignant neoplasm of skin of lip
C44.1121	Basal cell carcinoma of skin of right upper eyelid, including canthus ☑
C44.1122	Basal cell carcinoma of skin of right lower eyelid, including canthus ☑
C44.1221	Squamous cell carcinoma of skin of right upper eyelid, including canthus ☑
C44.1222	Squamous cell carcinoma of skin of right lower eyelid, including canthus ☑
C44.212	Basal cell carcinoma of skin of right ear and external auricular canal ☑
C44.219	Basal cell carcinoma of skin of left ear and external auricular canal ☑
C44.222	Squamous cell carcinoma of skin of right ear and external auricular canal ☑
C44.229	Squamous cell carcinoma of skin of left ear and external auricular canal ☑
C44.292	Other specified malignant neoplasm of skin of right ear and external auricular canal ☑
C44.311	Basal cell carcinoma of skin of nose
C44.319	Basal cell carcinoma of skin of other parts of face
C44.321	Squamous cell carcinoma of skin of nose
C44.391	Other specified malignant neoplasm of skin of nose
C44.399	Other specified malignant neoplasm of skin of other parts of face
C4A.0	Merkel cell carcinoma of lip
C4A.111	Merkel cell carcinoma of right upper eyelid, including canthus ☑
C4A.112	Merkel cell carcinoma of right lower eyelid, including canthus ☑
C4A.21	Merkel cell carcinoma of right ear and external auricular canal ☑
C4A.22	Merkel cell carcinoma of left ear and external auricular canal ☑
C4A.31	Merkel cell carcinoma of nose
C76.0	Malignant neoplasm of head, face and neck
D03.0	Melanoma in situ of lip
D03.111	Melanoma in situ of right upper eyelid, including canthus ☑
D03.112	Melanoma in situ of right lower eyelid, including canthus ☑
D03.22	Melanoma in situ of left ear and external auricular canal ☑
D04.0	Carcinoma in situ of skin of lip
D04.111	Carcinoma in situ of skin of right upper eyelid, including canthus ☑
D04.112	Carcinoma in situ of skin of right lower eyelid, including canthus ☑
D04.22	Carcinoma in situ of skin of left ear and external auricular canal ☑
D04.39	Carcinoma in situ of skin of other parts of face
D17.0	Benign lipomatous neoplasm of skin and subcutaneous tissue of head, face and neck
D22.0	Melanocytic nevi of lip
D22.111	Melanocytic nevi of right upper eyelid, including canthus ☑
D22.112	Melanocytic nevi of right lower eyelid, including canthus ☑
D22.21	Melanocytic nevi of right ear and external auricular canal ☑
D22.22	Melanocytic nevi of left ear and external auricular canal ☑
D22.39	Melanocytic nevi of other parts of face

Repair

D23.0	Other benign neoplasm of skin of lip
D23.111	Other benign neoplasm of skin of right upper eyelid, including canthus ☑
D23.112	Other benign neoplasm of skin of right lower eyelid, including canthus ☑
D23.22	Other benign neoplasm of skin of left ear and external auricular canal ☑
H02.821	Cysts of right upper eyelid ☑
S01.111A	Laceration without foreign body of right eyelid and periocular area, initial encounter ☑
S01.112A	Laceration without foreign body of left eyelid and periocular area, initial encounter ☑
S01.121A	Laceration with foreign body of right eyelid and periocular area, initial encounter ☑
S01.122A	Laceration with foreign body of left eyelid and periocular area, initial encounter ☑
S01.131A	Puncture wound without foreign body of right eyelid and periocular area, initial encounter ☑
S01.132A	Puncture wound without foreign body of left eyelid and periocular area, initial encounter ☑
S01.141A	Puncture wound with foreign body of right eyelid and periocular area, initial encounter ☑
S01.152A	Open bite of left eyelid and periocular area, initial encounter ☑
S01.21XA	Laceration without foreign body of nose, initial encounter
S01.22XA	Laceration with foreign body of nose, initial encounter
S01.23XA	Puncture wound without foreign body of nose, initial encounter
S01.24XA	Puncture wound with foreign body of nose, initial encounter
S01.25XA	Open bite of nose, initial encounter
S01.311A	Laceration without foreign body of right ear, initial encounter ☑
S01.312A	Laceration without foreign body of left ear, initial encounter ☑
S01.321A	Laceration with foreign body of right ear, initial encounter ☑
S01.322A	Laceration with foreign body of left ear, initial encounter ☑
S01.331A	Puncture wound without foreign body of right ear, initial encounter ☑
S01.332A	Puncture wound without foreign body of left ear, initial encounter ☑
S01.351A	Open bite of right ear, initial encounter ☑
S01.352A	Open bite of left ear, initial encounter ☑
S01.412A	Laceration without foreign body of left cheek and temporomandibular area, initial encounter ☑
S01.421A	Laceration with foreign body of right cheek and temporomandibular area, initial encounter ☑
S01.422A	Laceration with foreign body of left cheek and temporomandibular area, initial encounter ☑
S01.431A	Puncture wound without foreign body of right cheek and temporomandibular area, initial encounter ☑
S01.432A	Puncture wound without foreign body of left cheek and temporomandibular area, initial encounter ☑
S01.441A	Puncture wound with foreign body of right cheek and temporomandibular area, initial encounter ☑
S01.442A	Puncture wound with foreign body of left cheek and temporomandibular area, initial encounter ☑
S01.451A	Open bite of right cheek and temporomandibular area, initial encounter ☑
S01.452A	Open bite of left cheek and temporomandibular area, initial encounter ☑

S01.511A	Laceration without foreign body of lip, initial encounter
S01.521A	Laceration with foreign body of lip, initial encounter
S01.522A	Laceration with foreign body of oral cavity, initial encounter
S01.531A	Puncture wound without foreign body of lip, initial encounter
S01.532A	Puncture wound without foreign body of oral cavity, initial encounter
S01.541A	Puncture wound with foreign body of lip, initial encounter
S01.542A	Puncture wound with foreign body of oral cavity, initial encounter
S01.551A	Open bite of lip, initial encounter
S01.552A	Open bite of oral cavity, initial encounter

AMA: **12051** 2019,Nov,3; 2018,Sep,7; 2018,Jan,8; 2017,Jan,8; 2016,Jan,13; 2015,Jan,16 **12052** 2019,Nov,3; 2018,Sep,7; 2018,Jan,8; 2017,Jan,8; 2016,Jan,13; 2015,Jan,16 **12053** 2019,Nov,3; 2018,Sep,7; 2018,Jan,8; 2017,Jan,8; 2016,Jan,13; 2015,Jan,16 **12054** 2019,Nov,3; 2018,Sep,7; 2018,Jan,8; 2017,Jan,8; 2016,Jan,13; 2015,Jan,16 **12055** 2019,Nov,3; 2018,Sep,7; 2018,Jan,8; 2017,Jan,8; 2016,Jan,13; 2015,Jan,16 **12056** 2019,Nov,3; 2018,Sep,7; 2018,Jan,8; 2017,Jan,8; 2016,Jan,13; 2015,Jan,16 **12057** 2019,Nov,3; 2018,Sep,7; 2018,Jan,8; 2017,Jan,8; 2016,Jan,13; 2015,Jan,16

Relative Value Units/Medicare Edits

Non-Facility RVU	Work	PE	MP	Total
12051	2.33	5.76	0.28	8.37
12052	2.87	6.1	0.34	9.31
12053	3.17	7.28	0.43	10.88
12054	3.5	7.45	0.54	11.49
12055	4.5	9.72	0.79	15.01
12056	5.3	11.05	0.94	17.29
12057	6.0	11.25	1.07	18.32
Facility RVU	**Work**	**PE**	**MP**	**Total**
12051	2.33	2.29	0.28	4.9
12052	2.87	2.58	0.34	5.79
12053	3.17	2.66	0.43	6.26
12054	3.5	2.32	0.54	6.36
12055	4.5	3.43	0.79	8.72
12056	5.3	5.03	0.94	11.27
12057	6.0	5.28	1.07	12.35

	FUD	Status	MUE	Modifiers				IOM Reference
12051	10	A	1(2)	51	N/A	N/A	N/A	None
12052	10	A	1(2)	51	N/A	N/A	N/A	
12053	10	A	1(2)	51	N/A	N/A	N/A	
12054	10	A	1(2)	51	N/A	N/A	N/A	
12055	10	A	1(2)	51	N/A	N/A	N/A	
12056	10	A	1(2)	51	N/A	N/A	80*	
12057	10	A	1(2)	51	N/A	62*	80	

* with documentation

Repair

13100-13102

13100   Repair, complex, trunk; 1.1 cm to 2.5 cm
13101   2.6 cm to 7.5 cm
+   13102   each additional 5 cm or less (List separately in addition to code for primary procedure)

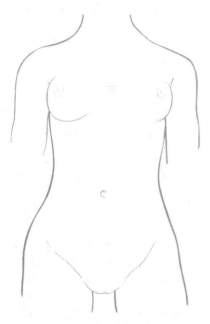

A complex repair in the general region
of the trunk is performed

Explanation

The physician repairs complex wounds of the trunk. The physician performs complex, layered suturing of torn, crushed, or deeply lacerated tissue. The physician debrides the wound by removing foreign material or damaged tissue. Irrigation of the wound is performed and antimicrobial solutions are used to decontaminate and cleanse the wound. The physician may trim skin margins with a scalpel or scissors to allow for proper closure. The wound is closed in layers. The physician may perform scar revision, which creates a complex defect requiring repair. Stents or retention sutures may also be used in complex repair of a wound. Reconstructive procedures, such as utilization of local flaps, may be required and are reported separately. Report 13100 for wounds 1.1 cm to 2.5 cm; 13101 for 2.6 cm to 7.5 cm; and 13102 for each additional 5 cm or less.

Coding Tips

Report 13102 in addition to 13101. When reporting the repair of wounds, the sum of the lengths of repair are added together and are listed as a total for each anatomical site. For wounds 1 cm or less, see simple or intermediate repair codes. Complex wounds require additional special treatment, such as the use of stent dressings, retention sutures, or extensive revision, which may involve removing sizable portions of skin or extensive undermining of the skin to loosen the tissues to close a defect. In addition, at least one of the following is required: 1) exposure of bone, cartilage, tendon, or a named neurovascular structure, 2) extensive undermining that is at least one entire edge of the defect but a distance greater than or equal to the maximum width of the defect, measured perpendicular to the closure line, 3) involvement of free margins of helical rim, nostril rim, or vermilion border in which retention sutures are placed. When more than one repair and/or another separately identifiable procedure is performed, the highest dollar value code is listed as the primary procedure and subsequent procedures are appended with modifier

51. Surgical trays, A4550, are not separately reimbursed by Medicare; however, other third-party payers may cover them. Check with the specific payer to determine coverage.

ICD-10-CM Diagnostic Codes

C43.52	Malignant melanoma of skin of breast
C43.59	Malignant melanoma of other part of trunk
C44.511	Basal cell carcinoma of skin of breast
C44.519	Basal cell carcinoma of skin of other part of trunk
C44.521	Squamous cell carcinoma of skin of breast
C44.529	Squamous cell carcinoma of skin of other part of trunk
C4A.52	Merkel cell carcinoma of skin of breast
C4A.59	Merkel cell carcinoma of other part of trunk
D03.52	Melanoma in situ of breast (skin) (soft tissue)
D03.59	Melanoma in situ of other part of trunk
D04.5	Carcinoma in situ of skin of trunk
D17.1	Benign lipomatous neoplasm of skin and subcutaneous tissue of trunk
D22.5	Melanocytic nevi of trunk
D24.1	Benign neoplasm of right breast ☑
D24.2	Benign neoplasm of left breast ☑
S21.011A	Laceration without foreign body of right breast, initial encounter ☑
S21.012A	Laceration without foreign body of left breast, initial encounter ☑
S21.021A	Laceration with foreign body of right breast, initial encounter ☑
S21.022A	Laceration with foreign body of left breast, initial encounter ☑
S21.031A	Puncture wound without foreign body of right breast, initial encounter ☑
S21.032A	Puncture wound without foreign body of left breast, initial encounter ☑
S21.041A	Puncture wound with foreign body of right breast, initial encounter ☑
S21.042A	Puncture wound with foreign body of left breast, initial encounter ☑
S21.051A	Open bite of right breast, initial encounter ☑
S21.052A	Open bite of left breast, initial encounter ☑
S21.112A	Laceration without foreign body of left front wall of thorax without penetration into thoracic cavity, initial encounter
S21.121A	Laceration with foreign body of right front wall of thorax without penetration into thoracic cavity, initial encounter
S21.122A	Laceration with foreign body of left front wall of thorax without penetration into thoracic cavity, initial encounter
S21.131A	Puncture wound without foreign body of right front wall of thorax without penetration into thoracic cavity, initial encounter
S21.142A	Puncture wound with foreign body of left front wall of thorax without penetration into thoracic cavity, initial encounter
S21.151A	Open bite of right front wall of thorax without penetration into thoracic cavity, initial encounter
S21.152A	Open bite of left front wall of thorax without penetration into thoracic cavity, initial encounter
S29.021A	Laceration of muscle and tendon of front wall of thorax, initial encounter
S31.010A	Laceration without foreign body of lower back and pelvis without penetration into retroperitoneum, initial encounter

Repair

S31.020A Laceration with foreign body of lower back and pelvis without penetration into retroperitoneum, initial encounter

S31.030A Puncture wound without foreign body of lower back and pelvis without penetration into retroperitoneum, initial encounter

S31.040A Puncture wound with foreign body of lower back and pelvis without penetration into retroperitoneum, initial encounter

S31.050A Open bite of lower back and pelvis without penetration into retroperitoneum, initial encounter

S31.110A Laceration without foreign body of abdominal wall, right upper quadrant without penetration into peritoneal cavity, initial encounter ☑

S31.112A Laceration without foreign body of abdominal wall, epigastric region without penetration into peritoneal cavity, initial encounter

S31.113A Laceration without foreign body of abdominal wall, right lower quadrant without penetration into peritoneal cavity, initial encounter ☑

S31.114A Laceration without foreign body of abdominal wall, left lower quadrant without penetration into peritoneal cavity, initial encounter ☑

S31.120A Laceration of abdominal wall with foreign body, right upper quadrant without penetration into peritoneal cavity, initial encounter ☑

S31.121A Laceration of abdominal wall with foreign body, left upper quadrant without penetration into peritoneal cavity, initial encounter ☑

S31.122A Laceration of abdominal wall with foreign body, epigastric region without penetration into peritoneal cavity, initial encounter

S31.123A Laceration of abdominal wall with foreign body, right lower quadrant without penetration into peritoneal cavity, initial encounter ☑

S31.124A Laceration of abdominal wall with foreign body, left lower quadrant without penetration into peritoneal cavity, initial encounter ☑

S31.130A Puncture wound of abdominal wall without foreign body, right upper quadrant without penetration into peritoneal cavity, initial encounter ☑

S31.131A Puncture wound of abdominal wall without foreign body, left upper quadrant without penetration into peritoneal cavity, initial encounter ☑

S31.132A Puncture wound of abdominal wall without foreign body, epigastric region without penetration into peritoneal cavity, initial encounter

S31.133A Puncture wound of abdominal wall without foreign body, right lower quadrant without penetration into peritoneal cavity, initial encounter ☑

S31.134A Puncture wound of abdominal wall without foreign body, left lower quadrant without penetration into peritoneal cavity, initial encounter ☑

S31.135A Puncture wound of abdominal wall without foreign body, periumbilic region without penetration into peritoneal cavity, initial encounter

S31.140A Puncture wound of abdominal wall with foreign body, right upper quadrant without penetration into peritoneal cavity, initial encounter ☑

S31.143A Puncture wound of abdominal wall with foreign body, right lower quadrant without penetration into peritoneal cavity, initial encounter ☑

S31.144A Puncture wound of abdominal wall with foreign body, left lower quadrant without penetration into peritoneal cavity, initial encounter ☑

S31.145A Puncture wound of abdominal wall with foreign body, periumbilic region without penetration into peritoneal cavity, initial encounter

S31.150A Open bite of abdominal wall, right upper quadrant without penetration into peritoneal cavity, initial encounter ☑

S31.151A Open bite of abdominal wall, left upper quadrant without penetration into peritoneal cavity, initial encounter ☑

S31.154A Open bite of abdominal wall, left lower quadrant without penetration into peritoneal cavity, initial encounter ☑

S31.155A Open bite of abdominal wall, periumbilic region without penetration into peritoneal cavity, initial encounter

S31.811A Laceration without foreign body of right buttock, initial encounter ☑

S31.812A Laceration with foreign body of right buttock, initial encounter ☑

S31.813A Puncture wound without foreign body of right buttock, initial encounter ☑

S31.814A Puncture wound with foreign body of right buttock, initial encounter ☑

S31.815A Open bite of right buttock, initial encounter ☑

S31.822A Laceration with foreign body of left buttock, initial encounter ☑

S31.823A Puncture wound without foreign body of left buttock, initial encounter ☑

S31.824A Puncture wound with foreign body of left buttock, initial encounter ☑

S31.825A Open bite of left buttock, initial encounter ☑

S31.831A Laceration without foreign body of anus, initial encounter

S31.832A Laceration with foreign body of anus, initial encounter

AMA: 13100 2019,Nov,3; 2019,Nov,14; 2018,Sep,7; 2018,Jan,8; 2017,Jan,8; 2017,Apr,9; 2016,Jan,13; 2015,Jan,16 **13101** 2019,Nov,3; 2019,Dec,14; 2018,Sep,7; 2018,Jan,8; 2017,Jan,8; 2017,Apr,9; 2016,Jan,13; 2015,Jan,16 **13102** 2019,Nov,14; 2019,Nov,3; 2018,Sep,7; 2018,Jan,8; 2017,Jan,8; 2017,Apr,9; 2016,Jan,13; 2015,Jan,16

Relative Value Units/Medicare Edits

Non-Facility RVU	Work	PE	MP	Total
13100	3.0	6.88	0.36	10.24
13101	3.5	8.05	0.39	11.94
13102	1.24	2.09	0.19	3.52
Facility RVU	**Work**	**PE**	**MP**	**Total**
13100	3.0	2.49	0.36	5.85
13101	3.5	3.38	0.39	7.27
13102	1.24	0.68	0.19	2.11

	FUD	Status	MUE	Modifiers				IOM Reference
13100	10	A	1(2)	51	N/A	N/A	N/A	None
13101	10	A	1(2)	51	N/A	N/A	N/A	
13102	N/A	A	9(3)	N/A	N/A	N/A	N/A	

* with documentation

13120-13122

13120   Repair, complex, scalp, arms, and/or legs; 1.1 cm to 2.5 cm
13121   2.6 cm to 7.5 cm
+   13122   each additional 5 cm or less (List separately in addition to code for primary procedure)

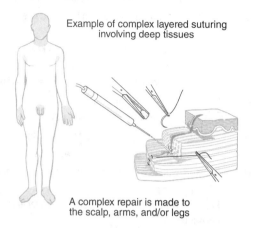

Example of complex layered suturing involving deep tissues

A complex repair is made to the scalp, arms, and/or legs

Explanation

The physician repairs wounds located on the scalp, arms, and/or legs. The physician performs complex, layered suturing of torn, crushed, or deeply lacerated tissue. The physician debrides the wound by removing foreign material or damaged tissue. Irrigation of the wound is performed and antimicrobial solutions are used to decontaminate and cleanse the wound. The physician may trim skin margins with a scalpel or scissors to allow for proper closure. The wound is closed in layers. The physician may perform scar revision, which creates a complex defect requiring repair. Stents or retention sutures may also be used in a complex repair of a wound. Reconstructive procedures, such as utilization of local flaps, may be required and are reported separately. Report 13120 for wounds 1.1 cm to 2.5 cm; 13121 for 2.6 cm to 7.5 cm; and 13122 for each additional 5 cm or less.

Coding Tips

Report 13122 in addition to 13121. When reporting the repair of wounds, the sum of the lengths of repair are added together and are listed as a total for each anatomical site. For wounds 1 cm or less, see simple or intermediate repair codes. Complex wounds require additional special treatment, such as the use of stent dressings, retention sutures, or extensive revision, which may involve removing sizable portions of skin or extensive undermining of the skin to loosen the tissues to close a defect. In addition, at least one of the following is required: 1) exposure of bone, cartilage, tendon, or a named neurovascular structure, 2) extensive undermining that is at least one entire edge of the defect but a distance greater than or equal to the maximum width of the defect, measured perpendicular to the closure line, 3) involvement of free margins of helical rim, nostril rim, or vermilion border in which retention sutures are placed. When more than one repair and/or another separately identifiable procedure is performed, the highest dollar value code is listed as the primary procedure and subsequent procedures are appended with modifier 51.

ICD-10-CM Diagnostic Codes

C43.4	Malignant melanoma of scalp and neck
C43.61	Malignant melanoma of right upper limb, including shoulder ☑
C43.62	Malignant melanoma of left upper limb, including shoulder ☑
C43.71	Malignant melanoma of right lower limb, including hip ☑
C43.72	Malignant melanoma of left lower limb, including hip ☑
C44.41	Basal cell carcinoma of skin of scalp and neck
C44.42	Squamous cell carcinoma of skin of scalp and neck
C44.49	Other specified malignant neoplasm of skin of scalp and neck
C44.612	Basal cell carcinoma of skin of right upper limb, including shoulder ☑
C44.619	Basal cell carcinoma of skin of left upper limb, including shoulder ☑
C44.622	Squamous cell carcinoma of skin of right upper limb, including shoulder ☑
C44.629	Squamous cell carcinoma of skin of left upper limb, including shoulder ☑
C44.692	Other specified malignant neoplasm of skin of right upper limb, including shoulder ☑
C44.712	Basal cell carcinoma of skin of right lower limb, including hip ☑
C44.719	Basal cell carcinoma of skin of left lower limb, including hip ☑
C44.722	Squamous cell carcinoma of skin of right lower limb, including hip ☑
C44.729	Squamous cell carcinoma of skin of left lower limb, including hip ☑
C4A.4	Merkel cell carcinoma of scalp and neck
C4A.61	Merkel cell carcinoma of right upper limb, including shoulder ☑
C4A.62	Merkel cell carcinoma of left upper limb, including shoulder ☑
C4A.71	Merkel cell carcinoma of right lower limb, including hip ☑
C4A.72	Merkel cell carcinoma of left lower limb, including hip ☑
C76.41	Malignant neoplasm of right upper limb ☑
C76.42	Malignant neoplasm of left upper limb ☑
C76.51	Malignant neoplasm of right lower limb ☑
C76.52	Malignant neoplasm of left lower limb ☑
D03.4	Melanoma in situ of scalp and neck
D03.61	Melanoma in situ of right upper limb, including shoulder ☑
D03.62	Melanoma in situ of left upper limb, including shoulder ☑
D03.71	Melanoma in situ of right lower limb, including hip ☑
D03.72	Melanoma in situ of left lower limb, including hip ☑
D04.4	Carcinoma in situ of skin of scalp and neck
D04.61	Carcinoma in situ of skin of right upper limb, including shoulder ☑
D04.62	Carcinoma in situ of skin of left upper limb, including shoulder ☑
D04.71	Carcinoma in situ of skin of right lower limb, including hip ☑
D04.72	Carcinoma in situ of skin of left lower limb, including hip ☑
D17.21	Benign lipomatous neoplasm of skin and subcutaneous tissue of right arm ☑
D17.22	Benign lipomatous neoplasm of skin and subcutaneous tissue of left arm ☑
D17.23	Benign lipomatous neoplasm of skin and subcutaneous tissue of right leg ☑
D17.24	Benign lipomatous neoplasm of skin and subcutaneous tissue of left leg ☑
D22.4	Melanocytic nevi of scalp and neck
D22.61	Melanocytic nevi of right upper limb, including shoulder ☑
D22.62	Melanocytic nevi of left upper limb, including shoulder ☑
D22.71	Melanocytic nevi of right lower limb, including hip ☑
D22.72	Melanocytic nevi of left lower limb, including hip ☑
D23.4	Other benign neoplasm of skin of scalp and neck
D23.61	Other benign neoplasm of skin of right upper limb, including shoulder ☑

Repair

D23.71	Other benign neoplasm of skin of right lower limb, including hip ☑
S01.02XA	Laceration with foreign body of scalp, initial encounter
S01.04XA	Puncture wound with foreign body of scalp, initial encounter
S01.05XA	Open bite of scalp, initial encounter
S08.0XXA	Avulsion of scalp, initial encounter
S41.111A	Laceration without foreign body of right upper arm, initial encounter ☑
S41.112A	Laceration without foreign body of left upper arm, initial encounter ☑
S41.121A	Laceration with foreign body of right upper arm, initial encounter ☑
S41.122A	Laceration with foreign body of left upper arm, initial encounter ☑
S41.141A	Puncture wound with foreign body of right upper arm, initial encounter ☑
S41.142A	Puncture wound with foreign body of left upper arm, initial encounter ☑
S41.151A	Open bite of right upper arm, initial encounter ☑
S41.152A	Open bite of left upper arm, initial encounter ☑
S51.011A	Laceration without foreign body of right elbow, initial encounter ☑
S51.012A	Laceration without foreign body of left elbow, initial encounter ☑
S51.021A	Laceration with foreign body of right elbow, initial encounter ☑
S51.022A	Laceration with foreign body of left elbow, initial encounter ☑
S51.031A	Puncture wound without foreign body of right elbow, initial encounter ☑
S51.032A	Puncture wound without foreign body of left elbow, initial encounter ☑
S51.042A	Puncture wound with foreign body of left elbow, initial encounter ☑
S51.051A	Open bite, right elbow, initial encounter ☑
S51.052A	Open bite, left elbow, initial encounter ☑
S51.812A	Laceration without foreign body of left forearm, initial encounter ☑
S51.821A	Laceration with foreign body of right forearm, initial encounter ☑
S51.822A	Laceration with foreign body of left forearm, initial encounter ☑
S51.831A	Puncture wound without foreign body of right forearm, initial encounter ☑
S51.842A	Puncture wound with foreign body of left forearm, initial encounter ☑
S51.851A	Open bite of right forearm, initial encounter ☑
S51.852A	Open bite of left forearm, initial encounter ☑
S71.012A	Laceration without foreign body, left hip, initial encounter ☑
S71.021A	Laceration with foreign body, right hip, initial encounter ☑
S71.031A	Puncture wound without foreign body, right hip, initial encounter ☑
S71.042A	Puncture wound with foreign body, left hip, initial encounter ☑
S71.051A	Open bite, right hip, initial encounter ☑
S71.052A	Open bite, left hip, initial encounter ☑
S71.121A	Laceration with foreign body, right thigh, initial encounter ☑
S71.122A	Laceration with foreign body, left thigh, initial encounter ☑
S71.132A	Puncture wound without foreign body, left thigh, initial encounter ☑
S71.141A	Puncture wound with foreign body, right thigh, initial encounter ☑
S71.142A	Puncture wound with foreign body, left thigh, initial encounter ☑
S71.152A	Open bite, left thigh, initial encounter ☑
S81.011A	Laceration without foreign body, right knee, initial encounter ☑
S81.021A	Laceration with foreign body, right knee, initial encounter ☑
S81.022A	Laceration with foreign body, left knee, initial encounter ☑
S81.032A	Puncture wound without foreign body, left knee, initial encounter ☑
S81.041A	Puncture wound with foreign body, right knee, initial encounter ☑
S81.042A	Puncture wound with foreign body, left knee, initial encounter ☑
S81.051A	Open bite, right knee, initial encounter ☑
S81.052A	Open bite, left knee, initial encounter ☑
S81.821A	Laceration with foreign body, right lower leg, initial encounter ☑
S81.822A	Laceration with foreign body, left lower leg, initial encounter ☑
S81.841A	Puncture wound with foreign body, right lower leg, initial encounter ☑
S81.842A	Puncture wound with foreign body, left lower leg, initial encounter ☑
S81.851A	Open bite, right lower leg, initial encounter ☑
S81.852A	Open bite, left lower leg, initial encounter ☑

AMA: **13120** 2019,Nov,3; 2018,Sep,7; 2018,Jan,8; 2017,Jan,8; 2016,Jan,13; 2015,Jan,16 **13121** 2019,Nov,3; 2018,Sep,7; 2018,Jan,8; 2017,Jan,8; 2016,Jan,13; 2015,Jan,16 **13122** 2019,Nov,3; 2018,Sep,7; 2018,Jan,8; 2017,Jan,8; 2016,Jan,13; 2015,Jan,16

Relative Value Units/Medicare Edits

Non-Facility RVU	Work	PE	MP	Total
13120	3.23	7.04	0.37	10.64
13121	4.0	8.34	0.43	12.77
13122	1.44	2.18	0.2	3.82
Facility RVU	Work	PE	MP	Total
13120	3.23	3.22	0.37	6.82
13121	4.0	3.08	0.43	7.51
13122	1.44	0.78	0.2	2.42

	FUD	Status	MUE	Modifiers				IOM Reference
13120	10	A	1(2)	51	N/A	N/A	N/A	None
13121	10	A	1(2)	51	N/A	N/A	N/A	
13122	N/A	A	9(3)	N/A	N/A	N/A	N/A	

* with documentation

Terms To Know

complex repair. Surgical closure of a wound requiring more than layered closure of the deeper subcutaneous tissue and fascia.

debride. To remove all foreign objects and devitalized or infected tissue from a burn or wound to prevent infection and promote healing.

irrigation. To wash out or cleanse a body cavity, wound, or tissue with water or other fluid.

reconstruction. Recreating, restoring, or rebuilding a body part or organ.

13131-13133

13131   Repair, complex, forehead, cheeks, chin, mouth, neck, axillae, genitalia, hands and/or feet; 1.1 cm to 2.5 cm

13132   2.6 cm to 7.5 cm

+ 13133   each additional 5 cm or less (List separately in addition to code for primary procedure)

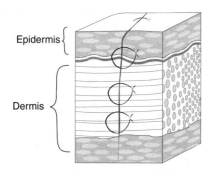

Schematic of complex layered suturing
of torn or deeply lacerated tissue

Explanation

The physician repairs wounds located on the forehead, cheeks, chin, mouth, neck, axillae, genitalia, hands, and/or feet. The physician performs complex, layered suturing of torn, crushed, or deeply lacerated tissue. The physician debrides the wound by removing foreign material or damaged tissue. Irrigation of the wound is performed and antimicrobial solutions are used to decontaminate and cleanse the wound. The physician may trim skin margins with a scalpel or scissors to allow for proper closure. The wound is closed in layers. The physician may perform scar revision, which creates a complex defect requiring repair. Stents or retention sutures may also be used in complex repair of a wound. Reconstructive procedures, such as utilization of local flaps, may be required and are reported separately. Report 13131 for wounds 1.1 cm to 2.5 cm; 13132 for 2.6 cm to 7.5 cm; and 13133 for each additional 5 cm or less.

Coding Tips

Report 13133 in addition to 13132. When reporting the repair of wounds, the sum of the lengths of repair are added together and are listed as a total for each anatomical site. For wounds 1 cm or less, see simple or intermediate repair codes. Complex wounds require additional special treatment, such as the use of stent dressings, retention sutures, or extensive revision, which may involve removing sizable portions of skin or extensive undermining of the skin to loosen the tissues to close a defect. In addition, at least one of the following is required: 1) exposure of bone, cartilage, tendon, or a named neurovascular structure, 2) extensive undermining that is at least one entire edge of the defect but a distance greater than or equal to the maximum width of the defect, measured perpendicular to the closure line, 3) involvement of free margins of helical rim, nostril rim, or vermilion border in which retention sutures are placed. When more than one repair and/or another separately identifiable procedure is performed, the highest dollar value code is listed as the primary procedure and subsequent procedures are appended with modifier 51.

ICD-10-CM Diagnostic Codes

C43.39	Malignant melanoma of other parts of face
C43.4	Malignant melanoma of scalp and neck
C44.41	Basal cell carcinoma of skin of scalp and neck
C44.42	Squamous cell carcinoma of skin of scalp and neck
C60.2	Malignant neoplasm of body of penis ♂
C60.8	Malignant neoplasm of overlapping sites of penis ♂
C63.2	Malignant neoplasm of scrotum ♂
C76.0	Malignant neoplasm of head, face and neck
D00.06	Carcinoma in situ of floor of mouth
D03.39	Melanoma in situ of other parts of face
D03.4	Melanoma in situ of scalp and neck
D07.2	Carcinoma in situ of vagina ♀
D07.4	Carcinoma in situ of penis ♂
D07.61	Carcinoma in situ of scrotum ♂
D22.39	Melanocytic nevi of other parts of face
D29.4	Benign neoplasm of scrotum ♂
N90.812	Female genital mutilation Type II status ♀
N90.813	Female genital mutilation Type III status ♀
S01.412A	Laceration without foreign body of left cheek and temporomandibular area, initial encounter ☑
S01.432A	Puncture wound without foreign body of left cheek and temporomandibular area, initial encounter ☑
S01.441A	Puncture wound with foreign body of right cheek and temporomandibular area, initial encounter ☑
S01.452A	Open bite of left cheek and temporomandibular area, initial encounter ☑
S01.542A	Puncture wound with foreign body of oral cavity, initial encounter
S01.552A	Open bite of oral cavity, initial encounter
S31.22XA	Laceration with foreign body of penis, initial encounter ♂
S31.31XA	Laceration without foreign body of scrotum and testes, initial encounter ♂
S31.33XA	Puncture wound without foreign body of scrotum and testes, initial encounter ♂
S31.34XA	Puncture wound with foreign body of scrotum and testes, initial encounter ♂
S31.35XA	Open bite of scrotum and testes, initial encounter ♂
S31.42XA	Laceration with foreign body of vagina and vulva, initial encounter ♀
S31.44XA	Puncture wound with foreign body of vagina and vulva, initial encounter ♀
S31.45XA	Open bite of vagina and vulva, initial encounter ♀
S61.012A	Laceration without foreign body of left thumb without damage to nail, initial encounter ☑
S61.031A	Puncture wound without foreign body of right thumb without damage to nail, initial encounter ☑
S61.042A	Puncture wound with foreign body of left thumb without damage to nail, initial encounter ☑
S61.051A	Open bite of right thumb without damage to nail, initial encounter ☑
S61.121A	Laceration with foreign body of right thumb with damage to nail, initial encounter ☑
S61.131A	Puncture wound without foreign body of right thumb with damage to nail, initial encounter ☑
S61.141A	Puncture wound with foreign body of right thumb with damage to nail, initial encounter ☑
S61.151A	Open bite of right thumb with damage to nail, initial encounter ☑
S61.210A	Laceration without foreign body of right index finger without damage to nail, initial encounter ☑

Repair

S61.212A Laceration without foreign body of right middle finger without damage to nail, initial encounter ☑

S61.217A Laceration without foreign body of left little finger without damage to nail, initial encounter ☑

S61.223A Laceration with foreign body of left middle finger without damage to nail, initial encounter ☑

S61.225A Laceration with foreign body of left ring finger without damage to nail, initial encounter ☑

S61.242A Puncture wound with foreign body of right middle finger without damage to nail, initial encounter ☑

S61.244A Puncture wound with foreign body of right ring finger without damage to nail, initial encounter ☑

S61.245A Puncture wound with foreign body of left ring finger without damage to nail, initial encounter ☑

S61.247A Puncture wound with foreign body of left little finger without damage to nail, initial encounter ☑

S61.250A Open bite of right index finger without damage to nail, initial encounter ☑

S61.252A Open bite of right middle finger without damage to nail, initial encounter ☑

S61.311A Laceration without foreign body of left index finger with damage to nail, initial encounter ☑

S61.316A Laceration without foreign body of right little finger with damage to nail, initial encounter ☑

S61.323A Laceration with foreign body of left middle finger with damage to nail, initial encounter ☑

S61.324A Laceration with foreign body of right ring finger with damage to nail, initial encounter ☑

S61.330A Puncture wound without foreign body of right index finger with damage to nail, initial encounter ☑

S61.334A Puncture wound without foreign body of right ring finger with damage to nail, initial encounter ☑

S61.337A Puncture wound without foreign body of left little finger with damage to nail, initial encounter ☑

S61.341A Puncture wound with foreign body of left index finger with damage to nail, initial encounter ☑

S61.342A Puncture wound with foreign body of right middle finger with damage to nail, initial encounter ☑

S61.351A Open bite of left index finger with damage to nail, initial encounter ☑

S61.352A Open bite of right middle finger with damage to nail, initial encounter ☑

S61.354A Open bite of right ring finger with damage to nail, initial encounter ☑

S61.357A Open bite of left little finger with damage to nail, initial encounter ☑

S61.431A Puncture wound without foreign body of right hand, initial encounter ☑

S61.442A Puncture wound with foreign body of left hand, initial encounter ☑

S61.451A Open bite of right hand, initial encounter ☑

S91.114A Laceration without foreign body of right lesser toe(s) without damage to nail, initial encounter ☑

S91.122A Laceration with foreign body of left great toe without damage to nail, initial encounter ☑

S91.124A Laceration with foreign body of right lesser toe(s) without damage to nail, initial encounter ☑

S91.132A Puncture wound without foreign body of left great toe without damage to nail, initial encounter ☑

S91.141A Puncture wound with foreign body of right great toe without damage to nail, initial encounter ☑

S91.145A Puncture wound with foreign body of left lesser toe(s) without damage to nail, initial encounter ☑

S91.152A Open bite of left great toe without damage to nail, initial encounter ☑

S91.212A Laceration without foreign body of left great toe with damage to nail, initial encounter ☑

S91.222A Laceration with foreign body of left great toe with damage to nail, initial encounter ☑

S91.241A Puncture wound with foreign body of right great toe with damage to nail, initial encounter ☑

S91.242A Puncture wound with foreign body of left great toe with damage to nail, initial encounter ☑

S91.245A Puncture wound with foreign body of left lesser toe(s) with damage to nail, initial encounter ☑

S91.251A Open bite of right great toe with damage to nail, initial encounter ☑

S91.311A Laceration without foreign body, right foot, initial encounter ☑

S91.321A Laceration with foreign body, right foot, initial encounter ☑

S91.322A Laceration with foreign body, left foot, initial encounter ☑

S91.331A Puncture wound without foreign body, right foot, initial encounter ☑

S91.341A Puncture wound with foreign body, right foot, initial encounter ☑

S91.342A Puncture wound with foreign body, left foot, initial encounter ☑

S91.351A Open bite, right foot, initial encounter ☑

AMA: **13131** 2019,Nov,3; 2018,Sep,7; 2018,Jan,8; 2017,Jan,8; 2017,Apr,9; 2016,Jan,13; 2015,Jan,16 **13132** 2019,Nov,3; 2018,Sep,7; 2018,Jan,8; 2017,Jan,8; 2017,Apr,9; 2016,Jan,13; 2015,Jan,16 **13133** 2019,Nov,3; 2018,Sep,7; 2018,Jan,8; 2017,Jan,8; 2017,Apr,9; 2016,Jan,13; 2015,Jan,16

Relative Value Units/Medicare Edits

Non-Facility RVU	Work	PE	MP	Total
13131	3.73	7.46	0.43	11.62
13132	4.78	8.81	0.49	14.08
13133	2.19	2.58	0.26	5.03
Facility RVU	Work	PE	MP	Total
13131	3.73	2.9	0.43	7.06
13132	4.78	3.52	0.49	8.79
13133	2.19	1.22	0.26	3.67

	FUD	Status	MUE	Modifiers				IOM Reference
13131	10	A	1(2)	51	N/A	N/A	N/A	None
13132	10	A	1(2)	51	N/A	N/A	N/A	
13133	N/A	A	7(3)	N/A	N/A	N/A	N/A	

* with documentation

13151-13153

13151 Repair, complex, eyelids, nose, ears and/or lips; 1.1 cm to 2.5 cm

13152 2.6 cm to 7.5 cm

+ 13153 each additional 5 cm or less (List separately in addition to code for primary procedure)

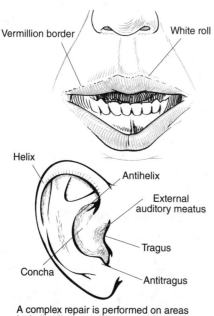

A complex repair is performed on areas including the eyelid, lips, nose, and ears

Explanation

The physician repairs complex wounds of the eyelids, nose, ears, and/or lips. The physician performs complex, layered suturing of torn, crushed, or deeply lacerated tissue. The physician debrides the wound by removing foreign material or damaged tissue. Wound irrigation is performed with an antimicrobial solution to decontaminate and cleanse the wound. The physician may trim skin margins to allow for proper closure. The wound is closed in layers. The physician may perform scar revision, which creates a complex defect requiring repair. Stents or retention sutures may also be used in complex repair. Reconstructive procedures, such as local flaps, may be required and are reported separately. Report 13151 for wounds 1.1 cm to 2.5 cm; 13152 for 2.6 cm to 7.5 cm; and 13153 for each additional 5 cm or less. A code for simple or intermediate repair is reported for wounds that are 1 cm or less.

Coding Tips

Report 13153 in addition to 13152. When reporting the repair of wounds, the sum of the lengths of repair are added together and are listed as a total for each anatomical site. For wounds 1 cm or less, see simple or intermediate repair codes. Complex wounds require additional special treatment, such as the use of stent dressings, retention sutures, or extensive revision, which may involve removing sizable portions of skin or extensive undermining of the skin to loosen the tissues to close a defect. In addition, at least one of the following is required: 1) exposure of bone, cartilage, tendon, or a named neurovascular structure, 2) extensive undermining that is at least one entire edge of the defect but a distance greater than or equal to the maximum width of the defect, measured perpendicular to the closure line, 3) involvement of free margins of helical rim, nostril rim, or vermilion border in which retention sutures are placed. When more than one repair and/or another separately identifiable procedure is performed, the highest dollar value code is listed as the primary procedure and subsequent procedures are appended with modifier 51.

ICD-10-CM Diagnostic Codes

C00.0	Malignant neoplasm of external upper lip	
C00.1	Malignant neoplasm of external lower lip	
C00.3	Malignant neoplasm of upper lip, inner aspect	
C00.4	Malignant neoplasm of lower lip, inner aspect	
C43.0	Malignant melanoma of lip	
C43.111	Malignant melanoma of right upper eyelid, including canthus	☑
C43.112	Malignant melanoma of right lower eyelid, including canthus	☑
C43.21	Malignant melanoma of right ear and external auricular canal	☑
C43.22	Malignant melanoma of left ear and external auricular canal	☑
C43.31	Malignant melanoma of nose	
C44.01	Basal cell carcinoma of skin of lip	
C44.02	Squamous cell carcinoma of skin of lip	
C44.09	Other specified malignant neoplasm of skin of lip	
C44.1121	Basal cell carcinoma of skin of right upper eyelid, including canthus ☑	
C44.1122	Basal cell carcinoma of skin of right lower eyelid, including canthus ☑	
C44.1221	Squamous cell carcinoma of skin of right upper eyelid, including canthus ☑	
C44.1222	Squamous cell carcinoma of skin of right lower eyelid, including canthus ☑	
C44.212	Basal cell carcinoma of skin of right ear and external auricular canal ☑	
C44.219	Basal cell carcinoma of skin of left ear and external auricular canal ☑	
C44.222	Squamous cell carcinoma of skin of right ear and external auricular canal ☑	
C44.229	Squamous cell carcinoma of skin of left ear and external auricular canal ☑	
C44.292	Other specified malignant neoplasm of skin of right ear and external auricular canal ☑	
C44.299	Other specified malignant neoplasm of skin of left ear and external auricular canal ☑	
C44.311	Basal cell carcinoma of skin of nose	
C44.321	Squamous cell carcinoma of skin of nose	
C44.391	Other specified malignant neoplasm of skin of nose	
C4A.0	Merkel cell carcinoma of lip	
C4A.111	Merkel cell carcinoma of right upper eyelid, including canthus ☑	
C4A.112	Merkel cell carcinoma of right lower eyelid, including canthus ☑	
C4A.21	Merkel cell carcinoma of right ear and external auricular canal ☑	
C4A.22	Merkel cell carcinoma of left ear and external auricular canal ☑	
C4A.31	Merkel cell carcinoma of nose	
D03.0	Melanoma in situ of lip	
D03.111	Melanoma in situ of right upper eyelid, including canthus ☑	
D03.112	Melanoma in situ of right lower eyelid, including canthus ☑	
D03.21	Melanoma in situ of right ear and external auricular canal ☑	
D03.22	Melanoma in situ of left ear and external auricular canal ☑	
D04.0	Carcinoma in situ of skin of lip	
D04.111	Carcinoma in situ of skin of right upper eyelid, including canthus ☑	
D04.112	Carcinoma in situ of skin of right lower eyelid, including canthus ☑	

Repair

D04.21	Carcinoma in situ of skin of right ear and external auricular canal ☑
D04.22	Carcinoma in situ of skin of left ear and external auricular canal ☑
D10.0	Benign neoplasm of lip
D22.0	Melanocytic nevi of lip
D22.111	Melanocytic nevi of right upper eyelid, including canthus ☑
D22.112	Melanocytic nevi of right lower eyelid, including canthus ☑
D22.21	Melanocytic nevi of right ear and external auricular canal ☑
D22.22	Melanocytic nevi of left ear and external auricular canal ☑
D23.0	Other benign neoplasm of skin of lip
D23.111	Other benign neoplasm of skin of right upper eyelid, including canthus ☑
D23.112	Other benign neoplasm of skin of right lower eyelid, including canthus ☑
D23.21	Other benign neoplasm of skin of right ear and external auricular canal ☑
D23.22	Other benign neoplasm of skin of left ear and external auricular canal ☑
D37.01	Neoplasm of uncertain behavior of lip
S01.111A	Laceration without foreign body of right eyelid and periocular area, initial encounter ☑
S01.112A	Laceration without foreign body of left eyelid and periocular area, initial encounter ☑
S01.121A	Laceration with foreign body of right eyelid and periocular area, initial encounter ☑
S01.122A	Laceration with foreign body of left eyelid and periocular area, initial encounter ☑
S01.131A	Puncture wound without foreign body of right eyelid and periocular area, initial encounter ☑
S01.132A	Puncture wound without foreign body of left eyelid and periocular area, initial encounter ☑
S01.141A	Puncture wound with foreign body of right eyelid and periocular area, initial encounter ☑
S01.142A	Puncture wound with foreign body of left eyelid and periocular area, initial encounter ☑
S01.151A	Open bite of right eyelid and periocular area, initial encounter ☑
S01.152A	Open bite of left eyelid and periocular area, initial encounter ☑
S01.21XA	Laceration without foreign body of nose, initial encounter
S01.22XA	Laceration with foreign body of nose, initial encounter
S01.23XA	Puncture wound without foreign body of nose, initial encounter
S01.24XA	Puncture wound with foreign body of nose, initial encounter
S01.25XA	Open bite of nose, initial encounter
S01.311A	Laceration without foreign body of right ear, initial encounter ☑
S01.312A	Laceration without foreign body of left ear, initial encounter ☑
S01.321A	Laceration with foreign body of right ear, initial encounter ☑
S01.322A	Laceration with foreign body of left ear, initial encounter ☑
S01.331A	Puncture wound without foreign body of right ear, initial encounter ☑
S01.332A	Puncture wound without foreign body of left ear, initial encounter ☑
S01.341A	Puncture wound with foreign body of right ear, initial encounter ☑
S01.342A	Puncture wound with foreign body of left ear, initial encounter ☑
S01.351A	Open bite of right ear, initial encounter ☑
S01.352A	Open bite of left ear, initial encounter ☑
S01.511A	Laceration without foreign body of lip, initial encounter
S01.521A	Laceration with foreign body of lip, initial encounter
S01.531A	Puncture wound without foreign body of lip, initial encounter
S01.541A	Puncture wound with foreign body of lip, initial/encounter
S01.551A	Open bite of lip, initial encounter
S08.111A	Complete traumatic amputation of right ear, initial encounter ☑
S08.112A	Complete traumatic amputation of left ear, initial encounter ☑
S08.121A	Partial traumatic amputation of right ear, initial encounter ☑
S08.122A	Partial traumatic amputation of left ear, initial encounter ☑
S08.811A	Complete traumatic amputation of nose, initial encounter
S08.812A	Partial traumatic amputation of nose, initial encounter
S09.311A	Primary blast injury of right ear, initial encounter ☑
S09.312A	Primary blast injury of left ear, initial encounter ☑
S09.313A	Primary blast injury of ear, bilateral, initial encounter ☑

AMA: **13151** 2019,Nov,3; 2018,Sep,7; 2018,Jan,8; 2017,Jan,8; 2016,Jan,13; 2015,Jan,16 **13152** 2019,Nov,3; 2018,Sep,7; 2018,Jan,8; 2017,Jan,8; 2016,Jan,13; 2015,Jan,16 **13153** 2019,Nov,3; 2018,Sep,7; 2018,Jan,8; 2017,Jan,8; 2016,Jan,13; 2015,Jan,16

Relative Value Units/Medicare Edits

Non-Facility RVU	Work	PE	MP	Total
13151	4.34	7.79	0.51	12.64
13152	5.34	8.93	0.61	14.88
13153	2.38	2.8	0.34	5.52
Facility RVU	Work	PE	MP	Total
13151	4.34	3.26	0.51	8.11
13152	5.34	3.83	0.61	9.78
13153	2.38	1.28	0.34	4.0

	FUD	Status	MUE	Modifiers				IOM Reference
13151	10	A	1(2)	51	N/A	N/A	N/A	None
13152	10	A	1(2)	51	N/A	N/A	N/A	
13153	N/A	A	2(3)	N/A	N/A	N/A	N/A	

* with documentation

Terms To Know

complex repair. Surgical closure of a wound requiring more than layered closure of the deeper subcutaneous tissue and fascia (i.e., exposed bone, cartilage, tendon, neurovascular structure, margins of helical rim, vermilion border or nostril rim, debridement, scar excision, placement of stents or retention sutures, and sometimes site preparation or extensive undermining that creates the defect requiring complex closure).

debride. To remove all foreign objects and devitalized or infected tissue from a burn or wound to prevent infection and promote healing.

irrigation. To wash out or cleanse a body cavity, wound, or tissue with water or other fluid.

reconstruction. Recreating, restoring, or rebuilding a body part or organ.

13160

13160 Secondary closure of surgical wound or dehiscence, extensive or complicated

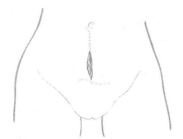

An extensive or complicated surgical wound is closed secondarily or extensive or complicated dehiscence is treated and closed

Explanation

The physician secondarily repairs a surgical skin closure after an infectious breakdown of the healing skin. After resolution of the infection, the wound is now ready for closure. The physician uses a scalpel to excise granulation and scar tissue. Skin margins are trimmed to bleeding edges. The wound is sutured in several layers.

Coding Tips

For simple closure of secondary wound dehiscence, see 12020; with packing, see 12021. If incision and drainage of a hematoma, seroma, or fluid collection is performed, see 10140. Do not report 13160 with 11960. Surgical trays, A4550, are not separately reimbursed by Medicare; however, other third-party payers may cover them. Check with the specific payer to determine coverage.

ICD-10-CM Diagnostic Codes

T81.31XA	Disruption of external operation (surgical) wound, not elsewhere classified, initial encounter
T81.32XA	Disruption of internal operation (surgical) wound, not elsewhere classified, initial encounter
Z48.1	Encounter for planned postprocedural wound closure

AMA: **13160** 2019,Nov,3; 2018,Jan,8; 2017,Jan,8; 2016,Jan,13; 2015,Jan,16

Relative Value Units/Medicare Edits

Non-Facility RVU	Work	PE	MP	Total
13160	12.04	9.29	2.07	23.4
Facility RVU	Work	PE	MP	Total
13160	12.04	9.29	2.07	23.4

	FUD	Status	MUE	Modifiers				IOM Reference
13160	90	A	2(3)	51	N/A	N/A	N/A	None

* with documentation

15002-15003

15002 Surgical preparation or creation of recipient site by excision of open wounds, burn eschar, or scar (including subcutaneous tissues), or incisional release of scar contracture, trunk, arms, legs; first 100 sq cm or 1% of body area of infants and children

+ **15003** each additional 100 sq cm, or part thereof, or each additional 1% of body area of infants and children (List separately in addition to code for primary procedure)

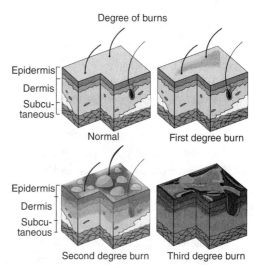

Degree of burns

Epidermis
Dermis
Subcu-
taneous

Normal   First degree burn

Epidermis
Dermis
Subcu-
taneous

Second degree burn   Third degree burn

Explanation

The physician prepares tissue to receive a free skin graft needed to close or repair a defect. Skin, subcutaneous tissue, scars, burn eschar, and lesions are excised to provide a healthy, vascular tissue bed (where new vessels have been formed) onto which a skin graft will be placed. Alternatively, the physician may prepare tissue by incising or excising a scar contracture that is causing excessive tightening of the skin. Simple debridement of granulations or of recent avulsion is included. Report 15002 for the first 100 sq cm or 1 percent of body area of infants and children for grafts of the trunk arms and legs. Report 15003 for each additional 100 sq cm (or part thereof) of graft area or each additional 1 percent of surface body area in infants and children within the same areas.

Coding Tips

Report 15003 in addition to 15002. These procedures are for preparation or creation of the recipient site only and should be reported with the appropriate skin graft/replacement codes, see 15050–15261 and 15271–15278. For linear scar revision, see 13100–13153. Surgical trays, A4550, are not separately reimbursed by Medicare; however, other third-party payers may cover them. Check with the specific payer to determine coverage.

ICD-10-CM Diagnostic Codes

C43.52	Malignant melanoma of skin of breast
C43.61	Malignant melanoma of right upper limb, including shoulder ☑
C43.71	Malignant melanoma of right lower limb, including hip ☑
C44.511	Basal cell carcinoma of skin of breast
C44.521	Squamous cell carcinoma of skin of breast
C44.591	Other specified malignant neoplasm of skin of breast
C44.612	Basal cell carcinoma of skin of right upper limb, including shoulder ☑

Repair

C44.622	Squamous cell carcinoma of skin of right upper limb, including shoulder ☑
C44.712	Basal cell carcinoma of skin of right lower limb, including hip ☑
C44.722	Squamous cell carcinoma of skin of right lower limb, including hip ☑
C4A.52	Merkel cell carcinoma of skin of breast
C4A.59	Merkel cell carcinoma of other part of trunk
C4A.61	Merkel cell carcinoma of right upper limb, including shoulder ☑
D03.61	Melanoma in situ of right upper limb, including shoulder ☑
D03.71	Melanoma in situ of right lower limb, including hip ☑
D04.5	Carcinoma in situ of skin of trunk
D22.71	Melanocytic nevi of right lower limb, including hip ☑
L89.013	Pressure ulcer of right elbow, stage 3 ☑
L89.014	Pressure ulcer of right elbow, stage 4 ☑
L89.113	Pressure ulcer of right upper back, stage 3 ☑
L89.114	Pressure ulcer of right upper back, stage 4 ☑
L89.116	Pressure-induced deep tissue damage of right upper back ☑
L89.133	Pressure ulcer of right lower back, stage 3 ☑
L89.134	Pressure ulcer of right lower back, stage 4 ☑
L89.153	Pressure ulcer of sacral region, stage 3
L89.154	Pressure ulcer of sacral region, stage 4
L89.216	Pressure-induced deep tissue damage of right hip ☑
L89.314	Pressure ulcer of right buttock, stage 4 ☑
L89.316	Pressure-induced deep tissue damage of right buttock ☑
L89.513	Pressure ulcer of right ankle, stage 3 ☑
L97.112	Non-pressure chronic ulcer of right thigh with fat layer exposed ☑
L97.113	Non-pressure chronic ulcer of right thigh with necrosis of muscle ☑
L97.212	Non-pressure chronic ulcer of right calf with fat layer exposed ☑
L97.213	Non-pressure chronic ulcer of right calf with necrosis of muscle ☑
L97.214	Non-pressure chronic ulcer of right calf with necrosis of bone ☑
L97.313	Non-pressure chronic ulcer of right ankle with necrosis of muscle ☑
L97.314	Non-pressure chronic ulcer of right ankle with necrosis of bone ☑
L97.812	Non-pressure chronic ulcer of other part of right lower leg with fat layer exposed ☑
L97.813	Non-pressure chronic ulcer of other part of right lower leg with necrosis of muscle ☑
L97.814	Non-pressure chronic ulcer of other part of right lower leg with necrosis of bone ☑
L98.413	Non-pressure chronic ulcer of buttock with necrosis of muscle
L98.414	Non-pressure chronic ulcer of buttock with necrosis of bone
L98.422	Non-pressure chronic ulcer of back with fat layer exposed
L98.423	Non-pressure chronic ulcer of back with necrosis of muscle
S21.041A	Puncture wound with foreign body of right breast, initial encounter ☑
S21.051A	Open bite of right breast, initial encounter ☑
S21.121A	Laceration with foreign body of right front wall of thorax without penetration into thoracic cavity, initial encounter
S21.151A	Open bite of right front wall of thorax without penetration into thoracic cavity, initial encounter
S21.211A	Laceration without foreign body of right back wall of thorax without penetration into thoracic cavity, initial encounter
S21.241A	Puncture wound with foreign body of right back wall of thorax without penetration into thoracic cavity, initial encounter
S28.1XXA	Traumatic amputation (partial) of part of thorax, except breast, initial encounter
S28.211A	Complete traumatic amputation of right breast, initial encounter ☑
S29.021A	Laceration of muscle and tendon of front wall of thorax, initial encounter
S31.815A	Open bite of right buttock, initial encounter ☑
S41.121A	Laceration with foreign body of right upper arm, initial encounter ☑
S41.141A	Puncture wound with foreign body of right upper arm, initial encounter ☑
S41.151A	Open bite of right upper arm, initial encounter ☑
S48.011A	Complete traumatic amputation at right shoulder joint, initial encounter ☑
S48.021A	Partial traumatic amputation at right shoulder joint, initial encounter ☑
S51.021A	Laceration with foreign body of right elbow, initial encounter ☑
S51.841A	Puncture wound with foreign body of right forearm, initial encounter ☑
S58.011A	Complete traumatic amputation at elbow level, right arm, initial encounter ☑
S58.021A	Partial traumatic amputation at elbow level, right arm, initial encounter ☑
S58.111A	Complete traumatic amputation at level between elbow and wrist, right arm, initial encounter ☑
S61.521A	Laceration with foreign body of right wrist, initial encounter ☑
S61.551A	Open bite of right wrist, initial encounter ☑
S68.411A	Complete traumatic amputation of right hand at wrist level, initial encounter ☑
S71.011A	Laceration without foreign body, right hip, initial encounter ☑
S71.021A	Laceration with foreign body, right hip, initial encounter ☑
S71.041A	Puncture wound with foreign body, right hip, initial encounter ☑
S71.111A	Laceration without foreign body, right thigh, initial encounter ☑
S71.151A	Open bite, right thigh, initial encounter ☑
S78.011A	Complete traumatic amputation at right hip joint, initial encounter ☑
S81.021A	Laceration with foreign body, right knee, initial encounter ☑
S81.031A	Puncture wound without foreign body, right knee, initial encounter ☑
S81.051A	Open bite, right knee, initial encounter ☑
S81.821A	Laceration with foreign body, right lower leg, initial encounter ☑
S81.831A	Puncture wound without foreign body, right lower leg, initial encounter ☑
S88.011A	Complete traumatic amputation at knee level, right lower leg, initial encounter ☑
S88.111A	Complete traumatic amputation at level between knee and ankle, right lower leg, initial encounter ☑
S88.121A	Partial traumatic amputation at level between knee and ankle, right lower leg, initial encounter ☑
S91.021A	Laceration with foreign body of right ankle, initial encounter ☑
S91.031A	Puncture wound without foreign body of right ankle, initial encounter ☑
T21.31XA	Burn of third degree of chest wall, initial encounter
T21.32XA	Burn of third degree of abdominal wall, initial encounter

T21.33XA	Burn of third degree of upper back, initial encounter
T21.71XA	Corrosion of third degree of chest wall, initial encounter
T21.72XA	Corrosion of third degree of abdominal wall, initial encounter
T21.74XA	Corrosion of third degree of lower back, initial encounter
T21.75XA	Corrosion of third degree of buttock, initial encounter
T22.321A	Burn of third degree of right elbow, initial encounter ☑
T22.331A	Burn of third degree of right upper arm, initial encounter ☑
T22.391A	Burn of third degree of multiple sites of right shoulder and upper limb, except wrist and hand, initial encounter ☑
T22.721A	Corrosion of third degree of right elbow, initial encounter ☑
T22.751A	Corrosion of third degree of right shoulder, initial encounter ☑
T24.321A	Burn of third degree of right knee, initial encounter ☑
T24.731A	Corrosion of third degree of right lower leg, initial encounter ☑

AMA: 15002 2019,Nov,3; 2018,Jan,8; 2017,Jan,8; 2016,Jan,13; 2015,Jan,16
15003 2019,Nov,3; 2018,Jan,8; 2017,Jan,8; 2016,Jan,13; 2015,Jan,16

Relative Value Units/Medicare Edits

Non-Facility RVU	Work	PE	MP	Total
15002	3.65	6.16	0.64	10.45
15003	0.8	1.16	0.16	2.12
Facility RVU	**Work**	**PE**	**MP**	**Total**
15002	3.65	2.17	0.64	6.46
15003	0.8	0.37	0.16	1.33

	FUD	Status	MUE	Modifiers				IOM Reference
15002	0	A	1(2)	N/A	N/A	N/A	80*	None
15003	N/A	A	60(3)	N/A	N/A	N/A	80*	

* with documentation

Terms To Know

contracture. Shortening of muscle or connective tissue.

debridement. Removal of dead or contaminated tissue and foreign matter from a wound.

eschar. Leathery slough produced by burns.

excision. Surgical removal of an organ or tissue.

free graft. Unattached piece of skin and tissue moved to another part of the body and sutured into place to repair a defect.

granulation. Formation of small, bead-like masses of cytoplasm or granules on the surface of healing wounds of an organ, membrane, or tissue.

scar tissue. Fibrous connective tissue that forms around a wounded area or injury, composed mainly of fibroblasts or collagen fibers.

subcutaneous tissue. Sheet or wide band of adipose (fat) and areolar connective tissue in two layers attached to the dermis.

15004-15005

15004 Surgical preparation or creation of recipient site by excision of open wounds, burn eschar, or scar (including subcutaneous tissues), or incisional release of scar contracture, face, scalp, eyelids, mouth, neck, ears, orbits, genitalia, hands, feet and/or multiple digits; first 100 sq cm or 1% of body area of infants and children

+ 15005 each additional 100 sq cm, or part thereof, or each additional 1% of body area of infants and children (List separately in addition to code for primary procedure)

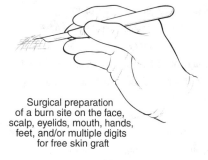

Surgical preparation of a burn site on the face, scalp, eyelids, mouth, hands, feet, and/or multiple digits for free skin graft

A recipient site is surgically prepared through excision of tissues

Explanation

The physician prepares tissue to receive a free skin graft needed to close or repair a defect. Skin, subcutaneous tissue, scars, burn eschar, and lesions are excised to provide a healthy, vascular tissue bed (where new vessels have been formed) onto which a skin graft will be placed. Alternatively, the physician may prepare tissue by incising or excising a scar contracture that is causing excessive tightening of the skin. Simple debridement of granulations or of recent avulsion is included. Report 15004 for the first 100 sq cm or 1 percent of body area in infants and children of the face, scalp, eyelids, mouth, neck, ears, orbits, genitalia, hands, and/or feet. Report 15005 for each additional 100 sq cm (or part thereof) or each additional 1 percent of body area in infants and children.

Coding Tips

Report 15005 in addition to 15004. These procedures are for preparation or creation of the recipient site only and should be reported with the appropriate skin graft/replacement codes, see 15050–15261 and 15271–15278. Surgical trays, A4550, are not separately reimbursed by Medicare; however, other third-party payers may cover them. Check with the specific payer to determine coverage.

ICD-10-CM Diagnostic Codes

C43.0	Malignant melanoma of lip
C43.111	Malignant melanoma of right upper eyelid, including canthus ☑
C43.112	Malignant melanoma of right lower eyelid, including canthus ☑
C43.21	Malignant melanoma of right ear and external auricular canal ☑
C43.31	Malignant melanoma of nose
C43.4	Malignant melanoma of scalp and neck
C44.01	Basal cell carcinoma of skin of lip
C44.02	Squamous cell carcinoma of skin of lip
C44.1121	Basal cell carcinoma of skin of right upper eyelid, including canthus ☑

Repair

C44.1122	Basal cell carcinoma of skin of right lower eyelid, including canthus ☑
C44.1221	Squamous cell carcinoma of skin of right upper eyelid, including canthus ☑
C44.1222	Squamous cell carcinoma of skin of right lower eyelid, including canthus ☑
C44.212	Basal cell carcinoma of skin of right ear and external auricular canal ☑
C44.222	Squamous cell carcinoma of skin of right ear and external auricular canal ☑
C44.292	Other specified malignant neoplasm of skin of right ear and external auricular canal ☑
C44.311	Basal cell carcinoma of skin of nose
C44.321	Squamous cell carcinoma of skin of nose
C44.41	Basal cell carcinoma of skin of scalp and neck
C44.42	Squamous cell carcinoma of skin of scalp and neck
C49.0	Malignant neoplasm of connective and soft tissue of head, face and neck
C4A.0	Merkel cell carcinoma of lip
C4A.111	Merkel cell carcinoma of right upper eyelid, including canthus ☑
C4A.112	Merkel cell carcinoma of right lower eyelid, including canthus ☑
C4A.21	Merkel cell carcinoma of right ear and external auricular canal ☑
C4A.31	Merkel cell carcinoma of nose
C4A.4	Merkel cell carcinoma of scalp and neck
C76.0	Malignant neoplasm of head, face and neck
D03.4	Melanoma in situ of scalp and neck
D04.0	Carcinoma in situ of skin of lip
D04.21	Carcinoma in situ of skin of right ear and external auricular canal ☑
D04.4	Carcinoma in situ of skin of scalp and neck
D10.0	Benign neoplasm of lip
D17.0	Benign lipomatous neoplasm of skin and subcutaneous tissue of head, face and neck
D21.0	Benign neoplasm of connective and other soft tissue of head, face and neck
D22.0	Melanocytic nevi of lip
D23.0	Other benign neoplasm of skin of lip
D23.4	Other benign neoplasm of skin of scalp and neck
S01.22XA	Laceration with foreign body of nose, initial encounter
S01.311A	Laceration without foreign body of right ear, initial encounter ☑
S01.321A	Laceration with foreign body of right ear, initial encounter ☑
S01.341A	Puncture wound with foreign body of right ear, initial encounter ☑
S01.351A	Open bite of right ear, initial encounter ☑
S01.411A	Laceration without foreign body of right cheek and temporomandibular area, initial encounter ☑
S01.431A	Puncture wound without foreign body of right cheek and temporomandibular area, initial encounter ☑
S01.521A	Laceration with foreign body of lip, initial encounter
S01.551A	Open bite of lip, initial encounter
S01.82XA	Laceration with foreign body of other part of head, initial encounter
S01.85XA	Open bite of other part of head, initial encounter
S08.111A	Complete traumatic amputation of right ear, initial encounter ☑
S31.21XA	Laceration without foreign body of penis, initial encounter ♂

S31.25XA	Open bite of penis, initial encounter ♂
S31.31XA	Laceration without foreign body of scrotum and testes, initial encounter ♂
S31.41XA	Laceration without foreign body of vagina and vulva, initial encounter ♀
S31.42XA	Laceration with foreign body of vagina and vulva, initial encounter ♀
S31.43XA	Puncture wound without foreign body of vagina and vulva, initial encounter ♀
S61.011A	Laceration without foreign body of right thumb without damage to nail, initial encounter ☑
S61.216A	Laceration without foreign body of right little finger without damage to nail, initial encounter ☑
S61.224A	Laceration with foreign body of right ring finger without damage to nail, initial encounter ☑
S61.242A	Puncture wound with foreign body of right middle finger without damage to nail, initial encounter ☑
S61.244A	Puncture wound with foreign body of right ring finger without damage to nail, initial encounter ☑
S61.310A	Laceration without foreign body of right index finger with damage to nail, initial encounter ☑
S61.312A	Laceration without foreign body of right middle finger with damage to nail, initial encounter ☑
S61.322A	Laceration with foreign body of right middle finger with damage to nail, initial encounter ☑
S61.326A	Laceration with foreign body of right little finger with damage to nail, initial encounter ☑
S61.340A	Puncture wound with foreign body of right index finger with damage to nail, initial encounter ☑
S61.350A	Open bite of right index finger with damage to nail, initial encounter ☑
S61.354A	Open bite of right ring finger with damage to nail, initial encounter ☑
S61.431A	Puncture wound without foreign body of right hand, initial encounter ☑
S66.091A	Other specified injury of long flexor muscle, fascia and tendon of right thumb at wrist and hand level, initial encounter ☑
S66.196A	Other injury of flexor muscle, fascia and tendon of right little finger at wrist and hand level, initial encounter ☑
S91.221A	Laceration with foreign body of right great toe with damage to nail, initial encounter ☑
S91.234A	Puncture wound without foreign body of right lesser toe(s) with damage to nail, initial encounter ☑
S91.244A	Puncture wound with foreign body of right lesser toe(s) with damage to nail, initial encounter ☑
S91.251A	Open bite of right great toe with damage to nail, initial encounter ☑
S91.254A	Open bite of right lesser toe(s) with damage to nail, initial encounter ☑
S91.331A	Puncture wound without foreign body, right foot, initial encounter ☑
S91.341A	Puncture wound with foreign body, right foot, initial encounter ☑
S96.091A	Other injury of muscle and tendon of long flexor muscle of toe at ankle and foot level, right foot, initial encounter ☑
S96.891A	Other specified injury of other specified muscles and tendons at ankle and foot level, right foot, initial encounter ☑

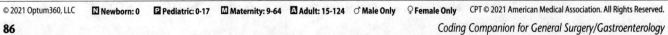

T20.311A	Burn of third degree of right ear [any part, except ear drum], initial encounter ☑
T20.32XA	Burn of third degree of lip(s), initial encounter
T20.33XA	Burn of third degree of chin, initial encounter
T20.36XA	Burn of third degree of forehead and cheek, initial encounter
T20.37XA	Burn of third degree of neck, initial encounter
T20.711A	Corrosion of third degree of right ear [any part, except ear drum], initial encounter ☑
T20.75XA	Corrosion of third degree of scalp [any part], initial encounter
T20.76XA	Corrosion of third degree of forehead and cheek, initial encounter
T21.37XA	Burn of third degree of female genital region, initial encounter ♀
T21.76XA	Corrosion of third degree of male genital region, initial encounter ♂
T22.341A	Burn of third degree of right axilla, initial encounter ☑
T23.321A	Burn of third degree of single right finger (nail) except thumb, initial encounter ☑
T23.331A	Burn of third degree of multiple right fingers (nail), not including thumb, initial encounter ☑
T23.351A	Burn of third degree of right palm, initial encounter ☑
T23.361A	Burn of third degree of back of right hand, initial encounter ☑
T25.321A	Burn of third degree of right foot, initial encounter ☑
T25.711A	Corrosion of third degree of right ankle, initial encounter ☑
T25.721A	Corrosion of third degree of right foot, initial encounter ☑
T25.731A	Corrosion of third degree of right toe(s) (nail), initial encounter ☑

AMA: 15004 2019,Nov,3; 2018,Jan,8; 2017,Jan,8; 2016,Jan,13; 2015,Jan,16
15005 2019,Nov,3; 2018,Jan,8; 2017,Jan,8; 2016,Jan,13; 2015,Jan,16

Relative Value Units/Medicare Edits

Non-Facility RVU	Work	PE	MP	Total
15004	4.58	6.61	0.64	11.83
15005	1.6	1.62	0.32	3.54
Facility RVU	**Work**	**PE**	**MP**	**Total**
15004	4.58	2.44	0.64	7.66
15005	1.6	0.75	0.32	2.67

	FUD	Status	MUE	Modifiers				IOM Reference
15004	0	A	1(2)	N/A	N/A	N/A	80*	None
15005	N/A	A	19(3)	N/A	N/A	N/A	80*	

* with documentation

Terms To Know

contracture. Shortening of muscle or connective tissue.

eschar. Leathery slough produced by burns.

granulation. Formation of small, bead-like masses of cytoplasm or granules on the surface of healing wounds of an organ, membrane, or tissue.

15100-15101

| 15100 | Split-thickness autograft, trunk, arms, legs; first 100 sq cm or less, or 1% of body area of infants and children (except 15050) |
| + 15101 | each additional 100 sq cm, or each additional 1% of body area of infants and children, or part thereof (List separately in addition to code for primary procedure) |

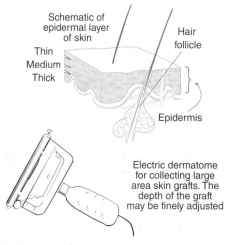

Schematic of epidermal layer of skin

Hair follicle

Thin
Medium
Thick

Epidermis

Electric dermatome for collecting large area skin grafts. The depth of the graft may be finely adjusted

A split thickness skin graft is harvested and applied

Explanation

The physician takes a split-thickness skin autograft from one area of the body and grafts it to an area needing repair. This procedure is performed when direct wound closure or adjacent tissue transfer is not possible. The physician harvests a split-thickness skin graft with a dermatome. The epidermis or top layer of skin is taken, along with a small portion of the dermis or bottom layer of the skin. This graft is applied to the recipient area on the trunk, arms, or legs. Report 15100 for the first 100 sq cm or less in adults or 1 percent of the total body area of infants and children. Report 15101 for each additional 100 sq cm or each additional 1 percent of the total body area in infants and children.

Coding Tips

Report 15101 in addition to 15100. Preparation of the recipient site is reported separately, see 15002–15003. Repair of the donor site requiring skin grafts or local flaps is added as an additional procedure. Surgical trays, A4550, are not separately reimbursed by Medicare; however, other third-party payers may cover them. Check with the specific payer to determine coverage.

ICD-10-CM Diagnostic Codes

C43.51	Malignant melanoma of anal skin
C43.52	Malignant melanoma of skin of breast
C43.59	Malignant melanoma of other part of trunk
C43.61	Malignant melanoma of right upper limb, including shoulder ☑
C44.510	Basal cell carcinoma of anal skin
C44.511	Basal cell carcinoma of skin of breast
C44.519	Basal cell carcinoma of skin of other part of trunk
C44.520	Squamous cell carcinoma of anal skin
C44.521	Squamous cell carcinoma of skin of breast
C44.529	Squamous cell carcinoma of skin of other part of trunk
C44.590	Other specified malignant neoplasm of anal skin
C44.591	Other specified malignant neoplasm of skin of breast

Repair

C44.599	Other specified malignant neoplasm of skin of other part of trunk
C44.629	Squamous cell carcinoma of skin of left upper limb, including shoulder ☑
C44.719	Basal cell carcinoma of skin of left lower limb, including hip ☑
C44.729	Squamous cell carcinoma of skin of left lower limb, including hip ☑
C4A.4	Merkel cell carcinoma of scalp and neck
C4A.51	Merkel cell carcinoma of anal skin
C4A.52	Merkel cell carcinoma of skin of breast
C4A.59	Merkel cell carcinoma of other part of trunk
D03.4	Melanoma in situ of scalp and neck
D03.51	Melanoma in situ of anal skin
D03.52	Melanoma in situ of breast (skin) (soft tissue)
D03.59	Melanoma in situ of other part of trunk
D04.5	Carcinoma in situ of skin of trunk
D22.5	Melanocytic nevi of trunk
D22.71	Melanocytic nevi of right lower limb, including hip ☑
L89.013	Pressure ulcer of right elbow, stage 3 ☑
L89.014	Pressure ulcer of right elbow, stage 4 ☑
L89.116	Pressure-induced deep tissue damage of right upper back ☑
L89.124	Pressure ulcer of left upper back, stage 4 ☑
L89.136	Pressure-induced deep tissue damage of right lower back ☑
L89.143	Pressure ulcer of left lower back, stage 3 ☑
L89.144	Pressure ulcer of left lower back, stage 4 ☑
L89.154	Pressure ulcer of sacral region, stage 4
L89.224	Pressure ulcer of left hip, stage 4 ☑
L89.313	Pressure ulcer of right buttock, stage 3 ☑
L89.314	Pressure ulcer of right buttock, stage 4 ☑
L89.316	Pressure-induced deep tissue damage of right buttock ☑
L89.323	Pressure ulcer of left buttock, stage 3 ☑
L89.324	Pressure ulcer of left buttock, stage 4 ☑
L89.43	Pressure ulcer of contiguous site of back, buttock and hip, stage 3
L89.44	Pressure ulcer of contiguous site of back, buttock and hip, stage 4
L89.513	Pressure ulcer of right ankle, stage 3 ☑
L89.514	Pressure ulcer of right ankle, stage 4 ☑
L89.516	Pressure-induced deep tissue damage of right ankle ☑
L97.115	Non-pressure chronic ulcer of right thigh with muscle involvement without evidence of necrosis ☑
L97.116	Non-pressure chronic ulcer of right thigh with bone involvement without evidence of necrosis ☑
L97.213	Non-pressure chronic ulcer of right calf with necrosis of muscle ☑
L97.214	Non-pressure chronic ulcer of right calf with necrosis of bone ☑
L97.225	Non-pressure chronic ulcer of left calf with muscle involvement without evidence of necrosis ☑
L97.226	Non-pressure chronic ulcer of left calf with bone involvement without evidence of necrosis ☑
L97.312	Non-pressure chronic ulcer of right ankle with fat layer exposed ☑
L97.313	Non-pressure chronic ulcer of right ankle with necrosis of muscle ☑
L97.314	Non-pressure chronic ulcer of right ankle with necrosis of bone ☑
L97.326	Non-pressure chronic ulcer of left ankle with bone involvement without evidence of necrosis ☑
L97.415	Non-pressure chronic ulcer of right heel and midfoot with muscle involvement without evidence of necrosis ☑
L97.416	Non-pressure chronic ulcer of right heel and midfoot with bone involvement without evidence of necrosis ☑
L98.411	Non-pressure chronic ulcer of buttock limited to breakdown of skin
L98.412	Non-pressure chronic ulcer of buttock with fat layer exposed
L98.413	Non-pressure chronic ulcer of buttock with necrosis of muscle
L98.414	Non-pressure chronic ulcer of buttock with necrosis of bone
L98.421	Non-pressure chronic ulcer of back limited to breakdown of skin
S21.021A	Laceration with foreign body of right breast, initial encounter ☑
S21.111A	Laceration without foreign body of right front wall of thorax without penetration into thoracic cavity, initial encounter
S21.222A	Laceration with foreign body of left back wall of thorax without penetration into thoracic cavity, initial encounter
S28.212A	Complete traumatic amputation of left breast, initial encounter ☑
S28.222A	Partial traumatic amputation of left breast, initial encounter ☑
S31.010A	Laceration without foreign body of lower back and pelvis without penetration into retroperitoneum, initial encounter
S31.115A	Laceration without foreign body of abdominal wall, periumbilic region without penetration into peritoneal cavity, initial encounter
S31.122A	Laceration of abdominal wall with foreign body, epigastric region without penetration into peritoneal cavity, initial encounter
S31.811A	Laceration without foreign body of right buttock, initial encounter ☑
S31.812A	Laceration with foreign body of right buttock, initial encounter ☑
S31.831A	Laceration without foreign body of anus, initial encounter
S31.832A	Laceration with foreign body of anus, initial encounter
S41.121A	Laceration with foreign body of right upper arm, initial encounter ☑
S61.511A	Laceration without foreign body of right wrist, initial encounter ☑
S61.512A	Laceration without foreign body of left wrist, initial encounter ☑
S61.521A	Laceration with foreign body of right wrist, initial encounter ☑
S61.522A	Laceration with foreign body of left wrist, initial encounter ☑
S61.541A	Puncture wound with foreign body of right wrist, initial encounter ☑
S61.542A	Puncture wound with foreign body of left wrist, initial encounter ☑
S61.551A	Open bite of right wrist, initial encounter ☑
S61.552A	Open bite of left wrist, initial encounter ☑
S71.022A	Laceration with foreign body, left hip, initial encounter ☑
S71.112A	Laceration without foreign body, left thigh, initial encounter ☑
S78.012A	Complete traumatic amputation at left hip joint, initial encounter ☑
S78.021A	Partial traumatic amputation at right hip joint, initial encounter ☑
S81.822A	Laceration with foreign body, left lower leg, initial encounter ☑
T21.35XA	Burn of third degree of buttock, initial encounter
T21.71XA	Corrosion of third degree of chest wall, initial encounter
T21.72XA	Corrosion of third degree of abdominal wall, initial encounter

Repair

T21.75XA	Corrosion of third degree of buttock, initial encounter
T22.332A	Burn of third degree of left upper arm, initial encounter ☑
T22.351A	Burn of third degree of right shoulder, initial encounter ☑
T22.711A	Corrosion of third degree of right forearm, initial encounter ☑
T22.721A	Corrosion of third degree of right elbow, initial encounter ☑
T22.732A	Corrosion of third degree of left upper arm, initial encounter ☑
T22.751A	Corrosion of third degree of right shoulder, initial encounter ☑
T24.321A	Burn of third degree of right knee, initial encounter ☑
T24.732A	Corrosion of third degree of left lower leg, initial encounter ☑

AMA: 15100 2018,Jan,8; 2017,Jan,8; 2016,Jun,8; 2016,Jan,13; 2015,Jan,16
15101 2018,Jan,8; 2017,Jan,8; 2016,Jun,8; 2016,Jan,13; 2015,Jan,16

Relative Value Units/Medicare Edits

Non-Facility RVU	Work	PE	MP	Total
15100	9.9	13.91	1.88	25.69
15101	1.72	3.61	0.34	5.67
Facility RVU	**Work**	**PE**	**MP**	**Total**
15100	9.9	9.16	1.88	20.94
15101	1.72	1.24	0.34	3.3

	FUD	Status	MUE	Modifiers				IOM Reference
15100	90	A	1(2)	51	N/A	N/A	N/A	None
15101	N/A	A	40(3)	N/A	N/A	N/A	N/A	

* with documentation

Terms To Know

adjacent tissue transfer. Rotation or advancement of skin from an adjacent area to repair or fill in a defect while maintaining attachment to original blood supply.

autograft. Any tissue harvested from one anatomical site of a person and grafted to another anatomical site of the same person. Most commonly, blood vessels, skin, tendons, fascia, and bone are used as autografts.

dermis. Skin layer found under the epidermis that contains a papillary upper layer and the deep reticular layer of collagen, vascular bed, and nerves.

epidermis. Outermost, nonvascular layer of skin that contains four to five differentiated layers depending on its body location: stratum corneum, lucidum, granulosum, spinosum, and basale.

graft. Tissue implant from another part of the body or another person.

harvest. Removal of cells or tissue from their native site to be used as a graft or transplant to another part of the donor's body or placed into another person.

15120-15121

15120 Split-thickness autograft, face, scalp, eyelids, mouth, neck, ears, orbits, genitalia, hands, feet, and/or multiple digits; first 100 sq cm or less, or 1% of body area of infants and children (except 15050)

+ 15121 each additional 100 sq cm, or each additional 1% of body area of infants and children, or part thereof (List separately in addition to code for primary procedure)

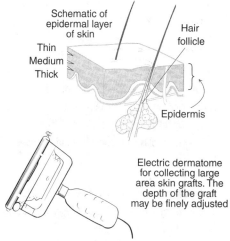

A split thickness skin graft is harvested and applied

Explanation

The physician takes a split-thickness skin autograft from one area of the body and grafts it to an area needing repair. This procedure is performed when direct wound closure or adjacent tissue transfer is not possible. The physician harvests a split-thickness skin graft with a dermatome. The epidermis or top layer of skin is taken, along with a small portion of the dermis or bottom layer of the skin. This graft is sutured or stapled onto the recipient area of the face, scalp, eyelids, neck, ears, orbits, mouth, genitalia, hands, feet, and/or multiple digits. Report 15120 for the first 100 sq cm or less in adults or children age 10 or over or 1 percent of the total body area of infants and children younger than age 10. Report 15121 for each additional 100 sq cm and each additional 1 percent of total body area of infants and children.

Coding Tips

Report 15121 in addition to 15120. Preparation of the recipient site is reported separately, see 15004–15005. Repair of the donor site requiring skin grafts or local flaps is added as an additional procedure. Local anesthesia is included in these services. However, these procedures may be performed under general anesthesia, depending on the age and/or condition of the patient. Surgical trays, A4550, are not separately reimbursed by Medicare; however, other third-party payers may cover them. Check with the specific payer to determine coverage.

ICD-10-CM Diagnostic Codes

C43.0	Malignant melanoma of lip
C43.111	Malignant melanoma of right upper eyelid, including canthus ☑
C43.112	Malignant melanoma of right lower eyelid, including canthus ☑
C43.21	Malignant melanoma of right ear and external auricular canal ☑
C43.22	Malignant melanoma of left ear and external auricular canal ☑
C43.31	Malignant melanoma of nose
C43.4	Malignant melanoma of scalp and neck

Repair

C44.01	Basal cell carcinoma of skin of lip
C44.02	Squamous cell carcinoma of skin of lip
C44.1121	Basal cell carcinoma of skin of right upper eyelid, including canthus ☑
C44.1122	Basal cell carcinoma of skin of right lower eyelid, including canthus ☑
C44.212	Basal cell carcinoma of skin of right ear and external auricular canal ☑
C44.219	Basal cell carcinoma of skin of left ear and external auricular canal ☑
C44.222	Squamous cell carcinoma of skin of right ear and external auricular canal ☑
C44.229	Squamous cell carcinoma of skin of left ear and external auricular canal ☑
C44.311	Basal cell carcinoma of skin of nose
C44.321	Squamous cell carcinoma of skin of nose
C44.41	Basal cell carcinoma of skin of scalp and neck
C44.42	Squamous cell carcinoma of skin of scalp and neck
C49.0	Malignant neoplasm of connective and soft tissue of head, face and neck
C4A.0	Merkel cell carcinoma of lip
C4A.111	Merkel cell carcinoma of right upper eyelid, including canthus ☑
C4A.112	Merkel cell carcinoma of right lower eyelid, including canthus ☑
C4A.21	Merkel cell carcinoma of right ear and external auricular canal ☑
C4A.22	Merkel cell carcinoma of left ear and external auricular canal ☑
C4A.31	Merkel cell carcinoma of nose
C4A.4	Merkel cell carcinoma of scalp and neck
C63.7	Malignant neoplasm of other specified male genital organs ♂
C76.0	Malignant neoplasm of head, face and neck
D03.0	Melanoma in situ of lip
D03.21	Melanoma in situ of right ear and external auricular canal ☑
D03.22	Melanoma in situ of left ear and external auricular canal ☑
D03.4	Melanoma in situ of scalp and neck
D04.0	Carcinoma in situ of skin of lip
D04.21	Carcinoma in situ of skin of right ear and external auricular canal ☑
D04.22	Carcinoma in situ of skin of left ear and external auricular canal ☑
D04.4	Carcinoma in situ of skin of scalp and neck
D10.0	Benign neoplasm of lip
D17.0	Benign lipomatous neoplasm of skin and subcutaneous tissue of head, face and neck
D21.0	Benign neoplasm of connective and other soft tissue of head, face and neck
D22.0	Melanocytic nevi of lip
D22.21	Melanocytic nevi of right ear and external auricular canal ☑
D22.22	Melanocytic nevi of left ear and external auricular canal ☑
D22.4	Melanocytic nevi of scalp and neck
D23.0	Other benign neoplasm of skin of lip
D37.01	Neoplasm of uncertain behavior of lip
S01.21XA	Laceration without foreign body of nose, initial encounter
S01.23XA	Puncture wound without foreign body of nose, initial encounter
S01.25XA	Open bite of nose, initial encounter
S01.311A	Laceration without foreign body of right ear, initial encounter ☑
S01.312A	Laceration without foreign body of left ear, initial encounter ☑
S01.331A	Puncture wound without foreign body of right ear, initial encounter ☑
S01.332A	Puncture wound without foreign body of left ear, initial encounter ☑
S01.351A	Open bite of right ear, initial encounter ☑
S01.352A	Open bite of left ear, initial encounter ☑
S01.412A	Laceration without foreign body of left cheek and temporomandibular area, initial encounter ☑
S01.452A	Open bite of left cheek and temporomandibular area, initial encounter ☑
S01.511A	Laceration without foreign body of lip, initial encounter
S01.531A	Puncture wound without foreign body of lip, initial encounter
S01.551A	Open bite of lip, initial encounter
S01.81XA	Laceration without foreign body of other part of head, initial encounter
S01.83XA	Puncture wound without foreign body of other part of head, initial encounter
S31.21XA	Laceration without foreign body of penis, initial encounter ♂
S31.25XA	Open bite of penis, initial encounter ♂
S31.31XA	Laceration without foreign body of scrotum and testes, initial encounter ♂
S31.35XA	Open bite of scrotum and testes, initial encounter ♂
S31.41XA	Laceration without foreign body of vagina and vulva, initial encounter ♀
S31.45XA	Open bite of vagina and vulva, initial encounter ♀
S61.011A	Laceration without foreign body of right thumb without damage to nail, initial encounter ☑
S61.031A	Puncture wound without foreign body of right thumb without damage to nail, initial encounter ☑
S61.052A	Open bite of left thumb without damage to nail, initial encounter ☑
S61.212A	Laceration without foreign body of right middle finger without damage to nail, initial encounter ☑
S61.216A	Laceration without foreign body of right little finger without damage to nail, initial encounter ☑
S61.225A	Laceration with foreign body of left ring finger without damage to nail, initial encounter ☑
S61.226A	Laceration with foreign body of right little finger without damage to nail, initial encounter ☑
S61.253A	Open bite of left middle finger without damage to nail, initial encounter ☑
S61.254A	Open bite of right ring finger without damage to nail, initial encounter ☑
S61.255A	Open bite of left ring finger without damage to nail, initial encounter ☑
S61.310A	Laceration without foreign body of right index finger with damage to nail, initial encounter ☑
S61.315A	Laceration without foreign body of left ring finger with damage to nail, initial encounter ☑
S61.355A	Open bite of left ring finger with damage to nail, initial encounter ☑
S61.356A	Open bite of right little finger with damage to nail, initial encounter ☑
S61.411A	Laceration without foreign body of right hand, initial encounter ☑
S61.452A	Open bite of left hand, initial encounter ☑

Repair

S91.112A	Laceration without foreign body of left great toe without damage to nail, initial encounter ☑	
S91.154A	Open bite of right lesser toe(s) without damage to nail, initial encounter ☑	
S91.211A	Laceration without foreign body of right great toe with damage to nail, initial encounter ☑	
S91.212A	Laceration without foreign body of left great toe with damage to nail, initial encounter ☑	
S91.252A	Open bite of left great toe with damage to nail, initial encounter ☑	
S91.254A	Open bite of right lesser toe(s) with damage to nail, initial encounter ☑	
S91.351A	Open bite, right foot, initial encounter ☑	
S91.352A	Open bite, left foot, initial encounter ☑	

AMA: 15120 2018,Jan,8; 2017,Jan,8; 2016,Jun,8; 2016,Jan,13; 2015,Jan,16 **15121** 2018,Jan,8; 2017,Jan,8; 2016,Jun,8; 2016,Jan,13; 2015,Jan,16

Relative Value Units/Medicare Edits

Non-Facility RVU	Work	PE	MP	Total
15120	10.15	13.24	1.59	24.98
15121	2.0	3.96	0.39	6.35
Facility RVU	**Work**	**PE**	**MP**	**Total**
15120	10.15	8.42	1.59	20.16
15121	2.0	1.6	0.39	3.99

	FUD	Status	MUE	Modifiers				IOM Reference
15120	90	A	1(2)	51	N/A	N/A	N/A	None
15121	N/A	A	8(3)	N/A	N/A	62*	N/A	

* with documentation

Terms To Know

autograft. Any tissue harvested from one anatomical site of a person and grafted to another anatomical site of the same person. Most commonly, blood vessels, skin, tendons, fascia, and bone are used as autografts.

dermis. Skin layer found under the epidermis that contains a papillary upper layer and the deep reticular layer of collagen, vascular bed, and nerves.

epidermis. Outermost, nonvascular layer of skin that contains four to five differentiated layers depending on its body location: stratum corneum, lucidum, granulosum, spinosum, and basale.

graft. Tissue implant from another part of the body or another person.

harvest. Removal of cells or tissue from their native site to be used as a graft or transplant to another part of the donor's body or placed into another person.

necrosis. Death of cells or tissue within a living organ or structure.

15200-15201

15200 Full thickness graft, free, including direct closure of donor site, trunk; 20 sq cm or less

+ 15201 each additional 20 sq cm, or part thereof (List separately in addition to code for primary procedure)

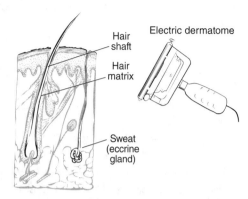

A full thickness graft (epidermis and dermis) is harvested, usually by dermatome, from a suitable area

Explanation

The physician harvests a full-thickness skin graft from one area of the body and grafts it to an area on the trunk needing repair. A full-thickness skin graft consists of the superficial and deeper layers of skin (epidermis and dermis). The resulting surgical wound at the donor site is closed by lifting the remaining skin edges and placing sutures to close directly. Residual adipose tissue is removed from the underside of the graft. The graft is sutured onto the wound bed to cover a defect of no more than 20 sq cm. Report 15201 for each additional 20 sq cm or part thereof.

Coding Tips

Report 15201 in addition to 15200. Preparation of the recipient site is reported separately, see 15002–15003. Repair of the donor site requiring skin grafts or local flaps is to be added as an additional procedure. If significant additional time and effort is documented, append modifier 22 and submit a cover letter and operative report. Local anesthesia is included in these services; however, these procedures may be performed with the patient under general anesthesia. For split-thickness grafts, see 15100 and 15101. Surgical trays, A4550, are not separately reimbursed by Medicare; however, other third-party payers may cover them. Check with the specific payer to determine coverage.

ICD-10-CM Diagnostic Codes

C43.52	Malignant melanoma of skin of breast
C44.511	Basal cell carcinoma of skin of breast
C44.519	Basal cell carcinoma of skin of other part of trunk
C44.521	Squamous cell carcinoma of skin of breast
C44.529	Squamous cell carcinoma of skin of other part of trunk
C4A.52	Merkel cell carcinoma of skin of breast
D03.52	Melanoma in situ of breast (skin) (soft tissue)
D03.59	Melanoma in situ of other part of trunk
D04.5	Carcinoma in situ of skin of trunk
D22.5	Melanocytic nevi of trunk
D23.5	Other benign neoplasm of skin of trunk
L89.113	Pressure ulcer of right upper back, stage 3 ☑
L89.114	Pressure ulcer of right upper back, stage 4 ☑
L89.116	Pressure-induced deep tissue damage of right upper back ☑

Repair

L89.133	Pressure ulcer of right lower back, stage 3 ☑	
L89.134	Pressure ulcer of right lower back, stage 4 ☑	
L89.136	Pressure-induced deep tissue damage of right lower back ☑	
L89.150	Pressure ulcer of sacral region, unstageable	
L89.153	Pressure ulcer of sacral region, stage 3	
L89.154	Pressure ulcer of sacral region, stage 4	
L89.43	Pressure ulcer of contiguous site of back, buttock and hip, stage 3	
L89.44	Pressure ulcer of contiguous site of back, buttock and hip, stage 4	
L89.45	Pressure ulcer of contiguous site of back, buttock and hip, unstageable	
L98.415	Non-pressure chronic ulcer of buttock with muscle involvement without evidence of necrosis	
L98.416	Non-pressure chronic ulcer of buttock with bone involvement without evidence of necrosis	
L98.421	Non-pressure chronic ulcer of back limited to breakdown of skin	
L98.423	Non-pressure chronic ulcer of back with necrosis of muscle	
L98.425	Non-pressure chronic ulcer of back with muscle involvement without evidence of necrosis	
L98.426	Non-pressure chronic ulcer of back with bone involvement without evidence of necrosis	
S21.011A	Laceration without foreign body of right breast, initial encounter ☑	
S21.021A	Laceration with foreign body of right breast, initial encounter ☑	
S21.051A	Open bite of right breast, initial encounter ☑	
S21.111A	Laceration without foreign body of right front wall of thorax without penetration into thoracic cavity, initial encounter	
S21.121A	Laceration with foreign body of right front wall of thorax without penetration into thoracic cavity, initial encounter	
S21.151A	Open bite of right front wall of thorax without penetration into thoracic cavity, initial encounter	
S21.211A	Laceration without foreign body of right back wall of thorax without penetration into thoracic cavity, initial encounter	
S21.212A	Laceration without foreign body of left back wall of thorax without penetration into thoracic cavity, initial encounter	
S21.221A	Laceration with foreign body of right back wall of thorax without penetration into thoracic cavity, initial encounter	
S21.251A	Open bite of right back wall of thorax without penetration into thoracic cavity, initial encounter	
S28.1XXA	Traumatic amputation (partial) of part of thorax, except breast, initial encounter	
S28.211A	Complete traumatic amputation of right breast, initial encounter ☑	
S28.221A	Partial traumatic amputation of right breast, initial encounter ☑	
S29.021A	Laceration of muscle and tendon of front wall of thorax, initial encounter	
S29.022A	Laceration of muscle and tendon of back wall of thorax, initial encounter	
S31.010A	Laceration without foreign body of lower back and pelvis without penetration into retroperitoneum, initial encounter	
S31.020A	Laceration with foreign body of lower back and pelvis without penetration into retroperitoneum, initial encounter	
S31.050A	Open bite of lower back and pelvis without penetration into retroperitoneum, initial encounter	

S31.110A	Laceration without foreign body of abdominal wall, right upper quadrant without penetration into peritoneal cavity, initial encounter ☑
S31.112A	Laceration without foreign body of abdominal wall, epigastric region without penetration into peritoneal cavity, initial encounter
S31.115A	Laceration without foreign body of abdominal wall, periumbilic region without penetration into peritoneal cavity, initial encounter
S31.120A	Laceration of abdominal wall with foreign body, right upper quadrant without penetration into peritoneal cavity, initial encounter ☑
S31.123A	Laceration of abdominal wall with foreign body, right lower quadrant without penetration into peritoneal cavity, initial encounter ☑
S31.125A	Laceration of abdominal wall with foreign body, periumbilic region without penetration into peritoneal cavity, initial encounter
S31.150A	Open bite of abdominal wall, right upper quadrant without penetration into peritoneal cavity, initial encounter ☑
S31.152A	Open bite of abdominal wall, epigastric region without penetration into peritoneal cavity, initial encounter
S39.021A	Laceration of muscle, fascia and tendon of abdomen, initial encounter
S39.022A	Laceration of muscle, fascia and tendon of lower back, initial encounter
S39.023A	Laceration of muscle, fascia and tendon of pelvis, initial encounter
T21.31XA	Burn of third degree of chest wall, initial encounter
T21.32XA	Burn of third degree of abdominal wall, initial encounter
T21.33XA	Burn of third degree of upper back, initial encounter
T21.34XA	Burn of third degree of lower back, initial encounter
T21.71XA	Corrosion of third degree of chest wall, initial encounter
T21.72XA	Corrosion of third degree of abdominal wall, initial encounter
T21.73XA	Corrosion of third degree of upper back, initial encounter
T21.74XA	Corrosion of third degree of lower back, initial encounter

AMA: 15200 2018,Jan,8; 2017,Jan,8; 2016,Jun,8; 2016,Jan,13; 2015,Jan,16
15201 2018,Jan,8; 2017,Jan,8; 2016,Jun,8; 2016,Jan,13; 2015,Jan,16

Relative Value Units/Medicare Edits

Non-Facility RVU	Work	PE	MP	Total
15200	9.15	14.02	1.52	24.69
15201	1.32	2.77	0.25	4.34
Facility RVU	Work	PE	MP	Total
15200	9.15	8.92	1.52	19.59
15201	1.32	0.7	0.25	2.27

	FUD	Status	MUE	Modifiers				IOM Reference
15200	90	A	1(2)	51	N/A	N/A	N/A	None
15201	N/A	A	7(3)	N/A	N/A	N/A	N/A	

* with documentation

Repair

15220-15221

15220 Full thickness graft, free, including direct closure of donor site, scalp, arms, and/or legs; 20 sq cm or less

+ 15221 each additional 20 sq cm, or part thereof (List separately in addition to code for primary procedure)

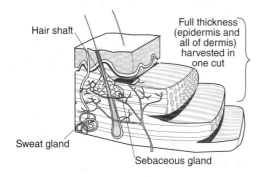

Hair shaft

Full thickness (epidermis and all of dermis) harvested in one cut

Sweat gland

Sebaceous gland

Explanation

The physician harvests a full-thickness skin graft from one area of the body and grafts it to an area on the scalp, arms, and/or legs needing repair. A full-thickness skin graft consists of the superficial and deeper layers of skin (epidermis and dermis). The resulting surgical wound at the donor site is closed by lifting the remaining skin edges and placing sutures to close directly. Residual adipose tissue is removed from the underside of the graft. The graft is sutured onto the wound bed to cover a defect of no more than 20 sq cm. Report 15221 for each additional 20 sq cm or part thereof.

Coding Tips

Report 15221 in addition to 15220. Preparation of the recipient site is reported separately, see 15002–15005. Repair of the donor site requiring skin grafts or local flaps is to be added as an additional procedure. If significant additional time and effort is documented, append modifier 22 and submit a cover letter and operative report. Local anesthesia is included in these services; however, these procedures may be performed with the patient under general anesthesia. For split-thickness grafts, see 15100 and 15101. Surgical trays, A4550, are not separately reimbursed by Medicare; however, other third-party payers may cover them. Check with the specific payer to determine coverage.

ICD-10-CM Diagnostic Codes

C43.4	Malignant melanoma of scalp and neck
C43.61	Malignant melanoma of right upper limb, including shoulder ☑
C43.71	Malignant melanoma of right lower limb, including hip ☑
C44.41	Basal cell carcinoma of skin of scalp and neck
C44.42	Squamous cell carcinoma of skin of scalp and neck
C44.612	Basal cell carcinoma of skin of right upper limb, including shoulder ☑
C44.712	Basal cell carcinoma of skin of right lower limb, including hip ☑
C44.719	Basal cell carcinoma of skin of left lower limb, including hip ☑
C44.722	Squamous cell carcinoma of skin of right lower limb, including hip ☑
C4A.61	Merkel cell carcinoma of right upper limb, including shoulder ☑
D03.4	Melanoma in situ of scalp and neck
D03.61	Melanoma in situ of right upper limb, including shoulder ☑
D03.71	Melanoma in situ of right lower limb, including hip ☑
D04.61	Carcinoma in situ of skin of right upper limb, including shoulder ☑
D04.62	Carcinoma in situ of skin of left upper limb, including shoulder ☑
D22.4	Melanocytic nevi of scalp and neck
D22.61	Melanocytic nevi of right upper limb, including shoulder ☑
D22.72	Melanocytic nevi of left lower limb, including hip ☑
L89.010	Pressure ulcer of right elbow, unstageable ☑
L89.014	Pressure ulcer of right elbow, stage 4 ☑
L89.216	Pressure-induced deep tissue damage of right hip ☑
L89.223	Pressure ulcer of left hip, stage 3 ☑
L89.316	Pressure-induced deep tissue damage of right buttock ☑
L89.43	Pressure ulcer of contiguous site of back, buttock and hip, stage 3
L89.513	Pressure ulcer of right ankle, stage 3 ☑
L97.123	Non-pressure chronic ulcer of left thigh with necrosis of muscle ☑
L97.212	Non-pressure chronic ulcer of right calf with fat layer exposed ☑
L97.313	Non-pressure chronic ulcer of right ankle with necrosis of muscle ☑
L97.314	Non-pressure chronic ulcer of right ankle with necrosis of bone ☑
L97.322	Non-pressure chronic ulcer of left ankle with fat layer exposed ☑
L97.324	Non-pressure chronic ulcer of left ankle with necrosis of bone ☑
L97.812	Non-pressure chronic ulcer of other part of right lower leg with fat layer exposed ☑
L97.814	Non-pressure chronic ulcer of other part of right lower leg with necrosis of bone ☑
L97.821	Non-pressure chronic ulcer of other part of left lower leg limited to breakdown of skin ☑
L97.824	Non-pressure chronic ulcer of other part of left lower leg with necrosis of bone ☑
S01.01XA	Laceration without foreign body of scalp, initial encounter
S01.02XA	Laceration with foreign body of scalp, initial encounter
S01.05XA	Open bite of scalp, initial encounter
S08.0XXA	Avulsion of scalp, initial encounter
S41.112A	Laceration without foreign body of left upper arm, initial encounter ☑
S41.122A	Laceration with foreign body of left upper arm, initial encounter ☑
S41.151A	Open bite of right upper arm, initial encounter ☑
S48.022A	Partial traumatic amputation at left shoulder joint, initial encounter ☑
S48.121A	Partial traumatic amputation at level between right shoulder and elbow, initial encounter ☑
S51.011A	Laceration without foreign body of right elbow, initial encounter ☑
S51.021A	Laceration with foreign body of right elbow, initial encounter ☑
S51.022A	Laceration with foreign body of left elbow, initial encounter ☑
S51.052A	Open bite, left elbow, initial encounter ☑
S51.812A	Laceration without foreign body of left forearm, initial encounter ☑
S51.821A	Laceration with foreign body of right forearm, initial encounter ☑
S51.851A	Open bite of right forearm, initial encounter ☑
S58.021A	Partial traumatic amputation at elbow level, right arm, initial encounter ☑
S58.121A	Partial traumatic amputation at level between elbow and wrist, right arm, initial encounter ☑

Repair

S61.511A	Laceration without foreign body of right wrist, initial encounter ☑	
S61.522A	Laceration with foreign body of left wrist, initial encounter ☑	
S61.552A	Open bite of left wrist, initial encounter ☑	
S68.422A	Partial traumatic amputation of left hand at wrist level, initial encounter ☑	
S71.021A	Laceration with foreign body, right hip, initial encounter ☑	
S71.051A	Open bite, right hip, initial encounter ☑	
S71.121A	Laceration with foreign body, right thigh, initial encounter ☑	
S71.152A	Open bite, left thigh, initial encounter ☑	
S78.022A	Partial traumatic amputation at left hip joint, initial encounter ☑	
S78.121A	Partial traumatic amputation at level between right hip and knee, initial encounter ☑	
S81.011A	Laceration without foreign body, right knee, initial encounter ☑	
S81.022A	Laceration with foreign body, left knee, initial encounter ☑	
S81.052A	Open bite, left knee, initial encounter ☑	
S81.812A	Laceration without foreign body, left lower leg, initial encounter ☑	
S81.851A	Open bite, right lower leg, initial encounter ☑	
S81.852A	Open bite, left lower leg, initial encounter ☑	
S88.021A	Partial traumatic amputation at knee level, right lower leg, initial encounter ☑	
S88.121A	Partial traumatic amputation at level between knee and ankle, right lower leg, initial encounter ☑	
S91.012A	Laceration without foreign body, left ankle, initial encounter ☑	
S91.022A	Laceration with foreign body, left ankle, initial encounter ☑	
S91.051A	Open bite, right ankle, initial encounter ☑	
T20.35XA	Burn of third degree of scalp [any part], initial encounter	
T22.311A	Burn of third degree of right forearm, initial encounter ☑	
T22.321A	Burn of third degree of right elbow, initial encounter ☑	
T22.332A	Burn of third degree of left upper arm, initial encounter ☑	
T22.351A	Burn of third degree of right shoulder, initial encounter ☑	
T22.711A	Corrosion of third degree of right forearm, initial encounter ☑	
T22.722A	Corrosion of third degree of left elbow, initial encounter ☑	
T22.731A	Corrosion of third degree of right upper arm, initial encounter ☑	
T24.711A	Corrosion of third degree of right thigh, initial encounter ☑	

AMA: 15220 2018,Jan,8; 2017,Jan,8; 2016,Jun,8; 2016,Jan,13; 2015,Jan,16
15221 2018,Jan,8; 2017,Jan,8; 2016,Jun,8; 2016,Jan,13; 2015,Jan,16

Relative Value Units/Medicare Edits

Non-Facility RVU	Work	PE	MP	Total
15220	8.09	13.42	1.1	22.61
15221	1.19	2.6	0.21	4.0
Facility RVU	Work	PE	MP	Total
15220	8.09	8.53	1.1	17.72
15221	1.19	0.64	0.21	2.04

	FUD	Status	MUE	Modifiers				IOM Reference
15220	90	A	1(2)	51	N/A	N/A	N/A	None
15221	N/A	A	9(3)	N/A	N/A	N/A	N/A	

* with documentation

15240-15241

	15240	Full thickness graft, free, including direct closure of donor site, forehead, cheeks, chin, mouth, neck, axillae, genitalia, hands, and/or feet; 20 sq cm or less
+	15241	each additional 20 sq cm, or part thereof (List separately in addition to code for primary procedure)

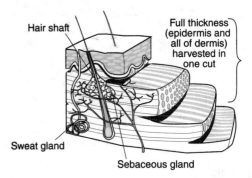

Explanation

The physician harvests a full-thickness skin graft from one area of the body and grafts it to an area on the forehead, cheeks, chin, mouth, neck, axillae, genitalia, hands, and/or feet needing repair. A full-thickness skin graft consists of the superficial and deeper layers of skin (epidermis and dermis). The resulting surgical wound at the donor site is closed by lifting the remaining skin edges and placing sutures to close directly. Residual adipose tissue is removed from the underside of the graft. The graft is sutured onto the wound bed to cover a defect of no more than 20 sq cm. Report 15241 for each additional 20 sq cm or part thereof.

Coding Tips

Report 15241 in addition to 15240. Preparation of the recipient site is reported separately, see 15004–15005. Repair of the donor site requiring skin graft or local flaps is to be added as an additional procedure. If significant additional time and effort is documented, append modifier 22 and submit a cover letter and operative report. Local anesthesia is included in these services; however, these procedures may be performed with the patient under general anesthesia. Pinch graft, single or multiple, is reported with 15050. Surgical trays, A4550, are not separately reimbursed by Medicare; however, other third-party payers may cover them. Check with the specific payer to determine coverage.

ICD-10-CM Diagnostic Codes

C43.4	Malignant melanoma of scalp and neck
C44.41	Basal cell carcinoma of skin of scalp and neck
C44.42	Squamous cell carcinoma of skin of scalp and neck
C49.0	Malignant neoplasm of connective and soft tissue of head, face and neck
C51.0	Malignant neoplasm of labium majus ♀
C51.1	Malignant neoplasm of labium minus ♀
C51.2	Malignant neoplasm of clitoris ♀
C52	Malignant neoplasm of vagina ♀
C60.2	Malignant neoplasm of body of penis ♂
C63.2	Malignant neoplasm of scrotum ♂
C76.0	Malignant neoplasm of head, face and neck
D03.4	Melanoma in situ of scalp and neck
D04.4	Carcinoma in situ of skin of scalp and neck

Repair

D17.0	Benign lipomatous neoplasm of skin and subcutaneous tissue of head, face and neck
D21.0	Benign neoplasm of connective and other soft tissue of head, face and neck
S01.411A	Laceration without foreign body of right cheek and temporomandibular area, initial encounter ☑
S01.451A	Open bite of right cheek and temporomandibular area, initial encounter ☑
S61.022A	Laceration with foreign body of left thumb without damage to nail, initial encounter ☑
S61.052A	Open bite of left thumb without damage to nail, initial encounter ☑
S61.111A	Laceration without foreign body of right thumb with damage to nail, initial encounter ☑
S61.151A	Open bite of right thumb with damage to nail, initial encounter ☑
S61.211A	Laceration without foreign body of left index finger without damage to nail, initial encounter ☑
S61.212A	Laceration without foreign body of right middle finger without damage to nail, initial encounter ☑
S61.216A	Laceration without foreign body of right little finger without damage to nail, initial encounter ☑
S61.255A	Open bite of left ring finger without damage to nail, initial encounter ☑
S61.256A	Open bite of right little finger without damage to nail, initial encounter ☑
S61.315A	Laceration without foreign body of left ring finger with damage to nail, initial encounter ☑
S61.356A	Open bite of right little finger with damage to nail, initial encounter ☑
S61.422A	Laceration with foreign body of left hand, initial encounter ☑
S91.112A	Laceration without foreign body of left great toe without damage to nail, initial encounter ☑
S91.152A	Open bite of left great toe without damage to nail, initial encounter ☑
S91.211A	Laceration without foreign body of right great toe with damage to nail, initial encounter ☑
S91.225A	Laceration with foreign body of left lesser toe(s) with damage to nail, initial encounter ☑
S91.252A	Open bite of left great toe with damage to nail, initial encounter ☑
S91.254A	Open bite of right lesser toe(s) with damage to nail, initial encounter ☑
S91.321A	Laceration with foreign body, right foot, initial encounter ☑
S91.352A	Open bite, left foot, initial encounter ☑
T20.33XA	Burn of third degree of chin, initial encounter
T20.36XA	Burn of third degree of forehead and cheek, initial encounter
T20.37XA	Burn of third degree of neck, initial encounter
T20.73XA	Corrosion of third degree of chin, initial encounter
T20.76XA	Corrosion of third degree of forehead and cheek, initial encounter
T20.79XA	Corrosion of third degree of multiple sites of head, face, and neck, initial encounter
T21.36XA	Burn of third degree of male genital region, initial encounter ♂
T21.77XA	Corrosion of third degree of female genital region, initial encounter ♀
T22.341A	Burn of third degree of right axilla, initial encounter ☑
T22.741A	Corrosion of third degree of right axilla, initial encounter ☑
T23.342A	Burn of third degree of multiple left fingers (nail), including thumb, initial encounter ☑
T23.352A	Burn of third degree of left palm, initial encounter ☑
T23.361A	Burn of third degree of back of right hand, initial encounter ☑
T23.371A	Burn of third degree of right wrist, initial encounter ☑
T23.711A	Corrosion of third degree of right thumb (nail), initial encounter ☑
T23.721A	Corrosion of third degree of single right finger (nail) except thumb, initial encounter ☑
T23.731A	Corrosion of third degree of multiple right fingers (nail), not including thumb, initial encounter ☑
T23.751A	Corrosion of third degree of right palm, initial encounter ☑
T23.762A	Corrosion of third degree of back of left hand, initial encounter ☑
T23.772A	Corrosion of third degree of left wrist, initial encounter ☑
T23.791A	Corrosion of third degree of multiple sites of right wrist and hand, initial encounter ☑
T25.311A	Burn of third degree of right ankle, initial encounter ☑
T25.322A	Burn of third degree of left foot, initial encounter ☑
T25.331A	Burn of third degree of right toe(s) (nail), initial encounter ☑
T25.391A	Burn of third degree of multiple sites of right ankle and foot, initial encounter ☑
T25.711A	Corrosion of third degree of right ankle, initial encounter ☑
T25.731A	Corrosion of third degree of right toe(s) (nail), initial encounter ☑
T25.791A	Corrosion of third degree of multiple sites of right ankle and foot, initial encounter ☑

AMA: **15240** 2018,Jan,8; 2017,Jan,8; 2016,Jun,8; 2016,Jan,13; 2015,Jan,16 **15241** 2018,Jan,8; 2017,Jan,8; 2016,Jun,8; 2016,Jan,13; 2015,Jan,16

Relative Value Units/Medicare Edits

Non-Facility RVU	Work	PE	MP	Total
15240	10.41	15.47	1.35	27.23
15241	1.86	3.11	0.27	5.24
Facility RVU	Work	PE	MP	Total
15240	10.41	11.3	1.35	23.06
15241	1.86	0.96	0.27	3.09

	FUD	Status	MUE	Modifiers				IOM Reference
15240	90	A	1(2)	51	N/A	N/A	N/A	None
15241	N/A	A	9(3)	N/A	N/A	N/A	N/A	

* with documentation

Repair

15260-15261

15260 Full thickness graft, free, including direct closure of donor site, nose, ears, eyelids, and/or lips; 20 sq cm or less

+ **15261** each additional 20 sq cm, or part thereof (List separately in addition to code for primary procedure)

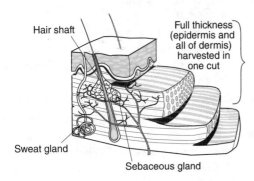

Hair shaft

Full thickness (epidermis and all of dermis) harvested in one cut

Sweat gland

Sebaceous gland

Explanation

The physician harvests a full-thickness skin graft from one area of the body and grafts it to an area on the nose, ears, eyelids, and/or lips needing repair. A full-thickness skin graft consists of both the superficial and deeper layers of skin (epidermis and dermis). The resulting surgical wound at the donor site is closed by lifting the remaining skin edges and placing sutures to close directly. Residual adipose tissue is removed from the underside of the graft. The graft is sutured onto the wound bed to cover a defect of the nose, ears, eyelids, and/or lips of no more than 20 sq cm. Report 15261 for each additional 20 sq cm or part thereof.

Coding Tips

Report 15261 in addition to 15260. Preparation of the recipient site is reported separately, see 15004-15005. Repair of the donor site requiring skin grafts or local flaps is to be added as an additional procedure. If significant additional time and effort is documented, append modifier 22 and submit a cover letter and operative report. Local anesthesia is included in these services; however, these procedures may be performed with the patient under general anesthesia.

ICD-10-CM Diagnostic Codes

C43.0	Malignant melanoma of lip
C43.111	Malignant melanoma of right upper eyelid, including canthus ☑
C43.112	Malignant melanoma of right lower eyelid, including canthus ☑
C43.21	Malignant melanoma of right ear and external auricular canal ☑
C43.22	Malignant melanoma of left ear and external auricular canal ☑
C43.31	Malignant melanoma of nose
C44.01	Basal cell carcinoma of skin of lip
C44.02	Squamous cell carcinoma of skin of lip
C44.09	Other specified malignant neoplasm of skin of lip
C44.1121	Basal cell carcinoma of skin of right upper eyelid, including canthus ☑
C44.1122	Basal cell carcinoma of skin of right lower eyelid, including canthus ☑
C44.1221	Squamous cell carcinoma of skin of right upper eyelid, including canthus ☑
C44.1222	Squamous cell carcinoma of skin of right lower eyelid, including canthus ☑
C44.212	Basal cell carcinoma of skin of right ear and external auricular canal ☑
C44.219	Basal cell carcinoma of skin of left ear and external auricular canal ☑
C44.222	Squamous cell carcinoma of skin of right ear and external auricular canal ☑
C44.229	Squamous cell carcinoma of skin of left ear and external auricular canal ☑
C44.311	Basal cell carcinoma of skin of nose
C44.321	Squamous cell carcinoma of skin of nose
C4A.0	Merkel cell carcinoma of lip
C4A.111	Merkel cell carcinoma of right upper eyelid, including canthus ☑
C4A.112	Merkel cell carcinoma of right lower eyelid, including canthus ☑
C4A.21	Merkel cell carcinoma of right ear and external auricular canal ☑
C4A.22	Merkel cell carcinoma of left ear and external auricular canal ☑
C4A.31	Merkel cell carcinoma of nose
D03.0	Melanoma in situ of lip
D03.111	Melanoma in situ of right upper eyelid, including canthus ☑
D03.112	Melanoma in situ of right lower eyelid, including canthus ☑
D03.21	Melanoma in situ of right ear and external auricular canal ☑
D03.22	Melanoma in situ of left ear and external auricular canal ☑
D04.0	Carcinoma in situ of skin of lip
D04.111	Carcinoma in situ of skin of right upper eyelid, including canthus ☑
D04.112	Carcinoma in situ of skin of right lower eyelid, including canthus ☑
D04.21	Carcinoma in situ of skin of right ear and external auricular canal ☑
D04.22	Carcinoma in situ of skin of left ear and external auricular canal ☑
D10.0	Benign neoplasm of lip
D22.0	Melanocytic nevi of lip
D22.111	Melanocytic nevi of right upper eyelid, including canthus ☑
D22.112	Melanocytic nevi of right lower eyelid, including canthus ☑
D22.21	Melanocytic nevi of right ear and external auricular canal ☑
D22.22	Melanocytic nevi of left ear and external auricular canal ☑
D23.0	Other benign neoplasm of skin of lip
D23.111	Other benign neoplasm of skin of right upper eyelid, including canthus ☑
D23.112	Other benign neoplasm of skin of right lower eyelid, including canthus ☑
D23.21	Other benign neoplasm of skin of right ear and external auricular canal ☑
D23.22	Other benign neoplasm of skin of left ear and external auricular canal ☑
D37.01	Neoplasm of uncertain behavior of lip
S01.111A	Laceration without foreign body of right eyelid and periocular area, initial encounter ☑
S01.112A	Laceration without foreign body of left eyelid and periocular area, initial encounter ☑
S01.121A	Laceration with foreign body of right eyelid and periocular area, initial encounter ☑
S01.122A	Laceration with foreign body of left eyelid and periocular area, initial encounter ☑
S01.151A	Open bite of right eyelid and periocular area, initial encounter ☑
S01.152A	Open bite of left eyelid and periocular area, initial encounter ☑
S01.21XA	Laceration without foreign body of nose, initial encounter
S01.22XA	Laceration with foreign body of nose, initial encounter

Repair

S01.25XA	Open bite of nose, initial encounter
S01.311A	Laceration without foreign body of right ear, initial encounter ☑
S01.312A	Laceration without foreign body of left ear, initial encounter ☑
S01.321A	Laceration with foreign body of right ear, initial encounter ☑
S01.322A	Laceration with foreign body of left ear, initial encounter ☑
S01.351A	Open bite of right ear, initial encounter ☑
S01.352A	Open bite of left ear, initial encounter ☑
S01.511A	Laceration without foreign body of lip, initial encounter
S01.521A	Laceration with foreign body of lip, initial encounter
S01.551A	Open bite of lip, initial encounter
S08.111A	Complete traumatic amputation of right ear, initial encounter ☑
S08.112A	Complete traumatic amputation of left ear, initial encounter ☑
S08.121A	Partial traumatic amputation of right ear, initial encounter ☑
S08.122A	Partial traumatic amputation of left ear, initial encounter ☑
T20.311A	Burn of third degree of right ear [any part, except ear drum], initial encounter ☑
T20.312A	Burn of third degree of left ear [any part, except ear drum], initial encounter ☑
T20.32XA	Burn of third degree of lip(s), initial encounter
T20.34XA	Burn of third degree of nose (septum), initial encounter
T20.711A	Corrosion of third degree of right ear [any part, except ear drum], initial encounter ☑
T20.712A	Corrosion of third degree of left ear [any part, except ear drum], initial encounter ☑
T20.72XA	Corrosion of third degree of lip(s), initial encounter
T20.74XA	Corrosion of third degree of nose (septum), initial encounter

AMA: 15260 2018,Jan,8; 2017,Jan,8; 2016,Jun,8; 2016,Jan,13; 2015,Jan,16
15261 2018,Jan,8; 2017,Jan,8; 2016,Jun,8; 2016,Jan,13; 2015,Jan,16

Relative Value Units/Medicare Edits

Non-Facility RVU	Work	PE	MP	Total
15260	11.64	16.23	1.28	29.15
15261	2.23	3.62	0.3	6.15
Facility RVU	**Work**	**PE**	**MP**	**Total**
15260	11.64	11.54	1.28	24.46
15261	2.23	1.46	0.3	3.99

	FUD	Status	MUE	Modifiers				IOM Reference
15260	90	A	1(2)	51	N/A	N/A	N/A	None
15261	N/A	A	6(3)	N/A	N/A	N/A	N/A	

* with documentation

15850-15851

15850 Removal of sutures under anesthesia (other than local), same surgeon
15851 Removal of sutures under anesthesia (other than local), other surgeon

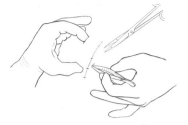

Sutures are removed under anesthesia

Explanation

The physician who completed the surgery on the patient now removes sutures on that patient with the aid of sedation or general anesthesia. Report 15851 for removal of sutures by another surgeon under anesthesia (not local).

Coding Tips

Under normal circumstances, suture removal is considered to be an inherent part of any surgery performed and is included in the global surgery package. When the same, or another, surgeon removes sutures under anesthesia (other than local), one of these codes may be selected to report the service. For secondary closure of a surgical wound or dehiscence, see 13160. For dressing change (other than burns) under non-local anesthesia, see 15852.

ICD-10-CM Diagnostic Codes

Z48.02   Encounter for removal of sutures

AMA: 15850 2018,Jan,8; 2017,Jan,8; 2016,Jan,13; 2015,Jan,16 **15851** 2018,Jan,8; 2017,Jan,8; 2016,Jan,13; 2015,Jan,16

Relative Value Units/Medicare Edits

Non-Facility RVU	Work	PE	MP	Total
15850	0.78	1.9	0.05	2.73
15851	0.86	2.21	0.1	3.17
Facility RVU	**Work**	**PE**	**MP**	**Total**
15850	0.78	0.3	0.05	1.13
15851	0.86	0.37	0.1	1.33

	FUD	Status	MUE	Modifiers				IOM Reference
15850	N/A	B	0(3)	N/A	N/A	N/A	N/A	None
15851	0	A	1(2)	51	N/A	N/A	N/A	

* with documentation

15852

15852   Dressing change (for other than burns) under anesthesia (other than local)

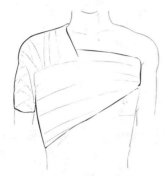

A dressing for a condition other than burn is changed under anesthesia

Explanation

The physician changes a dressing on a wound other than a burn while the patient is under sedation or general anesthesia. This is commonly done for severe crush injuries where serial tissue debridement is required and also for certain types of infection.

Coding Tips

For burn dressing and/or debridement, initial or subsequent, see 16020–16030. Supplies used when providing this procedure may be reported with the appropriate HCPCS Level II code. Check with the specific payer to determine coverage.

ICD-10-CM Diagnostic Codes

The application of this code is too broad to adequately present ICD-10-CM diagnostic code links here. Refer to your ICD-10-CM book.

AMA: 15852 1997,Nov,1

Relative Value Units/Medicare Edits

Non-Facility RVU	Work	PE	MP	Total
15852	0.86	0.35	0.15	1.36
Facility RVU	Work	PE	MP	Total
15852	0.86	0.35	0.15	1.36

	FUD	Status	MUE	Modifiers				IOM Reference
15852	0	A	1(3)	51	N/A	N/A	N/A	None

* with documentation

15920-15922

15920   Excision, coccygeal pressure ulcer, with coccygectomy; with primary suture
15922   with flap closure

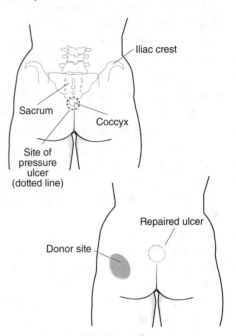

A coccygeal pressure ulcer is excised and the coccyx is also removed

Explanation

The physician excises a coccygeal pressure ulcer with coccygectomy. The patient is positioned prone (face down) and the physician makes an elliptical incision over the coccyx (tailbone), removing the strip of skin that contains the pressure sore. After freeing the coccyx from the surrounding soft tissues, it is separated from the sacrum and removed. The soft tissue is brought back together and the wound is closed with sutures. Report 15922 if the wound is closed using a skin flap from the groin or other donor site. The flap is sutured in place and covered with mesh petroleum gauze and loose bandages.

Coding Tips

Coccygectomy is included in this code and should not be reported separately. For primary coccygectomy (without excision of a pressure ulcer), see 27080. For excision of a sacral pressure ulcer with primary suture, see 15931; and ostectomy, see 15933. For excision of a sacral pressure ulcer with skin flap closure, see 15934; and ostectomy, see 15935. For excision of a sacral pressure ulcer, in preparation for muscle or myocutaneous flap or skin graft closure, see 15936; with ostectomy, see 15937.

ICD-10-CM Diagnostic Codes

L89.153	Pressure ulcer of sacral region, stage 3
L89.154	Pressure ulcer of sacral region, stage 4
L89.156	Pressure-induced deep tissue damage of sacral region
L89.43	Pressure ulcer of contiguous site of back, buttock and hip, stage 3
L89.44	Pressure ulcer of contiguous site of back, buttock and hip, stage 4
L89.46	Pressure-induced deep tissue damage of contiguous site of back, buttock and hip

Repair

AMA: **15920** 2011,May,3-5 **15922** 2011,May,3-5

Relative Value Units/Medicare Edits

Non-Facility RVU	Work	PE	MP	Total
15920	8.29	8.41	1.82	18.52
15922	10.38	11.1	1.84	23.32
Facility RVU	Work	PE	MP	Total
15920	8.29	8.41	1.82	18.52
15922	10.38	11.1	1.84	23.32

	FUD	Status	MUE	Modifiers				IOM Reference
15920	90	A	1(3)	51	N/A	N/A	80*	None
15922	90	A	1(3)	51	N/A	62*	80	

* with documentation

Terms To Know

chronic. Persistent, continuing, or recurring.

decubitus ulcer. Progressively eroding skin lesion produced by inflamed necrotic tissue as it sloughs off caused by continual pressure to a localized area, especially over bony areas, where blood circulation is cut off when a patient lies still for too long without changing position.

excision. Surgical removal of an organ or tissue.

flap. Mass of flesh and skin partially excised from its location but retaining its blood supply that is moved to another site to repair adjacent or distant defects.

gangrene. Death of tissue, usually resulting from a loss of vascular supply, followed by a bacterial attack or onset of disease.

harvest. Removal of cells or tissue from their native site to be used as a graft or transplant to another part of the donor's body or placed into another person.

osteomyelitis. Inflammation of bone that may remain localized or spread to the marrow, cortex, or periosteum, in response to an infecting organism, usually bacterial and pyogenic.

pressure ulcers. Progressively eroding skin lesion produced by inflamed necrotic tissue as it sloughs off, caused by continual pressure impeding blood circulation, especially over bony areas, when a patient lies still for too long without changing position.

15931-15933

15931	Excision, sacral pressure ulcer, with primary suture;
15933	with ostectomy

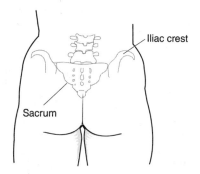

A sacral pressure ulcer is excised and a primary closure completes the procedure

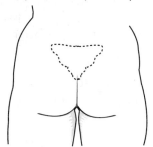

Ulcers may occur anywhere on the skin overlying the sacrum

Explanation

The physician excises a sacral pressure ulcer. The patient is positioned prone (face down) and the physician makes an elliptical incision over the sacrum, removing the strip of skin that contains the pressure sore. The wound is irrigated and the soft tissue is brought back together and closed with sutures. Report 15933 if bone below the wound is removed before the soft tissue is brought back together and closed.

Coding Tips

For excision of a sacral pressure ulcer with skin flap closure, see 15934; with ostectomy, see 15935. For excision of a sacral pressure ulcer, in preparation for muscle or myocutaneous flap or skin graft closure, see 15936; with ostectomy, see 15937.

ICD-10-CM Diagnostic Codes

L89.150	Pressure ulcer of sacral region, unstageable
L89.153	Pressure ulcer of sacral region, stage 3
L89.154	Pressure ulcer of sacral region, stage 4
L89.156	Pressure-induced deep tissue damage of sacral region
L89.43	Pressure ulcer of contiguous site of back, buttock and hip, stage 3
L89.44	Pressure ulcer of contiguous site of back, buttock and hip, stage 4
L89.45	Pressure ulcer of contiguous site of back, buttock and hip, unstageable
L89.46	Pressure-induced deep tissue damage of contiguous site of back, buttock and hip

AMA: **15931** 2011,May,3-5 **15933** 2011,May,3-5

Repair

Relative Value Units/Medicare Edits

Non-Facility RVU	Work	PE	MP	Total
15931	10.07	8.41	2.29	20.77
15933	11.77	11.21	2.53	25.51
Facility RVU	Work	PE	MP	Total
15931	10.07	8.41	2.29	20.77
15933	11.77	11.21	2.53	25.51

	FUD	Status	MUE	Modifiers				IOM Reference
15931	90	A	1(3)	51	N/A	N/A	N/A	None
15933	90	A	1(3)	51	N/A	N/A	80*	

* with documentation

Terms To Know

decubitus ulcer. Progressively eroding skin lesion produced by inflamed necrotic tissue as it sloughs off caused by continual pressure to a localized area, especially over bony areas, where blood circulation is cut off when a patient lies still for too long without changing position.

excision. Surgical removal of an organ or tissue.

myocutaneous flap. Skin, subcutaneous tissue, and intact muscle tissue that are transferred to a recipient site while retaining sufficient blood supply from its own vascular bed.

ostectomy. Excision of bone.

pressure ulcers. Progressively eroding skin lesion produced by inflamed necrotic tissue as it sloughs off, caused by continual pressure impeding blood circulation, especially over bony areas, when a patient lies still for too long without changing position.

sacrum. Lower portion of the spine composed of five fused vertebrae designated as S1-S5.

soft tissue. Nonepithelial tissues outside of the skeleton.

15934-15935

15934	Excision, sacral pressure ulcer, with skin flap closure;
15935	with ostectomy

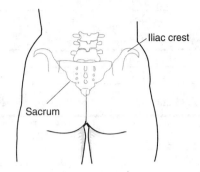

A sacral pressure ulcer is excised with a skin flap closure

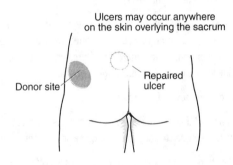

Ulcers may occur anywhere on the skin overlying the sacrum

Explanation

The physician excises a sacral pressure ulcer. The patient is positioned prone (face down) and the physician makes an elliptical incision over the sacrum, removing the strip of skin that contains the pressure sore. The wound is irrigated and closed using a skin flap from the groin or other donor site. The flap is sutured in place and covered with mesh petroleum gauze and loose bandages. Report 15935 if bone below the wound is removed before the wound is repaired with a skin flap.

Coding Tips

For excision of a coccygeal pressure ulcer, see 15920–15922. For excision of a sacral pressure ulcer with primary suture, see 15931; and ostectomy, see 15933. For excision of a sacral pressure ulcer, in preparation for muscle or myocutaneous flap or skin graft closure, see 15936; with ostectomy, see 15937.

ICD-10-CM Diagnostic Codes

L89.153	Pressure ulcer of sacral region, stage 3
L89.154	Pressure ulcer of sacral region, stage 4
L89.156	Pressure-induced deep tissue damage of sacral region
L89.43	Pressure ulcer of contiguous site of back, buttock and hip, stage 3
L89.44	Pressure ulcer of contiguous site of back, buttock and hip, stage 4
L89.46	Pressure-induced deep tissue damage of contiguous site of back, buttock and hip

AMA: 15934 2011,May,3-5 **15935** 2011,May,3-5

Repair

Relative Value Units/Medicare Edits

Non-Facility RVU	Work	PE	MP	Total
15934	13.68	11.46	2.75	27.89
15935	15.78	15.28	2.79	33.85
Facility RVU	Work	PE	MP	Total
15934	13.68	11.46	2.75	27.89
15935	15.78	15.28	2.79	33.85

	FUD	Status	MUE	Modifiers			IOM Reference
15934	90	A	1(3)	51	N/A	N/A	N/A	None
15935	90	A	1(3)	51	N/A	62*	80	

* with documentation

Terms To Know

chronic. Persistent, continuing, or recurring.

decubitus ulcer. Progressively eroding skin lesion produced by inflamed necrotic tissue as it sloughs off caused by continual pressure to a localized area, especially over bony areas, where blood circulation is cut off when a patient lies still for too long without changing position.

gangrene. Death of tissue, usually resulting from a loss of vascular supply, followed by a bacterial attack or onset of disease.

ostectomy. Excision of bone.

osteomyelitis. Inflammation of bone that may remain localized or spread to the marrow, cortex, or periosteum, in response to an infecting organism, usually bacterial and pyogenic.

pressure ulcers. Progressively eroding skin lesion produced by inflamed necrotic tissue as it sloughs off, caused by continual pressure impeding blood circulation, especially over bony areas, when a patient lies still for too long without changing position.

sacrum. Lower portion of the spine composed of five fused vertebrae designated as S1-S5.

subcutaneous tissue. Sheet or wide band of adipose (fat) and areolar connective tissue in two layers attached to the dermis.

suture. Numerous stitching techniques employed in wound closure.

buried suture. Continuous or interrupted suture placed under the skin for a layered closure.

continuous suture. Running stitch with tension evenly distributed across a single strand to provide a leakproof closure line.

interrupted suture. Series of single stitches with tension isolated at each stitch, in which all stitches are not affected if one becomes loose, and the isolated sutures cannot act as a wick to transport an infection.

purse-string suture. Continuous suture placed around a tubular structure and tightened, to reduce or close the lumen.

retention suture. Secondary stitching that bridges the primary suture, providing support for the primary repair; a plastic or rubber bolster may be placed over the primary repair and under the retention sutures.

15940-15941

15940 Excision, ischial pressure ulcer, with primary suture;
15941 with ostectomy (ischiectomy)

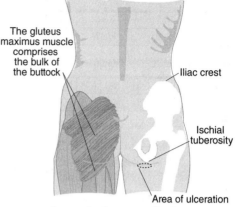

The gluteus maximus muscle comprises the bulk of the buttock

Iliac crest

Ischial tuberosity

Area of ulceration

A pressure ulcer caused by the ischial tuberosity is excised

Explanation

The physician excises an ischial pressure ulcer. An incision is made around the wound over the ischial tuberosity to remove the infected pressure sore. The remaining healthy tissues are irrigated, the wound is closed with sutures, and a soft dressing is applied. Report 15941 if a portion of bone from the ischium is removed before the wound is sutured closed.

Coding Tips

For excision of an ischial pressure ulcer with skin flap closure, see 15944–15945. For excision of an ischial pressure ulcer in preparation for muscle or myocutaneous flap or skin graft closure, see 15946. For excision of a sacral pressure ulcer with primary suture, see 15931– 15933; with skin flap closure, see 15934–15935. For excision of a coccygeal pressure ulcer, see 15920–15922.

ICD-10-CM Diagnostic Codes

L89.310	Pressure ulcer of right buttock, unstageable ☑
L89.313	Pressure ulcer of right buttock, stage 3 ☑
L89.314	Pressure ulcer of right buttock, stage 4 ☑
L89.316	Pressure-induced deep tissue damage of right buttock ☑
L89.320	Pressure ulcer of left buttock, unstageable ☑
L89.323	Pressure ulcer of left buttock, stage 3 ☑
L89.324	Pressure ulcer of left buttock, stage 4 ☑
L89.43	Pressure ulcer of contiguous site of back, buttock and hip, stage 3
L89.44	Pressure ulcer of contiguous site of back, buttock and hip, stage 4
L89.46	Pressure-induced deep tissue damage of contiguous site of back, buttock and hip

AMA: **15940** 2011,May,3-5 **15941** 2011,May,3-5

Repair

Relative Value Units/Medicare Edits

Non-Facility RVU	Work	PE	MP	Total
15940	10.2	8.39	2.14	20.73
15941	12.41	12.37	2.46	27.24
Facility RVU	Work	PE	MP	Total
15940	10.2	8.39	2.14	20.73
15941	12.41	12.37	2.46	27.24

	FUD	Status	MUE	Modifiers				IOM Reference
15940	90	A	2(3)	51	N/A	N/A	N/A	None
15941	90	A	2(3)	51	N/A	N/A	80*	

* with documentation

Terms To Know

lesion. Area of damaged tissue that has lost continuity or function, due to disease or trauma.

ostectomy. Excision of bone.

osteomyelitis. Inflammation of bone that may remain localized or spread to the marrow, cortex, or periosteum, in response to an infecting organism, usually bacterial and pyogenic.

pressure ulcers. Progressively eroding skin lesion produced by inflamed necrotic tissue as it sloughs off, caused by continual pressure impeding blood circulation, especially over bony areas, when a patient lies still for too long without changing position.

subcutaneous tissue. Sheet or wide band of adipose (fat) and areolar connective tissue in two layers attached to the dermis.

suture. Numerous stitching techniques employed in wound closure.

buried suture. Continuous or interrupted suture placed under the skin for a layered closure.

continuous suture. Running stitch with tension evenly distributed across a single strand to provide a leakproof closure line.

interrupted suture. Series of single stitches with tension isolated at each stitch, in which all stitches are not affected if one becomes loose, and the isolated sutures cannot act as a wick to transport an infection.

purse-string suture. Continuous suture placed around a tubular structure and tightened, to reduce or close the lumen.

retention suture. Secondary stitching that bridges the primary suture, providing support for the primary repair; a plastic or rubber bolster may be placed over the primary repair and under the retention sutures.

15944-15945

15944   Excision, ischial pressure ulcer, with skin flap closure;
15945   with ostectomy

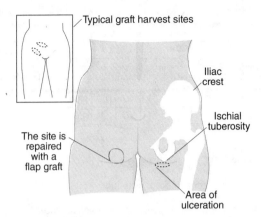

A pressure ulcer caused by the ischial tuberosity is excised and repaired with a flap graft

Explanation

The physician excises an ischial pressure ulcer, with skin flap closure. An incision is made around the wound over the ischial tuberosity in order to remove the infected pressure sore. The infected tissue is removed; however, the wound is large enough to require a flap of skin from another part of the body, such as the groin area at the front of the hip, to completely close the area. The physician makes an appropriate size flap from the donor area and sutures it in place following the removal of the infected tissue. The donor site is sutured closed and soft dressings are used to cover the wounds. Report 15945 if a portion of bone from the ischium is removed before the wound is closed with the flap.

Coding Tips

For excision of an ischial pressure ulcer with primary suture repair, see 15940–15941. For excision of an ischial pressure ulcer in preparation for muscle or myocutaneous flap or skin graft closure, see 15946. For excision of a sacral pressure ulcer with primary suture, see 15931; with skin flap closure, see 15934. For excision of a coccygeal pressure ulcer, with flap closure, see 15922.

ICD-10-CM Diagnostic Codes

L89.310	Pressure ulcer of right buttock, unstageable ☑
L89.313	Pressure ulcer of right buttock, stage 3 ☑
L89.314	Pressure ulcer of right buttock, stage 4 ☑
L89.316	Pressure-induced deep tissue damage of right buttock ☑
L89.320	Pressure ulcer of left buttock, unstageable ☑
L89.323	Pressure ulcer of left buttock, stage 3 ☑
L89.324	Pressure ulcer of left buttock, stage 4 ☑
L89.46	Pressure-induced deep tissue damage of contiguous site of back, buttock and hip

AMA: **15944** 2011,May,3-5 **15945** 2011,May,3-5

Relative Value Units/Medicare Edits

Non-Facility RVU	Work	PE	MP	Total
15944	12.44	12.2	2.36	27.0
15945	13.75	13.69	2.42	29.86
Facility RVU	**Work**	**PE**	**MP**	**Total**
15944	12.44	12.2	2.36	27.0
15945	13.75	13.69	2.42	29.86

	FUD	Status	MUE	Modifiers				IOM Reference
15944	90	A	2(3)	51	N/A	N/A	80*	None
15945	90	A	2(3)	51	N/A	N/A	80*	

* with documentation

Terms To Know

chronic. Persistent, continuing, or recurring.

decubitus ulcer. Progressively eroding skin lesion produced by inflamed necrotic tissue as it sloughs off caused by continual pressure to a localized area, especially over bony areas, where blood circulation is cut off when a patient lies still for too long without changing position.

excision. Surgical removal of an organ or tissue.

gangrene. Death of tissue, usually resulting from a loss of vascular supply, followed by a bacterial attack or onset of disease.

incision. Act of cutting into tissue or an organ.

infection. Presence of microorganisms in body tissues that may result in cellular damage.

ischial tuberosity. Bony projection of the lower end of the ischium easily identified as the weight-bearing point in a sitting position.

ostectomy. Excision of bone.

pressure ulcers. Progressively eroding skin lesion produced by inflamed necrotic tissue as it sloughs off, caused by continual pressure impeding blood circulation, especially over bony areas, when a patient lies still for too long without changing position.

subcutaneous tissue. Sheet or wide band of adipose (fat) and areolar connective tissue in two layers attached to the dermis.

15946

15946   Excision, ischial pressure ulcer, with ostectomy, in preparation for muscle or myocutaneous flap or skin graft closure

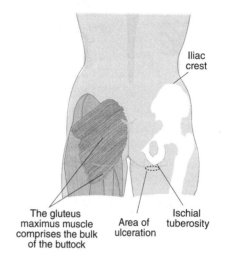

Iliac crest

The gluteus maximus muscle comprises the bulk of the buttock

Area of ulceration

Ischial tuberosity

A pressure ulcer caused by the ischial tuberosity is excised and a portion of the ischial tuberosity bone is removed. The site is then prepared to receive a muscle flap, a muscle-skin flap, or a skin graft closure

Explanation

The physician excises an ischial pressure ulcer and part of the ischial bone underlying the ulcer. The defect that remains is prepared for a graft that is reported separately, most commonly a gluteal thigh rotation flap, but it may also be a myocutaneous or muscle graft involving the gluteus maximus muscle. The graft is sutured in place and a soft dressing is applied.

Coding Tips

Muscle/myocutaneous flaps and skin grafts are reported in addition to this code, when performed, see 15734 or 15738 for flaps and 15100–15101 for grafts. For excision of an ischial pressure ulcer, with primary suture, see 15940; with ostectomy (ischiectomy), see 15941. For excision of an ischial pressure ulcer with skin flap closure, see 15944; with ostectomy, see 15945.

ICD-10-CM Diagnostic Codes

L89.314	Pressure ulcer of right buttock, stage 4 ☑
L89.316	Pressure-induced deep tissue damage of right buttock ☑
L89.324	Pressure ulcer of left buttock, stage 4 ☑

AMA: 15946 2018,Jan,8; 2017,Jan,8; 2016,Jan,13; 2015,Jan,16

Relative Value Units/Medicare Edits

Non-Facility RVU	Work	PE	MP	Total
15946	24.12	18.85	4.6	47.57
Facility RVU	**Work**	**PE**	**MP**	**Total**
15946	24.12	18.85	4.6	47.57

	FUD	Status	MUE	Modifiers			IOM Reference
15946	90	A	2(3)	51	N/A	62*	N/A	None

* with documentation

Repair

15950-15951

15950 Excision, trochanteric pressure ulcer, with primary suture;
15951   with ostectomy

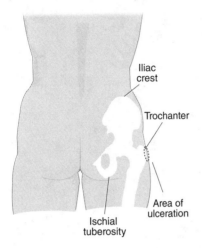

A pressure ulcer caused by the trochanter is excised
and the site closed with a primary suture

Explanation

The physician excises a trochanteric pressure ulcer, with primary suture closure. The physician makes an elliptical shaped incision around the wound, which is located over the outer hip bone. The infected pressure ulcer is removed and the wound is irrigated. The soft tissues are brought back together and closed with sutures. A soft dressing is applied. Report 15951 if a portion of the underlying bone is also removed because of the extent of the infection.

Coding Tips

For excision of a trochanteric pressure ulcer with skin flap closure, see 15952; and ostectomy, see 15953. For excision of an ischial pressure ulcer in preparation for muscle or myocutaneous flap or skin graft closure, with ostectomy, see 15946.

ICD-10-CM Diagnostic Codes

L89.210	Pressure ulcer of right hip, unstageable ☑
L89.213	Pressure ulcer of right hip, stage 3 ☑
L89.214	Pressure ulcer of right hip, stage 4 ☑
L89.216	Pressure-induced deep tissue damage of right hip ☑
L89.220	Pressure ulcer of left hip, unstageable ☑
L89.223	Pressure ulcer of left hip, stage 3 ☑
L89.224	Pressure ulcer of left hip, stage 4 ☑
L89.46	Pressure-induced deep tissue damage of contiguous site of back, buttock and hip

AMA: 15950 2011,May,3-5 **15951** 2011,May,3-5

Relative Value Units/Medicare Edits

Non-Facility RVU	Work	PE	MP	Total
15950	8.03	8.33	1.69	18.05
15951	11.58	12.71	2.05	26.34
Facility RVU	**Work**	**PE**	**MP**	**Total**
15950	8.03	8.33	1.69	18.05
15951	11.58	12.71	2.05	26.34

	FUD	Status	MUE	Modifiers			IOM Reference
15950	90	A	2(3)	51	N/A	N/A	N/A	None
15951	90	A	2(3)	51	N/A	62*	80*	

* with documentation

Terms To Know

closure. Repairing an incision or wound by suture or other means.

decubitus ulcer. Progressively eroding skin lesion produced by inflamed necrotic tissue as it sloughs off caused by continual pressure to a localized area, especially over bony areas, where blood circulation is cut off when a patient lies still for too long without changing position.

gangrene. Death of tissue, usually resulting from a loss of vascular supply, followed by a bacterial attack or onset of disease.

ostectomy. Excision of bone.

pressure ulcers. Progressively eroding skin lesion produced by inflamed necrotic tissue as it sloughs off, caused by continual pressure impeding blood circulation, especially over bony areas, when a patient lies still for too long without changing position.

primary. Principal or first in the order of occurrence or importance.

soft tissue. Nonepithelial tissues outside of the skeleton.

suture. Numerous stitching techniques employed in wound closure.

buried suture. Continuous or interrupted suture placed under the skin for a layered closure.

continuous suture. Running stitch with tension evenly distributed across a single strand to provide a leakproof closure line.

interrupted suture. Series of single stitches with tension isolated at each stitch, in which all stitches are not affected if one becomes loose, and the isolated sutures cannot act as a wick to transport an infection.

purse-string suture. Continuous suture placed around a tubular structure and tightened, to reduce or close the lumen.

retention suture. Secondary stitching that bridges the primary suture, providing support for the primary repair; a plastic or rubber bolster may be placed over the primary repair and under the retention sutures.

Repair

15952-15953

15952 Excision, trochanteric pressure ulcer, with skin flap closure;
15953 with ostectomy

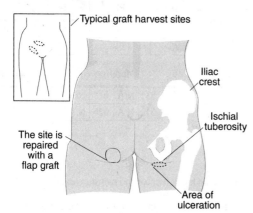

Typical graft harvest sites

Iliac crest

Ischial tuberosity

The site is repaired with a flap graft

Area of ulceration

A pressure ulcer caused by the trochanter is excised and repaired with a flap graft

Explanation

The physician excises a trochanteric pressure ulcer with skin flap closure. An incision is made around the wound over the trochanter (outer hip bone) in order to remove the infected pressure sore. The remaining defect requires skin flap closure. The most common skin flap donor sites are the groin area at the front of the hip, gluteal thigh, or anterior thigh. The physician takes an appropriate size graft from the donor area and sutures it in place covering the defect. The donor site is also sutured closed. Soft dressings are used to cover the wounds. Report 15953 if a portion or all of the trochanter is removed during the ulcer excision.

Coding Tips

For excision of a trochanteric pressure ulcer with primary suture, see 15950; with ostectomy, see 15951. For excision of an ischial pressure ulcer in preparation for muscle or myocutaneous flap or skin graft closure, with ostectomy, see 15946.

ICD-10-CM Diagnostic Codes

L89.210	Pressure ulcer of right hip, unstageable ☑
L89.213	Pressure ulcer of right hip, stage 3 ☑
L89.214	Pressure ulcer of right hip, stage 4 ☑
L89.216	Pressure-induced deep tissue damage of right hip ☑
L89.220	Pressure ulcer of left hip, unstageable ☑
L89.223	Pressure ulcer of left hip, stage 3 ☑
L89.224	Pressure ulcer of left hip, stage 4 ☑
L89.43	Pressure ulcer of contiguous site of back, buttock and hip, stage 3
L89.44	Pressure ulcer of contiguous site of back, buttock and hip, stage 4
L89.46	Pressure-induced deep tissue damage of contiguous site of back, buttock and hip

AMA: 15952 2011,May,3-5 **15953** 2011,May,3-5

Relative Value Units/Medicare Edits

Non-Facility RVU	Work	PE	MP	Total
15952	12.31	12.32	2.2	26.83
15953	13.57	13.58	2.41	29.56
Facility RVU	Work	PE	MP	Total
15952	12.31	12.32	2.2	26.83
15953	13.57	13.58	2.41	29.56

	FUD	Status	MUE	Modifiers				IOM Reference
15952	90	A	2(3)	51	N/A	62*	80	None
15953	90	A	2(3)	51	N/A	62*	N/A	

* with documentation

Terms To Know

decubitus ulcer. Progressively eroding skin lesion produced by inflamed necrotic tissue as it sloughs off caused by continual pressure to a localized area, especially over bony areas, where blood circulation is cut off when a patient lies still for too long without changing position.

excision. Surgical removal of an organ or tissue.

flap. Mass of flesh and skin partially excised from its location but retaining its blood supply that is moved to another site to repair adjacent or distant defects.

gangrene. Death of tissue, usually resulting from a loss of vascular supply, followed by a bacterial attack or onset of disease.

graft. Tissue implant from another part of the body or another person.

incision. Act of cutting into tissue or an organ.

infection. Presence of microorganisms in body tissues that may result in cellular damage.

ostectomy. Excision of bone.

pressure ulcers. Progressively eroding skin lesion produced by inflamed necrotic tissue as it sloughs off, caused by continual pressure impeding blood circulation, especially over bony areas, when a patient lies still for too long without changing position.

subcutaneous tissue. Sheet or wide band of adipose (fat) and areolar connective tissue in two layers attached to the dermis.

Repair

15956-15958

15956 Excision, trochanteric pressure ulcer, in preparation for muscle or myocutaneous flap or skin graft closure;

15958 with ostectomy

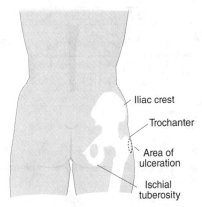

A pressure ulcer caused by the trochanter is excised and a portion of the trochanteric bone is removed. The site is then prepared for a muscle graft, muscle-skin graft, or a skin graft closure

Explanation

The physician excises a trochanteric pressure ulcer. The defect that remains is prepared for a myocutaneous or muscle graft that is reported separately, most commonly harvested from the tensor fasciae latae (AFT) muscle. The graft is sutured in place and a soft dressing is applied. Report 15958 if a portion or all of the trochanter is removed during the ulcer excision.

Coding Tips

Muscle/myocutaneous flaps and skin grafts are reported in addition to these codes, when performed, see 15734 or 15738 for flaps and 15100–15101 for grafts. For excision of an ischial pressure ulcer, with primary suture, see 15940; and ostectomy (ischiectomy), see 15941; with skin flap closure, see 15944; and ostectomy, see 15945.

ICD-10-CM Diagnostic Codes

L89.210	Pressure ulcer of right hip, unstageable ☑
L89.213	Pressure ulcer of right hip, stage 3 ☑
L89.214	Pressure ulcer of right hip, stage 4 ☑
L89.216	Pressure-induced deep tissue damage of right hip ☑
L89.220	Pressure ulcer of left hip, unstageable ☑
L89.223	Pressure ulcer of left hip, stage 3 ☑
L89.224	Pressure ulcer of left hip, stage 4 ☑
L89.226	Pressure-induced deep tissue damage of left hip ☑
L89.43	Pressure ulcer of contiguous site of back, buttock and hip, stage 3
L89.44	Pressure ulcer of contiguous site of back, buttock and hip, stage 4
L89.46	Pressure-induced deep tissue damage of contiguous site of back, buttock and hip

AMA: 15956 2011,May,3-5 **15958** 2011,May,3-5

Relative Value Units/Medicare Edits

Non-Facility RVU	Work	PE	MP	Total
15956	16.79	14.2	3.35	34.34
15958	16.75	15.01	3.11	34.87
Facility RVU	**Work**	**PE**	**MP**	**Total**
15956	16.79	14.2	3.35	34.34
15958	16.75	15.01	3.11	34.87

	FUD	Status	MUE	Modifiers				IOM Reference
15956	90	A	2(3)	51	N/A	62*	N/A	None
15958	90	A	2(3)	51	N/A	62*	N/A	

* with documentation

Terms To Know

closure. Repairing an incision or wound by suture or other means.

decubitus ulcer. Progressively eroding skin lesion produced by inflamed necrotic tissue as it sloughs off caused by continual pressure to a localized area, especially over bony areas, where blood circulation is cut off when a patient lies still for too long without changing position.

gangrene. Death of tissue, usually resulting from a loss of vascular supply, followed by a bacterial attack or onset of disease.

myocutaneous flap graft. Section of tissue containing muscle and attached skin is partially removed from its donor site so as to retain its own blood supply for transfer to a new recipient site.

ostectomy. Excision of bone.

pressure ulcers. Progressively eroding skin lesion produced by inflamed necrotic tissue as it sloughs off, caused by continual pressure impeding blood circulation, especially over bony areas, when a patient lies still for too long without changing position.

N Newborn: 0 **P** Pediatric: 0-17 **M** Maternity: 9-64 **A** Adult: 15-124 ♂ Male Only ♀ Female Only CPT © 2021 American Medical Association. All Rights Reserved.

Repair

16020-16030

16020 Dressings and/or debridement of partial-thickness burns, initial or subsequent; small (less than 5% total body surface area)

16025 medium (eg, whole face or whole extremity, or 5% to 10% total body surface area)

16030 large (eg, more than 1 extremity, or greater than 10% total body surface area)

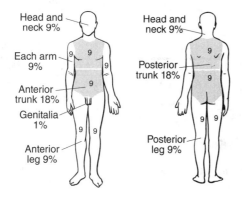

Explanation

The physician applies dressing material(s) and/or debrides a partial-thickness burn of blisters and nonviable or nonadherent tissue, initial or subsequent. The physician removes devitalized tissue or tissue that is contaminated by bacteria, foreign material, dead cells, or a crust. The wound is cleansed and a dressing is applied. Report 16020 for treatment of a small burn area, less than 5 percent of total body surface area; 16025 for a medium-sized area, 5 to 10 percent of total body surface area, such as the whole face or a whole extremity; and 16030 for a large burn area, greater than 10 percent of total body surface area, such as more than one extremity.

Coding Tips

These codes refer to local treatment of the burned surface only and include the application of materials, such as dressings, not described by codes 15100–15278. List the percentage of total body surface area (TBSA) involved and the depth of the burn. For additional medical procedures or related services, such as hospital visits, report separately using the appropriate procedure/evaluation and management code. Application of skin grafts/substitutes are reported with codes 15100–15278.

ICD-10-CM Diagnostic Codes

S00.222A	Blister (nonthermal) of left eyelid and periocular area, initial encounter ☑
S00.32XA	Blister (nonthermal) of nose, initial encounter
S00.421A	Blister (nonthermal) of right ear, initial encounter ☑
S00.521A	Blister (nonthermal) of lip, initial encounter
S10.12XA	Blister (nonthermal) of throat, initial encounter
S20.121A	Blister (nonthermal) of breast, right breast, initial encounter ☑
S20.321A	Blister (nonthermal) of right front wall of thorax, initial encounter
S30.820A	Blister (nonthermal) of lower back and pelvis, initial encounter
S30.822A	Blister (nonthermal) of penis, initial encounter ♂
S30.824A	Blister (nonthermal) of vagina and vulva, initial encounter ♀
S60.321A	Blister (nonthermal) of right thumb, initial encounter ☑
S60.427A	Blister (nonthermal) of left little finger, initial encounter ☑
S60.522A	Blister (nonthermal) of left hand, initial encounter ☑
S70.221A	Blister (nonthermal), right hip, initial encounter ☑

S80.222A	Blister (nonthermal), left knee, initial encounter ☑
S90.521A	Blister (nonthermal), right ankle, initial encounter ☑
S90.822A	Blister (nonthermal), left foot, initial encounter ☑
T20.212A	Burn of second degree of left ear [any part, except ear drum], initial encounter ☑
T20.22XA	Burn of second degree of lip(s), initial encounter
T20.23XA	Burn of second degree of chin, initial encounter
T20.25XA	Burn of second degree of scalp [any part], initial encounter
T20.26XA	Burn of second degree of forehead and cheek, initial encounter
T20.27XA	Burn of second degree of neck, initial encounter
T20.29XA	Burn of second degree of multiple sites of head, face, and neck, initial encounter
T20.611A	Corrosion of second degree of right ear [any part, except ear drum], initial encounter ☑
T20.62XA	Corrosion of second degree of lip(s), initial encounter
T20.64XA	Corrosion of second degree of nose (septum), initial encounter
T20.65XA	Corrosion of second degree of scalp [any part], initial encounter
T20.66XA	Corrosion of second degree of forehead and cheek, initial encounter
T20.69XA	Corrosion of second degree of multiple sites of head, face, and neck, initial encounter
T21.21XA	Burn of second degree of chest wall, initial encounter
T21.22XA	Burn of second degree of abdominal wall, initial encounter
T21.23XA	Burn of second degree of upper back, initial encounter
T21.24XA	Burn of second degree of lower back, initial encounter
T21.25XA	Burn of second degree of buttock, initial encounter
T21.26XA	Burn of second degree of male genital region, initial encounter ♂
T21.61XA	Corrosion of second degree of chest wall, initial encounter
T21.65XA	Corrosion of second degree of buttock, initial encounter
T21.67XA	Corrosion of second degree of female genital region, initial encounter ♀
T22.211A	Burn of second degree of right forearm, initial encounter ☑
T22.222A	Burn of second degree of left elbow, initial encounter ☑
T22.231A	Burn of second degree of right upper arm, initial encounter ☑
T22.232A	Burn of second degree of left upper arm, initial encounter ☑
T22.242A	Burn of second degree of left axilla, initial encounter ☑
T22.251A	Burn of second degree of right shoulder, initial encounter ☑
T22.261A	Burn of second degree of right scapular region, initial encounter ☑
T22.291A	Burn of second degree of multiple sites of right shoulder and upper limb, except wrist and hand, initial encounter ☑
T22.611A	Corrosion of second degree of right forearm, initial encounter ☑
T22.632A	Corrosion of second degree of left upper arm, initial encounter ☑
T22.641A	Corrosion of second degree of right axilla, initial encounter ☑
T22.652A	Corrosion of second degree of left shoulder, initial encounter ☑
T22.661A	Corrosion of second degree of right scapular region, initial encounter ☑
T22.692A	Corrosion of second degree of multiple sites of left shoulder and upper limb, except wrist and hand, initial encounter ☑
T23.211A	Burn of second degree of right thumb (nail), initial encounter ☑
T23.222A	Burn of second degree of single left finger (nail) except thumb, initial encounter ☑
T23.231A	Burn of second degree of multiple right fingers (nail), not including thumb, initial encounter ☑

T23.241A	Burn of second degree of multiple right fingers (nail), including thumb, initial encounter ☑
T23.242A	Burn of second degree of multiple left fingers (nail), including thumb, initial encounter ☑
T23.251A	Burn of second degree of right palm, initial encounter ☑
T23.262A	Burn of second degree of back of left hand, initial encounter ☑
T23.271A	Burn of second degree of right wrist, initial encounter ☑
T23.292A	Burn of second degree of multiple sites of left wrist and hand, initial encounter ☑
T23.611A	Corrosion of second degree of right thumb (nail), initial encounter ☑
T23.622A	Corrosion of second degree of single left finger (nail) except thumb, initial encounter ☑
T23.642A	Corrosion of second degree of multiple left fingers (nail), including thumb, initial encounter ☑
T23.651A	Corrosion of second degree of right palm, initial encounter ☑
T23.662A	Corrosion of second degree back of left hand, initial encounter ☑
T23.671A	Corrosion of second degree of right wrist, initial encounter ☑
T23.691A	Corrosion of second degree of multiple sites of right wrist and hand, initial encounter ☑
T24.211A	Burn of second degree of right thigh, initial encounter ☑
T24.212A	Burn of second degree of left thigh, initial encounter ☑
T24.221A	Burn of second degree of right knee, initial encounter ☑
T24.231A	Burn of second degree of right lower leg, initial encounter ☑
T24.292A	Burn of second degree of multiple sites of left lower limb, except ankle and foot, initial encounter ☑
T24.612A	Corrosion of second degree of left thigh, initial encounter ☑
T24.621A	Corrosion of second degree of right knee, initial encounter ☑
T24.631A	Corrosion of second degree of right lower leg, initial encounter ☑
T24.632A	Corrosion of second degree of left lower leg, initial encounter ☑
T25.211A	Burn of second degree of right ankle, initial encounter ☑
T25.222A	Burn of second degree of left foot, initial encounter ☑
T25.232A	Burn of second degree of left toe(s) (nail), initial encounter ☑
T25.291A	Burn of second degree of multiple sites of right ankle and foot, initial encounter ☑
T25.612A	Corrosion of second degree of left ankle, initial encounter ☑
T25.622A	Corrosion of second degree of left foot, initial encounter ☑
T25.691A	Corrosion of second degree of right ankle and foot, initial encounter ☑
T28.0XXA	Burn of mouth and pharynx, initial encounter
T28.5XXA	Corrosion of mouth and pharynx, initial encounter
T31.0	Burns involving less than 10% of body surface
T32.0	Corrosions involving less than 10% of body surface

AMA: **16020** 2018,Jan,8; 2017,Jan,8; 2016,Jan,13; 2015,Jan,16 **16025** 2018,Jan,8; 2017,Jan,8; 2016,Jan,13; 2015,Jan,16 **16030** 2018,Jan,8; 2017,Jan,8; 2016,Jan,13; 2015,Jan,16

Relative Value Units/Medicare Edits

Non-Facility RVU	Work	PE	MP	Total
16020	0.71	1.66	0.13	2.5
16025	1.74	2.58	0.26	4.58
16030	2.08	3.28	0.37	5.73
Facility RVU	**Work**	**PE**	**MP**	**Total**
16020	0.71	0.77	0.13	1.61
16025	1.74	1.22	0.26	3.22
16030	2.08	1.38	0.37	3.83

	FUD	Status	MUE	Modifiers				IOM Reference
16020	0	A	1(3)	51	N/A	N/A	N/A	None
16025	0	A	1(3)	51	N/A	N/A	N/A	
16030	0	A	1(3)	51	N/A	N/A	N/A	

* with documentation

Terms To Know

debridement. Removal of dead or contaminated tissue and foreign matter from a wound.

dressing. Material applied to a wound or surgical site for protection, absorption, or drainage of the area.

epidermal. Pertaining to or on the outer layer of skin.

rule of nines. Rapid measurement system used to calculate the total body surface area (TBSA) involved in burns, based upon dividing the total area into segments as multiples of 9 percent. The perineum or external genitals are 1 percent; each arm is 9 percent; the front and back of the trunk, and each leg are separately counted as 18 percent; and the head is another 9 percent in adults. For infants and children, the head is 18 percent involvement and the legs are 14 percent each, due to the larger surface area of a child's head in proportion to the body.

second-degree burn. Deep partial-thickness burn with destruction of the epidermis, the upper portion of the dermis, possibly some deeper dermal tissues, and blistering of the skin with fluid exudate.

TBSA. Total body surface area.

third-degree burn. Full-thickness burn with total destruction of the epidermis and dermis, while deeper underlying tissue may also be affected, including the loss of body parts (e.g., nose, ear, extremity).

tissue. Group of similar cells with a similar function that form definite structures and organs. Tissue types include epithelial tissue, muscle tissue, connective tissue, and nervous tissue.

Repair

16035-16036

16035 Escharotomy; initial incision
+ 16036 each additional incision (List separately in addition to code for primary procedure)

An escharotomy is performed

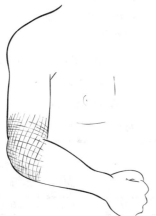

Eschar is the hardened skin caused by a thermal burn

Explanation

The physician performs an escharotomy. Eschar is a leathery slough produced by thermal burns. The physician makes an incision through the area of eschar and undermines it. With adequate incision of the eschar, the physician achieves release of movement for the underlying tissue. Report 16035 for the initial incision and 16036 for each additional incision.

Coding Tips

Report 16036 in addition to 16035. List the percentage of body surface area involved and the depth of the burn. These codes refer to the incision of eschar only. Additional medical procedures or related services, such as hospital visits, should be reported separately using the appropriate procedure/evaluation and management code. For dressing and/or debridement of a burn wound, see 16020–16030. For fractional ablative laser fenestration for functional improvement of scars resulting from trauma or burns, see 0479T-0480T.

ICD-10-CM Diagnostic Codes

T20.33XA	Burn of third degree of chin, initial encounter
T20.36XA	Burn of third degree of forehead and cheek, initial encounter
T20.37XA	Burn of third degree of neck, initial encounter
T20.711A	Corrosion of third degree of right ear [any part, except ear drum], initial encounter ☑
T20.72XA	Corrosion of third degree of lip(s), initial encounter
T20.74XA	Corrosion of third degree of nose (septum), initial encounter
T20.75XA	Corrosion of third degree of scalp [any part], initial encounter
T20.76XA	Corrosion of third degree of forehead and cheek, initial encounter
T20.79XA	Corrosion of third degree of multiple sites of head, face, and neck, initial encounter
T21.31XA	Burn of third degree of chest wall, initial encounter
T21.33XA	Burn of third degree of upper back, initial encounter
T21.34XA	Burn of third degree of lower back, initial encounter
T21.35XA	Burn of third degree of buttock, initial encounter
T21.36XA	Burn of third degree of male genital region, initial encounter ♂
T21.37XA	Burn of third degree of female genital region, initial encounter ♀

T21.71XA	Corrosion of third degree of chest wall, initial encounter
T21.74XA	Corrosion of third degree of lower back, initial encounter
T21.77XA	Corrosion of third degree of female genital region, initial encounter ♀
T22.312A	Burn of third degree of left forearm, initial encounter ☑
T22.331A	Burn of third degree of right upper arm, initial encounter ☑
T22.332A	Burn of third degree of left upper arm, initial encounter ☑
T22.342A	Burn of third degree of left axilla, initial encounter ☑
T22.352A	Burn of third degree of left shoulder, initial encounter ☑
T22.361A	Burn of third degree of right scapular region, initial encounter ☑
T22.391A	Burn of third degree of multiple sites of right shoulder and upper limb, except wrist and hand, initial encounter ☑
T22.712A	Corrosion of third degree of left forearm, initial encounter ☑
T22.732A	Corrosion of third degree of left upper arm, initial encounter ☑
T22.751A	Corrosion of third degree of right shoulder, initial encounter ☑
T22.761A	Corrosion of third degree of right scapular region, initial encounter ☑
T22.791A	Corrosion of third degree of multiple sites of right shoulder and upper limb, except wrist and hand, initial encounter ☑
T23.312A	Burn of third degree of left thumb (nail), initial encounter ☑
T23.321A	Burn of third degree of single right finger (nail) except thumb, initial encounter ☑
T23.332A	Burn of third degree of multiple left fingers (nail), not including thumb, initial encounter ☑
T23.362A	Burn of third degree of back of left hand, initial encounter ☑
T23.371A	Burn of third degree of right wrist, initial encounter ☑
T23.391A	Burn of third degree of multiple sites of right wrist and hand, initial encounter ☑
T23.722A	Corrosion of third degree of single left finger (nail) except thumb, initial encounter ☑
T23.741A	Corrosion of third degree of multiple right fingers (nail), including thumb, initial encounter ☑
T23.752A	Corrosion of third degree of left palm, initial encounter ☑
T23.762A	Corrosion of third degree of back of left hand, initial encounter ☑
T23.771A	Corrosion of third degree of right wrist, initial encounter ☑
T23.792A	Corrosion of third degree of multiple sites of left wrist and hand, initial encounter ☑
T24.311A	Burn of third degree of right thigh, initial encounter ☑
T24.322A	Burn of third degree of left knee, initial encounter ☑
T24.331A	Burn of third degree of right lower leg, initial encounter ☑
T24.391A	Burn of third degree of multiple sites of right lower limb, except ankle and foot, initial encounter ☑
T24.711A	Corrosion of third degree of right thigh, initial encounter ☑
T24.722A	Corrosion of third degree of left knee, initial encounter ☑
T24.731A	Corrosion of third degree of right lower leg, initial encounter ☑
T25.311A	Burn of third degree of right ankle, initial encounter ☑
T25.391A	Burn of third degree of multiple sites of right ankle and foot, initial encounter ☑
T25.711A	Corrosion of third degree of right ankle, initial encounter ☑
T25.731A	Corrosion of third degree of right toe(s) (nail), initial encounter ☑
T25.792A	Corrosion of third degree of multiple sites of left ankle and foot, initial encounter ☑
T31.11	Burns involving 10-19% of body surface with 10-19% third degree burns

T31.30	Burns involving 30-39% of body surface with 0% to 9% third degree burns
T31.32	Burns involving 30-39% of body surface with 20-29% third degree burns
T31.43	Burns involving 40-49% of body surface with 30-39% third degree burns
T31.50	Burns involving 50-59% of body surface with 0% to 9% third degree burns
T31.55	Burns involving 50-59% of body surface with 50-59% third degree burns
T31.64	Burns involving 60-69% of body surface with 40-49% third degree burns
T31.66	Burns involving 60-69% of body surface with 60-69% third degree burns
T31.72	Burns involving 70-79% of body surface with 20-29% third degree burns
T31.74	Burns involving 70-79% of body surface with 40-49% third degree burns
T31.76	Burns involving 70-79% of body surface with 60-69% third degree burns
T31.80	Burns involving 80-89% of body surface with 0% to 9% third degree burns
T31.82	Burns involving 80-89% of body surface with 20-29% third degree burns
T31.87	Burns involving 80-89% of body surface with 70-79% third degree burns
T31.92	Burns involving 90% or more of body surface with 20-29% third degree burns
T31.98	Burns involving 90% or more of body surface with 80-89% third degree burns
T32.10	Corrosions involving 10-19% of body surface with 0% to 9% third degree corrosion
T32.21	Corrosions involving 20-29% of body surface with 10-19% third degree corrosion
T32.32	Corrosions involving 30-39% of body surface with 20-29% third degree corrosion
T32.40	Corrosions involving 40-49% of body surface with 0% to 9% third degree corrosion
T32.42	Corrosions involving 40-49% of body surface with 20-29% third degree corrosion
T32.51	Corrosions involving 50-59% of body surface with 10-19% third degree corrosion
T32.54	Corrosions involving 50-59% of body surface with 40-49% third degree corrosion
T32.55	Corrosions involving 50-59% of body surface with 50-59% third degree corrosion
T32.60	Corrosions involving 60-69% of body surface with 0% to 9% third degree corrosion
T32.65	Corrosions involving 60-69% of body surface with 50-59% third degree corrosion
T32.72	Corrosions involving 70-79% of body surface with 20-29% third degree corrosion
T32.75	Corrosions involving 70-79% of body surface with 50-59% third degree corrosion
T32.83	Corrosions involving 80-89% of body surface with 30-39% third degree corrosion
T32.85	Corrosions involving 80-89% of body surface with 50-59% third degree corrosion
T32.88	Corrosions involving 80-89% of body surface with 80-89% third degree corrosion
T32.90	Corrosions involving 90% or more of body surface with 0% to 9% third degree corrosion
T32.95	Corrosions involving 90% or more of body surface with 50-59% third degree corrosion
T32.98	Corrosions involving 90% or more of body surface with 80-89% third degree corrosion

AMA: **16035** 2018,Jan,8; 2017,Jan,8; 2016,Jan,13; 2015,Jan,16 **16036** 2018,Jan,8; 2017,Jan,8; 2016,Jan,13; 2015,Jan,16

Relative Value Units/Medicare Edits

Non-Facility RVU	Work	PE	MP	Total
16035	3.74	1.36	0.56	5.66
16036	1.5	0.54	0.26	2.3
Facility RVU	**Work**	**PE**	**MP**	**Total**
16035	3.74	1.36	0.56	5.66
16036	1.5	0.54	0.26	2.3

	FUD	Status	MUE	Modifiers				IOM Reference
16035	0	A	1(2)	51	N/A	N/A	N/A	None
16036	N/A	A	8(3)	N/A	N/A	N/A	N/A	

* with documentation

Terms To Know

escharotomy. Surgical incision into the scab or crust resulting from a severe burn in order to relieve constriction and allow blood flow to the distal unburned tissue.

first-degree burn. Superficial partial-thickness burn in which only the epidermis or a portion of the dermis is involved, displaying redness but no blister formation.

second-degree burn. Deep partial-thickness burn with destruction of the epidermis, the upper portion of the dermis, possibly some deeper dermal tissues, and blistering of the skin with fluid exudate.

subcutaneous tissue. Sheet or wide band of adipose (fat) and areolar connective tissue in two layers attached to the dermis.

third-degree burn. Full-thickness burn with total destruction of the epidermis and dermis, while deeper underlying tissue may also be affected, including the loss of body parts (e.g., nose, ear, extremity).

Repair

17311-17312

17311 Mohs micrographic technique, including removal of all gross tumor, surgical excision of tissue specimens, mapping, color coding of specimens, microscopic examination of specimens by the surgeon, and histopathologic preparation including routine stain(s) (eg, hematoxylin and eosin, toluidine blue), head, neck, hands, feet, genitalia, or any location with surgery directly involving muscle, cartilage, bone, tendon, major nerves, or vessels; first stage, up to 5 tissue blocks

+ 17312 each additional stage after the first stage, up to 5 tissue blocks (List separately in addition to code for primary procedure)

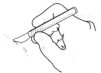

A thin, horizontal layer of tissue is removed. The wound is immediately mapped and a frozen slide prepared

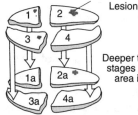

Lesion

Deeper tissue is removed in stages until each mapped area is free of disease

Mohs micrographic technique is often used for basal and squamous cell carcinoma. The incisions are repeated until review shows absence of disease. A single physician performs all aspects

Explanation

The physician performs chemosurgery using Mohs micrographic technique. The physician places a chemical agent on the lesion prior to excision. This chemical acts as a tissue fixative. The lesion is excised via serial tangential cuts, allowing the physician to more closely assess wound margins and the extent of the defect being excised. Report 17311 for first stage, fresh tissue, up to five specimens of the head, neck, hands, feet, genitalia, or any location with surgery directly involving muscle, cartilage, bone, tendon, major nerves, or vessels and 17312 for each additional stage, fixed or fresh tissue, up to five specimens.

Coding Tips

Report 17312 in addition to 17311. These procedures require the physician to act as both the surgeon and the pathologist. If either of these responsibilities is delegated to another physician who reports services separately, these codes are not applicable. If repair is performed, use separate repair, flap, or graft codes. Each additional tissue block after the first five is reported separately, see 17315. Do not report 88314 for routine frozen section stain performed in conjunction with Mohs surgery. Do not report surgical pathology codes 88302–88309 separately on the same specimen obtained as part of the Mohs surgery. For a non-routine stain or when a diagnostic skin biopsy (11102–11107) and frozen section (88331) are performed on the same day as Mohs surgery, append modifier 59 or an X{EPSU} modifier with 88314 to distinguish these services from the Mohs surgery. For Mohs surgery performed on the trunk, arms, or legs and not involving muscle, cartilage, bone, tendon, major nerves, or major vessels, see 17313 and 17314. For additional special pathology procedures, stains, or immunostains, see 88311–88314 and 88342.

ICD-10-CM Diagnostic Codes

C00.0	Malignant neoplasm of external upper lip
C00.1	Malignant neoplasm of external lower lip
C00.3	Malignant neoplasm of upper lip, inner aspect
C00.4	Malignant neoplasm of lower lip, inner aspect
C43.0	Malignant melanoma of lip
C43.111	Malignant melanoma of right upper eyelid, including canthus ☑
C43.112	Malignant melanoma of right lower eyelid, including canthus ☑
C43.21	Malignant melanoma of right ear and external auricular canal ☑
C43.22	Malignant melanoma of left ear and external auricular canal ☑
C43.31	Malignant melanoma of nose
C43.39	Malignant melanoma of other parts of face
C43.4	Malignant melanoma of scalp and neck
C43.51	Malignant melanoma of anal skin
C43.61	Malignant melanoma of right upper limb, including shoulder ☑
C43.71	Malignant melanoma of right lower limb, including hip ☑
C43.72	Malignant melanoma of left lower limb, including hip ☑
C43.8	Malignant melanoma of overlapping sites of skin
C44.01	Basal cell carcinoma of skin of lip
C44.02	Squamous cell carcinoma of skin of lip
C44.09	Other specified malignant neoplasm of skin of lip
C44.1121	Basal cell carcinoma of skin of right upper eyelid, including canthus ☑
C44.1122	Basal cell carcinoma of skin of right lower eyelid, including canthus ☑
C44.1221	Squamous cell carcinoma of skin of right upper eyelid, including canthus ☑
C44.1222	Squamous cell carcinoma of skin of right lower eyelid, including canthus ☑
C44.1321	Sebaceous cell carcinoma of skin of right upper eyelid, including canthus ☑
C44.1322	Sebaceous cell carcinoma of skin of right lower eyelid, including canthus ☑
C44.212	Basal cell carcinoma of skin of right ear and external auricular canal ☑
C44.219	Basal cell carcinoma of skin of left ear and external auricular canal ☑
C44.222	Squamous cell carcinoma of skin of right ear and external auricular canal ☑
C44.229	Squamous cell carcinoma of skin of left ear and external auricular canal ☑
C44.292	Other specified malignant neoplasm of skin of right ear and external auricular canal ☑
C44.299	Other specified malignant neoplasm of skin of left ear and external auricular canal ☑
C44.311	Basal cell carcinoma of skin of nose
C44.319	Basal cell carcinoma of skin of other parts of face
C44.321	Squamous cell carcinoma of skin of nose
C44.329	Squamous cell carcinoma of skin of other parts of face
C44.391	Other specified malignant neoplasm of skin of nose
C44.399	Other specified malignant neoplasm of skin of other parts of face
C44.41	Basal cell carcinoma of skin of scalp and neck
C44.42	Squamous cell carcinoma of skin of scalp and neck
C44.510	Basal cell carcinoma of anal skin
C44.519	Basal cell carcinoma of skin of other part of trunk

Destruction

C44.520	Squamous cell carcinoma of anal skin
C44.521	Squamous cell carcinoma of skin of breast
C44.612	Basal cell carcinoma of skin of right upper limb, including shoulder ☑
C44.619	Basal cell carcinoma of skin of left upper limb, including shoulder ☑
C44.622	Squamous cell carcinoma of skin of right upper limb, including shoulder ☑
C44.629	Squamous cell carcinoma of skin of left upper limb, including shoulder ☑
C44.692	Other specified malignant neoplasm of skin of right upper limb, including shoulder ☑
C44.699	Other specified malignant neoplasm of skin of left upper limb, including shoulder ☑
C44.712	Basal cell carcinoma of skin of right lower limb, including hip ☑
C44.719	Basal cell carcinoma of skin of left lower limb, including hip ☑
C44.722	Squamous cell carcinoma of skin of right lower limb, including hip ☑
C44.729	Squamous cell carcinoma of skin of left lower limb, including hip ☑
C44.792	Other specified malignant neoplasm of skin of right lower limb, including hip ☑
C44.799	Other specified malignant neoplasm of skin of left lower limb, including hip ☑
C44.82	Squamous cell carcinoma of overlapping sites of skin
C4A.0	Merkel cell carcinoma of lip
C4A.111	Merkel cell carcinoma of right upper eyelid, including canthus ☑
C4A.112	Merkel cell carcinoma of right lower eyelid, including canthus ☑
C4A.21	Merkel cell carcinoma of right ear and external auricular canal ☑
C4A.22	Merkel cell carcinoma of left ear and external auricular canal ☑
C4A.31	Merkel cell carcinoma of nose
C4A.39	Merkel cell carcinoma of other parts of face
C4A.4	Merkel cell carcinoma of scalp and neck
C4A.51	Merkel cell carcinoma of anal skin
C4A.52	Merkel cell carcinoma of skin of breast
C4A.59	Merkel cell carcinoma of other part of trunk
C4A.61	Merkel cell carcinoma of right upper limb, including shoulder ☑
C4A.62	Merkel cell carcinoma of left upper limb, including shoulder ☑
C4A.71	Merkel cell carcinoma of right lower limb, including hip ☑
C4A.72	Merkel cell carcinoma of left lower limb, including hip ☑
C51.0	Malignant neoplasm of labium majus ♀
C51.1	Malignant neoplasm of labium minus ♀
C51.2	Malignant neoplasm of clitoris ♀
C52	Malignant neoplasm of vagina ♀
C60.2	Malignant neoplasm of body of penis ♂
C63.2	Malignant neoplasm of scrotum ♂
C76.0	Malignant neoplasm of head, face and neck
C76.2	Malignant neoplasm of abdomen
C76.41	Malignant neoplasm of right upper limb ☑
C76.42	Malignant neoplasm of left upper limb ☑
C7B.1	Secondary Merkel cell carcinoma

AMA: **17311** 2018,Jan,8; 2017,Jan,8; 2016,Jan,13; 2015,Jan,16 **17312** 2018,Jan,8; 2017,Jan,8; 2016,Jan,13; 2015,Jan,16

Relative Value Units/Medicare Edits

Non-Facility RVU	Work	PE	MP	Total
17311	6.2	12.99	0.59	19.78
17312	3.3	8.41	0.31	12.02
Facility RVU	**Work**	**PE**	**MP**	**Total**
17311	6.2	3.57	0.59	10.36
17312	3.3	1.89	0.31	5.5

	FUD	Status	MUE	Modifiers				IOM Reference
17311	0	A	4(3)	51	N/A	N/A	N/A	None
17312	N/A	A	6(3)	N/A	N/A	N/A	N/A	

* with documentation

Terms To Know

chemosurgery. Application of chemical agents to destroy tissue, originally referring to the in situ chemical fixation of premalignant or malignant lesions to facilitate surgical excision.

lesion. Area of damaged tissue that has lost continuity or function, due to disease or trauma.

Mohs micrographic surgery. Special technique used to treat complex or ill-defined skin cancer and requires a single physician to provide two distinct services. The first service is surgical and involves the destruction of the lesion by a combination of chemosurgery and excision. The second service is that of a pathologist and includes mapping, color coding of specimens, microscopic examination of specimens, and complete histopathologic preparation.

specimen. Tissue cells or sample of fluid taken for analysis, pathologic examination, and diagnosis.

tissue. Group of similar cells with a similar function that form definite structures and organs. Tissue types include epithelial tissue, muscle tissue, connective tissue, and nervous tissue.

17313 Mohs micrographic technique, including removal of all gross tumor, surgical excision of tissue specimens, mapping, color coding of specimens, microscopic examination of specimens by the surgeon, and histopathologic preparation including routine stain(s) (eg, hematoxylin and eosin, toluidine blue), of the trunk, arms, or legs; first stage, up to 5 tissue blocks

+ **17314** each additional stage after the first stage, up to 5 tissue blocks (List separately in addition to code for primary procedure)

A thin, horizontal layer of tissue is removed. The wound is immediately mapped and a frozen slide prepared

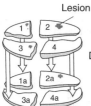

Lesion

Deeper tissue is removed in stages until each mapped area is free of disease

Mohs micrographic technique is often used for basal and squamous cell carcinoma. The incisions are repeated until review shows absence of disease. A single physician performs all aspects

Explanation

The physician performs chemosurgery using Mohs micrographic technique. The physician places a chemical agent on the lesion prior to excision. This chemical acts as a tissue fixative. The lesion is excised via serial tangential cuts, allowing the physician to more closely assess wound margins and the extent of the defect being excised. Report 17313 for first stage, fixed or fresh tissue, up to five specimens of the trunk, arms, or legs and 17314 for additional stages, each stage, up to five specimens.

Coding Tips

Report 17314 in addition to 17313. These procedures require the physician to act as the surgeon and the pathologist. If either of these responsibilities is delegated to another physician who reports services separately, these codes are not applicable. If repair is performed, use separate repair, flap, or graft codes. Each additional tissue block after the first five is reported separately, see 17315. For Mohs surgery performed on the head, neck, hands, feet, genitalia, or any location including the trunk, arms, or legs that involves muscle, cartilage, bone, tendon, major nerves, or major vessels, see 17311 and 17312. If additional special pathology procedures, stains, or immunostains are performed, see 88311–88314 and 88342. Do not report 88314 for routine frozen section stain performed in conjunction with Mohs surgery. Do not report surgical pathology codes 88302–88309 separately on the same specimen obtained as part of Mohs surgery. Append modifier 59 or an X{EPSU} modifier with 88314 if a non-routine stain is required or when a diagnostic skin biopsy (11102–11107) and frozen section (88331) are performed on the same day as the Mohs surgery to distinguish these services from the Mohs surgery.

ICD-10-CM Diagnostic Codes

C43.52	Malignant melanoma of skin of breast
C43.59	Malignant melanoma of other part of trunk
C43.61	Malignant melanoma of right upper limb, including shoulder ☑
C43.62	Malignant melanoma of left upper limb, including shoulder ☑
C43.71	Malignant melanoma of right lower limb, including hip ☑
C43.72	Malignant melanoma of left lower limb, including hip ☑
C43.8	Malignant melanoma of overlapping sites of skin
C44.510	Basal cell carcinoma of anal skin
C44.511	Basal cell carcinoma of skin of breast
C44.519	Basal cell carcinoma of skin of other part of trunk
C44.520	Squamous cell carcinoma of anal skin
C44.521	Squamous cell carcinoma of skin of breast
C44.529	Squamous cell carcinoma of skin of other part of trunk
C44.590	Other specified malignant neoplasm of anal skin
C44.591	Other specified malignant neoplasm of skin of breast
C44.599	Other specified malignant neoplasm of skin of other part of trunk
C44.612	Basal cell carcinoma of skin of right upper limb, including shoulder ☑
C44.619	Basal cell carcinoma of skin of left upper limb, including shoulder ☑
C44.622	Squamous cell carcinoma of skin of right upper limb, including shoulder ☑
C44.629	Squamous cell carcinoma of skin of left upper limb, including shoulder ☑
C44.692	Other specified malignant neoplasm of skin of right upper limb, including shoulder ☑
C44.699	Other specified malignant neoplasm of skin of left upper limb, including shoulder ☑
C44.712	Basal cell carcinoma of skin of right lower limb, including hip ☑
C44.719	Basal cell carcinoma of skin of left lower limb, including hip ☑
C44.722	Squamous cell carcinoma of skin of right lower limb, including hip ☑
C44.729	Squamous cell carcinoma of skin of left lower limb, including hip ☑
C44.792	Other specified malignant neoplasm of skin of right lower limb, including hip ☑
C44.799	Other specified malignant neoplasm of skin of left lower limb, including hip ☑
C44.81	Basal cell carcinoma of overlapping sites of skin
C44.82	Squamous cell carcinoma of overlapping sites of skin
C44.89	Other specified malignant neoplasm of overlapping sites of skin
C4A.52	Merkel cell carcinoma of skin of breast
C4A.59	Merkel cell carcinoma of other part of trunk
C4A.61	Merkel cell carcinoma of right upper limb, including shoulder ☑
C4A.62	Merkel cell carcinoma of left upper limb, including shoulder ☑
C4A.71	Merkel cell carcinoma of right lower limb, including hip ☑
C4A.72	Merkel cell carcinoma of left lower limb, including hip ☑
C4A.8	Merkel cell carcinoma of overlapping sites
C76.2	Malignant neoplasm of abdomen
C76.3	Malignant neoplasm of pelvis
C76.41	Malignant neoplasm of right upper limb ☑
C76.42	Malignant neoplasm of left upper limb ☑
C76.8	Malignant neoplasm of other specified ill-defined sites
C7B.1	Secondary Merkel cell carcinoma

AMA: 17313 2018,Jan,8; 2017,Jan,8; 2016,Jan,13; 2015,Jan,16 **17314** 2018,Jan,8; 2017,Jan,8; 2016,Jan,13; 2015,Jan,16

Destruction

Non-Facility RVU	Work	PE	MP	Total
17313	5.56	12.49	0.52	18.57
17314	3.06	8.16	0.28	11.5
Facility RVU	Work	PE	MP	Total
17313	5.56	3.2	0.52	9.28
17314	3.06	1.76	0.28	5.1

	FUD	Status	MUE	Modifiers				IOM Reference
17313	0	A	3(3)	51	N/A	N/A	N/A	None
17314	N/A	A	4(3)	N/A	N/A	N/A	N/A	

* with documentation

Terms To Know

chemosurgery. Application of chemical agents to destroy tissue, originally referring to the in situ chemical fixation of premalignant or malignant lesions to facilitate surgical excision.

defect. Imperfection, flaw, or absence.

lesion. Area of damaged tissue that has lost continuity or function, due to disease or trauma.

margin. Boundary, edge, or border, as of a surface or structure.

Mohs micrographic surgery. Special technique used to treat complex or ill-defined skin cancer and requires a single physician to provide two distinct services. The first service is surgical and involves the destruction of the lesion by a combination of chemosurgery and excision. The second service is that of a pathologist and includes mapping, color coding of specimens, microscopic examination of specimens, and complete histopathologic preparation.

specimen. Tissue cells or sample of fluid taken for analysis, pathologic examination, and diagnosis.

tissue. Group of similar cells with a similar function that form definite structures and organs. Tissue types include epithelial tissue, muscle tissue, connective tissue, and nervous tissue.

17315

+ 17315 Mohs micrographic technique, including removal of all gross tumor, surgical excision of tissue specimens, mapping, color coding of specimens, microscopic examination of specimens by the surgeon, and histopathologic preparation including routine stain(s) (eg, hematoxylin and eosin, toluidine blue), each additional block after the first 5 tissue blocks, any stage (List separately in addition to code for primary procedure)

A thin, horizontal layer of tissue is removed. The wound is immediately mapped and a frozen slide prepared

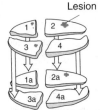

Lesion

Deeper tissue is removed in stages until each mapped area is free of disease

Mohs micrographic technique is often used for basal and squamous cell carcinoma. The incisions are repeated until review shows absence of disease. A single physician performs all aspects

Explanation

The physician performs chemosurgery using Mohs micrographic technique. The physician places a chemical agent on the lesion prior to excision. This chemical acts as a tissue fixative. The lesion is excised via serial tangential cuts, allowing the physician to more closely assess wound margins and the extent of the defect being excised. Report 17315 in addition to the code for the primary procedure for each additional block after the first five tissue blocks, any stage.

Coding Tips

Report 17315 in addition to 17311–17314. Mohs surgery requires the physician to act as both the surgeon and the pathologist. If either of these responsibilities is delegated to another physician who reports services separately, these codes are not applicable. If repair is performed, use separate repair, flap, or graft codes. For Mohs surgery performed on the head, neck, hands, feet, genitalia, or any location including the trunk, arms, or legs that involves muscle, cartilage, bone, tendon, major nerves, or major vessels, see 17311 and 17312. For Mohs surgery performed on the trunk, arms, or legs and not involving muscle, cartilage, bone, tendon, major nerves, or major vessels, see 17313 and 17314. If additional special pathology procedures, stains, or immunostains are performed, see 88311–88314 and 88342. Do not report 88314 for routine frozen section stain performed in conjunction with Mohs surgery. Do not report surgical pathology codes 88302–88309 separately on the same specimen obtained as part of the Mohs surgery. Append modifier 59 or an X{EPSU} modifier with 88314 if a non-routine stain is required or when a diagnostic skin biopsy (11102–11107) and frozen section (88331) are performed on the same day as the Mohs surgery to distinguish these services from the Mohs surgery.

ICD-10-CM Diagnostic Codes

C00.0	Malignant neoplasm of external upper lip
C00.1	Malignant neoplasm of external lower lip
C00.3	Malignant neoplasm of upper lip, inner aspect

Destruction

C00.4	Malignant neoplasm of lower lip, inner aspect
C43.0	Malignant melanoma of lip
C43.111	Malignant melanoma of right upper eyelid, including canthus ☑
C43.112	Malignant melanoma of right lower eyelid, including canthus ☑
C43.21	Malignant melanoma of right ear and external auricular canal ☑
C43.31	Malignant melanoma of nose
C43.39	Malignant melanoma of other parts of face
C43.4	Malignant melanoma of scalp and neck
C43.51	Malignant melanoma of anal skin
C43.52	Malignant melanoma of skin of breast
C43.59	Malignant melanoma of other part of trunk
C43.61	Malignant melanoma of right upper limb, including shoulder ☑
C43.71	Malignant melanoma of right lower limb, including hip ☑
C43.8	Malignant melanoma of overlapping sites of skin
C44.01	Basal cell carcinoma of skin of lip
C44.02	Squamous cell carcinoma of skin of lip
C44.1121	Basal cell carcinoma of skin of right upper eyelid, including canthus ☑
C44.1122	Basal cell carcinoma of skin of right lower eyelid, including canthus ☑
C44.1221	Squamous cell carcinoma of skin of right upper eyelid, including canthus ☑
C44.1222	Squamous cell carcinoma of skin of right lower eyelid, including canthus ☑
C44.1321	Sebaceous cell carcinoma of skin of right upper eyelid, including canthus ☑
C44.1322	Sebaceous cell carcinoma of skin of right lower eyelid, including canthus ☑
C44.212	Basal cell carcinoma of skin of right ear and external auricular canal ☑
C44.222	Squamous cell carcinoma of skin of right ear and external auricular canal ☑
C44.292	Other specified malignant neoplasm of skin of right ear and external auricular canal ☑
C44.311	Basal cell carcinoma of skin of nose
C44.319	Basal cell carcinoma of skin of other parts of face
C44.321	Squamous cell carcinoma of skin of nose
C44.329	Squamous cell carcinoma of skin of other parts of face
C44.41	Basal cell carcinoma of skin of scalp and neck
C44.42	Squamous cell carcinoma of skin of scalp and neck
C44.49	Other specified malignant neoplasm of skin of scalp and neck
C44.510	Basal cell carcinoma of anal skin
C44.511	Basal cell carcinoma of skin of breast
C44.519	Basal cell carcinoma of skin of other part of trunk
C44.520	Squamous cell carcinoma of anal skin
C44.521	Squamous cell carcinoma of skin of breast
C44.529	Squamous cell carcinoma of skin of other part of trunk
C44.590	Other specified malignant neoplasm of anal skin
C44.591	Other specified malignant neoplasm of skin of breast
C44.599	Other specified malignant neoplasm of skin of other part of trunk
C44.612	Basal cell carcinoma of skin of right upper limb, including shoulder ☑
C44.622	Squamous cell carcinoma of skin of right upper limb, including shoulder ☑
C44.692	Other specified malignant neoplasm of skin of right upper limb, including shoulder ☑
C44.712	Basal cell carcinoma of skin of right lower limb, including hip ☑
C44.722	Squamous cell carcinoma of skin of right lower limb, including hip ☑
C44.792	Other specified malignant neoplasm of skin of right lower limb, including hip ☑
C44.81	Basal cell carcinoma of overlapping sites of skin
C44.82	Squamous cell carcinoma of overlapping sites of skin
C44.89	Other specified malignant neoplasm of overlapping sites of skin
C4A.0	Merkel cell carcinoma of lip
C4A.111	Merkel cell carcinoma of right upper eyelid, including canthus ☑
C4A.112	Merkel cell carcinoma of right lower eyelid, including canthus ☑
C4A.21	Merkel cell carcinoma of right ear and external auricular canal ☑
C4A.31	Merkel cell carcinoma of nose
C4A.39	Merkel cell carcinoma of other parts of face
C4A.4	Merkel cell carcinoma of scalp and neck
C4A.51	Merkel cell carcinoma of anal skin
C4A.52	Merkel cell carcinoma of skin of breast
C4A.59	Merkel cell carcinoma of other part of trunk
C4A.61	Merkel cell carcinoma of right upper limb, including shoulder ☑
C4A.71	Merkel cell carcinoma of right lower limb, including hip ☑
C4A.8	Merkel cell carcinoma of overlapping sites
C51.1	Malignant neoplasm of labium minus ♀
C51.2	Malignant neoplasm of clitoris ♀
C52	Malignant neoplasm of vagina ♀
C60.0	Malignant neoplasm of prepuce ♂
C60.1	Malignant neoplasm of glans penis ♂
C60.2	Malignant neoplasm of body of penis ♂
C63.2	Malignant neoplasm of scrotum ♂
C76.0	Malignant neoplasm of head, face and neck
C76.2	Malignant neoplasm of abdomen
C76.3	Malignant neoplasm of pelvis
C76.41	Malignant neoplasm of right upper limb ☑
C76.8	Malignant neoplasm of other specified ill-defined sites
C7B.1	Secondary Merkel cell carcinoma

AMA: **17315** 2018,Jan,8; 2017,Jan,8; 2016,Jan,13; 2015,Jan,16

Relative Value Units/Medicare Edits

Non-Facility RVU	Work	PE	MP	Total
17315	0.87	1.3	0.09	2.26
Facility RVU	**Work**	**PE**	**MP**	**Total**
17315	0.87	0.5	0.09	1.46

	FUD	Status	MUE	Modifiers				IOM Reference
17315	N/A	A	15(3)	N/A	N/A	N/A	N/A	None

* with documentation

Destruction

19000-19001

19000 Puncture aspiration of cyst of breast;
+ 19001 each additional cyst (List separately in addition to code for primary procedure)

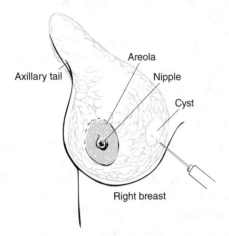

A breast cyst is punctured and needle aspirated

Explanation

The physician punctures with a syringe needle the skin of the breast overlying a cyst. The needle is inserted into the cyst and fluid is evacuated into the syringe, thus reducing the size of the cyst. The physician withdraws the needle and applies pressure to the puncture wound to stop the bleeding. Report 19001 for aspiration of each additional cyst of the breast.

Coding Tips

Report 19001 in addition to 19000. Imaging guidance is reported with 76942 or 77021, when performed. For puncture aspiration of a cyst, abscess, hematoma, or bulla, see 10160. For mastotomy with exploration or drainage of a deep abscess, see 19020. For excision of a breast cyst, fibroadenoma, or other benign or malignant tumor, aberrant breast tissue, duct, nipple, or areolar lesion, open, see 19120. Surgical trays, A4550, are not separately reimbursed by Medicare; however, other third-party payers may cover them. Check with the specific payer to determine coverage.</p>

ICD-10-CM Diagnostic Codes

N60.01 Solitary cyst of right breast ☑
N60.02 Solitary cyst of left breast ☑
N60.11 Diffuse cystic mastopathy of right breast 🅰 ☑
N60.12 Diffuse cystic mastopathy of left breast 🅰 ☑
N60.81 Other benign mammary dysplasias of right breast ☑
N60.82 Other benign mammary dysplasias of left breast ☑
N63.11 Unspecified lump in the right breast, upper outer quadrant ☑
N63.12 Unspecified lump in the right breast, upper inner quadrant ☑
N63.13 Unspecified lump in the right breast, lower outer quadrant ☑
N63.14 Unspecified lump in the right breast, lower inner quadrant ☑
N63.21 Unspecified lump in the left breast, upper outer quadrant ☑
N63.22 Unspecified lump in the left breast, upper inner quadrant ☑
N63.23 Unspecified lump in the left breast, lower outer quadrant ☑
N63.24 Unspecified lump in the left breast, lower inner quadrant ☑
N63.31 Unspecified lump in axillary tail of the right breast ☑
N63.32 Unspecified lump in axillary tail of the left breast ☑
N63.41 Unspecified lump in right breast, subareolar ☑
N63.42 Unspecified lump in left breast, subareolar ☑

AMA: **19000** 2018,Jan,8; 2017,Jan,8; 2016,Jan,13; 2015,Jan,16 **19001** 2018,Jan,8; 2017,Jan,8; 2016,Jan,13; 2015,Jan,16

Relative Value Units/Medicare Edits

Non-Facility RVU	Work	PE	MP	Total
19000	0.84	2.22	0.11	3.17
19001	0.42	0.32	0.05	0.79
Facility RVU	Work	PE	MP	Total
19000	0.84	0.31	0.11	1.26
19001	0.42	0.15	0.05	0.62

	FUD	Status	MUE	Modifiers				IOM Reference
19000	0	A	2(3)	51	N/A	N/A	N/A	100-04,13,80.1
19001	N/A	A	5(3)	N/A	N/A	N/A	N/A	

* with documentation

Terms To Know

axillary region. Area immediately surrounding the armpit.

benign mammary dysplasias. Noncancerous fibrous or cystic growths in the breast.

cyst. Elevated encapsulated mass containing fluid, semisolid, or solid material with a membranous lining.

diffuse cystic mastopathy. Condition in which benign cysts are scattered throughout the breast, thought to be associated with ovarian hormones.

dysplasia. Abnormality or alteration in the size, shape, and organization of cells from their normal pattern of development.

evacuation. Removal or purging of waste material.

exploration. Examination for diagnostic purposes.

galactocele. Tumor or cyst-like enlargement of the milk-containing gland in the breast.

insertion. Placement or implantation into a body part.

mastopathy. Disease or disorder of the breast or lactiferous (mammary) glands.

puncture aspiration. Use of a knife or needle to pierce a fluid-filled cavity and then withdraw the fluid using a syringe or suction device.

19020

19020 Mastotomy with exploration or drainage of abscess, deep

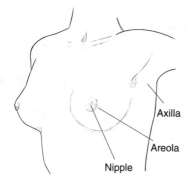

Breast tissue is incised and explored
or a deep abscess is drained

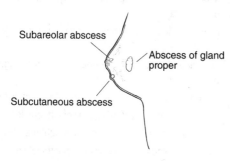

Subareolar abscess
Abscess of gland proper
Subcutaneous abscess

Explanation

The physician makes an incision in the skin of the breast over the site of an abscess or suspicious tissue for exploration or drainage. The infected cavity is accessed and specimens for culture are taken before the cavity is irrigated with warm saline solution. Bleeding vessels may be tied or cauterized. If no abscess or suspicious tissue is found, the wound is closed with sutures. In the case of an abscess, the wound is usually loosely packed with gauze to promote free drainage rather than being closed with sutures.

Coding Tips

This is a unilateral procedure. If performed bilaterally, some payers require that the service be reported twice with modifier 50 appended to the second code while others require identification of the service only once with modifier 50 appended. Check with individual payers. Modifier 50 identifies a procedure performed identically on the opposite side of the body (mirror image). For puncture aspiration of a breast cyst(s), see 19000–19001. For a percutaneous needle core breast biopsy without imaging guidance, see 19100; open incisional, see 19101. Breast biopsies with imaging guidance, including placement of localization devices, are reported with 19081–19086. For placement of localization devices without biopsy, see 19281–19288. Excision of a breast lesion may be reported with 19120. Surgical trays, A4550, are not separately reimbursed by Medicare; however, other third-party payers may cover them. Check with the specific payer to determine coverage.

ICD-10-CM Diagnostic Codes

N61.1	Abscess of the breast and nipple
N61.21	Granulomatous mastitis, right breast ☑
N61.22	Granulomatous mastitis, left breast ☑
N61.23	Granulomatous mastitis, bilateral breast ☑
O91.111	Abscess of breast associated with pregnancy, first trimester Ⓜ ♀
O91.112	Abscess of breast associated with pregnancy, second trimester Ⓜ ♀
O91.113	Abscess of breast associated with pregnancy, third trimester Ⓜ ♀
O91.12	Abscess of breast associated with the puerperium Ⓜ ♀
O91.13	Abscess of breast associated with lactation Ⓜ ♀

AMA: 19020 2018,Jan,8; 2017,Jan,8; 2016,Jan,13; 2015,Jan,16

Relative Value Units/Medicare Edits

Non-Facility RVU	Work	PE	MP	Total
19020	3.83	9.57	0.86	14.26
Facility RVU	**Work**	**PE**	**MP**	**Total**
19020	3.83	4.5	0.86	9.19

	FUD	Status	MUE	Modifiers				IOM Reference
19020	90	A	2(3)	51	50	N/A	N/A	None

* with documentation

Terms To Know

abscess. Circumscribed collection of pus resulting from bacteria, frequently associated with swelling and other signs of inflammation.

benign mammary dysplasias. Noncancerous fibrous or cystic growths in the breast.

cystic mastopathy. Mammary dysplasia involving inflammation and the formation of fluid-filled nodular cysts in the breast tissue.

infection. Presence of microorganisms in body tissues that may result in cellular damage.

mammary duct ectasia. Condition characterized by dilated ducts of the mammary gland.

mastitis. Inflammation of the breast. Acute mastitis is caused by a bacterial infection; chronic mastitis is caused by hormonal changes.

mastodynia. Pain, discomfort, or tenderness in the breast, often due to hormonal changes.

mastotomy. Incision of the breast, often performed for exploration of suspicious tissue or for drainage of an abscess.

nonpurulent mastitis. Inflammation of the breast without the formation of infected discharge.

Breast

19081-19082

19081 Biopsy, breast, with placement of breast localization device(s) (eg, clip, metallic pellet), when performed, and imaging of the biopsy specimen, when performed, percutaneous; first lesion, including stereotactic guidance

+ 19082 each additional lesion, including stereotactic guidance (List separately in addition to code for primary procedure)

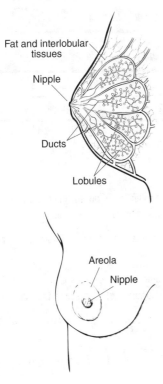

Fat and interlobular tissues
Nipple
Ducts
Lobules

Areola
Nipple

Explanation

The physician performs a breast biopsy with image guidance using a percutaneous needle core or automated vacuum assisted or rotating biopsy device and insertion of a localization device. Using image guidance, the physician places a metallic clip or pellet adjacent to a breast lesion to mark the site. A large gauge (e.g., 14 gauge), hollow core biopsy needle or the biopsy device is inserted through the skin of the breast and into the suspicious breast tissue. The physician takes multiple core tissue samples from a single lesion to obtain a sufficient amount of tissue for diagnosis. The needle or automated vacuum assisted or rotating biopsy device is withdrawn. Pressure and bandages are applied to the puncture site. Report 19081 for the first lesion and 19082 for each additional lesion removed using stereotactic guidance.

Coding Tips

Report 19082 in addition to 19081. These are unilateral procedures. If performed bilaterally, some payers require that the service be reported twice with modifier 50 appended to the second code while others require identification of the service only once with modifier 50 appended. Check with individual payers. Modifier 50 identifies a procedure performed identically on the opposite side of the body (mirror image). Do not report 19081 or 19082 in addition to 19281–19288, 76098, 76942, 77002, or 77021 when performed on the same lesion.

ICD-10-CM Diagnostic Codes

C50.011	Malignant neoplasm of nipple and areola, right female breast ♀ ☑
C50.012	Malignant neoplasm of nipple and areola, left female breast ♀ ☑
C50.021	Malignant neoplasm of nipple and areola, right male breast ♂ ☑
C50.022	Malignant neoplasm of nipple and areola, left male breast ♂ ☑
C50.111	Malignant neoplasm of central portion of right female breast ♀ ☑
C50.112	Malignant neoplasm of central portion of left female breast ♀ ☑
C50.121	Malignant neoplasm of central portion of right male breast ♂ ☑
C50.122	Malignant neoplasm of central portion of left male breast ♂ ☑
C50.211	Malignant neoplasm of upper-inner quadrant of right female breast ♀ ☑
C50.221	Malignant neoplasm of upper-inner quadrant of right male breast ♂ ☑
C50.311	Malignant neoplasm of lower-inner quadrant of right female breast ♀ ☑
C50.321	Malignant neoplasm of lower-inner quadrant of right male breast ♂ ☑
C50.411	Malignant neoplasm of upper-outer quadrant of right female breast ♀ ☑
C50.421	Malignant neoplasm of upper-outer quadrant of right male breast ♂ ☑
C50.511	Malignant neoplasm of lower-outer quadrant of right female breast ♀ ☑
C50.521	Malignant neoplasm of lower-outer quadrant of right male breast ♂ ☑
C50.611	Malignant neoplasm of axillary tail of right female breast ♀ ☑
C50.612	Malignant neoplasm of axillary tail of left female breast ♀ ☑
C50.621	Malignant neoplasm of axillary tail of right male breast ♂ ☑
C50.622	Malignant neoplasm of axillary tail of left male breast ♂ ☑
C50.811	Malignant neoplasm of overlapping sites of right female breast ♀ ☑
C50.812	Malignant neoplasm of overlapping sites of left female breast ♀ ☑
C50.821	Malignant neoplasm of overlapping sites of right male breast ♂ ☑
C50.822	Malignant neoplasm of overlapping sites of left male breast ♂ ☑
C79.81	Secondary malignant neoplasm of breast
D03.52	Melanoma in situ of breast (skin) (soft tissue)
D05.01	Lobular carcinoma in situ of right breast ☑
D05.02	Lobular carcinoma in situ of left breast ☑
D05.11	Intraductal carcinoma in situ of right breast ☑
D05.12	Intraductal carcinoma in situ of left breast ☑
D05.81	Other specified type of carcinoma in situ of right breast ☑
D05.82	Other specified type of carcinoma in situ of left breast ☑
D24.1	Benign neoplasm of right breast ☑
D24.2	Benign neoplasm of left breast ☑
D48.61	Neoplasm of uncertain behavior of right breast ☑
N60.01	Solitary cyst of right breast ☑
N60.11	Diffuse cystic mastopathy of right breast 🅐 ☑
N60.12	Diffuse cystic mastopathy of left breast 🅐 ☑
N60.21	Fibroadenosis of right breast ☑
N60.22	Fibroadenosis of left breast ☑
N60.31	Fibrosclerosis of right breast ☑
N60.32	Fibrosclerosis of left breast ☑
N60.41	Mammary duct ectasia of right breast ☑
N60.42	Mammary duct ectasia of left breast ☑
N60.81	Other benign mammary dysplasias of right breast ☑

N61.21	Granulomatous mastitis, right breast ☑	
N61.22	Granulomatous mastitis, left breast ☑	
N61.23	Granulomatous mastitis, bilateral breast ☑	
N62	Hypertrophy of breast	
N63.11	Unspecified lump in the right breast, upper outer quadrant ☑	
N63.12	Unspecified lump in the right breast, upper inner quadrant ☑	
N63.13	Unspecified lump in the right breast, lower outer quadrant ☑	
N63.14	Unspecified lump in the right breast, lower inner quadrant ☑	
N63.21	Unspecified lump in the left breast, upper outer quadrant ☑	
N63.22	Unspecified lump in the left breast, upper inner quadrant ☑	
N63.23	Unspecified lump in the left breast, lower outer quadrant ☑	
N63.24	Unspecified lump in the left breast, lower inner quadrant ☑	
N63.31	Unspecified lump in axillary tail of the right breast ☑	
N63.41	Unspecified lump in right breast, subareolar ☑	
N64.1	Fat necrosis of breast	
N64.51	Induration of breast	
N64.89	Other specified disorders of breast	
R92.0	Mammographic microcalcification found on diagnostic imaging of breast	
R92.1	Mammographic calcification found on diagnostic imaging of breast	
R92.8	Other abnormal and inconclusive findings on diagnostic imaging of breast	

AMA: **19081** 2019,Apr,4; 2018,Jan,8; 2017,Jan,8; 2016,Jun,3; 2016,Jan,13; 2015,May,8; 2015,Mar,5; 2015,Jan,16 **19082** 2019,Apr,4; 2018,Jan,8; 2017,Jan,8; 2016,Jun,3; 2016,Jan,13; 2015,May,8; 2015,Mar,5; 2015,Jan,16

Relative Value Units/Medicare Edits

Non-Facility RVU	Work	PE	MP	Total
19081	3.29	13.26	0.32	16.87
19082	1.65	11.7	0.16	13.51
Facility RVU	Work	PE	MP	Total
19081	3.29	1.19	0.32	4.8
19082	1.65	0.6	0.16	2.41

	FUD	Status	MUE	Modifiers				IOM Reference
19081	0	A	1(2)	51	50	N/A	80*	100-04,12,40.7; 100-04,13,80.1
19082	N/A	A	2(3)	N/A	N/A	N/A	80*	
* with documentation								

Terms To Know

core needle biopsy. Large-bore biopsy needle inserted into a mass and a core of tissue is removed for diagnostic study.

localization. Limitation to one area.

percutaneous. Through the skin.

stereotaxis. Three-dimensional method for precisely locating structures.

19083-19084

	19083	Biopsy, breast, with placement of breast localization device(s) (eg, clip, metallic pellet), when performed, and imaging of the biopsy specimen, when performed, percutaneous; first lesion, including ultrasound guidance
+	19084	each additional lesion, including ultrasound guidance (List separately in addition to code for primary procedure)

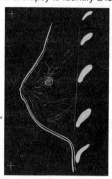

A metallic localization device is placed concurrently with a biopsy to identify a lesion

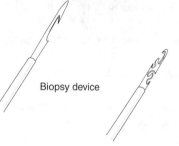

Biopsy device

Explanation

The physician performs a breast biopsy with image guidance using a percutaneous needle core or automated vacuum assisted or rotating biopsy device and insertion of a localization device. Using image guidance, the physician places a metallic clip or pellet adjacent to a breast lesion to mark the site. A large gauge (e.g., 14 gauge), hollow core biopsy needle or the biopsy device is inserted through the skin of the breast and into the suspicious breast tissue. The physician takes multiple core tissue samples from a single lesion to obtain a sufficient amount of tissue for diagnosis. The needle or automated vacuum assisted or rotating biopsy device is withdrawn. Pressure and bandages are applied to the puncture site. Report 19083 for the first lesion and 19084 for each additional lesion using ultrasound guidance.

Coding Tips

Report 19084 in conjunction with 19083. Do not report 19083 or 19084 in conjunction with 19281–19288, 76098, 76942, 77002, or 77021 when performed on the same lesion.

ICD-10-CM Diagnostic Codes

C50.011	Malignant neoplasm of nipple and areola, right female breast ♀ ☑	
C50.012	Malignant neoplasm of nipple and areola, left female breast ♀ ☑	
C50.021	Malignant neoplasm of nipple and areola, right male breast ♂ ☑	
C50.022	Malignant neoplasm of nipple and areola, left male breast ♂ ☑	
C50.111	Malignant neoplasm of central portion of right female breast ♀ ☑	
C50.112	Malignant neoplasm of central portion of left female breast ♀ ☑	
C50.121	Malignant neoplasm of central portion of right male breast ♂ ☑	

Breast

C50.122	Malignant neoplasm of central portion of left male breast ♂ ☑	D48.62	Neoplasm of uncertain behavior of left breast ☑
C50.211	Malignant neoplasm of upper-inner quadrant of right female breast ♀ ☑	N60.01	Solitary cyst of right breast ☑
C50.212	Malignant neoplasm of upper-inner quadrant of left female breast ♀ ☑	N60.02	Solitary cyst of left breast ☑

C50.122   Malignant neoplasm of central portion of left male breast ♂ ☑

C50.211   Malignant neoplasm of upper-inner quadrant of right female breast ♀ ☑

C50.212   Malignant neoplasm of upper-inner quadrant of left female breast ♀ ☑

C50.221   Malignant neoplasm of upper-inner quadrant of right male breast ♂ ☑

C50.222   Malignant neoplasm of upper-inner quadrant of left male breast ♂ ☑

C50.311   Malignant neoplasm of lower-inner quadrant of right female breast ♀ ☑

C50.312   Malignant neoplasm of lower-inner quadrant of left female breast ♀ ☑

C50.321   Malignant neoplasm of lower-inner quadrant of right male breast ♂ ☑

C50.322   Malignant neoplasm of lower-inner quadrant of left male breast ♂ ☑

C50.411   Malignant neoplasm of upper-outer quadrant of right female breast ♀ ☑

C50.412   Malignant neoplasm of upper-outer quadrant of left female breast ♀ ☑

C50.421   Malignant neoplasm of upper-outer quadrant of right male breast ♂ ☑

C50.422   Malignant neoplasm of upper-outer quadrant of left male breast ♂ ☑

C50.511   Malignant neoplasm of lower-outer quadrant of right female breast ♀ ☑

C50.512   Malignant neoplasm of lower-outer quadrant of left female breast ♀ ☑

C50.521   Malignant neoplasm of lower-outer quadrant of right male breast ♂ ☑

C50.522   Malignant neoplasm of lower-outer quadrant of left male breast ♂ ☑

C50.611   Malignant neoplasm of axillary tail of right female breast ♀ ☑

C50.612   Malignant neoplasm of axillary tail of left female breast ♀ ☑

C50.621   Malignant neoplasm of axillary tail of right male breast ♂ ☑

C50.622   Malignant neoplasm of axillary tail of left male breast ♂ ☑

C50.811   Malignant neoplasm of overlapping sites of right female breast ♀ ☑

C50.812   Malignant neoplasm of overlapping sites of left female breast ♀ ☑

C50.821   Malignant neoplasm of overlapping sites of right male breast ♂ ☑

C50.822   Malignant neoplasm of overlapping sites of left male breast ♂ ☑

C79.81   Secondary malignant neoplasm of breast

D03.52   Melanoma in situ of breast (skin) (soft tissue)

D05.01   Lobular carcinoma in situ of right breast ☑

D05.02   Lobular carcinoma in situ of left breast ☑

D05.11   Intraductal carcinoma in situ of right breast ☑

D05.12   Intraductal carcinoma in situ of left breast ☑

D05.81   Other specified type of carcinoma in situ of right breast ☑

D05.82   Other specified type of carcinoma in situ of left breast ☑

D24.1   Benign neoplasm of right breast ☑

D24.2   Benign neoplasm of left breast ☑

D48.61   Neoplasm of uncertain behavior of right breast ☑

D48.62   Neoplasm of uncertain behavior of left breast ☑

N60.01   Solitary cyst of right breast ☑

N60.02   Solitary cyst of left breast ☑

N60.11   Diffuse cystic mastopathy of right breast 🅰 ☑

N60.12   Diffuse cystic mastopathy of left breast 🅰 ☑

N60.21   Fibroadenosis of right breast ☑

N60.31   Fibrosclerosis of right breast ☑

N60.41   Mammary duct ectasia of right breast ☑

N60.81   Other benign mammary dysplasias of right breast ☑

N61.21   Granulomatous mastitis, right breast ☑

N61.22   Granulomatous mastitis, left breast ☑

N61.23   Granulomatous mastitis, bilateral breast ☑

N62   Hypertrophy of breast

N63.11   Unspecified lump in the right breast, upper outer quadrant ☑

N63.12   Unspecified lump in the right breast, upper inner quadrant ☑

N63.13   Unspecified lump in the right breast, lower outer quadrant ☑

N63.14   Unspecified lump in the right breast, lower inner quadrant ☑

N63.31   Unspecified lump in axillary tail of the right breast ☑

N63.41   Unspecified lump in right breast, subareolar ☑

N63.42   Unspecified lump in left breast, subareolar ☑

N64.1   Fat necrosis of breast

N64.51   Induration of breast

N64.89   Other specified disorders of breast

R92.0   Mammographic microcalcification found on diagnostic imaging of breast

R92.1   Mammographic calcification found on diagnostic imaging of breast

R92.8   Other abnormal and inconclusive findings on diagnostic imaging of breast

AMA: **19083** 2019,Apr,4; 2018,Jan,8; 2017,Jan,8; 2016,Jun,3; 2016,Jan,13; 2015,May,8; 2015,Mar,5; 2015,Jan,16 **19084** 2019,Apr,4; 2018,Jan,8; 2017,Jan,8; 2016,Jun,3; 2016,Jan,13; 2015,May,8; 2015,Mar,5; 2015,Jan,16

Relative Value Units/Medicare Edits

Non-Facility RVU	Work	PE	MP	Total
19083	3.1	13.47	0.32	16.89
19084	1.55	11.57	0.15	13.27
Facility RVU	Work	PE	MP	Total
19083	3.1	1.12	0.32	4.54
19084	1.55	0.56	0.15	2.26

	FUD	Status	MUE	Modifiers				IOM Reference
19083	0	A	1(2)	51	50	N/A	80*	None
19084	N/A	A	2(3)	N/A	N/A	N/A	80*	

* with documentation

19085-19086

19085 Biopsy, breast, with placement of breast localization device(s) (eg, clip, metallic pellet), when performed, and imaging of the biopsy specimen, when performed, percutaneous; first lesion, including magnetic resonance guidance

+ 19086 each additional lesion, including magnetic resonance guidance (List separately in addition to code for primary procedure)

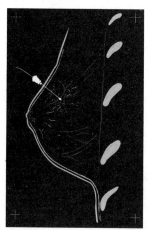

A metallic localization device is placed concurrently with a biopsy to identify a lesion

Explanation

The physician performs a breast biopsy with image guidance using a percutaneous needle core or automated vacuum assisted or rotating biopsy device and insertion of a localization device. Using image guidance, the physician places a metallic clip or pellet adjacent to a breast lesion to mark the site. A large gauge (e.g., 14 gauge), hollow core biopsy needle or the biopsy device is inserted through the skin of the breast and into the suspicious breast tissue. The physician takes multiple core tissue samples from a single lesion to obtain a sufficient amount of tissue for diagnosis. The needle or automated vacuum assisted or rotating biopsy device is withdrawn. Pressure and bandages are applied to the puncture site. Report 19085 for the first lesion and 19086 for each additional lesion using magnetic resonance imaging (MRI).

Coding Tips

Report 19086 in addition to 19085. These are unilateral procedures. If performed bilaterally, some payers require that the service be reported twice with modifier 50 appended to the second code while others require identification of the service only once with modifier 50 appended. Check with individual payers. Modifier 50 identifies a procedure performed identically on the opposite side of the body (mirror image). Do not report 19085 or 19086 in addition to 19281–19288, 76098, 76942, 77002, or 77021 when performed on the same lesion.

ICD-10-CM Diagnostic Codes

C50.011	Malignant neoplasm of nipple and areola, right female breast ♀ ☑
C50.012	Malignant neoplasm of nipple and areola, left female breast ♀ ☑
C50.021	Malignant neoplasm of nipple and areola, right male breast ♂ ☑
C50.022	Malignant neoplasm of nipple and areola, left male breast ♂ ☑
C50.111	Malignant neoplasm of central portion of right female breast ♀ ☑
C50.112	Malignant neoplasm of central portion of left female breast ♀ ☑
C50.121	Malignant neoplasm of central portion of right male breast ♂ ☑
C50.122	Malignant neoplasm of central portion of left male breast ♂ ☑
C50.211	Malignant neoplasm of upper-inner quadrant of right female breast ♀ ☑
C50.212	Malignant neoplasm of upper-inner quadrant of left female breast ♀ ☑
C50.221	Malignant neoplasm of upper-inner quadrant of right male breast ♂ ☑
C50.222	Malignant neoplasm of upper-inner quadrant of left male breast ♂ ☑
C50.311	Malignant neoplasm of lower-inner quadrant of right female breast ♀ ☑
C50.312	Malignant neoplasm of lower-inner quadrant of left female breast ♀ ☑
C50.321	Malignant neoplasm of lower-inner quadrant of right male breast ♂ ☑
C50.322	Malignant neoplasm of lower-inner quadrant of left male breast ♂ ☑
C50.411	Malignant neoplasm of upper-outer quadrant of right female breast ♀ ☑
C50.412	Malignant neoplasm of upper-outer quadrant of left female breast ♀ ☑
C50.421	Malignant neoplasm of upper-outer quadrant of right male breast ♂ ☑
C50.422	Malignant neoplasm of upper-outer quadrant of left male breast ♂ ☑
C50.511	Malignant neoplasm of lower-outer quadrant of right female breast ♀ ☑
C50.512	Malignant neoplasm of lower-outer quadrant of left female breast ♀ ☑
C50.521	Malignant neoplasm of lower-outer quadrant of right male breast ♂ ☑
C50.522	Malignant neoplasm of lower-outer quadrant of left male breast ♂ ☑
C50.611	Malignant neoplasm of axillary tail of right female breast ♀ ☑
C50.612	Malignant neoplasm of axillary tail of left female breast ♀ ☑
C50.621	Malignant neoplasm of axillary tail of right male breast ♂ ☑
C50.622	Malignant neoplasm of axillary tail of left male breast ♂ ☑
C50.811	Malignant neoplasm of overlapping sites of right female breast ♀ ☑
C50.812	Malignant neoplasm of overlapping sites of left female breast ♀ ☑
C50.821	Malignant neoplasm of overlapping sites of right male breast ♂ ☑
C50.822	Malignant neoplasm of overlapping sites of left male breast ♂ ☑
C79.81	Secondary malignant neoplasm of breast
D03.52	Melanoma in situ of breast (skin) (soft tissue)
D05.01	Lobular carcinoma in situ of right breast ☑
D05.02	Lobular carcinoma in situ of left breast ☑
D05.11	Intraductal carcinoma in situ of right breast ☑
D05.12	Intraductal carcinoma in situ of left breast ☑
D05.81	Other specified type of carcinoma in situ of right breast ☑
D05.82	Other specified type of carcinoma in situ of left breast ☑
D24.1	Benign neoplasm of right breast ☑
D24.2	Benign neoplasm of left breast ☑
D48.61	Neoplasm of uncertain behavior of right breast ☑

Breast

D48.62	Neoplasm of uncertain behavior of left breast ☑
N60.01	Solitary cyst of right breast ☑
N60.02	Solitary cyst of left breast ☑
N60.11	Diffuse cystic mastopathy of right breast A ☑
N60.12	Diffuse cystic mastopathy of left breast A ☑
N60.21	Fibroadenosis of right breast ☑
N60.22	Fibroadenosis of left breast ☑
N60.31	Fibrosclerosis of right breast ☑
N60.32	Fibrosclerosis of left breast ☑
N60.41	Mammary duct ectasia of right breast ☑
N60.42	Mammary duct ectasia of left breast ☑
N60.81	Other benign mammary dysplasias of right breast ☑
N60.82	Other benign mammary dysplasias of left breast ☑
N61.21	Granulomatous mastitis, right breast ☑
N61.22	Granulomatous mastitis, left breast ☑
N61.23	Granulomatous mastitis, bilateral breast ☑
N62	Hypertrophy of breast
N63.11	Unspecified lump in the right breast, upper outer quadrant ☑
N63.13	Unspecified lump in the right breast, lower outer quadrant ☑
N63.22	Unspecified lump in the left breast, upper inner quadrant ☑
N63.24	Unspecified lump in the left breast, lower inner quadrant ☑
N63.31	Unspecified lump in axillary tail of the right breast ☑
N63.42	Unspecified lump in left breast, subareolar ☑
N64.1	Fat necrosis of breast
N64.51	Induration of breast
N64.89	Other specified disorders of breast
R92.0	Mammographic microcalcification found on diagnostic imaging of breast
R92.1	Mammographic calcification found on diagnostic imaging of breast
R92.8	Other abnormal and inconclusive findings on diagnostic imaging of breast

AMA: **19085** 2019,Apr,4; 2018,Jan,8; 2017,Jan,8; 2016,Jun,3; 2016,Jan,13; 2015,May,8; 2015,Mar,5; 2015,Jan,16 **19086** 2019,Apr,4; 2018,Jan,8; 2017,Jan,8; 2016,Jun,3; 2016,Jan,13; 2015,May,8; 2015,Mar,5; 2015,Jan,16

Relative Value Units/Medicare Edits

Non-Facility RVU	Work	PE	MP	Total
19085	3.64	22.01	0.3	25.95
19086	1.82	18.59	0.15	20.56
Facility RVU	Work	PE	MP	Total
19085	3.64	1.32	0.3	5.26
19086	1.82	0.66	0.15	2.63

	FUD	Status	MUE	Modifiers				IOM Reference
19085	0	A	1(2)	51	50	N/A	80*	None
19086	N/A	A	2(3)	N/A	N/A	N/A	80*	

* with documentation

19100

19100   Biopsy of breast; percutaneous, needle core, not using imaging guidance (separate procedure)

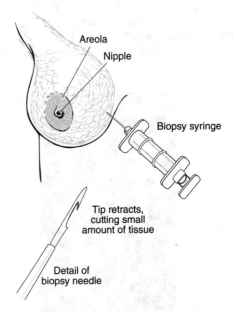

Explanation

The physician inserts a large gauge needle through the skin of the breast and into the suspect breast tissue. The needle is removed along with a core of breast tissue. Pressure is applied to the puncture site to stop any bleeding.

Coding Tips

This separate procedure by definition is usually a component of a more complex service and is not identified separately. When performed alone or with other unrelated procedures or services it may be reported. If performed alone, list the code; if performed with other procedures/services, list the code and append modifier 59 or an X{EPSU} modifier. This is a unilateral procedure. If performed bilaterally, some payers require that the service be reported twice with modifier 50 appended to the second code while others require identification of the service only once with modifier 50 appended. Check with individual payers. Modifier 50 identifies a procedure performed identically on the opposite side of the body (mirror image). For puncture aspiration of a breast cyst, see 19000. For open, incisional breast biopsy, see 19101. Breast biopsies with imaging guidance, including placement of localization devices, are reported with 19081–19086. For placement of localization devices under imaging guidance without biopsy, see 19281–19288. For excision of a breast lesion, see 19120. For a biopsy using fine needle aspiration, see 10004-10012 and 10021. Surgical trays, A4550, are not separately reimbursed by Medicare; however, other third-party payers may cover them. Check with the specific payer to determine coverage.

ICD-10-CM Diagnostic Codes

C50.011	Malignant neoplasm of nipple and areola, right female breast ♀ ☑
C50.021	Malignant neoplasm of nipple and areola, right male breast ♂ ☑
C50.111	Malignant neoplasm of central portion of right female breast ♀ ☑
C50.121	Malignant neoplasm of central portion of right male breast ♂ ☑
C50.211	Malignant neoplasm of upper-inner quadrant of right female breast ♀ ☑
C50.221	Malignant neoplasm of upper-inner quadrant of right male breast ♂ ☑

Breast

C50.311	Malignant neoplasm of lower-inner quadrant of right female breast ♀ ☑	N64.1	Fat necrosis of breast
C50.321	Malignant neoplasm of lower-inner quadrant of right male breast ♂ ☑	N64.51	Induration of breast

C50.311 Malignant neoplasm of lower-inner quadrant of right female breast ♀ ☑

C50.321 Malignant neoplasm of lower-inner quadrant of right male breast ♂ ☑

C50.411 Malignant neoplasm of upper-outer quadrant of right female breast ♀ ☑

C50.421 Malignant neoplasm of upper-outer quadrant of right male breast ♂ ☑

C50.511 Malignant neoplasm of lower-outer quadrant of right female breast ♀ ☑

C50.521 Malignant neoplasm of lower-outer quadrant of right male breast ♂ ☑

C50.611 Malignant neoplasm of axillary tail of right female breast ♀ ☑

C50.612 Malignant neoplasm of axillary tail of left female breast ♀ ☑

C50.621 Malignant neoplasm of axillary tail of right male breast ♂ ☑

C50.622 Malignant neoplasm of axillary tail of left male breast ♂ ☑

C50.811 Malignant neoplasm of overlapping sites of right female breast ♀ ☑

C50.812 Malignant neoplasm of overlapping sites of left female breast ♀ ☑

C50.821 Malignant neoplasm of overlapping sites of right male breast ♂ ☑

C50.822 Malignant neoplasm of overlapping sites of left male breast ♂ ☑

C79.81 Secondary malignant neoplasm of breast

D05.01 Lobular carcinoma in situ of right breast ☑

D05.02 Lobular carcinoma in situ of left breast ☑

D05.11 Intraductal carcinoma in situ of right breast ☑

D05.12 Intraductal carcinoma in situ of left breast ☑

D05.81 Other specified type of carcinoma in situ of right breast ☑

D05.82 Other specified type of carcinoma in situ of left breast ☑

D24.1 Benign neoplasm of right breast ☑

D24.2 Benign neoplasm of left breast ☑

D48.61 Neoplasm of uncertain behavior of right breast ☑

D48.62 Neoplasm of uncertain behavior of left breast ☑

N60.01 Solitary cyst of right breast ☑

N60.02 Solitary cyst of left breast ☑

N60.11 Diffuse cystic mastopathy of right breast 🅰 ☑

N60.12 Diffuse cystic mastopathy of left breast 🅰 ☑

N60.21 Fibroadenosis of right breast ☑

N60.22 Fibroadenosis of left breast ☑

N60.31 Fibrosclerosis of right breast ☑

N60.32 Fibrosclerosis of left breast ☑

N60.41 Mammary duct ectasia of right breast ☑

N60.42 Mammary duct ectasia of left breast ☑

N60.81 Other benign mammary dysplasias of right breast ☑

N60.82 Other benign mammary dysplasias of left breast ☑

N61.21 Granulomatous mastitis, right breast ☑

N61.22 Granulomatous mastitis, left breast ☑

N61.23 Granulomatous mastitis, bilateral breast ☑

N62 Hypertrophy of breast

N63.12 Unspecified lump in the right breast, upper inner quadrant ☑

N63.13 Unspecified lump in the right breast, lower outer quadrant ☑

N63.31 Unspecified lump in axillary tail of the right breast ☑

N63.41 Unspecified lump in right breast, subareolar ☑

N64.1 Fat necrosis of breast

N64.51 Induration of breast

N64.89 Other specified disorders of breast

R92.0 Mammographic microcalcification found on diagnostic imaging of breast

R92.1 Mammographic calcification found on diagnostic imaging of breast

R92.8 Other abnormal and inconclusive findings on diagnostic imaging of breast

AMA: 19100 2018,Jan,8; 2017,Jan,8; 2016,Jan,13; 2015,Jan,16

Relative Value Units/Medicare Edits

Non-Facility RVU	Work	PE	MP	Total
19100	1.27	3.11	0.3	4.68
Facility RVU	Work	PE	MP	Total
19100	1.27	0.48	0.3	2.05

	FUD	Status	MUE	Modifiers				IOM Reference
19100	0	A	4(3)	51	50	N/A	N/A	100-04,12,40.7; 100-04,13,80.1

* with documentation

Terms To Know

benign mammary dysplasias. Noncancerous fibrous or cystic growths in the breast.

carcinoma in situ of breast. Malignant neoplasm that has not invaded tissue beyond the epithelium of the breast.

cystic mastopathy. Mammary dysplasia involving inflammation and the formation of fluid-filled nodular cysts in the breast tissue.

Breast

19101

19101   Biopsy of breast; open, incisional

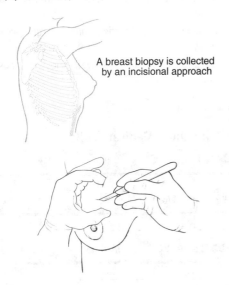

A breast biopsy is collected by an incisional approach

Explanation

The physician removes tissue for biopsy. The physician makes an incision in the skin of the breast near the site of the suspect mass. The mass is identified and a sample of the lesion is removed. This specimen is often examined immediately. If the lesion is benign, the incision is repaired with layered closure. If malignant, the incision may be closed pending a separate, more extensive surgical session, or a more extensive surgery may occur immediately, in which case this code would not be reported.

Coding Tips

This is a unilateral procedure. If performed bilaterally, some payers require that the service be reported twice with modifier 50 appended to the second code while others require identification of the service only once with modifier 50 appended. Check with individual payers. Modifier 50 identifies a procedure performed identically on the opposite side of the body (mirror image). For aspiration of a breast cyst, see 19000. For percutaneous needle core breast biopsy without imaging guidance, see 19100. Breast biopsies with imaging guidance, including placement of localization devices, are reported with 19081–19086. For placement of localization devices under imaging guidance without biopsy, see 19281–19288. For excision of a breast lesion, see 19120. Surgical trays, A4550, are not separately reimbursed by Medicare; however, other third-party payers may cover them. Check with the specific payer to determine coverage.

ICD-10-CM Diagnostic Codes

C50.011	Malignant neoplasm of nipple and areola, right female breast ♀ ☑
C50.012	Malignant neoplasm of nipple and areola, left female breast ♀ ☑
C50.021	Malignant neoplasm of nipple and areola, right male breast ♂ ☑
C50.022	Malignant neoplasm of nipple and areola, left male breast ♂ ☑
C50.111	Malignant neoplasm of central portion of right female breast ♀ ☑
C50.112	Malignant neoplasm of central portion of left female breast ♀ ☑
C50.121	Malignant neoplasm of central portion of right male breast ♂ ☑
C50.122	Malignant neoplasm of central portion of left male breast ♂ ☑
C50.211	Malignant neoplasm of upper-inner quadrant of right female breast ♀ ☑
C50.212	Malignant neoplasm of upper-inner quadrant of left female breast ♀ ☑
C50.221	Malignant neoplasm of upper-inner quadrant of right male breast ♂ ☑
C50.222	Malignant neoplasm of upper-inner quadrant of left male breast ♂ ☑
C50.311	Malignant neoplasm of lower-inner quadrant of right female breast ♀ ☑
C50.312	Malignant neoplasm of lower-inner quadrant of left female breast ♀ ☑
C50.321	Malignant neoplasm of lower-inner quadrant of right male breast ♂ ☑
C50.322	Malignant neoplasm of lower-inner quadrant of left male breast ♂ ☑
C50.411	Malignant neoplasm of upper-outer quadrant of right female breast ♀ ☑
C50.412	Malignant neoplasm of upper-outer quadrant of left female breast ♀ ☑
C50.421	Malignant neoplasm of upper-outer quadrant of right male breast ♂ ☑
C50.422	Malignant neoplasm of upper-outer quadrant of left male breast ♂ ☑
C50.511	Malignant neoplasm of lower-outer quadrant of right female breast ♀ ☑
C50.512	Malignant neoplasm of lower-outer quadrant of left female breast ♀ ☑
C50.521	Malignant neoplasm of lower-outer quadrant of right male breast ♂ ☑
C50.522	Malignant neoplasm of lower-outer quadrant of left male breast ♂ ☑
C50.611	Malignant neoplasm of axillary tail of right female breast ♀ ☑
C50.612	Malignant neoplasm of axillary tail of left female breast ♀ ☑
C50.621	Malignant neoplasm of axillary tail of right male breast ♂ ☑
C50.622	Malignant neoplasm of axillary tail of left male breast ♂ ☑
C50.811	Malignant neoplasm of overlapping sites of right female breast ♀ ☑
C50.812	Malignant neoplasm of overlapping sites of left female breast ♀ ☑
C50.821	Malignant neoplasm of overlapping sites of right male breast ♂ ☑
C50.822	Malignant neoplasm of overlapping sites of left male breast ♂ ☑
C79.81	Secondary malignant neoplasm of breast
C84.7A	Anaplastic large cell lymphoma, ALK-negative, breast
D05.01	Lobular carcinoma in situ of right breast ☑
D05.02	Lobular carcinoma in situ of left breast ☑
D05.11	Intraductal carcinoma in situ of right breast ☑
D05.12	Intraductal carcinoma in situ of left breast ☑
D05.81	Other specified type of carcinoma in situ of right breast ☑
D05.82	Other specified type of carcinoma in situ of left breast ☑
D24.1	Benign neoplasm of right breast ☑
D24.2	Benign neoplasm of left breast ☑
D48.61	Neoplasm of uncertain behavior of right breast ☑
D48.62	Neoplasm of uncertain behavior of left breast ☑
N60.01	Solitary cyst of right breast ☑
N60.02	Solitary cyst of left breast ☑

Breast

N60.11	Diffuse cystic mastopathy of right breast ⒜ ☑
N60.12	Diffuse cystic mastopathy of left breast ⒜ ☑
N60.21	Fibroadenosis of right breast ☑
N60.22	Fibroadenosis of left breast ☑
N60.31	Fibrosclerosis of right breast ☑
N60.32	Fibrosclerosis of left breast ☑
N60.41	Mammary duct ectasia of right breast ☑
N60.42	Mammary duct ectasia of left breast ☑
N60.81	Other benign mammary dysplasias of right breast ☑
N60.82	Other benign mammary dysplasias of left breast ☑
N61.21	Granulomatous mastitis, right breast ☑
N61.22	Granulomatous mastitis, left breast ☑
N61.23	Granulomatous mastitis, bilateral breast ☑
N62	Hypertrophy of breast
N63.11	Unspecified lump in the right breast, upper outer quadrant ☑
N63.12	Unspecified lump in the right breast, upper inner quadrant ☑
N63.13	Unspecified lump in the right breast, lower outer quadrant ☑
N63.14	Unspecified lump in the right breast, lower inner quadrant ☑
N63.31	Unspecified lump in axillary tail of the right breast ☑
N63.41	Unspecified lump in right breast, subareolar ☑
N64.1	Fat necrosis of breast
N64.51	Induration of breast
N64.89	Other specified disorders of breast
R92.0	Mammographic microcalcification found on diagnostic imaging of breast
R92.1	Mammographic calcification found on diagnostic imaging of breast
R92.8	Other abnormal and inconclusive findings on diagnostic imaging of breast

AMA: **19101** 2018,Jan,8; 2017,Jan,8; 2016,Jan,13; 2015,Jan,16

Relative Value Units/Medicare Edits

Non-Facility RVU	Work	PE	MP	Total
19101	3.23	6.19	0.74	10.16
Facility RVU	Work	PE	MP	Total
19101	3.23	2.63	0.74	6.6

	FUD	Status	MUE	Modifiers				IOM Reference
19101	10	A	3(3)	51	50	N/A	N/A	None

* with documentation

Terms To Know

calcification. Normal process of calcium salts deposition in bone. Calcification can also occur abnormally in fibroconnective soft tissues.

dysplasia. Abnormality or alteration in the size, shape, and organization of cells from their normal pattern of development.

hypertrophy. Overgrowth or enlargement of normal cells in tissue.

19105

| 19105 | Ablation, cryosurgical, of fibroadenoma, including ultrasound guidance, each fibroadenoma |

One lesion is treated

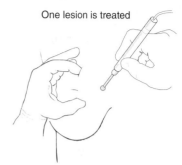

A fibroadenoma of the breast is destroyed with a freezing probe inserted through a small incision in the skin

Explanation

The physician uses cryotherapy to obliterate a fibroadenoma of the breast. The patient's skin is cleansed and the ablation site is anesthetized. Ultrasound is used to locate the tumor. A cryoprobe is inserted through a small incision and placed within the fibroadenoma under ultrasound. The device initiates ice ball formation. The cryoprobe is warmed before removal from the breast. This code reports treatment of one fibroadenoma.

Coding Tips

Ultrasound guidance (76940, 76942) is included in the code description and is not reported separately. If adjacent lesions are treated with one cryoprobe insertion, only report 19105 once. For excision of a breast cyst, fibroadenoma, or other benign or malignant tumor, aberrant breast tissue, duct, nipple, or areolar lesion, open, see 19120. For cryoablation of a malignant breast tumor, see 0581T.

ICD-10-CM Diagnostic Codes

| D24.1 | Benign neoplasm of right breast ☑ |
| D24.2 | Benign neoplasm of left breast ☑ |

AMA: **19105** 2007,Mar,7-8

Relative Value Units/Medicare Edits

Non-Facility RVU	Work	PE	MP	Total
19105	3.69	75.4	0.91	80.0
Facility RVU	Work	PE	MP	Total
19105	3.69	1.62	0.91	6.22

	FUD	Status	MUE	Modifiers				IOM Reference
19105	0	A	2(3)	51	50	N/A	N/A	100-04,13,80.1; 100-04,13,80.2

* with documentation

Breast

19110

19110 Nipple exploration, with or without excision of a solitary lactiferous duct or a papilloma lactiferous duct

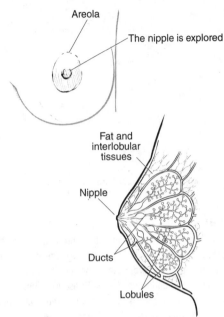

The nipple is explored
Areola

Fat and interlobular tissues

Nipple

Ducts

Lobules

The ducts deliver milk from the lobules through and out the nipples

Explanation

The physician makes an incision at the edge of the areola near the site of a suspect duct for nipple exploration, with or without excision of a solitary lactiferous duct or a papilloma lactiferous duct. The duct is dissected from surrounding tissue and examined. Surrounding ducts and tissue are also examined. The suspect duct may be excised. Bleeding vessels are controlled with electrocautery or ligated with sutures. The incision is sutured in layered closure and a light pressure dressing is applied.

Coding Tips

This is a unilateral procedure. If performed bilaterally, some payers require that the service be reported twice with modifier 50 appended to the second code while others require identification of the service only once with modifier 50 appended. Check with individual payers. Modifier 50 identifies a procedure performed identically on the opposite side of the body (mirror image). For excision of a lactiferous duct fistula, see 19112. For open excision of a duct, nipple, or areolar lesion (male or female), see 19120. Surgical trays, A4550, are not separately reimbursed by Medicare; however, other third-party payers may cover them. Check with the specific payer to determine coverage.

ICD-10-CM Diagnostic Codes

C50.011	Malignant neoplasm of nipple and areola, right female breast ♀ ☑
C50.012	Malignant neoplasm of nipple and areola, left female breast ♀ ☑
C50.811	Malignant neoplasm of overlapping sites of right female breast ♀ ☑
C50.812	Malignant neoplasm of overlapping sites of left female breast ♀ ☑
D05.01	Lobular carcinoma in situ of right breast ☑
D05.02	Lobular carcinoma in situ of left breast ☑
D05.11	Intraductal carcinoma in situ of right breast ☑
D05.12	Intraductal carcinoma in situ of left breast ☑
D05.81	Other specified type of carcinoma in situ of right breast ☑
D05.82	Other specified type of carcinoma in situ of left breast ☑
D24.1	Benign neoplasm of right breast ☑
D24.2	Benign neoplasm of left breast ☑
D48.61	Neoplasm of uncertain behavior of right breast ☑
D48.62	Neoplasm of uncertain behavior of left breast ☑
D49.3	Neoplasm of unspecified behavior of breast
N60.01	Solitary cyst of right breast ☑
N60.02	Solitary cyst of left breast ☑
N60.41	Mammary duct ectasia of right breast ☑
N60.42	Mammary duct ectasia of left breast ☑
N61.0	Mastitis without abscess
N61.1	Abscess of the breast and nipple
N63.41	Unspecified lump in right breast, subareolar ☑
N63.42	Unspecified lump in left breast, subareolar ☑
N64.52	Nipple discharge

AMA: 19110 2018,Jan,8; 2017,Jan,8; 2016,Jan,13; 2015,Jan,16

Relative Value Units/Medicare Edits

Non-Facility RVU	Work	PE	MP	Total
19110	4.44	9.33	1.09	14.86
Facility RVU	**Work**	**PE**	**MP**	**Total**
19110	4.44	4.86	1.09	10.39

	FUD	Status	MUE	Modifiers				IOM Reference
19110	90	A	1(3)	51	50	N/A	N/A	100-04,12,40.7

* with documentation

Terms To Know

benign. Mild or nonmalignant in nature.

carcinoma in situ. Malignancy that arises from the cells of the vessel, gland, or organ of origin that remains confined to that site or has not invaded neighboring tissue.

dissect. Cut apart or separate tissue for surgical purposes or for visual or microscopic study.

dressing. Material applied to a wound or surgical site for protection, absorption, or drainage of the area.

electrocautery. Division or cutting of tissue using high-frequency electrical current to produce heat, which destroys cells.

galactocele. Tumor or cyst-like enlargement of the milk-containing gland in the breast.

ligation. Tying off a blood vessel or duct with a suture or a soft, thin wire.

malignant neoplasm. Any cancerous tumor or lesion exhibiting uncontrolled tissue growth that can progressively invade other parts of the body with its disease-generating cells.

mammary duct ectasia. Condition characterized by dilated ducts of the mammary gland.

neoplasm. New abnormal growth, tumor.

Breast

19112

19112   Excision of lactiferous duct fistula

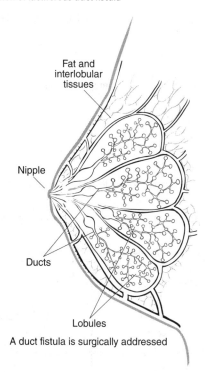

A duct fistula is surgically addressed

Labels on figure:
- Fat and interlobular tissues
- Nipple
- Ducts
- Lobules

Explanation

The physician makes an incision around the abnormal opening of a lactiferous duct fistula on the skin. The fistula is dissected down to the duct. The duct, fistula, and skin opening are all excised. The remaining portion of the duct may be ligated. The wound is irrigated with warm sterile saline and closed in layers.

Coding Tips

This is a unilateral procedure. If performed bilaterally, some payers require that the service be reported twice with modifier 50 appended to the second code while others require identification of the service only once with modifier 50 appended. Check with individual payers. Modifier 50 identifies a procedure performed identically on the opposite side of the body (mirror image). For other fistula excision codes, see the specific anatomic site. For nipple exploration, with or without excision of a solitary lactiferous duct or a papilloma lactiferous duct, see 19110. Surgical trays, A4550, are not separately reimbursed by Medicare; however, other third-party payers may cover them. Check with the specific payer to determine coverage.

ICD-10-CM Diagnostic Codes

N61.0   Mastitis without abscess
N61.1   Abscess of the breast and nipple

AMA: **19112** 2018,Jan,8; 2017,Jan,8; 2016,Jan,13; 2015,Jan,16

Relative Value Units/Medicare Edits

Non-Facility RVU	Work	PE	MP	Total
19112	3.81	9.28	0.93	14.02
Facility RVU	Work	PE	MP	Total
19112	3.81	4.73	0.93	9.47

	FUD	Status	MUE	Modifiers				IOM Reference
19112	90	A	2(3)	51	50	N/A	80*	None

* with documentation

Terms To Know

dissection. Separating by cutting tissue or body structures apart.

fistula. Abnormal tube-like passage between two body cavities or organs or from an organ to the outside surface.

irrigation. To wash out or cleanse a body cavity, wound, or tissue with water or other fluid.

lactiferous duct. Duct that drains the mammary glands of the breast.

ligation. Tying off a blood vessel or duct with a suture or a soft, thin wire.

mastitis. Inflammation of the breast. Acute mastitis is caused by a bacterial infection; chronic mastitis is caused by hormonal changes.

Breast

19120

19120 Excision of cyst, fibroadenoma, or other benign or malignant tumor, aberrant breast tissue, duct lesion, nipple or areolar lesion (except 19300), open, male or female, 1 or more lesions

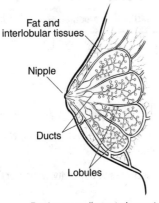

Fat and interlobular tissues
Nipple
Ducts
Lobules

Benign or malignant aberrant tissue is excised from a human breast

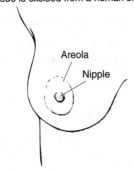

Areola
Nipple

Explanation

The physician excises breast tissue for biopsy. The physician makes an incision in the skin of the breast overlying the site of the mass. Skin and tissue are dissected from the abnormality. The lesion is removed. Bleeding vessels are controlled with electrocautery or ligated with sutures. A drain may be inserted into the wound. The incision is sutured in layered closure and a light pressure dressing is applied.

Coding Tips

This is a unilateral procedure. If performed bilaterally, some payers require that the service be reported twice with modifier 50 appended to the second code while others require identification of the service only once with modifier 50 appended. Check with individual payers. Modifier 50 identifies a procedure performed identically on the opposite side of the body (mirror image). For percutaneous needle core breast biopsy, see 19100; with imaging guidance, see 19081–19086. Lumpectomy is reported with 19301. Surgical trays, A4550, are not separately reimbursed by Medicare; however, other third-party payers may cover them. Check with the specific payer to determine coverage.

ICD-10-CM Diagnostic Codes

C50.011	Malignant neoplasm of nipple and areola, right female breast ♀ ☑
C50.012	Malignant neoplasm of nipple and areola, left female breast ♀ ☑
C50.021	Malignant neoplasm of nipple and areola, right male breast ♂ ☑
C50.022	Malignant neoplasm of nipple and areola, left male breast ♂ ☑
C50.111	Malignant neoplasm of central portion of right female breast ♀ ☑
C50.112	Malignant neoplasm of central portion of left female breast ♀ ☑
C50.121	Malignant neoplasm of central portion of right male breast ♂ ☑
C50.122	Malignant neoplasm of central portion of left male breast ♂ ☑
C50.211	Malignant neoplasm of upper-inner quadrant of right female breast ♀ ☑
C50.212	Malignant neoplasm of upper-inner quadrant of left female breast ♀ ☑
C50.221	Malignant neoplasm of upper-inner quadrant of right male breast ♂ ☑
C50.222	Malignant neoplasm of upper-inner quadrant of left male breast ♂ ☑
C50.311	Malignant neoplasm of lower-inner quadrant of right female breast ♀ ☑
C50.312	Malignant neoplasm of lower-inner quadrant of left female breast ♀ ☑
C50.321	Malignant neoplasm of lower-inner quadrant of right male breast ♂ ☑
C50.322	Malignant neoplasm of lower-inner quadrant of left male breast ♂ ☑
C50.411	Malignant neoplasm of upper-outer quadrant of right female breast ♀ ☑
C50.412	Malignant neoplasm of upper-outer quadrant of left female breast ♀ ☑
C50.421	Malignant neoplasm of upper-outer quadrant of right male breast ♂ ☑
C50.422	Malignant neoplasm of upper-outer quadrant of left male breast ♂ ☑
C50.511	Malignant neoplasm of lower-outer quadrant of right female breast ♀ ☑
C50.512	Malignant neoplasm of lower-outer quadrant of left female breast ♀ ☑
C50.521	Malignant neoplasm of lower-outer quadrant of right male breast ♂ ☑
C50.522	Malignant neoplasm of lower-outer quadrant of left male breast ♂ ☑
C50.611	Malignant neoplasm of axillary tail of right female breast ♀ ☑
C50.612	Malignant neoplasm of axillary tail of left female breast ♀ ☑
C50.621	Malignant neoplasm of axillary tail of right male breast ♂ ☑
C50.622	Malignant neoplasm of axillary tail of left male breast ♂ ☑
C50.811	Malignant neoplasm of overlapping sites of right female breast ♀ ☑
C50.812	Malignant neoplasm of overlapping sites of left female breast ♀ ☑
C50.821	Malignant neoplasm of overlapping sites of right male breast ♂ ☑
C50.822	Malignant neoplasm of overlapping sites of left male breast ♂ ☑
C79.81	Secondary malignant neoplasm of breast
D05.01	Lobular carcinoma in situ of right breast ☑
D05.02	Lobular carcinoma in situ of left breast ☑
D05.11	Intraductal carcinoma in situ of right breast ☑
D05.12	Intraductal carcinoma in situ of left breast ☑
D05.81	Other specified type of carcinoma in situ of right breast ☑
D05.82	Other specified type of carcinoma in situ of left breast ☑
D24.1	Benign neoplasm of right breast ☑
D24.2	Benign neoplasm of left breast ☑
D48.61	Neoplasm of uncertain behavior of right breast ☑

Breast

D48.62	Neoplasm of uncertain behavior of left breast ☑	
N60.01	Solitary cyst of right breast ☑	
N60.02	Solitary cyst of left breast ☑	
N60.11	Diffuse cystic mastopathy of right breast 🄰 ☑	
N60.12	Diffuse cystic mastopathy of left breast 🄰 ☑	
N60.21	Fibroadenosis of right breast ☑	
N60.22	Fibroadenosis of left breast ☑	
N60.31	Fibrosclerosis of right breast ☑	
N60.32	Fibrosclerosis of left breast ☑	
N60.41	Mammary duct ectasia of right breast ☑	
N60.42	Mammary duct ectasia of left breast ☑	
N60.81	Other benign mammary dysplasias of right breast ☑	
N60.82	Other benign mammary dysplasias of left breast ☑	
N61.21	Granulomatous mastitis, right breast ☑	
N61.22	Granulomatous mastitis, left breast ☑	
N61.23	Granulomatous mastitis, bilateral breast ☑	
N62	Hypertrophy of breast	
N63.11	Unspecified lump in the right breast, upper outer quadrant ☑	
N63.13	Unspecified lump in the right breast, lower outer quadrant ☑	
N63.22	Unspecified lump in the left breast, upper inner quadrant ☑	
N63.24	Unspecified lump in the left breast, lower inner quadrant ☑	
N63.31	Unspecified lump in axillary tail of the right breast ☑	
N63.32	Unspecified lump in axillary tail of the left breast ☑	
N63.41	Unspecified lump in right breast, subareolar ☑	
N63.42	Unspecified lump in left breast, subareolar ☑	
N64.1	Fat necrosis of breast	
N64.51	Induration of breast	
N64.89	Other specified disorders of breast	

AMA: 19120 2018,Jan,8; 2017,Jan,8; 2016,Jan,13; 2015,Mar,5; 2015,Jan,16

Relative Value Units/Medicare Edits

Non-Facility RVU	Work	PE	MP	Total
19120	5.92	7.99	1.41	15.32
Facility RVU	Work	PE	MP	Total
19120	5.92	4.97	1.41	12.3

	FUD	Status	MUE	Modifiers				IOM Reference
19120	90	A	1(2)	51	50	N/A	N/A	None

* with documentation

Terms To Know

cystic mastopathy. Mammary dysplasia involving inflammation and the formation of fluid-filled nodular cysts in the breast tissue.

fibroadenoma. Benign neoplasm of glandular epithelium frequently found in the breast.

mammary duct ectasia. Condition characterized by dilated ducts of the mammary gland.

unilateral. Located on or affecting one side.

19125-19126

19125 Excision of breast lesion identified by preoperative placement of radiological marker, open; single lesion

+ 19126 each additional lesion separately identified by a preoperative radiological marker (List separately in addition to code for primary procedure)

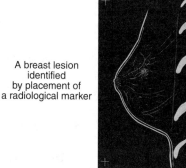

A breast lesion identified by placement of a radiological marker

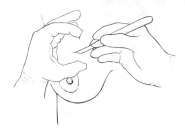

Explanation

The physician uses radiologic markers to identify breast tissue to be excised for biopsy. The physician makes an incision in the skin of the breast over the site of the lesion marked for excision by preoperative placement of a radiological marker. The lesion and marker are excised. Bleeding vessels are controlled with electrocautery or ligated with sutures. A drain may be inserted into the wound. The incision is sutured in layered closure and a light dressing is applied. Report 19126 for each additional lesion identified by a preoperative marker and removed during the same surgical session.

Coding Tips

Report 19126 in addition to 19125. For excision of a lesion without preoperative placement of a radiological marker, see 19120. For placement of localization devices under imaging guidance with image-guided breast biopsy, see 19081–19086; without image-guided biopsy, see 19281–19288. Intraoperative clip placement is included in these services and should not be separately reported.

ICD-10-CM Diagnostic Codes

C50.011	Malignant neoplasm of nipple and areola, right female breast ♀ ☑	
C50.012	Malignant neoplasm of nipple and areola, left female breast ♀ ☑	
C50.021	Malignant neoplasm of nipple and areola, right male breast ♂ ☑	
C50.022	Malignant neoplasm of nipple and areola, left male breast ♂ ☑	
C50.111	Malignant neoplasm of central portion of right female breast ♀ ☑	
C50.112	Malignant neoplasm of central portion of left female breast ♀ ☑	
C50.121	Malignant neoplasm of central portion of right male breast ♂ ☑	
C50.122	Malignant neoplasm of central portion of left male breast ♂ ☑	

Breast

C50.211 Malignant neoplasm of upper-inner quadrant of right female breast ♀ ☑

C50.212 Malignant neoplasm of upper-inner quadrant of left female breast ♀ ☑

C50.221 Malignant neoplasm of upper-inner quadrant of right male breast ♂ ☑

C50.222 Malignant neoplasm of upper-inner quadrant of left male breast ♂ ☑

C50.311 Malignant neoplasm of lower-inner quadrant of right female breast ♀ ☑

C50.312 Malignant neoplasm of lower-inner quadrant of left female breast ♀ ☑

C50.321 Malignant neoplasm of lower-inner quadrant of right male breast ♂ ☑

C50.322 Malignant neoplasm of lower-inner quadrant of left male breast ♂ ☑

C50.411 Malignant neoplasm of upper-outer quadrant of right female breast ♀ ☑

C50.412 Malignant neoplasm of upper-outer quadrant of left female breast ♀ ☑

C50.421 Malignant neoplasm of upper-outer quadrant of right male breast ♂ ☑

C50.422 Malignant neoplasm of upper-outer quadrant of left male breast ♂ ☑

C50.511 Malignant neoplasm of lower-outer quadrant of right female breast ♀ ☑

C50.512 Malignant neoplasm of lower-outer quadrant of left female breast ♀ ☑

C50.521 Malignant neoplasm of lower-outer quadrant of right male breast ♂ ☑

C50.522 Malignant neoplasm of lower-outer quadrant of left male breast ♂ ☑

C50.611 Malignant neoplasm of axillary tail of right female breast ♀ ☑

C50.612 Malignant neoplasm of axillary tail of left female breast ♀ ☑

C50.621 Malignant neoplasm of axillary tail of right male breast ♂ ☑

C50.622 Malignant neoplasm of axillary tail of left male breast ♂ ☑

C50.811 Malignant neoplasm of overlapping sites of right female breast ♀ ☑

C50.812 Malignant neoplasm of overlapping sites of left female breast ♀ ☑

C50.821 Malignant neoplasm of overlapping sites of right male breast ♂ ☑

C79.81 Secondary malignant neoplasm of breast

D05.01 Lobular carcinoma in situ of right breast ☑

D05.02 Lobular carcinoma in situ of left breast ☑

D05.11 Intraductal carcinoma in situ of right breast ☑

D05.12 Intraductal carcinoma in situ of left breast ☑

D24.1 Benign neoplasm of right breast ☑

D24.2 Benign neoplasm of left breast ☑

D48.61 Neoplasm of uncertain behavior of right breast ☑

D48.62 Neoplasm of uncertain behavior of left breast ☑

N60.01 Solitary cyst of right breast ☑

N60.02 Solitary cyst of left breast ☑

N60.21 Fibroadenosis of right breast ☑

N60.22 Fibroadenosis of left breast ☑

N60.81 Other benign mammary dysplasias of right breast ☑

N60.82 Other benign mammary dysplasias of left breast ☑

N61.21 Granulomatous mastitis, right breast ☑

N61.22 Granulomatous mastitis, left breast ☑

N61.23 Granulomatous mastitis, bilateral breast ☑

N63.11 Unspecified lump in the right breast, upper outer quadrant ☑

N63.13 Unspecified lump in the right breast, lower outer quadrant ☑

N63.31 Unspecified lump in axillary tail of the right breast ☑

N63.41 Unspecified lump in right breast, subareolar ☑

R92.0 Mammographic microcalcification found on diagnostic imaging of breast

R92.1 Mammographic calcification found on diagnostic imaging of breast

AMA: **19125** 2018,Jan,8; 2017,Jan,8; 2016,Jan,13; 2015,Mar,5; 2015,Jan,16 **19126** 2018,Jan,8; 2017,Jan,8; 2016,Jan,13; 2015,Jan,16

Relative Value Units/Medicare Edits

Non-Facility RVU	Work	PE	MP	Total
19125	6.69	8.58	1.62	16.89
19126	2.93	1.1	0.71	4.74
Facility RVU	**Work**	**PE**	**MP**	**Total**
19125	6.69	5.31	1.62	13.62
19126	2.93	1.1	0.71	4.74

	FUD	Status	MUE	Modifiers				IOM Reference
19125	90	A	1(2)	51	50	62*	N/A	None
19126	N/A	A	3(3)	N/A	N/A	62*	N/A	

* with documentation

Terms To Know

biopsy. Tissue or fluid removed for diagnostic purposes through analysis of the cells in the biopsy material.

calcification. Normal process of calcium salts deposition in bone. Calcification can also occur abnormally in fibroconnective soft tissues.

ligate. To tie off a blood vessel or duct with a suture or a soft, thin wire (ligature wire).

suture. Numerous stitching techniques employed in wound closure.

buried suture. Continuous or interrupted suture placed under the skin for a layered closure.

continuous suture. Running stitch with tension evenly distributed across a single strand to provide a leakproof closure line.

interrupted suture. Series of single stitches with tension isolated at each stitch, in which all stitches are not affected if one becomes loose, and the isolated sutures cannot act as a wick to transport an infection.

purse-string suture. Continuous suture placed around a tubular structure and tightened, to reduce or close the lumen.

retention suture. Secondary stitching that bridges the primary suture, providing support for the primary repair; a plastic or rubber bolster may be placed over the primary repair and under the retention sutures.

19294

+ **19294** Preparation of tumor cavity, with placement of a radiation therapy applicator for intraoperative radiation therapy (IORT) concurrent with partial mastectomy (List separately in addition to code for primary procedure)

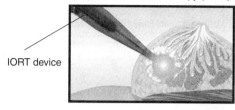
Concurrent intraoperative radiation therapy (IORT)

IORT device

Explanation

The radiation oncologist delivers intraoperative radiation therapy (IORT) at the same time as the patient is undergoing a lumpectomy or partial mastectomy. A miniature, low energy, isotope-free x-ray source is brought into the operating room at the time the lumpectomy is performed to deliver a precise and targeted dose of radiation directly to the lumpectomy cavity. The surgeon removes the malignant tumor and awaits the initial pathology report. Once the malignancy is confirmed, the physician prepares the tumor cavity for temporary insertion of a flexible balloon applicator. The radiation oncologist inserts the miniature x-ray source inside a balloon-shaped catheter device and a single dose of radiation is directed at the tumor cavity while medical personnel remain behind a rolling shield. The process takes eight to 12 minutes. Once the treatment is complete, the catheter is withdrawn and the applicator is removed. The incision is closed.

Coding Tips

Report 19294 in addition to 19301 or 19302 for partial mastectomy. This code describes the preparation of the tumor cavity and the intraoperative placement of a radiation therapy applicator at the time of a partial mastectomy.

ICD-10-CM Diagnostic Codes

C50.011	Malignant neoplasm of nipple and areola, right female breast ♀ ☑
C50.012	Malignant neoplasm of nipple and areola, left female breast ♀ ☑
C50.021	Malignant neoplasm of nipple and areola, right male breast ♂ ☑
C50.022	Malignant neoplasm of nipple and areola, left male breast ♂ ☑
C50.111	Malignant neoplasm of central portion of right female breast ♀ ☑
C50.112	Malignant neoplasm of central portion of left female breast ♀ ☑
C50.121	Malignant neoplasm of central portion of right male breast ♂ ☑
C50.122	Malignant neoplasm of central portion of left male breast ♂ ☑
C50.211	Malignant neoplasm of upper-inner quadrant of right female breast ♀ ☑
C50.212	Malignant neoplasm of upper-inner quadrant of left female breast ♀ ☑
C50.221	Malignant neoplasm of upper-inner quadrant of right male breast ♂ ☑
C50.222	Malignant neoplasm of upper-inner quadrant of left male breast ♂ ☑
C50.311	Malignant neoplasm of lower-inner quadrant of right female breast ♀ ☑
C50.312	Malignant neoplasm of lower-inner quadrant of left female breast ♀ ☑
C50.321	Malignant neoplasm of lower-inner quadrant of right male breast ♂ ☑
C50.322	Malignant neoplasm of lower-inner quadrant of left male breast ♂ ☑
C50.411	Malignant neoplasm of upper-outer quadrant of right female breast ♀ ☑
C50.412	Malignant neoplasm of upper-outer quadrant of left female breast ♀ ☑
C50.421	Malignant neoplasm of upper-outer quadrant of right male breast ♂ ☑
C50.422	Malignant neoplasm of upper-outer quadrant of left male breast ♂ ☑
C50.511	Malignant neoplasm of lower-outer quadrant of right female breast ♀ ☑
C50.512	Malignant neoplasm of lower-outer quadrant of left female breast ♀ ☑
C50.521	Malignant neoplasm of lower-outer quadrant of right male breast ♂ ☑
C50.522	Malignant neoplasm of lower-outer quadrant of left male breast ♂ ☑
C50.611	Malignant neoplasm of axillary tail of right female breast ♀ ☑
C50.612	Malignant neoplasm of axillary tail of left female breast ♀ ☑
C50.621	Malignant neoplasm of axillary tail of right male breast ♂ ☑
C50.622	Malignant neoplasm of axillary tail of left male breast ♂ ☑
D05.01	Lobular carcinoma in situ of right breast ☑
D05.02	Lobular carcinoma in situ of left breast ☑
D05.11	Intraductal carcinoma in situ of right breast ☑
D05.12	Intraductal carcinoma in situ of left breast ☑
D05.81	Other specified type of carcinoma in situ of right breast ☑
D05.82	Other specified type of carcinoma in situ of left breast ☑

AMA: **19294** 2020,May,9

Relative Value Units/Medicare Edits

Non-Facility RVU	Work	PE	MP	Total
19294	3.0	1.14	0.71	4.85
Facility RVU	**Work**	**PE**	**MP**	**Total**
19294	3.0	1.14	0.71	4.85

	FUD	Status	MUE	Modifiers				IOM Reference
19294	N/A	A	2(3)	N/A	N/A	N/A	80*	None

* with documentation

Breast

19296-19297

19296 Placement of radiotherapy afterloading expandable catheter (single or multichannel) into the breast for interstitial radioelement application following partial mastectomy, includes imaging guidance; on date separate from partial mastectomy

+ 19297 concurrent with partial mastectomy (List separately in addition to code for primary procedure)

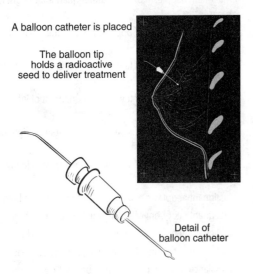

A balloon catheter is placed

The balloon tip holds a radioactive seed to deliver treatment

Detail of balloon catheter

Explanation

A remote single or multichannel afterloading expandable catheter for interstitial radiotherapy treatment is placed in the breast following partial mastectomy. A catheter is placed at a later date, separate from the lumpectomy surgery in 19296, and concurrently with the lumpectomy in 19297. This is a single catheter with an expandable balloon tip that holds the radioactive seed or treatment source, which is loaded and removed for each session. The catheter can be single or multichannel, depending on the treatment delivery requirements. During the lumpectomy surgery, an uninflated balloon catheter is inserted into the recently created tumor cavity and positioned under imaging with a portion of the catheter remaining outside of the body. If a separate procedure is done after surgery, a small incision is first made and the uninflated balloon catheter is guided into position under imaging. After correct placement is determined, the balloon is inflated with saline to fit snugly into the lumpectomy cavity, and the breast is bandaged. The catheter remains until radiotherapy treatment sessions are complete.

Coding Tips

Report 19297 in addition to 19301 or 19302 for partial mastectomy. These codes report only the radiotherapy balloon catheter placement and subsequent catheter removal for interstitial brachytherapy. Preparation of the isodose plan is reported separately, see 77316–77318. For remote afterloading of the actual radiotherapy source through the catheter, see 77770–77772.

ICD-10-CM Diagnostic Codes

C50.011	Malignant neoplasm of nipple and areola, right female breast ♀ ☑
C50.012	Malignant neoplasm of nipple and areola, left female breast ♀ ☑
C50.021	Malignant neoplasm of nipple and areola, right male breast ♂ ☑
C50.022	Malignant neoplasm of nipple and areola, left male breast ♂ ☑
C50.111	Malignant neoplasm of central portion of right female breast ♀ ☑
C50.112	Malignant neoplasm of central portion of left female breast ♀ ☑
C50.121	Malignant neoplasm of central portion of right male breast ♂ ☑
C50.122	Malignant neoplasm of central portion of left male breast ♂ ☑
C50.211	Malignant neoplasm of upper-inner quadrant of right female breast ♀ ☑
C50.212	Malignant neoplasm of upper-inner quadrant of left female breast ♀ ☑
C50.221	Malignant neoplasm of upper-inner quadrant of right male breast ♂ ☑
C50.222	Malignant neoplasm of upper-inner quadrant of left male breast ♂ ☑
C50.311	Malignant neoplasm of lower-inner quadrant of right female breast ♀ ☑
C50.312	Malignant neoplasm of lower-inner quadrant of left female breast ♀ ☑
C50.321	Malignant neoplasm of lower-inner quadrant of right male breast ♂ ☑
C50.322	Malignant neoplasm of lower-inner quadrant of left male breast ♂ ☑
C50.411	Malignant neoplasm of upper-outer quadrant of right female breast ♀ ☑
C50.412	Malignant neoplasm of upper-outer quadrant of left female breast ♀ ☑
C50.421	Malignant neoplasm of upper-outer quadrant of right male breast ♂ ☑
C50.422	Malignant neoplasm of upper-outer quadrant of left male breast ♂ ☑
C50.511	Malignant neoplasm of lower-outer quadrant of right female breast ♀ ☑
C50.512	Malignant neoplasm of lower-outer quadrant of left female breast ♀ ☑
C50.521	Malignant neoplasm of lower-outer quadrant of right male breast ♂ ☑
C50.522	Malignant neoplasm of lower-outer quadrant of left male breast ♂ ☑
C50.611	Malignant neoplasm of axillary tail of right female breast ♀ ☑
C50.612	Malignant neoplasm of axillary tail of left female breast ♀ ☑
C50.621	Malignant neoplasm of axillary tail of right male breast ♂ ☑
C50.622	Malignant neoplasm of axillary tail of left male breast ♂ ☑
C50.811	Malignant neoplasm of overlapping sites of right female breast ♀ ☑
C50.812	Malignant neoplasm of overlapping sites of left female breast ♀ ☑
C50.821	Malignant neoplasm of overlapping sites of right male breast ♂ ☑
C50.822	Malignant neoplasm of overlapping sites of left male breast ♂ ☑
C79.81	Secondary malignant neoplasm of breast
D05.01	Lobular carcinoma in situ of right breast ☑
D05.02	Lobular carcinoma in situ of left breast ☑
D05.11	Intraductal carcinoma in situ of right breast ☑
D05.12	Intraductal carcinoma in situ of left breast ☑
D05.81	Other specified type of carcinoma in situ of right breast ☑
D05.82	Other specified type of carcinoma in situ of left breast ☑
D48.61	Neoplasm of uncertain behavior of right breast ☑
D48.62	Neoplasm of uncertain behavior of left breast ☑

Breast

AMA: **19296** 2020,May,9; 2018,Jan,8; 2017,Jan,8; 2016,Jan,13; 2015,Jan,16
19297 2020,May,9; 2019,Apr,10; 2018,Jan,8; 2017,Jan,8; 2016,Jan,13; 2015,Jan,16

Relative Value Units/Medicare Edits

Non-Facility RVU	Work	PE	MP	Total
19296	3.63	119.04	0.84	123.51
19297	1.72	0.65	0.43	2.8
Facility RVU	Work	PE	MP	Total
19296	3.63	1.7	0.84	6.17
19297	1.72	0.65	0.43	2.8

	FUD	Status	MUE	Modifiers				IOM Reference
19296	0	A	1(3)	51	50	N/A	80*	100-04,12,40.7;
19297	N/A	A	2(3)	N/A	N/A	N/A	80*	100-04,13,80.2

* with documentation

Terms To Know

balloon catheter. Any catheter equipped with an inflatable balloon at the end to hold it in place in a body cavity or to be used for dilation of a vessel lumen.

imaging. Radiologic means of producing pictures for clinical study of the internal structures and functions of the body, such as x-ray, ultrasound, magnetic resonance, or positron emission tomography.

interstitial radiation. Radioactive source placed into the tissue being treated.

mastectomy. Surgical removal of one or both breasts.

19298

19298 Placement of radiotherapy after loading brachytherapy catheters (multiple tube and button type) into the breast for interstitial radioelement application following (at the time of or subsequent to) partial mastectomy, includes imaging guidance

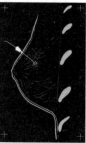

Afterloading catheters are placed into the breast, typically at the time of a lumpectomy, to deliver brachytherapy

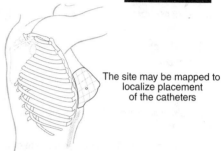

The site may be mapped to localize placement of the catheters

Explanation

Using imaging guidance, at the time of a partial mastectomy, or subsequent to a partial mastectomy having been performed, remote afterloading catheters are placed into the breast for interstitial radiotherapy application. The lumpectomy site is identified. A template with pre-drilled holes that function as coordinates for catheter placement around the surgical area may be applied for imaging. Brachytherapy needles are first inserted into the chosen coordinates. The brachytherapy catheters are fed into position through the needles, which are removed. A catheter button is positioned to hold each catheter in place and imaging confirms their position. These remain in place until the actual loading of the radioactive material for treatment. This code reports only the placement of the catheters.

Coding Tips

This code reports only the placement and subsequent removal of multiple tube and button type catheters for interstitial brachytherapy. Preparation of the isodose plan is reported separately with 77316–77318. For remote afterloading of the actual radiotherapy source through the catheter, see 77770–77772.

ICD-10-CM Diagnostic Codes

C50.011	Malignant neoplasm of nipple and areola, right female breast ♀ ☑
C50.012	Malignant neoplasm of nipple and areola, left female breast ♀ ☑
C50.021	Malignant neoplasm of nipple and areola, right male breast ♂ ☑
C50.022	Malignant neoplasm of nipple and areola, left male breast ♂ ☑
C50.111	Malignant neoplasm of central portion of right female breast ♀ ☑
C50.112	Malignant neoplasm of central portion of left female breast ♀ ☑
C50.121	Malignant neoplasm of central portion of right male breast ♂ ☑
C50.122	Malignant neoplasm of central portion of left male breast ♂ ☑
C50.211	Malignant neoplasm of upper-inner quadrant of right female breast ♀ ☑

Breast

Breast

C50.212	Malignant neoplasm of upper-inner quadrant of left female breast ♀ ☑
C50.221	Malignant neoplasm of upper-inner quadrant of right male breast ♂ ☑
C50.222	Malignant neoplasm of upper-inner quadrant of left male breast ♂ ☑
C50.311	Malignant neoplasm of lower-inner quadrant of right female breast ♀ ☑
C50.312	Malignant neoplasm of lower-inner quadrant of left female breast ♀ ☑
C50.321	Malignant neoplasm of lower-inner quadrant of right male breast ♂ ☑
C50.322	Malignant neoplasm of lower-inner quadrant of left male breast ♂ ☑
C50.411	Malignant neoplasm of upper-outer quadrant of right female breast ♀ ☑
C50.412	Malignant neoplasm of upper-outer quadrant of left female breast ♀ ☑
C50.421	Malignant neoplasm of upper-outer quadrant of right male breast ♂ ☑
C50.422	Malignant neoplasm of upper-outer quadrant of left male breast ♂ ☑
C50.511	Malignant neoplasm of lower-outer quadrant of right female breast ♀ ☑
C50.512	Malignant neoplasm of lower-outer quadrant of left female breast ♀ ☑
C50.521	Malignant neoplasm of lower-outer quadrant of right male breast ♂ ☑
C50.522	Malignant neoplasm of lower-outer quadrant of left male breast ♂ ☑
C50.611	Malignant neoplasm of axillary tail of right female breast ♀ ☑
C50.612	Malignant neoplasm of axillary tail of left female breast ♀ ☑
C50.621	Malignant neoplasm of axillary tail of right male breast ♂ ☑
C50.622	Malignant neoplasm of axillary tail of left male breast ♂ ☑
C50.811	Malignant neoplasm of overlapping sites of right female breast ♀ ☑
C50.812	Malignant neoplasm of overlapping sites of left female breast ♀ ☑
C50.821	Malignant neoplasm of overlapping sites of right male breast ♂ ☑
C50.822	Malignant neoplasm of overlapping sites of left male breast ♂ ☑
C79.81	Secondary malignant neoplasm of breast
D05.01	Lobular carcinoma in situ of right breast ☑
D05.02	Lobular carcinoma in situ of left breast ☑
D05.11	Intraductal carcinoma in situ of right breast ☑
D05.12	Intraductal carcinoma in situ of left breast ☑
D05.81	Other specified type of carcinoma in situ of right breast ☑
D05.82	Other specified type of carcinoma in situ of left breast ☑
D48.61	Neoplasm of uncertain behavior of right breast ☑
D48.62	Neoplasm of uncertain behavior of left breast ☑

AMA: **19298** 2020,May,9; 2018,Jan,8; 2017,Jan,8; 2016,Jan,13; 2015,Jan,16

Relative Value Units/Medicare Edits

Non-Facility RVU	Work	PE	MP	Total
19298	5.75	22.92	0.74	29.41
Facility RVU	Work	PE	MP	Total
19298	5.75	2.79	0.74	9.28

	FUD	Status	MUE	Modifiers				IOM Reference
19298	0	A	1(2)	51	50	N/A	80*	100-04,13,80.1; 100-04,13,80.2

* with documentation

Terms To Know

brachytherapy. Form of radiation therapy in which radioactive pellets or seeds are implanted directly into the tissue being treated to deliver their dose of radiation in a more directed fashion. Brachytherapy provides radiation to the prescribed body area while minimizing exposure to normal tissue.

imaging. Radiologic means of producing pictures for clinical study of the internal structures and functions of the body, such as x-ray, ultrasound, magnetic resonance, or positron emission tomography.

partial mastectomy. Removal of breast tissue with specific attention to surgical margins to remove a tumor or disease area, commonly referred to as a lumpectomy, tylectomy, quadrantectomy, or segmentectomy.

19300

19300   Mastectomy for gynecomastia

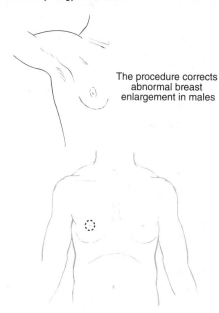

The procedure corrects abnormal breast enlargement in males

A common access may involve removal of the areola. Excess tissue is removed from the breast and the areola reattached

Explanation

The physician performs a mastectomy for gynecomastia on a male patient. The physician makes a circular incision in the skin of the breast at the edge of the areola or in the inframammary fold. Extraneous fat and breast tissue are dissected from the pectoral fascia and removed. Bleeding vessels are ligated with sutures or cauterized. The incision is sutured in layered closure and a dressing is applied.

Coding Tips

This code is for males only. This is a unilateral procedure. If performed bilaterally, some payers require that the service be reported twice with modifier 50 appended to the second code while others require identification of the service only once with modifier 50 appended. Check with individual payers. Modifier 50 identifies a procedure performed identically on the opposite side of the body (mirror image). For open excision of cyst, fibroadenoma, other benign or malignant tumor, aberrant breast tissue, duct lesion, nipple lesion, or areolar lesion, male or female, one or more lesions, see 19120. For mastectomies for other than gynecomastia, see 19301–19307. For breast reduction other than for gynecomastia, see 19318.

ICD-10-CM Diagnostic Codes

N62   Hypertrophy of breast

AMA: 19300 2020,May,9; 2018,Jan,8; 2017,Jan,8; 2016,Jan,13; 2015,Jan,16

Relative Value Units/Medicare Edits

Non-Facility RVU	Work	PE	MP	Total
19300	5.31	10.66	1.19	17.16
Facility RVU	**Work**	**PE**	**MP**	**Total**
19300	5.31	6.12	1.19	12.62

	FUD	Status	MUE	Modifiers				IOM Reference
19300	90	A	1(2)	51	50	N/A	N/A	100-04,12,40.7

* with documentation

Terms To Know

cauterization. Tissue destruction by means of a hot instrument, an electric current, or a caustic chemical.

dissect. Cut apart or separate tissue for surgical purposes or for visual or microscopic study.

fascia. Fibrous sheet or band of tissue that envelops organs, muscles, and groupings of muscles.

gynecomastia. Condition in which the male mammary glands are abnormally large.

hypertrophy of breast. Overgrowth of normal breast tissue.

ligate. To tie off a blood vessel or duct with a suture or a soft, thin wire (ligature wire).

19301-19302

19301 Mastectomy, partial (eg, lumpectomy, tylectomy, quadrantectomy, segmentectomy);
19302 with axillary lymphadenectomy

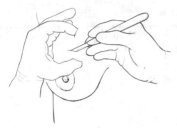

A partial breast removal is performed

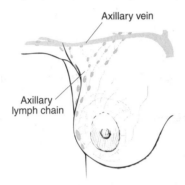

Axillary vein

Axillary lymph chain

Explanation

The physician excises a breast tumor and a margin of normal tissue by performing a partial mastectomy by making an incision through the skin and fascia over a breast malignancy and clamping any lymphatic and blood vessels. The physician excises the mass along with a margin or rim of healthy tissue. This procedure is often referred to as a segmental mastectomy or a quadrantectomy, but is also called a lumpectomy. In 19302, an axillary lymphadenectomy is also performed. The lymph nodes between the pectoralis major and the pectoralis minor muscles and the nodes in the axilla are removed through a separate incision. A drainage tube may be placed through a separate stab incision to enhance drainage from the wound or lymphatic system. The incision is repaired with layered closure and a dressing is applied.

Coding Tips

These are unilateral procedures. If performed bilaterally, some payers require that the service be reported twice with modifier 50 appended to the second code while others require identification of the service only once with modifier 50 appended. Check with individual payers. Modifier 50 identifies a procedure performed identically on the opposite side of the body (mirror image). Removal of axillary lymph nodes including the sentinel node is included in 19302 and should not be reported separately. Placement of intraoperative clips should not be reported separately. For other mastectomies, see 19303–19307. For mastectomy due to gynecomastia, see 19300. For preparation of a tumor cavity with placement of an intraoperative applicator used for radiation therapy when partial mastectomy is performed concurrently, see 19294. Partial mastectomy documentation should include information detailing the removal of sufficient surgical margins around the mass or lesion.

ICD-10-CM Diagnostic Codes

C50.011	Malignant neoplasm of nipple and areola, right female breast ♀ ☑
C50.012	Malignant neoplasm of nipple and areola, left female breast ♀ ☑

C50.021	Malignant neoplasm of nipple and areola, right male breast ♂ ☑
C50.022	Malignant neoplasm of nipple and areola, left male breast ♂ ☑
C50.111	Malignant neoplasm of central portion of right female breast ♀ ☑
C50.112	Malignant neoplasm of central portion of left female breast ♀ ☑
C50.121	Malignant neoplasm of central portion of right male breast ♂ ☑
C50.122	Malignant neoplasm of central portion of left male breast ♂ ☑
C50.211	Malignant neoplasm of upper-inner quadrant of right female breast ♀ ☑
C50.212	Malignant neoplasm of upper-inner quadrant of left female breast ♀ ☑
C50.221	Malignant neoplasm of upper-inner quadrant of right male breast ♂ ☑
C50.222	Malignant neoplasm of upper-inner quadrant of left male breast ♂ ☑
C50.311	Malignant neoplasm of lower-inner quadrant of right female breast ♀ ☑
C50.312	Malignant neoplasm of lower-inner quadrant of left female breast ♀ ☑
C50.321	Malignant neoplasm of lower-inner quadrant of right male breast ♂ ☑
C50.322	Malignant neoplasm of lower-inner quadrant of left male breast ♂ ☑
C50.411	Malignant neoplasm of upper-outer quadrant of right female breast ♀ ☑
C50.412	Malignant neoplasm of upper-outer quadrant of left female breast ♀ ☑
C50.421	Malignant neoplasm of upper-outer quadrant of right male breast ♂ ☑
C50.422	Malignant neoplasm of upper-outer quadrant of left male breast ♂ ☑
C50.511	Malignant neoplasm of lower-outer quadrant of right female breast ♀ ☑
C50.512	Malignant neoplasm of lower-outer quadrant of left female breast ♀ ☑
C50.521	Malignant neoplasm of lower-outer quadrant of right male breast ♂ ☑
C50.522	Malignant neoplasm of lower-outer quadrant of left male breast ♂ ☑
C50.611	Malignant neoplasm of axillary tail of right female breast ♀ ☑
C50.612	Malignant neoplasm of axillary tail of left female breast ♀ ☑
C50.621	Malignant neoplasm of axillary tail of right male breast ♂ ☑
C50.622	Malignant neoplasm of axillary tail of left male breast ♂ ☑
C50.811	Malignant neoplasm of overlapping sites of right female breast ♀ ☑
C50.812	Malignant neoplasm of overlapping sites of left female breast ♀ ☑
C50.821	Malignant neoplasm of overlapping sites of right male breast ♂ ☑
C50.822	Malignant neoplasm of overlapping sites of left male breast ♂ ☑
C79.81	Secondary malignant neoplasm of breast
D05.01	Lobular carcinoma in situ of right breast ☑
D05.02	Lobular carcinoma in situ of left breast ☑
D05.11	Intraductal carcinoma in situ of right breast ☑
D05.12	Intraductal carcinoma in situ of left breast ☑
D05.81	Other specified type of carcinoma in situ of right breast ☑

Breast

D05.82	Other specified type of carcinoma in situ of left breast ☑
D48.61	Neoplasm of uncertain behavior of right breast ☑
D48.62	Neoplasm of uncertain behavior of left breast ☑
N61.21	Granulomatous mastitis, right breast ☑
N61.22	Granulomatous mastitis, left breast ☑
N61.23	Granulomatous mastitis, bilateral breast ☑

AMA: **19301** 2020,May,9; 2018,Jan,8; 2017,Oct,9; 2017,Jan,8; 2016,Jan,13; 2015,Mar,5; 2015,Jan,16 **19302** 2020,Nov,12; 2020,May,9; 2019,Feb,8; 2018,Jan,8; 2017,Jan,8; 2016,Jan,13; 2015,Mar,5; 2015,Jan,16

Relative Value Units/Medicare Edits

Non-Facility RVU	Work	PE	MP	Total
19301	10.13	6.94	2.42	19.49
19302	13.99	9.43	3.37	26.79
Facility RVU	**Work**	**PE**	**MP**	**Total**
19301	10.13	6.94	2.42	19.49
19302	13.99	9.43	3.37	26.79

	FUD	Status	MUE	Modifiers				IOM Reference
19301	90	A	1(3)	51	50	N/A	80*	None
19302	90	A	1(2)	51	50	62*	80	

* with documentation

Terms To Know

axillary. Area under the arm.

lymphadenectomy. Dissection of lymph nodes free from the vessels and removal for examination by frozen section in a separate procedure to detect early-stage metastases.

lymphatic system. Lymphatic capillaries, vessels, lymph nodes, spleen, thymus gland, and bone marrow.

pectoralis major. Chest muscle connecting at the clavicle, upper ribs, sternum, and the axilla.

19303

| 19303 | Mastectomy, simple, complete |

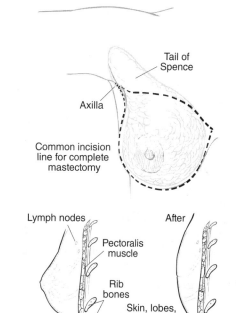

Explanation

The physician removes all subcutaneous breast tissue, with or without nipple and skin. The physician makes an elliptical incision around the breast that includes the tail of Spence, the extension of mammary tissue into the axillary region. The breast tissue is dissected from the pectoral fascia and sternum. The breast tissue is removed, along with a portion of skin, including the nipple. In a modification of the simple mastectomy, skin and nipple may be spared, but all subcutaneous breast tissue is removed. The physician ligates any bleeding vessels. A closed wound drainage catheter may be inserted and the edges of skin are approximated, sutured, and a dressing is applied.

Coding Tips

This is a unilateral procedure. If performed bilaterally, some payers require that the service be reported twice with modifier 50 appended to the second code while others require identification of the service only once with modifier 50 appended. Check with individual payers. Modifier 50 identifies a procedure performed identically on the opposite side of the body (mirror image). For immediate or delayed insertion of an implant, see 19340–19342. Placement of intraoperative clips should not be reported separately. Breast reconstruction should be reported separately. For mastectomy due to gynecomastia, see 19300.

ICD-10-CM Diagnostic Codes

C50.011	Malignant neoplasm of nipple and areola, right female breast ♀ ☑
C50.012	Malignant neoplasm of nipple and areola, left female breast ♀ ☑
C50.021	Malignant neoplasm of nipple and areola, right male breast ♂ ☑
C50.022	Malignant neoplasm of nipple and areola, left male breast ♂ ☑
C50.111	Malignant neoplasm of central portion of right female breast ♀ ☑
C50.112	Malignant neoplasm of central portion of left female breast ♀ ☑
C50.121	Malignant neoplasm of central portion of right male breast ♂ ☑

Breast

C50.122	Malignant neoplasm of central portion of left male breast ♂ ☑	
C50.211	Malignant neoplasm of upper-inner quadrant of right female breast ♀ ☑	
C50.212	Malignant neoplasm of upper-inner quadrant of left female breast ♀ ☑	
C50.221	Malignant neoplasm of upper-inner quadrant of right male breast ♂ ☑	
C50.222	Malignant neoplasm of upper-inner quadrant of left male breast ♂ ☑	
C50.311	Malignant neoplasm of lower-inner quadrant of right female breast ♀ ☑	
C50.312	Malignant neoplasm of lower-inner quadrant of left female breast ♀ ☑	
C50.321	Malignant neoplasm of lower-inner quadrant of right male breast ♂ ☑	
C50.322	Malignant neoplasm of lower-inner quadrant of left male breast ♂ ☑	
C50.411	Malignant neoplasm of upper-outer quadrant of right female breast ♀ ☑	
C50.412	Malignant neoplasm of upper-outer quadrant of left female breast ♀ ☑	
C50.421	Malignant neoplasm of upper-outer quadrant of right male breast ♂ ☑	
C50.422	Malignant neoplasm of upper-outer quadrant of left male breast ♂ ☑	
C50.511	Malignant neoplasm of lower-outer quadrant of right female breast ♀ ☑	
C50.512	Malignant neoplasm of lower-outer quadrant of left female breast ♀ ☑	
C50.611	Malignant neoplasm of axillary tail of right female breast ♀ ☑	
C50.612	Malignant neoplasm of axillary tail of left female breast ♀ ☑	
C50.621	Malignant neoplasm of axillary tail of right male breast ♂ ☑	
C50.622	Malignant neoplasm of axillary tail of left male breast ♂ ☑	
C50.811	Malignant neoplasm of overlapping sites of right female breast ♀ ☑	
C50.812	Malignant neoplasm of overlapping sites of left female breast ♀ ☑	
C50.821	Malignant neoplasm of overlapping sites of right male breast ♂ ☑	
C50.822	Malignant neoplasm of overlapping sites of left male breast ♂ ☑	
C79.81	Secondary malignant neoplasm of breast	
D05.11	Intraductal carcinoma in situ of right breast ☑	
D05.12	Intraductal carcinoma in situ of left breast ☑	
D05.81	Other specified type of carcinoma in situ of right breast ☑	
D05.82	Other specified type of carcinoma in situ of left breast ☑	
D48.61	Neoplasm of uncertain behavior of right breast ☑	
D48.62	Neoplasm of uncertain behavior of left breast ☑	
N61.21	Granulomatous mastitis, right breast ☑	
N61.22	Granulomatous mastitis, left breast ☑	
N61.23	Granulomatous mastitis, bilateral breast ☑	
Z40.01	Encounter for prophylactic removal of breast	

AMA: 19303 2020,May,9; 2019,Dec,4; 2018,Jan,8; 2017,Jan,8; 2016,Jan,13; 2015,Mar,5; 2015,Jan,16

Relative Value Units/Medicare Edits

Non-Facility RVU	Work	PE	MP	Total
19303	15.0	9.73	3.6	28.33
Facility RVU	**Work**	**PE**	**MP**	**Total**
19303	15.0	9.73	3.6	28.33

	FUD	Status	MUE	Modifiers				IOM Reference
19303	90	A	1(2)	51	50	62*	80	None

* with documentation

Terms To Know

ligate. To tie off a blood vessel or duct with a suture or a soft, thin wire (ligature wire).

malignant neoplasm. Any cancerous tumor or lesion exhibiting uncontrolled tissue growth that can progressively invade other parts of the body with its disease-generating cells.

simple mastectomy. Only breast tissue, nipple, and a small portion of overlying skin are removed.

subcutaneous tissue. Sheet or wide band of adipose (fat) and areolar connective tissue in two layers attached to the dermis.

19305

19305 Mastectomy, radical, including pectoral muscles, axillary lymph nodes

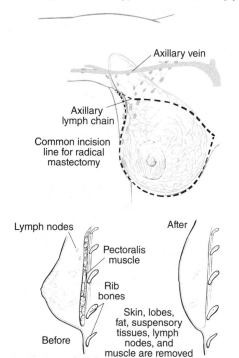

Explanation

The physician performs a radical mastectomy. The physician makes an elliptical incision that includes the nipple and the tail of Spence, the extension of mammary tissue into the axillary region. The breast, along with the overlying skin, the pectoralis major and minor muscles, and the lymph nodes in the axilla, are removed as a single specimen. Bleeding vessels are ligated or electrocauterized. In large-breasted patients, adequate skin may be available for primary closure. Patients with insufficient skin for coverage may require skin grafts or myocutaneous flaps. If no implant is to be inserted, a closed wound suction catheter may be inserted. The wound is closed and a pressure dressing is applied.

Coding Tips

This is a unilateral procedure. If performed bilaterally, some payers require that the service be reported twice with modifier 50 appended to the second code while others require identification of the service only once with modifier 50 appended. Check with individual payers. Modifier 50 identifies a procedure performed identically on the opposite side of the body (mirror image). Lymph node dissection is included in this code and should not be reported separately. Any breast reconstruction should be reported separately. For immediate or delayed insertion of an implant, see 19340–19342. Placement of intraoperative clips should not be reported separately.

ICD-10-CM Diagnostic Codes

C50.011	Malignant neoplasm of nipple and areola, right female breast ♀ ☑
C50.012	Malignant neoplasm of nipple and areola, left female breast ♀ ☑
C50.021	Malignant neoplasm of nipple and areola, right male breast ♂ ☑
C50.022	Malignant neoplasm of nipple and areola, left male breast ♂ ☑
C50.111	Malignant neoplasm of central portion of right female breast ♀ ☑
C50.112	Malignant neoplasm of central portion of left female breast ♀ ☑
C50.121	Malignant neoplasm of central portion of right male breast ♂ ☑
C50.122	Malignant neoplasm of central portion of left male breast ♂ ☑
C50.211	Malignant neoplasm of upper-inner quadrant of right female breast ♀ ☑
C50.212	Malignant neoplasm of upper-inner quadrant of left female breast ♀ ☑
C50.221	Malignant neoplasm of upper-inner quadrant of right male breast ♂ ☑
C50.222	Malignant neoplasm of upper-inner quadrant of left male breast ♂ ☑
C50.311	Malignant neoplasm of lower-inner quadrant of right female breast ♀ ☑
C50.312	Malignant neoplasm of lower-inner quadrant of left female breast ♀ ☑
C50.321	Malignant neoplasm of lower-inner quadrant of right male breast ♂ ☑
C50.322	Malignant neoplasm of lower-inner quadrant of left male breast ♂ ☑
C50.411	Malignant neoplasm of upper-outer quadrant of right female breast ♀ ☑
C50.412	Malignant neoplasm of upper-outer quadrant of left female breast ♀ ☑
C50.421	Malignant neoplasm of upper-outer quadrant of right male breast ♂ ☑
C50.422	Malignant neoplasm of upper-outer quadrant of left male breast ♂ ☑
C50.511	Malignant neoplasm of lower-outer quadrant of right female breast ♀ ☑
C50.512	Malignant neoplasm of lower-outer quadrant of left female breast ♀ ☑
C50.521	Malignant neoplasm of lower-outer quadrant of right male breast ♂ ☑
C50.522	Malignant neoplasm of lower-outer quadrant of left male breast ♂ ☑
C50.611	Malignant neoplasm of axillary tail of right female breast ♀ ☑
C50.612	Malignant neoplasm of axillary tail of left female breast ♀ ☑
C50.621	Malignant neoplasm of axillary tail of right male breast ♂ ☑
C50.622	Malignant neoplasm of axillary tail of left male breast ♂ ☑
C50.811	Malignant neoplasm of overlapping sites of right female breast ♀ ☑
C50.812	Malignant neoplasm of overlapping sites of left female breast ♀ ☑
C50.821	Malignant neoplasm of overlapping sites of right male breast ♂ ☑
C50.822	Malignant neoplasm of overlapping sites of left male breast ♂ ☑
C50.921	Malignant neoplasm of unspecified site of right male breast ♂ ☑
C50.922	Malignant neoplasm of unspecified site of left male breast ♂ ☑
C79.81	Secondary malignant neoplasm of breast
D05.01	Lobular carcinoma in situ of right breast ☑
D05.11	Intraductal carcinoma in situ of right breast ☑
D24.1	Benign neoplasm of right breast ☑
D48.61	Neoplasm of uncertain behavior of right breast ☑

AMA: 19305 2020,May,9; 2018,Jan,8; 2017,Jan,8; 2016,Jan,13; 2015,Jan,16

Breast

Relative Value Units/Medicare Edits

Non-Facility RVU	Work	PE	MP	Total
19305	17.46	12.2	4.18	33.84
Facility RVU	Work	PE	MP	Total
19305	17.46	12.2	4.18	33.84

	FUD	Status	MUE	Modifiers				IOM Reference
19305	90	A	1(2)	51	50	62*	80	None

* with documentation

Terms To Know

electrocautery. Division or cutting of tissue using high-frequency electrical current to produce heat, which destroys cells.

ligation. Tying off a blood vessel or duct with a suture or a soft, thin wire.

malignant neoplasm. Any cancerous tumor or lesion exhibiting uncontrolled tissue growth that can progressively invade other parts of the body with its disease-generating cells.

myocutaneous flap. Skin, subcutaneous tissue, and intact muscle tissue that are transferred to a recipient site while retaining sufficient blood supply from its own vascular bed.

pectoralis major. Chest muscle connecting at the clavicle, upper ribs, sternum, and the axilla.

radical mastectomy. Surgical removal of breast, lymph nodes of the axilla, some muscles of the chest wall, and sometimes the internal mammary nodes.

19306

19306   Mastectomy, radical, including pectoral muscles, axillary and internal mammary lymph nodes (Urban type operation)

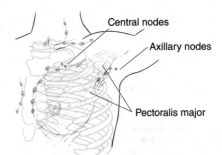

A radical mastectomy is performed, including removal of the pectoralis major and the underlying pectoralis minor muscles and lymph nodes

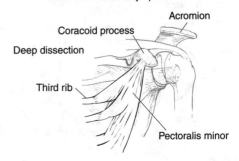

Explanation

The physician performs a radical Urban-type mastectomy. The physician makes an elliptical incision that includes the nipple and the tail of Spence, the extension of mammary tissue into the axillary region. The breast tissue, skin, and pectoral muscles are removed. All tissue within the parameters of the sternum, the rectus fascia, the latissimus dorsi muscle, and the clavicle are removed, including the axillary and internal mammary lymph nodes. Bleeding vessels are ligated or electrocauterized. In large-breasted patients, adequate skin may be available for primary closure. Patients with insufficient skin for coverage may require skin grafts or myocutaneous flaps. If no prosthesis is to be inserted, a closed wound suction catheter may be inserted. The wound is closed and a pressure dressing is applied.

Coding Tips

This is a unilateral procedure. If performed bilaterally, some payers require that the service be reported twice with modifier 50 appended to the second code while others require identification of the service only once with modifier 50 appended. Check with individual payers. Modifier 50 identifies a procedure performed identically on the opposite side of the body (mirror image). Lymph node dissection is included in this code and should not be reported separately. Any breast reconstruction should be reported separately. For immediate or delayed insertion of an implant, see 19340–19342. Placement of intraoperative clips should not be reported separately.

ICD-10-CM Diagnostic Codes

C50.011	Malignant neoplasm of nipple and areola, right female breast ♀ ☑
C50.012	Malignant neoplasm of nipple and areola, left female breast ♀ ☑
C50.021	Malignant neoplasm of nipple and areola, right male breast ♂ ☑
C50.022	Malignant neoplasm of nipple and areola, left male breast ♂ ☑
C50.111	Malignant neoplasm of central portion of right female breast ♀ ☑

C50.112	Malignant neoplasm of central portion of left female breast ♀ ☑
C50.121	Malignant neoplasm of central portion of right male breast ♂ ☑
C50.122	Malignant neoplasm of central portion of left male breast ♂ ☑
C50.211	Malignant neoplasm of upper-inner quadrant of right female breast ♀ ☑
C50.221	Malignant neoplasm of upper-inner quadrant of right male breast ♂ ☑
C50.222	Malignant neoplasm of upper-inner quadrant of left male breast ♂ ☑
C50.311	Malignant neoplasm of lower-inner quadrant of right female breast ♀ ☑
C50.312	Malignant neoplasm of lower-inner quadrant of left female breast ♀ ☑
C50.321	Malignant neoplasm of lower-inner quadrant of right male breast ♂ ☑
C50.411	Malignant neoplasm of upper-outer quadrant of right female breast ♀ ☑
C50.412	Malignant neoplasm of upper-outer quadrant of left female breast ♀ ☑
C50.421	Malignant neoplasm of upper-outer quadrant of right male breast ♂ ☑
C50.511	Malignant neoplasm of lower-outer quadrant of right female breast ♀ ☑
C50.512	Malignant neoplasm of lower-outer quadrant of left female breast ♀ ☑
C50.521	Malignant neoplasm of lower-outer quadrant of right male breast ♂ ☑
C50.522	Malignant neoplasm of lower-outer quadrant of left male breast ♂ ☑
C50.611	Malignant neoplasm of axillary tail of right female breast ♀ ☑
C50.612	Malignant neoplasm of axillary tail of left female breast ♀ ☑
C50.621	Malignant neoplasm of axillary tail of right male breast ♂ ☑
C50.622	Malignant neoplasm of axillary tail of left male breast ♂ ☑
C50.811	Malignant neoplasm of overlapping sites of right female breast ♀ ☑
C50.812	Malignant neoplasm of overlapping sites of left female breast ♀ ☑
C50.821	Malignant neoplasm of overlapping sites of right male breast ♂ ☑
C50.822	Malignant neoplasm of overlapping sites of left male breast ♂ ☑

AMA: **19306** 2020,May,9; 2018,Jan,8; 2017,Jan,8; 2016,Jan,13; 2015,Jan,16

Relative Value Units/Medicare Edits

Non-Facility RVU	Work	PE	MP	Total
19306	18.13	13.48	4.43	36.04
Facility RVU	**Work**	**PE**	**MP**	**Total**
19306	18.13	13.48	4.43	36.04

	FUD	Status	MUE	Modifiers				IOM Reference
19306	90	A	1(2)	51	50	62*	80	None

* with documentation

19307

| 19307 | Mastectomy, modified radical, including axillary lymph nodes, with or without pectoralis minor muscle, but excluding pectoralis major muscle |

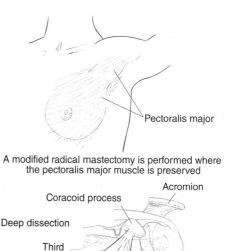

A modified radical mastectomy is performed where the pectoralis major muscle is preserved

Explanation

The physician performs a modified radical mastectomy. The physician makes an elliptical incision that includes the nipple and the tail of Spence, the extension of mammary tissue into the axillary region. The breast tissue and skin are dissected from the pectoral fascia and removed from the pectoral muscle. The pectoralis minor muscle may also be resected to facilitate the axillary dissection, but the pectoralis major muscle is left intact. Bleeding vessels are ligated or electrocauterized. The breast tissue and axillary tissue, including lymph nodes, are removed en bloc and the wound is irrigated. Adequate skin is usually available for primary closure. Patients with insufficient skin for coverage may require skin grafts or myocutaneous flaps. If no implant is to be inserted, a closed wound suction catheter may be inserted. The wound is closed and a pressure dressing is applied.

Coding Tips

This is a unilateral procedure. If performed bilaterally, some payers require that the service be reported twice with modifier 50 appended to the second code while others require identification of the service only once with modifier 50 appended. Check with individual payers. Modifier 50 identifies a procedure performed identically on the opposite side of the body (mirror image). Lymph node dissection is included in this code and should not be reported separately. Any breast reconstruction should be reported separately. For immediate or delayed insertion of an implant, see 19340–19342. Placement of intraoperative clips should not be reported separately.

ICD-10-CM Diagnostic Codes

C50.011	Malignant neoplasm of nipple and areola, right female breast ♀ ☑
C50.021	Malignant neoplasm of nipple and areola, right male breast ♂ ☑
C50.111	Malignant neoplasm of central portion of right female breast ♀ ☑
C50.121	Malignant neoplasm of central portion of right male breast ♂ ☑

Breast

● New   ▲ Revised   + Add On   ★ Telemedicine   AMA: CPT Assist   [Resequenced]   ☑ Laterality   © 2021 Optum360, LLC

Coding Companion for General Surgery/Gastroenterology   **141**

C50.211	Malignant neoplasm of upper-inner quadrant of right female breast ♀ ☑
C50.221	Malignant neoplasm of upper-inner quadrant of right male breast ♂ ☑
C50.311	Malignant neoplasm of lower-inner quadrant of right female breast ♀ ☑
C50.321	Malignant neoplasm of lower-inner quadrant of right male breast ♂ ☑
C50.411	Malignant neoplasm of upper-outer quadrant of right female breast ♀ ☑
C50.421	Malignant neoplasm of upper-outer quadrant of right male breast ♂ ☑
C50.511	Malignant neoplasm of lower-outer quadrant of right female breast ♀ ☑
C50.521	Malignant neoplasm of lower-outer quadrant of right male breast ♂ ☑
C50.611	Malignant neoplasm of axillary tail of right female breast ♀ ☑
C50.621	Malignant neoplasm of axillary tail of right male breast ♂ ☑
C50.811	Malignant neoplasm of overlapping sites of right female breast ♀ ☑
C50.821	Malignant neoplasm of overlapping sites of right male breast ♂ ☑
C79.81	Secondary malignant neoplasm of breast
D05.01	Lobular carcinoma in situ of right breast ☑
D05.11	Intraductal carcinoma in situ of right breast ☑
D05.81	Other specified type of carcinoma in situ of right breast ☑

AMA: 19307 2020,May,9; 2019,Feb,8; 2018,Jan,8; 2017,Jan,8; 2016,Jan,13; 2015,Mar,5; 2015,Jan,16

Relative Value Units/Medicare Edits

Non-Facility RVU	Work	PE	MP	Total
19307	17.99	12.69	4.33	35.01
Facility RVU	Work	PE	MP	Total
19307	17.99	12.69	4.33	35.01

	FUD	Status	MUE	Modifiers				IOM Reference
19307	90	A	1(2)	51	50	62*	80	None

* with documentation

Terms To Know

dissection. Separating by cutting tissue or body structures apart.

electrocautery. Division or cutting of tissue using high-frequency electrical current to produce heat, which destroys cells.

ligation. Tying off a blood vessel or duct with a suture or a soft, thin wire.

myocutaneous flap. Skin, subcutaneous tissue, and intact muscle tissue that are transferred to a recipient site while retaining sufficient blood supply from its own vascular bed.

Breast

20100-20103

20100	Exploration of penetrating wound (separate procedure); neck
20101	chest
20102	abdomen/flank/back
20103	extremity

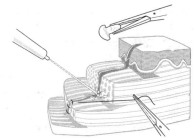

A penetrating wound is explored. The depth of the wound is assessed and the tissues debrided of fragments

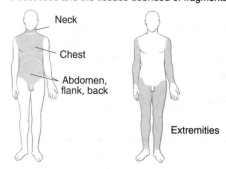

Neck

Chest

Abdomen, flank, back

Extremities

Explanation

The physician explores a penetrating wound in the operating room, such as a gunshot or stab wound, to help identify damaged structures. Nerve, organ, and blood vessel integrity is assessed. The wound may be enlarged to help assess the damage. Debridement, removal of foreign bodies, and ligation or coagulation of minor blood vessels in the subcutaneous tissues, fascia, and muscle are also included in this range of codes. Damaged tissues are debrided and repaired when possible. The wound is closed (if clean) or packed open if contaminated by the penetrating body. Report 20100 for exploration of a neck wound. Report 20101 for exploration of a chest wound. Report 20102 for exploration of an abdomen, flank, or back wound. Report 20103 for exploration of a wound to an extremity.

Coding Tips

This separate procedure by definition is usually a component of a more complex service and is not identified separately. When performed alone or with other unrelated procedures/services it may be reported. If performed alone, list the code; if performed with other procedures/services, list the code and append modifier 59 or an X{EPSU} modifier. This code identifies surgical exploration and enlargement of the defect, dissection, debridement, any foreign body removal, and cauterization of smaller blood vessels. If any extensive repairs are performed on structures, organs, muscles, major blood vessels, subcutaneous tissue, of the neck, they should be reported with the appropriate repair code.

ICD-10-CM Diagnostic Codes

S11.011A	Laceration without foreign body of larynx, initial encounter
S11.013A	Puncture wound without foreign body of larynx, initial encounter
S11.022A	Laceration with foreign body of trachea, initial encounter
S11.025A	Open bite of trachea, initial encounter

S11.14XA	Puncture wound with foreign body of thyroid gland, initial encounter
S11.15XA	Open bite of thyroid gland, initial encounter
S11.21XA	Laceration without foreign body of pharynx and cervical esophagus, initial encounter
S16.2XXA	Laceration of muscle, fascia and tendon at neck level, initial encounter
S21.122A	Laceration with foreign body of left front wall of thorax without penetration into thoracic cavity, initial encounter
S21.152A	Open bite of left front wall of thorax without penetration into thoracic cavity, initial encounter
S21.231A	Puncture wound without foreign body of right back wall of thorax without penetration into thoracic cavity, initial encounter
S21.241A	Puncture wound with foreign body of right back wall of thorax without penetration into thoracic cavity, initial encounter
S29.021A	Laceration of muscle and tendon of front wall of thorax, initial encounter
S31.010A	Laceration without foreign body of lower back and pelvis without penetration into retroperitoneum, initial encounter
S31.040A	Puncture wound with foreign body of lower back and pelvis without penetration into retroperitoneum, initial encounter
S31.110A	Laceration without foreign body of abdominal wall, right upper quadrant without penetration into peritoneal cavity, initial encounter ☑
S31.113A	Laceration without foreign body of abdominal wall, right lower quadrant without penetration into peritoneal cavity, initial encounter ☑
S31.115A	Laceration without foreign body of abdominal wall, periumbilic region without penetration into peritoneal cavity, initial encounter
S31.133A	Puncture wound of abdominal wall without foreign body, right lower quadrant without penetration into peritoneal cavity, initial encounter ☑
S31.142A	Puncture wound of abdominal wall with foreign body, epigastric region without penetration into peritoneal cavity, initial encounter
S31.150A	Open bite of abdominal wall, right upper quadrant without penetration into peritoneal cavity, initial encounter ☑
S31.153A	Open bite of abdominal wall, right lower quadrant without penetration into peritoneal cavity, initial encounter ☑
S31.812A	Laceration with foreign body of right buttock, initial encounter ☑
S39.021A	Laceration of muscle, fascia and tendon of abdomen, initial encounter
S39.022A	Laceration of muscle, fascia and tendon of lower back, initial encounter
S39.023A	Laceration of muscle, fascia and tendon of pelvis, initial encounter
S41.011A	Laceration without foreign body of right shoulder, initial encounter ☑
S41.021A	Laceration with foreign body of right shoulder, initial encounter ☑
S41.031A	Puncture wound without foreign body of right shoulder, initial encounter ☑
S41.041A	Puncture wound with foreign body of right shoulder, initial encounter ☑
S41.051A	Open bite of right shoulder, initial encounter ☑
S41.121A	Laceration with foreign body of right upper arm, initial encounter ☑

S41.141A	Puncture wound with foreign body of right upper arm, initial encounter ☑
S51.021A	Laceration with foreign body of right elbow, initial encounter ☑
S51.031A	Puncture wound without foreign body of right elbow, initial encounter ☑
S51.051A	Open bite, right elbow, initial encounter ☑
S51.821A	Laceration with foreign body of right forearm, initial encounter ☑
S51.831A	Puncture wound without foreign body of right forearm, initial encounter ☑
S56.495A	Other injury of extensor muscle, fascia and tendon of right ring finger at forearm level, initial encounter ☑
S61.011A	Laceration without foreign body of right thumb without damage to nail, initial encounter ☑
S61.051A	Open bite of right thumb without damage to nail, initial encounter ☑
S61.214A	Laceration without foreign body of right ring finger without damage to nail, initial encounter ☑
S61.220A	Laceration with foreign body of right index finger without damage to nail, initial encounter ☑
S61.232A	Puncture wound without foreign body of right middle finger without damage to nail, initial encounter ☑
S61.310A	Laceration without foreign body of right index finger with damage to nail, initial encounter ☑
S61.316A	Laceration without foreign body of right little finger with damage to nail, initial encounter ☑
S61.332A	Puncture wound without foreign body of right middle finger with damage to nail, initial encounter ☑
S61.342A	Puncture wound with foreign body of right middle finger with damage to nail, initial encounter ☑
S61.411A	Laceration without foreign body of right hand, initial encounter ☑
S61.431A	Puncture wound without foreign body of right hand, initial encounter ☑
S61.441A	Puncture wound with foreign body of right hand, initial encounter ☑
S61.451A	Open bite of right hand, initial encounter ☑
S61.521A	Laceration with foreign body of right wrist, initial encounter ☑
S61.551A	Open bite of right wrist, initial encounter ☑
S66.091A	Other specified injury of long flexor muscle, fascia and tendon of right thumb at wrist and hand level, initial encounter ☑
S66.291A	Other specified injury of extensor muscle, fascia and tendon of right thumb at wrist and hand level, initial encounter ☑
S71.111A	Laceration without foreign body, right thigh, initial encounter ☑
S71.121A	Laceration with foreign body, right thigh, initial encounter ☑
S71.141A	Puncture wound with foreign body, right thigh, initial encounter ☑
S81.011A	Laceration without foreign body, right knee, initial encounter ☑
S81.041A	Puncture wound with foreign body, right knee, initial encounter ☑
S81.051A	Open bite, right knee, initial encounter ☑
S81.821A	Laceration with foreign body, right lower leg, initial encounter ☑
S81.832A	Puncture wound without foreign body, left lower leg, initial encounter ☑
S86.191A	Other injury of other muscle(s) and tendon(s) of posterior muscle group at lower leg level, right leg, initial encounter ☑
S91.011A	Laceration without foreign body, right ankle, initial encounter ☑
S91.051A	Open bite, right ankle, initial encounter ☑
S91.124A	Laceration with foreign body of right lesser toe(s) without damage to nail, initial encounter ☑
S91.134A	Puncture wound without foreign body of right lesser toe(s) without damage to nail, initial encounter ☑
S91.151A	Open bite of right great toe without damage to nail, initial encounter ☑
S91.155A	Open bite of left lesser toe(s) without damage to nail, initial encounter ☑
S91.221A	Laceration with foreign body of right great toe with damage to nail, initial encounter ☑
S91.321A	Laceration with foreign body, right foot, initial encounter ☑
S91.341A	Puncture wound with foreign body, right foot, initial encounter ☑
S91.351A	Open bite, right foot, initial encounter ☑
S96.091A	Other injury of muscle and tendon of long flexor muscle of toe at ankle and foot level, right foot, initial encounter ☑

AMA: **20100** 2018,Jan,8; 2017,Jan,8; 2016,Jan,13; 2015,Jan,16 **20101** 2018,Jan,8; 2017,Jan,8; 2016,Jan,13; 2015,Jan,16 **20102** 2020,Jan,6; 2018,Jan,8; 2017,Jan,8; 2016,Jan,13; 2015,Jan,16 **20103** 2018,Jan,8; 2017,Jan,8; 2016,Jan,13; 2015,Jan,16

Relative Value Units/Medicare Edits

Non-Facility RVU	Work	PE	MP	Total
20100	10.38	5.3	2.04	17.72
20101	3.23	13.98	0.78	17.99
20102	3.98	13.79	0.9	18.67
20103	5.34	10.85	0.96	17.15
Facility RVU	Work	PE	MP	Total
20100	10.38	5.3	2.04	17.72
20101	3.23	2.2	0.78	6.21
20102	3.98	2.64	0.9	7.52
20103	5.34	3.85	0.96	10.15

	FUD	Status	MUE	Modifiers				IOM Reference
20100	10	A	2(3)	51	50	N/A	80	None
20101	10	A	2(3)	51	N/A	N/A	N/A	
20102	10	A	3(3)	51	N/A	N/A	N/A	
20103	10	A	3(3)	51	N/A	N/A	80*	

* with documentation

20200-20206

20200 Biopsy, muscle; superficial
20205   deep
20206 Biopsy, muscle, percutaneous needle

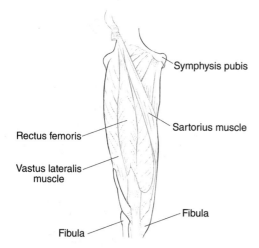

Symphysis pubis

Rectus femoris

Sartorius muscle

Vastus lateralis muscle

Fibula

Fibula

A biopsy sample is taken from muscle tissue

Explanation

The physician secures a sample of tissue from a muscle for biopsy. The physician incises the overlying skin and bluntly dissects to the suspect muscle. The muscle tissue is obtained. Bleeding is controlled and the wound is sutured in layers. Report 20200 if the muscle site sampled is superficial and 20205 if the muscle site sampled is deep. Report 20206 if the muscle biopsy is obtained using a bore needle to pierce the skin, fascia, and muscle in a percutaneous type procedure.

Coding Tips

An excisional biopsy is not reported separately when a therapeutic excision is performed during the same surgical session. Other biopsies should be reported by the appropriate anatomic site. Imaging guidance is reported with 76942, 77002, 77012, or 77021, when performed. For a biopsy using fine needle aspiration, see 10004-10012 and 10021. Surgical trays, A4550, are not separately reimbursed by Medicare; however, other third-party payers may cover them. Check with the specific payer to determine coverage.

ICD-10-CM Diagnostic Codes

C49.0	Malignant neoplasm of connective and soft tissue of head, face and neck
C49.11	Malignant neoplasm of connective and soft tissue of right upper limb, including shoulder ☑
C49.21	Malignant neoplasm of connective and soft tissue of right lower limb, including hip ☑
C49.3	Malignant neoplasm of connective and soft tissue of thorax
C49.4	Malignant neoplasm of connective and soft tissue of abdomen
C49.5	Malignant neoplasm of connective and soft tissue of pelvis
C49.8	Malignant neoplasm of overlapping sites of connective and soft tissue
C79.89	Secondary malignant neoplasm of other specified sites
C7A.098	Malignant carcinoid tumors of other sites
C96.5	Multifocal and unisystemic Langerhans-cell histiocytosis
C96.6	Unifocal Langerhans-cell histiocytosis
D19.7	Benign neoplasm of mesothelial tissue of other sites
D21.0	Benign neoplasm of connective and other soft tissue of head, face and neck
D21.11	Benign neoplasm of connective and other soft tissue of right upper limb, including shoulder ☑
D21.12	Benign neoplasm of connective and other soft tissue of left upper limb, including shoulder ☑
D21.21	Benign neoplasm of connective and other soft tissue of right lower limb, including hip ☑
D21.3	Benign neoplasm of connective and other soft tissue of thorax
D21.4	Benign neoplasm of connective and other soft tissue of abdomen
D21.5	Benign neoplasm of connective and other soft tissue of pelvis
D36.7	Benign neoplasm of other specified sites
D3A.098	Benign carcinoid tumors of other sites
D48.1	Neoplasm of uncertain behavior of connective and other soft tissue
D49.2	Neoplasm of unspecified behavior of bone, soft tissue, and skin
D86.3	Sarcoidosis of skin
D86.87	Sarcoid myositis
E71.39	Other disorders of fatty-acid metabolism
E71.41	Primary carnitine deficiency
E71.42	Carnitine deficiency due to inborn errors of metabolism
E71.43	Iatrogenic carnitine deficiency
E71.440	Ruvalcaba-Myhre-Smith syndrome
E71.448	Other secondary carnitine deficiency
E74.09	Other glycogen storage disease
E80.3	Defects of catalase and peroxidase
G71.01	Duchenne or Becker muscular dystrophy
G71.02	Facioscapulohumeral muscular dystrophy
G71.09	Other specified muscular dystrophies
G71.21	Nemaline myopathy
G71.220	X-linked myotubular myopathy
G71.228	Other centronuclear myopathy
G71.8	Other primary disorders of muscles
G72.49	Other inflammatory and immune myopathies, not elsewhere classified
G72.81	Critical illness myopathy
M05.412	Rheumatoid myopathy with rheumatoid arthritis of left shoulder ☑
M05.422	Rheumatoid myopathy with rheumatoid arthritis of left elbow ☑
M05.431	Rheumatoid myopathy with rheumatoid arthritis of right wrist ☑
M05.442	Rheumatoid myopathy with rheumatoid arthritis of left hand ☑
M05.451	Rheumatoid myopathy with rheumatoid arthritis of right hip ☑
M05.462	Rheumatoid myopathy with rheumatoid arthritis of left knee ☑
M05.471	Rheumatoid myopathy with rheumatoid arthritis of right ankle and foot ☑
M33.22	Polymyositis with myopathy
M35.03	Sjögren syndrome with myopathy
M60.011	Infective myositis, right shoulder ☑
M60.021	Infective myositis, right upper arm ☑
M60.031	Infective myositis, right forearm ☑
M60.042	Infective myositis, left hand ☑
M60.044	Infective myositis, right finger(s) ☑
M60.052	Infective myositis, left thigh ☑
M60.061	Infective myositis, right lower leg ☑

M60.071	Infective myositis, left ankle ☑	
M60.074	Infective myositis, left foot ☑	
M60.076	Infective myositis, right toe(s) ☑	
M60.111	Interstitial myositis, right shoulder ☑	
M60.132	Interstitial myositis, left forearm ☑	
M60.171	Interstitial myositis, right ankle and foot ☑	

M61.311   Calcification and ossification of muscles associated with burns, right shoulder ☑

M61.322   Calcification and ossification of muscles associated with burns, left upper arm ☑

M61.332   Calcification and ossification of muscles associated with burns, left forearm ☑

M61.342   Calcification and ossification of muscles associated with burns, left hand ☑

M61.351   Calcification and ossification of muscles associated with burns, right thigh ☑

M61.361   Calcification and ossification of muscles associated with burns, right lower leg ☑

M61.371   Calcification and ossification of muscles associated with burns, right ankle and foot ☑

M62.82   Rhabdomyolysis

M79.11   Myalgia of mastication muscle

M79.12   Myalgia of auxiliary muscles, head and neck

M79.18   Myalgia, other site

M79.7   Fibromyalgia

AMA: 20200 2020,Nov,1 **20206** 2019,Apr,4

Relative Value Units/Medicare Edits

Non-Facility RVU	Work	PE	MP	Total
20200	1.46	4.89	0.34	6.69
20205	2.35	6.27	0.62	9.24
20206	0.99	6.04	0.09	7.12
Facility RVU	Work	PE	MP	Total
20200	1.46	0.96	0.34	2.76
20205	2.35	1.57	0.62	4.54
20206	0.99	0.58	0.09	1.66

	FUD	Status	MUE	Modifiers				IOM Reference
20200	0	A	2(3)	51	N/A	N/A	N/A	100-04,13,80.1;
20205	0	A	3(3)	51	N/A	N/A	N/A	100-04,13,80.2
20206	0	A	3(3)	51	N/A	N/A	N/A	

* with documentation

20520-20525

20520   Removal of foreign body in muscle or tendon sheath; simple
20525   deep or complicated

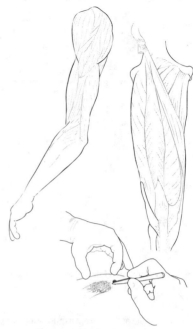

Removal of a foreign body from
muscle or tendon sheath

Explanation

The physician removes a foreign body in a muscle or tendon sheath. The physician incises the skin and dissects to the muscle or sheath. The foreign body is isolated by palpation or radiographic imagery (separately reported) and removed. The incision may be closed if clean or packed if contaminated by the object. Report 20520 if the removal is simple; report 20525 if the foreign object lies deep or requires a complicated procedure to remove it.

Coding Tips

For removal of a foreign body from the skin and subcutaneous tissues, see 10120–10121. For removal of a foreign body from soft tissues, or other sites, see the specific anatomical section.

ICD-10-CM Diagnostic Codes

M60.211   Foreign body granuloma of soft tissue, not elsewhere classified, right shoulder ☑

M60.222   Foreign body granuloma of soft tissue, not elsewhere classified, left upper arm ☑

M60.231   Foreign body granuloma of soft tissue, not elsewhere classified, right forearm ☑

M60.241   Foreign body granuloma of soft tissue, not elsewhere classified, right hand ☑

M60.242   Foreign body granuloma of soft tissue, not elsewhere classified, left hand ☑

M60.252   Foreign body granuloma of soft tissue, not elsewhere classified, left thigh ☑

M60.261   Foreign body granuloma of soft tissue, not elsewhere classified, right lower leg ☑

M60.272   Foreign body granuloma of soft tissue, not elsewhere classified, left ankle and foot ☑

M79.5	Residual foreign body in soft tissue
S01.421A	Laceration with foreign body of right cheek and temporomandibular area, initial encounter ☑
S01.441A	Puncture wound with foreign body of right cheek and temporomandibular area, initial encounter ☑
S01.521A	Laceration with foreign body of lip, initial encounter
S01.541A	Puncture wound with foreign body of lip, initial encounter
S21.121A	Laceration with foreign body of right front wall of thorax without penetration into thoracic cavity, initial encounter
S21.122A	Laceration with foreign body of left front wall of thorax without penetration into thoracic cavity, initial encounter
S21.141A	Puncture wound with foreign body of right front wall of thorax without penetration into thoracic cavity, initial encounter
S21.142A	Puncture wound with foreign body of left front wall of thorax without penetration into thoracic cavity, initial encounter
S21.242A	Puncture wound with foreign body of left back wall of thorax without penetration into thoracic cavity, initial encounter
S31.020A	Laceration with foreign body of lower back and pelvis without penetration into retroperitoneum, initial encounter
S31.040A	Puncture wound with foreign body of lower back and pelvis without penetration into retroperitoneum, initial encounter
S31.120A	Laceration of abdominal wall with foreign body, right upper quadrant without penetration into peritoneal cavity, initial encounter ☑
S31.121A	Laceration of abdominal wall with foreign body, left upper quadrant without penetration into peritoneal cavity, initial encounter ☑
S31.125A	Laceration of abdominal wall with foreign body, periumbilic region without penetration into peritoneal cavity, initial encounter
S31.143A	Puncture wound of abdominal wall with foreign body, right lower quadrant without penetration into peritoneal cavity, initial encounter ☑
S41.021A	Laceration with foreign body of right shoulder, initial encounter ☑
S41.122A	Laceration with foreign body of left upper arm, initial encounter ☑
S41.141A	Puncture wound with foreign body of right upper arm, initial encounter ☑
S51.022A	Laceration with foreign body of left elbow, initial encounter ☑
S51.821A	Laceration with foreign body of right forearm, initial encounter ☑
S51.842A	Puncture wound with foreign body of left forearm, initial encounter ☑
S61.021A	Laceration with foreign body of right thumb without damage to nail, initial encounter ☑
S61.041A	Puncture wound with foreign body of right thumb without damage to nail, initial encounter ☑
S61.042A	Puncture wound with foreign body of left thumb without damage to nail, initial encounter ☑
S61.121A	Laceration with foreign body of right thumb with damage to nail, initial encounter ☑
S61.142A	Puncture wound with foreign body of left thumb with damage to nail, initial encounter ☑
S61.220A	Laceration with foreign body of right index finger without damage to nail, initial encounter ☑
S61.223A	Laceration with foreign body of left middle finger without damage to nail, initial encounter ☑
S61.224A	Laceration with foreign body of right ring finger without damage to nail, initial encounter ☑
S61.226A	Laceration with foreign body of right little finger without damage to nail, initial encounter ☑
S61.227A	Laceration with foreign body of left little finger without damage to nail, initial encounter ☑
S61.242A	Puncture wound with foreign body of right middle finger without damage to nail, initial encounter ☑
S61.243A	Puncture wound with foreign body of left middle finger without damage to nail, initial encounter ☑
S61.247A	Puncture wound with foreign body of left little finger without damage to nail, initial encounter ☑
S61.321A	Laceration with foreign body of left index finger with damage to nail, initial encounter ☑
S61.322A	Laceration with foreign body of right middle finger with damage to nail, initial encounter ☑
S61.324A	Laceration with foreign body of right ring finger with damage to nail, initial encounter ☑
S61.326A	Laceration with foreign body of right little finger with damage to nail, initial encounter ☑
S61.341A	Puncture wound with foreign body of left index finger with damage to nail, initial encounter ☑
S61.342A	Puncture wound with foreign body of right middle finger with damage to nail, initial encounter ☑
S61.347A	Puncture wound with foreign body of left little finger with damage to nail, initial encounter ☑
S61.422A	Laceration with foreign body of left hand, initial encounter ☑
S61.441A	Puncture wound with foreign body of right hand, initial encounter ☑
S61.521A	Laceration with foreign body of right wrist, initial encounter ☑
S61.541A	Puncture wound with foreign body of right wrist, initial encounter ☑
S61.542A	Puncture wound with foreign body of left wrist, initial encounter ☑
S71.021A	Laceration with foreign body, right hip, initial encounter ☑
S71.042A	Puncture wound with foreign body, left hip, initial encounter ☑
S71.121A	Laceration with foreign body, right thigh, initial encounter ☑
S71.141A	Puncture wound with foreign body, right thigh, initial encounter ☑
S81.021A	Laceration with foreign body, right knee, initial encounter ☑
S81.022A	Laceration with foreign body, left knee, initial encounter ☑
S81.042A	Puncture wound with foreign body, left knee, initial encounter ☑
S81.821A	Laceration with foreign body, right lower leg, initial encounter ☑
S81.822A	Laceration with foreign body, left lower leg, initial encounter ☑
S81.842A	Puncture wound with foreign body, left lower leg, initial encounter ☑
S91.021A	Laceration with foreign body, right ankle, initial encounter ☑
S91.041A	Puncture wound with foreign body, right ankle, initial encounter ☑
S91.122A	Laceration with foreign body of left great toe without damage to nail, initial encounter ☑
S91.124A	Laceration with foreign body of right lesser toe(s) without damage to nail, initial encounter ☑
S91.141A	Puncture wound with foreign body of right great toe without damage to nail, initial encounter ☑

General Musculoskeletal

S91.144A	Puncture wound with foreign body of right lesser toe(s) without damage to nail, initial encounter ☑					
S91.145A	Puncture wound with foreign body of left lesser toe(s) without damage to nail, initial encounter ☑					
S91.222A	Laceration with foreign body of left great toe with damage to nail, initial encounter ☑					
S91.224A	Laceration with foreign body of right lesser toe(s) with damage to nail, initial encounter ☑					
S91.242A	Puncture wound with foreign body of left great toe with damage to nail, initial encounter ☑					
S91.244A	Puncture wound with foreign body of right lesser toe(s) with damage to nail, initial encounter ☑					
S91.321A	Laceration with foreign body, right foot, initial encounter ☑					
S91.322A	Laceration with foreign body, left foot, initial encounter ☑					
S91.342A	Puncture wound with foreign body, left foot, initial encounter ☑					

Relative Value Units/Medicare Edits

Non-Facility RVU	Work	PE	MP	Total
20520	1.9	4.24	0.27	6.41
20525	3.54	10.08	0.63	14.25
Facility RVU	Work	PE	MP	Total
20520	1.9	2.15	0.27	4.32
20525	3.54	3.09	0.63	7.26

	FUD	Status	MUE	Modifiers				IOM Reference
20520	10	A	2(3)	51	N/A	N/A	N/A	None
20525	10	A	4(3)	51	N/A	N/A	N/A	

* with documentation

Terms To Know

foreign body. Any object or substance found in an organ and tissue that does not belong under normal circumstances.

incise. To cut open or into.

palpate. Examination by feeling with the hand.

sheath. Covering enclosing an organ or part.

20550-20551

20550	Injection(s); single tendon sheath, or ligament, aponeurosis (eg, plantar "fascia")
20551	single tendon origin/insertion

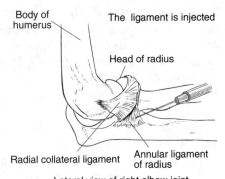

Body of humerus
The ligament is injected
Head of radius
Radial collateral ligament
Annular ligament of radius
Lateral view of right elbow joint

Explanation

The physician injects a therapeutic agent into a single tendon sheath, or ligament, aponeurosis such as the plantar fascia in 20550 and into a single tendon origin/insertion site in 20551. The physician identifies the injection site by palpation or radiographs (reported separately) and marks the injection site. The needle is inserted and the medicine is injected. After withdrawing the needle, the patient is monitored for reactions to the therapeutic agent.

Coding Tips

For injection of a therapeutic agent into single or multiple trigger points of one or two muscles, see 20552; three or more muscles, see 20553. If imaging guidance is performed, see 76942, 77002, and 77021. For aspiration or injection of a ganglion cyst, see 20612. Injection of Morton's neuroma is reported with 64455 or 64632. For platelet rich plasma injections, see Category III code 0232T. Do not report 20550–20551 with 0232T or 0481T. For injection of autologous adipose-derived regenerative cells, see 0489T-0490T.

ICD-10-CM Diagnostic Codes

D86.86	Sarcoid arthropathy
G89.0	Central pain syndrome
G89.11	Acute pain due to trauma
G89.12	Acute post-thoracotomy pain
G89.21	Chronic pain due to trauma
G89.22	Chronic post-thoracotomy pain
G89.28	Other chronic postprocedural pain
G89.29	Other chronic pain
G89.4	Chronic pain syndrome
M25.512	Pain in left shoulder ☑
M25.521	Pain in right elbow ☑
M25.532	Pain in left wrist ☑
M25.561	Pain in right knee ☑
M25.571	Pain in right ankle and joints of right foot ☑
M65.011	Abscess of tendon sheath, right shoulder ☑
M65.042	Abscess of tendon sheath, left hand ☑
M65.051	Abscess of tendon sheath, right thigh ☑
M65.062	Abscess of tendon sheath, left lower leg ☑
M65.071	Abscess of tendon sheath, right ankle and foot ☑
M65.111	Other infective (teno)synovitis, right shoulder ☑

M65.122	Other infective (teno)synovitis, left elbow ☑	
M65.221	Calcific tendinitis, right upper arm ☑	
M65.241	Calcific tendinitis, right hand ☑	
M65.261	Calcific tendinitis, right lower leg ☑	
M65.272	Calcific tendinitis, left ankle and foot ☑	
M65.311	Trigger thumb, right thumb ☑	
M65.331	Trigger finger, right middle finger ☑	
M65.341	Trigger finger, right ring finger ☑	
M65.811	Other synovitis and tenosynovitis, right shoulder ☑	
M65.852	Other synovitis and tenosynovitis, left thigh ☑	
M65.862	Other synovitis and tenosynovitis, left lower leg ☑	
M65.871	Other synovitis and tenosynovitis, right ankle and foot ☑	
M66.232	Spontaneous rupture of extensor tendons, left forearm ☑	
M66.241	Spontaneous rupture of extensor tendons, right hand ☑	
M66.261	Spontaneous rupture of extensor tendons, right lower leg ☑	
M66.312	Spontaneous rupture of flexor tendons, left shoulder ☑	
M66.332	Spontaneous rupture of flexor tendons, left forearm ☑	
M66.341	Spontaneous rupture of flexor tendons, right hand ☑	
M66.831	Spontaneous rupture of other tendons, right forearm ☑	
M66.841	Spontaneous rupture of other tendons, right hand ☑	
M66.852	Spontaneous rupture of other tendons, left thigh ☑	
M66.861	Spontaneous rupture of other tendons, right lower leg ☑	
M66.872	Spontaneous rupture of other tendons, left ankle and foot ☑	
M67.311	Transient synovitis, right shoulder ☑	
M67.341	Transient synovitis, right hand ☑	
M67.352	Transient synovitis, left hip ☑	
M67.361	Transient synovitis, right knee ☑	
M67.372	Transient synovitis, left ankle and foot ☑	
M70.031	Crepitant synovitis (acute) (chronic), right wrist ☑	
M70.041	Crepitant synovitis (acute) (chronic), right hand ☑	
M70.12	Bursitis, left hand ☑	
M70.22	Olecranon bursitis, left elbow ☑	
M70.31	Other bursitis of elbow, right elbow ☑	
M70.41	Prepatellar bursitis, right knee ☑	
M70.51	Other bursitis of knee, right knee ☑	
M71.121	Other infective bursitis, right elbow ☑	
M71.132	Other infective bursitis, left wrist ☑	
M71.161	Other infective bursitis, right knee ☑	
M72.2	Plantar fascial fibromatosis	
M75.21	Bicipital tendinitis, right shoulder ☑	
M75.31	Calcific tendinitis of right shoulder ☑	
M75.32	Calcific tendinitis of left shoulder ☑	
M75.42	Impingement syndrome of left shoulder ☑	
M75.51	Bursitis of right shoulder ☑	
M75.52	Bursitis of left shoulder ☑	
M76.02	Gluteal tendinitis, left hip ☑	
M76.11	Psoas tendinitis, right hip ☑	
M76.41	Tibial collateral bursitis [Pellegrini-Stieda], right leg ☑	
M76.52	Patellar tendinitis, left knee ☑	
M76.62	Achilles tendinitis, left leg ☑	
M76.71	Peroneal tendinitis, right leg ☑	
M76.822	Posterior tibial tendinitis, left leg ☑	
M77.12	Lateral epicondylitis, left elbow ☑	

M79.601	Pain in right arm ☑	
M79.621	Pain in right upper arm ☑	
M79.631	Pain in right forearm ☑	
M79.642	Pain in left hand ☑	
M79.662	Pain in left lower leg ☑	
M79.671	Pain in right foot ☑	
M79.675	Pain in left toe(s) ☑	

AMA: **20550** 2018,Jan,8; 2017,Jan,8; 2016,Jan,13; 2015,Jan,16 **20551** 2018,Jan,8; 2017,Jan,8; 2017,Dec,13; 2016,Jan,13; 2015,Jan,16

Relative Value Units/Medicare Edits

Non-Facility RVU	Work	PE	MP	Total
20550	0.75	0.8	0.09	1.64
20551	0.75	0.84	0.09	1.68
Facility RVU	Work	PE	MP	Total
20550	0.75	0.3	0.09	1.14
20551	0.75	0.31	0.09	1.15

	FUD	Status	MUE	Modifiers				IOM Reference
20550	0	A	5(3)	51	50	N/A	N/A	100-03,150.7;
20551	0	A	5(3)	51	N/A	N/A	N/A	100-04,13,80.1; 100-04,13,80.2

* with documentation

Terms To Know

aponeurosis. Flat expansion of white, ribbon-like tendinous tissue that functions as the connection of a muscle to its moving part.

fascia. Fibrous sheet or band of tissue that envelops organs, muscles, and groupings of muscles.

ligament. Band or sheet of fibrous tissue that connects the articular surfaces of bones or supports visceral organs.

sheath. Covering enclosing an organ or part.

tendon. Fibrous tissue that connects muscle to bone, consisting primarily of collagen and containing little vasculature.

[20560, 20561]

20560 Needle insertion(s) without injection(s); 1 or 2 muscle(s)
20561 Needle insertion(s) without injection(s); 3 or more muscles

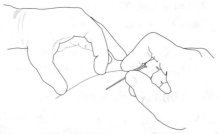

A needle is placed into the muscle

Explanation

The physician inserts a dry solid filament needle through the skin and into one or two muscles in 20560 and into three or more muscles in 20561. Indicated for myofascial pain relief and movement impairments, trigger points (focal, discrete spots of hypersensitive irritability identified within bands of muscle) are often the target of insertion. These points cause local or referred pain and may be formed by acute or repetitive trauma to the muscle tissue. This procedure, also known as dry needling or trigger-point acupuncture, does not involve the administration of injectable therapeutic agents.

Coding Tips

For trigger point injections, see 20550-20553. Do not report 20560 or 20561 with 20552-20553 for the same muscles.

ICD-10-CM Diagnostic Codes

G54.6	Phantom limb syndrome with pain
G89.0	Central pain syndrome
G89.21	Chronic pain due to trauma
G89.22	Chronic post-thoracotomy pain
G89.28	Other chronic postprocedural pain
G89.29	Other chronic pain
G89.4	Chronic pain syndrome
M54.51	Vertebrogenic low back pain
M65.4	Radial styloid tenosynovitis [de Quervain]
M65.811	Other synovitis and tenosynovitis, right shoulder ☑
M65.821	Other synovitis and tenosynovitis, right upper arm ☑
M65.831	Other synovitis and tenosynovitis, right forearm ☑
M65.851	Other synovitis and tenosynovitis, right thigh ☑
M65.861	Other synovitis and tenosynovitis, right lower leg ☑
M65.871	Other synovitis and tenosynovitis, right ankle and foot ☑
M70.811	Other soft tissue disorders related to use, overuse and pressure, right shoulder ☑
M70.821	Other soft tissue disorders related to use, overuse and pressure, right upper arm ☑
M70.831	Other soft tissue disorders related to use, overuse and pressure, right forearm ☑
M70.841	Other soft tissue disorders related to use, overuse and pressure, right hand ☑
M70.851	Other soft tissue disorders related to use, overuse and pressure, right thigh ☑
M70.861	Other soft tissue disorders related to use, overuse and pressure, right lower leg ☑
M70.871	Other soft tissue disorders related to use, overuse and pressure, right ankle and foot ☑
M79.601	Pain in right arm ☑
M79.604	Pain in right leg ☑
M79.631	Pain in right forearm ☑
M79.641	Pain in right hand ☑
M79.651	Pain in right thigh ☑
M79.661	Pain in right lower leg ☑
M79.671	Pain in right foot ☑
M79.7	Fibromyalgia

AMA: **20560** 2020,Feb,9 **20561** 2020,Feb,9

Relative Value Units/Medicare Edits

Non-Facility RVU	Work	PE	MP	Total
20560	0.32	0.41	0.04	0.77
20561	0.48	0.59	0.04	1.11
Facility RVU	**Work**	**PE**	**MP**	**Total**
20560	0.32	0.12	0.04	0.48
20561	0.48	0.19	0.04	0.71

	FUD	Status	MUE	Modifiers				IOM Reference
20560	N/A	A	1(2)	N/A	N/A	N/A	N/A	None
20561	N/A	A	1(2)	N/A	N/A	N/A	N/A	

* with documentation

Terms To Know

dry needling. Skilled intervention that uses a thin filiform needle to penetrate the skin and stimulate underlying myofascial trigger points, such as muscular and connective tissues, for the management of neuromusculoskeletal pain and movement impairments. Distinct from acupuncture, dry needling is based on western neuroanatomy and modern scientific study of the musculoskeletal and nervous systems.

trigger point. Focal, discrete spot of hypersensitivity identified within bands of muscle that causes local or referred pain. Trigger points may be formed by acute or repetitive trauma to the muscle tissue, which puts too much stress on the fibers.

20555

20555 Placement of needles or catheters into muscle and/or soft tissue for subsequent interstitial radioelement application (at the time of or subsequent to the procedure)

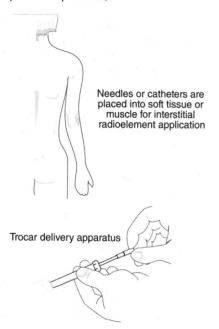

Needles or catheters are placed into soft tissue or muscle for interstitial radioelement application

Trocar delivery apparatus

Explanation

Interstitial radioelement application is a form of brachytherapy (treatment involving the placement of radioactive isotopes for internal radiation) in which the applicators are placed directly within the tissues of the body. The physician places needles or catheters into muscle and/or soft tissue close to the tumor bed for subsequent interstitial radioelement application to treat such tumors as soft tissue sarcoma. If the tumor bed is close to bone or neurovascular structures, materials such as gel-foam may be inserted between the catheters and the critical structures. Catheters may be secured to muscle with absorbable sutures. The radioactive isotopes, such as iridium-192, may be introduced directly after the needle or catheter insertion or on a subsequent visit. The isotopes are contained within tiny seeds (sources) that are left in place to deliver radiation over a period of weeks or months. They do not cause any harm after becoming inert. This method provides radiation to the prescribed body area while minimizing exposure to normal tissue.

Coding Tips

For device placement into the breast for interstitial radioelement application, see 19296–19298. For needle, catheter, or device placement into muscle or soft tissue of the head and neck for interstitial radioelement application, see 41019. For needle or catheter placement for interstitial radioelement application into pelvic organs or genitalia, see 55920. Interstitial radioelement application is reported with 77770-77772 or 77778. For imaging guidance, see 76942, 77002, 77012, or 77021.

ICD-10-CM Diagnostic Codes

C15.3	Malignant neoplasm of upper third of esophagus
C15.4	Malignant neoplasm of middle third of esophagus
C15.5	Malignant neoplasm of lower third of esophagus
C15.8	Malignant neoplasm of overlapping sites of esophagus
C18.8	Malignant neoplasm of overlapping sites of colon
C19	Malignant neoplasm of rectosigmoid junction
C20	Malignant neoplasm of rectum
C22.0	Liver cell carcinoma
C23	Malignant neoplasm of gallbladder
C26.1	Malignant neoplasm of spleen
C40.01	Malignant neoplasm of scapula and long bones of right upper limb ☑
C40.11	Malignant neoplasm of short bones of right upper limb ☑
C40.21	Malignant neoplasm of long bones of right lower limb ☑
C40.31	Malignant neoplasm of short bones of right lower limb ☑
C41.0	Malignant neoplasm of bones of skull and face
C41.1	Malignant neoplasm of mandible
C41.2	Malignant neoplasm of vertebral column
C41.3	Malignant neoplasm of ribs, sternum and clavicle
C41.4	Malignant neoplasm of pelvic bones, sacrum and coccyx
C43.0	Malignant melanoma of lip
C43.21	Malignant melanoma of right ear and external auricular canal ☑
C43.31	Malignant melanoma of nose
C43.4	Malignant melanoma of scalp and neck
C43.51	Malignant melanoma of anal skin
C43.61	Malignant melanoma of right upper limb, including shoulder ☑
C43.71	Malignant melanoma of right lower limb, including hip ☑
C45.0	Mesothelioma of pleura
C45.1	Mesothelioma of peritoneum
C45.2	Mesothelioma of pericardium
C47.0	Malignant neoplasm of peripheral nerves of head, face and neck
C47.11	Malignant neoplasm of peripheral nerves of right upper limb, including shoulder ☑
C47.12	Malignant neoplasm of peripheral nerves of left upper limb, including shoulder ☑
C47.21	Malignant neoplasm of peripheral nerves of right lower limb, including hip ☑
C47.22	Malignant neoplasm of peripheral nerves of left lower limb, including hip ☑
C47.3	Malignant neoplasm of peripheral nerves of thorax
C47.4	Malignant neoplasm of peripheral nerves of abdomen
C47.5	Malignant neoplasm of peripheral nerves of pelvis
C48.0	Malignant neoplasm of retroperitoneum
C48.1	Malignant neoplasm of specified parts of peritoneum
C49.0	Malignant neoplasm of connective and soft tissue of head, face and neck
C49.11	Malignant neoplasm of connective and soft tissue of right upper limb, including shoulder ☑
C49.21	Malignant neoplasm of connective and soft tissue of right lower limb, including hip ☑
C49.3	Malignant neoplasm of connective and soft tissue of thorax
C49.4	Malignant neoplasm of connective and soft tissue of abdomen
C49.5	Malignant neoplasm of connective and soft tissue of pelvis
C49.8	Malignant neoplasm of overlapping sites of connective and soft tissue
C49.A1	Gastrointestinal stromal tumor of esophagus
C49.A2	Gastrointestinal stromal tumor of stomach
C49.A3	Gastrointestinal stromal tumor of small intestine
C49.A4	Gastrointestinal stromal tumor of large intestine
C49.A5	Gastrointestinal stromal tumor of rectum

C49.A9	Gastrointestinal stromal tumor of other sites
C73	Malignant neoplasm of thyroid gland
C74.01	Malignant neoplasm of cortex of right adrenal gland ☑
C74.02	Malignant neoplasm of cortex of left adrenal gland ☑
C74.11	Malignant neoplasm of medulla of right adrenal gland ☑
C74.12	Malignant neoplasm of medulla of left adrenal gland ☑
C75.0	Malignant neoplasm of parathyroid gland
C75.1	Malignant neoplasm of pituitary gland
C75.2	Malignant neoplasm of craniopharyngeal duct
C75.3	Malignant neoplasm of pineal gland
C75.4	Malignant neoplasm of carotid body
C75.5	Malignant neoplasm of aortic body and other paraganglia
C75.8	Malignant neoplasm with pluriglandular involvement, unspecified
C76.1	Malignant neoplasm of thorax
C76.2	Malignant neoplasm of abdomen
C76.41	Malignant neoplasm of right upper limb ☑
C76.51	Malignant neoplasm of right lower limb ☑
C79.51	Secondary malignant neoplasm of bone
C79.52	Secondary malignant neoplasm of bone marrow
C79.89	Secondary malignant neoplasm of other specified sites

AMA: 20555 2018,Jan,8; 2017,Jan,8; 2016,Jan,13; 2015,Jan,16

Relative Value Units/Medicare Edits

Non-Facility RVU	Work	PE	MP	Total
20555	6.0	3.12	0.54	9.66
Facility RVU	**Work**	**PE**	**MP**	**Total**
20555	6.0	3.12	0.54	9.66

	FUD	Status	MUE	Modifiers				IOM Reference
20555	0	A	1(3)	51	N/A	N/A	80*	100-04,13,70.4

* with documentation

Terms To Know

absorbable sutures. Strands used for suture or repair of tissue prepared from collagen or a synthetic polymer and capable of being absorbed by tissue over time.

brachytherapy. Form of radiation therapy in which radioactive pellets or seeds are implanted directly into the tissue being treated to deliver their dose of radiation in a more directed fashion. Brachytherapy provides radiation to the prescribed body area while minimizing exposure to normal tissue.

interstitial radiation. Radioactive source placed into the tissue being treated.

isotope. Chemical element possessing the same atomic number (protons in the nucleus) as another, but with a different atomic weight (number of neutrons).

20600-20611

20600	Arthrocentesis, aspiration and/or injection, small joint or bursa (eg, fingers, toes); without ultrasound guidance
20604	with ultrasound guidance, with permanent recording and reporting
20605	Arthrocentesis, aspiration and/or injection, intermediate joint or bursa (eg, temporomandibular, acromioclavicular, wrist, elbow or ankle, olecranon bursa); without ultrasound guidance
20606	with ultrasound guidance, with permanent recording and reporting
20610	Arthrocentesis, aspiration and/or injection, major joint or bursa (eg, shoulder, hip, knee, subacromial bursa); without ultrasound guidance
20611	with ultrasound guidance, with permanent recording and reporting

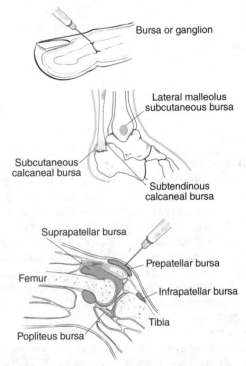

Aspiration/Injection of bursa
Bursa or ganglion
Lateral malleolus subcutaneous bursa
Subcutaneous calcaneal bursa
Subtendinous calcaneal bursa
Suprapatellar bursa
Prepatellar bursa
Femur
Infrapatellar bursa
Tibia
Popliteus bursa

Explanation

After administering a local anesthetic, the physician inserts a needle through the skin and into a joint or bursa. A fluid sample may be removed from the joint for examination or a fluid may be injected for lavage or drug therapy. The needle is withdrawn and pressure is applied to stop any bleeding. Report 20600 for arthrocentesis of a small joint or bursa, such as the fingers or toes, without ultrasound guidance; 20604 for arthrocentesis of a small joint or bursa, with ultrasound guidance, including permanent record and report; 20605 for an intermediate joint or bursa, such as the wrist, elbow, ankle, olecranon bursa, or temporomandibular or acromioclavicular area, without ultrasound guidance; 20606 for intermediate joint or bursa, with ultrasound guidance, including permanent record and report; 20610 for a major joint or bursa injection or aspiration, such as of the shoulder, hip, knee joint, or subacromial bursa, without ultrasound guidance; 20611 for a major joint or bursa, with ultrasound guidance, including permanent record and report.

Coding Tips

Code selection depends on the size of the joint and whether the procedure was performed with or without ultrasonic guidance. If fluoroscopic, CT, or MRI guidance is performed, see 77002, 77012, and 77021. Do not report 20600–20611 with 76942. Do not report 20600 or 20604 with 0489T-0490T. Do not report 20610–20611 with 27369. When more than one procedure is performed on the same joint, do not report separately. For aspiration or injection of a ganglion cyst, any location, see 20612. For injection of autologous, adipose-derived regenerative cells, see 0489T-0490T.

ICD-10-CM Diagnostic Codes

M00.041	Staphylococcal arthritis, right hand ☑
M00.042	Staphylococcal arthritis, left hand ☑
M00.071	Staphylococcal arthritis, right ankle and foot ☑
M00.072	Staphylococcal arthritis, left ankle and foot ☑
M00.141	Pneumococcal arthritis, right hand ☑
M00.142	Pneumococcal arthritis, left hand ☑
M00.171	Pneumococcal arthritis, right ankle and foot ☑
M00.172	Pneumococcal arthritis, left ankle and foot ☑
M00.841	Arthritis due to other bacteria, right hand ☑
M00.842	Arthritis due to other bacteria, left hand ☑
M05.041	Felty's syndrome, right hand ☑
M05.071	Felty's syndrome, right ankle and foot ☑
M05.072	Felty's syndrome, left ankle and foot ☑
M05.241	Rheumatoid vasculitis with rheumatoid arthritis of right hand ☑
M05.271	Rheumatoid vasculitis with rheumatoid arthritis of right ankle and foot ☑
M05.341	Rheumatoid heart disease with rheumatoid arthritis of right hand ☑
M05.342	Rheumatoid heart disease with rheumatoid arthritis of left hand ☑
M05.441	Rheumatoid myopathy with rheumatoid arthritis of right hand ☑
M05.442	Rheumatoid myopathy with rheumatoid arthritis of left hand ☑
M05.471	Rheumatoid myopathy with rheumatoid arthritis of right ankle and foot ☑
M05.641	Rheumatoid arthritis of right hand with involvement of other organs and systems ☑
M05.642	Rheumatoid arthritis of left hand with involvement of other organs and systems ☑
M05.741	Rheumatoid arthritis with rheumatoid factor of right hand without organ or systems involvement ☑
M05.841	Other rheumatoid arthritis with rheumatoid factor of right hand ☑
M05.842	Other rheumatoid arthritis with rheumatoid factor of left hand ☑
M06.241	Rheumatoid bursitis, right hand ☑
M06.242	Rheumatoid bursitis, left hand ☑
M07.641	Enteropathic arthropathies, right hand ☑
M07.642	Enteropathic arthropathies, left hand ☑
M08.241	Juvenile rheumatoid arthritis with systemic onset, right hand ☑
M08.242	Juvenile rheumatoid arthritis with systemic onset, left hand ☑
M08.271	Juvenile rheumatoid arthritis with systemic onset, right ankle and foot ☑
M08.441	Pauciarticular juvenile rheumatoid arthritis, right hand ☑
M08.442	Pauciarticular juvenile rheumatoid arthritis, left hand ☑
M08.841	Other juvenile arthritis, right hand ☑
M08.842	Other juvenile arthritis, left hand ☑
M08.871	Other juvenile arthritis, right ankle and foot ☑
M08.872	Other juvenile arthritis, left ankle and foot ☑
M10.041	Idiopathic gout, right hand ☑
M10.042	Idiopathic gout, left hand ☑
M10.171	Lead-induced gout, right ankle and foot ☑
M10.241	Drug-induced gout, right hand ☑
M10.271	Drug-induced gout, right ankle and foot ☑
M11.041	Hydroxyapatite deposition disease, right hand ☑
M11.042	Hydroxyapatite deposition disease, left hand ☑
M11.141	Familial chondrocalcinosis, right hand ☑
M11.142	Familial chondrocalcinosis, left hand ☑
M12.541	Traumatic arthropathy, right hand ☑
M12.542	Traumatic arthropathy, left hand ☑
M13.141	Monoarthritis, not elsewhere classified, right hand ☑
M13.142	Monoarthritis, not elsewhere classified, left hand ☑
M17.0	Bilateral primary osteoarthritis of knee
M17.11	Unilateral primary osteoarthritis, right knee ☑
M19.041	Primary osteoarthritis, right hand ☑
M19.042	Primary osteoarthritis, left hand ☑
M19.071	Primary osteoarthritis, right ankle and foot ☑
M19.072	Primary osteoarthritis, left ankle and foot ☑
M19.272	Secondary osteoarthritis, left ankle and foot ☑
M1A.0411	Idiopathic chronic gout, right hand, with tophus (tophi) ☑
M1A.0421	Idiopathic chronic gout, left hand, with tophus (tophi) ☑
M1A.0710	Idiopathic chronic gout, right ankle and foot, without tophus (tophi) ☑
M1A.0720	Idiopathic chronic gout, left ankle and foot, without tophus (tophi) ☑
M1A.2410	Drug-induced chronic gout, right hand, without tophus (tophi) ☑
M1A.2411	Drug-induced chronic gout, right hand, with tophus (tophi) ☑
M1A.2711	Drug-induced chronic gout, right ankle and foot, with tophus (tophi) ☑
M1A.3410	Chronic gout due to renal impairment, right hand, without tophus (tophi) ☑
M1A.3710	Chronic gout due to renal impairment, right ankle and foot, without tophus (tophi) ☑
M1A.3711	Chronic gout due to renal impairment, right ankle and foot, with tophus (tophi) ☑
M1A.4410	Other secondary chronic gout, right hand, without tophus (tophi) ☑
M25.041	Hemarthrosis, right hand ☑
M25.042	Hemarthrosis, left hand ☑
M25.074	Hemarthrosis, right foot ☑
M25.075	Hemarthrosis, left foot ☑
M25.474	Effusion, right foot ☑
M25.475	Effusion, left foot ☑
M25.541	Pain in joints of right hand ☑
M25.542	Pain in joints of left hand ☑
M67.341	Transient synovitis, right hand ☑
M67.371	Transient synovitis, right ankle and foot ☑
M67.372	Transient synovitis, left ankle and foot ☑
M70.041	Crepitant synovitis (acute) (chronic), right hand ☑
M71.341	Other bursal cyst, right hand ☑

M71.342	Other bursal cyst, left hand ☑	
M71.371	Other bursal cyst, right ankle and foot ☑	
M71.372	Other bursal cyst, left ankle and foot ☑	
M77.41	Metatarsalgia, right foot ☑	
M77.42	Metatarsalgia, left foot ☑	
M77.51	Other enthesopathy of right foot and ankle ☑	
M79.641	Pain in right hand ☑	
M79.642	Pain in left hand ☑	
M79.644	Pain in right finger(s) ☑	
M79.645	Pain in left finger(s) ☑	
M79.671	Pain in right foot ☑	
M79.672	Pain in left foot ☑	

AMA: 20600 2018,Sep,12; 2018,Jan,8; 2017,Jan,8; 2017,Aug,9; 2016,Jan,13; 2015,Nov,10; 2015,Jan,16; 2015,Feb,6 **20604** 2018,Sep,12; 2018,Jan,8; 2017,Jan,8; 2016,Jan,13; 2015,Jul,10; 2015,Feb,6 **20605** 2018,Jan,8; 2017,Jan,8; 2017,Aug,9; 2016,Jan,13; 2015,Nov,10; 2015,Jan,16; 2015,Feb,6 **20606** 2018,Jan,8; 2017,Jan,8; 2016,Jan,13; 2015,Jul,10; 2015,Feb,6 **20610** 2019,Aug,7; 2018,Jan,8; 2017,Jan,8; 2017,Apr,9; 2016,Jan,13; 2015,Nov,10; 2015,Jan,16; 2015,Feb,6; 2015,Aug,6 **20611** 2019,Aug,7; 2018,Jan,8; 2017,Jan,8; 2016,Jan,13; 2015,Nov,10; 2015,Jul,10; 2015,Feb,6; 2015,Aug,6

Relative Value Units/Medicare Edits

Non-Facility RVU	Work	PE	MP	Total
20600	0.66	0.77	0.09	1.52
20604	0.89	1.38	0.1	2.37
20605	0.68	0.81	0.09	1.58
20606	1.0	1.47	0.13	2.6
20610	0.79	0.96	0.13	1.88
20611	1.1	1.65	0.15	2.9
Facility RVU	**Work**	**PE**	**MP**	**Total**
20600	0.66	0.3	0.09	1.05
20604	0.89	0.36	0.1	1.35
20605	0.68	0.32	0.09	1.09
20606	1.0	0.42	0.13	1.55
20610	0.79	0.42	0.13	1.34
20611	1.1	0.51	0.15	1.76

	FUD	Status	MUE	Modifiers				IOM Reference
20600	0	A	6(3)	51	50	N/A	N/A	100-03,150.7; 100-04,13,80.2
20604	0	A	4(3)	51	50	N/A	N/A	
20605	0	A	2(3)	51	50	N/A	N/A	
20606	0	A	2(3)	51	50	N/A	N/A	
20610	0	A	2(3)	51	50	N/A	N/A	
20611	0	A	2(3)	51	50	N/A	N/A	

* with documentation

20612

20612 Aspiration and/or injection of ganglion cyst(s) any location

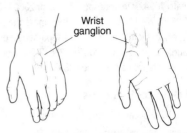

Wrist ganglion

Ganglion cysts can be found in numerous sites, particularly on the hands and feet

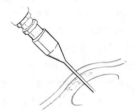

The cyst is aspirated or injected

Explanation

The physician aspirates and/or injects a ganglion cyst. After administering a local anesthetic, the physician inserts a needle through the skin and into the ganglion cyst. A ganglion cyst is a benign mass consisting of a thin capsule containing clear, mucinous fluid arising from an aponeurosis or tendon sheath, such as on the back of the wrist or foot. A fluid sample may be withdrawn from the cyst or a medicinal substance may be injected for therapy. The needle is withdrawn and pressure is applied to stop any bleeding.

Coding Tips

Multiple ganglion cyst aspirations/injections may be reported by appending modifier 59 or an X{EPSU} modifier to this code. For injection of a single tendon sheath or ligament, see 20550. To report arthrocentesis, aspiration and/or injection of a small joint or bursa, see 20600; intermediate joint or bursa, see 20605; major joint or bursa, see 20610. For aspiration and injection of a bone cyst, see 20615. Imaging guidance is reported with 76942, 77002, 77012, or 77021, when performed. Surgical trays, A4550, are not separately reimbursed by Medicare; however, other third-party payers may cover them. Supplies used when providing this procedure may be reported with the appropriate HCPCS Level II "J" code. Check with the specific payer to determine coverage.

ICD-10-CM Diagnostic Codes

M67.411	Ganglion, right shoulder ☑	
M67.412	Ganglion, left shoulder ☑	
M67.421	Ganglion, right elbow ☑	
M67.422	Ganglion, left elbow ☑	
M67.431	Ganglion, right wrist ☑	
M67.432	Ganglion, left wrist ☑	
M67.441	Ganglion, right hand ☑	
M67.442	Ganglion, left hand ☑	
M67.451	Ganglion, right hip ☑	
M67.452	Ganglion, left hip ☑	
M67.461	Ganglion, right knee ☑	
M67.462	Ganglion, left knee ☑	

M67.471	Ganglion, right ankle and foot ☑
M67.472	Ganglion, left ankle and foot ☑
M67.48	Ganglion, other site
M67.49	Ganglion, multiple sites

Relative Value Units/Medicare Edits

Non-Facility RVU	Work	PE	MP	Total
20612	0.7	1.06	0.1	1.86
Facility RVU	**Work**	**PE**	**MP**	**Total**
20612	0.7	0.41	0.1	1.21

	FUD	Status	MUE	Modifiers				IOM Reference
20612	0	A	2(3)	51	N/A	N/A	N/A	None

* with documentation

Terms To Know

anesthesia. Loss of feeling or sensation, usually induced to permit the performance of surgery or other painful procedures.

aponeurosis. Flat expansion of white, ribbon-like tendinous tissue that functions as the connection of a muscle to its moving part.

aspiration. Drawing fluid out by suction.

benign. Mild or nonmalignant in nature.

cyst. Elevated encapsulated mass containing fluid, semisolid, or solid material with a membranous lining.

excision. Surgical removal of an organ or tissue.

ganglion. Fluid-filled, benign cyst appearing on a tendon sheath or aponeurosis, frequently connecting to an underlying joint.

injection. Forcing a liquid substance into a body part such as a joint or muscle.

joint capsule. Sac-like enclosure enveloping the synovial joint cavity with a fibrous membrane attached to the articular ends of the bones in the joint.

synovia. Clear fluid lubricant of joints, bursae, and tendon sheaths, secreted by the synovial membrane.

tendon. Fibrous tissue that connects muscle to bone, consisting primarily of collagen and containing little vasculature.

therapeutic. Act meant to alleviate a medical or mental condition.

20700-20701

+ **20700** Manual preparation and insertion of drug-delivery device(s), deep (eg, subfascial) (List separately in addition to code for primary procedure)

+ **20701** Removal of drug-delivery device(s), deep (eg, subfascial) (List separately in addition to code for primary procedure)

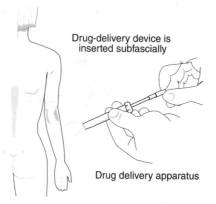

Drug-delivery device is inserted subfascially

Drug delivery apparatus

Explanation

In conjunction with procedures such as arthrotomy, excisional debridement, open bone biopsies/excisions, or incision and drainage of abscesses or hematomas of deep tissues, the physician or other qualified health care professional manually prepares and inserts a drug-delivery device that is not prefabricated into the deep tissues in 20700. Antibiotics or other therapeutic agents are mixed with a carrier substance, shaped into drug-delivery devices such as beads, nails, or spacers, and placed into the subfascial tissues. Device removal, also performed in conjunction with the aforementioned procedures, is reported with 20701.

Coding Tips

Report 20700 and 20701 in addition to 11010-11012, 11043-11047, 20240-20251, 21010, 21025-21026, 21501-21510, 21627, 21630, 22010, 22015, 23030-23044, 23170-23174, 23180-23184, 23334-23335, 23930-23935, 24000, 24134-24140, 24147, 24160, 25031-25040, 25145-25151, 26070, 26230-26236, 26990-26992, 27030, 27070-27071, 27090, 27301-27303, 27310, 27360, 27603-27604, 27610, 27640-27641, 28001-28003, 28020, and 28120-28122. Do not report 20700 with 11981. Do not report 20701 with 11982.

ICD-10-CM Diagnostic Codes

This/these CPT code(s) are add-on code(s). See the primary procedure code that this code is performed with for your ICD-10-CM code selections.

Relative Value Units/Medicare Edits

Non-Facility RVU	Work	PE	MP	Total
20700	1.5	0.68	0.26	2.44
20701	1.13	0.51	0.21	1.85
Facility RVU	**Work**	**PE**	**MP**	**Total**
20700	1.5	0.68	0.26	2.44
20701	1.13	0.51	0.21	1.85

	FUD	Status	MUE	Modifiers				IOM Reference
20700	N/A	A	1(3)	N/A	N/A	N/A	80*	None
20701	N/A	A	1(3)	N/A	N/A	N/A	80*	

* with documentation

21501-21502

21501 Incision and drainage, deep abscess or hematoma, soft tissues of neck or thorax;

21502 with partial rib ostectomy

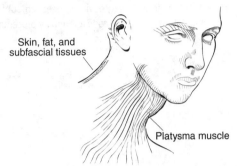

Skin, fat, and subfascial tissues

Platysma muscle

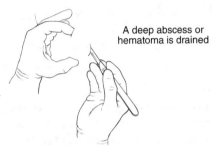

A deep abscess or hematoma is drained

Explanation

The physician performs surgery to remove or drain an abscess or hematoma from the deep soft tissues of the neck or thorax. With proper anesthesia administered, the physician makes an incision overlying the site of the abscess or hematoma of the neck or thorax. Dissection is carried down through the deep subcutaneous tissues and may be continued into the fascia or muscle to expose the abscess or hematoma. The incision may be extended if the mass is larger than expected. The abscess or hematoma is incised and the contents are drained. The area is irrigated and the incision is repaired in layers with sutures, staples, and/or Steri-strips; closed with drains in place; or simply left open to further facilitate drainage of infection. Report 21502 if a partial rib ostectomy is performed during this procedure.

Coding Tips

For posterior spine subfascial incision and drainage, see 22010–22015. If significant additional time and effort are documented, append modifier 22 and submit a cover letter and operative report. For a soft tissue biopsy of the of the neck or thorax, see 21550.

ICD-10-CM Diagnostic Codes

L03.221	Cellulitis of neck
L03.312	Cellulitis of back [any part except buttock]
L03.313	Cellulitis of chest wall
S10.83XA	Contusion of other specified part of neck, initial encounter
S20.211A	Contusion of right front wall of thorax, initial encounter
S20.212A	Contusion of left front wall of thorax, initial encounter
S20.214A	Contusion of middle front wall of thorax, initial encounter
S20.224A	Contusion of middle back wall of thorax, initial encounter
T81.42XA	Infection following a procedure, deep incisional surgical site, initial encounter

AMA: **21501** 2018,Sep,7; 2018,Jan,8; 2017,Jan,8; 2016,Jan,13; 2015,Jan,16
21502 2018,Sep,7

Relative Value Units/Medicare Edits

Non-Facility RVU	Work	PE	MP	Total
21501	3.98	9.62	0.76	14.36
21502	7.55	5.73	1.73	15.01
Facility RVU	**Work**	**PE**	**MP**	**Total**
21501	3.98	4.93	0.76	9.67
21502	7.55	5.73	1.73	15.01

	FUD	Status	MUE	Modifiers				IOM Reference
21501	90	A	3(3)	51	N/A	N/A	N/A	None
21502	90	A	1(3)	51	N/A	N/A	80	

* with documentation

Terms To Know

abscess. Circumscribed collection of pus resulting from bacteria, frequently associated with swelling and other signs of inflammation.

blunt dissection. Surgical technique used to expose an underlying area by separating along natural cleavage lines of tissue, without cutting.

cellulitis. Infection of the skin and subcutaneous tissues, most often caused by Staphylococcus or Streptococcus bacteria secondary to a cutaneous lesion. Progression of the inflammation may lead to abscess and tissue death, or even systemic infection-like bacteremia.

fascia. Fibrous sheet or band of tissue that envelops organs, muscles, and groupings of muscles.

hematoma. Tumor-like collection of blood in some part of the body caused by a break in a blood vessel wall, usually as a result of trauma.

incision and drainage. Cutting open body tissue for the removal of tissue fluids or infected discharge from a wound or cavity.

irrigation. To wash out or cleanse a body cavity, wound, or tissue with water or other fluid.

myotomy. Surgical cutting of a muscle to gain access to underlying tissues or for therapeutic reasons.

seroma. Swelling caused by the collection of serum, or clear fluid, in the tissues.

soft tissue. Nonepithelial tissues outside of the skeleton that includes subcutaneous adipose tissue, fibrous tissue, fascia, muscles, blood and lymph vessels, and peripheral nervous system tissue.

subcutaneous tissue. Sheet or wide band of adipose (fat) and areolar connective tissue in two layers attached to the dermis.

Neck

21550

21550   Biopsy, soft tissue of neck or thorax

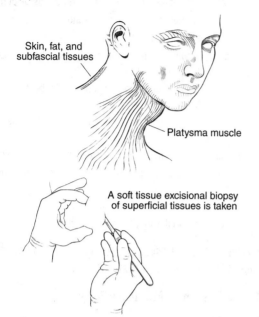

Skin, fat, and
subfascial tissues

Platysma muscle

A soft tissue excisional biopsy
of superficial tissues is taken

Explanation

The physician performs a biopsy of the soft tissues of the neck or thorax. With proper anesthesia administered, the physician identifies the mass through palpation and x-ray (reported separately), if needed. An incision is made over the site and dissection is taken down to the subcutaneous fat or further into the fascia or muscle to reach the lesion. A portion of the tissue mass is excised and submitted for pathology. The area is irrigated and the incision is closed with layered sutures.

Coding Tips

A biopsy is not reported separately when followed by an excisional removal during the same operative session. When 21550 is performed with another separately identifiable procedure, the highest dollar value code is listed as the primary procedure, and subsequent procedures are appended with modifier 51. For a needle biopsy of muscle, see 20206. Surgical trays, A4550, are not separately reimbursed by Medicare; however, other third-party payers may cover them. Check with the specific payer to determine coverage.

ICD-10-CM Diagnostic Codes

C49.0	Malignant neoplasm of connective and soft tissue of head, face and neck
C49.3	Malignant neoplasm of connective and soft tissue of thorax
C76.0	Malignant neoplasm of head, face and neck
C76.1	Malignant neoplasm of thorax
C79.89	Secondary malignant neoplasm of other specified sites
D09.8	Carcinoma in situ of other specified sites
D21.0	Benign neoplasm of connective and other soft tissue of head, face and neck
D21.3	Benign neoplasm of connective and other soft tissue of thorax
D49.89	Neoplasm of unspecified behavior of other specified sites
L03.221	Cellulitis of neck
L03.313	Cellulitis of chest wall
R22.1	Localized swelling, mass and lump, neck
R22.2	Localized swelling, mass and lump, trunk

AMA: 21550 2018,Sep,7

Relative Value Units/Medicare Edits

Non-Facility RVU	Work	PE	MP	Total
21550	2.11	5.63	0.27	8.01
Facility RVU	**Work**	**PE**	**MP**	**Total**
21550	2.11	2.17	0.27	4.55

	FUD	Status	MUE	Modifiers				IOM Reference
21550	10	A	2(3)	51	N/A	N/A	N/A	None

* with documentation

Terms To Know

benign. Mild or nonmalignant in nature.

biopsy. Tissue or fluid removed for diagnostic purposes through analysis of the cells in the biopsy material.

carcinoma in situ. Malignancy that arises from the cells of the vessel, gland, or organ of origin that remains confined to that site or has not invaded neighboring tissue.

malignant. Any condition tending to progress toward death, specifically an invasive tumor with a loss of cellular differentiation that has the ability to spread or metastasize to other body areas.

neoplasm. New abnormal growth, tumor.

secondary. Second in order of occurrence or importance, or appearing during the course of another disease or condition.

soft tissue. Nonepithelial tissues outside of the skeleton that includes subcutaneous adipose tissue, fibrous tissue, fascia, muscles, blood and lymph vessels, and peripheral nervous system tissue.

subcutaneous tissue. Sheet or wide band of adipose (fat) and areolar connective tissue in two layers attached to the dermis.

suture. Numerous stitching techniques employed in wound closure.

buried suture. Continuous or interrupted suture placed under the skin for a layered closure.

continuous suture. Running stitch with tension evenly distributed across a single strand to provide a leakproof closure line.

interrupted suture. Series of single stitches with tension isolated at each stitch, in which all stitches are not affected if one becomes loose, and the isolated sutures cannot act as a wick to transport an infection.

purse-string suture. Continuous suture placed around a tubular structure and tightened, to reduce or close the lumen.

retention suture. Secondary stitching that bridges the primary suture, providing support for the primary repair; a plastic or rubber bolster may be placed over the primary repair and under the retention sutures.

Neck

21555-21556 [21552, 21554]

21555 Excision, tumor, soft tissue of neck or anterior thorax, subcutaneous; less than 3 cm

21552 Excision, tumor, soft tissue of neck or anterior thorax, subcutaneous; 3 cm or greater

21556 Excision, tumor, soft tissue of neck or anterior thorax, subfascial (eg, intramuscular); less than 5 cm

21554 Excision, tumor, soft tissue of neck or anterior thorax, subfascial (eg, intramuscular); 5 cm or greater

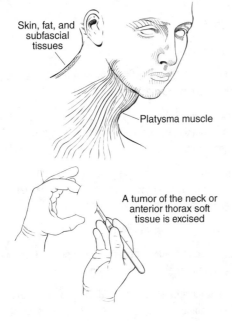

Skin, fat, and subfascial tissues

Platysma muscle

A tumor of the neck or anterior thorax soft tissue is excised

Explanation

The physician removes a tumor from the soft tissue of the neck or anterior thorax (chest) that is located in the subcutaneous tissue in 21552 or 21555 and in the deep soft tissue, below the fascial plane or within the muscle, in 21554 or 21556. With the proper anesthesia administered, the physician makes an incision in the skin overlying the mass and dissects down to the tumor. The extent of the tumor is identified and a dissection is undertaken all the way around the tumor. A portion of neighboring soft tissue may also be removed to ensure adequate removal of all tumor tissue. A drain may be inserted and the incision is repaired with layers of sutures, staples, or Steri-strips. Report 21555 for excision of subcutaneous tumors whose resected area is less than 3 cm and 21552 for excision of subcutaneous tumors 3 cm or greater. Report 21556 for excision of subfascial or intramuscular tumors whose resected area is less than 5 cm and 21554 for excision of subfascial or intramuscular tumors 5 cm or greater.

Coding Tips

When any of these procedures are performed with another separately identifiable procedure, the highest dollar value code is listed as the primary procedure and subsequent procedures are appended with modifier 51. An excisional biopsy is not reported separately when a therapeutic excision is performed during the same surgical session. Report any free grafts or flaps separately. For excision of cutaneous, benign lesions, see 11420–11426. Surgical trays, A4550, are not separately reimbursed by Medicare; however, other third-party payers may cover them. Check with the specific payer to determine coverage.

ICD-10-CM Diagnostic Codes

C49.0	Malignant neoplasm of connective and soft tissue of head, face and neck
C49.3	Malignant neoplasm of connective and soft tissue of thorax
C76.0	Malignant neoplasm of head, face and neck
C76.1	Malignant neoplasm of thorax
D17.0	Benign lipomatous neoplasm of skin and subcutaneous tissue of head, face and neck
D17.1	Benign lipomatous neoplasm of skin and subcutaneous tissue of trunk
D21.0	Benign neoplasm of connective and other soft tissue of head, face and neck
D21.3	Benign neoplasm of connective and other soft tissue of thorax
D48.1	Neoplasm of uncertain behavior of connective and other soft tissue
R22.1	Localized swelling, mass and lump, neck
R22.2	Localized swelling, mass and lump, trunk

AMA: **21552** 2018,Sep,7 **21554** 2018,Sep,7 **21555** 2018,Sep,7; 2018,Jan,8; 2017,Jan,8; 2016,Jan,13; 2015,Jan,16 **21556** 2018,Sep,7

Relative Value Units/Medicare Edits

Non-Facility RVU	Work	PE	MP	Total
21555	3.96	8.19	0.77	12.92
21552	6.49	5.24	1.45	13.18
21556	7.66	6.48	1.45	15.59
21554	11.13	8.06	2.31	21.5
Facility RVU	**Work**	**PE**	**MP**	**Total**
21555	3.96	4.26	0.77	8.99
21552	6.49	5.24	1.45	13.18
21556	7.66	6.48	1.45	15.59
21554	11.13	8.06	2.31	21.5

	FUD	Status	MUE	Modifiers				IOM Reference
21555	90	A	2(3)	51	N/A	N/A	N/A	None
21552	90	A	2(3)	51	N/A	N/A	80	
21556	90	A	2(3)	51	N/A	N/A	N/A	
21554	90	A	2(3)	51	N/A	N/A	80	

* with documentation

Terms To Know

soft tissue. Nonepithelial tissues outside of the skeleton that includes subcutaneous adipose tissue, fibrous tissue, fascia, muscles, blood and lymph vessels, and peripheral nervous system tissue.

subcutaneous tissue. Sheet or wide band of adipose (fat) and areolar connective tissue in two layers attached to the dermis.

subfascial. Beneath the band of fibrous tissue that lies deep to the skin, encloses muscles, and separates their layers.

21557-21558

21557 Radical resection of tumor (eg, sarcoma), soft tissue of neck or anterior thorax; less than 5 cm

21558 5 cm or greater

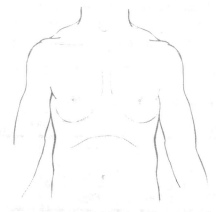

Radical resection of soft tissue
tumor of the neck or anterior thorax

Explanation

The physician performs a radical resection of a malignant soft tissue tumor (i.e., sarcoma) from the neck or anterior thorax, not involving bone. An incision is made over the tumor and dissection exposes it. The tumor and any adjacent tissue that may be affected by the spread of the neoplasm are excised. Large resections may be needed. The type and stage of the lesion determines the extent of the tumor margin resection area. Muscle or fascia may need to be repaired and drains may be placed. The surgical wound may be closed using simple or intermediate repair or separately reportable complex closure, adjacent tissue transfer, or graft. Report 21557 for excision of tumors whose resected area is less than 5 cm and 21558 for excision of tumors 5 cm or greater.

Coding Tips

An excisional biopsy is not reported separately when a therapeutic excision is performed during the same surgical session. Report any free grafts or flaps separately. For radical resection of cutaneous tumors, see 11600–11620.

ICD-10-CM Diagnostic Codes

C49.0	Malignant neoplasm of connective and soft tissue of head, face and neck
C49.3	Malignant neoplasm of connective and soft tissue of thorax
C76.0	Malignant neoplasm of head, face and neck
C76.1	Malignant neoplasm of thorax

AMA: 21557 2020,Apr,10; 2018,Sep,7; 2018,Jan,8; 2017,Jan,8; 2016,Jan,13; 2015,Jan,16 **21558** 2020,Apr,10; 2018,Sep,7

Relative Value Units/Medicare Edits

Non-Facility RVU	Work	PE	MP	Total
21557	14.75	10.39	2.91	28.05
21558	21.58	13.42	4.51	39.51
Facility RVU	**Work**	**PE**	**MP**	**Total**
21557	14.75	10.39	2.91	28.05
21558	21.58	13.42	4.51	39.51

	FUD	Status	MUE	Modifiers				IOM Reference
21557	90	A	1(3)	51	N/A	62*	80	None
21558	90	A	1(3)	51	N/A	62*	80	

* with documentation

Terms To Know

adjacent tissue transfer. Rotation or advancement of skin from an adjacent area to repair or fill in a defect while maintaining attachment to original blood supply.

dissection. Separating by cutting tissue or body structures apart.

excision. Surgical removal of an organ or tissue.

radical resection. Removal of an entire tumor (e.g., malignant neoplasm) along with a large area of surrounding tissue, including adjacent lymph nodes that may have been infiltrated.

soft tissue. Nonepithelial tissues outside of the skeleton.

subcutaneous tissue. Sheet or wide band of adipose (fat) and areolar connective tissue in two layers attached to the dermis.

subfascial. Beneath the band of fibrous tissue that lies deep to the skin, encloses muscles, and separates their layers.

21601-21603

21601 Excision of chest wall tumor including rib(s)
21602 Excision of chest wall tumor involving rib(s), with plastic reconstruction; without mediastinal lymphadenectomy
21603 with mediastinal lymphadenectomy

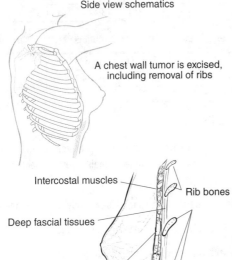

Side view schematics

A chest wall tumor is excised, including removal of ribs

Intercostal muscles

Rib bones

Deep fascial tissues

Pectoralis major muscle

Explanation

The physician excises a chest wall tumor, including ribs. An incision in the skin of the chest overlying the site of the tumor is made. The tumor and surrounding tissue are excised. The tissue removed includes at least one adjacent rib above or below the tumor site and any associated intercostal muscles. It may also include rib cage resection and/or an en bloc resection of muscles, including the pectoralis minor or major, the serratus anterior, or the latissimus dorsi. The physician ligates or cauterizes bleeding vessels. A chest tube may be placed to re-expand the lung. The incision is repaired with layered closure and a pressure dressing is applied to the wound. In 21602, the physician excises a chest wall tumor, involving ribs, with plastic reconstruction. The tumor and surrounding tissue are excised and includes at least one adjacent rib above and below the tumor site and all intervening intercostal muscles. It may also include an en bloc resection of muscles, including the pectoralis minor or major, the serratus anterior, or the latissimus dorsi. In 21603, lymphatic tissue lying within the mediastinum is also removed. The physician ligates or cauterizes bleeding vessels. A chest tube may be placed to re-expand the lung. Plastic reconstruction is done and may involve rib grafts and/or a myocutaneous flap. A pressure dressing is applied to the wound.

Coding Tips

For a tumor of the neck or thorax not involving the ribs, see 21555–21557. An excisional biopsy is not reported separately when a therapeutic excision is performed during the same surgical session. Do not report 21601–21603 with 32100, 32503-32504, 32551, or 32554-32555.

ICD-10-CM Diagnostic Codes

C41.3	Malignant neoplasm of ribs, sternum and clavicle
C49.3	Malignant neoplasm of connective and soft tissue of thorax
C76.1	Malignant neoplasm of thorax
D09.8	Carcinoma in situ of other specified sites
D16.7	Benign neoplasm of ribs, sternum and clavicle
D21.3	Benign neoplasm of connective and other soft tissue of thorax
D36.0	Benign neoplasm of lymph nodes
D48.0	Neoplasm of uncertain behavior of bone and articular cartilage
D48.1	Neoplasm of uncertain behavior of connective and other soft tissue
D48.7	Neoplasm of uncertain behavior of other specified sites
D49.2	Neoplasm of unspecified behavior of bone, soft tissue, and skin
D49.89	Neoplasm of unspecified behavior of other specified sites

AMA: **21601** 2019,Dec,4 **21602** 2019,Dec,4 **21603** 2019,Dec,4

Relative Value Units/Medicare Edits

Non-Facility RVU	Work	PE	MP	Total
21601	17.78	12.6	4.15	34.53
21602	22.19	19.28	5.08	46.55
21603	25.17	19.79	5.78	50.74
Facility RVU	Work	PE	MP	Total
21601	17.78	12.6	4.15	34.53
21602	22.19	19.28	5.08	46.55
21603	25.17	19.79	5.78	50.74

	FUD	Status	MUE	Modifiers				IOM Reference
21601	90	A	2(3)	51	N/A	62*	80	None
21602	90	A	1(3)	51	N/A	62*	80	
21603	90	A	1(3)	51	N/A	62*	80	

* with documentation

21920-21925

21920   Biopsy, soft tissue of back or flank; superficial
21925   deep

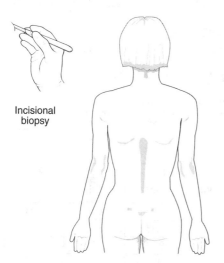

Incisional biopsy

The soft tissue of the back or flank is biopsied through an open incision

Explanation

The physician performs a biopsy of the soft tissues of the back or flank. The patient is positioned lying on the side or prone. With proper anesthesia administered, an incision is made over the biopsy area. Dissection is carried down within the superficial soft tissue layers in 21920, usually the subcutaneous fat to the uppermost fascial layer. In 21925, dissection is taken down deep within the soft tissue, such as into the fascial layer or within the muscle. A portion of the tissue is excised and submitted for pathology. The area is irrigated and the incision is closed with layered sutures, staples, or Steri-strips.

Coding Tips

An excisional biopsy is not reported separately when a therapeutic excision is performed during the same surgical session. For a soft tissue tumor excision of the back or flank, subcutaneous, less than 3 cm, see 21930; greater than 3 cm, see 21931; subfascial, less than 5 cm, see 21932; greater than 5 cm, see 21933. For radical resection of a soft tissue tumor of the back or flank, less than 5 cm, see 21935; 5 cm or greater, see 21936. Surgical trays, A4550, are not separately reimbursed by Medicare; however, other third-party payers may cover them. Check with the specific payer to determine coverage.

ICD-10-CM Diagnostic Codes

C43.59	Malignant melanoma of other part of trunk
C4A.59	Merkel cell carcinoma of other part of trunk
C76.8	Malignant neoplasm of other specified ill-defined sites
D03.59	Melanoma in situ of other part of trunk
D04.5	Carcinoma in situ of skin of trunk
D17.1	Benign lipomatous neoplasm of skin and subcutaneous tissue of trunk
D49.2	Neoplasm of unspecified behavior of bone, soft tissue, and skin
D49.89	Neoplasm of unspecified behavior of other specified sites
L03.312	Cellulitis of back [any part except buttock]
R22.2	Localized swelling, mass and lump, trunk

AMA: 21920 2018,Sep,7 **21925** 2018,Sep,7

Relative Value Units/Medicare Edits

Non-Facility RVU	Work	PE	MP	Total
21920	2.11	5.4	0.28	7.79
21925	4.63	8.73	0.99	14.35
Facility RVU	Work	PE	MP	Total
21920	2.11	2.17	0.28	4.56
21925	4.63	5.24	0.99	10.86

	FUD	Status	MUE	Modifiers				IOM Reference
21920	10	A	2(3)	51	N/A	N/A	N/A	None
21925	90	A	2(3)	51	N/A	N/A	N/A	

* with documentation

Terms To Know

benign. Mild or nonmalignant in nature.

biopsy. Tissue or fluid removed for diagnostic purposes through analysis of the cells in the biopsy material.

cyst. Elevated encapsulated mass containing fluid, semisolid, or solid material with a membranous lining.

fascia. Fibrous sheet or band of tissue that envelops organs, muscles, and groupings of muscles.

lipoma. Benign tumor containing fat cells and the most common of soft tissue lesions, which are usually painless and asymptomatic, with the exception of an angiolipoma.

malignant. Any condition tending to progress toward death, specifically an invasive tumor with a loss of cellular differentiation that has the ability to spread or metastasize to other body areas.

skin. Outer protective covering of the body composed of the epidermis and dermis, situated above the subcutaneous tissues.

soft tissue. Nonepithelial tissues outside of the skeleton.

suture. Numerous stitching techniques employed in wound closure.

buried suture. Continuous or interrupted suture placed under the skin for a layered closure.

continuous suture. Running stitch with tension evenly distributed across a single strand to provide a leakproof closure line.

interrupted suture. Series of single stitches with tension isolated at each stitch, in which all stitches are not affected if one becomes loose, and the isolated sutures cannot act as a wick to transport an infection.

purse-string suture. Continuous suture placed around a tubular structure and tightened, to reduce or close the lumen.

retention suture. Secondary stitching that bridges the primary suture, providing support for the primary repair; a plastic or rubber bolster may be placed over the primary repair and under the retention sutures.

21930-21933

21930 Excision, tumor, soft tissue of back or flank, subcutaneous; less than 3 cm
21931   3 cm or greater
21932 Excision, tumor, soft tissue of back or flank, subfascial (eg, intramuscular); less than 5 cm
21933   5 cm or greater

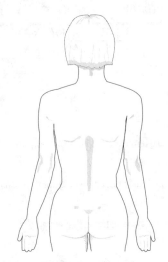

Excision of a soft tissue tumor of the back or flank

Explanation

The physician removes a tumor from the soft tissue of the back or flank that is located in the subcutaneous tissue in 21930–21931 and in the deep soft tissue, below the fascial plane or within the muscle, in 21932–21933. The patient is positioned lying on the side or prone. With the proper anesthesia administered, the physician makes an incision in the skin overlying the mass and dissects down to the tumor. The extent of the tumor is identified and a dissection is undertaken all the way around the tumor. A portion of neighboring soft tissue may also be removed to ensure adequate removal of all tumor tissue. A drain may be inserted and the incision is repaired with layers of sutures, staples, or Steri-strips. Report 21930 for excision of subcutaneous tumors whose resected area is less than 3 cm and 21931 for excision of subcutaneous tumors 3 cm or greater. Report 21932 for excision of subfascial or intramuscular tumors whose resected area is less than 5 cm and 21933 for excision of subfascial or intramuscular tumors 5 cm or greater.

Coding Tips

When any of these procedures are performed with another separately identifiable procedure, the highest dollar value code is listed as the primary procedure and subsequent procedures are appended with modifier 51. An excisional biopsy is not reported separately when a therapeutic excision is performed during the same surgical session. Report any free grafts or flaps separately. When medically necessary, report moderate (conscious) sedation provided by the performing physician with 99151–99153; another physician, see 99155–99157.

ICD-10-CM Diagnostic Codes

C43.59	Malignant melanoma of other part of trunk
C4A.59	Merkel cell carcinoma of other part of trunk
C76.8	Malignant neoplasm of other specified ill-defined sites
D03.59	Melanoma in situ of other part of trunk
D04.5	Carcinoma in situ of skin of trunk
D17.1	Benign lipomatous neoplasm of skin and subcutaneous tissue of trunk
D49.2	Neoplasm of unspecified behavior of bone, soft tissue, and skin
D49.89	Neoplasm of unspecified behavior of other specified sites
R22.2	Localized swelling, mass and lump, trunk

AMA: **21930** 2018,Sep,7; 2018,Jan,8; 2017,Jan,8; 2016,Jan,13; 2015,Jan,16 **21931** 2018,Sep,7 **21932** 2018,Sep,7 **21933** 2018,Sep,7

Relative Value Units/Medicare Edits

Non-Facility RVU	Work	PE	MP	Total
21930	4.94	8.94	1.03	14.91
21931	6.88	5.43	1.57	13.88
21932	9.82	7.56	2.17	19.55
21933	11.13	8.15	2.53	21.81
Facility RVU	**Work**	**PE**	**MP**	**Total**
21930	4.94	4.76	1.03	10.73
21931	6.88	5.43	1.57	13.88
21932	9.82	7.56	2.17	19.55
21933	11.13	8.15	2.53	21.81

	FUD	Status	MUE	Modifiers				IOM Reference
21930	90	A	5(3)	51	N/A	N/A	N/A	None
21931	90	A	3(3)	51	N/A	N/A	80	
21932	90	A	2(3)	51	N/A	N/A	80	
21933	90	A	2(3)	51	N/A	N/A	80	

* with documentation

Terms To Know

dissection. Separating by cutting tissue or body structures apart.

drain. Device that creates a channel to allow fluid from a cavity, wound, or infected area to exit the body.

excision. Surgical removal of an organ or tissue.

subcutaneous tissue. Sheet or wide band of adipose (fat) and areolar connective tissue in two layers attached to the dermis.

tumor. Pathological swelling or enlargement; a neoplastic growth of uncontrolled, abnormal multiplication of cells.

Back

21935-21936

21935 Radical resection of tumor (eg, sarcoma), soft tissue of back or flank; less than 5 cm

21936 5 cm or greater

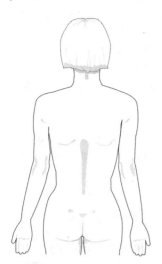

Radical resection of a soft tissue tumor of the back or flank

Explanation

The physician performs a radical resection of a malignant soft tissue tumor (i.e., sarcoma) from the back or flank, not involving bone. An incision is made over the tumor and dissection exposes it. The tumor and any adjacent tissue that may be affected by the spread of the neoplasm are excised. Large resections may be needed. The type and stage of the lesion determines the extent of the tumor margin resection area. Muscle or fascia may need to be repaired and drains may be placed. The surgical wound is closed using single or intermediate repair or separately reportable complex closure, adjacent tissue transfer, or graft. Report 21935 for excision of tumors whose resected area is less than 5 cm and 21936 for excision of tumors 5 cm or greater.

Coding Tips

An excisional biopsy is not reported separately when a therapeutic excision is performed during the same surgical session. Report any free grafts or flaps separately. For radical resection of cutaneous tumors, see 11600–11606.

ICD-10-CM Diagnostic Codes

C43.59	Malignant melanoma of other part of trunk
C4A.59	Merkel cell carcinoma of other part of trunk
C76.8	Malignant neoplasm of other specified ill-defined sites
C79.89	Secondary malignant neoplasm of other specified sites
D03.59	Melanoma in situ of other part of trunk
D17.1	Benign lipomatous neoplasm of skin and subcutaneous tissue of trunk

AMA: 21935 2018,Sep,7 **21936** 2018,Sep,7

Relative Value Units/Medicare Edits

Non-Facility RVU	Work	PE	MP	Total
21935	15.72	11.11	3.42	30.25
21936	22.55	14.01	5.07	41.63
Facility RVU	**Work**	**PE**	**MP**	**Total**
21935	15.72	11.11	3.42	30.25
21936	22.55	14.01	5.07	41.63

	FUD	Status	MUE	Modifiers			IOM Reference
21935	90	A	1(3)	51	N/A	62*	N/A	None
21936	90	A	1(3)	51	N/A	62*	80	

* with documentation

Terms To Know

adjacent tissue transfer. Rotation or advancement of skin from an adjacent area to repair or fill in a defect while maintaining attachment to original blood supply.

cutaneous. Relating to the skin.

dissection. Separating by cutting tissue or body structures apart.

malignant neoplasm. Any cancerous tumor or lesion exhibiting uncontrolled tissue growth that can progressively invade other parts of the body with its disease-generating cells.

radical resection. Removal of an entire tumor (e.g., malignant neoplasm) along with a large area of surrounding tissue, including adjacent lymph nodes that may have been infiltrated.

soft tissue. Nonepithelial tissues outside of the skeleton that includes subcutaneous adipose tissue, fibrous tissue, fascia, muscles, blood and lymph vessels, and peripheral nervous system tissue.

tumor. Pathological swelling or enlargement; a neoplastic growth of uncontrolled, abnormal multiplication of cells.

22010-22015

22010 Incision and drainage, open, of deep abscess (subfascial), posterior spine; cervical, thoracic, or cervicothoracic
22015   lumbar, sacral, or lumbosacral

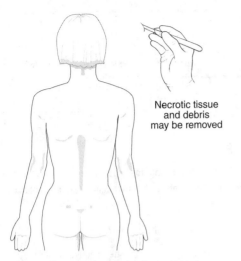

Open treatment of a deep abscess of the posterior spine

Necrotic tissue and debris may be removed

Spine

Explanation

The physician performs an open incision and drainage of a deep abscess of the posterior spine. Once a paraspinal soft tissue abscess or a lumbar psoas muscle abscess is identified by MRI or CT scan, an aspiration biopsy may be performed prior to open surgical drainage. The extent of the surgery depends on the size of the abscess and the area affected. The deep fascia is incised and the wound opened, irrigated, and debrided. Necrotic tissue and debris are removed and the cavity is irrigated with antibiotic solution. The wound is closed in layers and a drain or wound vacuum device may be placed. Report 22010 for incision and drainage of a deep abscess in the cervical, thoracic, or cervicothoracic region of the posterior spine and 22015 for the lumbar, sacral, or lumbosacral region.

Coding Tips

Do not report 22015 with 22010. For incision and drainage of an abscess, superficial, simple or single, see 10060; complicated or multiple, see 10061; for hematoma, seroma, or fluid collection, see 10140; for complex postoperative wound infection, see 10180. Instrumentation removal codes 22850 and 22852 should not be reported with 22015.

ICD-10-CM Diagnostic Codes

G06.1	Intraspinal abscess and granuloma
G07	Intracranial and intraspinal abscess and granuloma in diseases classified elsewhere
L02.212	Cutaneous abscess of back [any part, except buttock]
L03.221	Cellulitis of neck
L03.312	Cellulitis of back [any part except buttock]
M35.4	Diffuse (eosinophilic) fasciitis
M46.21	Osteomyelitis of vertebra, occipito-atlanto-axial region
M46.22	Osteomyelitis of vertebra, cervical region
M46.23	Osteomyelitis of vertebra, cervicothoracic region
M46.26	Osteomyelitis of vertebra, lumbar region
M46.27	Osteomyelitis of vertebra, lumbosacral region
M46.28	Osteomyelitis of vertebra, sacral and sacrococcygeal region

M46.31	Infection of intervertebral disc (pyogenic), occipito-atlanto-axial region
M46.32	Infection of intervertebral disc (pyogenic), cervical region
M46.33	Infection of intervertebral disc (pyogenic), cervicothoracic region
M46.36	Infection of intervertebral disc (pyogenic), lumbar region
M46.37	Infection of intervertebral disc (pyogenic), lumbosacral region
M46.38	Infection of intervertebral disc (pyogenic), sacral and sacrococcygeal region
M72.6	Necrotizing fasciitis
M72.8	Other fibroblastic disorders
M86.08	Acute hematogenous osteomyelitis, other sites
M86.18	Other acute osteomyelitis, other site
M86.28	Subacute osteomyelitis, other site
M86.38	Chronic multifocal osteomyelitis, other site
M86.48	Chronic osteomyelitis with draining sinus, other site
M86.58	Other chronic hematogenous osteomyelitis, other site
M86.68	Other chronic osteomyelitis, other site

AMA: **22010** 2018,Sep,7 **22015** 2018,Sep,7

Relative Value Units/Medicare Edits

Non-Facility RVU	Work	PE	MP	Total
22010	12.75	12.14	3.68	28.57
22015	12.64	12.01	3.35	28.0
Facility RVU	**Work**	**PE**	**MP**	**Total**
22010	12.75	12.14	3.68	28.57
22015	12.64	12.01	3.35	28.0

	FUD	Status	MUE	Modifiers				IOM Reference
22010	90	A	2(3)	51	N/A	N/A	80*	None
22015	90	A	2(3)	51	N/A	N/A	N/A	

* with documentation

Terms To Know

abscess. Circumscribed collection of pus resulting from bacteria, frequently associated with swelling and other signs of inflammation.

debridement. Removal of dead or contaminated tissue and foreign matter from a wound.

incision and drainage. Cutting open body tissue for the removal of tissue fluids or infected discharge from a wound or cavity.

irrigate. Washing out, lavage.

necrotic. Pathological condition of death occurring in a group of cells or tissues within a living part or organism.

tissue. Group of similar cells with a similar function that form definite structures and organs. Tissue types include epithelial tissue, muscle tissue, connective tissue, and nervous tissue.

22900-22903

22900   Excision, tumor, soft tissue of abdominal wall, subfascial (eg, intramuscular); less than 5 cm
22901   5 cm or greater
22902   Excision, tumor, soft tissue of abdominal wall, subcutaneous; less than 3 cm
22903   3 cm or greater

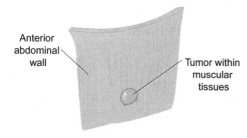

Anterior abdominal wall

Tumor within muscular tissues

An incision typically is made directly over the area of the tumor. Surrounding tissue may also be excised. Wound repair usually involves a layered closure

Explanation

The physician removes a tumor from the soft tissue of the abdominal wall that is located in the subcutaneous tissue in 22902–22903 and in the deep soft tissue, below the fascial plane or within the muscle, in 22900–22901. The patient is positioned supine on the operating table. With the proper anesthesia administered, the physician makes an incision in the skin overlying the mass and dissects down to the tumor. The extent of the tumor is identified and a dissection is undertaken all the way around the tumor. A portion of neighboring soft tissue may also be removed to ensure adequate removal of all tumor tissue. A drain may be inserted and the incision is repaired with layers of sutures, staples, or Steri-strips. Report 22902 for excision of subcutaneous tumors whose resected area is less than 3 cm and 22903 for excision of subcutaneous tumors 3 cm or greater. Report 22900 for excision of subfascial or intramuscular tumors whose resected area is less than 5 cm and 22901 for excision of subfascial or intramuscular tumors 5 cm or greater.

Coding Tips

An excisional biopsy is not reported separately when a therapeutic excision is performed during the same surgical session. When medically necessary, report moderate (conscious) sedation provided by the performing physician with 99151–99153; when provided by another physician report 99155–99157. For excision of cutaneous, benign lesions, see 11400–11406.

ICD-10-CM Diagnostic Codes

C49.4   Malignant neoplasm of connective and soft tissue of abdomen
D21.4   Benign neoplasm of connective and other soft tissue of abdomen
D48.1   Neoplasm of uncertain behavior of connective and other soft tissue

AMA: **22900** 2018,Sep,7 **22901** 2018,Sep,7 **22902** 2018,Sep,7 **22903** 2018,Sep,7

Relative Value Units/Medicare Edits

Non-Facility RVU	Work	PE	MP	Total
22900	8.32	6.48	1.89	16.69
22901	10.11	7.28	2.31	19.7
22902	4.42	8.6	1.02	14.04
22903	6.39	5.15	1.46	13.0
Facility RVU	Work	PE	MP	Total
22900	8.32	6.48	1.89	16.69
22901	10.11	7.28	2.31	19.7
22902	4.42	4.4	1.02	9.84
22903	6.39	5.15	1.46	13.0

	FUD	Status	MUE	Modifiers				IOM Reference
22900	90	A	3(3)	51	N/A	62*	80	None
22901	90	A	2(3)	51	N/A	62*	80	
22902	90	A	4(3)	51	N/A	62*	80	
22903	90	A	3(3)	51	N/A	62*	80	

* with documentation

Terms To Know

connective tissue. Body tissue made from fibroblasts, collagen, and elastic fibrils that connects, supports, and holds together other tissues and cells and includes cartilage, collagenous, fibrous, elastic, and osseous tissue.

dissection. Separating by cutting tissue or body structures apart.

malignant. Any condition tending to progress toward death, specifically an invasive tumor with a loss of cellular differentiation that has the ability to spread or metastasize to other body areas.

neoplasm. New abnormal growth, tumor.

soft tissue. Nonepithelial tissues outside of the skeleton that includes subcutaneous adipose tissue, fibrous tissue, fascia, muscles, blood and lymph vessels, and peripheral nervous system tissue.

subcutaneous tissue. Sheet or wide band of adipose (fat) and areolar connective tissue in two layers attached to the dermis.

subfascial. Beneath the band of fibrous tissue that lies deep to the skin, encloses muscles, and separates their layers.

Abdomen/Musculoskeletal

22904-22905

22904   Radical resection of tumor (eg, sarcoma), soft tissue of abdominal wall; less than 5 cm

22905   5 cm or greater

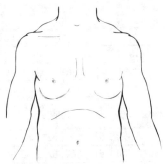

Radical excision of a soft tissue tumor of the abdomen

Explanation

The physician performs a radical resection of a malignant soft tissue tumor (i.e., sarcoma) from the abdominal wall, not involving bone. An incision is made over the tumor and dissection exposes it. The tumor and any adjacent tissue that may be affected by the spread of the neoplasm are excised. Large resections may be needed. The type and stage of the lesion determines the extent of the tumor margin resection area. Muscle or fascia may need to be repaired and drains may be placed. The surgical wound is closed using simple or intermediate repair or separately reportable complex closure, adjacent tissue transfer, or graft. Report 22904 for excision of tumors whose resected area is less than 5 cm and 22905 for excision of tumors 5 cm or greater.

Coding Tips

For excision of subfascial soft tissue abdominal wall tumors less than 5 cm, report 22900; greater than 5 cm, see 22901. For excision of subcutaneous soft tissue abdominal wall tumors less than 3 cm, see 22902; greater than 3 cm, see 22903. For radical resection of cutaneous tumors, see 11600–11606. An excisional biopsy is not reported separately when a therapeutic excision is performed during the same surgical session.

ICD-10-CM Diagnostic Codes

C49.4   Malignant neoplasm of connective and soft tissue of abdomen

AMA: **22904** 2018,Sep,7 **22905** 2018,Sep,7

Relative Value Units/Medicare Edits

Non-Facility RVU	Work	PE	MP	Total
22904	16.69	10.43	3.63	30.75
22905	21.58	12.6	4.74	38.92
Facility RVU	**Work**	**PE**	**MP**	**Total**
22904	16.69	10.43	3.63	30.75
22905	21.58	12.6	4.74	38.92

	FUD	Status	MUE	Modifiers				IOM Reference
22904	90	A	1(3)	51	N/A	62*	80	None
22905	90	A	1(3)	51	N/A	62*	80	

* with documentation

23930-23931

23930 Incision and drainage, upper arm or elbow area; deep abscess or hematoma
23931 bursa

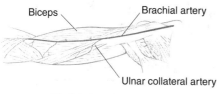

Biceps   Brachial artery

Ulnar collateral artery

Medial view of upper arm

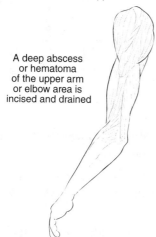

A deep abscess or hematoma of the upper arm or elbow area is incised and drained

Explanation

The physician drains a deep abscess or hematoma in 23930 or an infected bursa in 23931 from within the upper arm or elbow area. With proper anesthesia administered, the physician makes an incision in the upper arm or elbow overlying the site of the abscess, hematoma, or bursa to be incised. Dissection is carried down through the deep subcutaneous tissues and may be continued into the fascia or muscle to expose the abscess or hematoma. The incision may be extended if the mass is larger than expected. When the infected bursa, abscess, or hematoma is identified, it is incised and the contents are drained. The area is irrigated and the incision is repaired in layers with sutures, staples, and/or Steri-strips; closed with drains in place; or simply left open to further facilitate drainage of infection.

Coding Tips

For incision and drainage of an abscess, simple or single, see 10060; complicated or multiple, see 10061. For incision and drainage of a hematoma, seroma, or fluid collection, see 10140. Puncture aspiration of an abscess, hematoma, bulla, or cyst is reported with 10160.

ICD-10-CM Diagnostic Codes

L03.113	Cellulitis of right upper limb ☑
L03.114	Cellulitis of left upper limb ☑
L03.123	Acute lymphangitis of right upper limb ☑
L03.124	Acute lymphangitis of left upper limb ☑
M01.X21	Direct infection of right elbow in infectious and parasitic diseases classified elsewhere ☑
M01.X22	Direct infection of left elbow in infectious and parasitic diseases classified elsewhere ☑
M25.021	Hemarthrosis, right elbow ☑
M25.022	Hemarthrosis, left elbow ☑
M65.021	Abscess of tendon sheath, right upper arm ☑
M65.022	Abscess of tendon sheath, left upper arm ☑
M70.21	Olecranon bursitis, right elbow ☑
M70.22	Olecranon bursitis, left elbow ☑
M71.021	Abscess of bursa, right elbow ☑
M71.022	Abscess of bursa, left elbow ☑
S40.021A	Contusion of right upper arm, initial encounter ☑
S40.022A	Contusion of left upper arm, initial encounter ☑
S50.01XA	Contusion of right elbow, initial encounter ☑
S50.02XA	Contusion of left elbow, initial encounter ☑

AMA: 23930 2018,Sep,7 **23931** 2018,Sep,7

Relative Value Units/Medicare Edits

Non-Facility RVU	Work	PE	MP	Total
23930	2.99	7.38	0.62	10.99
23931	1.84	6.98	0.34	9.16
Facility RVU	**Work**	**PE**	**MP**	**Total**
23930	2.99	2.77	0.62	6.38
23931	1.84	2.53	0.34	4.71

	FUD	Status	MUE	Modifiers				IOM Reference
23930	10	A	2(3)	51	50	N/A	N/A	None
23931	10	A	2(3)	51	50	N/A	N/A	

* with documentation

Terms To Know

abscess. Circumscribed collection of pus resulting from bacteria, frequently associated with swelling and other signs of inflammation.

bursa. Cavity or sac containing fluid that occurs between articulating surfaces and serves to reduce friction from moving parts.

cellulitis. Infection of the skin and subcutaneous tissues, most often caused by Staphylococcus or Streptococcus bacteria secondary to a cutaneous lesion. Progression of the inflammation may lead to abscess and tissue death, or even systemic infection-like bacteremia.

deep dissection. Cutting through the skin to the subcutaneous fat just above the fascial plane and deeper structures, including fascia, muscle, and related structures.

fascia. Fibrous sheet or band of tissue that envelops organs, muscles, and groupings of muscles.

hemarthrosis. Occurrence of blood within a joint space.

hematoma. Tumor-like collection of blood in some part of the body caused by a break in a blood vessel wall, usually as a result of trauma.

incision and drainage. Cutting open body tissue for the removal of tissue fluids or infected discharge from a wound or cavity.

tendon. Fibrous tissue that connects muscle to bone, consisting primarily of collagen and containing little vasculature.

Humerus

24065-24066

24065 Biopsy, soft tissue of upper arm or elbow area; superficial
24066 deep (subfascial or intramuscular)

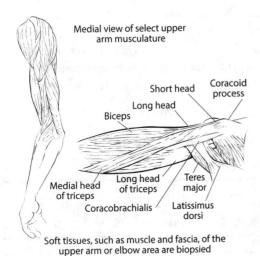

Medial view of select upper arm musculature

Short head
Coracoid process
Long head
Biceps
Long head of triceps
Teres major
Medial head of triceps
Coracobrachialis
Latissimus dorsi

Soft tissues, such as muscle and fascia, of the upper arm or elbow area are biopsied

Explanation

The physician performs a biopsy of the soft tissues of the upper arm or elbow area. With proper anesthesia administered, an incision is made over the biopsy area. Dissection is carried down within the superficial soft tissue layers in 24065, usually the subcutaneous fat to the uppermost fascial layer. In 24066, dissection is taken down deep within the soft tissue, such as into the fascial layer or within the muscle. A portion of the tissue is excised and submitted for pathology. The area is irrigated and the incision is closed with layered sutures, staples, or Steri-strips.

Coding Tips

An excisional biopsy is not reported separately when a therapeutic excision is performed during the same surgical session. For needle biopsy of soft tissue, see 20206. Local anesthesia is included in these services. However, these procedures may be performed under general anesthesia, depending on the age and/or condition of the patient. Surgical trays, A4550, are not separately reimbursed by Medicare; however, other third-party payers may cover them. Check with the specific payer to determine coverage.

ICD-10-CM Diagnostic Codes

C49.11	Malignant neoplasm of connective and soft tissue of right upper limb, including shoulder ☑
C49.12	Malignant neoplasm of connective and soft tissue of left upper limb, including shoulder ☑
D17.21	Benign lipomatous neoplasm of skin and subcutaneous tissue of right arm ☑
D17.22	Benign lipomatous neoplasm of skin and subcutaneous tissue of left arm ☑
D21.11	Benign neoplasm of connective and other soft tissue of right upper limb, including shoulder ☑
D21.12	Benign neoplasm of connective and other soft tissue of left upper limb, including shoulder ☑
D48.1	Neoplasm of uncertain behavior of connective and other soft tissue
M60.221	Foreign body granuloma of soft tissue, not elsewhere classified, right upper arm ☑

M60.222	Foreign body granuloma of soft tissue, not elsewhere classified, left upper arm ☑

AMA: **24065** 2018,Sep,7 **24066** 2018,Sep,7

Relative Value Units/Medicare Edits

Non-Facility RVU	Work	PE	MP	Total
24065	2.13	5.34	0.3	7.77
24066	5.35	12.29	1.13	18.77
Facility RVU	**Work**	**PE**	**MP**	**Total**
24065	2.13	2.36	0.3	4.79
24066	5.35	5.91	1.13	12.39

	FUD	Status	MUE	Modifiers				IOM Reference
24065	10	A	2(3)	51	50	N/A	N/A	None
24066	90	A	2(3)	51	50	N/A	N/A	

* with documentation

Terms To Know

biopsy. Tissue or fluid removed for diagnostic purposes through analysis of the cells in the biopsy material.

deep fascia. Sheet of dense, fibrous tissue holding muscle groups together below the hypodermis layer or subcutaneous fat layer that lines the extremities and trunk.

dissection. Separating by cutting tissue or body structures apart.

granuloma. Abnormal, dense collections of cells forming a mass or nodule of chronically inflamed tissue with granulations that is usually associated with an infective process.

lipoma. Benign tumor containing fat cells and the most common of soft tissue lesions, which are usually painless and asymptomatic, with the exception of an angiolipoma.

muscle tissue. Network of specialized cells for performing contraction to produce voluntary or involuntary movement of body parts, and skeletal, cardiac, or visceral muscles.

soft tissue. Nonepithelial tissues outside of the skeleton.

subcutaneous tissue. Sheet or wide band of adipose (fat) and areolar connective tissue in two layers attached to the dermis.

subfascial. Beneath the band of fibrous tissue that lies deep to the skin, encloses muscles, and separates their layers.

Coding Companion for General Surgery/Gastroenterology

Humerus

24075-24076 [24071, 24073]

24075 Excision, tumor, soft tissue of upper arm or elbow area, subcutaneous; less than 3 cm

24071 Excision, tumor, soft tissue of upper arm or elbow area, subcutaneous; 3 cm or greater

24076 Excision, tumor, soft tissue of upper arm or elbow area, subfascial (eg, intramuscular); less than 5 cm

24073 Excision, tumor, soft tissue of upper arm or elbow area, subfascial (eg, intramuscular); 5 cm or greater

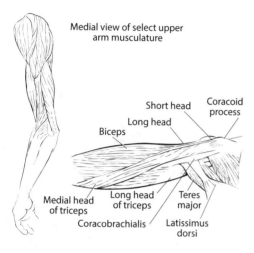

Medial view of select upper arm musculature

Explanation

The physician removes a tumor from the soft tissue of the upper arm or elbow area that is located in the subcutaneous tissue in 24071and 24075 and in the deep soft tissue, below the fascial plane or within the muscle, in 24073 and 24076. With the proper anesthesia administered, the physician makes an incision in the skin overlying the mass and dissects down to the tumor. The extent of the tumor is identified and a dissection is undertaken all the way around the tumor. A portion of neighboring soft tissue may also be removed to ensure adequate removal of all tumor tissue. A drain may be inserted and the incision is repaired with layers of sutures, staples, or Steri-strips. Report 24075 for excision of subcutaneous tumors whose resected area is less than 3 cm and 24071 for excision of subcutaneous tumors 3 cm or greater. Report 24076 for excision of subfascial or intramuscular tumors whose resected area is less than 5 cm and 24073 for excision of subfascial or intramuscular tumors 5 cm or greater.

Coding Tips

For excision of other soft tissues, see the specific anatomical section. An excisional biopsy is not reported separately when a therapeutic excision is performed during the same surgical session. Report any free grafts or flaps separately. When medically necessary, report moderate (conscious) sedation provided by the performing physician with 99151–99153. When provided by another physician report 99155–99157. For excision of cutaneous, benign lesions, see 11400–11406.

ICD-10-CM Diagnostic Codes

C49.11	Malignant neoplasm of connective and soft tissue of right upper limb, including shoulder ☑
C49.12	Malignant neoplasm of connective and soft tissue of left upper limb, including shoulder ☑
D17.21	Benign lipomatous neoplasm of skin and subcutaneous tissue of right arm ☑
D17.22	Benign lipomatous neoplasm of skin and subcutaneous tissue of left arm ☑
D21.11	Benign neoplasm of connective and other soft tissue of right upper limb, including shoulder ☑
D21.12	Benign neoplasm of connective and other soft tissue of left upper limb, including shoulder ☑
M60.221	Foreign body granuloma of soft tissue, not elsewhere classified, right upper arm ☑
M60.222	Foreign body granuloma of soft tissue, not elsewhere classified, left upper arm ☑

AMA: **24071** 2018,Sep,7 **24073** 2018,Sep,7 **24075** 2018,Sep,7 **24076** 2018,Sep,7

Relative Value Units/Medicare Edits

Non-Facility RVU	Work	PE	MP	Total
24075	4.24	10.86	0.86	15.96
24071	5.7	5.04	1.25	11.99
24076	7.41	7.14	1.51	16.06
24073	10.13	8.19	2.17	20.49
Facility RVU	**Work**	**PE**	**MP**	**Total**
24075	4.24	4.61	0.86	9.71
24071	5.7	5.04	1.25	11.99
24076	7.41	7.14	1.51	16.06
24073	10.13	8.19	2.17	20.49

	FUD	Status	MUE	Modifiers				IOM Reference
24075	90	A	5(3)	51	50	N/A	N/A	None
24071	90	A	2(3)	51	50	N/A	80	
24076	90	A	4(3)	51	50	N/A	N/A	
24073	90	A	2(3)	51	50	N/A	80	

* with documentation

Terms To Know

intramuscular. Within a muscle.

subcutaneous. Below the skin.

subfascial. Beneath the band of fibrous tissue that lies deep to the skin, encloses muscles, and separates their layers.

24077-24079

24077 Radical resection of tumor (eg, sarcoma), soft tissue of upper arm or elbow area; less than 5 cm

24079 5 cm or greater

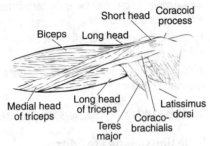

Radical resection of soft tissue tumor of the upper arm or elbow area

Explanation

The physician performs a radical resection of a malignant soft tissue tumor (i.e., sarcoma) from the upper arm or elbow area, not involving bone. An incision is made over the tumor and dissection exposes it. The tumor and any adjacent tissue that may be affected by the spread of the neoplasm are excised. Large resections may be needed. The type and stage of the lesion determines the extent of the tumor margin resection area. Muscle or fascia may need to be repaired and drains may be placed. The surgical wound is closed using simple or intermediate repair or separately reportable complex closure, adjacent tissue transfer, or graft. The arm may be placed in a posterior splint. Report 24077 for excision of tumors whose resected area is less than 5 cm and 24079 for excision of tumors 5 cm or greater.

Coding Tips

For radical resection of a forearm or wrist area soft tissue tumor, see 25077–25078; for shoulder area, see 23077–23078. For radical resection of cutaneous tumors, see 11600–11606. For resection of other soft tissues, see the specific anatomical section.

ICD-10-CM Diagnostic Codes

C49.11   Malignant neoplasm of connective and soft tissue of right upper limb, including shoulder ☑

C49.12   Malignant neoplasm of connective and soft tissue of left upper limb, including shoulder ☑

AMA: 24077 2018,Sep,7 **24079** 2018,Sep,7

Relative Value Units/Medicare Edits

Non-Facility RVU	Work	PE	MP	Total
24077	15.72	11.27	3.31	30.3
24079	20.61	13.83	4.49	38.93
Facility RVU	Work	PE	MP	Total
24077	15.72	11.27	3.31	30.3
24079	20.61	13.83	4.49	38.93

	FUD	Status	MUE	Modifiers					IOM Reference
24077	90	A	1(3)	51	50	62*	N/A		None
24079	90	A	1(3)	51	50	62*	80		

* with documentation

25065-25066

25065 Biopsy, soft tissue of forearm and/or wrist; superficial
25066   deep (subfascial or intramuscular)

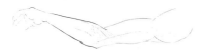

A biopsy of the forearm/wrist area is performed

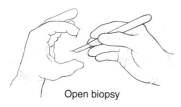

Open biopsy

Explanation

The physician performs a biopsy of the soft tissues of the forearm and/or wrist. With proper anesthesia administered, an incision is made over the biopsy area. Dissection is carried down within the superficial soft tissue layers in 25065, usually the subcutaneous fat to the uppermost fascial layer. In 25066, dissection is taken down deep within the soft tissue, such as into the fascial layer or within the muscle. A portion of the tissue is excised and submitted for pathology. The area is irrigated and the incision is closed with layered sutures, staples, or Steri-strips. If the wrist is involved, a splint may be applied to limit motion.

Coding Tips

For a needle biopsy of muscle, see 20206. Local anesthesia is included in these services. However, 25066 may be performed under general anesthesia, depending on the age and/or condition of the patient. Surgical trays, A4550, are not separately reimbursed by Medicare; however, other third-party payers may cover them. Check with the specific payer to determine coverage.

ICD-10-CM Diagnostic Codes

C49.11	Malignant neoplasm of connective and soft tissue of right upper limb, including shoulder ☑
C49.12	Malignant neoplasm of connective and soft tissue of left upper limb, including shoulder ☑
D17.21	Benign lipomatous neoplasm of skin and subcutaneous tissue of right arm ☑
D17.22	Benign lipomatous neoplasm of skin and subcutaneous tissue of left arm ☑
D21.11	Benign neoplasm of connective and other soft tissue of right upper limb, including shoulder ☑
D21.12	Benign neoplasm of connective and other soft tissue of left upper limb, including shoulder ☑
D48.1	Neoplasm of uncertain behavior of connective and other soft tissue
D49.2	Neoplasm of unspecified behavior of bone, soft tissue, and skin
M60.231	Foreign body granuloma of soft tissue, not elsewhere classified, right forearm ☑
M60.232	Foreign body granuloma of soft tissue, not elsewhere classified, left forearm ☑

AMA: **25065** 2018,Sep,7 **25066** 2018,Sep,7

Relative Value Units/Medicare Edits

Non-Facility RVU	Work	PE	MP	Total
25065	2.04	5.39	0.26	7.69
25066	4.27	5.64	0.78	10.69
Facility RVU	**Work**	**PE**	**MP**	**Total**
25065	2.04	2.34	0.26	4.64
25066	4.27	5.64	0.78	10.69

	FUD	Status	MUE	Modifiers				IOM Reference
25065	10	A	2(3)	51	50	N/A	N/A	None
25066	90	A	2(3)	51	50	N/A	N/A	

* with documentation

Terms To Know

benign. Mild or nonmalignant in nature.

biopsy. Tissue or fluid removed for diagnostic purposes through analysis of the cells in the biopsy material.

dissection. Separating by cutting tissue or body structures apart.

granuloma. Abnormal, dense collections of cells forming a mass or nodule of chronically inflamed tissue with granulations that is usually associated with an infective process.

irrigation. To wash out or cleanse a body cavity, wound, or tissue with water or other fluid.

malignant. Any condition tending to progress toward death, specifically an invasive tumor with a loss of cellular differentiation that has the ability to spread or metastasize to other body areas.

neoplasm. New abnormal growth, tumor.

soft tissue. Nonepithelial tissues outside of the skeleton.

subcutaneous. Below the skin.

subfascial. Beneath the band of fibrous tissue that lies deep to the skin, encloses muscles, and separates their layers.

tumor. Pathological swelling or enlargement; a neoplastic growth of uncontrolled, abnormal multiplication of cells.

Forearm/Wrist

25075-25076 [25071, 25073]

25075 Excision, tumor, soft tissue of forearm and/or wrist area, subcutaneous; less than 3 cm

25071 Excision, tumor, soft tissue of forearm and/or wrist area, subcutaneous; 3 cm or greater

25076 Excision, tumor, soft tissue of forearm and/or wrist area, subfascial (eg, intramuscular); less than 3 cm

25073 Excision, tumor, soft tissue of forearm and/or wrist area, subfascial (eg, intramuscular); 3 cm or greater

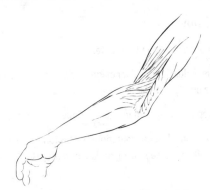

Soft tissue tumor of the forearm or wrist area

Explanation

The physician removes a tumor from the soft tissue of the forearm and/or wrist area that is located in the subcutaneous tissue in 25071 and 25075 and in the deep soft tissue, below the fascial plane or within the muscle, in 25073 and 25076. With the proper anesthesia administered, the physician makes an incision in the skin overlying the mass and dissects down to the tumor. The extent of the tumor is identified and a dissection is undertaken all the way around the tumor. A portion of neighboring soft tissue may also be removed to ensure adequate removal of all tumor tissue. A drain may be inserted and the incision is repaired with layers of sutures, staples, or Steri-strips. Report 25075 for excision of subcutaneous tumors whose resected area is less than 3 cm and 25071 for excision of subcutaneous tumors 3 cm or greater. Report 25076 for excision of subfascial or intramuscular tumors whose resected area is less than 3 cm and 25073 for excision of subfascial or intramuscular tumors 3 cm or greater.

Coding Tips

These codes include the use of local anesthesia. However, they may be performed under general anesthesia, depending on the age and/or condition of the patient. For needle biopsy of muscle, see 20206. For excision of cutaneous, benign lesions, see 11400–11406.

ICD-10-CM Diagnostic Codes

C49.11	Malignant neoplasm of connective and soft tissue of right upper limb, including shoulder ☑
C49.12	Malignant neoplasm of connective and soft tissue of left upper limb, including shoulder ☑
D17.21	Benign lipomatous neoplasm of skin and subcutaneous tissue of right arm ☑
D17.22	Benign lipomatous neoplasm of skin and subcutaneous tissue of left arm ☑
D21.11	Benign neoplasm of connective and other soft tissue of right upper limb, including shoulder ☑
D21.12	Benign neoplasm of connective and other soft tissue of left upper limb, including shoulder ☑
D48.1	Neoplasm of uncertain behavior of connective and other soft tissue
M60.231	Foreign body granuloma of soft tissue, not elsewhere classified, right forearm ☑
M60.232	Foreign body granuloma of soft tissue, not elsewhere classified, left forearm ☑

AMA: **25071** 2018,Sep,7 **25073** 2018,Sep,7 **25075** 2018,Sep,7 **25076** 2018,Sep,7

Relative Value Units/Medicare Edits

Non-Facility RVU	Work	PE	MP	Total
25075	3.96	10.85	0.77	15.58
25071	5.91	5.35	1.25	12.51
25076	6.74	7.27	1.25	15.26
25073	7.13	7.25	1.43	15.81

Facility RVU	Work	PE	MP	Total
25075	3.96	4.58	0.77	9.31
25071	5.91	5.35	1.25	12.51
25076	6.74	7.27	1.25	15.26
25073	7.13	7.25	1.43	15.81

	FUD	Status	MUE	Modifiers				IOM Reference
25075	90	A	6(3)	51	50	N/A	N/A	None
25071	90	A	3(3)	51	50	N/A	80	
25076	90	A	3(3)	51	50	N/A	N/A	
25073	90	A	2(3)	51	50	N/A	80	

* with documentation

Terms To Know

dissection. Separating by cutting tissue or body structures apart.

resect. Cutting out or removing a portion or all of a bone, organ, or other structure.

soft tissue. Nonepithelial tissues outside of the skeleton.

25077-25078

25077 Radical resection of tumor (eg, sarcoma), soft tissue of forearm and/or wrist area; less than 3 cm

25078 3 cm or greater

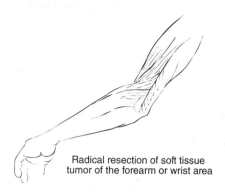

Radical resection of soft tissue tumor of the forearm or wrist area

Explanation

The physician performs a radical resection of a malignant soft tissue tumor (i.e., sarcoma) from the forearm and/or wrist area, not involving bone. An incision is made over the tumor and dissection exposes it. The tumor and any adjacent tissue that may be affected by the spread of the neoplasm are excised. Large resections may be needed. The type and stage of the lesion determine the extent of the tumor margin resection area. Muscle or fascia may need to be repaired and drains may be placed. The surgical wound is closed using simple or intermediate repair or separately reportable complex closure, adjacent tissue transfer, or graft. If the wrist is involved, a splint may be applied to limit motion. Report 25077 for excision of tumors whose resected area is less than 3 cm and 25078 for excision of tumors 3 cm or greater.

Coding Tips

For soft tissue tumor radical resection of the hand or finger, less than 3 cm, see 26117; greater than 3 cm, see 26118. For radical resection of cutaneous tumors, see 11600–11606. If significant additional time and effort is documented, append modifier 22 and submit a cover letter and operative report.

ICD-10-CM Diagnostic Codes

C49.11 Malignant neoplasm of connective and soft tissue of right upper limb, including shoulder ☑

C49.12 Malignant neoplasm of connective and soft tissue of left upper limb, including shoulder ☑

AMA: 25077 2018,Sep,7 **25078** 2018,Sep,7

Relative Value Units/Medicare Edits

Non-Facility RVU	Work	PE	MP	Total
25077	12.93	10.6	2.66	26.19
25078	17.69	12.72	3.82	34.23
Facility RVU	Work	PE	MP	Total
25077	12.93	10.6	2.66	26.19
25078	17.69	12.72	3.82	34.23

	FUD	Status	MUE	Modifiers				IOM Reference
25077	90	A	1(3)	51	50	N/A	N/A	None
25078	90	A	1(3)	51	50	N/A	80	

* with documentation

Terms To Know

adjacent tissue transfer. Rotation or advancement of skin from an adjacent area to repair or fill in a defect while maintaining attachment to original blood supply.

dissection. Separating by cutting tissue or body structures apart.

malignant neoplasm. Any cancerous tumor or lesion exhibiting uncontrolled tissue growth that can progressively invade other parts of the body with its disease-generating cells.

radical resection. Removal of an entire tumor (e.g., malignant neoplasm) along with a large area of surrounding tissue, including adjacent lymph nodes that may have been infiltrated.

soft tissue. Nonepithelial tissues outside of the skeleton that includes subcutaneous adipose tissue, fibrous tissue, fascia, muscles, blood and lymph vessels, and peripheral nervous system tissue.

tumor. Pathological swelling or enlargement; a neoplastic growth of uncontrolled, abnormal multiplication of cells.

25111-25112

25111 Excision of ganglion, wrist (dorsal or volar); primary
25112   recurrent

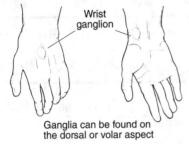

Ganglia can be found on the dorsal or volar aspect

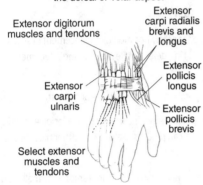

Select extensor muscles and tendons

Explanation

The physician removes a ganglion from the wrist in 25111 or a recurrent ganglion in 25112. An incision is made overlying the ganglion. The tissues are dissected around the ganglion, freeing it from surrounding tissue. (Scar tissue may be removed in 25112.) The physician may dissect deep within the wrist joint in order to excise all of the ganglion. The ganglion is removed. The joint or muscle tissue may be repaired in 25112. The physician irrigates the wound with antibiotic solution and closes the wound in layers.

Coding Tips

According to CPT guidelines, cast application or strapping (including removal) is only reported as a replacement procedure or when the cast application or strapping is an initial service performed without a restorative treatment or procedure. See "Application of Casts and Strapping" in the CPT book in the Surgery Section, under the Musculoskeletal system. Local anesthesia is included in these services. For excision of a hand or finger ganglion cyst, see 26160. For aspiration or injection of a ganglion cyst, any location, see 20612.

ICD-10-CM Diagnostic Codes

M67.431   Ganglion, right wrist ☑
M67.432   Ganglion, left wrist ☑

AMA: 25111 2018,Sep,7 **25112** 2018,Sep,7

Relative Value Units/Medicare Edits

Non-Facility RVU	Work	PE	MP	Total
25111	3.53	5.4	0.65	9.58
25112	4.67	5.98	0.86	11.51
Facility RVU	**Work**	**PE**	**MP**	**Total**
25111	3.53	5.4	0.65	9.58
25112	4.67	5.98	0.86	11.51

	FUD	Status	MUE	Modifiers				IOM Reference
25111	90	A	1(3)	51	50	N/A	N/A	None
25112	90	A	1(3)	51	50	N/A	N/A	

* with documentation

Terms To Know

dissection. Separating by cutting tissue or body structures apart.

dorsal. Pertaining to the back or posterior aspect.

ganglion. Fluid-filled, benign cyst appearing on a tendon sheath or aponeurosis, frequently connecting to an underlying joint.

irrigation. To wash out or cleanse a body cavity, wound, or tissue with water or other fluid.

scar tissue. Fibrous connective tissue that forms around a wounded area or injury, composed mainly of fibroblasts or collagenous fibers.

volar. Palm of the hand (palmar) or sole of the foot (plantar).

Forearm/Wrist

26115-26116 [26111, 26113]

26115 Excision, tumor or vascular malformation, soft tissue of hand or finger, subcutaneous; less than 1.5 cm

26111 Excision, tumor or vascular malformation, soft tissue of hand or finger, subcutaneous; 1.5 cm or greater

26116 Excision, tumor, soft tissue, or vascular malformation, of hand or finger, subfascial (eg, intramuscular); less than 1.5 cm

26113 Excision, tumor, soft tissue, or vascular malformation, of hand or finger, subfascial (eg, intramuscular); 1.5 cm or greater

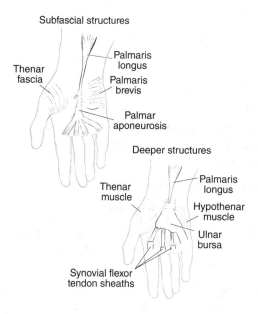

Subfascial structures

Thenar fascia
Palmaris longus
Palmaris brevis
Palmar aponeurosis

Deeper structures

Thenar muscle
Palmaris longus
Hypothenar muscle
Ulnar bursa
Synovial flexor tendon sheaths

Explanation

The physician removes a tumor or vascular malformation from the soft tissue of the hand or finger that is located in the subcutaneous tissue in 26111 and 26115 and in the deep soft tissue below the fascial plane, or within the muscle, in 26113 or 26116. With the proper anesthesia administered, the physician makes an incision in the skin overlying the mass and dissects down to the tumor or malformation. The extent of the tumor is identified and a dissection is undertaken all the way around the tumor. The blood vessels are ligated and the defective tissue of the vascular malformation is excised. A portion of neighboring soft tissue may also be removed to ensure adequate removal of all tumor tissue. A drain may be inserted, and the incision is repaired with layers of sutures, staples, or Steri-strips. Report 26115 for excision of subcutaneous tumors whose resected area is less than 1.5 cm and 26111 for excision of subcutaneous tumors 1.5 cm or greater. Report 26116 for excision of subfascial or intramuscular tumors whose resected area is less than 1.5 cm and 26113 for excision of subfascial or intramuscular tumors 1.5 cm or greater.

Coding Tips

If significant additional time and effort is documented, append modifier 22 and submit a cover letter and operative report. For excision of cutaneous, benign lesions, see 11420–11426.

ICD-10-CM Diagnostic Codes

C49.11	Malignant neoplasm of connective and soft tissue of right upper limb, including shoulder ☑
C49.12	Malignant neoplasm of connective and soft tissue of left upper limb, including shoulder ☑
D17.21	Benign lipomatous neoplasm of skin and subcutaneous tissue of right arm ☑
D17.22	Benign lipomatous neoplasm of skin and subcutaneous tissue of left arm ☑
D18.01	Hemangioma of skin and subcutaneous tissue
D21.11	Benign neoplasm of connective and other soft tissue of right upper limb, including shoulder ☑
D21.12	Benign neoplasm of connective and other soft tissue of left upper limb, including shoulder ☑
D48.1	Neoplasm of uncertain behavior of connective and other soft tissue
D49.2	Neoplasm of unspecified behavior of bone, soft tissue, and skin
M60.241	Foreign body granuloma of soft tissue, not elsewhere classified, right hand ☑
M60.242	Foreign body granuloma of soft tissue, not elsewhere classified, left hand ☑
Q27.31	Arteriovenous malformation of vessel of upper limb
Q27.8	Other specified congenital malformations of peripheral vascular system

AMA: **26111** 2018,Sep,7 **26113** 2018,Sep,7 **26115** 2018,Sep,7 **26116** 2018,Sep,7; 2018,Jan,8; 2017,Jan,8; 2016,Jan,13; 2015,Jan,16

Relative Value Units/Medicare Edits

Non-Facility RVU	Work	PE	MP	Total
26115	3.96	11.77	0.71	16.44
26111	5.42	5.84	1.02	12.28
26116	6.74	7.56	1.21	15.51
26113	7.13	7.73	1.28	16.14
Facility RVU	**Work**	**PE**	**MP**	**Total**
26115	3.96	5.11	0.71	9.78
26111	5.42	5.84	1.02	12.28
26116	6.74	7.56	1.21	15.51
26113	7.13	7.73	1.28	16.14

	FUD	Status	MUE	Modifiers				IOM Reference
26115	90	A	4(3)	51	N/A	N/A	N/A	None
26111	90	A	4(3)	51	N/A	N/A	80	
26116	90	A	2(3)	51	N/A	N/A	N/A	
26113	90	A	3(3)	51	N/A	N/A	80	

* with documentation

Terms To Know

subcutaneous. Below the skin.

subfascial. Beneath the band of fibrous tissue that lies deep to the skin, encloses muscles, and separates their layers.

Hands/Fingers

26117-26118

26117 Radical resection of tumor (eg, sarcoma), soft tissue of hand or finger; less than 3 cm

26118 3 cm or greater

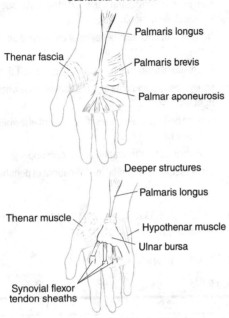

Radical resection of soft tissue tumor of the hand or fingers

Explanation

The physician removes a malignant soft tissue tumor (i.e., sarcoma) from the hand or finger, not involving bone. An incision is made over the tumor and dissection exposes it. The tumor and any adjacent tissue that may be affected by the spread of the neoplasm are excised. Large resections may be needed. The type and stage of the lesion determine the extent of the tumor margin resection area. Muscle or fascia may need to be repaired and drains may be placed. The surgical wound is closed using simple or intermediate repair or separately reportable complex closure, adjacent tissue transfer, or graft. Report 26117 for excision of tumors whose resected area is less than 3 cm and 26118 for excision of tumors 3 cm or greater.

Coding Tips

For soft tissue tumor excision of a hand or finger, subcutaneous, less than 1.5 cm, see 26115; greater than 1.5 cm, see 26111; subfascial, less than 1.5 cm, see 26116; greater than 1.5 cm, see 26113. For radical resection of a forearm or wrist area soft tissue tumor, see 25077–25078. For radical resection of cutaneous tumors, see 11620–11626.

ICD-10-CM Diagnostic Codes

C49.11 Malignant neoplasm of connective and soft tissue of right upper limb, including shoulder ☑

C49.12 Malignant neoplasm of connective and soft tissue of left upper limb, including shoulder ☑

AMA: 26117 2018,Sep,7 **26118** 2018,Sep,7

Relative Value Units/Medicare Edits

Non-Facility RVU	Work	PE	MP	Total
26117	10.13	9.81	1.88	21.82
26118	14.81	13.48	2.76	31.05
Facility RVU	**Work**	**PE**	**MP**	**Total**
26117	10.13	9.81	1.88	21.82
26118	14.81	13.48	2.76	31.05

	FUD	Status	MUE	Modifiers			IOM Reference
26117	90	A	2(3)	51	N/A	N/A	N/A	None
26118	90	A	1(3)	51	N/A	N/A	80	

* with documentation

Terms To Know

dissection. Separating by cutting tissue or body structures apart.

fascia. Fibrous sheet or band of tissue that envelops organs, muscles, and groupings of muscles.

malignant. Any condition tending to progress toward death, specifically an invasive tumor with a loss of cellular differentiation that has the ability to spread or metastasize to other body areas.

margin. Boundary, edge, or border, as of a surface or structure.

neoplasm. New abnormal growth, tumor.

radical resection. Removal of an entire tumor (e.g., malignant neoplasm) along with a large area of surrounding tissue, including adjacent lymph nodes that may have been infiltrated.

sarcoma. Malignant tumor arising in connective tissue, bone, cartilage, or striated muscle that spreads to neighboring tissue through the bloodstream.

soft tissue. Nonepithelial tissues outside of the skeleton that includes subcutaneous adipose tissue, fibrous tissue, fascia, muscles, blood and lymph vessels, and peripheral nervous system tissue.

tumor. Pathological swelling or enlargement; a neoplastic growth of uncontrolled, abnormal multiplication of cells.

Coding Companion for General Surgery/Gastroenterology

Hands/Fingers

26990

26990　Incision and drainage, pelvis or hip joint area; deep abscess or hematoma

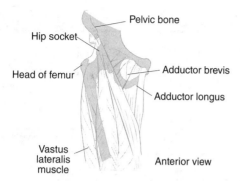

- Pelvic bone
- Hip socket
- Head of femur
- Adductor brevis
- Adductor longus
- Vastus lateralis muscle
- Anterior view

A deep abscess or hematoma of the hip/pelvis area is incised and drained

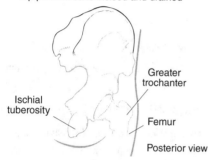

- Greater trochanter
- Ischial tuberosity
- Femur
- Posterior view

Explanation

The physician drains a deep abscess or hematoma from the pelvis or hip joint area. The physician makes an incision overlying the site of the abscess or hematoma. Dissection is carried through the deep subcutaneous tissues and may be continued into the fascia or muscle to expose the abscess or hematoma. The incision may be extended if the mass is larger than expected. When the abscess or hematoma is identified, it is incised and the contents are drained. The area is irrigated and the incision is repaired in layers with sutures, staples, and/or Steri-strips; closed with drains in place; or simply left open to further facilitate drainage of infection.

Coding Tips

For incision and drainage of an abscess, superficial, simple or single, see 10060; complicated or multiple, see 10061. Incision and drainage of an infected bursa in the pelvic or hip joint area is reported with 26991.

ICD-10-CM Diagnostic Codes

L03.115	Cellulitis of right lower limb ☑
L03.116	Cellulitis of left lower limb ☑
L03.125	Acute lymphangitis of right lower limb ☑
L03.126	Acute lymphangitis of left lower limb ☑
M01.X51	Direct infection of right hip in infectious and parasitic diseases classified elsewhere ☑
M01.X52	Direct infection of left hip in infectious and parasitic diseases classified elsewhere ☑
M70.61	Trochanteric bursitis, right hip ☑
M70.62	Trochanteric bursitis, left hip ☑
M70.71	Other bursitis of hip, right hip ☑
M70.72	Other bursitis of hip, left hip ☑
M71.051	Abscess of bursa, right hip ☑
M71.052	Abscess of bursa, left hip ☑
S30.0XXA	Contusion of lower back and pelvis, initial encounter
S70.01XA	Contusion of right hip, initial encounter ☑
S70.02XA	Contusion of left hip, initial encounter ☑

AMA: 26990 2018,Sep,7

Relative Value Units/Medicare Edits

Non-Facility RVU	Work	PE	MP	Total
26990	7.95	10.4	1.62	19.97
Facility RVU	**Work**	**PE**	**MP**	**Total**
26990	7.95	10.4	1.62	19.97

	FUD	Status	MUE	Modifiers				IOM Reference
26990	90	A	2(3)	51	N/A	N/A	N/A	None

* with documentation

Terms To Know

abscess. Circumscribed collection of pus resulting from bacteria, frequently associated with swelling and other signs of inflammation.

cellulitis. Infection of the skin and subcutaneous tissues, most often caused by Staphylococcus or Streptococcus bacteria secondary to a cutaneous lesion. Progression of the inflammation may lead to abscess and tissue death, or even systemic infection-like bacteremia.

contusion. Superficial injury (bruising) produced by impact without a break in the skin.

cyst. Elevated encapsulated mass containing fluid, semisolid, or solid material with a membranous lining.

dissection. Separating by cutting tissue or body structures apart.

fascia. Fibrous sheet or band of tissue that envelops organs, muscles, and groupings of muscles.

hematoma. Tumor-like collection of blood in some part of the body caused by a break in a blood vessel wall, usually as a result of trauma.

incision and drainage. Cutting open body tissue for the removal of tissue fluids or infected discharge from a wound or cavity.

infection. Presence of microorganisms in body tissues that may result in cellular damage.

lymphangitis. Inflammation of the lymph channels most often caused by streptococcus.

soft tissue. Nonepithelial tissues outside of the skeleton.

subcutaneous tissue. Sheet or wide band of adipose (fat) and areolar connective tissue in two layers attached to the dermis.

Pelvis/Hip

27040-27041

27040   Biopsy, soft tissue of pelvis and hip area; superficial
27041   deep, subfascial or intramuscular

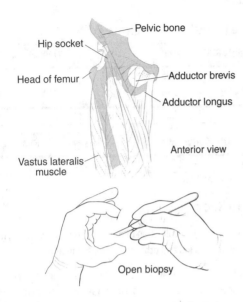

Anterior view

- Pelvic bone
- Hip socket
- Head of femur
- Adductor brevis
- Adductor longus
- Vastus lateralis muscle

Open biopsy

Soft tissue of the hip/pelvis area is biopsied

Explanation

The physician performs a biopsy to evaluate soft tissue. The area for biopsy is in the subcutaneous tissue between the muscle and skin layers in 27040. The suspect area is deeper and may be within muscle in 27041. An incision is made to expose the area. A tumor is typically surrounded by a capsule. The physician makes an incision through the capsule, removing a portion of the tumor for biopsy. The incision is repaired in layers using sutures, staples, and/or Steri-strips.

Coding Tips

An excisional biopsy is not reported separately when a therapeutic excision is performed during the same surgical session. For a needle biopsy of muscle, see 20206. Local anesthesia is included in these services. However, 27041 may be performed under general anesthesia, depending on the age and/or condition of the patient.

ICD-10-CM Diagnostic Codes

C49.21	Malignant neoplasm of connective and soft tissue of right lower limb, including hip ☑
C49.22	Malignant neoplasm of connective and soft tissue of left lower limb, including hip ☑
C49.5	Malignant neoplasm of connective and soft tissue of pelvis
C79.89	Secondary malignant neoplasm of other specified sites
D17.1	Benign lipomatous neoplasm of skin and subcutaneous tissue of trunk
D21.21	Benign neoplasm of connective and other soft tissue of right lower limb, including hip ☑
D21.22	Benign neoplasm of connective and other soft tissue of left lower limb, including hip ☑
D21.5	Benign neoplasm of connective and other soft tissue of pelvis
D48.1	Neoplasm of uncertain behavior of connective and other soft tissue

D49.2	Neoplasm of unspecified behavior of bone, soft tissue, and skin

AMA: **27040** 2018,Sep,7 **27041** 2018,Sep,7

Relative Value Units/Medicare Edits

Non-Facility RVU	Work	PE	MP	Total
27040	2.92	6.98	0.44	10.34
27041	10.18	8.66	1.92	20.76
Facility RVU	**Work**	**PE**	**MP**	**Total**
27040	2.92	2.48	0.44	5.84
27041	10.18	8.66	1.92	20.76

	FUD	Status	MUE	Modifiers				IOM Reference
27040	10	A	2(3)	51	50	N/A	N/A	None
27041	90	A	3(3)	51	50	N/A	N/A	

* with documentation

Terms To Know

benign. Mild or nonmalignant in nature.

biopsy. Tissue or fluid removed for diagnostic purposes through analysis of the cells in the biopsy material.

closure. Repairing an incision or wound by suture or other means.

granuloma. Abnormal, dense collections of cells forming a mass or nodule of chronically inflamed tissue with granulations that is usually associated with an infective process.

joint capsule. Sac-like enclosure enveloping the synovial joint cavity with a fibrous membrane attached to the articular ends of the bones in the joint.

lipoma. Benign tumor containing fat cells and the most common of soft tissue lesions, which are usually painless and asymptomatic, with the exception of an angiolipoma.

malignant. Any condition tending to progress toward death, specifically an invasive tumor with a loss of cellular differentiation that has the ability to spread or metastasize to other body areas.

neoplasm. New abnormal growth, tumor.

soft tissue. Nonepithelial tissues outside of the skeleton.

subcutaneous tissue. Sheet or wide band of adipose (fat) and areolar connective tissue in two layers attached to the dermis.

superficial. On the skin surface or near the surface of any involved structure or field of interest.

wound repair. Surgical closure of a wound is divided into three categories: simple, intermediate, and complex. *simple repair:* Surgical closure of a superficial wound, requiring single layer suturing of the skin epidermis, dermis, or subcutaneous tissue. *intermediate repair:* Surgical closure of a wound requiring closure of one or more of the deeper subcutaneous tissue and non-muscle fascia layers in addition to suturing the skin; contaminated wounds with single layer closure that need extensive cleaning or foreign body removal. *complex repair:* Repair of wounds requiring more than layered closure (debridement, scar revision, stents, retention sutures).

Pelvis/Hip

27047-27048 [27043, 27045]

27047 Excision, tumor, soft tissue of pelvis and hip area, subcutaneous; less than 3 cm

27043 Excision, tumor, soft tissue of pelvis and hip area, subcutaneous; 3 cm or greater

27048 Excision, tumor, soft tissue of pelvis and hip area, subfascial (eg, intramuscular); less than 5 cm

27045 Excision, tumor, soft tissue of pelvis and hip area, subfascial (eg, intramuscular); 5 cm or greater

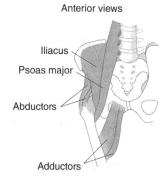

Anterior views

Iliacus
Psoas major
Abductors
Adductors

Excision of a soft tissue tumor of the pelvis or hip area

Explanation

The physician removes a tumor from the soft tissue of the pelvis and hip area that is located in the subcutaneous tissue in 27043 and 27047 and in the deep soft tissue, below the fascial plane, or within the muscle in 27045 and 27048. With the proper anesthesia administered, the physician makes an incision in the skin overlying the mass and dissects to the tumor. The extent of the tumor is identified and a dissection is undertaken all the way around the tumor. A portion of neighboring soft tissue may also be removed to ensure adequate removal of all tumor tissue. A drain may be inserted and the incision is repaired with layers of sutures, staples, or Steri-strips. Report 27047 for excision of a subcutaneous tumor whose resected area is less than 3 cm and 27043 for excision of a subcutaneous tumor 3 cm or greater. Report 27048 for excision of a subfascial or intramuscular tumor whose resected area is less than 5 cm and 27045 for excision of a subfascial or intramuscular tumor 5 cm or greater.

Coding Tips

If significant additional time and effort is documented, append modifier 22 and submit a cover letter and operative report. For soft tissue excision of other sites, see the specific anatomic site. An excisional biopsy is not reported separately when a therapeutic excision is performed during the same surgical session. For excision of cutaneous, benign lesions, see 11400–11406.

ICD-10-CM Diagnostic Codes

C49.21	Malignant neoplasm of connective and soft tissue of right lower limb, including hip ☑
C49.22	Malignant neoplasm of connective and soft tissue of left lower limb, including hip ☑
C49.5	Malignant neoplasm of connective and soft tissue of pelvis
C79.89	Secondary malignant neoplasm of other specified sites
D17.1	Benign lipomatous neoplasm of skin and subcutaneous tissue of trunk
D18.01	Hemangioma of skin and subcutaneous tissue
D21.21	Benign neoplasm of connective and other soft tissue of right lower limb, including hip ☑
D21.22	Benign neoplasm of connective and other soft tissue of left lower limb, including hip ☑
D21.5	Benign neoplasm of connective and other soft tissue of pelvis
D48.1	Neoplasm of uncertain behavior of connective and other soft tissue
D49.2	Neoplasm of unspecified behavior of bone, soft tissue, and skin
L92.3	Foreign body granuloma of the skin and subcutaneous tissue

AMA: **27043** 2018,Sep,7 **27045** 2018,Sep,7 **27047** 2018,Sep,7 **27048** 2018,Sep,7

Relative Value Units/Medicare Edits

Non-Facility RVU	Work	PE	MP	Total
27047	4.94	8.68	1.03	14.65
27043	6.88	5.38	1.57	13.83
27048	8.85	7.31	1.91	18.07
27045	11.13	8.26	2.32	21.71
Facility RVU	Work	PE	MP	Total
27047	4.94	4.63	1.03	10.6
27043	6.88	5.38	1.57	13.83
27048	8.85	7.31	1.91	18.07
27045	11.13	8.26	2.32	21.71

	FUD	Status	MUE	Modifiers				IOM Reference
27047	90	A	2(3)	51	50	N/A	N/A	None
27043	90	A	2(3)	51	50	N/A	N/A	
27048	90	A	2(3)	51	50	62*	80	
27045	90	A	3(3)	51	50	62*	80	

* with documentation

Terms To Know

dissection. Separating by cutting tissue or body structures apart.

fascia. Fibrous sheet or band of tissue that envelops organs, muscles, and groupings of muscles.

malignant. Any condition tending to progress toward death, specifically an invasive tumor with a loss of cellular differentiation that has the ability to spread or metastasize to other body areas.

soft tissue. Nonepithelial tissues outside of the skeleton.

subcutaneous tissue. Sheet or wide band of adipose (fat) and areolar connective tissue in two layers attached to the dermis.

tumor. Pathological swelling or enlargement; a neoplastic growth of uncontrolled, abnormal multiplication of cells.

Pelvis/Hip

27049 [27059]

27049 Radical resection of tumor (eg, sarcoma), soft tissue of pelvis and hip area; less than 5 cm

27059 Radical resection of tumor (eg, sarcoma), soft tissue of pelvis and hip area; 5 cm or greater

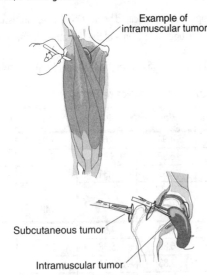

Example of intramuscular tumor

Subcutaneous tumor

Intramuscular tumor

Radical resection of soft tissue tumor of the pelvis or hip area

Explanation

The physician removes a malignant soft tissue tumor (i.e., sarcoma) from the pelvis and hip area, not involving bone. An incision is made over the tumor and dissection exposes it. The tumor and any adjacent tissue that may be affected by the spread of the neoplasm are excised. Large resections may be needed. The type and stage of the lesion determine the extent of the tumor margin resection area. Muscle or fascia may need to be repaired and drains may be placed. The surgical wound is closed using simple or intermediate repair or separately reportable complex closure, adjacent tissue transfer, or graft. Report 27049 if the resection area is less than 5 cm. Report 27059 if the resection area is 5 cm or greater.

Coding Tips

For excision of a soft tissue tumor, pelvic and hip area, subcutaneous, see 27043 and 27047; subfascial, see 27045 and 27048. For radical resection of cutaneous tumors, see 11600–11606.

ICD-10-CM Diagnostic Codes

C49.21	Malignant neoplasm of connective and soft tissue of right lower limb, including hip ☑
C49.22	Malignant neoplasm of connective and soft tissue of left lower limb, including hip ☑
C49.5	Malignant neoplasm of connective and soft tissue of pelvis
C79.89	Secondary malignant neoplasm of other specified sites

AMA: 27049 2018,Sep,7 **27059** 2018,Sep,7

Relative Value Units/Medicare Edits

Non-Facility RVU	Work	PE	MP	Total
27049	21.55	13.35	4.79	39.69
27059	29.35	17.98	5.89	53.22
Facility RVU	**Work**	**PE**	**MP**	**Total**
27049	21.55	13.35	4.79	39.69
27059	29.35	17.98	5.89	53.22

	FUD	Status	MUE	Modifiers				IOM Reference
27049	90	A	1(3)	51	50	62*	80	None
27059	90	A	1(3)	51	50	62*	80	

* with documentation

Terms To Know

dissection. Separating by cutting tissue or body structures apart.

lesion. Area of damaged tissue that has lost continuity or function, due to disease or trauma.

malignant neoplasm. Any cancerous tumor or lesion exhibiting uncontrolled tissue growth that can progressively invade other parts of the body with its disease-generating cells.

margin. Boundary, edge, or border, as of a surface or structure.

radical resection. Removal of an entire tumor (e.g., malignant neoplasm) along with a large area of surrounding tissue, including adjacent lymph nodes that may have been infiltrated.

sarcoma. Malignant tumor arising in connective tissue, bone, cartilage, or striated muscle that spreads to neighboring tissue through the bloodstream.

soft tissue. Nonepithelial tissues outside of the skeleton that includes subcutaneous adipose tissue, fibrous tissue, fascia, muscles, blood and lymph vessels, and peripheral nervous system tissue.

tumor. Pathological swelling or enlargement; a neoplastic growth of uncontrolled, abnormal multiplication of cells.

Pelvis/Hip

27075

27075 Radical resection of tumor; wing of ilium, 1 pubic or ischial ramus or symphysis pubis

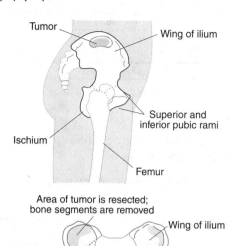

Tumor
Wing of ilium
Superior and inferior pubic rami
Ischium
Femur

Area of tumor is resected; bone segments are removed
Wing of ilium
Ischial ramus
Symphysis pubis

Explanation

The physician performs a radical resection (excision) of a tumor. The patient is positioned for a lithotomy with the buttock elevated. For resection of a tumor of the pubis and/or ischium, an incision is made from the pubic tubercle to the ischial tuberosity. The adductor and obturator muscles are detached from the pubis and ischium. Additional dissection is carried down to better expose the pubis and ischium. The remaining muscles and ligaments are released (freed by incision) while the pudendal and genital nerves and vessels are protected. The bone(s) is separated and cut with bone-cutting forceps and an osteotome or saw. The bone segments are removed. A separate incision is made to resect the ilium. The portion of the ilium needing resection is dissected out by releasing muscles, tendons, and ligaments. The incisions are repaired in layers.

Coding Tips

An excisional biopsy is not reported separately when a therapeutic excision is performed during the same surgical session. If significant additional time and effort is documented, append modifier 22 and submit a cover letter and operative report. For excision of a bone cyst or benign tumor, with or without autograft, superficial, see 27065; deep, see 27066; with autograft requiring separate incision, see 27067.

ICD-10-CM Diagnostic Codes

C41.4	Malignant neoplasm of pelvic bones, sacrum and coccyx
C79.51	Secondary malignant neoplasm of bone
C7B.03	Secondary carcinoid tumors of bone
D16.8	Benign neoplasm of pelvic bones, sacrum and coccyx

AMA: 27075 2019,May,7; 2018,Sep,7

Relative Value Units/Medicare Edits

Non-Facility RVU	Work	PE	MP	Total
27075	32.71	22.16	6.51	61.38
Facility RVU	**Work**	**PE**	**MP**	**Total**
27075	32.71	22.16	6.51	61.38

	FUD	Status	MUE	Modifiers				IOM Reference
27075	90	A	1(3)	51	N/A	62*	80	None

* with documentation

Terms To Know

dissection. Separating by cutting tissue or body structures apart.

ischial tuberosity. Bony projection of the lower end of the ischium easily identified as the weight-bearing point in a sitting position.

radical resection. Removal of an entire tumor (e.g., malignant neoplasm) along with a large area of surrounding tissue, including adjacent lymph nodes that may have been infiltrated.

symphysis. Joint that unifies two opposed bones by a junction of bony surfaces to a plate of fibrocartilage.

tumor. Pathological swelling or enlargement; a neoplastic growth of uncontrolled, abnormal multiplication of cells.

27076

27076 Radical resection of tumor; ilium, including acetabulum, both pubic rami, or ischium and acetabulum

Resected portion of pelvis is removed

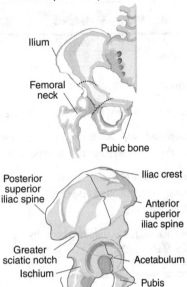

Lateral view of right hip and socket

Explanation

The physician performs a radical resection (excision) of a tumor. The patient is placed in a lateral decubitus (lying on the side) position. The physician makes an incision from the posterior crest of the ilium to the symphysis pubis. A vertical extension of this incision is made, extending into the proximal thigh. The physician carries dissection down, while protecting the femoral artery, vein, and nerve. The physician uses a saw to divide (separate) the ilium and the pubic bone. Any remaining soft tissue is released (freed by incision) from the segment of bone to be removed. The inguinal ligament is reattached to the iliopsoas tendon to prevent a hernia. The incision is repaired in layers over a suction drain.

Coding Tips

An excisional biopsy is not reported separately when a therapeutic excision is performed during the same surgical session. For excision of a bone cyst or benign tumor, with or without autograft, superficial, see 27065; deep, see 27066; with autograft requiring separate incision, see 27067. For radical resection of a tumor of the wing of ilium, one pubic or ischial ramus or symphysis pubis, see 27075. For excision of a soft tissue tumor, pelvic and hip area, subcutaneous, see 27047 and 27043; subfascial, see 27048 and 27045. For partial excision (craterization, saucerization) (e.g., for osteomyelitis or bone abscess), superficial, see 27070; deep, see 27071.

ICD-10-CM Diagnostic Codes

C41.4	Malignant neoplasm of pelvic bones, sacrum and coccyx
C79.51	Secondary malignant neoplasm of bone
C7B.03	Secondary carcinoid tumors of bone
D16.8	Benign neoplasm of pelvic bones, sacrum and coccyx

AMA: 27076 2019,May,7; 2018,Sep,7

Relative Value Units/Medicare Edits

Non-Facility RVU	Work	PE	MP	Total
27076	40.21	26.01	8.03	74.25
Facility RVU	**Work**	**PE**	**MP**	**Total**
27076	40.21	26.01	8.03	74.25

	FUD	Status	MUE	Modifiers				IOM Reference
27076	90	A	1(2)	51	N/A	62*	80	None

* with documentation

Terms To Know

acetabulum. Cup-shaped socket in the hipbone into which the head of the femur fits, forming a ball-and-socket joint.

iliopsoas tendon. Fibrous tissue that connects muscle to bone in the pelvic region, common to the iliacus and psoas major.

ilium. Part of the iliac bone. Superior part of the hip bone that expands.

radical resection. Removal of an entire tumor (e.g., malignant neoplasm) along with a large area of surrounding tissue, including adjacent lymph nodes that may have been infiltrated.

tumor. Pathological swelling or enlargement; a neoplastic growth of uncontrolled, abnormal multiplication of cells.

Pelvis/Hip

27077

27077   Radical resection of tumor; innominate bone, total

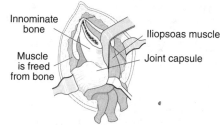

Joint capsule is incised and head of femur is freed from acetabulum

Innominate bone

Iliopsoas muscle

Muscle is freed from bone

Joint capsule

Innominate bone is removed from remainder of hip and sacrum

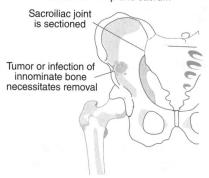

Sacroiliac joint is sectioned

Tumor or infection of innominate bone necessitates removal

Explanation

The physician performs a radical resection (excision) of a tumor of the innominate bone in which the bone is removed in total. The patient is placed in a supine position with the involved side elevated. The physician makes an incision extending from the posterosuperior iliac spine, along the iliac crest, to the symphysis pubis. A vertical incision is made extending into the upper thigh. The abdominal muscles are detached. All muscles that attach to the innominate bone are divided and detached. Vessels and nerves are also separated and/or ligated. The hip joint capsule is incised. The sacroiliac joint is exposed and divided with an osteotome. The innominate bone is removed. The incision is repaired in layers.

Coding Tips

An excisional biopsy is not reported separately when a therapeutic excision is performed during the same surgical session. For excision of a bone cyst or benign tumor, with or without autograft, superficial, see 27065; deep, see 27066; with autograft requiring separate incision, see 27067. For radical resection of a tumor of the wing of ilium, one pubic or ischial ramus or symphysis pubis, see 27075; ilium, including acetabulum, both pubic rami, or ischium and acetabulum, see 27076. For partial excision (craterization, saucerization) (e.g., for osteomyelitis or bone abscess), superficial, see 27070; deep, see 27071.

ICD-10-CM Diagnostic Codes

C41.4	Malignant neoplasm of pelvic bones, sacrum and coccyx
C79.51	Secondary malignant neoplasm of bone
C7B.03	Secondary carcinoid tumors of bone
D16.8	Benign neoplasm of pelvic bones, sacrum and coccyx

AMA: 27077 2019,May,7; 2018,Sep,7

Relative Value Units/Medicare Edits

Non-Facility RVU	Work	PE	MP	Total
27077	45.21	28.58	9.02	82.81
Facility RVU	Work	PE	MP	Total
27077	45.21	28.58	9.02	82.81

	FUD	Status	MUE	Modifiers				IOM Reference
27077	90	A	1(2)	51	N/A	62*	80	None

* with documentation

Terms To Know

excision. Surgical removal of an organ or tissue.

malignant neoplasm. Any cancerous tumor or lesion exhibiting uncontrolled tissue growth that can progressively invade other parts of the body with its disease-generating cells.

radical resection. Removal of an entire tumor (e.g., malignant neoplasm) along with a large area of surrounding tissue, including adjacent lymph nodes that may have been infiltrated.

supine. Lying on the back.

tumor. Pathological swelling or enlargement; a neoplastic growth of uncontrolled, abnormal multiplication of cells.

Pelvis/Hip

27078

27078 Radical resection of tumor; ischial tuberosity and greater trochanter of femur

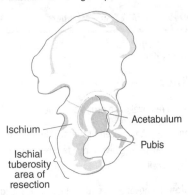

Lateral view of right hip and socket

Acetabulum
Ischium
Pubis
Ischial tuberosity area of resection

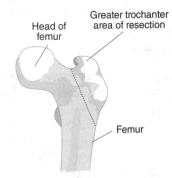

Head of femur
Greater trochanter area of resection
Femur

Explanation

The physician performs a radical resection (excision) of a tumor of the ischial tuberosity and greater trochanter of the femur. The patient is positioned prone to access the ischial tuberosity and a lateral decubitus position to access the greater trochanter. The physician makes an incision overlying the involved bone and dissects through the deep layers. The ischial tuberosity or greater trochanter is exposed and resected. The wound is closed in layers with sutures.

Coding Tips

An excisional biopsy is not reported separately when a therapeutic excision is performed during the same surgical session. Report any free grafts or flaps separately. Bone grafts from a distant site may be reported separately with codes 20900–20902. For radical resection of a tumor of the wing of ilium, one pubic or ischial ramus or symphysis pubis, see 27075; ilium, including acetabulum, both pubic rami, or ischium and acetabulum, see 27076; innominate bone, total, see 27077. For excision of a bone cyst or benign tumor, with or without autograft, superficial, see 27065; deep, see 27066; with autograft requiring separate incision, see 27067. For partial excision (craterization, saucerization) (e.g., for osteomyelitis or bone abscess), superficial, see 27070; deep, see 27071.

ICD-10-CM Diagnostic Codes

C40.21	Malignant neoplasm of long bones of right lower limb ☑
C40.22	Malignant neoplasm of long bones of left lower limb ☑
C41.4	Malignant neoplasm of pelvic bones, sacrum and coccyx
C79.51	Secondary malignant neoplasm of bone
C7B.03	Secondary carcinoid tumors of bone
D16.21	Benign neoplasm of long bones of right lower limb ☑
D16.22	Benign neoplasm of long bones of left lower limb ☑
D16.8	Benign neoplasm of pelvic bones, sacrum and coccyx

AMA: 27078 2019,May,7; 2018,Sep,7

Relative Value Units/Medicare Edits

Non-Facility RVU	Work	PE	MP	Total
27078	32.21	21.91	6.43	60.55
Facility RVU	**Work**	**PE**	**MP**	**Total**
27078	32.21	21.91	6.43	60.55

	FUD	Status	MUE	Modifiers				IOM Reference
27078	90	A	1(2)	51	50	62*	80	None

* with documentation

Terms To Know

decubitus. Patient lying on the side.

dissection. Separating by cutting tissue or body structures apart.

ischial tuberosity. Bony projection of the lower end of the ischium easily identified as the weight-bearing point in a sitting position.

malignant neoplasm. Any cancerous tumor or lesion exhibiting uncontrolled tissue growth that can progressively invade other parts of the body with its disease-generating cells.

radical resection. Removal of an entire tumor (e.g., malignant neoplasm) along with a large area of surrounding tissue, including adjacent lymph nodes that may have been infiltrated.

tumor. Pathological swelling or enlargement; a neoplastic growth of uncontrolled, abnormal multiplication of cells.

Pelvis/Hip

27323-27324

27323 Biopsy, soft tissue of thigh or knee area; superficial
27324   deep (subfascial or intramuscular)

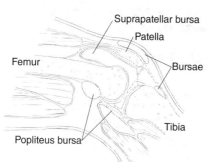

Side view schematic

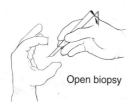

Open biopsy

A tumor in the soft tissue of the
thigh or knee is excised

Explanation

The physician performs a biopsy of the soft tissues of the thigh or knee area. With proper anesthesia administered, an incision is made over the biopsy area. Dissection is carried down within the superficial soft tissue layers in 27323, usually the subcutaneous fat to the uppermost fascial layer. In 27324, dissection is taken deep within the soft tissue, such as into the fascial layer or within the muscle. A portion of the tissue is excised and submitted for pathology. The area is irrigated and the incision is closed with layered sutures, staples, or Steri-strips.

Coding Tips

An excisional biopsy is not reported separately when a therapeutic excision is performed during the same surgical session. Local anesthesia is included in this service. However, 27324 may be performed under general anesthesia, depending on the age and/or condition of the patient. For needle biopsy of muscle, see 20206. Surgical trays, A4550, are not separately reimbursed by Medicare; however, other third-party payers may cover them. Check with the specific payer to determine coverage.

ICD-10-CM Diagnostic Codes

C49.21	Malignant neoplasm of connective and soft tissue of right lower limb, including hip ☑
C49.22	Malignant neoplasm of connective and soft tissue of left lower limb, including hip ☑
C76.51	Malignant neoplasm of right lower limb ☑
C76.52	Malignant neoplasm of left lower limb ☑
C79.89	Secondary malignant neoplasm of other specified sites
D21.21	Benign neoplasm of connective and other soft tissue of right lower limb, including hip ☑
D21.22	Benign neoplasm of connective and other soft tissue of left lower limb, including hip ☑
D36.7	Benign neoplasm of other specified sites
D48.1	Neoplasm of uncertain behavior of connective and other soft tissue
D48.7	Neoplasm of uncertain behavior of other specified sites
D49.2	Neoplasm of unspecified behavior of bone, soft tissue, and skin
D49.89	Neoplasm of unspecified behavior of other specified sites
R22.41	Localized swelling, mass and lump, right lower limb ☑
R22.42	Localized swelling, mass and lump, left lower limb ☑
R22.43	Localized swelling, mass and lump, lower limb, bilateral ☑

AMA: **27323** 2018,Sep,7; 2018,Jan,8; 2017,Jan,8; 2016,Jan,13; 2015,Jan,16
27324 2018,Sep,7; 2018,Jan,8; 2017,Jan,8; 2016,Jan,13; 2015,Jan,16

Relative Value Units/Medicare Edits

Non-Facility RVU	Work	PE	MP	Total
27323	2.33	5.53	0.34	8.2
27324	5.04	5.87	1.14	12.05
Facility RVU	**Work**	**PE**	**MP**	**Total**
27323	2.33	2.45	0.34	5.12
27324	5.04	5.87	1.14	12.05

	FUD	Status	MUE	Modifiers				IOM Reference
27323	10	A	2(3)	51	50	N/A	N/A	None
27324	90	A	3(3)	51	50	N/A	N/A	

* with documentation

Terms To Know

fascia. Fibrous sheet or band of tissue that envelops organs, muscles, and groupings of muscles.

soft tissue. Nonepithelial tissues outside of the skeleton that includes subcutaneous adipose tissue, fibrous tissue, fascia, muscles, blood and lymph vessels, and peripheral nervous system tissue.

subfascial. Beneath the band of fibrous tissue that lies deep to the skin, encloses muscles, and separates their layers.

superficial. On the skin surface or near the surface of any involved structure or field of interest.

Femur/Knee

27327-27328 [27337, 27339]

27327 Excision, tumor, soft tissue of thigh or knee area, subcutaneous; less than 3 cm

27337 Excision, tumor, soft tissue of thigh or knee area, subcutaneous; 3 cm or greater

27328 Excision, tumor, soft tissue of thigh or knee area, subfascial (eg, intramuscular); less than 5 cm

27339 Excision, tumor, soft tissue of thigh or knee area, subfascial (eg, intramuscular); 5 cm or greater

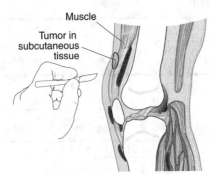

Excision of a soft tissue tumor
of the thigh or knee area

Explanation

The physician removes a tumor from the soft tissue of the thigh or knee area that is located in the subcutaneous tissue in 27327 and 27337 and in the deep soft tissue, below the fascial plane, or within the muscle in 27328 and 27339. With the proper anesthesia administered, the physician makes an incision in the skin overlying the mass and dissects to the tumor. The extent of the tumor is identified and a dissection is undertaken all the way around the tumor. A portion of neighboring soft tissue may also be removed to ensure adequate removal of all tumor tissue. A drain may be inserted and the incision is repaired with layers of sutures, staples, or Steri-strips. Report 27327 for excision of a subcutaneous tumor whose resected area is less than 3 cm, and 27337 for excision of a subcutaneous tumor that is 3 cm or greater. Report 27328 for excision of a subfascial or intramuscular tumor whose resected area is less than 5 cm, and 27339 for excision of a subfascial or intramuscular tumor that is 5 cm or greater.

Coding Tips

An excisional biopsy is not reported separately when a therapeutic excision is performed during the same surgical session. For radical resection of a soft tissue tumor, thigh or knee area, see 27329 and 27364; femur or knee tumor, see 27365. For excision of cutaneous, benign lesions, see 11400–11406.

ICD-10-CM Diagnostic Codes

C49.21	Malignant neoplasm of connective and soft tissue of right lower limb, including hip ☑
C49.22	Malignant neoplasm of connective and soft tissue of left lower limb, including hip ☑
D17.23	Benign lipomatous neoplasm of skin and subcutaneous tissue of right leg ☑
D17.24	Benign lipomatous neoplasm of skin and subcutaneous tissue of left leg ☑
D21.21	Benign neoplasm of connective and other soft tissue of right lower limb, including hip ☑
D21.22	Benign neoplasm of connective and other soft tissue of left lower limb, including hip ☑

AMA: **27327** 2018,Sep,7 **27328** 2018,Sep,7; 2018,Jan,8; 2017,Jan,8; 2016,Nov,9 **27337** 2018,Sep,7 **27339** 2018,Sep,7

Relative Value Units/Medicare Edits

Non-Facility RVU	Work	PE	MP	Total
27327	3.96	10.17	0.82	14.95
27337	5.91	5.14	1.34	12.39
27328	8.85	7.66	1.88	18.39
27339	11.13	8.68	2.42	22.23
Facility RVU	Work	PE	MP	Total
27327	3.96	4.44	0.82	9.22
27337	5.91	5.14	1.34	12.39
27328	8.85	7.66	1.88	18.39
27339	11.13	8.68	2.42	22.23

	FUD	Status	MUE	Modifiers				IOM Reference
27327	90	A	5(3)	51	50	N/A	N/A	None
27337	90	A	3(3)	51	50	N/A	80	
27328	90	A	3(3)	51	50	N/A	N/A	
27339	90	A	4(3)	51	50	N/A	80	

* with documentation

Terms To Know

deep fascia. Sheet of dense, fibrous tissue holding muscle groups together below the hypodermis layer or subcutaneous fat layer that lines the extremities and trunk.

dissection. Separating by cutting tissue or body structures apart.

intramuscular. Within a muscle.

ligament. Band or sheet of fibrous tissue that connects the articular surfaces of bones or supports visceral organs.

soft tissue. Nonepithelial tissues outside of the skeleton.

subfascial. Beneath the band of fibrous tissue that lies deep to the skin, encloses muscles, and separates their layers.

27364 [27329]

27329 Radical resection of tumor (eg, sarcoma), soft tissue of thigh or knee area; less than 5 cm
27364 5 cm or greater

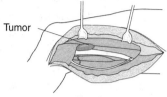

Radical resection of tumor includes extensive soft tissue removal, including nerves and muscle

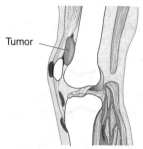

Radical resection of soft tissue tumor of the thigh or knee area

Explanation

The physician performs a radical resection (excision) of a malignant soft tissue tumor (i.e., sarcoma) from the thigh or knee area, not involving bone. An incision is made over the tumor and dissection exposes it. The tumor and any adjacent tissue that may be affected by the spread of the neoplasm are excised. Large resections may be needed. The type and stage of the lesion determines the extent of the tumor margin resection area. Muscle or fascia may need to be repaired and drains may be placed. The surgical wound is closed using simple or intermediate repair or separately reportable complex closure, adjacent tissue transfer, or graft. Report 27329 for a resection area of less than 5 cm and 27364 for a resection area 5 cm or greater.

Coding Tips

For soft tissue tumor excision, thigh or knee area, subcutaneous, see 27327 and 27337; subfascial, see 27328 and 27339. For radical resection of cutaneous tumors, see 11600–11606. An excisional biopsy is not reported separately when a therapeutic excision is performed during the same surgical session.

ICD-10-CM Diagnostic Codes

C49.21 Malignant neoplasm of connective and soft tissue of right lower limb, including hip ☑
C49.22 Malignant neoplasm of connective and soft tissue of left lower limb, including hip ☑

AMA: **27329** 2018,Sep,7 **27364** 2018,Sep,7

Relative Value Units/Medicare Edits

Non-Facility RVU	Work	PE	MP	Total
27329	15.72	11.49	3.42	30.63
27364	24.49	16.32	5.2	46.01
Facility RVU	Work	PE	MP	Total
27329	15.72	11.49	3.42	30.63
27364	24.49	16.32	5.2	46.01

	FUD	Status	MUE	Modifiers				IOM Reference
27329	90	A	1(3)	51	50	62*	80	None
27364	90	A	1(3)	51	50	62*	80	

* with documentation

Terms To Know

dissection. Separating by cutting tissue or body structures apart.

fascia. Fibrous sheet or band of tissue that envelops organs, muscles, and groupings of muscles.

malignant neoplasm. Any cancerous tumor or lesion exhibiting uncontrolled tissue growth that can progressively invade other parts of the body with its disease-generating cells.

margin. Boundary, edge, or border, as of a surface or structure.

radical resection. Removal of an entire tumor (e.g., malignant neoplasm) along with a large area of surrounding tissue, including adjacent lymph nodes that may have been infiltrated.

sarcoma. Malignant tumor arising in connective tissue, bone, cartilage, or striated muscle that spreads to neighboring tissue through the bloodstream.

soft tissue. Nonepithelial tissues outside of the skeleton that includes subcutaneous adipose tissue, fibrous tissue, fascia, muscles, blood and lymph vessels, and peripheral nervous system tissue.

tumor. Pathological swelling or enlargement; a neoplastic growth of uncontrolled, abnormal multiplication of cells.

27603-27604

27603 Incision and drainage, leg or ankle; deep abscess or hematoma
27604 infected bursa

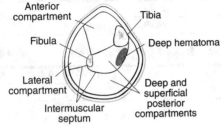

Cross section depicting compartments of lower leg

Anterior compartment
Tibia
Fibula
Deep hematoma
Lateral compartment
Deep and superficial posterior compartments
Intermuscular septum

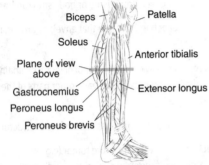

Select muscles and tendons

Biceps
Patella
Soleus
Plane of view above
Anterior tibialis
Gastrocnemius
Peroneus longus
Extensor longus
Peroneus brevis

A deep abscess or hematoma of the leg or ankle is incised and drained

Explanation

The physician drains an abscess or hematoma in 27603 or an infected bursa in 27604 from deep within the leg or ankle. The physician makes an incision in the leg or ankle overlying the site of the abscess, hematoma, or bursa to be incised. Dissection is carried through the deep subcutaneous tissues and may be continued into the fascia or muscle to expose the abscess or hematoma. The incision may be extended if the mass is larger than expected. When the infected bursa, abscess, or hematoma is identified, it is incised and the contents are drained. The area is irrigated and the incision is repaired in layers with sutures, staples, and/or Steri-strips; closed with drains in place; or simply left open to further facilitate drainage of infection.

Coding Tips

For incision and drainage of abscess, subcutaneous, simple or single, see 10060; complicated or multiple, see 10061. Incision and drainage of a hematoma, seroma, or fluid collection, superficial, see 10140. For incision and drainage procedures performed on the femur and knee joint area, see 27301.

ICD-10-CM Diagnostic Codes

L02.415	Cutaneous abscess of right lower limb ☑
L02.416	Cutaneous abscess of left lower limb ☑
L03.115	Cellulitis of right lower limb ☑
L03.116	Cellulitis of left lower limb ☑
L03.125	Acute lymphangitis of right lower limb ☑
L03.126	Acute lymphangitis of left lower limb ☑
L76.01	Intraoperative hemorrhage and hematoma of skin and subcutaneous tissue complicating a dermatologic procedure
L76.21	Postprocedural hemorrhage of skin and subcutaneous tissue following a dermatologic procedure
L76.31	Postprocedural hematoma of skin and subcutaneous tissue following a dermatologic procedure
L76.33	Postprocedural seroma of skin and subcutaneous tissue following a dermatologic procedure
L97.211	Non-pressure chronic ulcer of right calf limited to breakdown of skin ☑
L97.212	Non-pressure chronic ulcer of right calf with fat layer exposed ☑
L97.213	Non-pressure chronic ulcer of right calf with necrosis of muscle ☑
L97.214	Non-pressure chronic ulcer of right calf with necrosis of bone ☑
L97.215	Non-pressure chronic ulcer of right calf with muscle involvement without evidence of necrosis ☑
L97.216	Non-pressure chronic ulcer of right calf with bone involvement without evidence of necrosis ☑
L97.218	Non-pressure chronic ulcer of right calf with other specified severity ☑
L97.221	Non-pressure chronic ulcer of left calf limited to breakdown of skin ☑
L97.222	Non-pressure chronic ulcer of left calf with fat layer exposed ☑
L97.223	Non-pressure chronic ulcer of left calf with necrosis of muscle ☑
L97.224	Non-pressure chronic ulcer of left calf with necrosis of bone ☑
L97.312	Non-pressure chronic ulcer of right ankle with fat layer exposed ☑
L97.313	Non-pressure chronic ulcer of right ankle with necrosis of muscle ☑
L97.314	Non-pressure chronic ulcer of right ankle with necrosis of bone ☑
L97.315	Non-pressure chronic ulcer of right ankle with muscle involvement without evidence of necrosis ☑
L97.316	Non-pressure chronic ulcer of right ankle with bone involvement without evidence of necrosis ☑
L97.322	Non-pressure chronic ulcer of left ankle with fat layer exposed ☑
L97.323	Non-pressure chronic ulcer of left ankle with necrosis of muscle ☑
L97.324	Non-pressure chronic ulcer of left ankle with necrosis of bone ☑
M79.81	Nontraumatic hematoma of soft tissue
M96.810	Intraoperative hemorrhage and hematoma of a musculoskeletal structure complicating a musculoskeletal system procedure
M96.811	Intraoperative hemorrhage and hematoma of a musculoskeletal structure complicating other procedure
M96.830	Postprocedural hemorrhage of a musculoskeletal structure following a musculoskeletal system procedure
M96.831	Postprocedural hemorrhage of a musculoskeletal structure following other procedure
M96.840	Postprocedural hematoma of a musculoskeletal structure following a musculoskeletal system procedure
M96.842	Postprocedural seroma of a musculoskeletal structure following a musculoskeletal system procedure
S80.11XA	Contusion of right lower leg, initial encounter ☑
S81.821A	Laceration with foreign body, right lower leg, initial encounter ☑
S81.822A	Laceration with foreign body, left lower leg, initial encounter ☑
S81.841A	Puncture wound with foreign body, right lower leg, initial encounter ☑
S81.842A	Puncture wound with foreign body, left lower leg, initial encounter ☑
S90.01XA	Contusion of right ankle, initial encounter ☑
S91.021A	Laceration with foreign body, right ankle, initial encounter ☑
S91.022A	Laceration with foreign body, left ankle, initial encounter ☑

| S91.041A | Puncture wound with foreign body, right ankle, initial encounter ☑ |
| S91.042A | Puncture wound with foreign body, left ankle, initial encounter ☑ |

AMA: **27603** 2018,Sep,7 **27604** 2018,Sep,7

Relative Value Units/Medicare Edits

Non-Facility RVU	Work	PE	MP	Total
27603	5.23	9.79	1.0	16.02
27604	4.59	8.69	0.68	13.96
Facility RVU	Work	PE	MP	Total
27603	5.23	5.33	1.0	11.56
27604	4.59	4.42	0.68	9.69

	FUD	Status	MUE	Modifiers				IOM Reference
27603	90	A	2(3)	51	50	N/A	N/A	None
27604	90	A	2(3)	51	50	N/A	80*	

* with documentation

Terms To Know

abscess. Circumscribed collection of pus resulting from bacteria, frequently associated with swelling and other signs of inflammation.

bursa. Cavity or sac containing fluid that occurs between articulating surfaces and serves to reduce friction from moving parts.

hematoma. Tumor-like collection of blood in some part of the body caused by a break in a blood vessel wall, usually as a result of trauma.

pressure ulcers. Progressively eroding skin lesion produced by inflamed necrotic tissue as it sloughs off, caused by continual pressure impeding blood circulation, especially over bony areas, when a patient lies still for too long without changing position.

27613-27614

| 27613 | Biopsy, soft tissue of leg or ankle area; superficial |
| 27614 | deep (subfascial or intramuscular) |

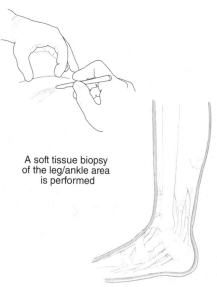

A soft tissue biopsy
of the leg/ankle area
is performed

Medial view

Explanation

The physician performs a biopsy of the soft tissues of the leg or ankle area. With proper anesthesia administered, an incision is made over the biopsy area. Dissection is carried down within the superficial soft tissue layers in 27613, usually the subcutaneous fat to the uppermost fascial layer. In 27614, dissection is taken deep within the soft tissue, such as into the fascial layer or within the muscle. A portion of the tissue is excised and submitted for pathology. The area is irrigated and the incision is closed with layered sutures, staples, or Steri-strips.

Coding Tips

A biopsy is not identified separately when followed by excisional removal during the same operative session. For a needle biopsy of muscle, see 20206. For radical resection of a soft tissue tumor, leg or ankle area, see 27615–27616. For excision of a soft tissue tumor, leg or ankle area, subcutaneous, see 27618 and 27632; subfascial, see 27619 and 27634.

ICD-10-CM Diagnostic Codes

C49.21	Malignant neoplasm of connective and soft tissue of right lower limb, including hip ☑
C49.22	Malignant neoplasm of connective and soft tissue of left lower limb, including hip ☑
C76.51	Malignant neoplasm of right lower limb ☑
C76.52	Malignant neoplasm of left lower limb ☑
C79.89	Secondary malignant neoplasm of other specified sites
D21.21	Benign neoplasm of connective and other soft tissue of right lower limb, including hip ☑
D36.7	Benign neoplasm of other specified sites
D48.1	Neoplasm of uncertain behavior of connective and other soft tissue
D48.2	Neoplasm of uncertain behavior of peripheral nerves and autonomic nervous system
D48.7	Neoplasm of uncertain behavior of other specified sites

D49.2	Neoplasm of unspecified behavior of bone, soft tissue, and skin			
D49.89	Neoplasm of unspecified behavior of other specified sites			
R22.41	Localized swelling, mass and lump, right lower limb ☑			
R22.42	Localized swelling, mass and lump, left lower limb ☑			
R22.43	Localized swelling, mass and lump, lower limb, bilateral ☑			

AMA: 27613 2018,Sep,7 **27614** 2018,Sep,7

Relative Value Units/Medicare Edits

Non-Facility RVU	Work	PE	MP	Total
27613	2.22	5.04	0.28	7.54
27614	5.8	10.68	0.94	17.42
Facility RVU	**Work**	**PE**	**MP**	**Total**
27613	2.22	2.17	0.28	4.67
27614	5.8	5.31	0.94	12.05

	FUD	Status	MUE	Modifiers				IOM Reference
27613	10	A	3(3)	51	50	N/A	N/A	None
27614	90	A	3(3)	51	50	N/A	N/A	

* with documentation

Terms To Know

benign. Mild or nonmalignant in nature.

biopsy. Tissue or fluid removed for diagnostic purposes through analysis of the cells in the biopsy material.

cellulitis. Infection of the skin and subcutaneous tissues, most often caused by Staphylococcus or Streptococcus bacteria secondary to a cutaneous lesion. Progression of the inflammation may lead to abscess and tissue death, or even systemic infection-like bacteremia.

lesion. Area of damaged tissue that has lost continuity or function, due to disease or trauma. Lesions may be located on internal structures such as the brain, nerves, or kidneys, or visible on the skin.

neoplasm. New abnormal growth, tumor.

soft tissue. Nonepithelial tissues outside of the skeleton that includes subcutaneous adipose tissue, fibrous tissue, fascia, muscles, blood and lymph vessels, and peripheral nervous system tissue.

wound repair. Surgical closure of a wound is divided into three categories: simple, intermediate, and complex. *simple repair:* Surgical closure of a superficial wound, requiring single layer suturing of the skin epidermis, dermis, or subcutaneous tissue. *intermediate repair:* Surgical closure of a wound requiring closure of one or more of the deeper subcutaneous tissue and non-muscle fascia layers in addition to suturing the skin; contaminated wounds with single layer closure that need extensive cleaning or foreign body removal. *complex repair:* Repair of wounds requiring more than layered closure (debridement, scar revision, stents, retention sutures).

27615-27616

27615	Radical resection of tumor (eg, sarcoma), soft tissue of leg or ankle area; less than 5 cm
27616	5 cm or greater

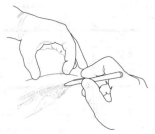

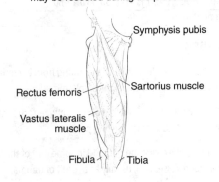

A radical resection of soft tissues of the leg/ankle region is performed to remove a tumor. Entire muscles and their compartments may be resected during the procedure

Symphysis pubis
Rectus femoris
Sartorius muscle
Vastus lateralis muscle
Fibula
Tibia

Explanation

The physician performs a radical resection (excision) of a malignant soft tissue tumor (i.e., sarcoma) from the leg or ankle area, not involving bone. An incision is made over the tumor and dissection exposes it. The tumor and any adjacent tissue that may be affected by the spread of the neoplasm are excised. Large resections may be needed. The type and stage of the lesion determine the extent of the tumor margin resection area. Muscle or fascia may need to be repaired and drains may be placed. The surgical wound is closed using simple or intermediate repair or separately reportable complex closure, adjacent tissue transfer, or graft. Report 27615 for a resected area that is less than 5 cm and 27616 for a resected area that is 5 cm or greater.

Coding Tips

An excisional biopsy is not reported separately when a therapeutic excision is performed during the same surgical session. For excision of a soft tissue tumor, leg or ankle area, subcutaneous, see 27618 and 27632; subfascial, see 27619 and 27634. For radical resection of cutaneous tumors, see 11600–11606. If significant additional time and effort is documented, append modifier 22 and submit a cover letter and operative report.

ICD-10-CM Diagnostic Codes

C49.21	Malignant neoplasm of connective and soft tissue of right lower limb, including hip ☑
C49.22	Malignant neoplasm of connective and soft tissue of left lower limb, including hip ☑

AMA: 27615 2018,Sep,7 **27616** 2018,Sep,7

Relative Value Units/Medicare Edits

Non-Facility RVU	Work	PE	MP	Total
27615	15.72	11.22	3.2	30.14
27616	19.63	13.66	4.14	37.43
Facility RVU	Work	PE	MP	Total
27615	15.72	11.22	3.2	30.14
27616	19.63	13.66	4.14	37.43

	FUD	Status	MUE	Modifiers				IOM Reference
27615	90	A	1(3)	51	50	62*	80*	None
27616	90	A	1(3)	51	50	62*	80*	

* with documentation

Terms To Know

dissection. Separating by cutting tissue or body structures apart.

fascia. Fibrous sheet or band of tissue that envelops organs, muscles, and groupings of muscles.

intermediate repair. *1)* Surgical closure of a wound requiring closure of one or more of the deeper subcutaneous tissue and non-muscle fascia layers in addition to the skin. *2)* Contaminated wounds with single layer closure that need extensive cleaning or foreign body removal. *3)* Wounds with limited undermining less than the width of the wound.

malignant neoplasm. Any cancerous tumor or lesion exhibiting uncontrolled tissue growth that can progressively invade other parts of the body with its disease-generating cells.

radical resection. Removal of an entire tumor (e.g., malignant neoplasm) along with a large area of surrounding tissue, including adjacent lymph nodes that may have been infiltrated.

sarcoma. Malignant tumor arising in connective tissue, bone, cartilage, or striated muscle that spreads to neighboring tissue through the bloodstream.

soft tissue. Nonepithelial tissues outside of the skeleton.

tumor. Pathological swelling or enlargement; a neoplastic growth of uncontrolled, abnormal multiplication of cells.

27618-27619 [27632, 27634]

27618 Excision, tumor, soft tissue of leg or ankle area, subcutaneous; less than 3 cm

27632 Excision, tumor, soft tissue of leg or ankle area, subcutaneous; 3 cm or greater

27619 Excision, tumor, soft tissue of leg or ankle area, subfascial (eg, intramuscular); less than 5 cm

27634 Excision, tumor, soft tissue of leg or ankle area, subfascial (eg, intramuscular); 5 cm or greater

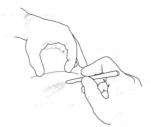

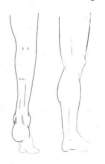

A tumor is removed from the leg/ankle region

Explanation

The physician removes a tumor from the soft tissue of the leg or ankle area that is located in the subcutaneous tissue in 27618 and 27632 and in the deep soft tissue, below the fascial plane, or within the muscle in 27619 and 27634. With the proper anesthesia administered, the physician makes an incision in the skin overlying the mass and dissects to the tumor. The extent of the tumor is identified and a dissection is undertaken all the way around the tumor. A portion of neighboring soft tissue may also be removed to ensure adequate removal of all tumor tissue. A drain may be inserted and the incision is repaired with layers of sutures, staples, or Steri-strips. Report 27618 for excision of a subcutaneous tumor whose resected area is less than 3 cm, and 27632 for a resected area 3 cm or greater. Report 27619 for excision of a subfascial or intramuscular tumor whose resected area is less than 5 cm, and 27634 for a resected area 5 cm or greater.

Coding Tips

Radical resection of a soft tissue tumor, leg or ankle area, is reported with 27615–27616. For excision of cutaneous, benign lesions, see 11400–11406. For excision of other soft tissue tumors, see the specific anatomic location. Excisional biopsy is not reported separately when performed with a therapeutic excision during the same surgical session.

ICD-10-CM Diagnostic Codes

C49.21	Malignant neoplasm of connective and soft tissue of right lower limb, including hip ☑
C49.22	Malignant neoplasm of connective and soft tissue of left lower limb, including hip ☑

D17.23	Benign lipomatous neoplasm of skin and subcutaneous tissue of right leg ☑	
D17.24	Benign lipomatous neoplasm of skin and subcutaneous tissue of left leg ☑	
D21.21	Benign neoplasm of connective and other soft tissue of right lower limb, including hip ☑	
D21.22	Benign neoplasm of connective and other soft tissue of left lower limb, including hip ☑	

AMA: **27618** 2018,Sep,7; 2018,Jan,8; 2017,Jan,8; 2016,Jan,13; 2015,Jan,16 **27619** 2018,Sep,7 **27632** 2018,Sep,7 **27634** 2018,Sep,7

Relative Value Units/Medicare Edits

Non-Facility RVU	Work	PE	MP	Total
27618	3.96	9.78	0.74	14.48
27632	5.91	5.02	1.25	12.18
27619	6.91	5.54	1.1	13.55
27634	10.13	7.92	1.93	19.98
Facility RVU	Work	PE	MP	Total
27618	3.96	4.27	0.74	8.97
27632	5.91	5.02	1.25	12.18
27619	6.91	5.54	1.1	13.55
27634	10.13	7.92	1.93	19.98

	FUD	Status	MUE	Modifiers				IOM Reference
27618	90	A	3(3)	51	50	N/A	N/A	None
27632	90	A	3(3)	51	50	N/A	80	
27619	90	A	2(3)	51	50	N/A	N/A	
27634	90	A	2(3)	51	50	N/A	80	

* with documentation

Terms To Know

soft tissue. Nonepithelial tissues outside of the skeleton.

subcutaneous tissue. Sheet or wide band of adipose (fat) and areolar connective tissue in two layers attached to the dermis.

subfascial. Beneath the band of fibrous tissue that lies deep to the skin, encloses muscles, and separates their layers.

tumor. Pathological swelling or enlargement; a neoplastic growth of uncontrolled, abnormal multiplication of cells.

28043-28045 [28039, 28041]

28043 Excision, tumor, soft tissue of foot or toe, subcutaneous; less than 1.5 cm

28039 Excision, tumor, soft tissue of foot or toe, subcutaneous; 1.5 cm or greater

28045 Excision, tumor, soft tissue of foot or toe, subfascial (eg, intramuscular); less than 1.5 cm

28041 Excision, tumor, soft tissue of foot or toe, subfascial (eg, intramuscular); 1.5 cm or greater

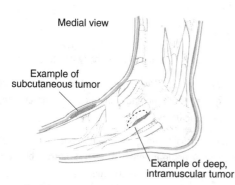

Medial view

Example of subcutaneous tumor

Example of deep, intramuscular tumor

Excision of a soft tissue tumor of the foot or toe

Explanation

The physician removes a tumor from the soft tissue of the foot or toe that is located in the subcutaneous tissue in 28039 and 28043 and in the deep soft tissue, below the fascial plane, or within the muscle in 28041 and 28045. With the proper anesthesia administered, the physician makes an incision in the skin overlying the mass and dissects down to the tumor. The extent of the tumor is identified and a dissection is undertaken all the way around the tumor. A portion of neighboring soft tissue may also be removed to ensure adequate removal of all tumor tissue. A drain may be inserted and the incision is repaired with layers of sutures, staples, or Steri-strips. Report 28043 for excision of a subcutaneous tumor whose resected area is less than 1.5 cm and 28039 for a resected area that is 1.5 cm or greater. Report 28045 for excision of a subfascial or intramuscular tumor whose resected area is less than 1.5 cm and 28041 for a resected area 1.5 cm or greater.

Coding Tips

For radical resection of a soft tissue tumor, foot or toe, see 28046–28047. For excision of cutaneous, benign lesions, see 11420-11426. An excisional biopsy is not reported separately when a therapeutic excision is performed during the same surgical session.

ICD-10-CM Diagnostic Codes

C43.71	Malignant melanoma of right lower limb, including hip ☑
C43.72	Malignant melanoma of left lower limb, including hip ☑
C49.21	Malignant neoplasm of connective and soft tissue of right lower limb, including hip ☑
C49.22	Malignant neoplasm of connective and soft tissue of left lower limb, including hip ☑
C4A.71	Merkel cell carcinoma of right lower limb, including hip ☑
C4A.72	Merkel cell carcinoma of left lower limb, including hip ☑
C76.51	Malignant neoplasm of right lower limb ☑
C76.52	Malignant neoplasm of left lower limb ☑
C79.89	Secondary malignant neoplasm of other specified sites
C7B.1	Secondary Merkel cell carcinoma
D03.71	Melanoma in situ of right lower limb, including hip ☑
D03.72	Melanoma in situ of left lower limb, including hip ☑
D17.23	Benign lipomatous neoplasm of skin and subcutaneous tissue of right leg ☑
D17.24	Benign lipomatous neoplasm of skin and subcutaneous tissue of left leg ☑
D17.39	Benign lipomatous neoplasm of skin and subcutaneous tissue of other sites
D21.21	Benign neoplasm of connective and other soft tissue of right lower limb, including hip ☑
D21.22	Benign neoplasm of connective and other soft tissue of left lower limb, including hip ☑
D48.1	Neoplasm of uncertain behavior of connective and other soft tissue
D48.2	Neoplasm of uncertain behavior of peripheral nerves and autonomic nervous system
D49.2	Neoplasm of unspecified behavior of bone, soft tissue, and skin

AMA: 28039 2018,Sep,7 **28041** 2018,Sep,7 **28043** 2018,Sep,7 **28045** 2018,Sep,7

Relative Value Units/Medicare Edits

Non-Facility RVU	Work	PE	MP	Total
28043	3.96	7.22	0.38	11.56
28039	5.42	8.57	0.74	14.73
28045	5.45	8.41	0.51	14.37
28041	7.13	5.22	0.81	13.16
Facility RVU	**Work**	**PE**	**MP**	**Total**
28043	3.96	3.25	0.38	7.59
28039	5.42	4.0	0.74	10.16
28045	5.45	4.15	0.51	10.11
28041	7.13	5.22	0.81	13.16

	FUD	Status	MUE	Modifiers				IOM Reference
28043	90	A	4(3)	51	50	N/A	N/A	None
28039	90	A	2(3)	51	50	N/A	80	
28045	90	A	4(3)	51	50	N/A	80*	
28041	90	A	2(3)	51	50	N/A	80*	

* with documentation

Terms To Know

deep fascia. Sheet of dense, fibrous tissue holding muscle groups together below the hypodermis layer or subcutaneous fat layer that lines the extremities and trunk.

soft tissue. Nonepithelial tissues outside of the skeleton that includes subcutaneous adipose tissue, fibrous tissue, fascia, muscles, blood and lymph vessels, and peripheral nervous system tissue.

subcutaneous tissue. Sheet or wide band of adipose (fat) and areolar connective tissue in two layers attached to the dermis.

subfascial. Beneath the band of fibrous tissue that lies deep to the skin, encloses muscles, and separates their layers.

28046-28047

28046   Radical resection of tumor (eg, sarcoma), soft tissue of foot or toe; less than 3 cm
28047   3 cm or greater

Select soft tissue structures of the medial foot

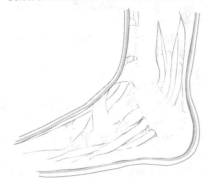

Radical resection of soft tissue
tumor of the foot or toe

Explanation

The physician performs a radical resection (excision) of a malignant soft tissue tumor (i.e., sarcoma) from the foot or toe, not involving bone. An incision is made over the tumor and dissection exposes it. The tumor and any adjacent tissue that may be affected by the spread of the neoplasm are excised. Large resections may be needed. The type and stage of the lesion determine the extent of the tumor margin resection area. Muscle or fascia may need to be repaired and drains may be placed. The surgical wound is closed using simple or intermediate repair or separately reportable complex closure, adjacent tissue transfer, or graft. Report 28046 for a resected area of less than 3 cm and 28047 for a resected area 3 cm or greater.

Coding Tips

An excisional biopsy is not reported separately when a therapeutic excision is performed during the same surgical session. For excision of a soft tissue tumor, foot or toe, subcutaneous, see 28039 and 28043; subfascial, see 28041 and 28045. For radical resection of cutaneous tumors, see 11620–11626. If significant additional time and effort is documented, append modifier 22 and submit a cover letter and operative report.

ICD-10-CM Diagnostic Codes

C49.21   Malignant neoplasm of connective and soft tissue of right lower limb, including hip ☑
C49.22   Malignant neoplasm of connective and soft tissue of left lower limb, including hip ☑

AMA: 28046 2018,Sep,7 **28047** 2018,Sep,7

Relative Value Units/Medicare Edits

Non-Facility RVU	Work	PE	MP	Total
28046	12.38	7.17	1.36	20.91
28047	17.45	10.22	2.59	30.26
Facility RVU	**Work**	**PE**	**MP**	**Total**
28046	12.38	7.17	1.36	20.91
28047	17.45	10.22	2.59	30.26

	FUD	Status	MUE	Modifiers				IOM Reference
28046	90	A	1(3)	51	50	62*	N/A	None
28047	90	A	1(3)	51	50	62*	80	

* with documentation

Terms To Know

dissection. Separating by cutting tissue or body structures apart.

radical resection. Removal of an entire tumor (e.g., malignant neoplasm) along with a large area of surrounding tissue, including adjacent lymph nodes that may have been infiltrated.

soft tissue. Nonepithelial tissues outside of the skeleton that includes subcutaneous adipose tissue, fibrous tissue, fascia, muscles, blood and lymph vessels, and peripheral nervous system tissue.

tumor. Pathological swelling or enlargement; a neoplastic growth of uncontrolled, abnormal multiplication of cells.

29848

29848 Endoscopy, wrist, surgical, with release of transverse carpal ligament

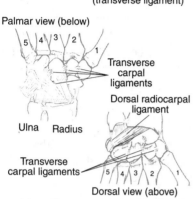

Arthroscopic equipment in place at the wrist

A wrist is scoped without entering the joint capsule (endoscopy) with release of a ligament binding the carpal bones across the hand (transverse ligament)

Palmar view (below)

Transverse carpal ligaments

Dorsal radiocarpal ligament

Ulna   Radius

Transverse carpal ligaments

Dorsal view (above)

Explanation

The patient is placed supine with the arm positioned on a hand table. Endoscopic release may be accomplished by a one or two portal technique. In a single portal technique, a small, 1 1/2 cm, horizontal incision is made at the wrist. Using a two portal technique, two small incisions are made, one in the palm and one at the wrist. The palmar skin, underlying cushioning fat, protective fascia, and muscle are not cut. The endoscope is introduced underneath the transverse carpal ligament. The endoscope allows the physician to view the procedure on a monitor. A blade attached to the arthroscope is used to incise the transverse carpal ligament from the inside of the carpal tunnel. The instruments are removed and the portal(s) closed with sutures or Steri-strips. A splint may be applied.

Coding Tips

Surgical arthroscopy always includes diagnostic arthroscopy. For open carpel tunnel release, see 64721. According to CPT guidelines, cast application or strapping (including removal) is only reported as a replacement procedure or when the cast application or strapping is an initial service performed without a restorative treatment or procedure. See "Application of Casts and Strapping" in the CPT book in the Surgery section, under the Musculoskeletal System. Do not report 29848 with 11960.

ICD-10-CM Diagnostic Codes

G56.01   Carpal tunnel syndrome, right upper limb ☑
G56.02   Carpal tunnel syndrome, left upper limb ☑
G56.03   Carpal tunnel syndrome, bilateral upper limbs ☑

AMA: 29848 2018,Jan,8; 2018,Apr,10; 2017,Jan,8; 2017,Jan,6; 2016,Jan,13; 2015,Jul,10; 2015,Jan,16

Relative Value Units/Medicare Edits

Non-Facility RVU	Work	PE	MP	Total
29848	6.39	7.53	1.16	15.08
Facility RVU	Work	PE	MP	Total
29848	6.39	7.53	1.16	15.08

	FUD	Status	MUE	Modifiers				IOM Reference
29848	90	A	1(2)	51	50	N/A	N/A	None

* with documentation

Terms To Know

arthroscopy. Use of an endoscope to examine the interior of a joint (diagnostic) or to perform surgery on joint structures (therapeutic).

carpal tunnel. Anatomical landmark referring to the space in the wrist on the palmar side that houses the median nerve and all nine of the flexor tendons serving the fingers and thumb. The space is created by the bones of the wrist on either side and a thick ligament called the transverse carpal ligament.

carpal tunnel syndrome. Swelling and inflammation in the tendons or bursa surrounding the median nerve caused by repetitive activity. The resulting compression on the nerve causes pain, numbness, and tingling especially to the palm, index, middle finger, and thumb.

closure. Repairing an incision or wound by suture or other means.

endoscopy. Visual inspection of the body using a fiberoptic scope.

fascia. Fibrous sheet or band of tissue that envelops organs, muscles, and groupings of muscles.

ligament. Band or sheet of fibrous tissue that connects the articular surfaces of bones or supports visceral organs.

release. Disconnection of a tendon or ligament.

skin. Outer protective covering of the body composed of the epidermis and dermis, situated above the subcutaneous tissues.

strapping. Application of overlapping strips of tape or bandaging to put pressure on and immobilize the affected area.

supine. Lying on the back.

tendon. Fibrous tissue that connects muscle to bone, consisting primarily of collagen and containing little vasculature.

transverse. Crosswise at right angles to the long axis of a structure or part.

Endoscopy

31500

31500 Intubation, endotracheal, emergency procedure

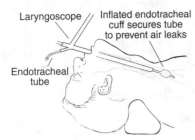

Laryngoscope — Inflated endotracheal cuff secures tube to prevent air leaks

Endotracheal tube

An emergency endotracheal intubation is performed

Explanation

The physician places an endotracheal tube to provide air passage in emergency situations. The patient is ventilated with a mask and bag and positioned by extending the neck anteriorly and the head posteriorly. The physician places the laryngoscope into the patient's mouth and advances the blade toward the epiglottis until the vocal cords are visible. An endotracheal tube is inserted between the vocal cords and advanced to the proper position. The cuff of the endotracheal tube is inflated.

Coding Tips

Emergency endotracheal intubation may be reported separately when performed in connection with critical care, see 99291 or 99292 for definitions of critical care and a list of other procedures that may be reported. Code 31500 is bundled into the neonatal (99468–99469) and pediatric (99471–99476) critical care service codes, as well as the neonatal and pediatric intensive care (99477–99480) codes.

ICD-10-CM Diagnostic Codes

I26.93	Single subsegmental pulmonary embolism without acute cor pulmonale
I26.94	Multiple subsegmental pulmonary emboli without acute cor pulmonale
I27.82	Chronic pulmonary embolism
I50.811	Acute right heart failure
I50.812	Chronic right heart failure
I50.813	Acute on chronic right heart failure
I50.814	Right heart failure due to left heart failure
J44.0	Chronic obstructive pulmonary disease with (acute) lower respiratory infection
J44.1	Chronic obstructive pulmonary disease with (acute) exacerbation
J45.22	Mild intermittent asthma with status asthmaticus
J45.32	Mild persistent asthma with status asthmaticus
J45.41	Moderate persistent asthma with (acute) exacerbation
J45.42	Moderate persistent asthma with status asthmaticus
J45.51	Severe persistent asthma with (acute) exacerbation
J45.52	Severe persistent asthma with status asthmaticus
J69.0	Pneumonitis due to inhalation of food and vomit
J81.0	Acute pulmonary edema
J82.81	Chronic eosinophilic pneumonia
J82.83	Eosinophilic asthma
J95.821	Acute postprocedural respiratory failure
J95.822	Acute and chronic postprocedural respiratory failure
J95.84	Transfusion-related acute lung injury (TRALI)
J96.01	Acute respiratory failure with hypoxia
J96.02	Acute respiratory failure with hypercapnia
J96.21	Acute and chronic respiratory failure with hypoxia
J96.22	Acute and chronic respiratory failure with hypercapnia

AMA: 31500 2018,Jan,8; 2017,Jan,8; 2016,Oct,8; 2016,May,3; 2016,Jan,13; 2015,Jan,16

Relative Value Units/Medicare Edits

Non-Facility RVU	Work	PE	MP	Total
31500	3.0	0.72	0.43	4.15
Facility RVU	**Work**	**PE**	**MP**	**Total**
31500	3.0	0.72	0.43	4.15

	FUD	Status	MUE	Modifiers				IOM Reference
31500	0	A	2(3)	N/A	N/A	N/A	N/A	None

* with documentation

Terms To Know

anterior. Situated in the front area or toward the belly surface of the body; an anatomical reference point used to show the position and relationship of one body structure to another.

epiglottis. Lid-like cartilaginous tissue that covers the entrance to the larynx and blocks food from entering the trachea.

intubation. Insertion of a tube into a hollow organ, canal, or cavity within the body.

larynx. Musculocartilaginous structure between the trachea and the pharynx that functions as the valve preventing food and other particles from entering the respiratory tract, as well as the voice mechanism. Also called the voicebox, the larynx is composed of three single cartilages: cricoid, epiglottis, and thyroid; and three paired cartilages: arytenoid, corniculate, and cuneiform.

posterior. Located in the back part or caudal end of the body.

tube. Long, hollow cylindrical instrument or body structure.

N Newborn: 0   **P** Pediatric: 0-17   **M** Maternity: 9-64   **A** Adult: 15-124   ♂ Male Only   ♀ Female Only   CPT © 2021 American Medical Association. All Rights Reserved.

Coding Companion for General Surgery/Gastroenterology

Respiratory

31592

31592　Cricotracheal resection

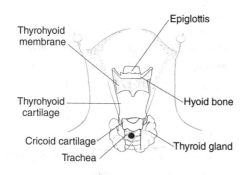

Epiglottis
Thyrohyoid membrane
Thyrohyoid cartilage
Hyoid bone
Cricoid cartilage
Trachea
Thyroid gland

Explanation

The physician removes a narrowed portion of the trachea usually below the larynx. A horizontal skin incision is made across the base of the neck or, in some cases, a sternotomy may be necessary. The prior tracheotomy stoma is removed when applicable. Flaps are lifted from the level of the hyoid bone to the suprasternal notch. The cricoid cartilage is split vertically and examined to be certain one intact ring between the area of resection and stoma is available in order for appropriate anastomosis between the trachea and larynx. Sutures are placed on both sides of the trachea just under the lowest level of the resection. Portions of the cricoid cartilage are removed from the anterior and lateral positions, avoiding the cricoarytenoid joint. The area of stenosis is removed with focus on avoiding the underlying esophagus. Upon removal of the narrowed portion, the ends are tied with absorbable sutures within the tracheal wall. Skin incisions are closed with sutures or staples. Sutures join the skin on the lower chin to the chest to prevent backward movement of the head or a neck brace may be utilized to keep sutures intact. This procedure may be performed as a single or double stage procedure depending on the exact location of the stenosis. In a single stage (SSCTR) procedure, a previously placed tracheotomy tube is removed and an endotracheal tube inserted. In a double stage (DSCTR) procedure, a stent may be inserted above the tracheotomy tube or a T-tube may be utilized instead of the tracheotomy tube. This allows the airway to remain open and is removed four to six weeks postop.

Coding Tips

If a graft is harvested through the cricotracheal resection incision it should not be reported separately. Local advancement or rotational flaps are not reported separately when performed through the same operative incision. For tracheostomy, see 31600-31601, 31603, 31605, and 31610. For excision and anastomosis of a tracheal stenosis, see 31780-31781.

ICD-10-CM Diagnostic Codes

J38.01	Paralysis of vocal cords and larynx, unilateral
J38.02	Paralysis of vocal cords and larynx, bilateral
J38.3	Other diseases of vocal cords
J38.6	Stenosis of larynx

AMA: **31592** 2018,Jan,8; 2017,Mar,10; 2017,Jul,7; 2017,Feb,14; 2017,Apr,5

Relative Value Units/Medicare Edits

Non-Facility RVU	Work	PE	MP	Total
31592	25.0	22.15	3.43	50.58
Facility RVU	**Work**	**PE**	**MP**	**Total**
31592	25.0	22.15	3.43	50.58

	FUD	Status	MUE	Modifiers				IOM Reference
31592	90	A	1(2)	51	N/A	62*	80*	None

* with documentation

Terms To Know

anastomosis. Surgically created connection between ducts, blood vessels, or bowel segments to allow flow from one to the other.

cartilage. Variety of fibrous connective tissue that is inherently nonvascular. Usually found in the joints, it aids in movement and provides a cushion to absorb jolts and shocks.

cricoid. Circular cartilage around the trachea.

larynx. Musculocartilaginous structure between the trachea and the pharynx that functions as the valve preventing food and other particles from entering the respiratory tract, as well as the voice mechanism.

resection. Surgical removal of a part or all of an organ or body part.

stenosis. Narrowing or constriction of a passage.

stent. Tube to provide support in a body cavity or lumen.

stoma. Opening created in the abdominal wall from an internal organ or structure for diversion of waste elimination, drainage, and access.

trachea. Tube descending from the larynx and branching into the right and left main bronchi.

tracheotomy. Formation of a tracheal opening on the neck surface with tube insertion to allow for respiration in cases of obstruction or decreased patency. A tracheotomy may be planned or performed on an emergency basis for temporary or long-term use.

Respiratory

31600-31610

31600 Tracheostomy, planned (separate procedure);
31601   younger than 2 years
31603 Tracheostomy, emergency procedure; transtracheal
31605   cricothyroid membrane
31610 Tracheostomy, fenestration procedure with skin flaps

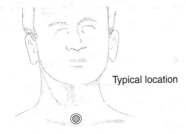

Typical location

An emergency tracheostomy is performed

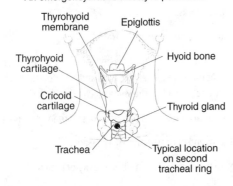

Explanation

The physician creates a tracheostomy. The physician makes a horizontal neck incision and dissects the muscles to expose the trachea. The thyroid isthmus is cut if necessary. The trachea is incised and an airway is inserted. After bleeding is controlled, a stoma is created by suturing the skin to the tissue layers. In 31600, the tracheostomy is a planned procedure. In 31601, it is a planned procedure performed on patients younger than 2 years of age. In 31603, it is performed under emergency conditions by puncturing the trachea and inserting a cannula. In 31605, it is performed under emergency conditions by puncturing the cricothyroid membrane located just above the cricoid and inserting a cannula. This is not a true tracheostomy and is usually converted to a tracheostomy once the situation is no longer emergent. In 31610, skin flaps are used to create a more permanent stoma.

Coding Tips

Note that 31600 and 31601, separate procedures by definition, are usually a component of a more complex service and are not identified separately. When performed alone or with other unrelated procedures/services they may be reported. If performed alone, list the code; if performed with other procedures/services, list the code and append modifier 59 or an X{EPSU} modifier. For endotracheal intubation, see 31500. For direct laryngoscopy with or without tracheoscopy, for aspiration under direct vision, see 31515. Tracheostoma revision, simple, without flap rotation, is reported with 31613; complex, with flap rotation, see 31614. For surgical closure of a tracheostomy or fistula, without plastic repair, see 31820; with plastic repair, see 31825. Revision of a tracheostomy scar is reported with 31830.

ICD-10-CM Diagnostic Codes

A80.0	Acute paralytic poliomyelitis, vaccine-associated
C01	Malignant neoplasm of base of tongue
C02.4	Malignant neoplasm of lingual tonsil
C09.0	Malignant neoplasm of tonsillar fossa
C09.1	Malignant neoplasm of tonsillar pillar (anterior) (posterior)
C09.8	Malignant neoplasm of overlapping sites of tonsil
C10.0	Malignant neoplasm of vallecula
C10.1	Malignant neoplasm of anterior surface of epiglottis
C10.2	Malignant neoplasm of lateral wall of oropharynx
C10.3	Malignant neoplasm of posterior wall of oropharynx
C10.4	Malignant neoplasm of branchial cleft
C10.8	Malignant neoplasm of overlapping sites of oropharynx
C12	Malignant neoplasm of pyriform sinus
C13.0	Malignant neoplasm of postcricoid region
C13.1	Malignant neoplasm of aryepiglottic fold, hypopharyngeal aspect
C13.2	Malignant neoplasm of posterior wall of hypopharynx
C13.8	Malignant neoplasm of overlapping sites of hypopharynx
C32.0	Malignant neoplasm of glottis
C32.1	Malignant neoplasm of supraglottis
C32.2	Malignant neoplasm of subglottis
C32.3	Malignant neoplasm of laryngeal cartilage
C32.8	Malignant neoplasm of overlapping sites of larynx
G12.0	Infantile spinal muscular atrophy, type I [Werdnig-Hoffman]
G12.1	Other inherited spinal muscular atrophy
G12.22	Progressive bulbar palsy
G46.3	Brain stem stroke syndrome
G80.0	Spastic quadriplegic cerebral palsy
G93.1	Anoxic brain damage, not elsewhere classified
J38.6	Stenosis of larynx
J95.821	Acute postprocedural respiratory failure
J95.822	Acute and chronic postprocedural respiratory failure
J96.01	Acute respiratory failure with hypoxia
J96.02	Acute respiratory failure with hypercapnia
J96.11	Chronic respiratory failure with hypoxia
J96.12	Chronic respiratory failure with hypercapnia
J96.21	Acute and chronic respiratory failure with hypoxia
J96.22	Acute and chronic respiratory failure with hypercapnia
P07.01	Extremely low birth weight newborn, less than 500 grams ℕ
P07.02	Extremely low birth weight newborn, 500-749 grams ℕ
P07.03	Extremely low birth weight newborn, 750-999 grams ℕ
P07.14	Other low birth weight newborn, 1000-1249 grams ℕ
P07.15	Other low birth weight newborn, 1250-1499 grams ℕ
P07.16	Other low birth weight newborn, 1500-1749 grams ℕ
P07.21	Extreme immaturity of newborn, gestational age less than 23 completed weeks ℕ
P07.22	Extreme immaturity of newborn, gestational age 23 completed weeks ℕ
P07.23	Extreme immaturity of newborn, gestational age 24 completed weeks ℕ
P07.24	Extreme immaturity of newborn, gestational age 25 completed weeks ℕ
P07.25	Extreme immaturity of newborn, gestational age 26 completed weeks ℕ
P07.26	Extreme immaturity of newborn, gestational age 27 completed weeks ℕ
P22.0	Respiratory distress syndrome of newborn ℕ

Respiratory

P22.8	Other respiratory distress of newborn ⒩	
P27.0	Wilson-Mikity syndrome	
P27.1	Bronchopulmonary dysplasia originating in the perinatal period	
P28.2	Cyanotic attacks of newborn ⒩	
P28.5	Respiratory failure of newborn ⒩	
P28.89	Other specified respiratory conditions of newborn ⒩	
Q31.1	Congenital subglottic stenosis	
Q31.2	Laryngeal hypoplasia	
Q31.3	Laryngocele	
Q31.5	Congenital laryngomalacia	
Q31.8	Other congenital malformations of larynx	
Q32.0	Congenital tracheomalacia	
Q32.1	Other congenital malformations of trachea	
Q32.2	Congenital bronchomalacia	
Q32.3	Congenital stenosis of bronchus	
Q32.4	Other congenital malformations of bronchus	
R06.03	Acute respiratory distress	
R06.89	Other abnormalities of breathing	
S11.011A	Laceration without foreign body of larynx, initial encounter	
S11.012A	Laceration with foreign body of larynx, initial encounter	
S11.013A	Puncture wound without foreign body of larynx, initial encounter	
S11.014A	Puncture wound with foreign body of larynx, initial encounter	
S11.015A	Open bite of larynx, initial encounter	
S11.032A	Laceration with foreign body of vocal cord, initial encounter	
S11.034A	Puncture wound with foreign body of vocal cord, initial encounter	
S12.8XXA	Fracture of other parts of neck, initial encounter	
S17.0XXA	Crushing injury of larynx and trachea, initial encounter	
S19.81XA	Other specified injuries of larynx, initial encounter	
S19.83XA	Other specified injuries of vocal cord, initial encounter	
T17.310A	Gastric contents in larynx causing asphyxiation, initial encounter	
T17.320A	Food in larynx causing asphyxiation, initial encounter	
T17.390A	Other foreign object in larynx causing asphyxiation, initial encounter	
T17.410A	Gastric contents in trachea causing asphyxiation, initial encounter	
T17.420A	Food in trachea causing asphyxiation, initial encounter	
T17.490A	Other foreign object in trachea causing asphyxiation, initial encounter	
T17.498A	Other foreign object in trachea causing other injury, initial encounter	
T17.810A	Gastric contents in other parts of respiratory tract causing asphyxiation, initial encounter	
T17.818A	Gastric contents in other parts of respiratory tract causing other injury, initial encounter	
T17.820A	Food in other parts of respiratory tract causing asphyxiation, initial encounter	
T17.890A	Other foreign object in other parts of respiratory tract causing asphyxiation, initial encounter	
T17.898A	Other foreign object in other parts of respiratory tract causing other injury, initial encounter	
T27.0XXA	Burn of larynx and trachea, initial encounter	
T27.1XXA	Burn involving larynx and trachea with lung, initial encounter	
T27.2XXA	Burn of other parts of respiratory tract, initial encounter	
T27.4XXA	Corrosion of larynx and trachea, initial encounter	
T27.5XXA	Corrosion involving larynx and trachea with lung, initial encounter	
T27.6XXA	Corrosion of other parts of respiratory tract, initial encounter	
T28.0XXA	Burn of mouth and pharynx, initial encounter	
T28.5XXA	Corrosion of mouth and pharynx, initial encounter	

AMA: **31600** 2020,Dec,11; 2019,Sep,10; 2017,Apr,5 **31601** 2020,Dec,11; 2017,Apr,5 **31603** 2020,Dec,11; 2017,Apr,5 **31605** 2017,Apr,5 **31610** 2020,Dec,11; 2017,Apr,5

Relative Value Units/Medicare Edits

Non-Facility RVU	Work	PE	MP	Total
31600	5.56	2.38	1.03	8.97
31601	8.0	3.93	1.1	13.03
31603	6.0	2.34	1.03	9.37
31605	6.45	2.02	1.26	9.73
31610	12.0	14.66	1.76	28.42
Facility RVU	**Work**	**PE**	**MP**	**Total**
31600	5.56	2.38	1.03	8.97
31601	8.0	3.93	1.1	13.03
31603	6.0	2.34	1.03	9.37
31605	6.45	2.02	1.26	9.73
31610	12.0	14.66	1.76	28.42

	FUD	Status	MUE	Modifiers				IOM Reference
31600	0	A	1(2)	51	N/A	N/A	N/A	None
31601	0	A	1(2)	51	N/A	62*	80	
31603	0	A	1(2)	51	N/A	N/A	N/A	
31605	0	A	1(2)	51	N/A	N/A	N/A	
31610	90	A	1(2)	51	N/A	N/A	N/A	

* with documentation

Terms To Know

cricoid. Circular cartilage around the trachea.

dissect. Cut apart or separate tissue for surgical purposes or for visual or microscopic study.

epiglottis. Lid-like cartilaginous tissue that covers the entrance to the larynx and blocks food from entering the trachea.

incision. Act of cutting into tissue or an organ.

stoma. Opening created in the abdominal wall from an internal organ or structure for diversion of waste elimination, drainage, and access.

trachea. Tube descending from the larynx and branching into the right and left main bronchi.

tracheostomy. Formation of a tracheal opening on the neck surface with tube insertion to allow for respiration in cases of obstruction or decreased patency. A tracheostomy may be planned or performed on an emergency basis for temporary or long-term use.

32503-32504

32503 Resection of apical lung tumor (eg, Pancoast tumor), including chest wall resection, rib(s) resection(s), neurovascular dissection, when performed; without chest wall reconstruction(s)

32504 with chest wall reconstruction

A Pancoast tumor is a tumor at the apex of the lung

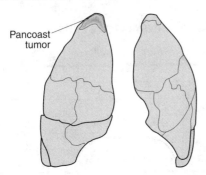

Pancoast tumor

Explanation

The physician removes a tumor from the apex of the lung, such as a Pancoast tumor, as well as a portion of the chest wall. The patient may be intubated with a double lumen endotracheal tube to verify correct positioning and to evaluate endobronchial disease. The chest cavity is entered using an anterior or posterior incision. The posterior incision is made along the outline of the scapula, entering the pleural space at the third or fourth intercostal space. In some cases, an anterior transcervical approach is used. The necessary extended en bloc resection of the chest wall includes posterior portions of the first three ribs, part of the upper thoracic vertebrae (including the transverse process), the intercostal nerves, the lower trunk of the brachial plexus, the stellate ganglion, a section of the dorsal sympathetic ganglion, and the portion of the involved lung. For tumors that are situated peripherally, the apical segment of the upper lobe of the lung is separated from the remaining superior lobe. The apex of the lung is left attached to the chest wall. The first through third, fourth, or fifth ribs are sectioned anteriorly. The subclavian artery is sharply dissected from the surrounding structures. A subperiosteal dissection is performed around the first rib, which is transected, and the subclavian vessels are mobilized superiorly. If preoperative magnetic resonance imaging demonstrated vessel involvement, an initial anterior approach is performed to dissect or graft the vessels. The ribs are disarticulated and the tumor, along with the involved chest wall, is gradually mobilized. Next, the segmental vessels are identified, doubly ligated, and transected. The parietal pleura are bluntly dissected along the anterior border of the spinal column. The tumor and the involved chest wall that has remained attached to the inferior trunk of the brachial plexus is excised, using caution to spare the T1 nerve root as it crosses beneath the angle of the first rib to join the C8 nerve root. If a tumor has invaded the vertebral bodies, the subclavian artery, or the C8 to T1 nerve routes, a multidisciplinary approach may be necessary. At the completion of the procedure, two large chest tubes are placed: one at the apex of the chest to drain any residual air and the other to drain fluids. Report 32504 when chest wall reconstruction is performed.

Coding Tips

Thoracentesis with tube insertion, thoracostomy or thoracotomy, and chest wall resection are included in these codes and should not be reported with 21601-21603, 32100, 32551, or 32554–32555. For excision of a chest wall tumor with rib involvement, without lung resection, see 21601-21603. Lung resection without chest wall resection is reported with 32480–32491 and 32505–32507.

ICD-10-CM Diagnostic Codes

C34.11	Malignant neoplasm of upper lobe, right bronchus or lung ☑
C34.12	Malignant neoplasm of upper lobe, left bronchus or lung ☑

AMA: **32503** 2019,Dec,4 **32504** 2019,Dec,4

Relative Value Units/Medicare Edits

Non-Facility RVU	Work	PE	MP	Total
32503	31.74	13.46	7.28	52.48
32504	36.54	14.85	8.38	59.77
Facility RVU	**Work**	**PE**	**MP**	**Total**
32503	31.74	13.46	7.28	52.48
32504	36.54	14.85	8.38	59.77

	FUD	Status	MUE	Modifiers				IOM Reference
32503	90	A	1(2)	51	N/A	62*	80	None
32504	90	A	1(2)	51	N/A	62*	80	

* with documentation

Terms To Know

brachial plexus. Large bundle of nerves originating in the C5 to T2 spinal segments, located in the neck, axilla, and subclavicular area, and an anatomic landmark and site of administration of medication for pain management.

en bloc removal. Take out as a whole or all in one mass.

reconstruction. Recreating, restoring, or rebuilding a body part or organ.

resection. Surgical removal of a part or all of an organ or body part.

Respiratory

32550

32550 Insertion of indwelling tunneled pleural catheter with cuff

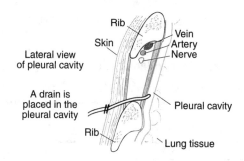

A tunneled indwelling catheter
is placed in the pleural cavity

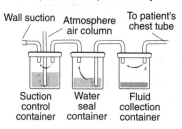

Explanation

The physician inserts a tunneled, indwelling pleural catheter to aid quality of life and long-term management of malignant effusion. The catheter allows drainage on an outpatient or home basis and consists of flexible rubber tubing with a safety drainage valve to provide access to the pleural cavity and prevent air and fluid entering. A polyester cuff secures the catheter in place and helps prevent infection. Using separately reportable imaging guidance, the physician inserts the catheter percutaneously through a small incision in the anterior axillary area. The pleural catheter is threaded over a guidewire to access the pleural cavity, tunneled under the skin along the chest wall, and brought out that side in the lower chest. After placement, the patient may drain pleural fluid at home periodically into vacuum bottles by connecting the matching drainage line access tip to the valve.

Coding Tips

Do not report 32550 with 32554–32557 when performed on the same side of the chest. Imaging guidance is reported with 75989, when performed.

ICD-10-CM Diagnostic Codes

J91.0   Malignant pleural effusion

AMA: **32550** 2018,Jan,8; 2017,Jan,8; 2016,Jan,13; 2015,Jan,16

Relative Value Units/Medicare Edits

Non-Facility RVU	Work	PE	MP	Total
32550	3.92	20.18	0.53	24.63
Facility RVU	**Work**	**PE**	**MP**	**Total**
32550	3.92	1.54	0.53	5.99

	FUD	Status	MUE	Modifiers				IOM Reference
32550	0	A	2(3)	N/A	N/A	N/A	N/A	None

* with documentation

32551

32551 Tube thoracostomy, includes connection to drainage system (eg, water seal), when performed, open (separate procedure)

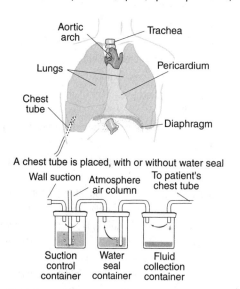

A chest tube is placed, with or without water seal

The conventional three-chamber water seal system
evacuates the pleural space without back pressure

Explanation

The physician removes fluid and/or air from the chest cavity by puncturing through the space between the ribs. To enter the chest cavity, the physician passes a trocar over the top of a rib, punctures through the chest tissues between the ribs, and enters the pleural cavity. Separately reportable imaging guidance may be used. With the end of the trocar in the chest cavity, the physician advances the plastic tube into the chest cavity. The sharp trocar is removed leaving one end of the plastic catheter in place within the chest cavity. A large syringe is attached to the outside end of the catheter and the fluid (blood or pus) is removed from the chest cavity by pulling back on the plunger of the syringe. The outside end of the tube may be connected to a drainage system, such as a water seal, to prevent air from being sucked into the chest cavity and to allow continuous or intermittent removal of air or fluid.

Coding Tips

This separate procedure by definition is usually a component of a more complex service and is not identified separately. When performed alone or with other unrelated procedures/services it may be reported. If performed alone, list the code; if performed with other procedures/services, list the code and append modifier 59 or an X{EPSU} modifier. This is a unilateral procedure. If performed bilaterally, some payers require that the service be reported twice with modifier 50 appended to the second code while others require identification of the service only once with modifier 50 appended. Check with individual payers. Modifier 50 identifies a procedure performed identically on the opposite side of the body (mirror image). Do not report 32551 in addition to 33020 or 33025 if a chest tube/pleural drain is placed on the ipsilateral side.

ICD-10-CM Diagnostic Codes

J86.0   Pyothorax with fistula
J86.9   Pyothorax without fistula
J90   Pleural effusion, not elsewhere classified
J91.0   Malignant pleural effusion
J91.8   Pleural effusion in other conditions classified elsewhere
J93.0   Spontaneous tension pneumothorax

J93.11	Primary spontaneous pneumothorax		S27.1XXA	Traumatic hemothorax, initial encounter
J93.12	Secondary spontaneous pneumothorax		S27.2XXA	Traumatic hemopneumothorax, initial encounter
J93.81	Chronic pneumothorax		S27.63XA	Laceration of pleura, initial encounter
J93.82	Other air leak		S27.69XA	Other injury of pleura, initial encounter

J93.11 Primary spontaneous pneumothorax
J93.12 Secondary spontaneous pneumothorax
J93.81 Chronic pneumothorax
J93.82 Other air leak
J93.83 Other pneumothorax
J94.0 Chylous effusion
J94.2 Hemothorax
J94.8 Other specified pleural conditions
J95.811 Postprocedural pneumothorax
P26.0 Tracheobronchial hemorrhage originating in the perinatal period N
P26.1 Massive pulmonary hemorrhage originating in the perinatal period N
P26.8 Other pulmonary hemorrhages originating in the perinatal period N
S21.311A Laceration without foreign body of right front wall of thorax with penetration into thoracic cavity, initial encounter
S21.312A Laceration without foreign body of left front wall of thorax with penetration into thoracic cavity, initial encounter
S21.321A Laceration with foreign body of right front wall of thorax with penetration into thoracic cavity, initial encounter
S21.322A Laceration with foreign body of left front wall of thorax with penetration into thoracic cavity, initial encounter
S21.331A Puncture wound without foreign body of right front wall of thorax with penetration into thoracic cavity, initial encounter
S21.332A Puncture wound without foreign body of left front wall of thorax with penetration into thoracic cavity, initial encounter
S21.341A Puncture wound with foreign body of right front wall of thorax with penetration into thoracic cavity, initial encounter
S21.342A Puncture wound with foreign body of left front wall of thorax with penetration into thoracic cavity, initial encounter
S21.351A Open bite of right front wall of thorax with penetration into thoracic cavity, initial encounter
S21.352A Open bite of left front wall of thorax with penetration into thoracic cavity, initial encounter
S21.411A Laceration without foreign body of right back wall of thorax with penetration into thoracic cavity, initial encounter
S21.412A Laceration without foreign body of left back wall of thorax with penetration into thoracic cavity, initial encounter
S21.421A Laceration with foreign body of right back wall of thorax with penetration into thoracic cavity, initial encounter
S21.422A Laceration with foreign body of left back wall of thorax with penetration into thoracic cavity, initial encounter
S21.431A Puncture wound without foreign body of right back wall of thorax with penetration into thoracic cavity, initial encounter
S21.432A Puncture wound without foreign body of left back wall of thorax with penetration into thoracic cavity, initial encounter
S21.441A Puncture wound with foreign body of right back wall of thorax with penetration into thoracic cavity, initial encounter
S21.442A Puncture wound with foreign body of left back wall of thorax with penetration into thoracic cavity, initial encounter
S21.451A Open bite of right back wall of thorax with penetration into thoracic cavity, initial encounter
S21.452A Open bite of left back wall of thorax with penetration into thoracic cavity, initial encounter
S27.0XXA Traumatic pneumothorax, initial encounter

S27.1XXA Traumatic hemothorax, initial encounter
S27.2XXA Traumatic hemopneumothorax, initial encounter
S27.63XA Laceration of pleura, initial encounter
S27.69XA Other injury of pleura, initial encounter

AMA: 32551 2019,Dec,4; 2018,Jul,7; 2018,Jan,8; 2017,Jun,10; 2017,Jan,8; 2016,Jan,13; 2015,Jan,16

Relative Value Units/Medicare Edits

Non-Facility RVU	Work	PE	MP	Total
32551	3.04	1.01	0.52	4.57
Facility RVU	Work	PE	MP	Total
32551	3.04	1.01	0.52	4.57

	FUD	Status	MUE	Modifiers				IOM Reference
32551	0	A	2(3)	51	50	N/A	N/A	None

* with documentation

Terms To Know

catheter. Flexible tube inserted into an area of the body for introducing or withdrawing fluid.

hemothorax. Blood collecting in the pleural cavity.

imaging. Radiologic means of producing pictures for clinical study of the internal structures and functions of the body, such as x-ray, ultrasound, magnetic resonance, or positron emission tomography.

pneumothorax. Collapsed lung due to air or gas trapped in the pleural space formed by the membrane that encloses the lungs and lines the thoracic cavity.

thoracostomy. Creation of an opening in the chest wall for drainage.

trocar. Cannula or a sharp pointed instrument used to puncture and aspirate fluid from cavities.

tube. Long, hollow cylindrical instrument or body structure.

32554-32555

32554 Thoracentesis, needle or catheter, aspiration of the pleural space; without imaging guidance

32555   with imaging guidance

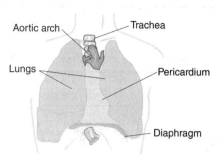

The pleural space is aspirated

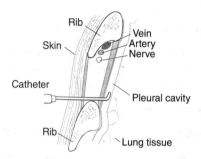

Explanation

The physician removes fluid and/or air from the chest cavity by puncturing through the space between the ribs with a hollow needle (cannula) and entering the chest cavity. The fluid (blood or pus) is removed from the chest cavity by pulling back on the plunger of the syringe attached to the cannula. Report 32554 if the procedure is performed without imaging guidance. Report 32555 when imaging guidance is used during the procedure.

Coding Tips

These are unilateral procedures. If performed bilaterally, some payers require that the service be reported twice with modifier 50 appended to the second code while others require identification of the service only once with modifier 50 appended. Check with individual payers. Modifier 50 identifies a procedure performed identically on the opposite side of the body (mirror image). When medically necessary, report moderate (conscious) sedation provided by the performing physician with 99151–99153. When provided by another physician, report 99155–99157. Imaging guidance is included in 32555 and is not reported separately. Do not report 32554-32555 with 75989, 76942, 77002, 77012, or 77021. These codes should not be reported with 32550 and 32551 when procedures are performed on the same side of the chest. For percutaneous insertion of an indwelling pleural catheter, see 32556 and 33557. For insertion of an indwelling tunneled pleural catheter with cuff, see 32550.

ICD-10-CM Diagnostic Codes

A15.6	Tuberculous pleurisy
J86.0	Pyothorax with fistula
J86.9	Pyothorax without fistula
J90	Pleural effusion, not elsewhere classified
J91.0	Malignant pleural effusion
J91.8	Pleural effusion in other conditions classified elsewhere
J93.0	Spontaneous tension pneumothorax
J93.11	Primary spontaneous pneumothorax
J94.0	Chylous effusion
J94.2	Hemothorax
J94.8	Other specified pleural conditions
J95.4	Chemical pneumonitis due to anesthesia
M32.13	Lung involvement in systemic lupus erythematosus
M35.02	Sjögren syndrome with lung involvement

AMA: **32554** 2019,Dec,4; 2018,Jan,8; 2017,Jan,8; 2016,Jan,13; 2015,Jan,16
32555 2019,Dec,4; 2018,Jan,8; 2017,Jan,8; 2016,Jan,13; 2015,Jan,16

Relative Value Units/Medicare Edits

Non-Facility RVU	Work	PE	MP	Total
32554	1.82	5.07	0.19	7.08
32555	2.27	7.14	0.2	9.61
Facility RVU	**Work**	**PE**	**MP**	**Total**
32554	1.82	0.6	0.19	2.61
32555	2.27	0.75	0.2	3.22

	FUD	Status	MUE	Modifiers				IOM Reference
32554	0	A	2(3)	51	50	N/A	N/A	None
32555	0	A	2(3)	51	50	N/A	N/A	

* with documentation

Terms To Know

hemothorax. Blood collecting in the pleural cavity.

malignant pleural effusion. Severe build-up of fluid in the pleural space from a disturbance of the normal processes that regulate fluid reabsorption. It is caused by an obstruction of the lymph that normally drains the parietal pleura or the transfer of a malignancy from a primary site to the lining of the lung, not to be confused with nonmalignant pleural effusion.

pleurisy. Inflammation of the serous membrane that lines the lungs and the thoracic cavity. Pleurisy may cause effusion within the cavity or have exudate in the pleural space or on the membrane surface.

pneumothorax. Collapsed lung due to air or gas trapped in the pleural space formed by the membrane that encloses the lungs and lines the thoracic cavity.

Respiratory

32556-32557

32556 Pleural drainage, percutaneous, with insertion of indwelling catheter; without imaging guidance
32557   with imaging guidance

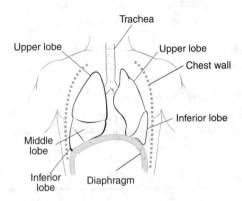

Explanation

The physician removes fluid and/or air from the chest cavity. The patient is positioned dependent upon the location of the fluid (blood or pus) on preprocedural imaging. The chest cavity is accessed by puncturing through the space between the ribs with a needle. Once the fluid is accessed via the needle(s), a guidewire is inserted to the most distal point of the fluid in the pleural cavity. A catheter (i.e., pigtail catheter) is inserted the length of the guidewire and the chest cavity is drained. In some instances, the catheter is connected to a water seal system. Report 32556 if the procedure is performed without imaging guidance. Report 32557 when imaging guidance is used during the procedure.

Coding Tips

These are unilateral procedures. If performed bilaterally, some payers require that the service be reported twice with modifier 50 appended to the second code while others require identification of the service only once with modifier 50 appended. Check with individual payers. Modifier 50 identifies a procedure performed identically on the opposite side of the body (mirror image). When medically necessary, report moderate (conscious) sedation provided by the performing physician with 99151–99153. When provided by another physician, report 99155–99157. Imaging guidance is included in 32557 and is not reported separately. Do not report 32556–32557 with 75989, 76942, 77002, 77012, or 77021. These codes should not be reported with 32550 and 32551 when procedures are performed on the same side of the chest. For needle or catheter aspiration of the pleural space via thoracentesis, without imaging, see 32554; with imaging, see 33555. For an indwelling tunneled pleural catheter with cuff, see 32550.

ICD-10-CM Diagnostic Codes

J90	Pleural effusion, not elsewhere classified
J91.0	Malignant pleural effusion
J91.8	Pleural effusion in other conditions classified elsewhere

AMA: 32556 2018,Jan,8; 2017,Jan,8; 2016,Jan,13; 2015,Jan,16 **32557** 2018,Jan,8; 2017,Jan,8; 2016,Jan,13; 2015,Jan,16

Relative Value Units/Medicare Edits

Non-Facility RVU	Work	PE	MP	Total
32556	2.5	19.31	0.3	22.11
32557	3.12	16.44	0.26	19.82
Facility RVU	**Work**	**PE**	**MP**	**Total**
32556	2.5	0.8	0.3	3.6
32557	3.12	0.98	0.26	4.36

	FUD	Status	MUE	Modifiers				IOM Reference
32556	0	A	2(3)	51	50	N/A	N/A	None
32557	0	A	2(3)	51	50	N/A	N/A	

* with documentation

Terms To Know

catheter. Flexible tube inserted into an area of the body for introducing or withdrawing fluid.

empyema. Accumulation of pus within the respiratory or pleural cavity.

imaging. Radiologic means of producing pictures for clinical study of the internal structures and functions of the body, such as x-ray, ultrasound, magnetic resonance, or positron emission tomography.

percutaneous. Through the skin.

pleural effusion. Collection of lymph and other fluid within the pleural space.

pneumothorax. Collapsed lung due to air or gas trapped in the pleural space formed by the membrane that encloses the lungs and lines the thoracic cavity.

Respiratory

35840

35840 Exploration for postoperative hemorrhage, thrombosis or infection; abdomen

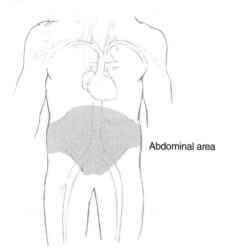

Abdominal area

A surgical exploration is performed in the abdominal cavity to find and identify postoperative hemorrhage, thrombosis (clotting), or infection

Explanation

The physician reopens the original incision site and inspects the operative area for active bleeding, hematoma, thrombus, and exudate. The physician removes or debrides any observed hematoma, thrombus, and infected tissues. The physician looks for and corrects any active bleeding sites using electrocautery or ligation of bleeding vessels. The physician may leave an infected wound open, but generally closes the incision, leaving drains in place.

Coding Tips

This code is used to report exploration for postoperative hemorrhage, thrombosis, or infection of veins and arteries of the abdomen only and is not used for exploration of vessels not followed by surgical repair. If performed during the postoperative period for a prior procedure, modifier 78 may be appended.

ICD-10-CM Diagnostic Codes

D78.21	Postprocedural hemorrhage of the spleen following a procedure on the spleen
D78.22	Postprocedural hemorrhage of the spleen following other procedure
D78.31	Postprocedural hematoma of the spleen following a procedure on the spleen
D78.32	Postprocedural hematoma of the spleen following other procedure
D78.33	Postprocedural seroma of the spleen following a procedure on the spleen
D78.34	Postprocedural seroma of the spleen following other procedure
G89.18	Other acute postprocedural pain
G89.28	Other chronic postprocedural pain
I77.2	Rupture of artery
K68.11	Postprocedural retroperitoneal abscess
K91.31	Postprocedural partial intestinal obstruction
K91.32	Postprocedural complete intestinal obstruction
K91.82	Postprocedural hepatic failure
K91.83	Postprocedural hepatorenal syndrome

K91.840	Postprocedural hemorrhage of a digestive system organ or structure following a digestive system procedure
K91.841	Postprocedural hemorrhage of a digestive system organ or structure following other procedure
K91.870	Postprocedural hematoma of a digestive system organ or structure following a digestive system procedure
K91.871	Postprocedural hematoma of a digestive system organ or structure following other procedure
K91.872	Postprocedural seroma of a digestive system organ or structure following a digestive system procedure
K91.873	Postprocedural seroma of a digestive system organ or structure following other procedure
K91.89	Other postprocedural complications and disorders of digestive system
N99.0	Postprocedural (acute) (chronic) kidney failure
N99.520	Hemorrhage of incontinent external stoma of urinary tract
N99.521	Infection of incontinent external stoma of urinary tract
N99.522	Malfunction of incontinent external stoma of urinary tract
N99.523	Herniation of incontinent stoma of urinary tract
N99.524	Stenosis of incontinent stoma of urinary tract
N99.528	Other complication of incontinent external stoma of urinary tract
N99.530	Hemorrhage of continent stoma of urinary tract
N99.531	Infection of continent stoma of urinary tract
N99.532	Malfunction of continent stoma of urinary tract
N99.533	Herniation of continent stoma of urinary tract
N99.534	Stenosis of continent stoma of urinary tract
N99.538	Other complication of continent stoma of urinary tract
N99.820	Postprocedural hemorrhage of a genitourinary system organ or structure following a genitourinary system procedure
N99.821	Postprocedural hemorrhage of a genitourinary system organ or structure following other procedure
N99.840	Postprocedural hematoma of a genitourinary system organ or structure following a genitourinary system procedure
N99.841	Postprocedural hematoma of a genitourinary system organ or structure following other procedure
N99.842	Postprocedural seroma of a genitourinary system organ or structure following a genitourinary system procedure
N99.843	Postprocedural seroma of a genitourinary system organ or structure following other procedure
N99.89	Other postprocedural complications and disorders of genitourinary system
T81.31XA	Disruption of external operation (surgical) wound, not elsewhere classified, initial encounter
T81.32XA	Disruption of internal operation (surgical) wound, not elsewhere classified, initial encounter
T81.41XA	Infection following a procedure, superficial incisional surgical site, initial encounter
T81.42XA	Infection following a procedure, deep incisional surgical site, initial encounter
T81.43XA	Infection following a procedure, organ and space surgical site, initial encounter
T81.44XA	Sepsis following a procedure, initial encounter
T81.710A	Complication of mesenteric artery following a procedure, not elsewhere classified, initial encounter
T81.711A	Complication of renal artery following a procedure, not elsewhere classified, initial encounter

T81.718A	Complication of other artery following a procedure, not elsewhere classified, initial encounter		
T81.72XA	Complication of vein following a procedure, not elsewhere classified, initial encounter		
T82.7XXA	Infection and inflammatory reaction due to other cardiac and vascular devices, implants and grafts, initial encounter		
T82.818A	Embolism due to vascular prosthetic devices, implants and grafts, initial encounter		
T82.828A	Fibrosis due to vascular prosthetic devices, implants and grafts, initial encounter		
T82.838A	Hemorrhage due to vascular prosthetic devices, implants and grafts, initial encounter		
T82.848A	Pain due to vascular prosthetic devices, implants and grafts, initial encounter		
T82.856A	Stenosis of peripheral vascular stent, initial encounter		
T82.858A	Stenosis of other vascular prosthetic devices, implants and grafts, initial encounter		
T82.868A	Thrombosis due to vascular prosthetic devices, implants and grafts, initial encounter		
T82.898A	Other specified complication of vascular prosthetic devices, implants and grafts, initial encounter		
T88.8XXA	Other specified complications of surgical and medical care, not elsewhere classified, initial encounter		

AMA: 35840 1997,Nov,1; 1997,May,4

Relative Value Units/Medicare Edits

Non-Facility RVU	Work	PE	MP	Total
35840	20.75	9.82	4.75	35.32
Facility RVU	**Work**	**PE**	**MP**	**Total**
35840	20.75	9.82	4.75	35.32

	FUD	Status	MUE	Modifiers				IOM Reference
35840	90	A	2(3)	51	N/A	62*	80	None

* with documentation

35870

35870	Repair of graft-enteric fistula

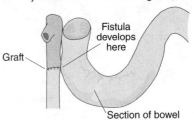

Fistulas sometimes develop at the site of an anastomosis or graft with the communication allowing blood to enter the bowel and digestive juices to further erode the graft site

Explanation

The physician opens the abdomen under antibiotic cover and exposes the graft-enteric fistula site by careful dissection (most often aortic/Dacron anastomosis with a fistulous connection to the duodenum). The fistula is disconnected and the enteric defect is repaired using two layers of suture. The vascular prosthesis is examined and removed with an appropriate new bypass graft sewn in if there is obvious graft infection. If there is no obvious infection, the graft is repaired with local sutures. The wound is closed, leaving drains in place.

Coding Tips

When 35870 is performed with another separately identifiable procedure, the highest dollar value code is listed as the primary procedure, and subsequent procedures are appended with modifier 51. For arteriovenous fistula repairs, see 35180–35190.

ICD-10-CM Diagnostic Codes

I77.2	Rupture of artery
T82.818A	Embolism due to vascular prosthetic devices, implants and grafts, initial encounter
T82.828A	Fibrosis due to vascular prosthetic devices, implants and grafts, initial encounter
T82.838A	Hemorrhage due to vascular prosthetic devices, implants and grafts, initial encounter
T82.848A	Pain due to vascular prosthetic devices, implants and grafts, initial encounter
T82.858A	Stenosis of other vascular prosthetic devices, implants and grafts, initial encounter
T82.868A	Thrombosis due to vascular prosthetic devices, implants and grafts, initial encounter
T82.898A	Other specified complication of vascular prosthetic devices, implants and grafts, initial encounter

AMA: 35870 1997,Nov,1

Relative Value Units/Medicare Edits

Non-Facility RVU	Work	PE	MP	Total
35870	24.5	5.81	5.93	36.24
Facility RVU	Work	PE	MP	Total
35870	24.5	5.81	5.93	36.24

	FUD	Status	MUE	Modifiers				IOM Reference
35870	90	A	1(3)	51	N/A	62*	80	None

* with documentation

Terms To Know

anastomosis. Surgically created connection between ducts, blood vessels, or bowel segments to allow flow from one to the other.

dissect. Cut apart or separate tissue for surgical purposes or for visual or microscopic study.

duodenum. First portion of the small intestine connected to the stomach at the pylorus and extending to the jejunum.

embolism. Obstruction of a blood vessel resulting from a clot or foreign substance.

fistula. Abnormal tube-like passage between two body cavities or organs or from an organ to the outside surface.

graft. Tissue implant from another part of the body or another person.

prosthesis. Man-made substitute for a missing body part.

small intestine. First portion of intestine connecting to the pylorus at the proximal end and consisting of the duodenum, jejunum, and ileum.

stenosis. Narrowing or constriction of a passage.

thrombus. Stationary blood clot inside a blood vessel.

35907

35907   Excision of infected graft; abdomen

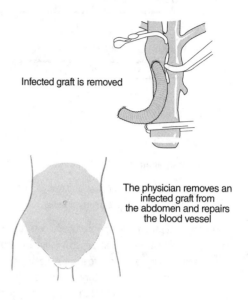

Infected graft is removed

The physician removes an infected graft from the abdomen and repairs the blood vessel

Explanation

Through an incision in the skin of the abdomen overlying the graft, the physician dissects around any muscle, vessels or other structures to access the graft site. The physician dissects around the vessel, and applies vessel clamps above and below the graft. The physician excises above and below the existing infected graft. The blood vessel is repaired with sutures. A catheter may be left in place to help drain infection. The skin is loosely closed. If the excised graft is replaced with a new graft, report the appropriate revascularization code.

Coding Tips

For initial placement of a bypass graft using a vein, see 35501–35571; in-situ vein, see 35583–35587. For initial placement of a bypass graft other than vein, see 35601–35671; composite grafts, see 35681–35683.

ICD-10-CM Diagnostic Codes

T81.41XA	Infection following a procedure, superficial incisional surgical site, initial encounter
T81.42XA	Infection following a procedure, deep incisional surgical site, initial encounter
T81.43XA	Infection following a procedure, organ and space surgical site, initial encounter
T81.44XA	Sepsis following a procedure, initial encounter
T82.7XXA	Infection and inflammatory reaction due to other cardiac and vascular devices, implants and grafts, initial encounter
T82.898A	Other specified complication of vascular prosthetic devices, implants and grafts, initial encounter

AMA: 35907 1997,Nov,1

Relative Value Units/Medicare Edits

Non-Facility RVU	Work	PE	MP	Total
35907	37.27	9.15	8.96	55.38
Facility RVU	Work	PE	MP	Total
35907	37.27	9.15	8.96	55.38

	FUD	Status	MUE	Modifiers				IOM Reference
35907	90	A	1(3)	51	N/A	62*	80	None

* with documentation

Terms To Know

dissection. Separating by cutting tissue or body structures apart.

graft. Tissue implant from another part of the body or another person.

revascularization. Restoration of blood flow and oxygen supply to a body part. This may apply to an extremity, the heart, or penis.

sepsis. Phase following septicemia in the infectious illness continuum, not to be used interchangeably with septicemia. Sepsis is defined for clinical coding purposes as septicemia that has advanced to involve the presence of two or more manifestations of systemic inflammatory response syndrome (SIRS), without organ dysfunction. This is a different clinical picture than septicemia, which has a different outcome.

suture. Numerous stitching techniques employed in wound closure.

buried suture. Continuous or interrupted suture placed under the skin for a layered closure.

continuous suture. Running stitch with tension evenly distributed across a single strand to provide a leakproof closure line.

interrupted suture. Series of single stitches with tension isolated at each stitch, in which all stitches are not affected if one becomes loose, and the isolated sutures cannot act as a wick to transport an infection.

purse-string suture. Continuous suture placed around a tubular structure and tightened, to reduce or close the lumen.

retention suture. Secondary stitching that bridges the primary suture, providing support for the primary repair; a plastic or rubber bolster may be placed over the primary repair and under the retention sutures.

36473-36474

36473 Endovenous ablation therapy of incompetent vein, extremity, inclusive of all imaging guidance and monitoring, percutaneous, mechanochemical; first vein treated

+ **36474** subsequent vein(s) treated in a single extremity, each through separate access sites (List separately in addition to code for primary procedure)

Incompetent veins are treated with endovenous ablation including imaging guidance and monitoring

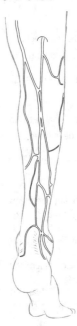

Explanation

The physician uses endovenous ablation therapy to treat venous incompetence in an extremity vein. Mechanochemical endovenous ablation (MOCA) uses a rotating wire in conjunction with an infused sclerosing agent to damage the wall of the vein. The most common site of treatment is the greater saphenous vein. The procedure includes any imaging guidance and monitoring. The leg is prepared and draped and a local anesthetic is applied to the puncture site. A needle is inserted into the access site. A guidewire is placed into the vessel using ultrasound guidance. An introducer sheath is placed over the guidewire and the guidewire is removed. A wire catheter system is introduced and the tip is advanced to the site of the venous incompetence under ultrasound guidance. The wire catheter system is connected to a handle with a motor that provides the rotation to the wire. The system is started for about 10 seconds to create vasospasm and slowly withdrawn with continuous infusion of sclerosing agent. The ablation catheter and introducer sheath are removed and pressure is applied to the puncture site. A compression stocking is applied for the immediate 24 hours and replaced daily for the following two weeks. Report 36473 for the initial vein treated and 36474 for subsequent veins treated in the same extremity via different access sites.

Coding Tips

Report 36474 in addition to 36473. When performed in the office setting, all local anesthesia, supplies, and equipment are included in these services, as well as the application of compression dressings, stockings, or bandages, when provided. Do not report these codes with 36000, 36002, 36005, 36410, 36425, 36475-36476, 36478-36479, 37241, 75894, 76000, 76937, 76942, 76998, 77022, 93970, or 93971 in the same surgical field. Do not report 36473-36474 with 29520-29584 for the same extremity. Report 36474 only once per extremity regardless of the number of veins treated. For catheter injection of an adhesive or sclerosant without concomitant endovascular mechanical disruption of the vein intima, see 37799.

ICD-10-CM Diagnostic Codes

I83.011	Varicose veins of right lower extremity with ulcer of thigh ▲ ☑
I83.012	Varicose veins of right lower extremity with ulcer of calf ▲ ☑
I83.013	Varicose veins of right lower extremity with ulcer of ankle ▲ ☑
I83.014	Varicose veins of right lower extremity with ulcer of heel and midfoot ▲ ☑
I83.015	Varicose veins of right lower extremity with ulcer other part of foot ▲ ☑
I83.018	Varicose veins of right lower extremity with ulcer other part of lower leg ▲ ☑
I83.021	Varicose veins of left lower extremity with ulcer of thigh ▲ ☑
I83.022	Varicose veins of left lower extremity with ulcer of calf ▲ ☑
I83.023	Varicose veins of left lower extremity with ulcer of ankle ▲ ☑
I83.024	Varicose veins of left lower extremity with ulcer of heel and midfoot ▲ ☑
I83.025	Varicose veins of left lower extremity with ulcer other part of foot ▲ ☑
I83.028	Varicose veins of left lower extremity with ulcer other part of lower leg ▲ ☑
I83.11	Varicose veins of right lower extremity with inflammation ▲ ☑
I83.12	Varicose veins of left lower extremity with inflammation ▲ ☑
I83.211	Varicose veins of right lower extremity with both ulcer of thigh and inflammation ▲ ☑
I83.212	Varicose veins of right lower extremity with both ulcer of calf and inflammation ▲ ☑
I83.213	Varicose veins of right lower extremity with both ulcer of ankle and inflammation ▲ ☑
I83.214	Varicose veins of right lower extremity with both ulcer of heel and midfoot and inflammation ▲ ☑
I83.215	Varicose veins of right lower extremity with both ulcer other part of foot and inflammation ▲ ☑
I83.218	Varicose veins of right lower extremity with both ulcer of other part of lower extremity and inflammation ▲ ☑
I83.221	Varicose veins of left lower extremity with both ulcer of thigh and inflammation ▲ ☑
I83.222	Varicose veins of left lower extremity with both ulcer of calf and inflammation ▲ ☑
I83.223	Varicose veins of left lower extremity with both ulcer of ankle and inflammation ▲ ☑
I83.224	Varicose veins of left lower extremity with both ulcer of heel and midfoot and inflammation ▲ ☑
I83.225	Varicose veins of left lower extremity with both ulcer other part of foot and inflammation ▲ ☑
I83.228	Varicose veins of left lower extremity with both ulcer of other part of lower extremity and inflammation ▲ ☑
I83.811	Varicose veins of right lower extremity with pain ▲ ☑
I83.812	Varicose veins of left lower extremity with pain ▲ ☑
I83.813	Varicose veins of bilateral lower extremities with pain ▲ ☑
I83.891	Varicose veins of right lower extremity with other complications ▲ ☑
I83.892	Varicose veins of left lower extremity with other complications ▲ ☑
I83.893	Varicose veins of bilateral lower extremities with other complications ▲ ☑
I83.91	Asymptomatic varicose veins of right lower extremity ▲ ☑
I83.92	Asymptomatic varicose veins of left lower extremity ▲ ☑
I83.93	Asymptomatic varicose veins of bilateral lower extremities ▲ ☑
I86.8	Varicose veins of other specified sites ▲

AMA: **36473** 2019,Feb,9; 2018,Mar,3; 2018,Jan,8; 2017,Jan,8; 2016,Nov,3
36474 2019,Feb,9; 2018,Mar,3; 2018,Jan,8; 2017,Jan,8; 2016,Nov,3

Relative Value Units/Medicare Edits

Non-Facility RVU	Work	PE	MP	Total
36473	3.5	37.12	0.69	41.31
36474	1.75	6.37	0.34	8.46
Facility RVU	**Work**	**PE**	**MP**	**Total**
36473	3.5	1.03	0.69	5.22
36474	1.75	0.53	0.34	2.62

	FUD	Status	MUE	Modifiers				IOM Reference
36473	0	A	1(3)	51	50	N/A	N/A	None
36474	N/A	A	1(3)	N/A	50	N/A	N/A	

* with documentation

Terms To Know

guidewire. Flexible metal instrument designed to lead another instrument in its proper course.

sclerotherapy. Injection of a chemical agent that will irritate, inflame, and cause fibrosis in a vein, eventually obliterating hemorrhoids or varicose veins.

varicose vein. Abnormal, permanently distended or stretched vein.

Arteries and Veins

36475-36476

36475   Endovenous ablation therapy of incompetent vein, extremity, inclusive of all imaging guidance and monitoring, percutaneous, radiofrequency; first vein treated

+   36476   subsequent vein(s) treated in a single extremity, each through separate access sites (List separately in addition to code for primary procedure)

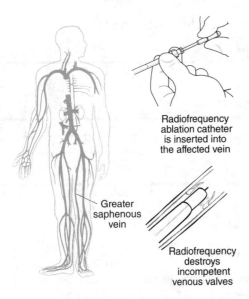

Radiofrequency ablation catheter is inserted into the affected vein

Greater saphenous vein

Radiofrequency destroys incompetent venous valves

Radiofrequency endovenous ablation therapy is performed on a site in an extremity

Explanation

The physician uses percutaneous, radiofrequency, endovenous ablation therapy to treat venous incompetence in an extremity vein. Radiofrequency energy is used to heat and seal the vein closed. The most common site of treatment is the greater saphenous vein. The procedure includes any imaging guidance and monitoring. The leg is prepared and draped and a local anesthetic is applied to the puncture site. A needle is inserted into the access site. A guidewire is placed into the vessel using ultrasound guidance. An introducer sheath is placed over the guidewire and the guidewire is removed. The radiofrequency ablation catheter system is introduced and the tip is advanced to the site of the venous incompetence under ultrasound guidance. A local anesthetic agent is injected into the tissues surrounding the vein within its fascial sheath along the course of the vein. Ultrasonography is used to position the catheter tip at the level of the terminal valve and the catheter electrodes are deployed. The electrodes should be just distal to the valve cusps of the terminal valve. Radiofrequency energy is applied until the thermocouple temperature rises to 80° to 85°C and remains at this temperature for 10 to 15 seconds. Once this temperature is reached, the catheter tip is slowly withdrawn until it reaches the introducer sheath in the distal vein. The ablation catheter and introducer sheath are removed and pressure is applied to the puncture site. Report 36475 for the first vein treated in a single extremity and 36476 for each additional vein treated through a separate access site in the same extremity.

Coding Tips

Report 36476 in addition to 36475. When these procedures are performed in the office setting, all local anesthesia, supplies, and equipment are included, as well as the application of compression dressings, stockings, or bandages, when provided. Do not report these codes with 36000, 36002, 36005, 36410, 36425, 36478-36479, 36482-36483, 37241–37244, 75894, 76000, 76937, 76942,

76998, 77022, or 93970–93971 in the same surgical field. Do not report 36475-36476 with 29520-29584 for the same extremity. Code 36476 should not be reported more than once per extremity regardless of the number of veins treated.

ICD-10-CM Diagnostic Codes

I83.011	Varicose veins of right lower extremity with ulcer of thigh 🅰 ☑
I83.012	Varicose veins of right lower extremity with ulcer of calf 🅰 ☑
I83.013	Varicose veins of right lower extremity with ulcer of ankle 🅰 ☑
I83.014	Varicose veins of right lower extremity with ulcer of heel and midfoot 🅰 ☑
I83.015	Varicose veins of right lower extremity with ulcer other part of foot 🅰 ☑
I83.018	Varicose veins of right lower extremity with ulcer other part of lower leg 🅰 ☑
I83.021	Varicose veins of left lower extremity with ulcer of thigh 🅰 ☑
I83.022	Varicose veins of left lower extremity with ulcer of calf 🅰 ☑
I83.023	Varicose veins of left lower extremity with ulcer of ankle 🅰 ☑
I83.024	Varicose veins of left lower extremity with ulcer of heel and midfoot 🅰 ☑
I83.025	Varicose veins of left lower extremity with ulcer other part of foot 🅰 ☑
I83.028	Varicose veins of left lower extremity with ulcer other part of lower leg 🅰 ☑
I83.11	Varicose veins of right lower extremity with inflammation 🅰 ☑
I83.12	Varicose veins of left lower extremity with inflammation 🅰 ☑
I83.211	Varicose veins of right lower extremity with both ulcer of thigh and inflammation 🅰 ☑
I83.212	Varicose veins of right lower extremity with both ulcer of calf and inflammation 🅰 ☑
I83.213	Varicose veins of right lower extremity with both ulcer of ankle and inflammation 🅰 ☑
I83.214	Varicose veins of right lower extremity with both ulcer of heel and midfoot and inflammation 🅰 ☑
I83.215	Varicose veins of right lower extremity with both ulcer other part of foot and inflammation 🅰 ☑
I83.218	Varicose veins of right lower extremity with both ulcer of other part of lower extremity and inflammation 🅰 ☑
I83.221	Varicose veins of left lower extremity with both ulcer of thigh and inflammation 🅰 ☑
I83.222	Varicose veins of left lower extremity with both ulcer of calf and inflammation 🅰 ☑
I83.223	Varicose veins of left lower extremity with both ulcer of ankle and inflammation 🅰 ☑
I83.224	Varicose veins of left lower extremity with both ulcer of heel and midfoot and inflammation 🅰 ☑
I83.225	Varicose veins of left lower extremity with both ulcer other part of foot and inflammation 🅰 ☑
I83.228	Varicose veins of left lower extremity with both ulcer of other part of lower extremity and inflammation 🅰 ☑
I83.811	Varicose veins of right lower extremity with pain 🅰 ☑
I83.812	Varicose veins of left lower extremity with pain 🅰 ☑
I83.813	Varicose veins of bilateral lower extremities with pain 🅰 ☑
I83.891	Varicose veins of right lower extremity with other complications 🅰 ☑

Ⓝ Newborn: 0   Ⓟ Pediatric: 0-17   Ⓜ Maternity: 9-64   🅰 Adult: 15-124   ♂ Male Only   ♀ Female Only

Arteries and Veins

I83.892	Varicose veins of left lower extremity with other complications 🅰 ☑
I83.893	Varicose veins of bilateral lower extremities with other complications 🅰 ☑
I83.91	Asymptomatic varicose veins of right lower extremity 🅰 ☑
I83.92	Asymptomatic varicose veins of left lower extremity 🅰 ☑
I83.93	Asymptomatic varicose veins of bilateral lower extremities 🅰 ☑
I86.8	Varicose veins of other specified sites 🅰

AMA: 36475 2018,Mar,3; 2018,Jan,8; 2017,Jan,8; 2016,Nov,3; 2016,Jan,13; 2016,Aug,3; 2015,Jan,16; 2015,Apr,10 **36476** 2018,Mar,3; 2018,Jan,8; 2017,Jan,8; 2016,Nov,3; 2016,Jan,13; 2016,Aug,3; 2015,Jan,16; 2015,Apr,10

Relative Value Units/Medicare Edits

Non-Facility RVU	Work	PE	MP	Total
36475	5.3	31.36	1.1	37.76
36476	2.65	5.77	0.54	8.96
Facility RVU	**Work**	**PE**	**MP**	**Total**
36475	5.3	1.73	1.1	8.13
36476	2.65	0.72	0.54	3.91

	FUD	Status	MUE	Modifiers				IOM Reference
36475	0	A	1(3)	51	50	N/A	N/A	None
36476	N/A	A	2(3)	N/A	50	N/A	N/A	

* with documentation

Terms To Know

catheter. Flexible tube inserted into an area of the body for introducing or withdrawing fluid.

guidewire. Flexible metal instrument designed to lead another instrument in its proper course.

imaging. Radiologic means of producing pictures for clinical study of the internal structures and functions of the body, such as x-ray, ultrasound, magnetic resonance, or positron emission tomography.

inflammation. Cytologic and chemical reactions that occur in affected blood vessels and adjacent tissues in response to injury or abnormal stimulation from a physical, chemical, or biologic agent.

percutaneous. Through the skin.

radiofrequency ablation. To destroy by electromagnetic wave frequencies.

ulcer. Open sore or excavating lesion of skin or the tissue on the surface of an organ from the sloughing of chronically inflamed and necrosing tissue.

ultrasound. Imaging using ultra-high sound frequency bounced off body structures.

varicose vein. Abnormal, permanently distended or stretched vein.

36478-36479

| 36478 | Endovenous ablation therapy of incompetent vein, extremity, inclusive of all imaging guidance and monitoring, percutaneous, laser; first vein treated |
| + 36479 | subsequent vein(s) treated in a single extremity, each through separate access sites (List separately in addition to code for primary procedure) |

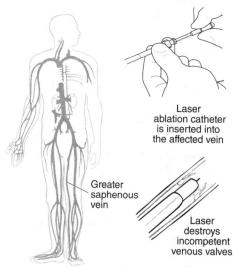

Laser ablation catheter is inserted into the affected vein

Greater saphenous vein

Laser destroys incompetent venous valves

Laser endovenous ablation therapy is performed on a site in an extremity

Explanation

The physician uses percutaneous, laser, endovenous ablation therapy to treat venous incompetence in an extremity vein. Laser energy is used to heat the vein and seal the vein closed. The most common site of treatment is the greater saphenous vein. The procedure includes any imaging guidance and monitoring. The leg is prepared and draped and a local anesthetic is applied to the puncture site. A needle is inserted into the access site. A guidewire is placed into the vessel using ultrasound guidance. An introducer sheath is placed over the guidewire and the guidewire is removed. The laser ablation catheter system is introduced and the tip is advanced to the site of the venous incompetence under ultrasound guidance. A local anesthetic agent is injected into the tissues surrounding the vein within its fascial sheath. The anesthetic is injected along the course of the vein. Ultrasonography is used to position the catheter tip at the level of the terminal valve and laser energy is applied via a laser fiber along the length of the vein as the catheter is slowly withdrawn. When the laser catheter tip reaches the introducer sheath in the distal vein, the laser energy is terminated. The ablation catheter and introducer sheath are removed and pressure is applied at the puncture site. Report 36478 for the first vein treated in a single extremity and 36479 for each additional vein treated through a separate access site in the same extremity.

Coding Tips

Report 36479 in addition to 36478. When these procedures are performed in the office setting, all local anesthesia, supplies, and equipment are included, as well as the application of compression dressings, stockings, or bandages, when provided. Do not report these codes with 36000, 36002, 36005, 36410, 36425, 36475–36476, 36482-36483, 37241, 75894, 76000, 76937, 76942, 76998, 77022, or 93970–93971. Do not report 36478-36479 with 29520-29584 for the same extremity. Code 36479 should not be reported more than once per extremity regardless of the number of additional veins treated.

Arteries and Veins

ICD-10-CM Diagnostic Codes

I83.011	Varicose veins of right lower extremity with ulcer of thigh 🅰 ☑
I83.012	Varicose veins of right lower extremity with ulcer of calf 🅰 ☑
I83.013	Varicose veins of right lower extremity with ulcer of ankle 🅰 ☑
I83.014	Varicose veins of right lower extremity with ulcer of heel and midfoot 🅰 ☑
I83.015	Varicose veins of right lower extremity with ulcer other part of foot 🅰 ☑
I83.018	Varicose veins of right lower extremity with ulcer other part of lower leg 🅰 ☑
I83.021	Varicose veins of left lower extremity with ulcer of thigh 🅰 ☑
I83.022	Varicose veins of left lower extremity with ulcer of calf 🅰 ☑
I83.023	Varicose veins of left lower extremity with ulcer of ankle 🅰 ☑
I83.024	Varicose veins of left lower extremity with ulcer of heel and midfoot 🅰 ☑
I83.025	Varicose veins of left lower extremity with ulcer other part of foot 🅰 ☑
I83.028	Varicose veins of left lower extremity with ulcer other part of lower leg 🅰 ☑
I83.11	Varicose veins of right lower extremity with inflammation 🅰 ☑
I83.12	Varicose veins of left lower extremity with inflammation 🅰 ☑
I83.211	Varicose veins of right lower extremity with both ulcer of thigh and inflammation 🅰 ☑
I83.212	Varicose veins of right lower extremity with both ulcer of calf and inflammation 🅰 ☑
I83.213	Varicose veins of right lower extremity with both ulcer of ankle and inflammation 🅰 ☑
I83.214	Varicose veins of right lower extremity with both ulcer of heel and midfoot and inflammation 🅰 ☑
I83.215	Varicose veins of right lower extremity with both ulcer other part of foot and inflammation 🅰 ☑
I83.218	Varicose veins of right lower extremity with both ulcer of other part of lower extremity and inflammation 🅰 ☑
I83.221	Varicose veins of left lower extremity with both ulcer of thigh and inflammation 🅰 ☑
I83.222	Varicose veins of left lower extremity with both ulcer of calf and inflammation 🅰 ☑
I83.223	Varicose veins of left lower extremity with both ulcer of ankle and inflammation 🅰 ☑
I83.224	Varicose veins of left lower extremity with both ulcer of heel and midfoot and inflammation 🅰 ☑
I83.225	Varicose veins of left lower extremity with both ulcer other part of foot and inflammation 🅰 ☑
I83.228	Varicose veins of left lower extremity with both ulcer of other part of lower extremity and inflammation 🅰 ☑
I83.811	Varicose veins of right lower extremity with pain 🅰 ☑
I83.812	Varicose veins of left lower extremity with pain 🅰 ☑
I83.813	Varicose veins of bilateral lower extremities with pain 🅰 ☑
I83.891	Varicose veins of right lower extremity with other complications 🅰 ☑
I83.892	Varicose veins of left lower extremity with other complications 🅰 ☑
I83.893	Varicose veins of bilateral lower extremities with other complications 🅰 ☑
I83.91	Asymptomatic varicose veins of right lower extremity 🅰 ☑
I83.92	Asymptomatic varicose veins of left lower extremity 🅰 ☑
I83.93	Asymptomatic varicose veins of bilateral lower extremities 🅰 ☑
I86.8	Varicose veins of other specified sites 🅰

AMA: **36478** 2020,May,13; 2018,Mar,3; 2018,Jan,8; 2017,Jan,8; 2016,Nov,3; 2016,Jan,13; 2016,Aug,3; 2015,Jan,16; 2015,Apr,10 **36479** 2020,May,13; 2018,Mar,3; 2018,Jan,8; 2017,Jan,8; 2016,Nov,3; 2016,Jan,13; 2016,Aug,3; 2015,Jan,16; 2015,Apr,10

Relative Value Units/Medicare Edits

Non-Facility RVU	Work	PE	MP	Total
36478	5.3	25.42	1.02	31.74
36479	2.65	6.26	0.52	9.43
Facility RVU	**Work**	**PE**	**MP**	**Total**
36478	5.3	1.76	1.02	8.08
36479	2.65	0.78	0.52	3.95

	FUD	Status	MUE	Modifiers				IOM Reference
36478	0	A	1(3)	51	50	N/A	N/A	None
36479	N/A	A	2(3)	N/A	50	N/A	N/A	

* with documentation

Terms To Know

ablation. Removal or destruction of tissue by cutting, electrical energy, chemical substances, or excessive heat application.

catheter. Flexible tube inserted into an area of the body for introducing or withdrawing fluid.

imaging. Radiologic means of producing pictures for clinical study of the internal structures and functions of the body, such as x-ray, ultrasound, magnetic resonance, or positron emission tomography.

introducer. Instrument, such as a catheter, needle, or tube, through which another instrument or device is introduced into the body.

laser surgery. Use of concentrated, sharply defined light beams to cut, cauterize, coagulate, seal, or vaporize tissue.

percutaneous. Through the skin.

varicose vein. Abnormal, permanently distended or stretched vein.

36555-36556

36555 Insertion of non-tunneled centrally inserted central venous catheter; younger than 5 years of age

36556 age 5 years or older

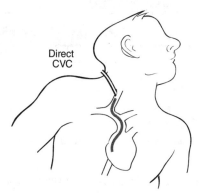

A non-tunneled centrally inserted CVC is inserted

Direct CVC

Explanation

A central venous access device (CVAD) or catheter is one in which the tip terminates in the subclavian, brachiocephalic, or iliac vein; the superior or inferior vena cava; or the right atrium. A centrally inserted CVAD has an entry site in the inferior vena cava or the jugular, subclavian, or femoral vein. For insertion of a non-tunneled, centrally inserted CVAD, the site over the access vein (e.g., subclavian, jugular) is injected with local anesthesia and punctured with a needle. A guidewire is inserted. The central venous catheter is placed over the guidewire. Ultrasound guidance may be used to gain venous access and/or fluoroscopy to check the positioning of the catheter tip. The catheter is secured into position and dressed. Non-tunneled catheters are percutaneously inserted for short term (five to seven days) use; to infuse medications, fluids, blood products, and parenteral nutrition; and to take blood draws. Report 36555 for insertion for children younger than 5 years of age and 36556 for a patient 5 years of age or older.

Coding Tips

If imaging guidance is used for obtaining access to the venous site or for manipulating the catheter into the final end position, see 76937 or 77001. For a peripherally inserted, central venous catheter for a patient younger than 5 years of age, see 36568; 5 years of age or older, see 36569.

ICD-10-CM Diagnostic Codes

The application of this code is too broad to adequately present ICD-10-CM diagnostic code links here. Refer to your ICD-10-CM book.

AMA: 36555 2019,May,3; 2018,Jan,8; 2017,Jan,8; 2016,Jan,13; 2015,Jan,16
36556 2019,May,3; 2018,Nov,11; 2018,Jan,8; 2017,Jan,8; 2016,Jan,13; 2015,Jan,16

Relative Value Units/Medicare Edits

Non-Facility RVU	Work	PE	MP	Total
36555	1.93	3.7	0.15	5.78
36556	1.75	4.6	0.21	6.56
Facility RVU	**Work**	**PE**	**MP**	**Total**
36555	1.93	0.37	0.15	2.45
36556	1.75	0.5	0.21	2.46

	FUD	Status	MUE	Modifiers				IOM Reference
36555	0	A	2(3)	N/A	N/A	N/A	N/A	None
36556	0	A	2(3)	N/A	N/A	N/A	N/A	

* with documentation

Terms To Know

catheter. Flexible tube inserted into an area of the body for introducing or withdrawing fluid.

central venous catheter. Catheter positioned in the superior vena cava or right atrium and introduced through a large vein, such as the jugular or subclavian, and used to measure venous pressure or administer fluids or medication.

fluoroscopy. Radiology technique that allows visual examination of part of the body or a function of an organ using a device that projects an x-ray image on a fluorescent screen.

guidewire. Flexible metal instrument designed to lead another instrument in its proper course.

injection. Forcing a liquid substance into a body part such as a joint or muscle.

jugular vein. Two pairs of veins on either side of the neck that open into the subclavian, sending blood from the head and neck to the heart.

parenteral nutrition. Nutrients provided subcutaneously, intravenously, intramuscularly, or intradermally for patients during the postoperative period and in other conditions, such as shock, coma, and renal failure.

percutaneous. Through the skin.

ultrasound. Imaging using ultra-high sound frequency bounced off body structures.

vein. Vessel through which oxygen-depleted blood passes back to the heart.

vena cava. Main venous trunk that empties into the right atrium from both the lower and upper regions, beginning at the junction of the common iliac veins inferiorly and the two brachiocephalic veins superiorly.

Arteries and Veins

36557-36558

36557 Insertion of tunneled centrally inserted central venous catheter, without subcutaneous port or pump; younger than 5 years of age
36558 age 5 years or older

A tunneled centrally inserted CVC is inserted

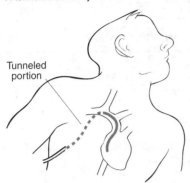

Tunneled portion

Explanation

A central venous access device (CVAD) or catheter is one in which the tip terminates in the subclavian, brachiocephalic, or iliac vein; the superior or inferior vena cava; or the right atrium. A centrally inserted CVAD has an entry site in the inferior vena cava or the jugular, subclavian, or femoral vein. A tunneled catheter has an entrance site at a distance from its entrance into the vascular system; they are "tunneled" through the skin and subcutaneous tissue to a great vein. For insertion of a tunneled, centrally inserted CVAD, without subcutaneous port or pump, standard preparations are made and the site over the access vein (e.g., subclavian, jugular) is injected with local anesthesia and punctured with a needle or accessed by cutdown approach. A guidewire is inserted. A subcutaneous tunnel is created using a blunt pair of forceps or sharp tunneling tools, over the clavicle from the anterior chest wall to the venotomy site, which is dilated to the right size. The catheter is passed through this tunnel over the guidewire and into the target vein. Ultrasound guidance may be used to gain venous access and/or fluoroscopy to check the positioning of the catheter tip. The catheter is secured into position and any incisions are sutured. Report 36557 for insertion for children younger than 5 years of age and 36558 for a patient 5 years of age or older.

Coding Tips

If imaging guidance is used for obtaining access to the venous site or for manipulating the catheter into final end position, see 76937 and 77001. For a peripherally inserted central venous catheter with port, less than 5 years of age, see 36570; 5 years of age or older, see 36571.

ICD-10-CM Diagnostic Codes

The application of this code is too broad to adequately present ICD-10-CM diagnostic code links here. Refer to your ICD-10-CM book.

AMA: 36557 2018,Jan,8; 2017,Jan,8; 2016,Jan,13; 2015,Jan,16 **36558** 2018,Jan,8; 2017,Jan,8; 2016,Jan,13; 2015,Jan,13; 2015,Jan,16

Relative Value Units/Medicare Edits

Non-Facility RVU	Work	PE	MP	Total
36557	4.89	29.6	1.2	35.69
36558	4.59	20.34	0.61	25.54
Facility RVU	Work	PE	MP	Total
36557	4.89	3.34	1.2	9.43
36558	4.59	2.37	0.61	7.57

	FUD	Status	MUE	Modifiers				IOM Reference
36557	10	A	2(3)	51	50	N/A	80*	None
36558	10	A	2(3)	51	50	N/A	80*	

* with documentation

Terms To Know

catheter. Flexible tube inserted into an area of the body for introducing or withdrawing fluid.

central venous catheter. Catheter positioned in the superior vena cava or right atrium and introduced through a large vein, such as the jugular or subclavian, and used to measure venous pressure or administer fluids or medication.

dilation. Artificial increase in the diameter of an opening or lumen made by medication or by instrumentation.

fluoroscopy. Radiology technique that allows visual examination of part of the body or a function of an organ using a device that projects an x-ray image on a fluorescent screen.

guidewire. Flexible metal instrument designed to lead another instrument in its proper course.

jugular vein. Two pairs of veins on either side of the neck that open into the subclavian, sending blood from the head and neck to the heart.

parenteral nutrition. Nutrients provided subcutaneously, intravenously, intramuscularly, or intradermally for patients during the postoperative period and in other conditions, such as shock, coma, and renal failure.

ultrasound. Imaging using ultra-high sound frequency bounced off body structures.

vena cava. Main venous trunk that empties into the right atrium from both the lower and upper regions, beginning at the junction of the common iliac veins inferiorly and the two brachiocephalic veins superiorly.

36560-36561

36560 Insertion of tunneled centrally inserted central venous access device, with subcutaneous port; younger than 5 years of age

36561 age 5 years or older

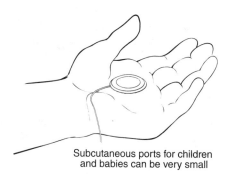

Subcutaneous ports for children and babies can be very small

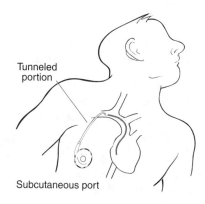

Tunneled portion

Subcutaneous port

Explanation

For insertion of a tunneled, centrally inserted CVAD, with subcutaneous port/pump, the site over the access vein (e.g., subclavian, jugular) is injected with local anesthesia and punctured with a needle or accessed by cutdown approach. A guidewire is inserted. A subcutaneous tunnel is created using a blunt pair of forceps or sharp tunneling tools, over the clavicle, from the anterior chest wall to the venotomy site, which is dilated to the right size. The catheter is passed through this tunnel over the guidewire and into the target vein. The subcutaneous pocket for the port/pump is created with an incision through the skin overlying the second rib, a few centimeters from the midline. Blunt dissection and cautery are used to create the pocket in the chest wall and the port/pump is placed. The catheter is connected to the port/pump and checked by injection. Ultrasound guidance may be used to gain venous access and/or fluoroscopy to check the positioning of the catheter tip. The catheter and port/pump are secured into position and any incisions are sutured. Report 36560 for insertion with a port for children younger than 5 years of age and 36561 for a patient 5 years of age or older.

Coding Tips

For a peripherally inserted central venous access device with a subcutaneous port, patient 5 years of age or less, see 36570; 5 years or older, see 36571. When imaging is used for gaining access to the venous entry site or for manipulating the catheter into final central position, see 76937 or 77001.

ICD-10-CM Diagnostic Codes

The application of this code is too broad to adequately present ICD-10-CM diagnostic code links here. Refer to your ICD-10-CM book.

AMA: 36560 2018,Jan,8; 2017,Jan,8; 2016,Jan,13; 2015,Jan,16 **36561** 2018,Jan,8; 2017,Jan,8; 2016,Jan,13; 2015,Jan,16

Relative Value Units/Medicare Edits

Non-Facility RVU	Work	PE	MP	Total
36560	6.04	32.51	1.47	40.02
36561	5.79	25.18	0.93	31.9
Facility RVU	Work	PE	MP	Total
36560	6.04	3.77	1.47	11.28
36561	5.79	3.05	0.93	9.77

	FUD	Status	MUE	Modifiers				IOM Reference
36560	10	A	2(3)	51	50	N/A	80*	None
36561	10	A	2(3)	51	50	N/A	80*	

* with documentation

Terms To Know

cautery. Destruction or burning of tissue by means of a hot instrument, an electric current, or a caustic chemical, such as silver nitrate.

fluoroscopy. Radiology technique that allows visual examination of part of the body or a function of an organ using a device that projects an x-ray image on a fluorescent screen.

guidewire. Flexible metal instrument designed to lead another instrument in its proper course.

jugular vein. Two pairs of veins on either side of the neck that open into the subclavian, sending blood from the head and neck to the heart.

parenteral nutrition. Nutrients provided subcutaneously, intravenously, intramuscularly, or intradermally for patients during the postoperative period and in other conditions, such as shock, coma, and renal failure.

subcutaneous pocket. Small space created under the skin in a suitable location for holding an implantable device, such as the pulse generator of a pacemaker or cardioverter defibrillator.

subcutaneous tissue. Sheet or wide band of adipose (fat) and areolar connective tissue in two layers attached to the dermis.

ultrasound. Imaging using ultra-high sound frequency bounced off body structures.

vena cava. Main venous trunk that empties into the right atrium from both the lower and upper regions, beginning at the junction of the common iliac veins inferiorly and the two brachiocephalic veins superiorly.

Arteries and Veins

36563

36563 Insertion of tunneled centrally inserted central venous access device with subcutaneous pump

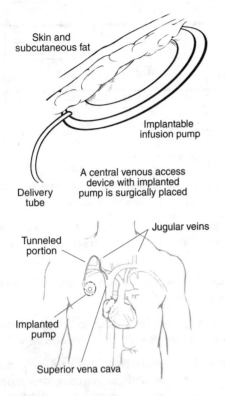

Skin and subcutaneous fat

Implantable infusion pump

A central venous access device with implanted pump is surgically placed

Delivery tube

Jugular veins

Tunneled portion

Implanted pump

Superior vena cava

Explanation

For insertion of a tunneled, centrally inserted CVAD, with subcutaneous port/pump, the site over the access vein (e.g., subclavian, jugular) is injected with local anesthesia and punctured with a needle or accessed by cutdown approach. A guidewire is inserted. A subcutaneous tunnel is created using a blunt pair of forceps or sharp tunneling tools, over the clavicle, from the anterior chest wall to the venotomy site, which is dilated to the right size. The catheter is passed through this tunnel over the guidewire and into the target vein. The subcutaneous pocket for the port/pump is created with an incision through the skin overlying the second rib, a few centimeters from the midline. Blunt dissection and cautery are used to create the pocket in the chest wall and the port/pump is placed. The catheter is connected to the port/pump and checked by injection. Ultrasound guidance may be used to gain venous access and/or fluoroscopy to check the positioning of the catheter tip. The catheter and port/pump are secured into position and any incisions are sutured. Report 36563 for insertion with a pump.

Coding Tips

When imaging is used to gain access to the venous entry site or for manipulating the catheter into final central position, see 76937 or 77001. For peripherally inserted central venous access device with subcutaneous port, under 5 years of age, see 36570; 5 years or older, see 36571.

ICD-10-CM Diagnostic Codes

The application of this code is too broad to adequately present ICD-10-CM diagnostic code links here. Refer to your ICD-10-CM book.

AMA: 36563 2018,Jan,8; 2017,Jan,8; 2016,Jan,13; 2015,Jan,16

Relative Value Units/Medicare Edits

Non-Facility RVU	Work	PE	MP	Total
36563	5.99	28.8	1.36	36.15
Facility RVU	Work	PE	MP	Total
36563	5.99	3.37	1.36	10.72

	FUD	Status	MUE	Modifiers				IOM Reference
36563	10	A	1(3)	51	N/A	N/A	80*	None

* with documentation

Terms To Know

anterior. Situated in the front area or toward the belly surface of the body; an anatomical reference point used to show the position and relationship of one body structure to another.

blunt dissection. Surgical technique used to expose an underlying area by separating along natural cleavage lines of tissue, without cutting.

cautery. Destruction or burning of tissue by means of a hot instrument, an electric current, or a caustic chemical, such as silver nitrate.

central venous access device. Catheter or other device introduced through a large vein, such as the subclavian or femoral vein, terminating in the superior or inferior vena cava or the right atrium and used to measure venous pressure or administer medication or fluids.

cutdown. Small, incised opening in the skin to expose a blood vessel, especially over a vein (venous cutdown) to allow venipuncture and permit a needle or cannula to be inserted for the withdrawal of blood or administration of fluids.

forceps. Tool used for grasping or compressing tissue.

infusion pump. Device that delivers a measured amount of drug or intravenous solution through injection over a period of time.

jugular vein. Two pairs of veins on either side of the neck that open into the subclavian, sending blood from the head and neck to the heart.

skin. Outer protective covering of the body composed of the epidermis and dermis, situated above the subcutaneous tissues.

subcutaneous pocket. Small space created under the skin in a suitable location for holding an implantable device, such as the pulse generator of a pacemaker or cardioverter defibrillator.

subcutaneous tissue. Sheet or wide band of adipose (fat) and areolar connective tissue in two layers attached to the dermis.

vein. Vessel through which oxygen-depleted blood passes back to the heart.

venotomy. Incision or puncture of a vein.

36568-36569 [36572, 36573]

36568 Insertion of peripherally inserted central venous catheter (PICC), without subcutaneous port or pump, without imaging guidance; younger than 5 years of age

36569 age 5 years or older

36572 Insertion of peripherally inserted central venous catheter (PICC), without subcutaneous port or pump, including all imaging guidance, image documentation, and all associated radiological supervision and interpretation required to perform the insertion; younger than 5 years of age

36573 Insertion of peripherally inserted central venous catheter (PICC), without subcutaneous port or pump, including all imaging guidance, image documentation, and all associated radiological supervision and interpretation required to perform the insertion; age 5 years or older

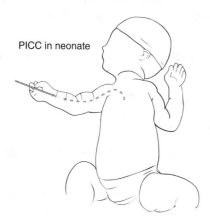

PICC in neonate

A central venous catheter is inserted from a periphery

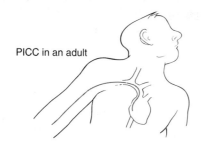

PICC in an adult

Explanation

A central venous access device or catheter is one in which the tip terminates in the subclavian, brachiocephalic, or iliac vein; the superior or inferior vena cava; or the right atrium. A peripherally inserted central venous catheter (PICC) has an entry site in the basilic or cephalic vein in the arm and is threaded into the superior vena cava above the right atrium. PICC lines are used for antibiotic therapy, chemotherapy, total parenteral nutrition, lab work, pain medications, blood transfusions, and hydration the same as a central line. For insertion of a (non-tunneled) peripherally inserted central venous catheter, without subcutaneous port or pump, the access vein (basilic or cephalic) is injected with local anesthesia and punctured with a needle. A guidewire is inserted. The central venous catheter is placed over the guidewire. The catheter is

secured into position and dressed. Report 36568 for insertion of a PICC, without imaging, for children younger than 5 years of age; for a patient 5 years of age or older, report 36569. Report 36572 for insertion of a PICC, with imaging, for children younger than 5 years age; for a patient 5 years of age or older, report 36573.

Coding Tips

For placement of a centrally inserted, non-tunneled central venous catheter, younger than 5 years of age, see 36555; 5 years of age or older, see 36556.

ICD-10-CM Diagnostic Codes

The application of this code is too broad to adequately present ICD-10-CM diagnostic code links here. Refer to your ICD-10-CM book.

AMA: 36568 2019,May,3; 2018,Jan,8; 2017,Jan,8; 2016,Jan,13; 2015,Jan,16 **36569** 2019,May,3; 2018,Jan,8; 2017,Jan,8; 2016,Jan,13; 2015,Jan,16 **36572** 2019,May,3; 2019,Mar,10 **36573** 2019,May,3; 2019,Mar,10

Relative Value Units/Medicare Edits

Non-Facility RVU	Work	PE	MP	Total
36568	2.11	0.34	0.21	2.66
36569	1.9	0.61	0.21	2.72
36572	1.82	11.35	0.17	13.34
36573	1.7	10.27	0.19	12.16
Facility RVU	**Work**	**PE**	**MP**	**Total**
36568	2.11	0.34	0.21	2.66
36569	1.9	0.61	0.21	2.72
36572	1.82	0.65	0.17	2.64
36573	1.7	0.56	0.19	2.45

	FUD	Status	MUE	Modifiers				IOM Reference
36568	0	A	2(3)	N/A	N/A	N/A	N/A	None
36569	0	A	2(3)	N/A	N/A	N/A	N/A	
36572	0	A	1(3)	N/A	N/A	N/A	N/A	
36573	0	A	1(3)	N/A	N/A	N/A	N/A	

* with documentation

Terms To Know

central venous catheter. Catheter positioned in the superior vena cava or right atrium and introduced through a large vein, such as the jugular or subclavian, and used to measure venous pressure or administer fluids or medication.

fluoroscopy. Radiology technique that allows visual examination of part of the body or a function of an organ using a device that projects an x-ray image on a fluorescent screen.

guidewire. Flexible metal instrument designed to lead another instrument in its proper course.

peripheral. Outside of a structure or organ.

subcutaneous tissue. Sheet or wide band of adipose (fat) and areolar connective tissue in two layers attached to the dermis.

vena cava. Main venous trunk that empties into the right atrium from both the lower and upper regions, beginning at the junction of the common iliac veins inferiorly and the two brachiocephalic veins superiorly.

36570-36571

36570 Insertion of peripherally inserted central venous access device, with subcutaneous port; younger than 5 years of age
36571 age 5 years or older

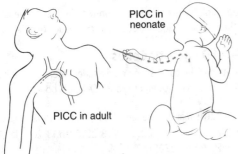

A central venous access device is inserted from a periphery, with use of a subcutaneous port

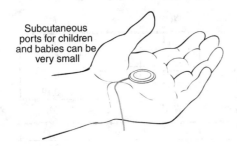

Subcutaneous ports for children and babies can be very small

Explanation

A central venous access device or catheter is one in which the tip terminates in the subclavian, brachiocephalic, or iliac vein; the superior or inferior vena cava; or the right atrium. A peripherally inserted central venous catheter (PICC) has an entry site in the basilic or cephalic vein in the arm and is threaded into the superior vena cava above the right atrium. PICC lines are used for antibiotic therapy, chemotherapy, total parenteral nutrition, lab work, pain medications, blood transfusions, and hydration the same as a central line. For insertion of a peripherally inserted central venous catheter with a subcutaneous port, the site over the access vein (basilic or cephalic) is injected with local anesthesia and punctured with a needle. A guidewire is inserted. The central venous catheter is placed over the guidewire and fed through the vein in the arm into the superior vena cava. The port may be placed in the chest in a subcutaneous pocket created through an incision in the chest wall, or placed in the arm through a small incision just above or halfway between the elbow crease and the shoulder on the inside of the arm. The port is attached to the catheter and checked. Ultrasound guidance may be used to gain venous access and/or fluoroscopy to check the positioning of the catheter tip. The catheter and port are secured into position and incisions are closed and dressed. Report 36570 for insertion for children younger than 5 years of age and 36571 for a patient 5 years of age or older.

Coding Tips

For insertion of a tunneled, centrally inserted central venous access device, with subcutaneous port, younger than 5 years of age, see 36560; 5 years or older, see 36561. When imaging is used for gaining access to the venous entry site or for manipulating the catheter into final central position, see 76937 or 77001.

ICD-10-CM Diagnostic Codes

The application of this code is too broad to adequately present ICD-10-CM diagnostic code links here. Refer to your ICD-10-CM book.

AMA: **36570** 2018,Jan,8; 2017,Jan,8; 2016,Jan,13; 2015,Jan,16 **36571** 2018,Jan,8; 2017,Jan,8; 2016,Jan,13; 2015,Jan,16

Relative Value Units/Medicare Edits

Non-Facility RVU	Work	PE	MP	Total
36570	5.11	40.19	1.25	46.55
36571	5.09	34.5	0.99	40.58
Facility RVU	**Work**	**PE**	**MP**	**Total**
36570	5.11	3.42	1.25	9.78
36571	5.09	3.11	0.99	9.19

	FUD	Status	MUE	Modifiers				IOM Reference
36570	10	A	2(3)	51	50	N/A	80*	None
36571	10	A	2(3)	51	50	N/A	80*	

* with documentation

Terms To Know

central venous access device. Catheter or other device introduced through a large vein, such as the subclavian or femoral vein, terminating in the superior or inferior vena cava or the right atrium and used to measure venous pressure or administer medication or fluids.

chemotherapy. Treatment of disease, especially cancerous conditions, using chemical agents.

fluoroscopy. Radiology technique that allows visual examination of part of the body or a function of an organ using a device that projects an x-ray image on a fluorescent screen.

guidewire. Flexible metal instrument designed to lead another instrument in its proper course.

ultrasound. Imaging using ultra-high sound frequency bounced off body structures.

vena cava. Main venous trunk that empties into the right atrium from both the lower and upper regions, beginning at the junction of the common iliac veins inferiorly and the two brachiocephalic veins superiorly.

36575-36576

36575 Repair of tunneled or non-tunneled central venous access catheter, without subcutaneous port or pump, central or peripheral insertion site

36576 Repair of central venous access device, with subcutaneous port or pump, central or peripheral insertion site

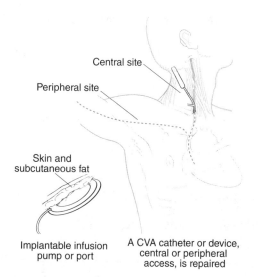

Central site

Peripheral site

Skin and subcutaneous fat

Implantable infusion pump or port

A CVA catheter or device, central or peripheral access, is repaired

Explanation

Code 36575 reports repair of a central venous access device (CVAD) that has external catheters with the access ports outside the body, and no subcutaneous ports or pumps, whether centrally or peripherally inserted, tunneled or non-tunneled. The repair is done on the catheter that is placed without any replacement of components. A Hickman catheter is an example of a tunneled CVAD with an external port. In 36576, the physician repairs a central venous access device (CVAD) that has an internal access port/pump in a subcutaneous pocket that is connected to the catheter, whether centrally or peripherally inserted. The repair is done on the device as it is placed within the patient, without any replacement of components, catheter or subcutaneous port/pump.

Coding Tips

Mechanical removal of pericatheter obstructive material is reported with 36595; intracatheter obstructive material, see 36596. If imaging guidance is used for obtaining access to the venous access site or for manipulating the catheter into final end position, see 76937 or 77001. Partial replacement of a central venous access device (catheter only) with subcutaneous port or pump, central or peripheral, is reported with 36578.

ICD-10-CM Diagnostic Codes

T80.211A	Bloodstream infection due to central venous catheter, initial encounter
T80.212A	Local infection due to central venous catheter, initial encounter
T80.218A	Other infection due to central venous catheter, initial encounter
T82.41XA	Breakdown (mechanical) of vascular dialysis catheter, initial encounter
T82.42XA	Displacement of vascular dialysis catheter, initial encounter
T82.43XA	Leakage of vascular dialysis catheter, initial encounter
T82.49XA	Other complication of vascular dialysis catheter, initial encounter
T82.514A	Breakdown (mechanical) of infusion catheter, initial encounter
T82.524A	Displacement of infusion catheter, initial encounter
T82.534A	Leakage of infusion catheter, initial encounter
T82.594A	Other mechanical complication of infusion catheter, initial encounter
T82.598A	Other mechanical complication of other cardiac and vascular devices and implants, initial encounter
T82.7XXA	Infection and inflammatory reaction due to other cardiac and vascular devices, implants and grafts, initial encounter
T82.818A	Embolism due to vascular prosthetic devices, implants and grafts, initial encounter
T82.828A	Fibrosis due to vascular prosthetic devices, implants and grafts, initial encounter
T82.838A	Hemorrhage due to vascular prosthetic devices, implants and grafts, initial encounter
T82.848A	Pain due to vascular prosthetic devices, implants and grafts, initial encounter
T82.858A	Stenosis of other vascular prosthetic devices, implants and grafts, initial encounter
T82.868A	Thrombosis due to vascular prosthetic devices, implants and grafts, initial encounter
T82.898A	Other specified complication of vascular prosthetic devices, implants and grafts, initial encounter
Z45.2	Encounter for adjustment and management of vascular access device

AMA: **36575** 2018,Jan,8; 2017,Jan,8; 2016,Jan,13; 2015,Jan,16 **36576** 2018,Jan,8; 2017,Jan,8; 2016,Jan,13; 2015,Jan,16

Relative Value Units/Medicare Edits

Non-Facility RVU	Work	PE	MP	Total
36575	0.67	4.04	0.09	4.8
36576	2.99	7.01	0.54	10.54
Facility RVU	**Work**	**PE**	**MP**	**Total**
36575	0.67	0.24	0.09	1.0
36576	2.99	1.86	0.54	5.39

	FUD	Status	MUE	Modifiers				IOM Reference
36575	0	A	2(3)	51	N/A	N/A	80*	None
36576	10	A	2(3)	51	N/A	N/A	80*	

* with documentation

Terms To Know

central venous access device. Catheter or other device introduced through a large vein, such as the subclavian or femoral vein, terminating in the superior or inferior vena cava or the right atrium and used to measure venous pressure or administer medication or fluids.

Hickman catheter. Central venous catheter used for long-term delivery of medications, such as antibiotics, nutritional substances, or chemotherapeutic agents.

36578

36578 Replacement, catheter only, of central venous access device, with subcutaneous port or pump, central or peripheral insertion site

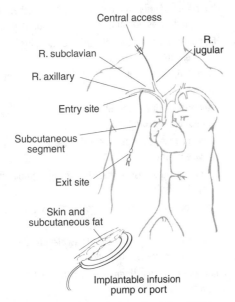

The catheter alone is replaced in a CVA device, with subcutaneous port or pump, central or peripheral access site

Explanation

The catheter only of a central venous access device with a subcutaneous port or pump is replaced, whether centrally or peripherally inserted. Local anesthesia is given and the subcutaneous pocket over the port is incised. The catheter is disconnected. A guidewire is placed through the existing catheter, which is removed over the guidewire. A new central venous catheter of correct length is placed into position and connected to the port/pump device that has not been removed or replaced. The connection with the new catheter is checked, as well as the catheter and port secured, and the wound is dressed.

Coding Tips

For complete replacement of an entire device through the same venous access, see 36582 or 36583. If imaging guidance is used for obtaining access to the venous access site or for manipulating the catheter into final end position, see 76937 or 77001.

ICD-10-CM Diagnostic Codes

T80.211A	Bloodstream infection due to central venous catheter, initial encounter
T80.212A	Local infection due to central venous catheter, initial encounter
T80.218A	Other infection due to central venous catheter, initial encounter
T82.43XA	Leakage of vascular dialysis catheter, initial encounter
T82.49XA	Other complication of vascular dialysis catheter, initial encounter
T82.514A	Breakdown (mechanical) of infusion catheter, initial encounter
T82.524A	Displacement of infusion catheter, initial encounter
T82.534A	Leakage of infusion catheter, initial encounter
T82.594A	Other mechanical complication of infusion catheter, initial encounter
T82.598A	Other mechanical complication of other cardiac and vascular devices and implants, initial encounter

T82.7XXA	Infection and inflammatory reaction due to other cardiac and vascular devices, implants and grafts, initial encounter
T82.818A	Embolism due to vascular prosthetic devices, implants and grafts, initial encounter
T82.828A	Fibrosis due to vascular prosthetic devices, implants and grafts, initial encounter
T82.838A	Hemorrhage due to vascular prosthetic devices, implants and grafts, initial encounter
T82.848A	Pain due to vascular prosthetic devices, implants and grafts, initial encounter
T82.858A	Stenosis of other vascular prosthetic devices, implants and grafts, initial encounter
T82.868A	Thrombosis due to vascular prosthetic devices, implants and grafts, initial encounter
T82.898A	Other specified complication of vascular prosthetic devices, implants and grafts, initial encounter
Z45.2	Encounter for adjustment and management of vascular access device

AMA: 36578 2018,Jan,8; 2017,Jan,8; 2016,Jan,13; 2015,Jan,16

Relative Value Units/Medicare Edits

Non-Facility RVU	Work	PE	MP	Total
36578	3.29	9.96	0.59	13.84
Facility RVU	**Work**	**PE**	**MP**	**Total**
36578	3.29	2.04	0.59	5.92

	FUD	Status	MUE	Modifiers				IOM Reference
36578	10	A	2(3)	51	N/A	N/A	80*	None

* with documentation

Terms To Know

catheter. Flexible tube inserted into an area of the body for introducing or withdrawing fluid.

central venous access device. Catheter or other device introduced through a large vein, such as the subclavian or femoral vein, terminating in the superior or inferior vena cava or the right atrium and used to measure venous pressure or administer medication or fluids.

peripheral. Outside of a structure or organ.

subcutaneous. Below the skin.

36580-36581

36580 Replacement, complete, of a non-tunneled centrally inserted central venous catheter, without subcutaneous port or pump, through same venous access

36581 Replacement, complete, of a tunneled centrally inserted central venous catheter, without subcutaneous port or pump, through same venous access

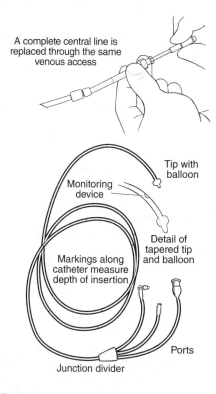

A complete central line is replaced through the same venous access

Tip with balloon
Monitoring device
Detail of tapered tip and balloon
Markings along catheter measure depth of insertion
Ports
Junction divider

Explanation

A non-tunneled, 36580, or tunneled, 36581, centrally inserted central venous catheter, without subcutaneous port or pump, is replaced through the same venous access site. Local anesthesia is given. A guidewire is passed through the existing central line catheter and the catheter is removed. A new central venous catheter is placed back into position over the guidewire, secured into position, and the wound dressed.

Coding Tips

If imaging guidance is used for obtaining access to the venous access site or for manipulating the replacement catheter into its final end position, see 76937 or 77001. Complete replacement of a tunneled central venous access device with subcutaneous port, see 36582; pump, see 36583.

ICD-10-CM Diagnostic Codes

T80.211A	Bloodstream infection due to central venous catheter, initial encounter
T80.212A	Local infection due to central venous catheter, initial encounter
T80.218A	Other infection due to central venous catheter, initial encounter
T82.41XA	Breakdown (mechanical) of vascular dialysis catheter, initial encounter
T82.42XA	Displacement of vascular dialysis catheter, initial encounter
T82.43XA	Leakage of vascular dialysis catheter, initial encounter
T82.49XA	Other complication of vascular dialysis catheter, initial encounter
T82.514A	Breakdown (mechanical) of infusion catheter, initial encounter
T82.524A	Displacement of infusion catheter, initial encounter
T82.534A	Leakage of infusion catheter, initial encounter
T82.594A	Other mechanical complication of infusion catheter, initial encounter
T82.598A	Other mechanical complication of other cardiac and vascular devices and implants, initial encounter
T82.7XXA	Infection and inflammatory reaction due to other cardiac and vascular devices, implants and grafts, initial encounter
T82.818A	Embolism due to vascular prosthetic devices, implants and grafts, initial encounter
T82.828A	Fibrosis due to vascular prosthetic devices, implants and grafts, initial encounter
T82.838A	Hemorrhage due to vascular prosthetic devices, implants and grafts, initial encounter
T82.848A	Pain due to vascular prosthetic devices, implants and grafts, initial encounter
T82.858A	Stenosis of other vascular prosthetic devices, implants and grafts, initial encounter
T82.868A	Thrombosis due to vascular prosthetic devices, implants and grafts, initial encounter
T82.898A	Other specified complication of vascular prosthetic devices, implants and grafts, initial encounter
Z45.2	Encounter for adjustment and management of vascular access device

AMA: 36580 2018,Jan,8; 2017,Jan,8; 2016,Jan,13; 2015,Jan,16 **36581** 2018,Jan,8; 2017,Jan,8; 2016,Jan,13; 2015,Jan,16

Relative Value Units/Medicare Edits

Non-Facility RVU	Work	PE	MP	Total
36580	1.31	4.79	0.15	6.25
36581	3.23	21.09	0.39	24.71
Facility RVU	**Work**	**PE**	**MP**	**Total**
36580	1.31	0.45	0.15	1.91
36581	3.23	1.72	0.39	5.34

	FUD	Status	MUE	Modifiers				IOM Reference
36580	0	A	2(3)	N/A	N/A	N/A	N/A	None
36581	10	A	2(3)	51	N/A	N/A	80*	

* with documentation

Terms To Know

central venous catheter. Catheter positioned in the superior vena cava or right atrium and introduced through a large vein, such as the jugular or subclavian, and used to measure venous pressure or administer fluids or medication.

peripheral. Outside of a structure or organ.

subcutaneous. Below the skin.

subcutaneous tissue. Sheet or wide band of adipose (fat) and areolar connective tissue in two layers attached to the dermis.

36582-36583

36582 Replacement, complete, of a tunneled centrally inserted central venous access device, with subcutaneous port, through same venous access

36583 Replacement, complete, of a tunneled centrally inserted central venous access device, with subcutaneous pump, through same venous access

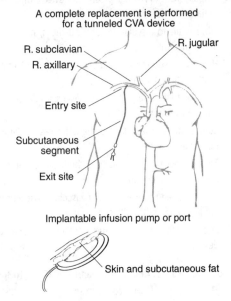

A complete replacement is performed for a tunneled CVA device

R. subclavian
R. jugular
R. axillary
Entry site
Subcutaneous segment
Exit site

Implantable infusion pump or port

Skin and subcutaneous fat

Explanation

A tunneled, centrally inserted central venous catheter, along with a subcutaneous port (36582) or pump (36583) device is replaced. Local anesthesia is given and the subcutaneous pocket over the port/pump device is incised. The pump/port is dissected free and tested. The catheter is disconnected and the pump/port device is removed from its pocket. A guidewire is placed over the existing catheter, which is removed, and a new central venous catheter is threaded into position over the guidewire. A new pump/port device is inserted into the subcutaneous pocket and the catheter is connected. The connection is checked with an injection. The new pump/port is secured into the pocket, incisions are closed, and the wound is dressed.

Coding Tips

If imaging guidance is used for obtaining access to the venous access site or for manipulating the catheter into final end position, see 76937 or 77001. For complete replacement of a peripherally inserted central venous catheter (PICC) without subcutaneous port or pump, see 36584; with subcutaneous port, see 36585.

ICD-10-CM Diagnostic Codes

T80.211A	Bloodstream infection due to central venous catheter, initial encounter
T80.212A	Local infection due to central venous catheter, initial encounter
T80.218A	Other infection due to central venous catheter, initial encounter
T82.41XA	Breakdown (mechanical) of vascular dialysis catheter, initial encounter
T82.42XA	Displacement of vascular dialysis catheter, initial encounter
T82.43XA	Leakage of vascular dialysis catheter, initial encounter
T82.49XA	Other complication of vascular dialysis catheter, initial encounter
T82.514A	Breakdown (mechanical) of infusion catheter, initial encounter
T82.524A	Displacement of infusion catheter, initial encounter
T82.534A	Leakage of infusion catheter, initial encounter
T82.594A	Other mechanical complication of infusion catheter, initial encounter
T82.598A	Other mechanical complication of other cardiac and vascular devices and implants, initial encounter
T82.7XXA	Infection and inflammatory reaction due to other cardiac and vascular devices, implants and grafts, initial encounter
T82.818A	Embolism due to vascular prosthetic devices, implants and grafts, initial encounter
T82.828A	Fibrosis due to vascular prosthetic devices, implants and grafts, initial encounter
T82.838A	Hemorrhage due to vascular prosthetic devices, implants and grafts, initial encounter
T82.848A	Pain due to vascular prosthetic devices, implants and grafts, initial encounter
T82.858A	Stenosis of other vascular prosthetic devices, implants and grafts, initial encounter
T82.868A	Thrombosis due to vascular prosthetic devices, implants and grafts, initial encounter
T82.898A	Other specified complication of vascular prosthetic devices, implants and grafts, initial encounter
Z45.2	Encounter for adjustment and management of vascular access device

AMA: 36582 2018,Jan,8; 2017,Jan,8; 2016,Jan,13; 2015,Jan,16 **36583** 2018,Jan,8; 2017,Jan,8; 2016,Jan,13; 2015,Jan,16

Relative Value Units/Medicare Edits

Non-Facility RVU	Work	PE	MP	Total
36582	4.99	23.24	0.81	29.04
36583	5.04	31.7	1.25	37.99
Facility RVU	**Work**	**PE**	**MP**	**Total**
36582	4.99	2.62	0.81	8.42
36583	5.04	3.4	1.25	9.69

	FUD	Status	MUE	Modifiers				IOM Reference
36582	10	A	2(3)	51	N/A	N/A	80*	None
36583	10	A	2(3)	51	N/A	N/A	80*	

* with documentation

Terms To Know

central venous access device. Catheter or other device introduced through a large vein, such as the subclavian or femoral vein, terminating in the superior or inferior vena cava or the right atrium and used to measure venous pressure or administer medication or fluids.

subcutaneous. Below the skin.

tunneled catheter. Catheter inserted into a central vein via a chest incision and maneuvered under the skin to a distal outlet location enabling secure placement with decreased risk of infection and can stay in place for extended periods of time. This procedure is commonly performed in an operating room.

Arteries and Veins

36584

36584 Replacement, complete, of a peripherally inserted central venous catheter (PICC), without subcutaneous port or pump, through same venous access, including all imaging guidance, image documentation, and all associated radiological supervision and interpretation required to perform the replacement

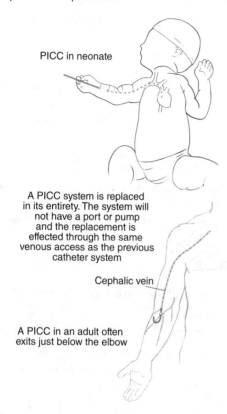

PICC in neonate

A PICC system is replaced in its entirety. The system will not have a port or pump and the replacement is effected through the same venous access as the previous catheter system

Cephalic vein

A PICC in an adult often exits just below the elbow

Explanation

A peripherally inserted central venous catheter (PICC), without subcutaneous port or pump, is replaced through the same venous access site. Local anesthesia is given and the sutures securing the cuff of the catheter with external port are freed from the skin and it is partially withdrawn. A sheath is placed over the nonfunctioning catheter and it is completely withdrawn. A guidewire is inserted into the access site through the sheath and advanced. A new catheter of correct length is placed over the guidewire and the sheath and guidewire are removed. The catheter is fastened in position and the wound is dressed. This service includes all imaging guidance and documentation, as well as the supervision and interpretation.

Coding Tips

For complete replacement of a non-tunneled central venous catheter, without subcutaneous port or pump, see 36580; tunneled central venous catheter, see 36581. For complete replacement of a tunneled, central venous access device with subcutaneous port, see 36582; for subcutaneous pump, see 36583. When this service is performed without imaging guidance, see 37799.

ICD-10-CM Diagnostic Codes

T80.211A	Bloodstream infection due to central venous catheter, initial encounter
T80.212A	Local infection due to central venous catheter, initial encounter
T80.218A	Other infection due to central venous catheter, initial encounter

T82.41XA	Breakdown (mechanical) of vascular dialysis catheter, initial encounter
T82.42XA	Displacement of vascular dialysis catheter, initial encounter
T82.43XA	Leakage of vascular dialysis catheter, initial encounter
T82.49XA	Other complication of vascular dialysis catheter, initial encounter
T82.514A	Breakdown (mechanical) of infusion catheter, initial encounter
T82.524A	Displacement of infusion catheter, initial encounter
T82.534A	Leakage of infusion catheter, initial encounter
T82.594A	Other mechanical complication of infusion catheter, initial encounter
T82.598A	Other mechanical complication of other cardiac and vascular devices and implants, initial encounter
T82.7XXA	Infection and inflammatory reaction due to other cardiac and vascular devices, implants and grafts, initial encounter
T82.818A	Embolism due to vascular prosthetic devices, implants and grafts, initial encounter
T82.828A	Fibrosis due to vascular prosthetic devices, implants and grafts, initial encounter
T82.838A	Hemorrhage due to vascular prosthetic devices, implants and grafts, initial encounter
T82.848A	Pain due to vascular prosthetic devices, implants and grafts, initial encounter
T82.858A	Stenosis of other vascular prosthetic devices, implants and grafts, initial encounter
T82.868A	Thrombosis due to vascular prosthetic devices, implants and grafts, initial encounter
T82.898A	Other specified complication of vascular prosthetic devices, implants and grafts, initial encounter
Z45.2	Encounter for adjustment and management of vascular access device

AMA: 36584 2019,May,3; 2019,Mar,10; 2018,Jan,8; 2017,Jan,8; 2016,Jan,13; 2015,Jan,16

Relative Value Units/Medicare Edits

Non-Facility RVU	Work	PE	MP	Total
36584	1.2	9.21	0.13	10.54
Facility RVU	**Work**	**PE**	**MP**	**Total**
36584	1.2	0.41	0.13	1.74

	FUD	Status	MUE	Modifiers				IOM Reference
36584	0	A	2(3)	N/A	N/A	N/A	N/A	None

* with documentation

Terms To Know

catheter. Flexible tube inserted into an area of the body for introducing or withdrawing fluid.

guidewire. Flexible metal instrument designed to lead another instrument in its proper course.

infection. Presence of microorganisms in body tissues that may result in cellular damage.

peripheral. Outside of a structure or organ.

36585

36585 Replacement, complete, of a peripherally inserted central venous access device, with subcutaneous port, through same venous access

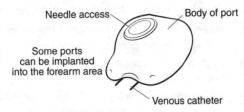

Needle access — Body of port

Some ports can be implanted into the forearm area

Venous catheter

A PICC system is replaced in its entirety

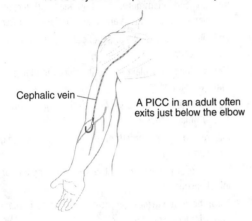

Cephalic vein

A PICC in an adult often exits just below the elbow

Explanation

A peripherally inserted central venous catheter (PICC), along with a subcutaneous port, is replaced through the same venous access site. Local anesthesia is given, the skin over the subcutaneous pocket is incised, and the port is dissected free. A sheath is placed over the nonfunctioning catheter and it is completely withdrawn. A guidewire is inserted into the access site through the sheath and advanced. A new catheter of correct length is placed over the guidewire and the sheath and guidewire are removed. The catheter is fastened in position and the wound is dressed.

Coding Tips

For complete replacement of a non-tunneled central venous catheter, without subcutaneous port or pump, see 36580; tunneled central venous catheter, see 36581. For complete replacement of a tunneled, central venous access device with subcutaneous port, see 36582; for subcutaneous pump, see 36583. If imaging guidance is used for obtaining access to the venous access site or for manipulating the catheter into final end position, see 76937 or 77001.

ICD-10-CM Diagnostic Codes

T80.211A	Bloodstream infection due to central venous catheter, initial encounter
T80.212A	Local infection due to central venous catheter, initial encounter
T80.218A	Other infection due to central venous catheter, initial encounter
T82.41XA	Breakdown (mechanical) of vascular dialysis catheter, initial encounter
T82.42XA	Displacement of vascular dialysis catheter, initial encounter
T82.43XA	Leakage of vascular dialysis catheter, initial encounter
T82.49XA	Other complication of vascular dialysis catheter, initial encounter
T82.514A	Breakdown (mechanical) of infusion catheter, initial encounter
T82.524A	Displacement of infusion catheter, initial encounter
T82.534A	Leakage of infusion catheter, initial encounter

T82.594A	Other mechanical complication of infusion catheter, initial encounter
T82.598A	Other mechanical complication of other cardiac and vascular devices and implants, initial encounter
T82.7XXA	Infection and inflammatory reaction due to other cardiac and vascular devices, implants and grafts, initial encounter
T82.818A	Embolism due to vascular prosthetic devices, implants and grafts, initial encounter
T82.828A	Fibrosis due to vascular prosthetic devices, implants and grafts, initial encounter
T82.838A	Hemorrhage due to vascular prosthetic devices, implants and grafts, initial encounter
T82.848A	Pain due to vascular prosthetic devices, implants and grafts, initial encounter
T82.858A	Stenosis of other vascular prosthetic devices, implants and grafts, initial encounter
T82.868A	Thrombosis due to vascular prosthetic devices, implants and grafts, initial encounter
T82.898A	Other specified complication of vascular prosthetic devices, implants and grafts, initial encounter
Z45.2	Encounter for adjustment and management of vascular access device

AMA: 36585 2018,Jan,8; 2017,Jan,8; 2016,Jan,13; 2015,Jan,16

Relative Value Units/Medicare Edits

Non-Facility RVU	Work	PE	MP	Total
36585	4.59	29.09	0.79	34.47
Facility RVU	**Work**	**PE**	**MP**	**Total**
36585	4.59	2.57	0.79	7.95

	FUD	Status	MUE	Modifiers				IOM Reference
36585	10	A	2(3)	51	N/A	N/A	80*	None

* with documentation

Terms To Know

guidewire. Flexible metal instrument designed to lead another instrument in its proper course.

infection. Presence of microorganisms in body tissues that may result in cellular damage.

peripheral. Outside of a structure or organ.

sheath. Covering enclosing an organ or part.

36589-36590

36589 Removal of tunneled central venous catheter, without subcutaneous port or pump

36590 Removal of tunneled central venous access device, with subcutaneous port or pump, central or peripheral insertion

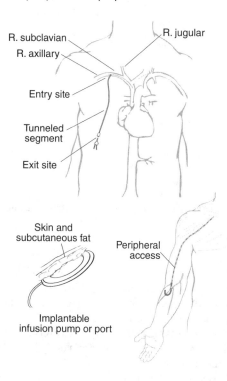

Explanation

In 36589, a tunneled central venous catheter without subcutaneous port or pump is removed. Local anesthesia is given and the sutures securing the cuff of the tunneled catheter's external port are freed from the skin. In 36590, a tunneled central venous access device, both catheter and subcutaneous port or pump, is removed. Local anesthesia is given and the subcutaneous pocket over the port/pump device is incised and the pump/port is dissected free. The catheter is disconnected and the pump/port device is removed from its pocket. In both cases, a guidewire is placed over the existing catheter, which is withdrawn over the guidewire, and the guidewire is removed. The incisions are closed and the wound is dressed.

Coding Tips

Do not report these codes for removal of non-tunneled central venous catheters. If imaging guidance is used for obtaining access to the venous access site or for manipulating the catheter into final end position, see 76937 and 77001.

ICD-10-CM Diagnostic Codes

T80.211A	Bloodstream infection due to central venous catheter, initial encounter
T80.212A	Local infection due to central venous catheter, initial encounter
T80.218A	Other infection due to central venous catheter, initial encounter
T82.41XA	Breakdown (mechanical) of vascular dialysis catheter, initial encounter
T82.42XA	Displacement of vascular dialysis catheter, initial encounter
T82.43XA	Leakage of vascular dialysis catheter, initial encounter
T82.49XA	Other complication of vascular dialysis catheter, initial encounter
T82.514A	Breakdown (mechanical) of infusion catheter, initial encounter
T82.524A	Displacement of infusion catheter, initial encounter
T82.534A	Leakage of infusion catheter, initial encounter
T82.594A	Other mechanical complication of infusion catheter, initial encounter
T82.598A	Other mechanical complication of other cardiac and vascular devices and implants, initial encounter
T82.7XXA	Infection and inflammatory reaction due to other cardiac and vascular devices, implants and grafts, initial encounter
T82.818A	Embolism due to vascular prosthetic devices, implants and grafts, initial encounter
T82.828A	Fibrosis due to vascular prosthetic devices, implants and grafts, initial encounter
T82.838A	Hemorrhage due to vascular prosthetic devices, implants and grafts, initial encounter
T82.848A	Pain due to vascular prosthetic devices, implants and grafts, initial encounter
T82.858A	Stenosis of other vascular prosthetic devices, implants and grafts, initial encounter
T82.868A	Thrombosis due to vascular prosthetic devices, implants and grafts, initial encounter
T82.898A	Other specified complication of vascular prosthetic devices, implants and grafts, initial encounter
Z45.2	Encounter for adjustment and management of vascular access device

AMA: **36589** 2018,Jan,8; 2017,Jan,8; 2016,Jan,13; 2015,Nov,10; 2015,Jan,16
36590 2018,Jan,8; 2017,Jan,8; 2016,Jan,13; 2015,Jan,16

Relative Value Units/Medicare Edits

Non-Facility RVU	Work	PE	MP	Total
36589	2.28	2.33	0.33	4.94
36590	3.1	3.05	0.53	6.68
Facility RVU	**Work**	**PE**	**MP**	**Total**
36589	2.28	1.42	0.33	4.03
36590	3.1	1.92	0.53	5.55

	FUD	Status	MUE	Modifiers				IOM Reference
36589	10	A	2(3)	51	N/A	N/A	80*	None
36590	10	A	2(3)	51	N/A	N/A	80*	

* with documentation

Terms To Know

central venous catheter. Catheter positioned in the superior vena cava or right atrium and introduced through a large vein, such as the jugular or subclavian, and used to measure venous pressure or administer fluids or medication.

36591

36591 Collection of blood specimen from a completely implantable venous access device

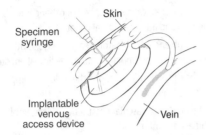

A blood specimen is collected from a partially or completely implantable venous access device

Explanation

The physician obtains a blood specimen from a previously placed, completely implantable venous access device. Completely implanted devices are those that have access through a subcutaneous port (e.g., Port-A-Cath, Infusaport). An implantable access device requires a percutaneous noncoring needle to accomplish the blood draw. The skin is cleansed with alcohol or iodine solution. The needle is placed into the port. Heparin is withdrawn. A second needle is inserted and the blood specimen obtained. The port is flushed with heparin solution.

Coding Tips

Do not report 36591 with any other service. Collection of venous blood specimen by venipuncture is reported with 36415. Medicare and some payers may require G0471 to report this service when provided in a federally qualified health center (FQHC). For collection of capillary blood specimen, see 36416. For arterial puncture, see 36600. Surgical trays, A4550, are not separately reimbursed by Medicare; however, other third-party payers may cover them. Check with the specific payer to determine coverage.

ICD-10-CM Diagnostic Codes

The application of this code is too broad to adequately present ICD-10-CM diagnostic code links here. Refer to your ICD-10-CM book.

AMA: 36591 2019,Aug,8; 2018,Jan,8; 2017,Jan,8; 2016,Jan,13; 2015,Jan,16

Relative Value Units/Medicare Edits

Non-Facility RVU	Work	PE	MP	Total
36591	0.0	0.76	0.01	0.77
Facility RVU	Work	PE	MP	Total
36591	0.0	0.76	0.01	0.77

	FUD	Status	MUE	Modifiers				IOM Reference
36591	N/A	T	2(3)	N/A	N/A	N/A	80*	None

* with documentation

36592

36592 Collection of blood specimen using established central or peripheral catheter, venous, not otherwise specified

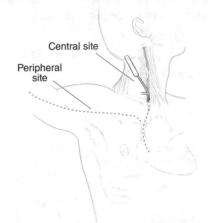

Blood specimen is collected from established catheter

Explanation

The physician obtains a blood specimen from an established central venous or peripheral venous catheter. A central venous catheter (CVC) is one that is inserted through the skin into central veins, such as the femoral, internal jugular, or subclavian veins. Peripheral catheters include those inserted in the arm veins (basilic or cephalic), such as a PICC line, saline lock, or heparin lock. In order to clear the catheter of any material that could contaminate the sample and affect the test results, a specific volume of infusing fluid and blood must be discarded before a blood specimen is obtained; this volume varies depending on the type of catheter utilized. With a central venous catheter, a three-way stopcock is attached to the catheter's hub and two syringes attached to the stopcock. Using one syringe, the catheter is flushed with normal saline. A specific amount of blood is aspirated into the same syringe used for the saline flush and discarded. The blood sample is then withdrawn using the other syringe and placed into an appropriate tube for laboratory analysis. If using a peripheral venous catheter, a specific amount of blood is also aspirated and discarded before the blood sample is drawn.

Coding Tips

Do not report 36592 with any other service. Collection of a specimen from a completely implantable venous access device is reported with code 36591. For collection of capillary blood specimen, see 36416. For blood collection from an established arterial catheter, see 37799.

ICD-10-CM Diagnostic Codes

The application of this code is too broad to adequately present ICD-10-CM diagnostic code links here. Refer to your ICD-10-CM book.

AMA: 36592 2018,Jan,8; 2017,Jan,8; 2016,Jan,13; 2015,Jan,16

Relative Value Units/Medicare Edits

Non-Facility RVU	Work	PE	MP	Total
36592	0.0	0.86	0.01	0.87
Facility RVU	Work	PE	MP	Total
36592	0.0	0.86	0.01	0.87

	FUD	Status	MUE	Modifiers				IOM Reference
36592	N/A	T	1(3)	N/A	N/A	N/A	80*	None

* with documentation

Terms To Know

analysis. Study of body fluid, tissue, section, or parts.

aspiration. Drawing fluid out by suction.

central venous catheter. Catheter positioned in the superior vena cava or right atrium and introduced through a large vein, such as the jugular or subclavian, and used to measure venous pressure or administer fluids or medication.

jugular vein. Two pairs of veins on either side of the neck that open into the subclavian, sending blood from the head and neck to the heart.

peripheral. Outside of a structure or organ.

PICC. Peripherally inserted central catheter. PICC is inserted into one of the large veins of the arm and threaded through the vein until the tip sits in a large vein just above the heart.

specimen. Tissue cells or sample of fluid taken for analysis, pathologic examination, and diagnosis.

venous. Relating to the veins.

36593

36593 Declotting by thrombolytic agent of implanted vascular access device or catheter

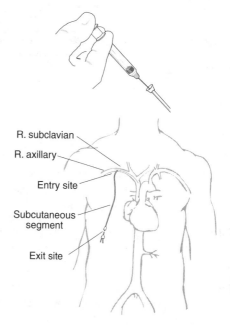

R. subclavian
R. axillary
Entry site
Subcutaneous segment
Exit site

A thrombolytic agent is used to declot a catheter or implanted vascular access device

Explanation

To remove a clot from an implanted vascular access device or catheter, the physician injects a thrombolytic agent (e.g., Streptokinase) into the catheter to dissolve the clot. The patient is observed for any abnormal signs of bleeding.

Coding Tips

When 36593 is performed with another separately identifiable procedure, the highest dollar value code is listed as the primary procedure and subsequent procedures are appended with modifier 51. Supplies used when providing this procedure may be reported with the appropriate HCPCS Level II "J" code. Check with the specific payer to determine coverage.

ICD-10-CM Diagnostic Codes

T82.818A	Embolism due to vascular prosthetic devices, implants and grafts, initial encounter
T82.848A	Pain due to vascular prosthetic devices, implants and grafts, initial encounter
T82.856A	Stenosis of peripheral vascular stent, initial encounter
T82.858A	Stenosis of other vascular prosthetic devices, implants and grafts, initial encounter
T82.868A	Thrombosis due to vascular prosthetic devices, implants and grafts, initial encounter
T82.898A	Other specified complication of vascular prosthetic devices, implants and grafts, initial encounter

AMA: 36593 2018,Jan,8; 2017,Jan,8; 2016,Jan,13; 2015,Jan,16

Arteries and Veins

Relative Value Units/Medicare Edits

Non-Facility RVU	Work	PE	MP	Total
36593	0.0	0.94	0.02	0.96
Facility RVU	Work	PE	MP	Total
36593	0.0	0.94	0.02	0.96

	FUD	Status	MUE	Modifiers				IOM Reference
36593	N/A	A	2(3)	N/A	N/A	N/A	80*	None

* with documentation

Terms To Know

blood clot. Semisolidified, coagulated mass of mainly platelets and fibrin in the bloodstream.

implantable venous access device. Catheter implanted for continuous access to the venous system for long-term parenteral feeding or for the administration of fluids or medications.

thrombolysis. Chemical process of dissolving or breaking down a blood clot by inducing a complex chain of events involving the action of plasminogen to solubilize fibrin clots and degrade fibrinogen.

thrombosis. Condition arising from the presence or formation of blood clots within a blood vessel that may cause vascular obstruction and insufficient oxygenation.

vascular. Pertaining to blood vessels.

36595-36596

36595 Mechanical removal of pericatheter obstructive material (eg, fibrin sheath) from central venous device via separate venous access

36596 Mechanical removal of intraluminal (intracatheter) obstructive material from central venous device through device lumen

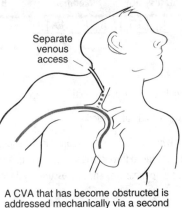

Separate venous access

A CVA that has become obstructed is addressed mechanically via a second venous access site. The obstructive matter is on the exterior of the catheter lumen

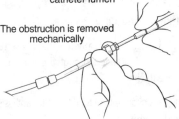

The obstruction is removed mechanically

Explanation

In 36595, pericatheter obstructive material such as a fibrin sheath is removed from around a central venous device via a separate venous access. Central venous catheters often fail because of the accumulation of an obstructing thrombus or fibrin sheath around the tip of the catheter. The catheter is first checked that it can aspirate and flush forward. The pericatheter material is identified by contrast material injection. Generally, a right femoral vein access is used. A guidewire followed by an angiographic catheter are advanced into the superior vena cava and exchanged for a loop snare with its catheter, which are advanced cephalad along the length of the central venous catheter beyond the ports. The loop snare is tightly closed about the central venous catheter to encircle it and slowly pulled down and off the tip of the catheter, stripping off the pericatheter obstructive material. This is repeated a few times and the catheter is rechecked for infusion and injection ability of the ports. A contrast study is done again to identify any fibrin and the process may be repeated until the fibrin sheath is completely removed. In 36596, intraluminal obstructive material, such as a thrombus or fibrin sheath, is removed from inside a central venous device through the lumen of the device. This does not require a separate access incision. The central venous catheter is first checked that it can aspirate and flush forward. The obstructing material is disrupted and removed mechanically by using an angioplasty balloon or other catheter introduced into the central venous catheter through its entry site on the skin. The catheter is checked for unimpeded, restored flow and the process may be repeated until the central venous catheter is cleared.

Coding Tips

Do not report these codes with 36593. Venous catheterization is reported with codes 36010–36012. Radiological supervision and interpretation for 36595 is reported with code 75901; for 36596, see 75902.

ICD-10-CM Diagnostic Codes

T82.49XA	Other complication of vascular dialysis catheter, initial encounter
T82.594A	Other mechanical complication of infusion catheter, initial encounter
T82.598A	Other mechanical complication of other cardiac and vascular devices and implants, initial encounter
T82.818A	Embolism due to vascular prosthetic devices, implants and grafts, initial encounter
T82.828A	Fibrosis due to vascular prosthetic devices, implants and grafts, initial encounter
T82.858A	Stenosis of other vascular prosthetic devices, implants and grafts, initial encounter
T82.868A	Thrombosis due to vascular prosthetic devices, implants and grafts, initial encounter
T82.898A	Other specified complication of vascular prosthetic devices, implants and grafts, initial encounter
Z45.2	Encounter for adjustment and management of vascular access device

AMA: 36595 2018,Jan,8; 2017,Jan,8; 2016,Jan,13; 2015,Jan,16 **36596** 2018,Jan,8; 2017,Jan,8; 2016,Jan,13; 2015,Jan,16

Relative Value Units/Medicare Edits

Non-Facility RVU	Work	PE	MP	Total
36595	3.59	14.89	0.39	18.87
36596	0.75	2.67	0.1	3.52
Facility RVU	Work	PE	MP	Total
36595	3.59	1.32	0.39	5.3
36596	0.75	0.42	0.1	1.27

	FUD	Status	MUE	Modifiers				IOM Reference
36595	0	A	2(3)	51	N/A	N/A	N/A	None
36596	0	A	2(3)	51	N/A	N/A	N/A	

* with documentation

Terms To Know

aspirate. To withdraw fluid or air from a body cavity by suction.

complication. Condition arising after the beginning of observation and treatment that modifies the course of the patient's illness or the medical care required, or an undesired result or misadventure in medical care.

contrast material. Any internally administered substance that has a different opacity from soft tissue on radiography or computed tomograph; includes barium, used to opacify parts of the gastrointestinal tract; water-soluble iodinated compounds, used to opacify blood vessels or the genitourinary tract; may refer to air occurring naturally or introduced into the body; also, paramagnetic substances used in magnetic resonance imaging. Substances may also be documented as contrast agent or contrast medium.

intra. Within.

36597

36597	Repositioning of previously placed central venous catheter under fluoroscopic guidance

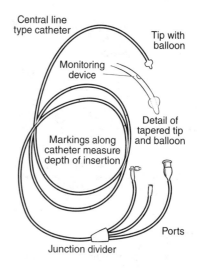

Explanation

A previously placed central venous catheter needs to be repositioned. It is possible for a catheter position to change significantly after the procedure is completed. Catheter position change and tip migration occur most often with subclavian venous access in women and obese patients, because the soft tissues of the chest wall move inferiorly with standing and often cause the catheter to get pulled back. When a catheter tip is incorrectly placed, it can increase the risks of thrombosis, fibrin sheath formation, perforation of the vein, and even arrhythmias. Fluoroscopy is used to check the positioning of the catheter tip and guide it to its correct position. Local anesthesia is given, and the sutures securing the cuff of the catheter may be freed from the skin. The catheter is partially withdrawn, and a sheath may be placed over the catheter at the existing venous access site. A guidewire is inserted through the catheter and advanced. The central venous catheter is maneuvered back into correct position and monitored with fluoroscopy to view correct placement of the tip.

Coding Tips

For fluoroscopic guidance, see 76000.

ICD-10-CM Diagnostic Codes

T82.41XA	Breakdown (mechanical) of vascular dialysis catheter, initial encounter
T82.42XA	Displacement of vascular dialysis catheter, initial encounter
T82.43XA	Leakage of vascular dialysis catheter, initial encounter
T82.49XA	Other complication of vascular dialysis catheter, initial encounter
T82.514A	Breakdown (mechanical) of infusion catheter, initial encounter
T82.524A	Displacement of infusion catheter, initial encounter
T82.534A	Leakage of infusion catheter, initial encounter
T82.594A	Other mechanical complication of infusion catheter, initial encounter
T82.598A	Other mechanical complication of other cardiac and vascular devices and implants, initial encounter
T82.898A	Other specified complication of vascular prosthetic devices, implants and grafts, initial encounter

Z45.2   Encounter for adjustment and management of vascular access device

Z45.89   Encounter for adjustment and management of other implanted devices

Z46.89   Encounter for fitting and adjustment of other specified devices

AMA: 36597 2018,Jan,8; 2017,Jan,8; 2016,Jan,13; 2015,Jan,16

Relative Value Units/Medicare Edits

Non-Facility RVU	Work	PE	MP	Total
36597	1.21	2.29	0.14	3.64
Facility RVU	**Work**	**PE**	**MP**	**Total**
36597	1.21	0.41	0.14	1.76

	FUD	Status	MUE	Modifiers			IOM Reference
36597	0	A	2(3)	51	N/A	N/A	N/A	None

* with documentation

Terms To Know

anesthesia. Loss of feeling or sensation, usually induced to permit the performance of surgery or other painful procedures.

central venous catheter. Catheter positioned in the superior vena cava or right atrium and introduced through a large vein, such as the jugular or subclavian, and used to measure venous pressure or administer fluids or medication.

fibrin sheath. Obstructive material or thrombus that forms around or within the lumen of an indwelling catheter or central venous access device.

fluoroscopy. Radiology technique that allows visual examination of part of the body or a function of an organ using a device that projects an x-ray image on a fluorescent screen.

guidewire. Flexible metal instrument designed to lead another instrument in its proper course.

subcutaneous tissue. Sheet or wide band of adipose (fat) and areolar connective tissue in two layers attached to the dermis.

thrombosis. Condition arising from the presence or formation of blood clots within a blood vessel that may cause vascular obstruction and insufficient oxygenation.

36598

36598   Contrast injection(s) for radiologic evaluation of existing central venous access device, including fluoroscopy, image documentation and report

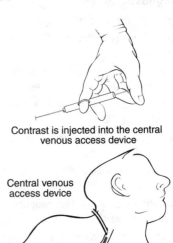

Contrast is injected into the central venous access device

Central venous access device

Explanation

A previously placed central venous access device is evaluated for complications that may be interfering with its proper functioning or the ability to draw blood from the catheter. Complications may include the presence of a fibrin sheath around the end of the catheter, migration of the catheter tip, patency of the tubing, kinking, fracture, or leaks. A small amount of contrast agent is injected into the catheter and the central venous access device is examined under fluoroscopy as the flow is evaluated. Images are documented and a radiological report is prepared.

Coding Tips

Fluoroscopy is included in this service and is not reported separately. Do not report this code with 36595–36596. Complete diagnostic studies (venography) are reported with codes 75820, 75825, or 75827.

ICD-10-CM Diagnostic Codes

T80.211A   Bloodstream infection due to central venous catheter, initial encounter

T80.212A   Local infection due to central venous catheter, initial encounter

T80.218A   Other infection due to central venous catheter, initial encounter

T82.41XA   Breakdown (mechanical) of vascular dialysis catheter, initial encounter

T82.42XA   Displacement of vascular dialysis catheter, initial encounter

T82.43XA   Leakage of vascular dialysis catheter, initial encounter

T82.49XA   Other complication of vascular dialysis catheter, initial encounter

T82.514A   Breakdown (mechanical) of infusion catheter, initial encounter

T82.524A   Displacement of infusion catheter, initial encounter

T82.534A   Leakage of infusion catheter, initial encounter

T82.594A   Other mechanical complication of infusion catheter, initial encounter

Arteries and Veins

T82.598A	Other mechanical complication of other cardiac and vascular devices and implants, initial encounter			
T82.7XXA	Infection and inflammatory reaction due to other cardiac and vascular devices, implants and grafts, initial encounter			
T82.818A	Embolism due to vascular prosthetic devices, implants and grafts, initial encounter			
T82.828A	Fibrosis due to vascular prosthetic devices, implants and grafts, initial encounter			
T82.838A	Hemorrhage due to vascular prosthetic devices, implants and grafts, initial encounter			
T82.848A	Pain due to vascular prosthetic devices, implants and grafts, initial encounter			
T82.858A	Stenosis of other vascular prosthetic devices, implants and grafts, initial encounter			
T82.868A	Thrombosis due to vascular prosthetic devices, implants and grafts, initial encounter			
T82.898A	Other specified complication of vascular prosthetic devices, implants and grafts, initial encounter			
Z45.2	Encounter for adjustment and management of vascular access device			

AMA: 36598 2014,Jan,11

Relative Value Units/Medicare Edits

Non-Facility RVU	Work	PE	MP	Total
36598	0.74	2.86	0.06	3.66
Facility RVU	**Work**	**PE**	**MP**	**Total**
36598	0.74	0.24	0.06	1.04

	FUD	Status	MUE	Modifiers				IOM Reference
36598	0	T	2(3)	51	50	N/A	80*	None

* with documentation

Terms To Know

central venous access device. Catheter or other device introduced through a large vein, such as the subclavian or femoral vein, terminating in the superior or inferior vena cava or the right atrium and used to measure venous pressure or administer medication or fluids.

complication. Condition arising after the beginning of observation and treatment that modifies the course of the patient's illness or the medical care required, or an undesired result or misadventure in medical care.

contrast material. Radiopaque substance placed into the body to enable a system or body structure to be visualized, such as nonionic and low osmolar contrast media (LOCM), ionic and high osmolar contrast media (HOCM), barium, and gadolinium.

fluoroscopy. Radiology technique that allows visual examination of part of the body or a function of an organ using a device that projects an x-ray image on a fluorescent screen.

imaging. Radiologic means of producing pictures for clinical study of the internal structures and functions of the body, such as x-ray, ultrasound, magnetic resonance, or positron emission tomography.

radiopaque dye. Medium injected into the body that is impenetrable by x-rays.

36620-36625

36620	Arterial catheterization or cannulation for sampling, monitoring or transfusion (separate procedure); percutaneous
36625	cutdown

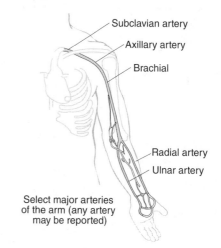

Select major arteries of the arm (any artery may be reported)

- Subclavian artery
- Axillary artery
- Brachial
- Radial artery
- Ulnar artery

Explanation

The physician accesses, in most cases, the ulnar or radial artery to insert a cannula, or tube-shaped portal. In 36620, the physician inserts a needle through the skin to puncture the artery and inserts a cannula. In 36625, the physician makes an incision in the skin overlying the artery and dissects the surrounding tissue to access it. The artery is sometimes nicked with a thin-bladed scalpel before the physician inserts the cannula. This cannula acts as a portal for sampling, monitoring or transfusion. Once the procedure is complete, the cannula is removed. In an open procedure, the opening in the artery may be sutured and the incision repaired with a layered closure. Pressure is applied to the puncture if a percutaneous approach is used.

Coding Tips

These separate procedures, by definition, are usually a component of a more complex service and are not identified separately. When performed alone or with other unrelated procedures/services, they may be reported. If performed alone, list the code; if performed with other unrelated procedures/services, list the code and append modifier 59 or an X{EPSU} modifier. These codes include only the insertion of the tube for giving the transfusion. For transfusion, see 36430–36460. For arterial catheterization for prolonged infusion therapy (chemotherapy) by cutdown, see 36640.

ICD-10-CM Diagnostic Codes

The application of this code is too broad to adequately present ICD-10-CM diagnostic code links here. Refer to your ICD-10-CM book.

AMA: 36620 2018,Jan,8; 2017,Jan,8; 2016,Jan,13; 2015,Jan,16 **36625** 2018,Jan,8; 2017,Jan,8; 2016,Jan,13; 2015,Jan,16

Arteries and Veins

Relative Value Units/Medicare Edits

Non-Facility RVU	Work	PE	MP	Total
36620	1.0	0.2	0.09	1.29
36625	2.11	0.63	0.34	3.08
Facility RVU	Work	PE	MP	Total
36620	1.0	0.2	0.09	1.29
36625	2.11	0.63	0.34	3.08

	FUD	Status	MUE	Modifiers				IOM Reference
36620	0	A	3(3)	N/A	N/A	N/A	N/A	100-03,110.7;
36625	0	A	2(3)	N/A	N/A	N/A	N/A	100-03,110.8

* with documentation

Terms To Know

artery. Vessel through which oxygenated blood passes away from the heart to any part of the body.

cannula. Tube inserted into a blood vessel, duct, or body cavity to facilitate passage.

catheter. Flexible tube inserted into an area of the body for introducing or withdrawing fluid.

cutdown. Small, incised opening in the skin to expose a blood vessel, especially over a vein (venous cutdown) to allow venipuncture and permit a needle or cannula to be inserted for the withdrawal of blood or administration of fluids.

dissection. Separating by cutting tissue or body structures apart.

incision. Act of cutting into tissue or an organ.

percutaneous. Through the skin.

repair. Surgical closure of a wound. The wound may be a result of injury/trauma or it may be a surgically created defect. Repairs are divided into three categories: simple, intermediate, and complex.

skin. Outer protective covering of the body composed of the epidermis and dermis, situated above the subcutaneous tissues.

transfusion. Process of transferring whole blood or blood components from one person, the donor, to another person, the recipient, or the process of taking liquid from one vessel and putting it into another.

36640

36640   Arterial catheterization for prolonged infusion therapy (chemotherapy), cutdown

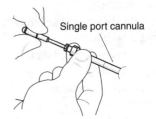

Cannulization is accomplished for prolonged chemotherapy infusion

Single port cannula

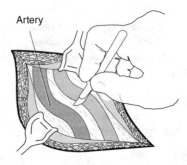

Artery

Cutdown is performed to isolate artery

Explanation

The physician accesses the artery supplying the area to be treated. To insert a cannula, or tube-shaped portal for prolonged infusion therapy, the physician makes an incision above the artery and dissects the surrounding tissue to access it. The artery is sometimes nicked with a thin-bladed scalpel before the physician inserts the catheter. The catheter may be advanced to a site immediately upstream of the site to be treated. This catheter acts as a portal for the infusion of chemotherapy drugs and will remain in place until chemotherapy is completed. The catheter is removed, the hole in the artery is repaired, and the incision is repaired with a layered closure.

Coding Tips

Report 36640 in addition to the code for chemotherapy treatment (96420–96425). When 36640 is performed with another separately identifiable procedure, the highest dollar value code is listed as the primary procedure and subsequent procedures are appended with modifier 51. Supplies used when providing this procedure may be reported with the appropriate HCPCS Level II code. Check with the specific payer to determine coverage. Arterial catheterization for occlusion therapy is reported with code 75894.

ICD-10-CM Diagnostic Codes

The application of this code is too broad to adequately present ICD-10-CM diagnostic code links here. Refer to your ICD-10-CM book.

AMA: 36640 2018,Jan,8; 2017,Jan,8; 2016,Jan,13; 2015,Jan,16

Arteries and Veins

Relative Value Units/Medicare Edits

Non-Facility RVU	Work	PE	MP	Total
36640	2.1	1.12	0.17	3.39
Facility RVU	Work	PE	MP	Total
36640	2.1	1.12	0.17	3.39

	FUD	Status	MUE	Modifiers				IOM Reference
36640	0	A	1(3)	51	N/A	N/A	N/A	None

* with documentation

Terms To Know

artery. Vessel through which oxygenated blood passes away from the heart to any part of the body.

cannula. Tube inserted into a blood vessel, duct, or body cavity to facilitate passage.

catheter. Flexible tube inserted into an area of the body for introducing or withdrawing fluid.

catheterization. Use or insertion of a tubular device into a duct, blood vessel, hollow organ, or body cavity for injecting or withdrawing fluids for diagnostic or therapeutic purposes.

chemotherapy. Treatment of disease, especially cancerous conditions, using chemical agents.

closure. Repairing an incision or wound by suture or other means.

cutdown. Small, incised opening in the skin to expose a blood vessel, especially over a vein (venous cutdown) to allow venipuncture and permit a needle or cannula to be inserted for the withdrawal of blood or administration of fluids.

dissect. Cut apart or separate tissue for surgical purposes or for visual or microscopic study.

incision. Act of cutting into tissue or an organ.

infusion. Introduction of a therapeutic fluid, other than blood, into the bloodstream.

repair. Surgical closure of a wound. The wound may be a result of injury/trauma or it may be a surgically created defect. Repairs are divided into three categories: simple, intermediate, and complex.

36800

36800 Insertion of cannula for hemodialysis, other purpose (separate procedure); vein to vein

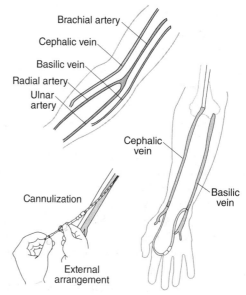

Vein-to-vein cannulization is established

Explanation

The physician isolates two veins, usually in the nondominant forearm, and inserts a needle through the skin and into each vessel. A guidance wire may be threaded through the needle into each vessel. The needle is removed. An end of a single cannula is inserted into each puncture, and any guidance wire removed. The cannula remains external, and may be left in place for several days. (This hemodialysis cannula is used to remove blood from the vein, route it through the dialysis machine, then reinfuse it.)

Coding Tips

This type of hemodialysis cannula is infrequently used; verify from the medical record that this is the type of procedure performed. This procedure includes venipuncture, when performed by the physician. For creation of an arteriovenous fistula, see 36825–36830. For open arteriovenous anastomosis, see 36818–36821.

ICD-10-CM Diagnostic Codes

D59.3	Hemolytic-uremic syndrome
E87.2	Acidosis
E87.5	Hyperkalemia
I12.0	Hypertensive chronic kidney disease with stage 5 chronic kidney disease or end stage renal disease
I12.9	Hypertensive chronic kidney disease with stage 1 through stage 4 chronic kidney disease, or unspecified chronic kidney disease
I13.0	Hypertensive heart and chronic kidney disease with heart failure and stage 1 through stage 4 chronic kidney disease, or unspecified chronic kidney disease
I13.10	Hypertensive heart and chronic kidney disease without heart failure, with stage 1 through stage 4 chronic kidney disease, or unspecified chronic kidney disease

Arteries and Veins

I13.11	Hypertensive heart and chronic kidney disease without heart failure, with stage 5 chronic kidney disease, or end stage renal disease
I13.2	Hypertensive heart and chronic kidney disease with heart failure and with stage 5 chronic kidney disease, or end stage renal disease
I16.0	Hypertensive urgency
I16.1	Hypertensive emergency
I82.3	Embolism and thrombosis of renal vein
M35.04	Sjögren syndrome with tubulo-interstitial nephropathy
M35.0A	Sjögren syndrome with glomerular disease
N00.0	Acute nephritic syndrome with minor glomerular abnormality
N00.1	Acute nephritic syndrome with focal and segmental glomerular lesions
N00.2	Acute nephritic syndrome with diffuse membranous glomerulonephritis
N00.3	Acute nephritic syndrome with diffuse mesangial proliferative glomerulonephritis
N00.4	Acute nephritic syndrome with diffuse endocapillary proliferative glomerulonephritis
N00.5	Acute nephritic syndrome with diffuse mesangiocapillary glomerulonephritis
N00.6	Acute nephritic syndrome with dense deposit disease
N00.7	Acute nephritic syndrome with diffuse crescentic glomerulonephritis
N00.8	Acute nephritic syndrome with other morphologic changes
N00.A	Acute nephritic syndrome with C3 glomerulonephritis
N01.0	Rapidly progressive nephritic syndrome with minor glomerular abnormality
N01.1	Rapidly progressive nephritic syndrome with focal and segmental glomerular lesions
N01.2	Rapidly progressive nephritic syndrome with diffuse membranous glomerulonephritis
N01.3	Rapidly progressive nephritic syndrome with diffuse mesangial proliferative glomerulonephritis
N01.4	Rapidly progressive nephritic syndrome with diffuse endocapillary proliferative glomerulonephritis
N01.5	Rapidly progressive nephritic syndrome with diffuse mesangiocapillary glomerulonephritis
N01.6	Rapidly progressive nephritic syndrome with dense deposit disease
N01.7	Rapidly progressive nephritic syndrome with diffuse crescentic glomerulonephritis
N01.8	Rapidly progressive nephritic syndrome with other morphologic changes
N01.A	Rapidly progressive nephritic syndrome with C3 glomerulonephritis
N03.0	Chronic nephritic syndrome with minor glomerular abnormality
N03.1	Chronic nephritic syndrome with focal and segmental glomerular lesions
N03.2	Chronic nephritic syndrome with diffuse membranous glomerulonephritis
N03.3	Chronic nephritic syndrome with diffuse mesangial proliferative glomerulonephritis
N03.4	Chronic nephritic syndrome with diffuse endocapillary proliferative glomerulonephritis
N03.5	Chronic nephritic syndrome with diffuse mesangiocapillary glomerulonephritis
N03.6	Chronic nephritic syndrome with dense deposit disease
N03.7	Chronic nephritic syndrome with diffuse crescentic glomerulonephritis
N03.8	Chronic nephritic syndrome with other morphologic changes
N03.A	Chronic nephritic syndrome with C3 glomerulonephritis
N04.0	Nephrotic syndrome with minor glomerular abnormality
N04.1	Nephrotic syndrome with focal and segmental glomerular lesions
N04.2	Nephrotic syndrome with diffuse membranous glomerulonephritis
N04.3	Nephrotic syndrome with diffuse mesangial proliferative glomerulonephritis
N04.4	Nephrotic syndrome with diffuse endocapillary proliferative glomerulonephritis
N04.5	Nephrotic syndrome with diffuse mesangiocapillary glomerulonephritis
N04.6	Nephrotic syndrome with dense deposit disease
N04.7	Nephrotic syndrome with diffuse crescentic glomerulonephritis
N04.8	Nephrotic syndrome with other morphologic changes
N04.A	Nephrotic syndrome with C3 glomerulonephritis
N07.0	Hereditary nephropathy, not elsewhere classified with minor glomerular abnormality
N07.1	Hereditary nephropathy, not elsewhere classified with focal and segmental glomerular lesions
N07.2	Hereditary nephropathy, not elsewhere classified with diffuse membranous glomerulonephritis
N07.3	Hereditary nephropathy, not elsewhere classified with diffuse mesangial proliferative glomerulonephritis
N07.4	Hereditary nephropathy, not elsewhere classified with diffuse endocapillary proliferative glomerulonephritis
N07.5	Hereditary nephropathy, not elsewhere classified with diffuse mesangiocapillary glomerulonephritis
N07.6	Hereditary nephropathy, not elsewhere classified with dense deposit disease
N07.7	Hereditary nephropathy, not elsewhere classified with diffuse crescentic glomerulonephritis
N07.8	Hereditary nephropathy, not elsewhere classified with other morphologic lesions
N07.A	Hereditary nephropathy, not elsewhere classified with C3 glomerulonephritis
N08	Glomerular disorders in diseases classified elsewhere
N10	Acute pyelonephritis
N11.0	Nonobstructive reflux-associated chronic pyelonephritis
N11.1	Chronic obstructive pyelonephritis
N11.8	Other chronic tubulo-interstitial nephritis
N12	Tubulo-interstitial nephritis, not specified as acute or chronic
N15.8	Other specified renal tubulo-interstitial diseases
N16	Renal tubulo-interstitial disorders in diseases classified elsewhere
N17.0	Acute kidney failure with tubular necrosis
N17.1	Acute kidney failure with acute cortical necrosis
N17.2	Acute kidney failure with medullary necrosis
N17.8	Other acute kidney failure
N18.1	Chronic kidney disease, stage 1
N18.2	Chronic kidney disease, stage 2 (mild)

N18.31	Chronic kidney disease, stage 3a	
N18.32	Chronic kidney disease, stage 3b	
N18.4	Chronic kidney disease, stage 4 (severe)	
N18.5	Chronic kidney disease, stage 5	
N18.6	End stage renal disease	

AMA: 36800 2018,Jan,8; 2017,Jan,8; 2016,Jan,13; 2015,Jan,16

Relative Value Units/Medicare Edits

Non-Facility RVU	Work	PE	MP	Total
36800	2.43	0.83	0.31	3.57
Facility RVU	**Work**	**PE**	**MP**	**Total**
36800	2.43	0.83	0.31	3.57

	FUD	Status	MUE	Modifiers				IOM Reference
36800	0	A	1(3)	51	N/A	N/A	N/A	None

* with documentation

Terms To Know

chronic. Persistent, continuing, or recurring.

ESRD. End stage renal disease. Progression of chronic renal failure to lasting and irreparable kidney damage that requires dialysis or renal transplant for survival.

glomerulonephritis. Disease of the kidney with diffuse inflammation of the capillary loops of the glomeruli. It may be a complication of bacterial infection or immune disorders and can lead to renal failure and may be associated with hypertension or diabetes.

hemodialysis. Cleansing of wastes and contaminating elements from the blood by virtue of different diffusion rates through a semipermeable membrane, which separates blood from a filtration solution that diffuses other elements out of the blood.

nephropathy. Disease or abnormality of the kidney.

nephrotic syndrome. Condition where levels of albumin in the blood and urine are far below the norm.

renal. Referring to the kidney.

renal failure. Inability of a kidney to eliminate metabolites and retain electrolytes at a normal level.

36810

36810   Insertion of cannula for hemodialysis, other purpose (separate procedure); arteriovenous, external (Scribner type)

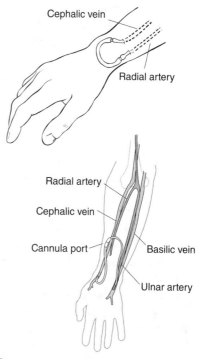

One end of the cannula is inserted into the artery and the other end is inserted into the vein to create a portal for hemodialysis

Explanation

The physician isolates an artery and a vein, usually in the nondominant forearm, and inserts a needle through the skin and into each vessel. A guidewire may be threaded through the needle into each vessel. The needle is removed. An end of a single cannula is inserted into each puncture, and any guidance wire removed. The Scribner cannula remains external, and may be left in place for several days. (This hemodialysis cannula is used to remove blood from the vessel, route it through the dialysis machine, then reinfuse it.)

Coding Tips

This type of hemodialysis cannula is infrequently used; verify from the medical record that this is the type of procedure performed. This procedure includes venipuncture when performed by the physician. For creation of an arteriovenous fistula, see 36825–36830. For open arteriovenous anastomosis, see 36818–36821.

ICD-10-CM Diagnostic Codes

D59.3	Hemolytic-uremic syndrome
E87.2	Acidosis
E87.5	Hyperkalemia
I12.0	Hypertensive chronic kidney disease with stage 5 chronic kidney disease or end stage renal disease
I13.0	Hypertensive heart and chronic kidney disease with heart failure and stage 1 through stage 4 chronic kidney disease, or unspecified chronic kidney disease
I13.11	Hypertensive heart and chronic kidney disease without heart failure, with stage 5 chronic kidney disease, or end stage renal disease

I13.2	Hypertensive heart and chronic kidney disease with heart failure and with stage 5 chronic kidney disease, or end stage renal disease
I16.0	Hypertensive urgency
I16.1	Hypertensive emergency
I82.3	Embolism and thrombosis of renal vein
M35.04	Sjögren syndrome with tubulo-interstitial nephropathy
M35.0A	Sjögren syndrome with glomerular disease
N00.0	Acute nephritic syndrome with minor glomerular abnormality
N00.1	Acute nephritic syndrome with focal and segmental glomerular lesions
N00.2	Acute nephritic syndrome with diffuse membranous glomerulonephritis
N00.3	Acute nephritic syndrome with diffuse mesangial proliferative glomerulonephritis
N00.4	Acute nephritic syndrome with diffuse endocapillary proliferative glomerulonephritis
N00.5	Acute nephritic syndrome with diffuse mesangiocapillary glomerulonephritis
N00.6	Acute nephritic syndrome with dense deposit disease
N00.7	Acute nephritic syndrome with diffuse crescentic glomerulonephritis
N00.8	Acute nephritic syndrome with other morphologic changes
N01.0	Rapidly progressive nephritic syndrome with minor glomerular abnormality
N01.1	Rapidly progressive nephritic syndrome with focal and segmental glomerular lesions
N01.2	Rapidly progressive nephritic syndrome with diffuse membranous glomerulonephritis
N01.3	Rapidly progressive nephritic syndrome with diffuse mesangial proliferative glomerulonephritis
N01.4	Rapidly progressive nephritic syndrome with diffuse endocapillary proliferative glomerulonephritis
N01.5	Rapidly progressive nephritic syndrome with diffuse mesangiocapillary glomerulonephritis
N01.6	Rapidly progressive nephritic syndrome with dense deposit disease
N01.7	Rapidly progressive nephritic syndrome with diffuse crescentic glomerulonephritis
N01.8	Rapidly progressive nephritic syndrome with other morphologic changes
N01.A	Rapidly progressive nephritic syndrome with C3 glomerulonephritis
N03.0	Chronic nephritic syndrome with minor glomerular abnormality
N03.1	Chronic nephritic syndrome with focal and segmental glomerular lesions
N03.2	Chronic nephritic syndrome with diffuse membranous glomerulonephritis
N03.3	Chronic nephritic syndrome with diffuse mesangial proliferative glomerulonephritis
N03.4	Chronic nephritic syndrome with diffuse endocapillary proliferative glomerulonephritis
N03.5	Chronic nephritic syndrome with diffuse mesangiocapillary glomerulonephritis
N03.6	Chronic nephritic syndrome with dense deposit disease
N03.7	Chronic nephritic syndrome with diffuse crescentic glomerulonephritis
N03.8	Chronic nephritic syndrome with other morphologic changes
N03.A	Chronic nephritic syndrome with C3 glomerulonephritis
N04.0	Nephrotic syndrome with minor glomerular abnormality
N04.1	Nephrotic syndrome with focal and segmental glomerular lesions
N04.2	Nephrotic syndrome with diffuse membranous glomerulonephritis
N04.3	Nephrotic syndrome with diffuse mesangial proliferative glomerulonephritis
N04.4	Nephrotic syndrome with diffuse endocapillary proliferative glomerulonephritis
N04.5	Nephrotic syndrome with diffuse mesangiocapillary glomerulonephritis
N04.6	Nephrotic syndrome with dense deposit disease
N04.7	Nephrotic syndrome with diffuse crescentic glomerulonephritis
N04.8	Nephrotic syndrome with other morphologic changes
N04.A	Nephrotic syndrome with C3 glomerulonephritis
N07.0	Hereditary nephropathy, not elsewhere classified with minor glomerular abnormality
N07.1	Hereditary nephropathy, not elsewhere classified with focal and segmental glomerular lesions
N07.2	Hereditary nephropathy, not elsewhere classified with diffuse membranous glomerulonephritis
N07.3	Hereditary nephropathy, not elsewhere classified with diffuse mesangial proliferative glomerulonephritis
N07.4	Hereditary nephropathy, not elsewhere classified with diffuse endocapillary proliferative glomerulonephritis
N07.5	Hereditary nephropathy, not elsewhere classified with diffuse mesangiocapillary glomerulonephritis
N07.6	Hereditary nephropathy, not elsewhere classified with dense deposit disease
N07.7	Hereditary nephropathy, not elsewhere classified with diffuse crescentic glomerulonephritis
N07.8	Hereditary nephropathy, not elsewhere classified with other morphologic lesions
N07.A	Hereditary nephropathy, not elsewhere classified with C3 glomerulonephritis
N08	Glomerular disorders in diseases classified elsewhere
N10	Acute pyelonephritis
N11.0	Nonobstructive reflux-associated chronic pyelonephritis
N11.1	Chronic obstructive pyelonephritis
N11.8	Other chronic tubulo-interstitial nephritis
N12	Tubulo-interstitial nephritis, not specified as acute or chronic
N15.8	Other specified renal tubulo-interstitial diseases
N16	Renal tubulo-interstitial disorders in diseases classified elsewhere
N17.0	Acute kidney failure with tubular necrosis
N17.1	Acute kidney failure with acute cortical necrosis
N17.2	Acute kidney failure with medullary necrosis
N17.8	Other acute kidney failure
N18.1	Chronic kidney disease, stage 1
N18.2	Chronic kidney disease, stage 2 (mild)
N18.31	Chronic kidney disease, stage 3a
N18.32	Chronic kidney disease, stage 3b
N18.4	Chronic kidney disease, stage 4 (severe)

| N18.5 | Chronic kidney disease, stage 5 |
| N18.6 | End stage renal disease |

AMA: 36810 2018,Jan,8; 2017,Jan,8; 2016,Jan,13; 2015,Jan,16

Relative Value Units/Medicare Edits

Non-Facility RVU	Work	PE	MP	Total
36810	3.96	1.8	0.48	6.24
Facility RVU	**Work**	**PE**	**MP**	**Total**
36810	3.96	1.8	0.48	6.24

	FUD	Status	MUE	Modifiers				IOM Reference
36810	0	A	1(3)	51	N/A	N/A	N/A	None

* with documentation

Terms To Know

acidosis. Reduction of alkaline in the blood and tissues caused by an increase in acid and decrease in bicarbonate.

chronic kidney disease. Decreased renal efficiency resulting in reduced ability of the kidney to filter waste. The National Kidney Foundation's classification includes clinical stages based on the glomerular filtration rate (GFR). The stages of CKD are as follows: stage 1, some kidney damage with a normal GFR of 90 or above; stage 2, mild kidney damage with a GFR of 60 to 89; stage 3a, mild to moderate kidney damage with a GFR of 45 to 59; stage 3b, moderate to severe kidney damage with a GFR of 30 to 44; stage 4, severe kidney damage with a GFR of 15 to 29; and stage 5, kidney failure with a GFR of less than 15. Dialysis or transplantation is required when kidney failure progresses to end stage renal disease.

ESRD. End stage renal disease. Progression of chronic renal failure to lasting and irreparable kidney damage that requires dialysis or renal transplant for survival.

glomerulonephritis. Disease of the kidney with diffuse inflammation of the capillary loops of the glomeruli. It may be a complication of bacterial infection or immune disorders and can lead to renal failure and may be associated with hypertension or diabetes.

hemodialysis. Cleansing of wastes and contaminating elements from the blood by virtue of different diffusion rates through a semipermeable membrane, which separates blood from a filtration solution that diffuses other elements out of the blood.

hemolytic-uremic syndrome. Enlargement of the liver and spleen and many erythroblasts in circulation.

nephrotic syndrome. Condition where levels of albumin in the blood and urine are far below the norm.

renal sclerosis. Atrophy, fibrosis, or other hardening of tissue in the kidney caused by inflammation, mineral deposits, or other causes.

Scribner type arteriovenous access. External cannula or shunt with the ends inserted into both an artery and a vein, at a puncture site made into the vessels through the skin, usually in the forearm. The Scribner cannula remains external and may be left in place for several days and is generally placed to route blood outside the body for hemodialysis purposes.

36815

| 36815 | Insertion of cannula for hemodialysis, other purpose (separate procedure); arteriovenous, external revision, or closure |

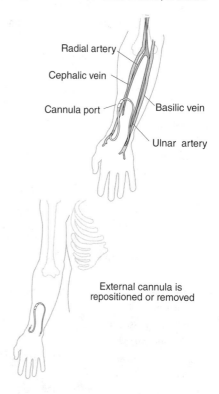

Radial artery
Cephalic vein
Cannula port
Basilic vein
Ulnar artery

External cannula is repositioned or removed

Explanation

The physician repositions an external cannula or removes it. The cannula forms a ready connection between the artery and vein or vein and vein for hemodialysis or another purpose. Closure of the insertion site is performed using sutures on the vessels or skin as necessary.

Coding Tips

This type of hemodialysis cannula is infrequently used; verify from the medical record that this is the type of procedure performed. This procedure includes venipuncture when performed by the physician. For creation of an arteriovenous fistula, see 36825–36830. For open arteriovenous anastomosis, see 36818–36821.

ICD-10-CM Diagnostic Codes

D59.3	Hemolytic-uremic syndrome
E87.2	Acidosis
E87.5	Hyperkalemia
I12.0	Hypertensive chronic kidney disease with stage 5 chronic kidney disease or end stage renal disease
I13.0	Hypertensive heart and chronic kidney disease with heart failure and stage 1 through stage 4 chronic kidney disease, or unspecified chronic kidney disease
I13.11	Hypertensive heart and chronic kidney disease without heart failure, with stage 5 chronic kidney disease, or end stage renal disease
I13.2	Hypertensive heart and chronic kidney disease with heart failure and with stage 5 chronic kidney disease, or end stage renal disease
I16.0	Hypertensive urgency

Arteries and Veins

I16.1	Hypertensive emergency
I82.3	Embolism and thrombosis of renal vein
M35.04	Sjögren syndrome with tubulo-interstitial nephropathy
M35.0A	Sjögren syndrome with glomerular disease
N00.0	Acute nephritic syndrome with minor glomerular abnormality
N00.1	Acute nephritic syndrome with focal and segmental glomerular lesions
N00.2	Acute nephritic syndrome with diffuse membranous glomerulonephritis
N00.3	Acute nephritic syndrome with diffuse mesangial proliferative glomerulonephritis
N00.4	Acute nephritic syndrome with diffuse endocapillary proliferative glomerulonephritis
N00.5	Acute nephritic syndrome with diffuse mesangiocapillary glomerulonephritis
N00.6	Acute nephritic syndrome with dense deposit disease
N00.7	Acute nephritic syndrome with diffuse crescentic glomerulonephritis
N00.A	Acute nephritic syndrome with C3 glomerulonephritis
N01.0	Rapidly progressive nephritic syndrome with minor glomerular abnormality
N01.1	Rapidly progressive nephritic syndrome with focal and segmental glomerular lesions
N01.2	Rapidly progressive nephritic syndrome with diffuse membranous glomerulonephritis
N01.3	Rapidly progressive nephritic syndrome with diffuse mesangial proliferative glomerulonephritis
N01.4	Rapidly progressive nephritic syndrome with diffuse endocapillary proliferative glomerulonephritis
N01.5	Rapidly progressive nephritic syndrome with diffuse mesangiocapillary glomerulonephritis
N01.6	Rapidly progressive nephritic syndrome with dense deposit disease
N01.7	Rapidly progressive nephritic syndrome with diffuse crescentic glomerulonephritis
N01.8	Rapidly progressive nephritic syndrome with other morphologic changes
N01.A	Rapidly progressive nephritic syndrome with C3 glomerulonephritis
N03.0	Chronic nephritic syndrome with minor glomerular abnormality
N03.1	Chronic nephritic syndrome with focal and segmental glomerular lesions
N03.2	Chronic nephritic syndrome with diffuse membranous glomerulonephritis
N03.3	Chronic nephritic syndrome with diffuse mesangial proliferative glomerulonephritis
N03.4	Chronic nephritic syndrome with diffuse endocapillary proliferative glomerulonephritis
N03.5	Chronic nephritic syndrome with diffuse mesangiocapillary glomerulonephritis
N03.6	Chronic nephritic syndrome with dense deposit disease
N03.7	Chronic nephritic syndrome with diffuse crescentic glomerulonephritis
N03.A	Chronic nephritic syndrome with C3 glomerulonephritis
N04.0	Nephrotic syndrome with minor glomerular abnormality
N04.1	Nephrotic syndrome with focal and segmental glomerular lesions
N04.2	Nephrotic syndrome with diffuse membranous glomerulonephritis
N04.3	Nephrotic syndrome with diffuse mesangial proliferative glomerulonephritis
N04.4	Nephrotic syndrome with diffuse endocapillary proliferative glomerulonephritis
N04.5	Nephrotic syndrome with diffuse mesangiocapillary glomerulonephritis
N04.6	Nephrotic syndrome with dense deposit disease
N04.7	Nephrotic syndrome with diffuse crescentic glomerulonephritis
N04.A	Nephrotic syndrome with C3 glomerulonephritis
N07.0	Hereditary nephropathy, not elsewhere classified with minor glomerular abnormality
N07.1	Hereditary nephropathy, not elsewhere classified with focal and segmental glomerular lesions
N07.2	Hereditary nephropathy, not elsewhere classified with diffuse membranous glomerulonephritis
N07.3	Hereditary nephropathy, not elsewhere classified with diffuse mesangial proliferative glomerulonephritis
N07.4	Hereditary nephropathy, not elsewhere classified with diffuse endocapillary proliferative glomerulonephritis
N07.5	Hereditary nephropathy, not elsewhere classified with diffuse mesangiocapillary glomerulonephritis
N07.6	Hereditary nephropathy, not elsewhere classified with dense deposit disease
N07.7	Hereditary nephropathy, not elsewhere classified with diffuse crescentic glomerulonephritis
N07.A	Hereditary nephropathy, not elsewhere classified with C3 glomerulonephritis
N08	Glomerular disorders in diseases classified elsewhere
N10	Acute pyelonephritis
N11.0	Nonobstructive reflux-associated chronic pyelonephritis
N11.1	Chronic obstructive pyelonephritis
N11.8	Other chronic tubulo-interstitial nephritis
N12	Tubulo-interstitial nephritis, not specified as acute or chronic
N16	Renal tubulo-interstitial disorders in diseases classified elsewhere
N17.0	Acute kidney failure with tubular necrosis
N17.1	Acute kidney failure with acute cortical necrosis
N17.2	Acute kidney failure with medullary necrosis
N18.1	Chronic kidney disease, stage 1
N18.2	Chronic kidney disease, stage 2 (mild)
N18.31	Chronic kidney disease, stage 3a
N18.32	Chronic kidney disease, stage 3b
N18.4	Chronic kidney disease, stage 4 (severe)
N18.5	Chronic kidney disease, stage 5
N18.6	End stage renal disease

AMA: **36815** 2018,Jan,8; 2017,Jan,8; 2016,Jan,13; 2015,Jan,16

N18.5   Chronic kidney disease, stage 5
N18.6   End stage renal disease

AMA: 36810 2018,Jan,8; 2017,Jan,8; 2016,Jan,13; 2015,Jan,16

Relative Value Units/Medicare Edits

Non-Facility RVU	Work	PE	MP	Total
36810	3.96	1.8	0.48	6.24
Facility RVU	**Work**	**PE**	**MP**	**Total**
36810	3.96	1.8	0.48	6.24

	FUD	Status	MUE	Modifiers			IOM Reference
36810	0	A	1(3)	51	N/A	N/A N/A	None

* with documentation

Terms To Know

acidosis. Reduction of alkaline in the blood and tissues caused by an increase in acid and decrease in bicarbonate.

chronic kidney disease. Decreased renal efficiency resulting in reduced ability of the kidney to filter waste. The National Kidney Foundation's classification includes clinical stages based on the glomerular filtration rate (GFR). The stages of CKD are as follows: stage 1, some kidney damage with a normal GFR of 90 or above; stage 2, mild kidney damage with a GFR of 60 to 89; stage 3a, mild to moderate kidney damage with a GFR of 45 to 59; stage 3b, moderate to severe kidney damage with a GFR of 30 to 44; stage 4, severe kidney damage with a GFR of 15 to 29; and stage 5, kidney failure with a GFR of less than 15. Dialysis or transplantation is required when kidney failure progresses to end stage renal disease.

ESRD. End stage renal disease. Progression of chronic renal failure to lasting and irreparable kidney damage that requires dialysis or renal transplant for survival.

glomerulonephritis. Disease of the kidney with diffuse inflammation of the capillary loops of the glomeruli. It may be a complication of bacterial infection or immune disorders and can lead to renal failure and may be associated with hypertension or diabetes.

hemodialysis. Cleansing of wastes and contaminating elements from the blood by virtue of different diffusion rates through a semipermeable membrane, which separates blood from a filtration solution that diffuses other elements out of the blood.

hemolytic-uremic syndrome. Enlargement of the liver and spleen and many erythroblasts in circulation.

nephrotic syndrome. Condition where levels of albumin in the blood and urine are far below the norm.

renal sclerosis. Atrophy, fibrosis, or other hardening of tissue in the kidney caused by inflammation, mineral deposits, or other causes.

Scribner type arteriovenous access. External cannula or shunt with the ends inserted into both an artery and a vein, at a puncture site made into the vessels through the skin, usually in the forearm. The Scribner cannula remains external and may be left in place for several days and is generally placed to route blood outside the body for hemodialysis purposes.

36815

36815   Insertion of cannula for hemodialysis, other purpose (separate procedure); arteriovenous, external revision, or closure

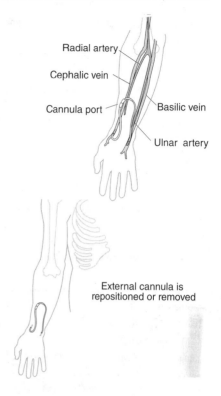

Radial artery
Cephalic vein
Cannula port
Basilic vein
Ulnar artery

External cannula is repositioned or removed

Explanation

The physician repositions an external cannula or removes it. The cannula forms a ready connection between the artery and vein or vein and vein for hemodialysis or another purpose. Closure of the insertion site is performed using sutures on the vessels or skin as necessary.

Coding Tips

This type of hemodialysis cannula is infrequently used; verify from the medical record that this is the type of procedure performed. This procedure includes venipuncture when performed by the physician. For creation of an arteriovenous fistula, see 36825–36830. For open arteriovenous anastomosis, see 36818–36821.

ICD-10-CM Diagnostic Codes

D59.3	Hemolytic-uremic syndrome
E87.2	Acidosis
E87.5	Hyperkalemia
I12.0	Hypertensive chronic kidney disease with stage 5 chronic kidney disease or end stage renal disease
I13.0	Hypertensive heart and chronic kidney disease with heart failure and stage 1 through stage 4 chronic kidney disease, or unspecified chronic kidney disease
I13.11	Hypertensive heart and chronic kidney disease without heart failure, with stage 5 chronic kidney disease, or end stage renal disease
I13.2	Hypertensive heart and chronic kidney disease with heart failure and with stage 5 chronic kidney disease, or end stage renal disease
I16.0	Hypertensive urgency

Arteries and Veins

I16.1	Hypertensive emergency
I82.3	Embolism and thrombosis of renal vein
M35.04	Sjögren syndrome with tubulo-interstitial nephropathy
M35.0A	Sjögren syndrome with glomerular disease
N00.0	Acute nephritic syndrome with minor glomerular abnormality
N00.1	Acute nephritic syndrome with focal and segmental glomerular lesions
N00.2	Acute nephritic syndrome with diffuse membranous glomerulonephritis
N00.3	Acute nephritic syndrome with diffuse mesangial proliferative glomerulonephritis
N00.4	Acute nephritic syndrome with diffuse endocapillary proliferative glomerulonephritis
N00.5	Acute nephritic syndrome with diffuse mesangiocapillary glomerulonephritis
N00.6	Acute nephritic syndrome with dense deposit disease
N00.7	Acute nephritic syndrome with diffuse crescentic glomerulonephritis
N00.A	Acute nephritic syndrome with C3 glomerulonephritis
N01.0	Rapidly progressive nephritic syndrome with minor glomerular abnormality
N01.1	Rapidly progressive nephritic syndrome with focal and segmental glomerular lesions
N01.2	Rapidly progressive nephritic syndrome with diffuse membranous glomerulonephritis
N01.3	Rapidly progressive nephritic syndrome with diffuse mesangial proliferative glomerulonephritis
N01.4	Rapidly progressive nephritic syndrome with diffuse endocapillary proliferative glomerulonephritis
N01.5	Rapidly progressive nephritic syndrome with diffuse mesangiocapillary glomerulonephritis
N01.6	Rapidly progressive nephritic syndrome with dense deposit disease
N01.7	Rapidly progressive nephritic syndrome with diffuse crescentic glomerulonephritis
N01.8	Rapidly progressive nephritic syndrome with other morphologic changes
N01.A	Rapidly progressive nephritic syndrome with C3 glomerulonephritis
N03.0	Chronic nephritic syndrome with minor glomerular abnormality
N03.1	Chronic nephritic syndrome with focal and segmental glomerular lesions
N03.2	Chronic nephritic syndrome with diffuse membranous glomerulonephritis
N03.3	Chronic nephritic syndrome with diffuse mesangial proliferative glomerulonephritis
N03.4	Chronic nephritic syndrome with diffuse endocapillary proliferative glomerulonephritis
N03.5	Chronic nephritic syndrome with diffuse mesangiocapillary glomerulonephritis
N03.6	Chronic nephritic syndrome with dense deposit disease
N03.7	Chronic nephritic syndrome with diffuse crescentic glomerulonephritis
N03.A	Chronic nephritic syndrome with C3 glomerulonephritis
N04.0	Nephrotic syndrome with minor glomerular abnormality
N04.1	Nephrotic syndrome with focal and segmental glomerular lesions
N04.2	Nephrotic syndrome with diffuse membranous glomerulonephritis
N04.3	Nephrotic syndrome with diffuse mesangial proliferative glomerulonephritis
N04.4	Nephrotic syndrome with diffuse endocapillary proliferative glomerulonephritis
N04.5	Nephrotic syndrome with diffuse mesangiocapillary glomerulonephritis
N04.6	Nephrotic syndrome with dense deposit disease
N04.7	Nephrotic syndrome with diffuse crescentic glomerulonephritis
N04.A	Nephrotic syndrome with C3 glomerulonephritis
N07.0	Hereditary nephropathy, not elsewhere classified with minor glomerular abnormality
N07.1	Hereditary nephropathy, not elsewhere classified with focal and segmental glomerular lesions
N07.2	Hereditary nephropathy, not elsewhere classified with diffuse membranous glomerulonephritis
N07.3	Hereditary nephropathy, not elsewhere classified with diffuse mesangial proliferative glomerulonephritis
N07.4	Hereditary nephropathy, not elsewhere classified with diffuse endocapillary proliferative glomerulonephritis
N07.5	Hereditary nephropathy, not elsewhere classified with diffuse mesangiocapillary glomerulonephritis
N07.6	Hereditary nephropathy, not elsewhere classified with dense deposit disease
N07.7	Hereditary nephropathy, not elsewhere classified with diffuse crescentic glomerulonephritis
N07.A	Hereditary nephropathy, not elsewhere classified with C3 glomerulonephritis
N08	Glomerular disorders in diseases classified elsewhere
N10	Acute pyelonephritis
N11.0	Nonobstructive reflux-associated chronic pyelonephritis
N11.1	Chronic obstructive pyelonephritis
N11.8	Other chronic tubulo-interstitial nephritis
N12	Tubulo-interstitial nephritis, not specified as acute or chronic
N16	Renal tubulo-interstitial disorders in diseases classified elsewhere
N17.0	Acute kidney failure with tubular necrosis
N17.1	Acute kidney failure with acute cortical necrosis
N17.2	Acute kidney failure with medullary necrosis
N18.1	Chronic kidney disease, stage 1
N18.2	Chronic kidney disease, stage 2 (mild)
N18.31	Chronic kidney disease, stage 3a
N18.32	Chronic kidney disease, stage 3b
N18.4	Chronic kidney disease, stage 4 (severe)
N18.5	Chronic kidney disease, stage 5
N18.6	End stage renal disease

AMA: 36815 2018,Jan,8; 2017,Jan,8; 2016,Jan,13; 2015,Jan,16

AMA: 36818 2018,Jan,8; 2017,Mar,3; 2017,Jan,8; 2016,Mar,10; 2016,Jan,13; 2015,Jan,16 **36819** 2018,Jan,8; 2017,Mar,3; 2017,Jan,8; 2016,Jan,13; 2015,Jan,16

Relative Value Units/Medicare Edits

Non-Facility RVU	Work	PE	MP	Total
36818	12.39	4.81	2.95	20.15
36819	13.29	4.87	3.18	21.34
Facility RVU	**Work**	**PE**	**MP**	**Total**
36818	12.39	4.81	2.95	20.15
36819	13.29	4.87	3.18	21.34

	FUD	Status	MUE	Modifiers				IOM Reference
36818	90	A	1(3)	51	N/A	62*	80	None
36819	90	A	1(3)	51	N/A	62*	80	

* with documentation

Terms To Know

anastomosis. Surgically created connection between ducts, blood vessels, or bowel segments to allow flow from one to the other.

chronic kidney disease. Decreased renal efficiency resulting in reduced ability of the kidney to filter waste. The National Kidney Foundation's classification includes clinical stages based on the glomerular filtration rate (GFR). The stages of CKD are as follows: stage 1, some kidney damage with a normal GFR of 90 or above; stage 2, mild kidney damage with a GFR of 60 to 89; stage 3a, mild to moderate kidney damage with a GFR of 45 to 59; stage 3b, moderate to severe kidney damage with a GFR of 30 to 44; stage 4, severe kidney damage with a GFR of 15 to 29; and stage 5, kidney failure with a GFR of less than 15. Dialysis or transplantation is required when kidney failure progresses to end stage renal disease.

ESRD. End stage renal disease. Progression of chronic renal failure to lasting and irreparable kidney damage that requires dialysis or renal transplant for survival.

hemodialysis. Cleansing of wastes and contaminating elements from the blood by virtue of different diffusion rates through a semipermeable membrane, which separates blood from a filtration solution that diffuses other elements out of the blood.

nephritis. Inflammation of the kidney, often due to infection, metabolic disorder, or an autoimmune process.

pyelonephritis. Infection of the renal pelvis and ureters that may be acute or chronic, often occurring as a result of a urinary tract infection, particularly in instances of vesicoureteric reflux, the backflow of urine from the bladder into the kidney pelvis or ureters.

renal failure. Inability of a kidney to eliminate metabolites and retain electrolytes at a normal level.

transposition. Removal or exchange from one side to another; change of position from one place to another.

36821

36821   Arteriovenous anastomosis, open; direct, any site (eg, Cimino type) (separate procedure)

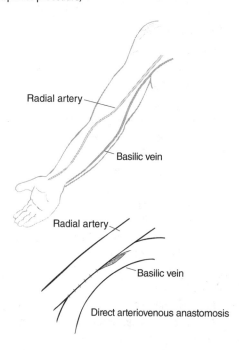

Radial artery

Basilic vein

Radial artery

Basilic vein

Direct arteriovenous anastomosis

Explanation

Through an incision, usually in the skin over an artery in the nondominant wrist or antecubital fossa, the physician isolates a desired section of artery and neighboring vein. Vessel clamps are placed on the vein and adjacent artery. The vein is dissected free, divided, and the downstream portion of the vein is sutured to an opening created in the adjacent artery, usually in an end-to-side fashion, allowing blood to flow both down the artery and into the vein. Large branches of the vein may be tied off to cause flow down a single vein. The skin incision is repaired with a layered closure. This arteriovenous anastomosis will allow an increased blood flow through the vein, usually for hemodialysis.

Coding Tips

This separate procedure by definition is usually a component of a more complex service and is not identified separately. When performed alone or with other unrelated procedures/services, it may be reported. If performed alone, list the code; if performed with other unrelated procedures/services, list the code and append modifier 59 or an X{EPSU} modifier. For insertion of a cannula for hemodialysis, other purpose, see 36800–36815. For creation of an arteriovenous fistula, by other than direct anastomosis, see 36825–36830.

ICD-10-CM Diagnostic Codes

D59.3	Hemolytic-uremic syndrome
E87.2	Acidosis
E87.5	Hyperkalemia
I12.0	Hypertensive chronic kidney disease with stage 5 chronic kidney disease or end stage renal disease
I13.0	Hypertensive heart and chronic kidney disease with heart failure and stage 1 through stage 4 chronic kidney disease, or unspecified chronic kidney disease

Arteries and Veins

I13.11	Hypertensive heart and chronic kidney disease without heart failure, with stage 5 chronic kidney disease, or end stage renal disease
I13.2	Hypertensive heart and chronic kidney disease with heart failure and with stage 5 chronic kidney disease, or end stage renal disease
I16.0	Hypertensive urgency
I16.1	Hypertensive emergency
I82.3	Embolism and thrombosis of renal vein
M35.04	Sjögren syndrome with tubulo-interstitial nephropathy
M35.0A	Sjögren syndrome with glomerular disease
N00.0	Acute nephritic syndrome with minor glomerular abnormality
N00.1	Acute nephritic syndrome with focal and segmental glomerular lesions
N00.2	Acute nephritic syndrome with diffuse membranous glomerulonephritis
N00.3	Acute nephritic syndrome with diffuse mesangial proliferative glomerulonephritis
N00.4	Acute nephritic syndrome with diffuse endocapillary proliferative glomerulonephritis
N00.5	Acute nephritic syndrome with diffuse mesangiocapillary glomerulonephritis
N00.6	Acute nephritic syndrome with dense deposit disease
N00.7	Acute nephritic syndrome with diffuse crescentic glomerulonephritis
N00.8	Acute nephritic syndrome with other morphologic changes
N01.0	Rapidly progressive nephritic syndrome with minor glomerular abnormality
N01.1	Rapidly progressive nephritic syndrome with focal and segmental glomerular lesions
N01.2	Rapidly progressive nephritic syndrome with diffuse membranous glomerulonephritis
N01.3	Rapidly progressive nephritic syndrome with diffuse mesangial proliferative glomerulonephritis
N01.4	Rapidly progressive nephritic syndrome with diffuse endocapillary proliferative glomerulonephritis
N01.5	Rapidly progressive nephritic syndrome with diffuse mesangiocapillary glomerulonephritis
N01.6	Rapidly progressive nephritic syndrome with dense deposit disease
N01.7	Rapidly progressive nephritic syndrome with diffuse crescentic glomerulonephritis
N01.8	Rapidly progressive nephritic syndrome with other morphologic changes
N01.A	Rapidly progressive nephritic syndrome with C3 glomerulonephritis
N03.0	Chronic nephritic syndrome with minor glomerular abnormality
N03.1	Chronic nephritic syndrome with focal and segmental glomerular lesions
N03.2	Chronic nephritic syndrome with diffuse membranous glomerulonephritis
N03.3	Chronic nephritic syndrome with diffuse mesangial proliferative glomerulonephritis
N03.4	Chronic nephritic syndrome with diffuse endocapillary proliferative glomerulonephritis
N03.5	Chronic nephritic syndrome with diffuse mesangiocapillary glomerulonephritis
N03.6	Chronic nephritic syndrome with dense deposit disease
N03.7	Chronic nephritic syndrome with diffuse crescentic glomerulonephritis
N03.8	Chronic nephritic syndrome with other morphologic changes
N03.A	Chronic nephritic syndrome with C3 glomerulonephritis
N04.0	Nephrotic syndrome with minor glomerular abnormality
N04.1	Nephrotic syndrome with focal and segmental glomerular lesions
N04.2	Nephrotic syndrome with diffuse membranous glomerulonephritis
N04.3	Nephrotic syndrome with diffuse mesangial proliferative glomerulonephritis
N04.4	Nephrotic syndrome with diffuse endocapillary proliferative glomerulonephritis
N04.5	Nephrotic syndrome with diffuse mesangiocapillary glomerulonephritis
N04.6	Nephrotic syndrome with dense deposit disease
N04.7	Nephrotic syndrome with diffuse crescentic glomerulonephritis
N04.8	Nephrotic syndrome with other morphologic changes
N04.A	Nephrotic syndrome with C3 glomerulonephritis
N07.0	Hereditary nephropathy, not elsewhere classified with minor glomerular abnormality
N07.1	Hereditary nephropathy, not elsewhere classified with focal and segmental glomerular lesions
N07.2	Hereditary nephropathy, not elsewhere classified with diffuse membranous glomerulonephritis
N07.3	Hereditary nephropathy, not elsewhere classified with diffuse mesangial proliferative glomerulonephritis
N07.4	Hereditary nephropathy, not elsewhere classified with diffuse endocapillary proliferative glomerulonephritis
N07.5	Hereditary nephropathy, not elsewhere classified with diffuse mesangiocapillary glomerulonephritis
N07.6	Hereditary nephropathy, not elsewhere classified with dense deposit disease
N07.7	Hereditary nephropathy, not elsewhere classified with diffuse crescentic glomerulonephritis
N07.8	Hereditary nephropathy, not elsewhere classified with other morphologic lesions
N07.A	Hereditary nephropathy, not elsewhere classified with C3 glomerulonephritis
N08	Glomerular disorders in diseases classified elsewhere
N10	Acute pyelonephritis
N11.0	Nonobstructive reflux-associated chronic pyelonephritis
N11.1	Chronic obstructive pyelonephritis
N11.8	Other chronic tubulo-interstitial nephritis
N12	Tubulo-interstitial nephritis, not specified as acute or chronic
N15.8	Other specified renal tubulo-interstitial diseases
N16	Renal tubulo-interstitial disorders in diseases classified elsewhere
N17.0	Acute kidney failure with tubular necrosis
N17.1	Acute kidney failure with acute cortical necrosis
N17.2	Acute kidney failure with medullary necrosis
N17.8	Other acute kidney failure
N18.1	Chronic kidney disease, stage 1
N18.2	Chronic kidney disease, stage 2 (mild)

N18.31	Chronic kidney disease, stage 3a
N18.32	Chronic kidney disease, stage 3b
N18.4	Chronic kidney disease, stage 4 (severe)
N18.5	Chronic kidney disease, stage 5
N18.6	End stage renal disease

AMA: 36821 2018,Jan,8; 2017,Mar,3; 2017,Jan,8; 2016,Jan,13; 2015,Jan,16; 2015,Aug,8

Relative Value Units/Medicare Edits

Non-Facility RVU	Work	PE	MP	Total
36821	11.9	4.61	2.84	19.35
Facility RVU	**Work**	**PE**	**MP**	**Total**
36821	11.9	4.61	2.84	19.35

	FUD	Status	MUE	Modifiers				IOM Reference
36821	90	A	2(3)	51	N/A	62*	80	None

* with documentation

Terms To Know

chronic kidney disease. Decreased renal efficiency resulting in reduced ability of the kidney to filter waste. The National Kidney Foundation's classification includes clinical stages based on the glomerular filtration rate (GFR). The stages of CKD are as follows: stage 1, some kidney damage with a normal GFR of 90 or above; stage 2, mild kidney damage with a GFR of 60 to 89; stage 3a, mild to moderate kidney damage with a GFR of 45 to 59; stage 3b, moderate to severe kidney damage with a GFR of 30 to 44; stage 4, severe kidney damage with a GFR of 15 to 29; and stage 5, kidney failure with a GFR of less than 15. Dialysis or transplantation is required when kidney failure progresses to end stage renal disease.

Cimino type arteriovenous anastomosis. Direct anastomosis of a vein to an artery, usually at the wrist of the nondominant hand. Using only a moderate amount of arterial and venous dissection, a portion of the vein is sutured in an end-to-side fashion to the adjacent artery, allowing blood to flow both down the artery and into the vein. The increased blood flow through the vein is used for hemodialysis.

ESRD. End stage renal disease. Progression of chronic renal failure to lasting and irreparable kidney damage that requires dialysis or renal transplant for survival.

hemodialysis. Cleansing of wastes and contaminating elements from the blood by virtue of different diffusion rates through a semipermeable membrane, which separates blood from a filtration solution that diffuses other elements out of the blood.

nephropathy. Disease or abnormality of the kidney.

renal failure. Inability of a kidney to eliminate metabolites and retain electrolytes at a normal level.

renal sclerosis. Atrophy, fibrosis, or other hardening of tissue in the kidney caused by inflammation, mineral deposits, or other causes.

36825-36830

| 36825 | Creation of arteriovenous fistula by other than direct arteriovenous anastomosis (separate procedure); autogenous graft |
| 36830 | nonautogenous graft (eg, biological collagen, thermoplastic graft) |

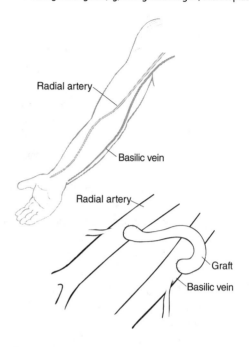

Radial artery

Basilic vein

Radial artery

Graft

Basilic vein

Explanation

The physician creates an arteriovenous fistula by other than direct anastomosis. The physician makes an incision in the skin over an artery and vein, and the vein and artery are dissected free. A vessel clamp is affixed to each. A length of harvested vein from the patient is used for an autogenous graft in 36825 and is sutured to the incised artery and vein, usually in an end-to-side fashion. The graft is passed in a superficial subcutaneous tunnel that is created bluntly and connects the arterial and venous sites. The clamps are removed, allowing the blood to flow through the graft, creating an arteriovenous fistula. The skin incision is repaired with a layered closure. Report 36830 if a nonautogenous graft, such as biological collagen or a thermoplastic graft, is used.

Coding Tips

These separate procedures by definition are usually a component of a more complex service and are not identified separately. When performed alone or with other unrelated procedures/services, they may be reported. If performed alone, list the code; if performed with other unrelated procedures/services, list the code and append modifier 59 or an X{EPSU} modifier. For direct arteriovenous anastomosis, see 36821.

ICD-10-CM Diagnostic Codes

D59.3	Hemolytic-uremic syndrome
E87.2	Acidosis
E87.5	Hyperkalemia
I12.0	Hypertensive chronic kidney disease with stage 5 chronic kidney disease or end stage renal disease
I13.0	Hypertensive heart and chronic kidney disease with heart failure and stage 1 through stage 4 chronic kidney disease, or unspecified chronic kidney disease

Arteries and Veins

I13.11	Hypertensive heart and chronic kidney disease without heart failure, with stage 5 chronic kidney disease, or end stage renal disease
I13.2	Hypertensive heart and chronic kidney disease with heart failure and with stage 5 chronic kidney disease, or end stage renal disease
I16.0	Hypertensive urgency
I16.1	Hypertensive emergency
I82.3	Embolism and thrombosis of renal vein
M35.04	Sjögren syndrome with tubulo-interstitial nephropathy
M35.0A	Sjögren syndrome with glomerular disease
N00.0	Acute nephritic syndrome with minor glomerular abnormality
N00.1	Acute nephritic syndrome with focal and segmental glomerular lesions
N00.2	Acute nephritic syndrome with diffuse membranous glomerulonephritis
N00.3	Acute nephritic syndrome with diffuse mesangial proliferative glomerulonephritis
N00.4	Acute nephritic syndrome with diffuse endocapillary proliferative glomerulonephritis
N00.5	Acute nephritic syndrome with diffuse mesangiocapillary glomerulonephritis
N00.6	Acute nephritic syndrome with dense deposit disease
N00.7	Acute nephritic syndrome with diffuse crescentic glomerulonephritis
N00.8	Acute nephritic syndrome with other morphologic changes
N00.A	Acute nephritic syndrome with C3 glomerulonephritis
N01.0	Rapidly progressive nephritic syndrome with minor glomerular abnormality
N01.1	Rapidly progressive nephritic syndrome with focal and segmental glomerular lesions
N01.2	Rapidly progressive nephritic syndrome with diffuse membranous glomerulonephritis
N01.3	Rapidly progressive nephritic syndrome with diffuse mesangial proliferative glomerulonephritis
N01.4	Rapidly progressive nephritic syndrome with diffuse endocapillary proliferative glomerulonephritis
N01.5	Rapidly progressive nephritic syndrome with diffuse mesangiocapillary glomerulonephritis
N01.6	Rapidly progressive nephritic syndrome with dense deposit disease
N01.7	Rapidly progressive nephritic syndrome with diffuse crescentic glomerulonephritis
N01.8	Rapidly progressive nephritic syndrome with other morphologic changes
N01.A	Rapidly progressive nephritic syndrome with C3 glomerulonephritis
N03.0	Chronic nephritic syndrome with minor glomerular abnormality
N03.1	Chronic nephritic syndrome with focal and segmental glomerular lesions
N03.2	Chronic nephritic syndrome with diffuse membranous glomerulonephritis
N03.3	Chronic nephritic syndrome with diffuse mesangial proliferative glomerulonephritis
N03.4	Chronic nephritic syndrome with diffuse endocapillary proliferative glomerulonephritis
N03.5	Chronic nephritic syndrome with diffuse mesangiocapillary glomerulonephritis
N03.6	Chronic nephritic syndrome with dense deposit disease
N03.7	Chronic nephritic syndrome with diffuse crescentic glomerulonephritis
N03.8	Chronic nephritic syndrome with other morphologic changes
N03.A	Chronic nephritic syndrome with C3 glomerulonephritis
N04.0	Nephrotic syndrome with minor glomerular abnormality
N04.1	Nephrotic syndrome with focal and segmental glomerular lesions
N04.2	Nephrotic syndrome with diffuse membranous glomerulonephritis
N04.3	Nephrotic syndrome with diffuse mesangial proliferative glomerulonephritis
N04.4	Nephrotic syndrome with diffuse endocapillary proliferative glomerulonephritis
N04.5	Nephrotic syndrome with diffuse mesangiocapillary glomerulonephritis
N04.6	Nephrotic syndrome with dense deposit disease
N04.7	Nephrotic syndrome with diffuse crescentic glomerulonephritis
N04.8	Nephrotic syndrome with other morphologic changes
N04.A	Nephrotic syndrome with C3 glomerulonephritis
N07.0	Hereditary nephropathy, not elsewhere classified with minor glomerular abnormality
N07.1	Hereditary nephropathy, not elsewhere classified with focal and segmental glomerular lesions
N07.2	Hereditary nephropathy, not elsewhere classified with diffuse membranous glomerulonephritis
N07.3	Hereditary nephropathy, not elsewhere classified with diffuse mesangial proliferative glomerulonephritis
N07.4	Hereditary nephropathy, not elsewhere classified with diffuse endocapillary proliferative glomerulonephritis
N07.5	Hereditary nephropathy, not elsewhere classified with diffuse mesangiocapillary glomerulonephritis
N07.6	Hereditary nephropathy, not elsewhere classified with dense deposit disease
N07.7	Hereditary nephropathy, not elsewhere classified with diffuse crescentic glomerulonephritis
N07.8	Hereditary nephropathy, not elsewhere classified with other morphologic lesions
N07.A	Hereditary nephropathy, not elsewhere classified with C3 glomerulonephritis
N08	Glomerular disorders in diseases classified elsewhere
N10	Acute pyelonephritis
N11.0	Nonobstructive reflux-associated chronic pyelonephritis
N11.1	Chronic obstructive pyelonephritis
N11.8	Other chronic tubulo-interstitial nephritis
N12	Tubulo-interstitial nephritis, not specified as acute or chronic
N15.8	Other specified renal tubulo-interstitial diseases
N16	Renal tubulo-interstitial disorders in diseases classified elsewhere
N17.0	Acute kidney failure with tubular necrosis
N17.1	Acute kidney failure with acute cortical necrosis
N17.2	Acute kidney failure with medullary necrosis
N17.8	Other acute kidney failure
N18.1	Chronic kidney disease, stage 1
N18.2	Chronic kidney disease, stage 2 (mild)

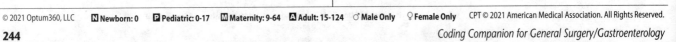

N18.31	Chronic kidney disease, stage 3a
N18.32	Chronic kidney disease, stage 3b
N18.4	Chronic kidney disease, stage 4 (severe)
N18.5	Chronic kidney disease, stage 5
N18.6	End stage renal disease

AMA: 36825 2018,Jan,8; 2017,Mar,3; 2017,Jan,8; 2016,Jan,13; 2015,Jan,16
36830 2018,Jan,8; 2017,Mar,3; 2017,Jan,8; 2016,Jan,13; 2015,Jan,13; 2015,Jan,16

Relative Value Units/Medicare Edits

Non-Facility RVU	Work	PE	MP	Total
36825	14.17	5.66	3.41	23.24
36830	12.03	4.56	2.87	19.46
Facility RVU	Work	PE	MP	Total
36825	14.17	5.66	3.41	23.24
36830	12.03	4.56	2.87	19.46

	FUD	Status	MUE	Modifiers				IOM Reference
36825	90	A	1(3)	51	N/A	62*	80	None
36830	90	A	2(3)	51	N/A	62*	80	

* with documentation

Terms To Know

anastomosis. Surgically created connection between ducts, blood vessels, or bowel segments to allow flow from one to the other.

arteriovenous fistula. Connecting passage between an artery and a vein.

chronic kidney disease. Decreased renal efficiency resulting in reduced ability of the kidney to filter waste. The National Kidney Foundation's classification includes clinical stages based on the glomerular filtration rate (GFR). The stages of CKD are as follows: stage 1, some kidney damage with a normal GFR of 90 or above; stage 2, mild kidney damage with a GFR of 60 to 89; stage 3a, mild to moderate kidney damage with a GFR of 45 to 59; stage 3b, moderate to severe kidney damage with a GFR of 30 to 44; stage 4, severe kidney damage with a GFR of 15 to 29; and stage 5, kidney failure with a GFR of less than 15. Dialysis or transplantation is required when kidney failure progresses to end stage renal disease.

ESRD. End stage renal disease. Progression of chronic renal failure to lasting and irreparable kidney damage that requires dialysis or renal transplant for survival.

glomerulonephritis. Disease of the kidney with diffuse inflammation of the capillary loops of the glomeruli. It may be a complication of bacterial infection or immune disorders and can lead to renal failure and may be associated with hypertension or diabetes.

hydronephrosis. Distension of the kidney caused by an accumulation of urine that cannot flow out due to an obstruction that may be caused by conditions such as kidney stones or vesicoureteral reflux.

nephropathy. Disease or abnormality of the kidney.

nonautogenous. Derived from a source other than the same individual or recipient (e.g., cells, tissue, blood vessels, and other organs donated from another human).

36831

36831 Thrombectomy, open, arteriovenous fistula without revision, autogenous or nonautogenous dialysis graft (separate procedure)

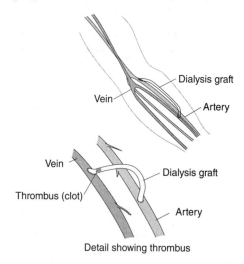

Detail showing thrombus

Explanation

The physician removes a blood clot from a surgically created connection between an artery and a vein (arteriovenous fistula). The procedure involves making an incision over the site of an existing fistula. The fistula is isolated and dissected free. Vessel clamps are affixed above and below the fistula. The blood clot is removed, the clamps are taken off, and the incision is repaired by layered sutures. The procedure may involve a vein acquired from the patient or the construction of a synthetic graft.

Coding Tips

This separate procedure, by definition, is usually a component of a more complex service and is not identified separately. When performed alone or with other unrelated procedures/services it may be reported. If performed alone, list the code; if performed with other procedures/services, list the code and append modifier 59 or an X{EPSU} modifier. Use this procedure for thrombectomy associated with reduced flow. This code reports open thrombectomy. For percutaneous thrombectomy, arteriovenous fistula, see 36904-36906. For external cannula declotting without balloon catheter, see 36860; with balloon catheter, see 36861. For thrombectomy with revision of an arteriovenous fistula, see 36833.

ICD-10-CM Diagnostic Codes

T82.818A	Embolism due to vascular prosthetic devices, implants and grafts, initial encounter
T82.828A	Fibrosis due to vascular prosthetic devices, implants and grafts, initial encounter
T82.848A	Pain due to vascular prosthetic devices, implants and grafts, initial encounter
T82.858A	Stenosis of other vascular prosthetic devices, implants and grafts, initial encounter
T82.868A	Thrombosis due to vascular prosthetic devices, implants and grafts, initial encounter
T82.898A	Other specified complication of vascular prosthetic devices, implants and grafts, initial encounter

AMA: 36831 2018,Jan,8; 2017,Mar,3; 2017,Jan,8; 2016,Jan,13; 2015,Jan,16

Relative Value Units/Medicare Edits

Non-Facility RVU	Work	PE	MP	Total
36831	11.0	4.32	2.63	17.95
Facility RVU	Work	PE	MP	Total
36831	11.0	4.32	2.63	17.95

	FUD	Status	MUE	Modifiers				IOM Reference
36831	90	A	1(3)	51	N/A	62*	80	None

* with documentation

Terms To Know

arteriovenous fistula. Connecting passage between an artery and a vein.

artery. Vessel through which oxygenated blood passes away from the heart to any part of the body.

autogenous transplant. Tissue, such as bone, that is harvested from the patient and used for transplantation back into the same patient.

blood clot. Semisolidified, coagulated mass of mainly platelets and fibrin in the bloodstream.

complication. Condition arising after the beginning of observation and treatment that modifies the course of the patient's illness or the medical care required, or an undesired result or misadventure in medical care.

dialysis. Artificial filtering of the blood to remove contaminating waste elements and restore normal balance.

dissect. Cut apart or separate tissue for surgical purposes or for visual or microscopic study.

graft. Tissue implant from another part of the body or another person.

nonautogenous. Derived from a source other than the same individual or recipient (e.g., cells, tissue, blood vessels, and other organs donated from another human).

thrombus. Stationary blood clot inside a blood vessel.

vein. Vessel through which oxygen-depleted blood passes back to the heart.

36832-36833

36832   Revision, open, arteriovenous fistula; without thrombectomy, autogenous or nonautogenous dialysis graft (separate procedure)

36833   with thrombectomy, autogenous or nonautogenous dialysis graft (separate procedure)

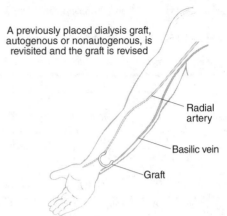

A previously placed dialysis graft, autogenous or nonautogenous, is revisited and the graft is revised

Radial artery

Basilic vein

Graft

Explanation

In 36832, the physician makes an incision at the site of an already existing artificial fistula between an artery and a vein. The fistula is dissected free. Vessel clamps are affixed above and below the fistula, which is incised. Revisions are made to the fistula at its juncture to the vein and/or artery and may require creating a new anastomosis with a graft obtained from a separate site or created with synthetic material. After the repair has been made, the fistula is sutured, the clamps removed, and the skin incision repaired with a layered closure. Report 36833 when the physician removes a blood clot at the fistula site in addition to revising the existing arteriovenous fistula.

Coding Tips

These separate procedures, by definition, are usually a component of a more complex service and are not identified separately. When performed alone or with other unrelated procedures/services they may be reported. If performed alone, list the code; if performed with other procedures/services, list the code and append modifier 59 or an X{EPSU} modifier. These codes should be reported only for open revision of an arteriovenous fistula. For external cannula declotting without balloon catheter, see 36860; with balloon catheter, see 36861. For open thrombectomy without revision of an arteriovenous fistula, see 36831. For percutaneous thrombectomy, arteriovenous fistula, within the dialysis circuit, see 36904–36906. For angioplasties of the central dialysis segment performed with 36818–36833, see 36907; for stent placement in conjunction with these codes, see 36908. Do not report these codes with 36901–36906 for revision of the dialysis circuit.

ICD-10-CM Diagnostic Codes

T82.510A	Breakdown (mechanical) of surgically created arteriovenous fistula, initial encounter
T82.520A	Displacement of surgically created arteriovenous fistula, initial encounter
T82.530A	Leakage of surgically created arteriovenous fistula, initial encounter
T82.590A	Other mechanical complication of surgically created arteriovenous fistula, initial encounter
T82.7XXA	Infection and inflammatory reaction due to other cardiac and vascular devices, implants and grafts, initial encounter

Coding Companion for General Surgery/Gastroenterology

T82.818A	Embolism due to vascular prosthetic devices, implants and grafts, initial encounter
T82.828A	Fibrosis due to vascular prosthetic devices, implants and grafts, initial encounter
T82.848A	Pain due to vascular prosthetic devices, implants and grafts, initial encounter
T82.858A	Stenosis of other vascular prosthetic devices, implants and grafts, initial encounter
T82.868A	Thrombosis due to vascular prosthetic devices, implants and grafts, initial encounter
T82.898A	Other specified complication of vascular prosthetic devices, implants and grafts, initial encounter
Z45.89	Encounter for adjustment and management of other implanted devices
Z46.89	Encounter for fitting and adjustment of other specified devices

AMA: 36832 2018,Jan,8; 2017,Mar,3; 2017,Jan,8; 2016,Jan,13; 2015,Jan,16
36833 2018,Jan,8; 2017,Mar,3; 2017,Jan,8; 2016,Jan,13; 2015,Jan,16

Relative Value Units/Medicare Edits

Non-Facility RVU	Work	PE	MP	Total
36832	13.5	5.34	3.23	22.07
36833	14.5	5.65	3.48	23.63
Facility RVU	Work	PE	MP	Total
36832	13.5	5.34	3.23	22.07
36833	14.5	5.65	3.48	23.63

	FUD	Status	MUE	Modifiers				IOM Reference
36832	90	A	2(3)	51	N/A	62*	80	None
36833	90	A	1(3)	51	N/A	62*	80	

* with documentation

Terms To Know

arteriovenous fistula. Connecting passage between an artery and a vein.

revision. Reordering or rearrangement of tissue to suit a particular need or function.

thrombectomy. Removal of a clot (thrombus) from a blood vessel utilizing various methods.

36835

36835   Insertion of Thomas shunt (separate procedure)

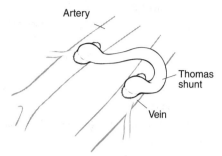

The Thomas shunt is a specialized synthetic graft and is typically used for infant and pediatric patients

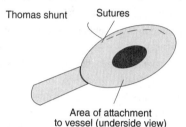

Area of attachment to vessel (underside view)

Explanation

Through an incision in the skin overlying a large vein or artery of a child, the physician dissects the vessel that will receive a synthetic shunt. The vessel may be clamped. The vessel is nicked, and a needle threads a guidance wire into the vein or artery. The shunt follows, and the wire is removed. The physician sutures the synthetic shunt end-to-end, or end-to-side, to the vein or artery. The shunt is most often used for access in hemodialysis.

Coding Tips

This type of shunt is infrequently used; verify this is the correct code by obtaining a copy of the shunt label from the medical record. This code includes venipuncture performed by the physician.

ICD-10-CM Diagnostic Codes

D59.3	Hemolytic-uremic syndrome
E87.2	Acidosis
E87.5	Hyperkalemia
I12.0	Hypertensive chronic kidney disease with stage 5 chronic kidney disease or end stage renal disease
I13.0	Hypertensive heart and chronic kidney disease with heart failure and stage 1 through stage 4 chronic kidney disease, or unspecified chronic kidney disease
I13.11	Hypertensive heart and chronic kidney disease without heart failure, with stage 5 chronic kidney disease, or end stage renal disease
I13.2	Hypertensive heart and chronic kidney disease with heart failure and with stage 5 chronic kidney disease, or end stage renal disease
I16.0	Hypertensive urgency
I16.1	Hypertensive emergency
I82.3	Embolism and thrombosis of renal vein
M35.04	Sjögren syndrome with tubulo-interstitial nephropathy
M35.0A	Sjögren syndrome with glomerular disease

N00.0	Acute nephritic syndrome with minor glomerular abnormality
N00.1	Acute nephritic syndrome with focal and segmental glomerular lesions
N00.2	Acute nephritic syndrome with diffuse membranous glomerulonephritis
N00.3	Acute nephritic syndrome with diffuse mesangial proliferative glomerulonephritis
N00.4	Acute nephritic syndrome with diffuse endocapillary proliferative glomerulonephritis
N00.5	Acute nephritic syndrome with diffuse mesangiocapillary glomerulonephritis
N00.6	Acute nephritic syndrome with dense deposit disease
N00.7	Acute nephritic syndrome with diffuse crescentic glomerulonephritis
N00.8	Acute nephritic syndrome with other morphologic changes
N00.A	Acute nephritic syndrome with C3 glomerulonephritis
N01.0	Rapidly progressive nephritic syndrome with minor glomerular abnormality
N01.1	Rapidly progressive nephritic syndrome with focal and segmental glomerular lesions
N01.2	Rapidly progressive nephritic syndrome with diffuse membranous glomerulonephritis
N01.3	Rapidly progressive nephritic syndrome with diffuse mesangial proliferative glomerulonephritis
N01.4	Rapidly progressive nephritic syndrome with diffuse endocapillary proliferative glomerulonephritis
N01.5	Rapidly progressive nephritic syndrome with diffuse mesangiocapillary glomerulonephritis
N01.6	Rapidly progressive nephritic syndrome with dense deposit disease
N01.7	Rapidly progressive nephritic syndrome with diffuse crescentic glomerulonephritis
N01.8	Rapidly progressive nephritic syndrome with other morphologic changes
N01.A	Rapidly progressive nephritic syndrome with C3 glomerulonephritis
N03.0	Chronic nephritic syndrome with minor glomerular abnormality
N03.1	Chronic nephritic syndrome with focal and segmental glomerular lesions
N03.2	Chronic nephritic syndrome with diffuse membranous glomerulonephritis
N03.3	Chronic nephritic syndrome with diffuse mesangial proliferative glomerulonephritis
N03.4	Chronic nephritic syndrome with diffuse endocapillary proliferative glomerulonephritis
N03.5	Chronic nephritic syndrome with diffuse mesangiocapillary glomerulonephritis
N03.6	Chronic nephritic syndrome with dense deposit disease
N03.7	Chronic nephritic syndrome with diffuse crescentic glomerulonephritis
N03.8	Chronic nephritic syndrome with other morphologic changes
N03.A	Chronic nephritic syndrome with C3 glomerulonephritis
N04.0	Nephrotic syndrome with minor glomerular abnormality
N04.1	Nephrotic syndrome with focal and segmental glomerular lesions
N04.2	Nephrotic syndrome with diffuse membranous glomerulonephritis
N04.3	Nephrotic syndrome with diffuse mesangial proliferative glomerulonephritis
N04.4	Nephrotic syndrome with diffuse endocapillary proliferative glomerulonephritis
N04.5	Nephrotic syndrome with diffuse mesangiocapillary glomerulonephritis
N04.6	Nephrotic syndrome with dense deposit disease
N04.7	Nephrotic syndrome with diffuse crescentic glomerulonephritis
N04.8	Nephrotic syndrome with other morphologic changes
N04.A	Nephrotic syndrome with C3 glomerulonephritis
N07.0	Hereditary nephropathy, not elsewhere classified with minor glomerular abnormality
N07.1	Hereditary nephropathy, not elsewhere classified with focal and segmental glomerular lesions
N07.2	Hereditary nephropathy, not elsewhere classified with diffuse membranous glomerulonephritis
N07.3	Hereditary nephropathy, not elsewhere classified with diffuse mesangial proliferative glomerulonephritis
N07.4	Hereditary nephropathy, not elsewhere classified with diffuse endocapillary proliferative glomerulonephritis
N07.5	Hereditary nephropathy, not elsewhere classified with diffuse mesangiocapillary glomerulonephritis
N07.6	Hereditary nephropathy, not elsewhere classified with dense deposit disease
N07.7	Hereditary nephropathy, not elsewhere classified with diffuse crescentic glomerulonephritis
N07.8	Hereditary nephropathy, not elsewhere classified with other morphologic lesions
N07.A	Hereditary nephropathy, not elsewhere classified with C3 glomerulonephritis
N08	Glomerular disorders in diseases classified elsewhere
N10	Acute pyelonephritis
N11.0	Nonobstructive reflux-associated chronic pyelonephritis
N11.1	Chronic obstructive pyelonephritis
N12	Tubulo-interstitial nephritis, not specified as acute or chronic
N16	Renal tubulo-interstitial disorders in diseases classified elsewhere
N17.0	Acute kidney failure with tubular necrosis
N17.1	Acute kidney failure with acute cortical necrosis
N17.2	Acute kidney failure with medullary necrosis
N17.8	Other acute kidney failure
N18.1	Chronic kidney disease, stage 1
N18.2	Chronic kidney disease, stage 2 (mild)
N18.31	Chronic kidney disease, stage 3a
N18.32	Chronic kidney disease, stage 3b
N18.4	Chronic kidney disease, stage 4 (severe)
N18.5	Chronic kidney disease, stage 5
N18.6	End stage renal disease
T80.211A	Bloodstream infection due to central venous catheter, initial encounter
T80.212A	Local infection due to central venous catheter, initial encounter
T80.218A	Other infection due to central venous catheter, initial encounter
T82.318A	Breakdown (mechanical) of other vascular grafts, initial encounter
T82.328A	Displacement of other vascular grafts, initial encounter
T82.338A	Leakage of other vascular grafts, initial encounter

T82.398A	Other mechanical complication of other vascular grafts, initial encounter	
T82.41XA	Breakdown (mechanical) of vascular dialysis catheter, initial encounter	
T82.42XA	Displacement of vascular dialysis catheter, initial encounter	
T82.43XA	Leakage of vascular dialysis catheter, initial encounter	
T82.49XA	Other complication of vascular dialysis catheter, initial encounter	
T82.510A	Breakdown (mechanical) of surgically created arteriovenous fistula, initial encounter	
T82.518A	Breakdown (mechanical) of other cardiac and vascular devices and implants, initial encounter	
T82.520A	Displacement of surgically created arteriovenous fistula, initial encounter	
T82.528A	Displacement of other cardiac and vascular devices and implants, initial encounter	
T82.530A	Leakage of surgically created arteriovenous fistula, initial encounter	
T82.538A	Leakage of other cardiac and vascular devices and implants, initial encounter	
T82.590A	Other mechanical complication of surgically created arteriovenous fistula, initial encounter	
T82.598A	Other mechanical complication of other cardiac and vascular devices and implants, initial encounter	
T82.7XXA	Infection and inflammatory reaction due to other cardiac and vascular devices, implants and grafts, initial encounter	
T82.818A	Embolism due to vascular prosthetic devices, implants and grafts, initial encounter	
T82.828A	Fibrosis due to vascular prosthetic devices, implants and grafts, initial encounter	
T82.838A	Hemorrhage due to vascular prosthetic devices, implants and grafts, initial encounter	
T82.858A	Stenosis of other vascular prosthetic devices, implants and grafts, initial encounter	
T82.868A	Thrombosis due to vascular prosthetic devices, implants and grafts, initial encounter	
T82.898A	Other specified complication of vascular prosthetic devices, implants and grafts, initial encounter	

AMA: 36835 2014,Jan,11

Relative Value Units/Medicare Edits

Non-Facility RVU	Work	PE	MP	Total
36835	7.51	4.96	1.73	14.2
Facility RVU	Work	PE	MP	Total
36835	7.51	4.96	1.73	14.2

	FUD	Status	MUE	Modifiers				IOM Reference
36835	90	A	1(3)	51	N/A	N/A	N/A	None

* with documentation

36838

36838   Distal revascularization and interval ligation (DRIL), upper extremity hemodialysis access (steal syndrome)

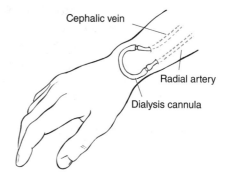

An artery distal to the hemodialysis access site is ligated. The procedure stops retrograde diastolic inflow into the surgically created fistula, a condition known as steal syndrome

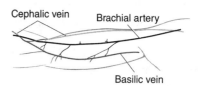

Explanation

A DRIL procedure, distal revascularization and interval ligation, is done to treat Steal syndrome occurring in patients with a permanent indwelling access site in the arm for hemodialysis. In Steal syndrome, the hand becomes cold and painful due to ischemia because the hemodialysis access is taking the arm's blood supply. The DRIL procedure restores blood flow to the hand and preserves the access site. It is a two-step procedure. The surgeon first creates a bypass graft around the access site, using a harvested vein conduit, usually the greater saphenous. An incision is made in the upper arm for the proximal anastomosis, which is placed above the dialysis access site, nearer to the axilla. Soft tissue is dissected to expose the brachial artery. An incision is also made lower in the arm for the site of the distal anastomosis, which is placed below the dialysis access site, down in the forearm. A tunnel is created from one site to the other and the graft is completed using the harvested vein. This is the revascularization portion of the procedure and allows a good flow of blood around the access site. The second part of the procedure is the ligation. The brachial artery is tied off at a point between the dialysis access and the distal anastomosis site of the bypass graft. Now the arterial blood flow being pumped from the heart runs through the bypass, supplying the hand with oxygen before entering the access site. The incisions are closed and pulses are checked for good perfusion before applying dressings.

Coding Tips

Do not report 36838 with 35512, 35522–35523, 36832, 37607, or 37618.

ICD-10-CM Diagnostic Codes

T80.211A	Bloodstream infection due to central venous catheter, initial encounter
T80.212A	Local infection due to central venous catheter, initial encounter
T80.218A	Other infection due to central venous catheter, initial encounter
T82.318A	Breakdown (mechanical) of other vascular grafts, initial encounter
T82.328A	Displacement of other vascular grafts, initial encounter

T82.338A	Leakage of other vascular grafts, initial encounter
T82.398A	Other mechanical complication of other vascular grafts, initial encounter
T82.41XA	Breakdown (mechanical) of vascular dialysis catheter, initial encounter
T82.42XA	Displacement of vascular dialysis catheter, initial encounter
T82.43XA	Leakage of vascular dialysis catheter, initial encounter
T82.49XA	Other complication of vascular dialysis catheter, initial encounter
T82.510A	Breakdown (mechanical) of surgically created arteriovenous fistula, initial encounter
T82.520A	Displacement of surgically created arteriovenous fistula, initial encounter
T82.530A	Leakage of surgically created arteriovenous fistula, initial encounter
T82.590A	Other mechanical complication of surgically created arteriovenous fistula, initial encounter
T82.818A	Embolism due to vascular prosthetic devices, implants and grafts, initial encounter
T82.838A	Hemorrhage due to vascular prosthetic devices, implants and grafts, initial encounter
T82.848A	Pain due to vascular prosthetic devices, implants and grafts, initial encounter
T82.858A	Stenosis of other vascular prosthetic devices, implants and grafts, initial encounter
T82.868A	Thrombosis due to vascular prosthetic devices, implants and grafts, initial encounter
T82.898A	Other specified complication of vascular prosthetic devices, implants and grafts, initial encounter
Z45.89	Encounter for adjustment and management of other implanted devices

AMA: 36838 2014,Jan,11

Relative Value Units/Medicare Edits

Non-Facility RVU	Work	PE	MP	Total
36838	21.69	6.38	5.2	33.27
Facility RVU	Work	PE	MP	Total
36838	21.69	6.38	5.2	33.27

	FUD	Status	MUE	Modifiers				IOM Reference
36838	90	A	1(3)	51	50	62*	80	None

* with documentation

Terms To Know

bypass graft. Surgically created alternative blood vessel used to reroute blood flow around an area of obstruction or disease.

fistula. Abnormal tube-like passage between two body cavities or organs or from an organ to the outside surface.

harvest. Removal of cells or tissue from their native site to be used as a graft or transplant to another part of the donor's body or placed into another person.

36860-36861

| 36860 | External cannula declotting (separate procedure); without balloon catheter |
| 36861 | with balloon catheter |

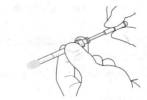

Port and catheter serve to infuse chemotherapy drugs

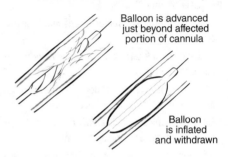

Cannula has been established in artery

Balloon is advanced just beyond affected portion of cannula

Balloon is inflated and withdrawn

Explanation

To remove a blood clot lodged in a previously placed cannula, the physician may inject a solution containing enzymes into the cannula to dissolve the clot (in 36860) or the physician may, after injecting a solution containing enzymes, insert a balloon catheter (in 36861) into the cannula to retrieve a clot there. The balloon is inserted and inflated beyond the clot. Then the catheter is slowly pulled out, capturing and retrieving the clot. Once the clot is dissolved or retrieved, the catheter is removed and the cannula is left in place.

Coding Tips

These separate procedures, by definition, are usually a component of a more complex service and are not identified separately. When performed alone or with other unrelated procedures/services, they may be reported. If performed alone, list the code; if performed with other unrelated procedures/services, list the code and append modifier 59 or an X{EPSU} modifier. For declotting of implanted vascular access device or catheter by thrombolytic agent, see 36593.

ICD-10-CM Diagnostic Codes

T82.49XA	Other complication of vascular dialysis catheter, initial encounter
T82.594A	Other mechanical complication of infusion catheter, initial encounter
T82.818A	Embolism due to vascular prosthetic devices, implants and grafts, initial encounter
T82.828A	Fibrosis due to vascular prosthetic devices, implants and grafts, initial encounter
T82.848A	Pain due to vascular prosthetic devices, implants and grafts, initial encounter
T82.858A	Stenosis of other vascular prosthetic devices, implants and grafts, initial encounter
T82.868A	Thrombosis due to vascular prosthetic devices, implants and grafts, initial encounter

Arteries and Veins

T82.898A   Other specified complication of vascular prosthetic devices, implants and grafts, initial encounter

AMA: **36860** 2018,Jan,8; 2017,Jan,8; 2016,Jan,13; 2015,Jan,16 **36861** 2018,Jan,8; 2017,Jan,8; 2016,Jan,13; 2015,Jan,16

Relative Value Units/Medicare Edits

Non-Facility RVU	Work	PE	MP	Total
36860	2.01	4.71	0.48	7.2
36861	2.52	0.94	0.63	4.09
Facility RVU	**Work**	**PE**	**MP**	**Total**
36860	2.01	0.75	0.48	3.24
36861	2.52	0.94	0.63	4.09

	FUD	Status	MUE	Modifiers				IOM Reference
36860	0	A	2(3)	51	N/A	N/A	N/A	None
36861	0	A	2(3)	51	N/A	N/A	N/A	

* with documentation

Terms To Know

artery. Vessel through which oxygenated blood passes away from the heart to any part of the body.

balloon catheter. Any catheter equipped with an inflatable balloon at the end to hold it in place in a body cavity or to be used for dilation of a vessel lumen.

blood clot. Semisolidified, coagulated mass of mainly platelets and fibrin in the bloodstream.

cannula. Tube inserted into a blood vessel, duct, or body cavity to facilitate passage.

complication. Condition arising after the beginning of observation and treatment that modifies the course of the patient's illness or the medical care required, or an undesired result or misadventure in medical care.

embolism. Obstruction of a blood vessel resulting from a clot or foreign substance.

fibrosis. Formation of fibrous tissue as part of the restorative process.

thrombosis. Condition arising from the presence or formation of blood clots within a blood vessel that may cause vascular obstruction and insufficient oxygenation.

thrombus. Stationary blood clot inside a blood vessel.

vascular. Pertaining to blood vessels.

36901-36903

36901 Introduction of needle(s) and/or catheter(s), dialysis circuit, with diagnostic angiography of the dialysis circuit, including all direct puncture(s) and catheter placement(s), injection(s) of contrast, all necessary imaging from the arterial anastomosis and adjacent artery through entire venous outflow including the inferior or superior vena cava, fluoroscopic guidance, radiological supervision and interpretation and image documentation and report;

36902   with transluminal balloon angioplasty, peripheral dialysis segment, including all imaging and radiological supervision and interpretation necessary to perform the angioplasty

36903   with transcatheter placement of intravascular stent(s), peripheral dialysis segment, including all imaging and radiological supervision and interpretation necessary to perform the stenting, and all angioplasty within the peripheral dialysis segment

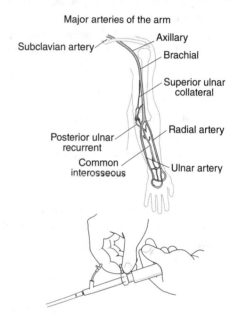

Major arteries of the arm

Subclavian artery
Axillary
Brachial
Superior ulnar collateral
Posterior ulnar recurrent
Radial artery
Common interosseous
Ulnar artery

Explanation

The physician inserts a needle or catheter into a dialysis circuit via a puncture in the skin overlying the circuit of a dialysis patient. The catheter is guided into the circuit and vessel to an area upstream of the site under investigation, and contrast material is injected into it. Report 36901 for the initial access, including shunt access, contrast injections, and all fluoroscopic imaging deemed necessary from the arterial anastomosis and adjacent artery through the entire venous outflow (inferior and superior vena cava included). In 36902, a catheter with a balloon attached is inserted into the peripheral dialysis segment and fed into the narrowed portion where its balloon may be inflated several times in order to stretch the diameter, allowing a more normal flow of blood through the area. In 36903, a catheter with a stent-transporting tip is threaded over the guidewire into the peripheral dialysis segment and the wire is extracted. The catheter travels to the point where the vessel needs additional support. The compressed stent is passed from the catheter into the vessel, where it deploys, expanding to support the vessel walls. Once the procedure is complete, the catheter is removed and pressure is applied over the puncture site.

Coding Tips

Direct access, imaging of the dialysis circuit, catheter manipulation, catheter advancement to the vena cava for imaging, dialysis circuit punctures, and venous side branches communicating with the dialysis circuit that require catheterization are included in these services. If ultrasound guidance is required to safely puncture the dialysis circuit for evaluation this may be reported separately, see 76937. Do not report these codes more than once per operative session. Do not report 36901 or 36903 with 36833, 36904–36906, or each other. Do not report 36902 with 36903.

ICD-10-CM Diagnostic Codes

D3A.093	Benign carcinoid tumor of the kidney
I12.0	Hypertensive chronic kidney disease with stage 5 chronic kidney disease or end stage renal disease
I12.9	Hypertensive chronic kidney disease with stage 1 through stage 4 chronic kidney disease, or unspecified chronic kidney disease
I13.0	Hypertensive heart and chronic kidney disease with heart failure and stage 1 through stage 4 chronic kidney disease, or unspecified chronic kidney disease
I13.10	Hypertensive heart and chronic kidney disease without heart failure, with stage 1 through stage 4 chronic kidney disease, or unspecified chronic kidney disease
I13.11	Hypertensive heart and chronic kidney disease without heart failure, with stage 5 chronic kidney disease, or end stage renal disease
N17.0	Acute kidney failure with tubular necrosis
N17.1	Acute kidney failure with acute cortical necrosis
N17.2	Acute kidney failure with medullary necrosis
N17.8	Other acute kidney failure
N18.4	Chronic kidney disease, stage 4 (severe)
N18.5	Chronic kidney disease, stage 5
N18.6	End stage renal disease
T82.43XA	Leakage of vascular dialysis catheter, initial encounter
T82.49XA	Other complication of vascular dialysis catheter, initial encounter
T82.510A	Breakdown (mechanical) of surgically created arteriovenous fistula, initial encounter
T82.520A	Displacement of surgically created arteriovenous fistula, initial encounter
T82.530A	Leakage of surgically created arteriovenous fistula, initial encounter
T82.590A	Other mechanical complication of surgically created arteriovenous fistula, initial encounter
T82.818A	Embolism due to vascular prosthetic devices, implants and grafts, initial encounter
T82.828A	Fibrosis due to vascular prosthetic devices, implants and grafts, initial encounter
T82.838A	Hemorrhage due to vascular prosthetic devices, implants and grafts, initial encounter
T82.848A	Pain due to vascular prosthetic devices, implants and grafts, initial encounter

AMA: **36901** 2018,Jan,8; 2017,Mar,3 **36902** 2018,Jan,8; 2017,Mar,3; 2017,Jul,3 **36903** 2018,Jan,8; 2017,Mar,3; 2017,Jul,3

Relative Value Units/Medicare Edits

Non-Facility RVU	Work	PE	MP	Total
36901	3.36	17.84	0.48	21.68
36902	4.83	33.47	0.66	38.96
36903	6.39	140.3	0.96	147.65
Facility RVU	**Work**	**PE**	**MP**	**Total**
36901	3.36	1.05	0.48	4.89
36902	4.83	1.47	0.66	6.96
36903	6.39	1.82	0.96	9.17

	FUD	Status	MUE	Modifiers				IOM Reference
36901	0	A	1(3)	51	N/A	N/A	N/A	None
36902	0	A	1(3)	51	N/A	N/A	N/A	
36903	0	A	1(3)	51	N/A	N/A	N/A	

* with documentation

Terms To Know

angiography. Radiographic imaging of the arteries.

contrast material. Any internally administered substance that has a different opacity from soft tissue on radiography or computed tomograph; includes barium, used to opacify parts of the gastrointestinal tract; water-soluble iodinated compounds, used to opacify blood vessels or the genitourinary tract; may refer to air occurring naturally or introduced into the body; also, paramagnetic substances used in magnetic resonance imaging. Substances may also be documented as contrast agent or contrast medium.

hemodialysis. Cleansing of wastes and contaminating elements from the blood by virtue of different diffusion rates through a semipermeable membrane, which separates blood from a filtration solution that diffuses other elements out of the blood.

stent. Tube to provide support in a body cavity or lumen.

transluminal balloon angioplasty. Balloon-tipped catheter is placed within a narrowed artery or vein and the balloon is inflated to stretch the vessel to a larger diameter for increased blood flow.

36904-36906

36904 Percutaneous transluminal mechanical thrombectomy and/or infusion for thrombolysis, dialysis circuit, any method, including all imaging and radiological supervision and interpretation, diagnostic angiography, fluoroscopic guidance, catheter placement(s), and intraprocedural pharmacological thrombolytic injection(s);

36905 with transluminal balloon angioplasty, peripheral dialysis segment, including all imaging and radiological supervision and interpretation necessary to perform the angioplasty

36906 with transcatheter placement of intravascular stent(s), peripheral dialysis segment, including all imaging and radiological supervision and interpretation necessary to perform the stenting, and all angioplasty within the peripheral dialysis circuit

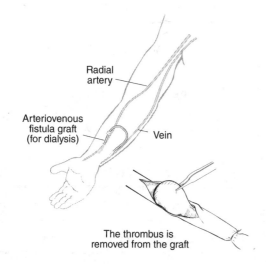

Radial artery

Arteriovenous fistula graft (for dialysis)

Vein

The thrombus is removed from the graft

Explanation

The physician treats the dialysis circuit occlusion with mechanical thrombectomy and/or thrombolysis infusion. The devices used for mechanical thrombectomy include those that fragment the thrombus with or without removal of the clot, as well as those that come into contact with the vessel wall. The dialysis circuit is cannulated to gain access and 5,000 units of heparin are administered. Angiography is performed to confirm the occluded segment. A hydrophilic wire is passed across the occlusion, followed by passing of the Trellis device over a stiff exchange length wire. The distal and proximal balloons are inflated in the segment on either side of a treatment zone containing infusion to isolate the treatment zone and to sustain the fluid concentration that is infused. One milligram of tissue plasminogen activator (TPA) is infused into the treatment zone. The Turbo Trellis is run at 4,000 rpm for five minutes. After the proximal balloon is deflated, small clots are removed via the integral aspiration port to prevent embolization. Thrombolysis infusion may be performed with a catheter threaded over the wire for pharmaceutical administration directly within the thrombosis. When the procedure is complete, the instruments are removed and pressure is applied over the puncture site to stop the bleeding. This procedure is reported with 36904 and includes imaging guidance, diagnostic angiography, catheter placement, and intraprocedural pharmacological thrombolytic injections. Report 36905 when the peripheral dialysis segment is treated with balloon angioplasty. A catheter with a balloon attached is inserted into the segment and fed into the narrowed portion, where its balloon may be inflated several times in order to stretch the diameter allowing a more normal flow of blood through the area. Report 36906 when the peripheral dialysis segment is treated with an intravascular stent. A catheter with a stent-transporting tip is threaded over the guidewire into the vessel and the wire is extracted. The catheter travels to the point where the vessel needs additional support. The compressed stent is passed from the catheter into the vessel, where it deploys, expanding to support the vessel walls. Once the procedure is complete, the catheter is removed and pressure is applied over the puncture site.

Coding Tips

Diagnostic angiography, fluoroscopy, all manipulation required to remove a thrombus, and catheter placement(s) are included in these services. Do not report these codes more than once per operative session. Do not report 36905 with 36904. Do not report 36906 with 36901–36905. For transluminal balloon angioplasty, see 36907. For transcatheter placement of intravascular stents, when performed within the central vein of the dialysis circuit, see 36908.

ICD-10-CM Diagnostic Codes

T82.41XA	Breakdown (mechanical) of vascular dialysis catheter, initial encounter
T82.42XA	Displacement of vascular dialysis catheter, initial encounter
T82.43XA	Leakage of vascular dialysis catheter, initial encounter
T82.49XA	Other complication of vascular dialysis catheter, initial encounter
T82.510A	Breakdown (mechanical) of surgically created arteriovenous fistula, initial encounter
T82.520A	Displacement of surgically created arteriovenous fistula, initial encounter
T82.530A	Leakage of surgically created arteriovenous fistula, initial encounter
T82.590A	Other mechanical complication of surgically created arteriovenous fistula, initial encounter
T82.818A	Embolism due to vascular prosthetic devices, implants and grafts, initial encounter
T82.828A	Fibrosis due to vascular prosthetic devices, implants and grafts, initial encounter
T82.838A	Hemorrhage due to vascular prosthetic devices, implants and grafts, initial encounter
T82.848A	Pain due to vascular prosthetic devices, implants and grafts, initial encounter
T82.858A	Stenosis of other vascular prosthetic devices, implants and grafts, initial encounter
T82.868A	Thrombosis due to vascular prosthetic devices, implants and grafts, initial encounter

AMA: **36904** 2018,Jan,8; 2017,Mar,3; 2017,Jul,3 **36905** 2018,Jan,8; 2017,Mar,3; 2017,Jul,3 **36906** 2018,Jan,8; 2017,Mar,3; 2017,Jul,3

Relative Value Units/Medicare Edits

Non-Facility RVU	Work	PE	MP	Total
36904	7.5	48.72	1.03	57.25
36905	9.0	63.02	1.16	73.18
36906	10.42	173.18	1.41	185.01
Facility RVU	Work	PE	MP	Total
36904	7.5	2.16	1.03	10.69
36905	9.0	2.73	1.16	12.89
36906	10.42	3.02	1.41	14.85

	FUD	Status	MUE	Modifiers				IOM Reference
36904	0	A	1(3)	51	N/A	62*	N/A	None
36905	0	A	1(3)	51	N/A	62*	N/A	
36906	0	A	1(3)	51	N/A	62*	N/A	

* with documentation

Arteries and Veins

36907-36908

+ **36907** Transluminal balloon angioplasty, central dialysis segment, performed through dialysis circuit, including all imaging and radiological supervision and interpretation required to perform the angioplasty (List separately in addition to code for primary procedure)

+ **36908** Transcatheter placement of intravascular stent(s), central dialysis segment, performed through dialysis circuit, including all imaging and radiological supervision and interpretation required to perform the stenting, and all angioplasty in the central dialysis segment (List separately in addition to code for primary procedure)

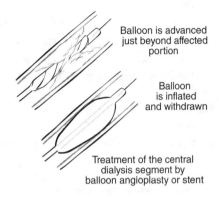

Balloon is advanced just beyond affected portion

Balloon is inflated and withdrawn

Treatment of the central dialysis segment by balloon angioplasty or stent

Explanation

The physician inserts a needle or catheter into a dialysis circuit via a puncture in the skin. The catheter is guided into the circuit to an area upstream of the investigation site and contrast material is injected. In 36907, a catheter with a balloon attached is inserted into the central dialysis segment and fed into the narrowed portion, where its balloon may be inflated several times in order to stretch the diameter, allowing a more normal blood flow through the area. In 36908, a catheter with a stent-transporting tip is threaded over the guidewire into the central dialysis segment and the wire is extracted. The catheter travels to the point where the vessel needs additional support. The compressed stent is passed from the catheter out into the vessel, where it deploys, expanding to support the vessel walls. Once the procedure is complete, the catheter is removed and pressure is applied over the puncture site. All imaging and radiological supervision and interpretation is included.

Coding Tips

Report 36907 and 36908 in addition to 36818-36833 and 36901-36906. Report 36907 once per encounter for all angioplasty performed within the central dialysis segment regardless of how many discrete lesions are treated in the central dialysis segment when reported with 36901-36906. Report 36908 once per encounter regardless of the number of stents placed or discrete lesions treated in the central dialysis segment when reported with 36901-36906. Do not report these codes with each other during the same session.

ICD-10-CM Diagnostic Codes

T82.41XA	Breakdown (mechanical) of vascular dialysis catheter, initial encounter
T82.42XA	Displacement of vascular dialysis catheter, initial encounter
T82.43XA	Leakage of vascular dialysis catheter, initial encounter
T82.49XA	Other complication of vascular dialysis catheter, initial encounter
T82.510A	Breakdown (mechanical) of surgically created arteriovenous fistula, initial encounter

T82.520A	Displacement of surgically created arteriovenous fistula, initial encounter
T82.530A	Leakage of surgically created arteriovenous fistula, initial encounter
T82.590A	Other mechanical complication of surgically created arteriovenous fistula, initial encounter
T82.818A	Embolism due to vascular prosthetic devices, implants and grafts, initial encounter
T82.828A	Fibrosis due to vascular prosthetic devices, implants and grafts, initial encounter
T82.838A	Hemorrhage due to vascular prosthetic devices, implants and grafts, initial encounter
T82.848A	Pain due to vascular prosthetic devices, implants and grafts, initial encounter
T82.858A	Stenosis of other vascular prosthetic devices, implants and grafts, initial encounter

AMA: **36907** 2018,Jan,8; 2017,Mar,3; 2017,Jul,3 **36908** 2018,Jan,8; 2017,Mar,3; 2017,Jul,3

Relative Value Units/Medicare Edits

Non-Facility RVU	Work	PE	MP	Total
36907	3.0	16.34	0.43	19.77
36908	4.25	49.5	0.64	54.39
Facility RVU	**Work**	**PE**	**MP**	**Total**
36907	3.0	0.83	0.43	4.26
36908	4.25	1.13	0.64	6.02

	FUD	Status	MUE	Modifiers				IOM Reference
36907	N/A	A	1(3)	N/A	N/A	N/A	N/A	None
36908	N/A	A	1(3)	N/A	N/A	N/A	N/A	

* with documentation

Terms To Know

stenosis. Narrowing or constriction of a passage.

stent. Tube to provide support in a body cavity or lumen.

supervision and interpretation. Radiology services that usually contain an invasive component and are reported by the radiologist for supervision of the procedure and the personnel involved with performing the examination, reading the film, and preparing the written report.

transluminal balloon angioplasty. Balloon-tipped catheter is placed within a narrowed artery or vein and the balloon is inflated to stretch the vessel to a larger diameter for increased blood flow.

Coding Companion for General Surgery/Gastroenterology

Arteries and Veins

36909

+ **36909** Dialysis circuit permanent vascular embolization or occlusion (including main circuit or any accessory veins), endovascular, including all imaging and radiological supervision and interpretation necessary to complete the intervention (List separately in addition to code for primary procedure)

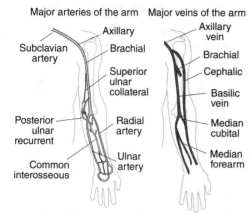

Major arteries of the arm | Major veins of the arm

Endovascular embolization or occlusion of dialysis circuit

Explanation

The physician performs embolization or occlusion of a dialysis circuit (main circuit or any accessory vein) due to complications or to assist in circuit maturity and/or patency. A needle is inserted through the skin and into a blood vessel. A guidewire is threaded through the needle into the vessel. The needle is removed. A catheter is threaded into the vessel and the wire is extracted. The catheter travels to the appropriate blood vessel and beads, coils, or another vessel-blocking device are released. The beads or other device block the vessel. The catheter is removed and pressure is applied over the puncture site to stop bleeding.

Coding Tips

Report 36909 in addition to 36901-36906. Code 36909 includes all permanent vascular occlusions within the dialysis circuit and may only be reported once per encounter per day. For open ligation/occlusion of dialysis access, see 37607.

ICD-10-CM Diagnostic Codes

T82.818A	Embolism due to vascular prosthetic devices, implants and grafts, initial encounter
T82.828A	Fibrosis due to vascular prosthetic devices, implants and grafts, initial encounter
T82.858A	Stenosis of other vascular prosthetic devices, implants and grafts, initial encounter
T82.868A	Thrombosis due to vascular prosthetic devices, implants and grafts, initial encounter

AMA: 36909 2018,Jan,8; 2017,Mar,3

Relative Value Units/Medicare Edits

Non-Facility RVU	Work	PE	MP	Total
36909	4.12	57.02	0.63	61.77
Facility RVU	**Work**	**PE**	**MP**	**Total**
36909	4.12	1.11	0.63	5.86

	FUD	Status	MUE	Modifiers				IOM Reference
36909	N/A	A	1(3)	N/A	N/A	N/A	N/A	None

* with documentation

Terms To Know

embolization. Placement of a clotting agent, such as a coil, plastic particles, gel, foam, etc., into an area of hemorrhage to stop the bleeding or to block blood flow to a problem area, such as an aneurysm or a tumor.

guidewire. Flexible metal instrument designed to lead another instrument in its proper course.

imaging. Radiologic means of producing pictures for clinical study of the internal structures and functions of the body, such as x-ray, ultrasound, magnetic resonance, or positron emission tomography.

patency. State of a tube-like structure or conduit being open and unobstructed.

supervision and interpretation. Radiology services that usually contain an invasive component and are reported by the radiologist for supervision of the procedure and the personnel involved with performing the examination, reading the film, and preparing the written report.

37140

37140   Venous anastomosis, open; portocaval

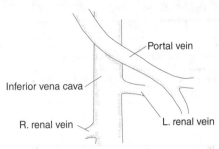

Portal vein
Inferior vena cava
R. renal vein
L. renal vein

Schematic of portocaval anatomy

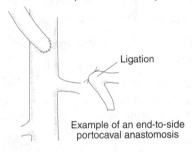

Ligation

Example of an end-to-side
portocaval anastomosis

Explanation

The physician performs portocaval venous anastomosis. The physician places a long right thoracoabdominal incision and exposes the liver. The physician exposes the inferior vena cava and portal vein through careful dissection. The physician places a plastic sling around the portal vein and ties it closed, just proximal to its bifurcation. The physician clamps and divides the portal vein. The physician applies a partial exclusion vascular clamp to the front of the vena cava and removes a small oval of tissue from the vena cava to allow end-to-side anastomosis of portal vein to the inferior vena cava. The physician removes the clamps and checks for appropriate flow without anastomotic leakage. The physician closes the incision, leaving a chest tube in place (but no abdominal drains, as this may lead to protein loss from postoperative drainage of ascites).

Coding Tips

When this code is performed with another separately identifiable procedure, the highest dollar value code is listed as the primary procedure and subsequent procedures are appended with modifier 51. An open venous anastomosis, renoportal, is reported with code 37145. For TIPS (percutaneous) procedure, see 37182. For peritoneal-venous shunt, see 49425.

ICD-10-CM Diagnostic Codes

I81	Portal vein thrombosis
I82.0	Budd-Chiari syndrome
I85.11	Secondary esophageal varices with bleeding
I87.1	Compression of vein
K70.0	Alcoholic fatty liver △
K70.30	Alcoholic cirrhosis of liver without ascites △
K70.31	Alcoholic cirrhosis of liver with ascites △
K74.69	Other cirrhosis of liver
K75.1	Phlebitis of portal vein
K76.0	Fatty (change of) liver, not elsewhere classified
K76.1	Chronic passive congestion of liver
K76.3	Infarction of liver
K76.5	Hepatic veno-occlusive disease
K76.6	Portal hypertension
K76.89	Other specified diseases of liver

AMA: **37140** 2014,Jan,11

Relative Value Units/Medicare Edits

Non-Facility RVU	Work	PE	MP	Total
37140	40.0	18.75	9.79	68.54
Facility RVU	**Work**	**PE**	**MP**	**Total**
37140	40.0	18.75	9.79	68.54

	FUD	Status	MUE	Modifiers				IOM Reference
37140	90	A	1(2)	51	N/A	62*	N/A	None

* with documentation

Terms To Know

anastomosis. Surgically created connection between ducts, blood vessels, or bowel segments to allow flow from one to the other.

ascites. Abnormal accumulation of free fluid in the abdominal cavity, causing distention and tightness in addition to shortness of breath as the fluid accumulates. Ascites is usually an underlying disorder and can be a manifestation of any number of diseases.

bifurcated. Having two branches or divisions, such as the left pulmonary veins that split off from the left atrium to carry oxygenated blood away from the heart.

Budd-Chiari syndrome. Thrombus or other obstruction of the hepatic vein, with an enlarged liver, intractable ascites, portal hypertension, and the growth of extensive collateral vessels.

hepatic portal vein. Blood vessel that delivers unoxygenated blood from the gastrointestinal tract, spleen, pancreas, and gallbladder to the liver.

inferior. Located toward the feet or lower part of the body.

ligation. Tying off a blood vessel or duct with a suture or a soft, thin wire.

portal hypertension. Abnormally high blood pressure in the portal vein.

thrombosis. Condition arising from the presence or formation of blood clots within a blood vessel that may cause vascular obstruction and insufficient oxygenation.

thrombus. Stationary blood clot inside a blood vessel.

varices. Enlarged, dilated, or twisted turning veins.

vena cava. Main venous trunk that empties into the right atrium from both the lower and upper regions, beginning at the junction of the common iliac veins inferiorly and the two brachiocephalic veins superiorly.

Arteries and Veins

37145

37145   Venous anastomosis, open; renoportal

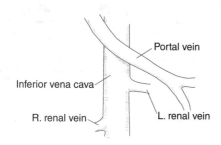

Inferior vena cava
Portal vein
R. renal vein
L. renal vein

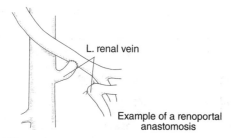

L. renal vein

Example of a renoportal anastomosis

Explanation

The physician performs an abdominal incision and exposes the left renal vein and inferior vena cava. The physician transects the left renal vein and attaches it to the portal circulation by sewing the vena caval end to the portal vein, the superior mesenteric vein, or the splenic vein. Alternatively, the physician may divide the portal vein and attach its splanchnic end to the end of the transected renal vein. The physician assesses patency of the anastomosis and may measure venous pressures before closing the abdomen.

Coding Tips

When this code is performed with another separately identifiable procedure, the highest dollar value code is listed as the primary procedure and subsequent procedures are appended with modifier 51. For venous anastomosis, portocaval, see 37140. For TIPS procedure, see 37182. For peritoneal-venous shunt, see 49425.

ICD-10-CM Diagnostic Codes

I81	Portal vein thrombosis
I82.0	Budd-Chiari syndrome
I82.3	Embolism and thrombosis of renal vein
I85.11	Secondary esophageal varices with bleeding
N28.0	Ischemia and infarction of kidney
Q27.34	Arteriovenous malformation of renal vessel
Q27.8	Other specified congenital malformations of peripheral vascular system
S35.311A	Laceration of portal vein, initial encounter
S35.318A	Other specified injury of portal vein, initial encounter

AMA: **37145** 2014,Jan,11

Relative Value Units/Medicare Edits

Non-Facility RVU	Work	PE	MP	Total
37145	37.0	17.53	9.05	63.58
Facility RVU	**Work**	**PE**	**MP**	**Total**
37145	37.0	17.53	9.05	63.58

	FUD	Status	MUE	Modifiers				IOM Reference
37145	90	A	1(3)	51	N/A	N/A	80	None

* with documentation

Terms To Know

anastomosis. Surgically created connection between ducts, blood vessels, or bowel segments to allow flow from one to the other.

anomaly. Irregularity in the structure or position of an organ or tissue.

arteriovenous malformation. Connecting passage between an artery and a vein.

blood clot. Semisolidified, coagulated mass of mainly platelets and fibrin in the bloodstream.

Budd-Chiari syndrome. Thrombus or other obstruction of the hepatic vein, with an enlarged liver, intractable ascites, portal hypertension, and the growth of extensive collateral vessels.

embolus. Any substance, such as air bubbles, cellular masses, calcium fragments, or blood clots, carried through the bloodstream that has become lodged in a vessel, resulting in an obstruction of circulation.

hepatic portal vein. Blood vessel that delivers unoxygenated blood from the gastrointestinal tract, spleen, pancreas, and gallbladder to the liver.

incision. Act of cutting into tissue or an organ.

patency. State of a tube-like structure or conduit being open and unobstructed.

renal failure. Inability of a kidney to eliminate metabolites and retain electrolytes at a normal level.

shunt. Surgically created passage between blood vessels or other natural passages, such as an arteriovenous anastomosis, to divert or bypass blood flow from the normal channel.

thrombosis. Condition arising from the presence or formation of blood clots within a blood vessel that may cause vascular obstruction and insufficient oxygenation.

thrombus. Stationary blood clot inside a blood vessel.

transection. Transverse dissection; to cut across a long axis; cross section.

vein. Vessel through which oxygen-depleted blood passes back to the heart.

Arteries and Veins

37160

37160   Venous anastomosis, open; caval-mesenteric

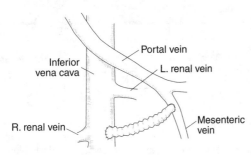

Example of a synthetic side-to-side
caval-mesenteric anastomosis

Explanation

The physician performs an upper midline vertical abdominal incision and retracts the transverse colon in a cephalad direction. The physician exposes the anterior surface of the inferior vena cava and frees the posterior surface of the superior mesenteric vein after careful dissection through the root of the transverse mesocolon. The physician isolates a long segment of the superior mesenteric vein with ties and partially occludes the inferior vena cava. The physician removes an ellipse of tissue from the inferior vena cava and performs and end-to-side anastomosis of Dacron graft to the inferior vena cava. The physician occludes the superior mesenteric vein, cuts an ellipse from its anterior surface, and sews the end of the Dacron graft to the side of the superior mesenteric vein. The physician assesses patency of the anastomosis and may measure venous pressures before closing the abdomen.

Coding Tips

When this code is performed with another separately identifiable procedure, the highest dollar value code is listed as the primary procedure and subsequent procedures are appended with modifier 51. For venous anastomosis, portocaval, see 37140; renoportal, see 37145.

ICD-10-CM Diagnostic Codes

I81	Portal vein thrombosis
I82.890	Acute embolism and thrombosis of other specified veins
I82.891	Chronic embolism and thrombosis of other specified veins
I85.11	Secondary esophageal varices with bleeding
I87.1	Compression of vein
K70.0	Alcoholic fatty liver 🅰
K70.30	Alcoholic cirrhosis of liver without ascites 🅰
K70.31	Alcoholic cirrhosis of liver with ascites 🅰
K74.69	Other cirrhosis of liver
K76.0	Fatty (change of) liver, not elsewhere classified
K76.1	Chronic passive congestion of liver
K76.3	Infarction of liver
K76.5	Hepatic veno-occlusive disease
K76.6	Portal hypertension
K76.89	Other specified diseases of liver
R16.0	Hepatomegaly, not elsewhere classified
R16.2	Hepatomegaly with splenomegaly, not elsewhere classified

AMA: 37160 2014,Jan,11

Relative Value Units/Medicare Edits

Non-Facility RVU	Work	PE	MP	Total
37160	38.0	18.01	9.28	65.29
Facility RVU	**Work**	**PE**	**MP**	**Total**
37160	38.0	18.01	9.28	65.29

	FUD	Status	MUE	Modifiers				IOM Reference
37160	90	A	1(3)	51	N/A	62*	80	None

* with documentation

Terms To Know

acute. Sudden, severe. Documentation and reporting of an acute condition is important to establishing medical necessity.

anastomosis. Surgically created connection between ducts, blood vessels, or bowel segments to allow flow from one to the other.

chronic. Persistent, continuing, or recurring.

dissection. Separating by cutting tissue or body structures apart.

embolus. Any substance, such as air bubbles, cellular masses, calcium fragments, or blood clots, carried through the bloodstream that has become lodged in a vessel, resulting in an obstruction of circulation.

graft. Tissue implant from another part of the body or another person.

hepatic portal vein. Blood vessel that delivers unoxygenated blood from the gastrointestinal tract, spleen, pancreas, and gallbladder to the liver.

patency. State of a tube-like structure or conduit being open and unobstructed.

shunt. Surgically created passage between blood vessels or other natural passages, such as an arteriovenous anastomosis, to divert or bypass blood flow from the normal channel.

thrombosis. Condition arising from the presence or formation of blood clots within a blood vessel that may cause vascular obstruction and insufficient oxygenation.

varices. Enlarged, dilated, or twisted turning veins.

vena cava. Main venous trunk that empties into the right atrium from both the lower and upper regions, beginning at the junction of the common iliac veins inferiorly and the two brachiocephalic veins superiorly.

Arteries and Veins

37180-37181

37180 Venous anastomosis, open; splenorenal, proximal
37181 splenorenal, distal (selective decompression of esophagogastric varices, any technique)

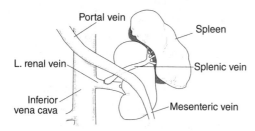

Example of a splenorenal anastomosis

Explanation

The physician performs a bilateral subcostal incision from the right midrectus position extending into the left flank, and dissects past bowel and pancreas to expose the splenic vein. The physician dissects the splenic vein free, ligating or clipping any vessels in continuity to the vein. The left renal vein is exposed by dissecting through the posterior parietal peritoneum, partially clamped, and an ellipse of renal vein at its upper border is excised. The physician performs an end-to-side anastomosis of the splenic vein to the renal vein, using harvested vein graft material if extension is required. The physician removes the clamps. In 37180, the vein is ligated toward the left, using the central (right) end of the vein for anastomosis. In 37181, the physician removes the clamps and divides the coronary (right gastric) vein, left gastric vein, and gastroepiploic veins. In both procedures, the physician may measure superior mesenteric (portal), renal, and splenic venous pressures. The physician may perform venography to establish patency of the graft. The physician closes the abdominal wound.

Coding Tips

When these codes are performed with another separately identifiable procedure, the highest dollar value code is listed as the primary procedure and subsequent procedures are appended with modifier 51. For venous anastomosis, portocaval, see 37140; renoportal, see 37145; caval-mesenteric, see 37160.

ICD-10-CM Diagnostic Codes

D73.1	Hypersplenism
I81	Portal vein thrombosis
I85.11	Secondary esophageal varices with bleeding
I87.1	Compression of vein
K70.0	Alcoholic fatty liver 🅰
K70.30	Alcoholic cirrhosis of liver without ascites 🅰
K70.31	Alcoholic cirrhosis of liver with ascites 🅰
K74.69	Other cirrhosis of liver
K76.0	Fatty (change of) liver, not elsewhere classified
K76.1	Chronic passive congestion of liver
K76.3	Infarction of liver
K76.5	Hepatic veno-occlusive disease
K76.6	Portal hypertension
K76.89	Other specified diseases of liver
R16.0	Hepatomegaly, not elsewhere classified
R16.1	Splenomegaly, not elsewhere classified
R16.2	Hepatomegaly with splenomegaly, not elsewhere classified

AMA: **37180** 2014,Jan,11 **37181** 2014,Jan,11

Relative Value Units/Medicare Edits

Non-Facility RVU	Work	PE	MP	Total
37180	36.5	17.32	8.94	62.76
37181	40.0	18.75	9.79	68.54
Facility RVU	**Work**	**PE**	**MP**	**Total**
37180	36.5	17.32	8.94	62.76
37181	40.0	18.75	9.79	68.54

	FUD	Status	MUE	Modifiers				IOM Reference
37180	90	A	1(2)	51	N/A	62*	80	None
37181	90	A	1(2)	51	N/A	62*	80	

* with documentation

Terms To Know

anastomosis. Surgically created connection between ducts, blood vessels, or bowel segments to allow flow from one to the other.

cirrhosis of liver. Chronic disease of the liver that characteristically produces intertwining bands of fibrotic tissue that change the normal structure of the lobes of the liver and destroys normal cells, which then regenerate into nodules and cause the liver to stop functioning over time. This form of cirrhosis is not alcohol related.

dissect. Cut apart or separate tissue for surgical purposes or for visual or microscopic study.

hepatomegaly. Enlarged liver.

posterior. Located in the back part or caudal end of the body.

proximal. Located closest to a specified reference point, usually the midline or trunk.

superior. Located toward the head or top of the body.

venography. Radiographic study of the veins.

venous. Relating to the veins.

Arteries and Veins

37182-37183

37182 Insertion of transvenous intrahepatic portosystemic shunt(s) (TIPS) (includes venous access, hepatic and portal vein catheterization, portography with hemodynamic evaluation, intrahepatic tract formation/dilatation, stent placement and all associated imaging guidance and documentation)

37183 Revision of transvenous intrahepatic portosystemic shunt(s) (TIPS) (includes venous access, hepatic and portal vein catheterization, portography with hemodynamic evaluation, intrahepatic tract recanulization/dilatation, stent placement and all associated imaging guidance and documentation)

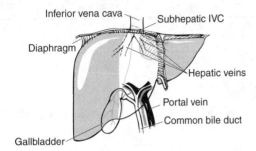

A transvenous shunt is performed between the portal and hepatic vessels. Vessel catheterization may be employed and stents may be placed to support the vessels

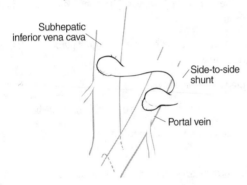

Explanation

A transvenous intrahepatic portosystemic shunt (TIPS) is inserted in 37182 and replaced in 37183. Shunts are placed percutaneously to manage the complications of portal hypertension and control variceal bleeding and ascites. Once the patient is under general anesthesia or conscious sedation, the right internal jugular vein is accessed and a catheter is placed into the right hepatic vein. Catheter placement is verified using venography. A Colapinto needle is advanced through the catheter into the wall of the right hepatic vein to access the right portal vein. A guidewire and catheter are advanced along this route into the portal vein and venography is performed again to verify placement. A self-expanding metallic stent is deployed through the catheter and dilated to the desired diameter where it bridges the portal and hepatic veins, using an angioplastic balloon. Postplacement venography and pressure measurements confirm adequate position and flow through the TIPS. The balloon, catheter, and other endoscopic tools are removed and pressure is applied to the insertion site, which may require suture. In 37183, the existing shunt is collapsed and removed through the catheter before a new one is inserted and dilated.

Coding Tips

Do not report these codes with 75885 or 75887. Report open TIPS procedure with 37140. For repair of arteriorvenous aneurysm, see 36832.

ICD-10-CM Diagnostic Codes

I81	Portal vein thrombosis
I82.0	Budd-Chiari syndrome
I85.01	Esophageal varices with bleeding
I85.11	Secondary esophageal varices with bleeding
I87.1	Compression of vein
K70.0	Alcoholic fatty liver 🅰
K70.10	Alcoholic hepatitis without ascites 🅰
K70.11	Alcoholic hepatitis with ascites 🅰
K70.2	Alcoholic fibrosis and sclerosis of liver 🅰
K70.30	Alcoholic cirrhosis of liver without ascites 🅰
K70.31	Alcoholic cirrhosis of liver with ascites 🅰
K70.40	Alcoholic hepatic failure without coma 🅰
K70.41	Alcoholic hepatic failure with coma 🅰
K71.0	Toxic liver disease with cholestasis
K71.10	Toxic liver disease with hepatic necrosis, without coma
K71.11	Toxic liver disease with hepatic necrosis, with coma
K71.2	Toxic liver disease with acute hepatitis
K71.3	Toxic liver disease with chronic persistent hepatitis
K71.4	Toxic liver disease with chronic lobular hepatitis
K71.50	Toxic liver disease with chronic active hepatitis without ascites
K71.51	Toxic liver disease with chronic active hepatitis with ascites
K71.6	Toxic liver disease with hepatitis, not elsewhere classified
K71.7	Toxic liver disease with fibrosis and cirrhosis of liver
K71.8	Toxic liver disease with other disorders of liver
K72.10	Chronic hepatic failure without coma
K72.11	Chronic hepatic failure with coma
K74.02	Hepatic fibrosis, advanced fibrosis
K74.1	Hepatic sclerosis
K74.2	Hepatic fibrosis with hepatic sclerosis
K74.69	Other cirrhosis of liver
K75.1	Phlebitis of portal vein
K75.89	Other specified inflammatory liver diseases
K76.0	Fatty (change of) liver, not elsewhere classified
K76.1	Chronic passive congestion of liver
K76.2	Central hemorrhagic necrosis of liver
K76.3	Infarction of liver
K76.5	Hepatic veno-occlusive disease
K76.6	Portal hypertension
K76.7	Hepatorenal syndrome
K76.89	Other specified diseases of liver
K91.82	Postprocedural hepatic failure
K91.83	Postprocedural hepatorenal syndrome
K91.89	Other postprocedural complications and disorders of digestive system
R18.0	Malignant ascites
R18.8	Other ascites
T82.7XXA	Infection and inflammatory reaction due to other cardiac and vascular devices, implants and grafts, initial encounter
T82.818A	Embolism due to vascular prosthetic devices, implants and grafts, initial encounter
T82.828A	Fibrosis due to vascular prosthetic devices, implants and grafts, initial encounter

Arteries and Veins

T82.838A	Hemorrhage due to vascular prosthetic devices, implants and grafts, initial encounter
T82.848A	Pain due to vascular prosthetic devices, implants and grafts, initial encounter
T82.856A	Stenosis of peripheral vascular stent, initial encounter
T82.858A	Stenosis of other vascular prosthetic devices, implants and grafts, initial encounter
T82.868A	Thrombosis due to vascular prosthetic devices, implants and grafts, initial encounter
T82.898A	Other specified complication of vascular prosthetic devices, implants and grafts, initial encounter

AMA: 37182 2018,Jan,8; 2017,Jan,8; 2016,Jan,13; 2015,Jan,16 **37183**
2018,Jan,8; 2017,Jan,8; 2016,Jan,13; 2015,Jan,16

Relative Value Units/Medicare Edits

Non-Facility RVU	Work	PE	MP	Total
37182	16.97	5.11	1.49	23.57
37183	7.74	180.49	0.69	188.92
Facility RVU	**Work**	**PE**	**MP**	**Total**
37182	16.97	5.11	1.49	23.57
37183	7.74	2.36	0.69	10.79

	FUD	Status	MUE	Modifiers				IOM Reference
37182	0	A	1(2)	51	N/A	N/A	80*	None
37183	0	A	1(2)	51	N/A	N/A	80*	

* with documentation

Terms To Know

anastomosis. Surgically created connection between ducts, blood vessels, or bowel segments to allow flow from one to the other.

revision. Reordering or rearrangement of tissue to suit a particular need or function.

shunt. Surgically created passage between blood vessels or other natural passages, such as an arteriovenous anastomosis, to divert or bypass blood flow from the normal channel.

stent. Tube to provide support in a body cavity or lumen.

TIPS. Transvenous intrahepatic portosystemic shunt. Life-saving procedure to improve blood flow, prevent hemorrhage, and manage the complications of portal hypertension, such as recurrent variceal bleeding and refractory ascites. The shunt may be portocaval, placed between the portal vein and the subhepatic inferior vena cava (IVC) or mesocaval, between the superior mesenteric vein (SMV) and the IVC.

37184-37185

	37184	Primary percutaneous transluminal mechanical thrombectomy, noncoronary, non-intracranial, arterial or arterial bypass graft, including fluoroscopic guidance and intraprocedural pharmacological thrombolytic injection(s); initial vessel
+	37185	second and all subsequent vessel(s) within the same vascular family (List separately in addition to code for primary mechanical thrombectomy procedure)

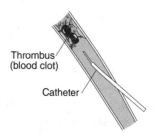

Thrombus (blood clot)

Catheter

A transluminal device removes a blood clot from an artery or artery graft other than from the heart

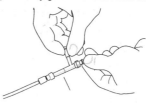

Explanation

The physician treats an acute noncoronary, nonintracranial arterial occlusion with a combination of thrombolytic drugs and percutaneous mechanical thrombectomy. The devices used for mechanical thrombectomy include those that fragment the thrombus with or without removal of the clot, as well as those that come into contact with the wall of the vessel. For the procedure using the Trellis device, the artery is cannulated to gain access and 5,000 units of heparin are administered. Angiography is performed to confirm the occluded arteries. A hydrophilic wire is passed across the occlusion, followed by passing of the Trellis device over a stiff exchange length wire. The distal and proximal balloons are inflated in the artery on either side of a treatment zone containing infusion to isolate the treatment zone and to sustain the fluid concentration that is infused. One milligram of tissue plasminogen activator (TPA) is infused into the treatment zone. The Turbo Trellis is run at 4,000 rpm for five minutes. After the proximal balloon is deflated, small clots are removed via the integral aspiration port to prevent embolization. Fluoroscopic guidance services and injections administered during the course of the procedure are included in the service. Separately reportable procedures include other percutaneous interventions such as stent placement and diagnostic studies. Report 37184 for the first vessel and 37185 for the second and subsequent vessels in the same vascular family.

Coding Tips

Report these codes in addition to 76000 or 96375 or with 61645 for treatment performed within the same vascular area.

ICD-10-CM Diagnostic Codes

I26.01	Septic pulmonary embolism with acute cor pulmonale
I26.02	Saddle embolus of pulmonary artery with acute cor pulmonale
I26.09	Other pulmonary embolism with acute cor pulmonale
I26.90	Septic pulmonary embolism without acute cor pulmonale

I26.92	Saddle embolus of pulmonary artery without acute cor pulmonale	
I26.93	Single subsegmental pulmonary embolism without acute cor pulmonale	
I26.94	Multiple subsegmental pulmonary emboli without acute cor pulmonale	
I26.99	Other pulmonary embolism without acute cor pulmonale	
I74.01	Saddle embolus of abdominal aorta	
I74.09	Other arterial embolism and thrombosis of abdominal aorta	
I74.11	Embolism and thrombosis of thoracic aorta	
I74.19	Embolism and thrombosis of other parts of aorta	
I74.2	Embolism and thrombosis of arteries of the upper extremities	
I74.3	Embolism and thrombosis of arteries of the lower extremities	
I74.5	Embolism and thrombosis of iliac artery	
I74.8	Embolism and thrombosis of other arteries	
I75.011	Atheroembolism of right upper extremity ☑	
I75.012	Atheroembolism of left upper extremity ☑	
I75.013	Atheroembolism of bilateral upper extremities ☑	
I75.021	Atheroembolism of right lower extremity ☑	
I75.022	Atheroembolism of left lower extremity ☑	
I75.023	Atheroembolism of bilateral lower extremities ☑	
I75.81	Atheroembolism of kidney	
I76	Septic arterial embolism	
T82.818A	Embolism due to vascular prosthetic devices, implants and grafts, initial encounter	
T82.868A	Thrombosis due to vascular prosthetic devices, implants and grafts, initial encounter	

AMA: 37184 2019,Sep,5; 2018,Jan,8; 2017,Jan,8; 2016,Mar,3; 2016,Jul,6; 2016,Jan,13; 2015,Nov,3; 2015,Jan,16; 2015,Apr,10 **37185** 2019,Sep,5; 2018,Jan,8; 2017,Jan,8; 2016,Jul,6; 2016,Jan,13; 2015,Nov,3; 2015,Jan,16; 2015,Apr,10

Relative Value Units/Medicare Edits

Non-Facility RVU	Work	PE	MP	Total
37184	8.41	46.67	1.62	56.7
37185	3.28	12.3	0.65	16.23
Facility RVU	**Work**	**PE**	**MP**	**Total**
37184	8.41	2.5	1.62	12.53
37185	3.28	0.81	0.65	4.74

	FUD	Status	MUE	Modifiers				IOM Reference
37184	0	A	1(2)	51	50	62	N/A	None
37185	N/A	A	2(3)	N/A	N/A	62	N/A	

* with documentation

Terms To Know

percutaneous. Through the skin.

thrombectomy. Removal of a clot (thrombus) from a blood vessel utilizing various methods.

thrombolytic agent. Drugs or other substances used to dissolve blood clots in blood vessels or in tubes that have been placed into the body.

37186

+ **37186** Secondary percutaneous transluminal thrombectomy (eg, nonprimary mechanical, snare basket, suction technique), noncoronary, non-intracranial, arterial or arterial bypass graft, including fluoroscopic guidance and intraprocedural pharmacological thrombolytic injections, provided in conjunction with another percutaneous intervention other than primary mechanical thrombectomy (List separately in addition to code for primary procedure)

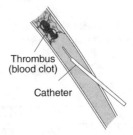

Thrombus (blood clot)

Catheter

Secondary percutaneous transluminal thrombectomy occurs prior to, or after, the primary procedure

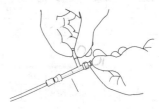

The thrombus may be removed using suction, a snare basket, or mechanical device. Thrombolytic injections may be employed

Explanation

The physician performs a secondary thrombectomy of a noncoronary, nonintracranial arterial occlusion. Prior to or after a percutaneous intervention is performed, such as balloon angioplasty or placement of a stent, the transcatheter removal of small sections of the thrombus or embolism is performed using suction, a snare basket, or a mechanical thrombectomy device under fluoroscopic guidance. Thrombolytic injections may also be used during the procedure.

Coding Tips

Do not report 37186 with 76000 or 96375. This code should not be reported with 61645 if the procedure is performed in the same vascular area.

ICD-10-CM Diagnostic Codes

This/these CPT code(s) are add-on code(s). See the primary procedure code that this code is performed with for your ICD-10-CM code selections.

AMA: 37186 2019,Sep,5; 2018,Jan,8; 2017,Jan,8; 2016,Jul,6; 2016,Jan,13; 2015,Nov,3; 2015,Jan,16

Relative Value Units/Medicare Edits

Non-Facility RVU	Work	PE	MP	Total
37186	4.92	33.37	0.94	39.23
Facility RVU	Work	PE	MP	Total
37186	4.92	1.24	0.94	7.1

	FUD	Status	MUE	Modifiers				IOM Reference
37186	N/A	A	2(3)	N/A	N/A	62	N/A	None

*with documentation

Terms To Know

angioplasty balloon. Balloon-tipped medical device used to clear the blockage of an artery. After insertion into the clogged artery, the balloon is inflated to expand a narrowing arterial section.

bypass graft. Surgically created alternative blood vessel used to reroute blood flow around an area of obstruction or disease.

embolism. Obstruction of a blood vessel resulting from a clot or foreign substance.

fluoroscopy. Radiology technique that allows visual examination of part of the body or a function of an organ using a device that projects an x-ray image on a fluorescent screen.

occlusion. Constriction, closure, or blockage of a passage.

percutaneous. Through the skin.

secondary. Second in order of occurrence or importance, or appearing during the course of another disease or condition.

stent. Tube to provide support in a body cavity or lumen.

thrombectomy. Removal of a clot (thrombus) from a blood vessel utilizing various methods.

thrombolytic agent. Drugs or other substances used to dissolve blood clots in blood vessels or in tubes that have been placed into the body.

37187-37188

37187 Percutaneous transluminal mechanical thrombectomy, vein(s), including intraprocedural pharmacological thrombolytic injections and fluoroscopic guidance

37188 Percutaneous transluminal mechanical thrombectomy, vein(s), including intraprocedural pharmacological thrombolytic injections and fluoroscopic guidance, repeat treatment on subsequent day during course of thrombolytic therapy

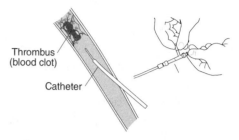

Thrombus (blood clot)

Catheter

A transluminal device is used for thrombolytic injections and fluoroscopic guidance

Explanation

The physician performs a percutaneous transluminal mechanical venous thrombectomy. A catheter sheath is inserted through a small incision in the vein, most commonly a groin incision in the femoral vein or an incision below the knee in the popliteal vein. Contrast is injected through the sheath and a separately reportable venography is performed to visualize the area of the vein being treated. Fluoroscopic guidance may be used. A guidewire is inserted through the sheath and advanced past the clot. A catheter is passed over the wire to the blocked area. A device at the tip of the catheter, a mechanical tool or a high-velocity liquid jet, is used to break the clot. A thrombolytic agent may be injected. When the procedure is completed, all instruments are removed and a compression bandage is applied. Report 37187 for the initial treatment. Report 37188 for repeat treatment on a subsequent day during the course of thrombolytic therapy.

Coding Tips

Do not report these codes with 76000 or 96375.

ICD-10-CM Diagnostic Codes

I80.01	Phlebitis and thrombophlebitis of superficial vessels of right lower extremity ☑
I80.02	Phlebitis and thrombophlebitis of superficial vessels of left lower extremity ☑
I80.03	Phlebitis and thrombophlebitis of superficial vessels of lower extremities, bilateral ☑
I80.11	Phlebitis and thrombophlebitis of right femoral vein ☑
I80.12	Phlebitis and thrombophlebitis of left femoral vein ☑
I80.13	Phlebitis and thrombophlebitis of femoral vein, bilateral ☑
I80.211	Phlebitis and thrombophlebitis of right iliac vein ☑
I80.212	Phlebitis and thrombophlebitis of left iliac vein ☑
I80.213	Phlebitis and thrombophlebitis of iliac vein, bilateral ☑
I80.221	Phlebitis and thrombophlebitis of right popliteal vein ☑
I80.222	Phlebitis and thrombophlebitis of left popliteal vein ☑
I80.223	Phlebitis and thrombophlebitis of popliteal vein, bilateral ☑
I80.231	Phlebitis and thrombophlebitis of right tibial vein ☑
I80.232	Phlebitis and thrombophlebitis of left tibial vein ☑

Arteries and Veins

I80.233	Phlebitis and thrombophlebitis of tibial vein, bilateral ☑
I80.241	Phlebitis and thrombophlebitis of right peroneal vein ☑
I80.251	Phlebitis and thrombophlebitis of right calf muscular vein ☑
I80.291	Phlebitis and thrombophlebitis of other deep vessels of right lower extremity ☑
I80.292	Phlebitis and thrombophlebitis of other deep vessels of left lower extremity ☑
I80.293	Phlebitis and thrombophlebitis of other deep vessels of lower extremity, bilateral ☑
I80.8	Phlebitis and thrombophlebitis of other sites
I82.0	Budd-Chiari syndrome
I82.1	Thrombophlebitis migrans
I82.210	Acute embolism and thrombosis of superior vena cava
I82.211	Chronic embolism and thrombosis of superior vena cava
I82.220	Acute embolism and thrombosis of inferior vena cava
I82.290	Acute embolism and thrombosis of other thoracic veins
I82.291	Chronic embolism and thrombosis of other thoracic veins
I82.3	Embolism and thrombosis of renal vein
I82.411	Acute embolism and thrombosis of right femoral vein ☑
I82.412	Acute embolism and thrombosis of left femoral vein ☑
I82.413	Acute embolism and thrombosis of femoral vein, bilateral ☑
I82.421	Acute embolism and thrombosis of right iliac vein ☑
I82.422	Acute embolism and thrombosis of left iliac vein ☑
I82.423	Acute embolism and thrombosis of iliac vein, bilateral ☑
I82.432	Acute embolism and thrombosis of left popliteal vein ☑
I82.433	Acute embolism and thrombosis of popliteal vein, bilateral ☑
I82.442	Acute embolism and thrombosis of left tibial vein ☑
I82.443	Acute embolism and thrombosis of tibial vein, bilateral ☑
I82.511	Chronic embolism and thrombosis of right femoral vein ☑
I82.512	Chronic embolism and thrombosis of left femoral vein ☑
I82.521	Chronic embolism and thrombosis of right iliac vein ☑
I82.522	Chronic embolism and thrombosis of left iliac vein ☑
I82.523	Chronic embolism and thrombosis of iliac vein, bilateral ☑
I82.532	Chronic embolism and thrombosis of left popliteal vein ☑
I82.533	Chronic embolism and thrombosis of popliteal vein, bilateral ☑
I82.541	Chronic embolism and thrombosis of right tibial vein ☑
I82.543	Chronic embolism and thrombosis of tibial vein, bilateral ☑
I82.551	Chronic embolism and thrombosis of right peroneal vein ☑
I82.561	Chronic embolism and thrombosis of right calf muscular vein ☑
I82.593	Chronic embolism and thrombosis of other specified deep vein of lower extremity, bilateral ☑
I82.611	Acute embolism and thrombosis of superficial veins of right upper extremity ☑
I82.612	Acute embolism and thrombosis of superficial veins of left upper extremity ☑
I82.621	Acute embolism and thrombosis of deep veins of right upper extremity ☑
I82.622	Acute embolism and thrombosis of deep veins of left upper extremity ☑
I82.713	Chronic embolism and thrombosis of superficial veins of upper extremity, bilateral ☑
I82.722	Chronic embolism and thrombosis of deep veins of left upper extremity ☑
I82.723	Chronic embolism and thrombosis of deep veins of upper extremity, bilateral ☑
I82.812	Embolism and thrombosis of superficial veins of left lower extremity ☑
I82.813	Embolism and thrombosis of superficial veins of lower extremities, bilateral ☑
I82.A11	Acute embolism and thrombosis of right axillary vein ☑
I82.A12	Acute embolism and thrombosis of left axillary vein ☑
I82.A21	Chronic embolism and thrombosis of right axillary vein ☑
I82.A23	Chronic embolism and thrombosis of axillary vein, bilateral ☑
I82.B12	Acute embolism and thrombosis of left subclavian vein ☑
I82.B13	Acute embolism and thrombosis of subclavian vein, bilateral ☑
I82.B22	Chronic embolism and thrombosis of left subclavian vein ☑
I82.B23	Chronic embolism and thrombosis of subclavian vein, bilateral ☑
I82.C12	Acute embolism and thrombosis of left internal jugular vein ☑
I82.C13	Acute embolism and thrombosis of internal jugular vein, bilateral ☑
I82.C21	Chronic embolism and thrombosis of right internal jugular vein ☑
I82.C23	Chronic embolism and thrombosis of internal jugular vein, bilateral ☑

AMA: **37187** 2018,Jan,8; 2017,Jan,8; 2016,Mar,3; 2016,Jul,6; 2016,Jan,13; 2015,Nov,3; 2015,Jan,16 **37188** 2018,Jan,8; 2017,Jan,8; 2016,Mar,3; 2016,Jul,6; 2016,Jan,13; 2015,Nov,3; 2015,Jan,16

Relative Value Units/Medicare Edits

Non-Facility RVU	Work	PE	MP	Total
37187	7.78	47.64	1.16	56.58
37188	5.46	42.21	0.84	48.51
Facility RVU	**Work**	**PE**	**MP**	**Total**
37187	7.78	2.45	1.16	11.39
37188	5.46	1.76	0.84	8.06

	FUD	Status	MUE	Modifiers				IOM Reference
37187	0	A	1(3)	51	50	62	N/A	None
37188	0	A	1(3)	N/A	50	62	N/A	

* with documentation

Terms To Know

fluoroscopy. Radiology technique that allows visual examination of part of the body or a function of an organ using a device that projects an x-ray image on a fluorescent screen.

thrombolytic agent. Drugs or other substances used to dissolve blood clots in blood vessels or in tubes that have been placed into the body.

37700

37700 Ligation and division of long saphenous vein at saphenofemoral junction, or distal interruptions

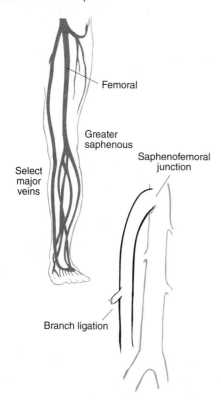

Femoral

Greater saphenous

Saphenofemoral junction

Select major veins

Branch ligation

Explanation

Through multiple small incisions in the skin of the upper thigh and along the femoral vein or its branches lower in the thigh, the physician isolates and separates the saphenous vein at the point it joins the femoral vein or at several points farther down the leg. The physician affixes vessel clamps and ligates sections of the saphenous vein along the leg as necessary. Once the ligations are completed, each skin incision is repaired with a layered closure.

Coding Tips

This is a unilateral procedure. If performed bilaterally, some payers require that the service be reported twice with modifier 50 appended to the second code while others require identification of the service only once with modifier 50 appended. Check with individual payers. Modifier 50 identifies a procedure performed identically on the opposite side of the body (mirror image). Do not report this code with 37718 or 37722. For ligation and stripping, short saphenous vein, see 37718; greater saphenous veins from saphenofemoral junction to knee or below, see 37722.

ICD-10-CM Diagnostic Codes

I80.01	Phlebitis and thrombophlebitis of superficial vessels of right lower extremity ☑
I80.02	Phlebitis and thrombophlebitis of superficial vessels of left lower extremity ☑
I80.03	Phlebitis and thrombophlebitis of superficial vessels of lower extremities, bilateral ☑
I80.11	Phlebitis and thrombophlebitis of right femoral vein ☑
I80.12	Phlebitis and thrombophlebitis of left femoral vein ☑
I80.13	Phlebitis and thrombophlebitis of femoral vein, bilateral ☑
I80.201	Phlebitis and thrombophlebitis of unspecified deep vessels of right lower extremity ☑
I80.202	Phlebitis and thrombophlebitis of unspecified deep vessels of left lower extremity ☑
I80.203	Phlebitis and thrombophlebitis of unspecified deep vessels of lower extremities, bilateral ☑
I80.291	Phlebitis and thrombophlebitis of other deep vessels of right lower extremity ☑
I80.292	Phlebitis and thrombophlebitis of other deep vessels of left lower extremity ☑
I80.293	Phlebitis and thrombophlebitis of other deep vessels of lower extremity, bilateral ☑
I83.011	Varicose veins of right lower extremity with ulcer of thigh 🅰 ☑
I83.012	Varicose veins of right lower extremity with ulcer of calf 🅰 ☑
I83.013	Varicose veins of right lower extremity with ulcer of ankle 🅰 ☑
I83.014	Varicose veins of right lower extremity with ulcer of heel and midfoot 🅰 ☑
I83.015	Varicose veins of right lower extremity with ulcer other part of foot 🅰 ☑
I83.018	Varicose veins of right lower extremity with ulcer other part of lower leg 🅰 ☑
I83.021	Varicose veins of left lower extremity with ulcer of thigh 🅰 ☑
I83.022	Varicose veins of left lower extremity with ulcer of calf 🅰 ☑
I83.023	Varicose veins of left lower extremity with ulcer of ankle 🅰 ☑
I83.024	Varicose veins of left lower extremity with ulcer of heel and midfoot 🅰 ☑
I83.025	Varicose veins of left lower extremity with ulcer other part of foot 🅰 ☑
I83.028	Varicose veins of left lower extremity with ulcer other part of lower leg 🅰 ☑
I83.11	Varicose veins of right lower extremity with inflammation 🅰 ☑
I83.12	Varicose veins of left lower extremity with inflammation 🅰 ☑
I83.211	Varicose veins of right lower extremity with both ulcer of thigh and inflammation 🅰 ☑
I83.212	Varicose veins of right lower extremity with both ulcer of calf and inflammation 🅰 ☑
I83.213	Varicose veins of right lower extremity with both ulcer of ankle and inflammation 🅰 ☑
I83.214	Varicose veins of right lower extremity with both ulcer of heel and midfoot and inflammation 🅰 ☑
I83.215	Varicose veins of right lower extremity with both ulcer other part of foot and inflammation 🅰 ☑
I83.218	Varicose veins of right lower extremity with both ulcer of other part of lower extremity and inflammation 🅰 ☑
I83.221	Varicose veins of left lower extremity with both ulcer of thigh and inflammation 🅰 ☑
I83.222	Varicose veins of left lower extremity with both ulcer of calf and inflammation 🅰 ☑
I83.223	Varicose veins of left lower extremity with both ulcer of ankle and inflammation 🅰 ☑
I83.224	Varicose veins of left lower extremity with both ulcer of heel and midfoot and inflammation 🅰 ☑
I83.225	Varicose veins of left lower extremity with both ulcer other part of foot and inflammation 🅰 ☑
I83.228	Varicose veins of left lower extremity with both ulcer of other part of lower extremity and inflammation 🅰 ☑

I83.811	Varicose veins of right lower extremity with pain Ⓐ ☑
I83.812	Varicose veins of left lower extremity with pain Ⓐ ☑
I83.813	Varicose veins of bilateral lower extremities with pain Ⓐ ☑
I83.891	Varicose veins of right lower extremity with other complications Ⓐ ☑
I83.892	Varicose veins of left lower extremity with other complications Ⓐ ☑
I83.893	Varicose veins of bilateral lower extremities with other complications Ⓐ ☑
I83.91	Asymptomatic varicose veins of right lower extremity Ⓐ ☑
I83.92	Asymptomatic varicose veins of left lower extremity Ⓐ ☑
I83.93	Asymptomatic varicose veins of bilateral lower extremities Ⓐ ☑
I87.2	Venous insufficiency (chronic) (peripheral)

AMA: 37700 2018,Mar,3; 2018,Jan,8; 2017,Jan,8; 2016,Jan,13; 2015,Jan,16

Relative Value Units/Medicare Edits

Non-Facility RVU	Work	PE	MP	Total
37700	3.82	2.46	0.9	7.18
Facility RVU	Work	PE	MP	Total
37700	3.82	2.46	0.9	7.18

	FUD	Status	MUE	Modifiers				IOM Reference
37700	90	A	1(2)	51	50	N/A	N/A	None

* with documentation

Terms To Know

bilateral. Consisting of or affecting two sides.

distal. Located farther away from a specified reference point or the trunk.

division. Separating into two or more parts.

ligation. Tying off a blood vessel or duct with a suture or a soft, thin wire.

occlusion. Constriction, closure, or blockage of a passage.

peripheral. Outside of a structure or organ.

ulcer. Open sore or excavating lesion of skin or the tissue on the surface of an organ from the sloughing of chronically inflamed and necrosing tissue.

unilateral. Located on or affecting one side.

varicose vein. Abnormal, permanently distended or stretched vein.

vascular insufficiency. Inadequate blood flow and oxygenation.

37718-37722

| 37718 | Ligation, division, and stripping, short saphenous vein |
| 37722 | Ligation, division, and stripping, long (greater) saphenous veins from saphenofemoral junction to knee or below |

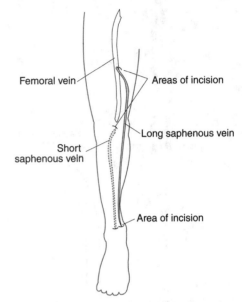

A vein stripper is commonly used in this procedure

Explanation

The physician makes a skin incision in the upper thigh or upper leg exposing the short saphenous vein (37718) or the long saphenous veins (37722). Additional skin incisions are made at the knee and the ankle and along the leg as necessary. A long wire is threaded through the length of the vein and brought out at the ankle. The vein is tied to the end of the wire and the wire is pulled out along with the vein. Once the vein has been removed, the skin incisions are repaired with layered closures. The leg is wrapped with an elastic pressure dressing postoperatively.

Coding Tips

These are unilateral procedures. If performed bilaterally, some payers require that the service be reported twice with modifier 50 appended to the second code while others require identification of the service only once with modifier 50 appended. Check with individual payers. Modifier 50 identifies a procedure performed identically on the opposite side of the body (mirror image). These codes are components of 37735 and should not be reported together. Code 37718 should not be reported with 37780; 37722 should not be reported with 37700.

ICD-10-CM Diagnostic Codes

I80.01	Phlebitis and thrombophlebitis of superficial vessels of right lower extremity ☑
I80.02	Phlebitis and thrombophlebitis of superficial vessels of left lower extremity ☑
I80.03	Phlebitis and thrombophlebitis of superficial vessels of lower extremities, bilateral ☑
I80.11	Phlebitis and thrombophlebitis of right femoral vein ☑
I80.12	Phlebitis and thrombophlebitis of left femoral vein ☑
I80.13	Phlebitis and thrombophlebitis of femoral vein, bilateral ☑
I80.291	Phlebitis and thrombophlebitis of other deep vessels of right lower extremity ☑

Arteries and Veins

I80.292	Phlebitis and thrombophlebitis of other deep vessels of left lower extremity ☑
I80.293	Phlebitis and thrombophlebitis of other deep vessels of lower extremity, bilateral ☑
I83.011	Varicose veins of right lower extremity with ulcer of thigh 🅐 ☑
I83.012	Varicose veins of right lower extremity with ulcer of calf 🅐 ☑
I83.013	Varicose veins of right lower extremity with ulcer of ankle 🅐 ☑
I83.014	Varicose veins of right lower extremity with ulcer of heel and midfoot 🅐 ☑
I83.015	Varicose veins of right lower extremity with ulcer other part of foot 🅐 ☑
I83.018	Varicose veins of right lower extremity with ulcer other part of lower leg 🅐 ☑
I83.021	Varicose veins of left lower extremity with ulcer of thigh 🅐 ☑
I83.022	Varicose veins of left lower extremity with ulcer of calf 🅐 ☑
I83.023	Varicose veins of left lower extremity with ulcer of ankle 🅐 ☑
I83.024	Varicose veins of left lower extremity with ulcer of heel and midfoot 🅐 ☑
I83.025	Varicose veins of left lower extremity with ulcer other part of foot 🅐 ☑
I83.028	Varicose veins of left lower extremity with ulcer other part of lower leg 🅐 ☑
I83.11	Varicose veins of right lower extremity with inflammation 🅐 ☑
I83.12	Varicose veins of left lower extremity with inflammation 🅐 ☑
I83.211	Varicose veins of right lower extremity with both ulcer of thigh and inflammation 🅐 ☑
I83.212	Varicose veins of right lower extremity with both ulcer of calf and inflammation 🅐 ☑
I83.213	Varicose veins of right lower extremity with both ulcer of ankle and inflammation 🅐 ☑
I83.214	Varicose veins of right lower extremity with both ulcer of heel and midfoot and inflammation 🅐 ☑
I83.215	Varicose veins of right lower extremity with both ulcer other part of foot and inflammation 🅐 ☑
I83.218	Varicose veins of right lower extremity with both ulcer of other part of lower extremity and inflammation 🅐 ☑
I83.221	Varicose veins of left lower extremity with both ulcer of thigh and inflammation 🅐 ☑
I83.222	Varicose veins of left lower extremity with both ulcer of calf and inflammation 🅐 ☑
I83.223	Varicose veins of left lower extremity with both ulcer of ankle and inflammation 🅐 ☑
I83.224	Varicose veins of left lower extremity with both ulcer of heel and midfoot and inflammation 🅐 ☑
I83.225	Varicose veins of left lower extremity with both ulcer other part of foot and inflammation 🅐 ☑
I83.228	Varicose veins of left lower extremity with both ulcer of other part of lower extremity and inflammation 🅐 ☑
I83.811	Varicose veins of right lower extremity with pain 🅐 ☑
I83.812	Varicose veins of left lower extremity with pain 🅐 ☑
I83.813	Varicose veins of bilateral lower extremities with pain 🅐 ☑
I83.891	Varicose veins of right lower extremity with other complications 🅐 ☑
I83.892	Varicose veins of left lower extremity with other complications 🅐 ☑

I83.893	Varicose veins of bilateral lower extremities with other complications 🅐 ☑
I83.91	Asymptomatic varicose veins of right lower extremity 🅐 ☑
I83.92	Asymptomatic varicose veins of left lower extremity 🅐 ☑
I83.93	Asymptomatic varicose veins of bilateral lower extremities 🅐 ☑
I87.2	Venous insufficiency (chronic) (peripheral)

AMA: 37718 2018,Mar,3; 2018,Jan,8; 2017,Jan,8 **37722** 2018,Mar,3; 2018,Jan,8; 2017,Jan,8

Relative Value Units/Medicare Edits

Non-Facility RVU	Work	PE	MP	Total
37718	7.13	3.57	1.71	12.41
37722	8.16	3.66	1.93	13.75
Facility RVU	Work	PE	MP	Total
37718	7.13	3.57	1.71	12.41
37722	8.16	3.66	1.93	13.75

	FUD	Status	MUE	Modifiers				IOM Reference
37718	90	A	1(2)	51	50	62*	N/A	None
37722	90	A	1(2)	51	50	62*	N/A	

* with documentation

Terms To Know

closure. Repairing an incision or wound by suture or other means.

division. Separating into two or more parts.

incision. Act of cutting into tissue or an organ.

ligation. Tying off a blood vessel or duct with a suture or a soft, thin wire.

pressure dressing. Wound dressing used to apply pressure to the injured area, often used after skin grafting procedures.

varicose vein. Abnormal, permanently distended or stretched vein.

vascular insufficiency. Inadequate blood flow and oxygenation.

37735

37735 Ligation and division and complete stripping of long or short saphenous veins with radical excision of ulcer and skin graft and/or interruption of communicating veins of lower leg, with excision of deep fascia

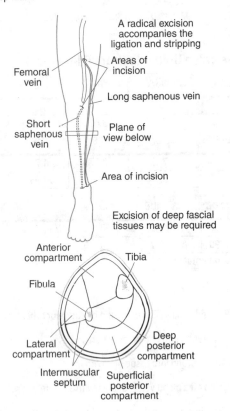

A radical excision accompanies the ligation and stripping

Areas of incision

Femoral vein

Long saphenous vein

Short saphenous vein

Plane of view below

Area of incision

Excision of deep fascial tissues may be required

Anterior compartment

Tibia

Fibula

Lateral compartment

Deep posterior compartment

Intermuscular septum

Superficial posterior compartment

Explanation

The physician makes a skin incision in the upper thigh and the upper leg exposing the long and short saphenous veins. Additional skin incisions are made at the ankle and along the leg as necessary. A long wire is passed through the length of the vein and brought out at the ankle. Each vein is tied to the end of the wire and the vein is pulled out along with the wire. The physician uses a scalpel to remove the skin ulcer from the leg. The ulcer site is covered with a piece of skin that has been shaved from another part of the patient's body. Veins that connect superficial veins with deep veins may be tied off. The tough, fibrous envelope containing the muscle of the leg is split and removed at points where the superficial and deep veins connect. The skin incisions are repaired with layered closures. The leg is wrapped with an elastic pressure dressing postoperatively.

Coding Tips

This is a unilateral procedure. If performed bilaterally, some payers require that the service be reported twice with modifier 50 appended to the second code while others require identification of the service only once with modifier 50 appended. Check with individual payers. Modifier 50 identifies a procedure performed identically on the opposite side of the body (mirror image). Do not report this code with 37700, 37718, 37722, or 37780.

ICD-10-CM Diagnostic Codes

I26.01	Septic pulmonary embolism with acute cor pulmonale
I26.09	Other pulmonary embolism with acute cor pulmonale
I26.90	Septic pulmonary embolism without acute cor pulmonale
I26.99	Other pulmonary embolism without acute cor pulmonale
I27.82	Chronic pulmonary embolism
I80.01	Phlebitis and thrombophlebitis of superficial vessels of right lower extremity ☑
I80.03	Phlebitis and thrombophlebitis of superficial vessels of lower extremities, bilateral ☑
I80.11	Phlebitis and thrombophlebitis of right femoral vein ☑
I80.13	Phlebitis and thrombophlebitis of femoral vein, bilateral ☑
I80.291	Phlebitis and thrombophlebitis of other deep vessels of right lower extremity ☑
I80.293	Phlebitis and thrombophlebitis of other deep vessels of lower extremity, bilateral ☑
I83.011	Varicose veins of right lower extremity with ulcer of thigh 🅰 ☑
I83.012	Varicose veins of right lower extremity with ulcer of calf 🅰 ☑
I83.013	Varicose veins of right lower extremity with ulcer of ankle 🅰 ☑
I83.014	Varicose veins of right lower extremity with ulcer of heel and midfoot 🅰 ☑
I83.015	Varicose veins of right lower extremity with ulcer other part of foot 🅰 ☑
I83.018	Varicose veins of right lower extremity with ulcer other part of lower leg 🅰 ☑
I83.11	Varicose veins of right lower extremity with inflammation 🅰 ☑
I83.211	Varicose veins of right lower extremity with both ulcer of thigh and inflammation 🅰 ☑
I83.212	Varicose veins of right lower extremity with both ulcer of calf and inflammation 🅰 ☑
I83.213	Varicose veins of right lower extremity with both ulcer of ankle and inflammation 🅰 ☑
I83.214	Varicose veins of right lower extremity with both ulcer of heel and midfoot and inflammation 🅰 ☑
I83.215	Varicose veins of right lower extremity with both ulcer other part of foot and inflammation 🅰 ☑
I83.218	Varicose veins of right lower extremity with both ulcer of other part of lower extremity and inflammation 🅰 ☑
I83.811	Varicose veins of right lower extremity with pain 🅰 ☑
I83.813	Varicose veins of bilateral lower extremities with pain 🅰 ☑
I83.891	Varicose veins of right lower extremity with other complications 🅰 ☑
I83.893	Varicose veins of bilateral lower extremities with other complications 🅰 ☑
I83.91	Asymptomatic varicose veins of right lower extremity 🅰 ☑
I83.93	Asymptomatic varicose veins of bilateral lower extremities 🅰 ☑
I87.2	Venous insufficiency (chronic) (peripheral)
L97.111	Non-pressure chronic ulcer of right thigh limited to breakdown of skin ☑
L97.112	Non-pressure chronic ulcer of right thigh with fat layer exposed ☑
L97.113	Non-pressure chronic ulcer of right thigh with necrosis of muscle ☑
L97.114	Non-pressure chronic ulcer of right thigh with necrosis of bone ☑
L97.211	Non-pressure chronic ulcer of right calf limited to breakdown of skin ☑
L97.212	Non-pressure chronic ulcer of right calf with fat layer exposed ☑
L97.213	Non-pressure chronic ulcer of right calf with necrosis of muscle ☑
L97.214	Non-pressure chronic ulcer of right calf with necrosis of bone ☑

Arteries and Veins

L97.311	Non-pressure chronic ulcer of right ankle limited to breakdown of skin ☑
L97.312	Non-pressure chronic ulcer of right ankle with fat layer exposed ☑
L97.313	Non-pressure chronic ulcer of right ankle with necrosis of muscle ☑
L97.314	Non-pressure chronic ulcer of right ankle with necrosis of bone ☑
L97.411	Non-pressure chronic ulcer of right heel and midfoot limited to breakdown of skin ☑
L97.412	Non-pressure chronic ulcer of right heel and midfoot with fat layer exposed ☑
L97.413	Non-pressure chronic ulcer of right heel and midfoot with necrosis of muscle ☑
L97.414	Non-pressure chronic ulcer of right heel and midfoot with necrosis of bone ☑
L97.511	Non-pressure chronic ulcer of other part of right foot limited to breakdown of skin ☑
L97.512	Non-pressure chronic ulcer of other part of right foot with fat layer exposed ☑
L97.513	Non-pressure chronic ulcer of other part of right foot with necrosis of muscle ☑
L97.514	Non-pressure chronic ulcer of other part of right foot with necrosis of bone ☑
L97.811	Non-pressure chronic ulcer of other part of right lower leg limited to breakdown of skin ☑
L97.812	Non-pressure chronic ulcer of other part of right lower leg with fat layer exposed ☑
L97.813	Non-pressure chronic ulcer of other part of right lower leg with necrosis of muscle ☑
L97.814	Non-pressure chronic ulcer of other part of right lower leg with necrosis of bone ☑

AMA: **37735** 2018,Mar,3; 2018,Jan,8; 2017,Jan,8; 2016,Jan,13; 2015,Jan,16

Relative Value Units/Medicare Edits

Non-Facility RVU	Work	PE	MP	Total
37735	10.9	3.4	2.62	16.92
Facility RVU	Work	PE	MP	Total
37735	10.9	3.4	2.62	16.92

	FUD	Status	MUE	Modifiers				IOM Reference
37735	90	A	1(2)	51	50	62*	N/A	None

* with documentation

Terms To Know

embolism. Obstruction of a blood vessel resulting from a clot or foreign substance.

ligation. Tying off a blood vessel or duct with a suture or a soft, thin wire.

ulcer. Open sore or excavating lesion of skin or the tissue on the surface of an organ from the sloughing of chronically inflamed and necrosing tissue.

varicose vein. Abnormal, permanently distended or stretched vein.

37765-37766

| 37765 | Stab phlebectomy of varicose veins, 1 extremity; 10-20 stab incisions |
| 37766 | more than 20 incisions |

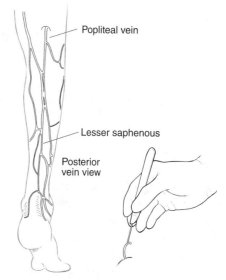

Stab incisions are made over the varicose vein and a hooked device retrieves the section of vein

Explanation

Stab phlebectomy for varicose veins is an ambulatory procedure that permits removal of nearly any incompetent vein below the saphenofemoral and saphenopopliteal junction. The varicose veins are identified with an indelible marking pen while the patient is standing. The patient is placed supine for further marking. Diluted lidocaine is injected into the tissues in large volumes until the perivenous tissues are engorged and distended with the anesthetic. Regional nerve blocks may be used for extensive areas. Tiny stab incisions are made with a scalpel or 18-gauge needle. The varicose vein is dissected with the phlebectomy hook. The vein is undermined along its course, all fibroadipose attachments to the vein are freed, and the vein is grasped with the hook and removed with mosquito forceps. Hemostasis is achieved by applying local compression to the veins already removed. The varicose vein is progressively extracted from one stab incision to the next. No skin closure is needed. Bandages are applied. Large pads are placed along the site of vein removal and covered with an inelastic bandage, followed by a second bandage of highly elastic material. Report 37765 when 10 to 20 stab incisions are made and 37766 when more than 20 are reported.

Coding Tips

To report less than 10 incisions, see 37799; more than 20 incisions, see 37766. These codes are unilateral procedures. If performed bilaterally, some payers require that the service be reported twice with modifier 50 appended to the second code while others require identification of the service only once with modifier 50 appended. Check with individual payers. Modifier 50 identifies a procedure performed identically on the opposite side of the body (mirror image).

ICD-10-CM Diagnostic Codes

I83.011	Varicose veins of right lower extremity with ulcer of thigh ▲ ☑
I83.012	Varicose veins of right lower extremity with ulcer of calf ▲ ☑
I83.013	Varicose veins of right lower extremity with ulcer of ankle ▲ ☑

Arteries and Veins

I83.014	Varicose veins of right lower extremity with ulcer of heel and midfoot △ ☑
I83.015	Varicose veins of right lower extremity with ulcer other part of foot △ ☑
I83.018	Varicose veins of right lower extremity with ulcer other part of lower leg △ ☑
I83.021	Varicose veins of left lower extremity with ulcer of thigh △ ☑
I83.022	Varicose veins of left lower extremity with ulcer of calf △ ☑
I83.023	Varicose veins of left lower extremity with ulcer of ankle △ ☑
I83.024	Varicose veins of left lower extremity with ulcer of heel and midfoot △ ☑
I83.025	Varicose veins of left lower extremity with ulcer other part of foot △ ☑
I83.028	Varicose veins of left lower extremity with ulcer other part of lower leg △ ☑
I83.11	Varicose veins of right lower extremity with inflammation △ ☑
I83.12	Varicose veins of left lower extremity with inflammation △ ☑
I83.211	Varicose veins of right lower extremity with both ulcer of thigh and inflammation △ ☑
I83.212	Varicose veins of right lower extremity with both ulcer of calf and inflammation △ ☑
I83.213	Varicose veins of right lower extremity with both ulcer of ankle and inflammation △ ☑
I83.214	Varicose veins of right lower extremity with both ulcer of heel and midfoot and inflammation △ ☑
I83.215	Varicose veins of right lower extremity with both ulcer other part of foot and inflammation △ ☑
I83.218	Varicose veins of right lower extremity with both ulcer of other part of lower extremity and inflammation △ ☑
I83.221	Varicose veins of left lower extremity with both ulcer of thigh and inflammation △ ☑
I83.222	Varicose veins of left lower extremity with both ulcer of calf and inflammation △ ☑
I83.223	Varicose veins of left lower extremity with both ulcer of ankle and inflammation △ ☑
I83.224	Varicose veins of left lower extremity with both ulcer of heel and midfoot and inflammation △ ☑
I83.225	Varicose veins of left lower extremity with both ulcer other part of foot and inflammation △ ☑
I83.228	Varicose veins of left lower extremity with both ulcer of other part of lower extremity and inflammation △ ☑
I83.811	Varicose veins of right lower extremity with pain △ ☑
I83.812	Varicose veins of left lower extremity with pain △ ☑
I83.813	Varicose veins of bilateral lower extremities with pain △ ☑
I83.891	Varicose veins of right lower extremity with other complications △ ☑
I83.892	Varicose veins of left lower extremity with other complications △ ☑
I83.893	Varicose veins of bilateral lower extremities with other complications △ ☑
I83.91	Asymptomatic varicose veins of right lower extremity △ ☑
I83.92	Asymptomatic varicose veins of left lower extremity △ ☑
I83.93	Asymptomatic varicose veins of bilateral lower extremities △ ☑
I87.2	Venous insufficiency (chronic) (peripheral)

AMA: **37765** 2018,Mar,3; 2018,Jan,8; 2017,Jan,8; 2016,Nov,3; 2016,Jan,13; 2015,Jan,16 **37766** 2018,Mar,3; 2018,Jan,8; 2017,Jan,8; 2016,Nov,3; 2016,Jan,13; 2015,Jan,16

Relative Value Units/Medicare Edits

Non-Facility RVU	Work	PE	MP	Total
37765	4.8	7.22	1.03	13.05
37766	6.0	7.92	1.25	15.17
Facility RVU	**Work**	**PE**	**MP**	**Total**
37765	4.8	2.08	1.03	7.91
37766	6.0	2.42	1.25	9.67

	FUD	Status	MUE	Modifiers				IOM Reference
37765	10	A	1(2)	51	50	62*	N/A	None
37766	10	A	1(2)	51	50	62*	N/A	

* with documentation

Terms To Know

dissect. Cut apart or separate tissue for surgical purposes or for visual or microscopic study.

distention. Enlarged or expanded due to pressure from inside.

hemostasis. Interruption of blood flow or the cessation or arrest of bleeding.

inflammation. Cytologic and chemical reactions that occur in affected blood vessels and adjacent tissues in response to injury or abnormal stimulation from a physical, chemical, or biologic agent.

ligation. Tying off a blood vessel or duct with a suture or a soft, thin wire.

posterior. Located in the back part or caudal end of the body.

ulcer. Open sore or excavating lesion of skin or the tissue on the surface of an organ from the sloughing of chronically inflamed and necrosing tissue.

varicose vein. Abnormal, permanently distended or stretched vein.

vein. Vessel through which oxygen-depleted blood passes back to the heart.

37785

37785 Ligation, division, and/or excision of varicose vein cluster(s), 1 leg

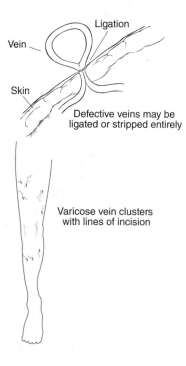

Ligation
Vein
Skin
Defective veins may be ligated or stripped entirely

Varicose vein clusters with lines of incision

Explanation

The physician ligates, divides, and/or excises a varicose vein cluster(s) in one leg. The physician makes small incisions in the skin over localized areas of superficial varicose veins along the leg. These veins are isolated and dissected free of neighboring tissue, tied with sutures and divided, or stripped out bluntly. Pressure is applied over the site to stop bleeding. All incisions are repaired with a layered closure. The legs are wrapped in an elastic pressure dressing postoperatively.

Coding Tips

This is a unilateral procedure. If performed bilaterally, some payers require that the service be reported twice with modifier 50 appended to the second code while others require identification of the service only once with modifier 50 appended. Check with individual payers. Modifier 50 identifies a procedure performed identically on the opposite side of the body (mirror image).

ICD-10-CM Diagnostic Codes

I83.011	Varicose veins of right lower extremity with ulcer of thigh 🅰 ☑
I83.012	Varicose veins of right lower extremity with ulcer of calf 🅰 ☑
I83.013	Varicose veins of right lower extremity with ulcer of ankle 🅰 ☑
I83.014	Varicose veins of right lower extremity with ulcer of heel and midfoot 🅰 ☑
I83.015	Varicose veins of right lower extremity with ulcer other part of foot 🅰 ☑
I83.018	Varicose veins of right lower extremity with ulcer other part of lower leg 🅰 ☑
I83.021	Varicose veins of left lower extremity with ulcer of thigh 🅰 ☑
I83.022	Varicose veins of left lower extremity with ulcer of calf 🅰 ☑
I83.023	Varicose veins of left lower extremity with ulcer of ankle 🅰 ☑
I83.024	Varicose veins of left lower extremity with ulcer of heel and midfoot 🅰 ☑
I83.025	Varicose veins of left lower extremity with ulcer other part of foot 🅰 ☑
I83.028	Varicose veins of left lower extremity with ulcer other part of lower leg 🅰 ☑
I83.11	Varicose veins of right lower extremity with inflammation 🅰 ☑
I83.12	Varicose veins of left lower extremity with inflammation 🅰 ☑
I83.211	Varicose veins of right lower extremity with both ulcer of thigh and inflammation 🅰 ☑
I83.212	Varicose veins of right lower extremity with both ulcer of calf and inflammation 🅰 ☑
I83.213	Varicose veins of right lower extremity with both ulcer of ankle and inflammation 🅰 ☑
I83.214	Varicose veins of right lower extremity with both ulcer of heel and midfoot and inflammation 🅰 ☑
I83.215	Varicose veins of right lower extremity with both ulcer other part of foot and inflammation 🅰 ☑
I83.218	Varicose veins of right lower extremity with both ulcer of other part of lower extremity and inflammation 🅰 ☑
I83.221	Varicose veins of left lower extremity with both ulcer of thigh and inflammation 🅰 ☑
I83.222	Varicose veins of left lower extremity with both ulcer of calf and inflammation 🅰 ☑
I83.223	Varicose veins of left lower extremity with both ulcer of ankle and inflammation 🅰 ☑
I83.224	Varicose veins of left lower extremity with both ulcer of heel and midfoot and inflammation 🅰 ☑
I83.225	Varicose veins of left lower extremity with both ulcer other part of foot and inflammation 🅰 ☑
I83.228	Varicose veins of left lower extremity with both ulcer of other part of lower extremity and inflammation 🅰 ☑
I83.811	Varicose veins of right lower extremity with pain 🅰 ☑
I83.812	Varicose veins of left lower extremity with pain 🅰 ☑
I83.813	Varicose veins of bilateral lower extremities with pain 🅰 ☑
I83.891	Varicose veins of right lower extremity with other complications 🅰 ☑
I83.892	Varicose veins of left lower extremity with other complications 🅰 ☑
I83.893	Varicose veins of bilateral lower extremities with other complications 🅰 ☑
I83.91	Asymptomatic varicose veins of right lower extremity 🅰 ☑
I83.92	Asymptomatic varicose veins of left lower extremity 🅰 ☑
I83.93	Asymptomatic varicose veins of bilateral lower extremities 🅰 ☑
I87.2	Venous insufficiency (chronic) (peripheral)

AMA: 37785 2018,Jan,8; 2017,Jan,8; 2016,Jan,13; 2015,Jan,16

Relative Value Units/Medicare Edits

Non-Facility RVU	Work	PE	MP	Total
37785	3.93	5.8	0.91	10.64
Facility RVU	**Work**	**PE**	**MP**	**Total**
37785	3.93	2.69	0.91	7.53

	FUD	Status	MUE	Modifiers				IOM Reference
37785	90	A	1(2)	51	50	N/A	N/A	None

* with documentation

● New   ▲ Revised   + Add On   ★ Telemedicine   AMA: CPT Assist   [Resequenced]   ☑ Laterality   © 2021 Optum360, LLC

38100-38102

38100 Splenectomy; total (separate procedure)
38101   partial (separate procedure)
+ 38102   total, en bloc for extensive disease, in conjunction with other procedure (List in addition to code for primary procedure)

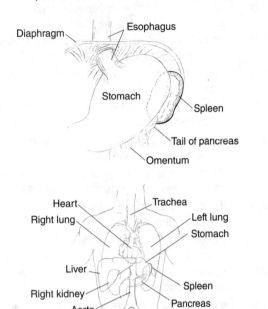

Explanation

The physician makes a midline incision and dissects tissue around the spleen. The short stomach vessels are doubly ligated and cut. The splenic recess is dissected and the splenic artery and vein are divided and cut individually. The physician removes the spleen. A drain may be placed and the wound is irrigated. The incision is closed with sutures or staples and a dry dressing is applied. Report 38101 if performing a partial splenectomy; report 38102 if performing a total splenectomy in conjunction with another procedure.

Coding Tips

Codes 38100 and 38101 are separate procedures by definition and are usually a component of a more complex service and are not identified separately. When performed alone or with other unrelated procedures/services they may be reported. If performed alone, list the code; if performed with other procedures/services, list the code and append modifier 59 or an X{EPSU} modifier. Report 38102 with the primary procedure, as appropriate. For laparoscopic splenectomy, see 38120.

ICD-10-CM Diagnostic Codes

A18.85	Tuberculosis of spleen
C26.1	Malignant neoplasm of spleen
C78.89	Secondary malignant neoplasm of other digestive organs
C81.07	Nodular lymphocyte predominant Hodgkin lymphoma, spleen
C81.17	Nodular sclerosis Hodgkin lymphoma, spleen
C81.27	Mixed cellularity Hodgkin lymphoma, spleen
C81.37	Lymphocyte depleted Hodgkin lymphoma, spleen
C81.47	Lymphocyte-rich Hodgkin lymphoma, spleen
C81.77	Other Hodgkin lymphoma, spleen
C82.07	Follicular lymphoma grade I, spleen
C82.17	Follicular lymphoma grade II, spleen
C82.37	Follicular lymphoma grade IIIa, spleen
C82.47	Follicular lymphoma grade IIIb, spleen
C82.57	Diffuse follicle center lymphoma, spleen
C82.67	Cutaneous follicle center lymphoma, spleen
C83.07	Small cell B-cell lymphoma, spleen
C83.37	Diffuse large B-cell lymphoma, spleen
C83.57	Lymphoblastic (diffuse) lymphoma, spleen
C83.77	Burkitt lymphoma, spleen
C84.07	Mycosis fungoides, spleen
C84.17	Sezary disease, spleen
C84.47	Peripheral T-cell lymphoma, not classified, spleen
C84.67	Anaplastic large cell lymphoma, ALK-positive, spleen
C84.77	Anaplastic large cell lymphoma, ALK-negative, spleen
C84.Z7	Other mature T/NK-cell lymphomas, spleen
C85.27	Mediastinal (thymic) large B-cell lymphoma, spleen
C86.1	Hepatosplenic T-cell lymphoma
C91.40	Hairy cell leukemia not having achieved remission
C96.0	Multifocal and multisystemic (disseminated) Langerhans-cell histiocytosis
C96.21	Aggressive systemic mastocytosis
C96.22	Mast cell sarcoma
C96.A	Histiocytic sarcoma
C96.Z	Other specified malignant neoplasms of lymphoid, hematopoietic and related tissue
D49.0	Neoplasm of unspecified behavior of digestive system
D56.0	Alpha thalassemia
D56.1	Beta thalassemia
D56.2	Delta-beta thalassemia
D56.3	Thalassemia minor
D56.5	Hemoglobin E-beta thalassemia
D57.02	Hb-SS disease with splenic sequestration
D57.212	Sickle-cell/Hb-C disease with splenic sequestration
D57.412	Sickle-cell thalassemia, unspecified, with splenic sequestration
D57.432	Sickle-cell thalassemia beta zero with splenic sequestration
D57.452	Sickle-cell thalassemia beta plus with splenic sequestration
D57.812	Other sickle-cell disorders with splenic sequestration
D58.0	Hereditary spherocytosis
D59.0	Drug-induced autoimmune hemolytic anemia
D59.11	Warm autoimmune hemolytic anemia
D69.3	Immune thrombocytopenic purpura
D69.41	Evans syndrome
D69.42	Congenital and hereditary thrombocytopenia purpura
D73.0	Hyposplenism
D73.1	Hypersplenism
D73.2	Chronic congestive splenomegaly
D73.3	Abscess of spleen
D73.4	Cyst of spleen
D73.5	Infarction of spleen
D73.81	Neutropenic splenomegaly
D75.82	Heparin induced thrombocytopenia (HIT)
D78.01	Intraoperative hemorrhage and hematoma of the spleen complicating a procedure on the spleen
D78.02	Intraoperative hemorrhage and hematoma of the spleen complicating other procedure

D78.11	Accidental puncture and laceration of the spleen during a procedure on the spleen
D78.12	Accidental puncture and laceration of the spleen during other procedure
D78.21	Postprocedural hemorrhage of the spleen following a procedure on the spleen
D78.22	Postprocedural hemorrhage of the spleen following other procedure
D78.31	Postprocedural hematoma of the spleen following a procedure on the spleen
D78.32	Postprocedural hematoma of the spleen following other procedure
D78.33	Postprocedural seroma of the spleen following a procedure on the spleen
D78.34	Postprocedural seroma of the spleen following other procedure
D78.81	Other intraoperative complications of the spleen
D78.89	Other postprocedural complications of the spleen
D86.89	Sarcoidosis of other sites
D89.41	Monoclonal mast cell activation syndrome
D89.42	Idiopathic mast cell activation syndrome
D89.43	Secondary mast cell activation
D89.82	Autoimmune lymphoproliferative syndrome [ALPS]
E75.22	Gaucher disease
K74.69	Other cirrhosis of liver
K76.6	Portal hypertension
M05.00	Felty's syndrome, unspecified site
P15.1	Birth injury to spleen N
Q89.09	Congenital malformations of spleen
R16.2	Hepatomegaly with splenomegaly, not elsewhere classified
S36.021A	Major contusion of spleen, initial encounter
S36.029A	Unspecified contusion of spleen, initial encounter
S36.031A	Moderate laceration of spleen, initial encounter
S36.032A	Major laceration of spleen, initial encounter

AMA: **38100** 2018,Jan,8; 2017,Jan,8; 2016,Jan,13; 2015,Jan,16 **38101** 2018,Jan,8; 2017,Jan,8; 2016,Jan,13; 2015,Jan,16 **38102** 2018,Jan,8; 2017,Jan,8; 2016,Jan,13; 2015,Jan,16

Relative Value Units/Medicare Edits

Non-Facility RVU	Work	PE	MP	Total
38100	19.55	9.91	4.54	34.0
38101	19.55	10.11	4.78	34.44
38102	4.79	1.85	1.03	7.67
Facility RVU	Work	PE	MP	Total
38100	19.55	9.91	4.54	34.0
38101	19.55	10.11	4.78	34.44
38102	4.79	1.85	1.03	7.67

	FUD	Status	MUE	Modifiers				IOM Reference
38100	90	A	1(2)	51	N/A	62*	80	None
38101	90	A	1(3)	51	N/A	62*	80	
38102	N/A	A	1(2)	N/A	N/A	62*	80	

* with documentation

38115

38115	Repair of ruptured spleen (splenorrhaphy) with or without partial splenectomy

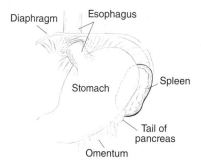

Any lacerations of the spleen are repaired

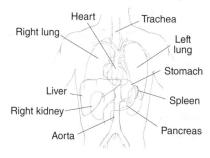

Explanation

The physician makes an upper midline incision and dissects around the spleen until it is exposed. Lacerations are sutured. The damaged segment of the spleen is resected and removed and the edges are sutured. The wound is irrigated and the incision is closed using sutures or staples and a dry dressing.

Coding Tips

For total splenectomy via an open approach, see 38100; partial, see 38101; laparoscopic, see 38120.

ICD-10-CM Diagnostic Codes

D78.11	Accidental puncture and laceration of the spleen during a procedure on the spleen
D78.12	Accidental puncture and laceration of the spleen during other procedure
P15.1	Birth injury to spleen N
S36.020A	Minor contusion of spleen, initial encounter
S36.021A	Major contusion of spleen, initial encounter
S36.030A	Superficial (capsular) laceration of spleen, initial encounter
S36.031A	Moderate laceration of spleen, initial encounter
S36.032A	Major laceration of spleen, initial encounter
S36.09XA	Other injury of spleen, initial encounter

AMA: **38115** 2018,Jan,8; 2017,Jan,8; 2016,Jan,13; 2015,Jan,16

Relative Value Units/Medicare Edits

Non-Facility RVU	Work	PE	MP	Total
38115	21.88	10.85	4.84	37.57
Facility RVU	**Work**	**PE**	**MP**	**Total**
38115	21.88	10.85	4.84	37.57

	FUD	Status	MUE	Modifiers				IOM Reference
38115	90	A	1(3)	51	N/A	62*	80	None

* with documentation

Terms To Know

absorbable sutures. Strands used for suture or repair of tissue prepared from collagen or a synthetic polymer and capable of being absorbed by tissue over time.

closure. Repairing an incision or wound by suture or other means.

dissect. Cut apart or separate tissue for surgical purposes or for visual or microscopic study.

hematoma. Tumor-like collection of blood in some part of the body caused by a break in a blood vessel wall, usually as a result of trauma.

incision. Act of cutting into tissue or an organ.

irrigate. Washing out, lavage.

lymphatic system. Lymphatic capillaries, vessels, lymph nodes, spleen, thymus gland, and bone marrow.

nonabsorbable sutures. Strands of natural or synthetic material that resist absorption into living tissue and are removed once healing is under way. Nonabsorbable sutures are commonly used to close skin wounds and repair tendons or collagenous tissue.

omentum. Fold of peritoneal tissue suspended between the stomach and neighboring visceral organs of the abdominal cavity.

resection. Surgical removal of a part or all of an organ or body part.

spleen. Largest organ of the lymph system located in the upper left side of the abdomen that disintegrates red blood cells and releases hemoglobin; rids the body of worn-out, damaged red blood cells and platelets; produces plasma cells and lymphocytes; and has other functions not fully understood.

38120

38120   Laparoscopy, surgical, splenectomy

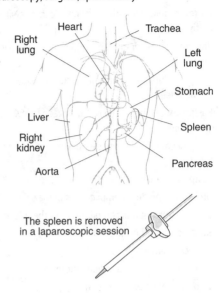

The spleen is removed in a laparoscopic session

Explanation

The physician performs a laparoscopic splenectomy. The patient is placed in a right lateral decubitus position, left arm over the head. With the patient under anesthesia, the physician makes a small incision in the abdominal wall and inserts a trocar just below or above the umbilicus. The physician insufflates the abdominal cavity and places the laparoscope through the umbilical incision. Dissection is carried down to the level of the spleen with care taken to identify the tail of the pancreas. Electrocautery is used to divide ligaments and the spleen is mobilized. Short gastric vessels may be transected to gain additional exposure. The splenic vessels are transected and the spleen is excised and hemostasis is ensured. The freed spleen is isolated and a surgical "retrieval bag" is inserted through a trocar into the abdomen. The spleen is placed into the bag, the bag is closed, and the neck of the bag is brought through the abdominal wall. The spleen is morcellized (unless pathological purposes require an intact specimen) within the bag and the bag containing the spleen is removed. The abdomen is evaluated for accessory spleens and hemostasis. The laparoscope and trocars are removed and the incisions are closed with sutures.

Coding Tips

Surgical laparoscopy always includes diagnostic laparoscopy. For splenectomy via an open approach, see 38100; partial, see 38101; total, en bloc, in conjunction with another procedure, see 38102. For repair of a ruptured spleen, with or without partial splenectomy, see 38115. For a diagnostic laparoscopy of the abdomen, peritoneum, and omentum, with or without specimen collection, see 49320.

ICD-10-CM Diagnostic Codes

A18.85	Tuberculosis of spleen
C26.1	Malignant neoplasm of spleen
C78.89	Secondary malignant neoplasm of other digestive organs
C81.07	Nodular lymphocyte predominant Hodgkin lymphoma, spleen
C81.17	Nodular sclerosis Hodgkin lymphoma, spleen
C81.27	Mixed cellularity Hodgkin lymphoma, spleen
C81.37	Lymphocyte depleted Hodgkin lymphoma, spleen
C81.47	Lymphocyte-rich Hodgkin lymphoma, spleen

Spleen

C81.77	Other Hodgkin lymphoma, spleen
C82.07	Follicular lymphoma grade I, spleen
C82.17	Follicular lymphoma grade II, spleen
C82.37	Follicular lymphoma grade IIIa, spleen
C82.47	Follicular lymphoma grade IIIb, spleen
C82.57	Diffuse follicle center lymphoma, spleen
C82.67	Cutaneous follicle center lymphoma, spleen
C82.87	Other types of follicular lymphoma, spleen
C83.07	Small cell B-cell lymphoma, spleen
C83.37	Diffuse large B-cell lymphoma, spleen
C83.57	Lymphoblastic (diffuse) lymphoma, spleen
C83.77	Burkitt lymphoma, spleen
C83.87	Other non-follicular lymphoma, spleen
C84.07	Mycosis fungoides, spleen
C84.17	Sezary disease, spleen
C84.47	Peripheral T-cell lymphoma, not classified, spleen
C84.67	Anaplastic large cell lymphoma, ALK-positive, spleen
C84.77	Anaplastic large cell lymphoma, ALK-negative, spleen
C84.Z7	Other mature T/NK-cell lymphomas, spleen
C85.27	Mediastinal (thymic) large B-cell lymphoma, spleen
C85.87	Other specified types of non-Hodgkin lymphoma, spleen
C86.1	Hepatosplenic T-cell lymphoma
C91.40	Hairy cell leukemia not having achieved remission
C96.0	Multifocal and multisystemic (disseminated) Langerhans-cell histiocytosis
C96.21	Aggressive systemic mastocytosis
C96.22	Mast cell sarcoma
C96.A	Histiocytic sarcoma
C96.Z	Other specified malignant neoplasms of lymphoid, hematopoietic and related tissue
D49.0	Neoplasm of unspecified behavior of digestive system
D56.0	Alpha thalassemia
D56.1	Beta thalassemia
D56.2	Delta-beta thalassemia
D56.3	Thalassemia minor
D56.5	Hemoglobin E-beta thalassemia
D56.8	Other thalassemias
D57.02	Hb-SS disease with splenic sequestration
D57.212	Sickle-cell/Hb-C disease with splenic sequestration
D57.412	Sickle-cell thalassemia, unspecified, with splenic sequestration
D57.432	Sickle-cell thalassemia beta zero with splenic sequestration
D57.452	Sickle-cell thalassemia beta plus with splenic sequestration
D58.0	Hereditary spherocytosis
D59.0	Drug-induced autoimmune hemolytic anemia
D59.12	Cold autoimmune hemolytic anemia
D69.3	Immune thrombocytopenic purpura
D69.41	Evans syndrome
D69.42	Congenital and hereditary thrombocytopenia purpura
D73.0	Hyposplenism
D73.1	Hypersplenism
D73.2	Chronic congestive splenomegaly
D73.3	Abscess of spleen
D73.4	Cyst of spleen

D73.5	Infarction of spleen
D73.81	Neutropenic splenomegaly
D73.89	Other diseases of spleen
D75.82	Heparin induced thrombocytopenia (HIT)
D78.01	Intraoperative hemorrhage and hematoma of the spleen complicating a procedure on the spleen
D78.02	Intraoperative hemorrhage and hematoma of the spleen complicating other procedure
D78.11	Accidental puncture and laceration of the spleen during a procedure on the spleen
D78.12	Accidental puncture and laceration of the spleen during other procedure
D78.21	Postprocedural hemorrhage of the spleen following a procedure on the spleen
D78.22	Postprocedural hemorrhage of the spleen following other procedure
D78.31	Postprocedural hematoma of the spleen following a procedure on the spleen
D78.32	Postprocedural hematoma of the spleen following other procedure
D78.33	Postprocedural seroma of the spleen following a procedure on the spleen
D78.34	Postprocedural seroma of the spleen following other procedure
D78.81	Other intraoperative complications of the spleen
D78.89	Other postprocedural complications of the spleen
D86.89	Sarcoidosis of other sites
D89.41	Monoclonal mast cell activation syndrome
D89.42	Idiopathic mast cell activation syndrome
D89.43	Secondary mast cell activation
D89.82	Autoimmune lymphoproliferative syndrome [ALPS]
E75.22	Gaucher disease
I72.8	Aneurysm of other specified arteries
K74.69	Other cirrhosis of liver
K76.6	Portal hypertension
P15.1	Birth injury to spleen ◨
Q89.09	Congenital malformations of spleen
S36.021A	Major contusion of spleen, initial encounter
S36.031A	Moderate laceration of spleen, initial encounter
S36.032A	Major laceration of spleen, initial encounter

AMA: 38120 2018,Jan,8; 2017,Jan,8; 2016,Jan,13; 2015,Jan,16

Relative Value Units/Medicare Edits

Non-Facility RVU	Work	PE	MP	Total
38120	17.07	10.06	4.06	31.19
Facility RVU	Work	PE	MP	Total
38120	17.07	10.06	4.06	31.19

	FUD	Status	MUE	Modifiers				IOM Reference
38120	90	A	1(2)	51	N/A	62*	80	None

* with documentation

38300-38305

38300 Drainage of lymph node abscess or lymphadenitis; simple
38305   extensive

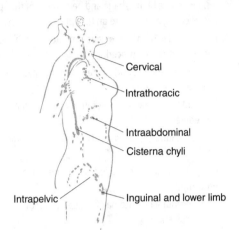

An abscess of a lymph node, or an inflamed
lymph node (lymphadenitis) is drained

Explanation

The physician performs this procedure to drain inflamed lymph nodes. The physician makes an incision over the affected lymph node and the abscess or infection is drained. The wound is irrigated and closed with sutures or Steri-strips. Report 38305 if the procedure is extensive.

Coding Tips

For biopsy or excision of lymph nodes, superficial, open, see 38500; by needle, see 38505; open deep cervical, see 38510; if excision of deep scalene fat pad is also performed, see 38520; deep axillary, see 38525; deep internal mammary, see 38530. Injection for sentinel node identification is reported with 38792.

ICD-10-CM Diagnostic Codes

I88.1	Chronic lymphadenitis, except mesenteric
I88.8	Other nonspecific lymphadenitis
I89.1	Lymphangitis
I89.8	Other specified noninfective disorders of lymphatic vessels and lymph nodes
L03.121	Acute lymphangitis of right axilla ☑
L03.122	Acute lymphangitis of left axilla ☑
L03.123	Acute lymphangitis of right upper limb ☑
L03.124	Acute lymphangitis of left upper limb ☑
L03.125	Acute lymphangitis of right lower limb ☑
L03.126	Acute lymphangitis of left lower limb ☑
L03.212	Acute lymphangitis of face
L03.222	Acute lymphangitis of neck
L03.321	Acute lymphangitis of abdominal wall
L03.322	Acute lymphangitis of back [any part except buttock]
L03.323	Acute lymphangitis of chest wall
L03.324	Acute lymphangitis of groin
L03.325	Acute lymphangitis of perineum
L03.326	Acute lymphangitis of umbilicus
L03.327	Acute lymphangitis of buttock
L03.891	Acute lymphangitis of head [any part, except face]
L03.898	Acute lymphangitis of other sites

L04.0	Acute lymphadenitis of face, head and neck
L04.1	Acute lymphadenitis of trunk
L04.2	Acute lymphadenitis of upper limb
L04.3	Acute lymphadenitis of lower limb
L04.8	Acute lymphadenitis of other sites
R59.0	Localized enlarged lymph nodes
R59.1	Generalized enlarged lymph nodes

AMA: 38300 2014,Jan,11 **38305** 2014,Jan,11

Relative Value Units/Medicare Edits

Non-Facility RVU	Work	PE	MP	Total
38300	2.36	7.31	0.59	10.26
38305	6.68	6.23	1.63	14.54
Facility RVU	**Work**	**PE**	**MP**	**Total**
38300	2.36	3.21	0.59	6.16
38305	6.68	6.23	1.63	14.54

	FUD	Status	MUE	Modifiers				IOM Reference
38300	10	A	1(3)	51	N/A	N/A	N/A	None
38305	90	A	1(3)	51	N/A	N/A	N/A	

* with documentation

Terms To Know

acute. Sudden, severe. Documentation and reporting of an acute condition is important to establishing medical necessity.

acute lymphadenitis. Sudden, severe inflammation, infection, and swelling in lymphatic tissue.

chronic. Persistent, continuing, or recurring.

closure. Repairing an incision or wound by suture or other means.

drain. Device that creates a channel to allow fluid from a cavity, wound, or infected area to exit the body.

incision. Act of cutting into tissue or an organ.

infection. Presence of microorganisms in body tissues that may result in cellular damage.

irrigate. Washing out, lavage.

lymph. Clear, sometimes yellow fluid that flows through the tissues in the body, through the lymphatic system, and into the blood stream.

lymph nodes. Bean-shaped structures along the lymphatic vessels that intercept and destroy foreign materials in the tissue and bloodstream.

lymphangitis. Inflammation of the lymph channels most often caused by streptococcus.

lymphatic system. Lymphatic capillaries, vessels, lymph nodes, spleen, thymus gland, and bone marrow.

38308

38308   Lymphangiotomy or other operations on lymphatic channels

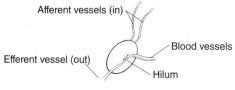

Schematic of lymph node

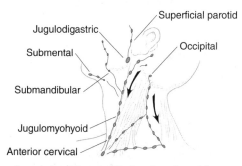

Lymphatic drainage of the head, neck, and face

Explanation

This procedure is performed to correct lymphangiomas, which are primarily found in the neck. The physician makes an incision over the site of the tumor. The tissue, muscles, nerves, and blood vessels are dissected away from the tumor. The tumor is removed. The incision is closed with sutures, wound drains are placed, and a sterile dressing is applied.

Coding Tips

For biopsy or excision of lymph nodes, superficial, open, see 38500; by needle, see 38505; open deep cervical, see 38510; if excision of deep scalene fat pad is also performed, see 38520; deep axillary, see 38525; deep internal mammary, see 38530. Injection for sentinel node identification is reported with 38792.

ICD-10-CM Diagnostic Codes

D18.1   Lymphangioma, any site

AMA: 38308 2014,Jan,11

Relative Value Units/Medicare Edits

Non-Facility RVU	Work	PE	MP	Total
38308	6.81	5.27	1.51	13.59
Facility RVU	Work	PE	MP	Total
38308	6.81	5.27	1.51	13.59

	FUD	Status	MUE	Modifiers				IOM Reference
38308	90	A	1(3)	51	N/A	62*	80	None

* with documentation

38380-38382

38380   Suture and/or ligation of thoracic duct; cervical approach
38381   thoracic approach
38382   abdominal approach

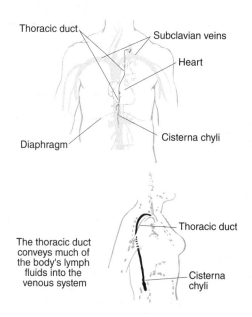

The thoracic duct conveys much of the body's lymph fluids into the venous system

Explanation

The thoracic duct is sutured or ligated. The thoracic duct is a tubular structure, approximately 2 to 3 mm in diameter, that originates in the cisterna chyli, which lies above the second lumbar vertebral body. It ascends on the right, anterior to the vertebral bodies, entering the chest through the aortic hiatus. At the fourth or fifth thoracic vertebra, it crosses to the left and empties into the left jugulosubclavian venous junction. Tears or injury can occur in any segment (cervical, thoracic, abdominal) and the approach is dependent on the site of the leak. An incision is made in the left neck, right or left chest, or abdomen. The involved compartment is drained of all effluent and the leak identified. The duct is ligated a few centimeters below the leak and also a few centimeters above it. Dry gauze is placed at the site of the leak to ensure that the ligation has completely sealed the leak. When it has been determined that the leak is completely sealed, the gauze is removed and glue or other sealant is applied to the area. If the leak is repaired by thoracotomy, chest tubes are placed. Incisions are closed. Report 38380 for a cervical approach; 38381 for a thoracic approach; or 38382 for an abdominal approach.

Coding Tips

When one of these procedures is performed with another separately identifiable procedure, the highest dollar value code is listed as the primary procedure and subsequent procedures are appended with modifier 51. For lymphangiotomy or other operations on the lymphatic channels, see 38308.

ICD-10-CM Diagnostic Codes

I89.8   Other specified noninfective disorders of lymphatic vessels and lymph nodes
S27.898A   Other injury of other specified intrathoracic organs, initial encounter

AMA: 38380 2014,Jan,11 38381 2014,Jan,11 38382 2014,Jan,11

Lymph Nodes

Relative Value Units/Medicare Edits

Non-Facility RVU	Work	PE	MP	Total
38380	8.46	6.85	1.36	16.67
38381	13.38	7.06	3.05	23.49
38382	10.65	7.0	2.44	20.09
Facility RVU	Work	PE	MP	Total
38380	8.46	6.85	1.36	16.67
38381	13.38	7.06	3.05	23.49
38382	10.65	7.0	2.44	20.09

	FUD	Status	MUE	Modifiers				IOM Reference
38380	90	A	1(2)	51	N/A	62*	80	None
38381	90	A	1(2)	51	N/A	62*	80	
38382	90	A	1(2)	51	N/A	62*	80	

* with documentation

Terms To Know

acute lymphadenitis. Sudden, severe inflammation, infection, and swelling in lymphatic tissue.

approach. Method or anatomical location used to gain access to a body organ or specific area for procedures.

chronic. Persistent, continuing, or recurring.

chylous. Pertaining to chyle, a white or yellowish fluid transferred into the lymphatic system from the intestines as a part of the digestion process.

dissect. Cut apart or separate tissue for surgical purposes or for visual or microscopic study.

ligation. Tying off a blood vessel or duct with a suture or a soft, thin wire.

lymphangitis. Inflammation of the lymph channels most often caused by streptococcus.

pleura. One of the two membranes that surround the lungs. The visceral pleura encases the lung and the parietal pleura lines the inner chest walls.

thoracic duct. Large vessel that drains lymph from the lymphatic vessels and trunks of the left side of the body, lower abdomen and pelvic area, and lower extremities.

38500-38531

38500	Biopsy or excision of lymph node(s); open, superficial
38505	by needle, superficial (eg, cervical, inguinal, axillary)
38510	open, deep cervical node(s)
38520	open, deep cervical node(s) with excision scalene fat pad
38525	open, deep axillary node(s)
38530	open, internal mammary node(s)
38531	open, inguinofemoral node(s)

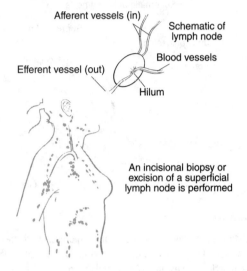

An incisional biopsy or excision of a superficial lymph node is performed

Explanation

The physician performs a biopsy on or removes one or more superficial lymph nodes. The physician makes a small incision through the skin overlying the lymph node. The tissue is dissected to the node. A small piece of the node and surrounding tissue are removed, or the node may be removed. The incision is repaired with a layered closure. Report 38505 if a needle is used; report 38510 if deep cervical nodes are biopsied; report 38520 if deep cervical nodes with excision scalene fat pads are checked; report 38525 if deep axillary nodes are biopsied. For examination of the internal mammary nodes, report 38530; for biopsy or excision of the inguinofemoral nodes, report 38531.

Coding Tips

Do not report 38500 with 38700–38780. Do not report 38530 with 38720–38746. When imaging guidance is performed, see 76942, 77002, 77012, or 77021. For fine needle aspiration, see 10004–10012 and 10021. For evaluation of fine needle aspirate, see 88172–88173. For injection of a sentinel node for identification, see 38792.

ICD-10-CM Diagnostic Codes

A15.4	Tuberculosis of intrathoracic lymph nodes
A18.2	Tuberculous peripheral lymphadenopathy
A50.06	Early cutaneous congenital syphilis
A50.07	Early mucocutaneous congenital syphilis
A50.1	Early congenital syphilis, latent
B20	Human immunodeficiency virus [HIV] disease
C43.51	Malignant melanoma of anal skin
C43.52	Malignant melanoma of skin of breast
C43.59	Malignant melanoma of other part of trunk
C43.61	Malignant melanoma of right upper limb, including shoulder ☑
C4A.0	Merkel cell carcinoma of lip

Lymph Nodes

C4A.4	Merkel cell carcinoma of scalp and neck
C4A.52	Merkel cell carcinoma of skin of breast
C4A.59	Merkel cell carcinoma of other part of trunk
C4A.61	Merkel cell carcinoma of right upper limb, including shoulder ☑
C50.011	Malignant neoplasm of nipple and areola, right female breast ♀ ☑
C50.111	Malignant neoplasm of central portion of right female breast ♀ ☑
C50.121	Malignant neoplasm of central portion of right male breast ♂ ☑
C50.211	Malignant neoplasm of upper-inner quadrant of right female breast ♀ ☑
C50.221	Malignant neoplasm of upper-inner quadrant of right male breast ♂ ☑
C50.311	Malignant neoplasm of lower-inner quadrant of right female breast ♀ ☑
C50.321	Malignant neoplasm of lower-inner quadrant of right male breast ♂ ☑
C50.411	Malignant neoplasm of upper-outer quadrant of right female breast ♀ ☑
C50.421	Malignant neoplasm of upper-outer quadrant of right male breast ♂ ☑
C50.511	Malignant neoplasm of lower-outer quadrant of right female breast ♀ ☑
C50.521	Malignant neoplasm of lower-outer quadrant of right male breast ♂ ☑
C50.611	Malignant neoplasm of axillary tail of right female breast ♀ ☑
C50.811	Malignant neoplasm of overlapping sites of right female breast ♀ ☑
C81.04	Nodular lymphocyte predominant Hodgkin lymphoma, lymph nodes of axilla and upper limb
C81.05	Nodular lymphocyte predominant Hodgkin lymphoma, lymph nodes of inguinal region and lower limb
C81.09	Nodular lymphocyte predominant Hodgkin lymphoma, extranodal and solid organ sites
C81.15	Nodular sclerosis Hodgkin lymphoma, lymph nodes of inguinal region and lower limb
C81.31	Lymphocyte depleted Hodgkin lymphoma, lymph nodes of head, face, and neck
C81.34	Lymphocyte depleted Hodgkin lymphoma, lymph nodes of axilla and upper limb
C81.39	Lymphocyte depleted Hodgkin lymphoma, extranodal and solid organ sites
C81.44	Lymphocyte-rich Hodgkin lymphoma, lymph nodes of axilla and upper limb
C81.49	Lymphocyte-rich Hodgkin lymphoma, extranodal and solid organ sites
C82.04	Follicular lymphoma grade I, lymph nodes of axilla and upper limb
C82.14	Follicular lymphoma grade II, lymph nodes of axilla and upper limb
C82.19	Follicular lymphoma grade II, extranodal and solid organ sites
C82.31	Follicular lymphoma grade IIIa, lymph nodes of head, face, and neck
C82.34	Follicular lymphoma grade IIIa, lymph nodes of axilla and upper limb
C82.54	Diffuse follicle center lymphoma, lymph nodes of axilla and upper limb
C82.59	Diffuse follicle center lymphoma, extranodal and solid organ sites
C82.61	Cutaneous follicle center lymphoma, lymph nodes of head, face, and neck
C82.69	Cutaneous follicle center lymphoma, extranodal and solid organ sites
C83.14	Mantle cell lymphoma, lymph nodes of axilla and upper limb
C83.19	Mantle cell lymphoma, extranodal and solid organ sites
C83.31	Diffuse large B-cell lymphoma, lymph nodes of head, face, and neck
C83.34	Diffuse large B-cell lymphoma, lymph nodes of axilla and upper limb
C83.39	Diffuse large B-cell lymphoma, extranodal and solid organ sites
C83.54	Lymphoblastic (diffuse) lymphoma, lymph nodes of axilla and upper limb
C83.55	Lymphoblastic (diffuse) lymphoma, lymph nodes of inguinal region and lower limb
C83.59	Lymphoblastic (diffuse) lymphoma, extranodal and solid organ sites
C83.71	Burkitt lymphoma, lymph nodes of head, face, and neck
C83.74	Burkitt lymphoma, lymph nodes of axilla and upper limb
C83.75	Burkitt lymphoma, lymph nodes of inguinal region and lower limb
C84.04	Mycosis fungoides, lymph nodes of axilla and upper limb
C84.19	Sezary disease, extranodal and solid organ sites
C84.44	Peripheral T-cell lymphoma, not classified, lymph nodes of axilla and upper limb
C84.49	Peripheral T-cell lymphoma, not classified, extranodal and solid organ sites
C84.61	Anaplastic large cell lymphoma, ALK-positive, lymph nodes of head, face, and neck
C84.64	Anaplastic large cell lymphoma, ALK-positive, lymph nodes of axilla and upper limb
C84.74	Anaplastic large cell lymphoma, ALK-negative, lymph nodes of axilla and upper limb
C84.79	Anaplastic large cell lymphoma, ALK-negative, extranodal and solid organ sites
C85.21	Mediastinal (thymic) large B-cell lymphoma, lymph nodes of head, face, and neck
C85.29	Mediastinal (thymic) large B-cell lymphoma, extranodal and solid organ sites
C88.4	Extranodal marginal zone B-cell lymphoma of mucosa-associated lymphoid tissue [MALT-lymphoma]
D03.52	Melanoma in situ of breast (skin) (soft tissue)
D03.59	Melanoma in situ of other part of trunk
D03.61	Melanoma in situ of right upper limb, including shoulder ☑
D05.11	Intraductal carcinoma in situ of right breast ☑
D36.0	Benign neoplasm of lymph nodes
D86.1	Sarcoidosis of lymph nodes
D86.2	Sarcoidosis of lung with sarcoidosis of lymph nodes
I88.1	Chronic lymphadenitis, except mesenteric
R59.0	Localized enlarged lymph nodes
R59.1	Generalized enlarged lymph nodes

AMA: **38500** 2019,Feb,8; 2018,Jan,8; 2017,Jan,8; 2016,Jan,13; 2015,Jan,16 **38505** 2019,Feb,8; 2018,Jan,8; 2017,Jan,8; 2016,Jan,13; 2015,Jan,16 **38510**

Lymph Nodes

2020,Dec,11; 2019,Feb,8; 2018,Jan,8; 2017,Jan,8; 2016,Jan,13; 2015,Jan,16
38520 2019,Feb,8; 2018,Jan,8; 2017,Jan,8; 2016,Jan,13; 2015,Jan,16 **38525**
2019,Feb,8; 2018,Jan,8; 2017,Jan,8; 2016,Jan,13; 2015,Mar,5; 2015,Jan,16 **38530**
2019,Feb,8; 2018,Jan,8; 2017,Jan,8; 2016,Jan,13; 2015,Jan,16 **38531** 2019,Feb,8

Relative Value Units/Medicare Edits

Non-Facility RVU	Work	PE	MP	Total
38500	3.79	5.4	0.86	10.05
38505	1.14	2.36	0.11	3.61
38510	6.74	7.63	1.25	15.62
38520	7.03	5.22	1.46	13.71
38525	6.43	5.03	1.53	12.99
38530	8.34	6.6	1.67	16.61
38531	6.74	4.91	1.46	13.11

Facility RVU	Work	PE	MP	Total
38500	3.79	2.88	0.86	7.53
38505	1.14	0.77	0.11	2.02
38510	6.74	4.28	1.25	12.27
38520	7.03	5.22	1.46	13.71
38525	6.43	5.03	1.53	12.99
38530	8.34	6.6	1.67	16.61
38531	6.74	4.91	1.46	13.11

	FUD	Status	MUE	Modifiers				IOM Reference
38500	10	A	2(3)	51	50	N/A	N/A	None
38505	0	A	2(3)	51	50	N/A	N/A	
38510	10	A	1(2)	51	50	N/A	N/A	
38520	90	A	1(2)	51	50	N/A	N/A	
38525	90	A	1(2)	51	50	N/A	N/A	
38530	90	A	1(2)	51	50	62*	80	
38531	90	A	1(2)	51	50	N/A	80*	

* with documentation

38542

38542   Dissection, deep jugular node(s)

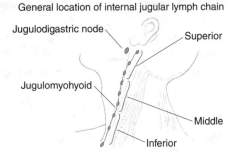

General location of internal jugular lymph chain

Jugulodigastric node

Superior

Jugulomyohyoid

Middle

Inferior

Explanation

The physician makes an incision over one of three jugular groups and retracts tissue. The nodes are isolated and excised. The incision is closed by sutures.

Coding Tips

If significant additional time and effort is documented, append modifier 22 and submit a cover letter and operative report. For excision of a cystic hygroma, axillary or cervical, see 38550; with deep neurovascular dissection, see 38555. For complete cervical lymphadenectomy, see 38720.

ICD-10-CM Diagnostic Codes

C08.0	Malignant neoplasm of submandibular gland
C32.0	Malignant neoplasm of glottis
C32.1	Malignant neoplasm of supraglottis
C32.3	Malignant neoplasm of laryngeal cartilage
C4A.4	Merkel cell carcinoma of scalp and neck
C73	Malignant neoplasm of thyroid gland
C75.0	Malignant neoplasm of parathyroid gland
C77.0	Secondary and unspecified malignant neoplasm of lymph nodes of head, face and neck
C7B.01	Secondary carcinoid tumors of distant lymph nodes
C7B.09	Secondary carcinoid tumors of other sites
C7B.1	Secondary Merkel cell carcinoma
C7B.8	Other secondary neuroendocrine tumors
C81.71	Other Hodgkin lymphoma, lymph nodes of head, face, and neck
C83.11	Mantle cell lymphoma, lymph nodes of head, face, and neck
C83.31	Diffuse large B-cell lymphoma, lymph nodes of head, face, and neck
C83.51	Lymphoblastic (diffuse) lymphoma, lymph nodes of head, face, and neck
C83.81	Other non-follicular lymphoma, lymph nodes of head, face, and neck
C84.41	Peripheral T-cell lymphoma, not classified, lymph nodes of head, face, and neck
C84.61	Anaplastic large cell lymphoma, ALK-positive, lymph nodes of head, face, and neck
C84.71	Anaplastic large cell lymphoma, ALK-negative, lymph nodes of head, face, and neck
C85.21	Mediastinal (thymic) large B-cell lymphoma, lymph nodes of head, face, and neck

C88.4	Extranodal marginal zone B-cell lymphoma of mucosa-associated lymphoid tissue [MALT-lymphoma]		
D18.1	Lymphangioma, any site		
R59.0	Localized enlarged lymph nodes		
R59.1	Generalized enlarged lymph nodes		

AMA: 38542 2019,Feb,8; 2018,Jan,8; 2017,Jan,8; 2016,Jan,13; 2015,Jan,16

Relative Value Units/Medicare Edits

Non-Facility RVU	Work	PE	MP	Total
38542	7.95	5.9	1.3	15.15
Facility RVU	Work	PE	MP	Total
38542	7.95	5.9	1.3	15.15

	FUD	Status	MUE	Modifiers				IOM Reference
38542	90	A	1(2)	51	50	62*	80	None

* with documentation

Terms To Know

dissection. Separating by cutting tissue or body structures apart.

lymph nodes. Bean-shaped structures along the lymphatic vessels that intercept and destroy foreign materials in the tissue and bloodstream.

lymphangioma. Benign, malformed lymph channels.

malignant. Any condition tending to progress toward death, specifically an invasive tumor with a loss of cellular differentiation that has the ability to spread or metastasize to other body areas.

neoplasm. New abnormal growth, tumor.

radical. Extensive surgery.

secondary. Second in order of occurrence or importance, or appearing during the course of another disease or condition.

38550-38555

38550	Excision of cystic hygroma, axillary or cervical; without deep neurovascular dissection
38555	with deep neurovascular dissection

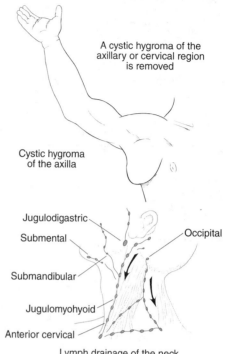

A cystic hygroma of the axillary or cervical region is removed

Cystic hygroma of the axilla

Jugulodigastric
Submental
Submandibular
Jugulomyohyoid
Anterior cervical
Occipital

Lymph drainage of the neck

Explanation

The physician removes a cystic hygroma, also called a lymphangioma, from the neck or axilla. A cystic hygroma is a congenital anomaly typically found in the neck or axilla, sometimes extending into the head or chest. Cystic hygromas may be diagnosed during fetal ultrasound or evident at birth. The majority are evident by age 2. Rarely, they are diagnosed into adulthood. Because cystic hygromas can be very large and can extend into multiple areas of the head, neck, and chest, the location and size of the incision will vary. A surgical incision is made in the area of the cyst. If the hygroma does not involve deeper neurovascular structures, the physician dissects away the surrounding tissue and exposes the sac. The sac is excised. The incision is closed and a dry, sterile dressing applied. A larger cystic hygroma may not have a defined capsule and may wrap around blood vessels, nerves, and muscles. In that case, the surgeon dissects the tissue around these vital structures before removing the cystic hygroma. Cystic hygromas may be removed in part or in full depending on whether excision would compromise nerves or blood vessels. If the entire cystic hygroma cannot be excised, the surgeon may cauterize the part remaining. Report 38550 for excision of a cystic hygroma without deep neurovascular dissection; report 38555 when deep neurovascular dissection is required.

Coding Tips

These procedures may be performed during multiple surgical sessions as staged procedures. To indicate that a staged or related procedure is performed during the postoperative period by the same physician, append modifier 58. When 38550 or 38555 is performed on a neonate or infant with a body weight less than or equal to 4 kg, append modifier 63 to account for the additional complexity and work associated with the procedure. If significant additional time and effort is documented, append modifier 22 and submit a cover letter and operative report.

Lymph Nodes

ICD-10-CM Diagnostic Codes

D18.1   Lymphangioma, any site

AMA: 38550 2014,Jan,11 **38555** 2014,Jan,11

Relative Value Units/Medicare Edits

Non-Facility RVU	Work	PE	MP	Total
38550	7.11	6.53	1.74	15.38
38555	15.59	10.85	3.82	30.26
Facility RVU	**Work**	**PE**	**MP**	**Total**
38550	7.11	6.53	1.74	15.38
38555	15.59	10.85	3.82	30.26

	FUD	Status	MUE	Modifiers				IOM Reference
38550	90	A	1(3)	51	N/A	N/A	80*	None
38555	90	A	1(3)	51	N/A	62*	80	

* with documentation

Terms To Know

anomaly. Irregularity in the structure or position of an organ or tissue.

axillary. Area under the arm.

cauterize. Heat or chemicals used to burn or cut.

cervical. Relation to the cervical spine or to the cervix.

congenital. Present at birth, occurring through heredity or an influence during gestation up to the moment of birth.

cystic hygroma. Large watery cyst of the lymphatic channel that frequently occurs in the neck and shoulder region.

dissection. Separating by cutting tissue or body structures apart.

drain. Device that creates a channel to allow fluid from a cavity, wound, or infected area to exit the body.

excision. Surgical removal of an organ or tissue.

lymphangioma. Benign, malformed lymph channels.

tissue. Group of similar cells with a similar function that form definite structures and organs. Tissue types include epithelial tissue, muscle tissue, connective tissue, and nervous tissue.

38562-38564

38562   Limited lymphadenectomy for staging (separate procedure); pelvic and para-aortic

38564   retroperitoneal (aortic and/or splenic)

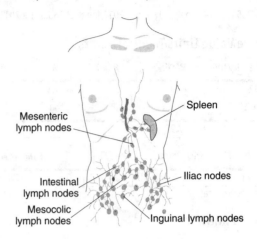

Explanation

The physician makes a midline abdominal incision just below the navel. The surrounding tissue, nerves, and blood vessels are dissected away, and the pelvic and/or para-aortic lymph nodes are visualized. The nodes are removed. The wound is closed with sutures or staples. Report 38564 if retroperitoneal lymphadenectomy is performed.

Coding Tips

These separate procedures, by definition, are usually a component of a more complex service and are not identified separately. When performed alone or with other unrelated procedures/services they may be reported. If performed alone, list the code; if performed with other procedures/services, list the code and append modifier 59 or an X{EPSU} modifier. For a laparoscopic retroperitoneal biopsy, see 38570; with bilateral total pelvic lymphadenectomy, see 38571; if periaortic lymph node sampling is also performed, see 38572.

ICD-10-CM Diagnostic Codes

C17.0   Malignant neoplasm of duodenum
C18.5   Malignant neoplasm of splenic flexure
C19   Malignant neoplasm of rectosigmoid junction
C20   Malignant neoplasm of rectum
C24.0   Malignant neoplasm of extrahepatic bile duct
C26.1   Malignant neoplasm of spleen
C45.1   Mesothelioma of peritoneum
C48.0   Malignant neoplasm of retroperitoneum
C48.1   Malignant neoplasm of specified parts of peritoneum
C48.8   Malignant neoplasm of overlapping sites of retroperitoneum and peritoneum
C53.0   Malignant neoplasm of endocervix ♀
C53.1   Malignant neoplasm of exocervix ♀
C53.8   Malignant neoplasm of overlapping sites of cervix uteri ♀
C54.0   Malignant neoplasm of isthmus uteri ♀
C54.1   Malignant neoplasm of endometrium ♀
C54.2   Malignant neoplasm of myometrium ♀
C54.8   Malignant neoplasm of overlapping sites of corpus uteri ♀
C56.1   Malignant neoplasm of right ovary ♀ ☑

Lymph Nodes

C56.2	Malignant neoplasm of left ovary ♀ ☑
C56.3	Malignant neoplasm of bilateral ovaries ♀ ☑
C57.01	Malignant neoplasm of right fallopian tube ♀ ☑
C57.02	Malignant neoplasm of left fallopian tube ♀ ☑
C57.21	Malignant neoplasm of right round ligament ♀ ☑
C57.22	Malignant neoplasm of left round ligament ♀ ☑
C57.3	Malignant neoplasm of parametrium ♀
C60.0	Malignant neoplasm of prepuce ♂
C60.1	Malignant neoplasm of glans penis ♂
C61	Malignant neoplasm of prostate ♂
C62.11	Malignant neoplasm of descended right testis ♂ ☑
C62.12	Malignant neoplasm of descended left testis ♂ ☑
C63.2	Malignant neoplasm of scrotum ♂
C64.1	Malignant neoplasm of right kidney, except renal pelvis ☑
C64.2	Malignant neoplasm of left kidney, except renal pelvis ☑
C66.1	Malignant neoplasm of right ureter ☑
C66.2	Malignant neoplasm of left ureter ☑
C67.0	Malignant neoplasm of trigone of bladder
C67.1	Malignant neoplasm of dome of bladder
C67.2	Malignant neoplasm of lateral wall of bladder
C67.3	Malignant neoplasm of anterior wall of bladder
C67.4	Malignant neoplasm of posterior wall of bladder
C67.5	Malignant neoplasm of bladder neck
C67.6	Malignant neoplasm of ureteric orifice
C67.8	Malignant neoplasm of overlapping sites of bladder
C68.0	Malignant neoplasm of urethra
C68.1	Malignant neoplasm of paraurethral glands
C68.8	Malignant neoplasm of overlapping sites of urinary organs
C76.3	Malignant neoplasm of pelvis
C7B.04	Secondary carcinoid tumors of peritoneum
C81.46	Lymphocyte-rich Hodgkin lymphoma, intrapelvic lymph nodes
C81.76	Other Hodgkin lymphoma, intrapelvic lymph nodes
C82.06	Follicular lymphoma grade I, intrapelvic lymph nodes
C82.16	Follicular lymphoma grade II, intrapelvic lymph nodes
C82.36	Follicular lymphoma grade IIIa, intrapelvic lymph nodes
C82.46	Follicular lymphoma grade IIIb, intrapelvic lymph nodes
C82.56	Diffuse follicle center lymphoma, intrapelvic lymph nodes
C82.66	Cutaneous follicle center lymphoma, intrapelvic lymph nodes
C82.86	Other types of follicular lymphoma, intrapelvic lymph nodes
C83.06	Small cell B-cell lymphoma, intrapelvic lymph nodes
C83.16	Mantle cell lymphoma, intrapelvic lymph nodes
C83.36	Diffuse large B-cell lymphoma, intrapelvic lymph nodes
C83.56	Lymphoblastic (diffuse) lymphoma, intrapelvic lymph nodes
C83.76	Burkitt lymphoma, intrapelvic lymph nodes
C83.86	Other non-follicular lymphoma, intrapelvic lymph nodes
C84.06	Mycosis fungoides, intrapelvic lymph nodes
C84.16	Sezary disease, intrapelvic lymph nodes
C84.46	Peripheral T-cell lymphoma, not classified, intrapelvic lymph nodes
C84.66	Anaplastic large cell lymphoma, ALK-positive, intrapelvic lymph nodes
C84.76	Anaplastic large cell lymphoma, ALK-negative, intrapelvic lymph nodes
C84.Z6	Other mature T/NK-cell lymphomas, intrapelvic lymph nodes
C85.26	Mediastinal (thymic) large B-cell lymphoma, intrapelvic lymph nodes
C85.86	Other specified types of non-Hodgkin lymphoma, intrapelvic lymph nodes
C85.89	Other specified types of non-Hodgkin lymphoma, extranodal and solid organ sites
D01.1	Carcinoma in situ of rectosigmoid junction
D01.2	Carcinoma in situ of rectum
D12.7	Benign neoplasm of rectosigmoid junction
D12.8	Benign neoplasm of rectum
D12.9	Benign neoplasm of anus and anal canal
D37.5	Neoplasm of uncertain behavior of rectum
D3A.026	Benign carcinoid tumor of the rectum
D48.3	Neoplasm of uncertain behavior of retroperitoneum

AMA: **38562** 2019,Feb,8; 2018,Jan,8; 2017,Jan,8; 2016,Jan,13; 2015,Jan,16
38564 2019,Feb,8

Relative Value Units/Medicare Edits

Non-Facility RVU	Work	PE	MP	Total
38562	11.06	7.76	1.93	20.75
38564	11.38	7.04	2.4	20.82
Facility RVU	Work	PE	MP	Total
38562	11.06	7.76	1.93	20.75
38564	11.38	7.04	2.4	20.82

	FUD	Status	MUE	Modifiers				IOM Reference
38562	90	A	1(2)	51	N/A	62*	80	None
38564	90	A	1(2)	51	N/A	62*	80	

* with documentation

Terms To Know

dissect. Cut apart or separate tissue for surgical purposes or for visual or microscopic study.

lymph nodes. Bean-shaped structures along the lymphatic vessels that intercept and destroy foreign materials in the tissue and bloodstream.

lymphadenectomy. Dissection of lymph nodes free from the vessels and removal for examination by frozen section in a separate procedure to detect early-stage metastases.

retroperitoneal. Located behind the peritoneum, the membrane that lines the abdominopelvic walls and forms a covering for the internal organs.

staging. Determination of the course of a disease, as in the case of a malignancy, to determine whether the malignancy is confined to the primary tumor, has spread to one or more lymph nodes, or has metastasized.

Lymph Nodes

38570-38573

38570 Laparoscopy, surgical; with retroperitoneal lymph node sampling (biopsy), single or multiple
38571 with bilateral total pelvic lymphadenectomy
38572 with bilateral total pelvic lymphadenectomy and peri-aortic lymph node sampling (biopsy), single or multiple
38573 Laparoscopy, surgical; with bilateral total pelvic lymphadenectomy and peri-aortic lymph node sampling, peritoneal washings, peritoneal biopsy(ies), omentectomy, and diaphragmatic washings, including diaphragmatic and other serosal biopsy(ies), when performed

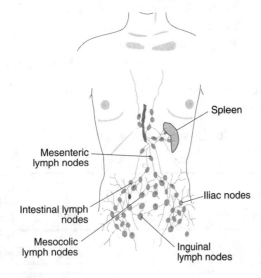

Spleen

Mesenteric lymph nodes

Intestinal lymph nodes

Iliac nodes

Mesocolic lymph nodes

Inguinal lymph nodes

Explanation

The physician performs a surgical laparoscopy. A trocar is placed at the umbilicus into the abdominal or retroperitoneal space to insufflate the abdominal, peritoneal, or retroperitoneal space. The laparoscope is placed through the umbilical trocar and additional trocars are placed into the peritoneal or retroperitoneal space. In 38570, retroperitoneal lymph node sampling is also performed. The lymph nodes are identified, dissected free of surrounding structures, and sampled for further separately reported analysis. In 38571, a bilateral pelvic lymphadenectomy is performed. The iliac vessels are identified and the lymph nodes are dissected from the surrounding structures and removed. When dissection is continued to the aorta for periaortic lymph node sampling, report 38572. In 38573, the services from 38571 and 38572 are performed, as well as peritoneal washing and biopsies, an omentectomy (removal of the membrane containing fat, lymph, and blood vessels that acts as a protective layer extending from the stomach to the transverse colon), and diaphragmatic washings. Diaphragmatic and other serosal biopsies are included in the procedure, when performed. When each procedure is complete, the trocars are removed and the incisions are closed.

Coding Tips

Surgical laparoscopy always includes diagnostic laparoscopy. Codes 38571–38573 are bilateral procedures and as such are reported once even if the procedure is performed on both sides. For a diagnostic laparoscopy (peritoneoscopy), see 49320. For biopsy or excision of lymph nodes, see 38500–38542. For drainage of lymphocele to peritoneal cavity, see 49323. Do not report 38573 with 38562, 38564, 38570-38572, 38589, 38770, 38780, 49255, 49320, 49326, 58541-58544, 58548, 58550, or 58552-58554.

ICD-10-CM Diagnostic Codes

C16.8	Malignant neoplasm of overlapping sites of stomach
C17.0	Malignant neoplasm of duodenum
C18.5	Malignant neoplasm of splenic flexure
C19	Malignant neoplasm of rectosigmoid junction
C20	Malignant neoplasm of rectum
C48.1	Malignant neoplasm of specified parts of peritoneum
C54.1	Malignant neoplasm of endometrium ♀
C54.2	Malignant neoplasm of myometrium ♀
C54.3	Malignant neoplasm of fundus uteri ♀
C56.1	Malignant neoplasm of right ovary ♀ ☑
C56.2	Malignant neoplasm of left ovary ♀ ☑
C56.3	Malignant neoplasm of bilateral ovaries ♀ ☑
C61	Malignant neoplasm of prostate ♂
C7B.01	Secondary carcinoid tumors of distant lymph nodes
C7B.04	Secondary carcinoid tumors of peritoneum
C7B.1	Secondary Merkel cell carcinoma
C7B.8	Other secondary neuroendocrine tumors
C82.03	Follicular lymphoma grade I, intra-abdominal lymph nodes
C82.13	Follicular lymphoma grade II, intra-abdominal lymph nodes
C82.33	Follicular lymphoma grade IIIa, intra-abdominal lymph nodes
C82.43	Follicular lymphoma grade IIIb, intra-abdominal lymph nodes
C82.53	Diffuse follicle center lymphoma, intra-abdominal lymph nodes
C82.63	Cutaneous follicle center lymphoma, intra-abdominal lymph nodes
C82.83	Other types of follicular lymphoma, intra-abdominal lymph nodes
C83.13	Mantle cell lymphoma, intra-abdominal lymph nodes
C83.33	Diffuse large B-cell lymphoma, intra-abdominal lymph nodes
C83.53	Lymphoblastic (diffuse) lymphoma, intra-abdominal lymph nodes
C83.83	Other non-follicular lymphoma, intra-abdominal lymph nodes
C84.43	Peripheral T-cell lymphoma, not classified, intra-abdominal lymph nodes
C84.63	Anaplastic large cell lymphoma, ALK-positive, intra-abdominal lymph nodes
C84.73	Anaplastic large cell lymphoma, ALK-negative, intra-abdominal lymph nodes
C84.Z3	Other mature T/NK-cell lymphomas, intra-abdominal lymph nodes
C85.23	Mediastinal (thymic) large B-cell lymphoma, intra-abdominal lymph nodes
C85.83	Other specified types of non-Hodgkin lymphoma, intra-abdominal lymph nodes
C86.2	Enteropathy-type (intestinal) T-cell lymphoma
C86.3	Subcutaneous panniculitis-like T-cell lymphoma
C88.4	Extranodal marginal zone B-cell lymphoma of mucosa-associated lymphoid tissue [MALT-lymphoma]
D48.7	Neoplasm of uncertain behavior of other specified sites
D49.89	Neoplasm of unspecified behavior of other specified sites
D72.89	Other specified disorders of white blood cells
I88.1	Chronic lymphadenitis, except mesenteric
I88.8	Other nonspecific lymphadenitis
I89.8	Other specified noninfective disorders of lymphatic vessels and lymph nodes
R59.0	Localized enlarged lymph nodes
R59.1	Generalized enlarged lymph nodes

Lymph Nodes

AMA: **38570** 2019,Feb,8; 2018,Jan,8; 2017,Jan,8; 2016,Jan,13; 2015,Jan,16 **38571** 2019,Feb,8; 2018,Jan,8; 2017,Jan,8; 2016,Jan,13; 2015,Jan,16 **38572** 2019,Feb,8; 2018,Jan,8; 2017,Jan,8; 2016,Jan,13; 2015,Jan,13; 2015,Jan,16 **38573** 2019,Mar,5; 2018,Apr,10

Relative Value Units/Medicare Edits

Non-Facility RVU	Work	PE	MP	Total
38570	8.49	5.18	1.44	15.11
38571	12.0	5.87	1.49	19.36
38572	15.6	8.67	2.38	26.65
38573	20.0	11.09	3.11	34.2
Facility RVU	Work	PE	MP	Total
38570	8.49	5.18	1.44	15.11
38571	12.0	5.87	1.49	19.36
38572	15.6	8.67	2.38	26.65
38573	20.0	11.09	3.11	34.2

	FUD	Status	MUE	Modifiers				IOM Reference
38570	10	A	1(2)	51	N/A	62	80	None
38571	10	A	1(2)	51	N/A	62	80	
38572	10	A	1(2)	51	N/A	62	80	
38573	10	A	1(2)	51	N/A	62	80	

* with documentation

Terms To Know

biopsy. Tissue or fluid removed for diagnostic purposes through analysis of the cells in the biopsy material.

dissection. (dis. apart; -section, act of cutting) Separating by cutting tissue or body structures apart.

lymphadenectomy. Dissection of lymph nodes free from the vessels and removal for examination by frozen section in a separate procedure to detect early-stage metastases.

peritoneal. Space between the lining of the abdominal wall, or parietal peritoneum, and the surface layer of the abdominal organs, or visceral peritoneum. It contains a thin, watery fluid that keeps the peritoneal surfaces moist.

retroperitoneal. Located behind the peritoneum, the membrane that lines the abdominopelvic walls and forms a covering for the internal organs.

trocar. Cannula or a sharp pointed instrument used to puncture and aspirate fluid from cavities.

38700

38700 Suprahyoid lymphadenectomy

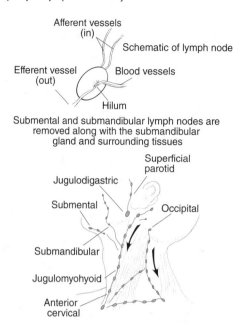

Submental and submandibular lymph nodes are removed along with the submandibular gland and surrounding tissues

Explanation

The physician makes a curved incision beginning below the ear curving down to the top of the hyoid bone and continuing toward the chin. The tissues are dissected and the targeted structures are exposed. The submental and submandibular lymph nodes are removed along with the submandibular gland and surrounding tissues. The incision is sutured with drain if necessary.

Coding Tips

This is a unilateral procedure. If performed bilaterally, some payers require that the service be reported twice with modifier 50 appended to the second code while others require identification of the service only once with modifier 50 appended. Check with individual payers. Modifier 50 identifies a procedure performed identically on the opposite side of the body (mirror image). For complete cervical lymphadenectomy, see 38720; for modified radical neck dissection, see 38724. If significant additional time and effort is documented, append modifier 22 and submit a cover letter and operative report.

ICD-10-CM Diagnostic Codes

C00.8	Malignant neoplasm of overlapping sites of lip
C06.0	Malignant neoplasm of cheek mucosa
C08.0	Malignant neoplasm of submandibular gland
C08.1	Malignant neoplasm of sublingual gland
C32.0	Malignant neoplasm of glottis
C32.1	Malignant neoplasm of supraglottis
C32.3	Malignant neoplasm of laryngeal cartilage
C32.8	Malignant neoplasm of overlapping sites of larynx
C41.0	Malignant neoplasm of bones of skull and face
C41.1	Malignant neoplasm of mandible
C4A.0	Merkel cell carcinoma of lip
C4A.111	Merkel cell carcinoma of right upper eyelid, including canthus ☑
C4A.112	Merkel cell carcinoma of right lower eyelid, including canthus ☑
C4A.121	Merkel cell carcinoma of left upper eyelid, including canthus ☑

Lymph Nodes

C4A.122 Merkel cell carcinoma of left lower eyelid, including canthus ☑

C4A.21 Merkel cell carcinoma of right ear and external auricular canal ☑

C4A.22 Merkel cell carcinoma of left ear and external auricular canal ☑

C4A.31 Merkel cell carcinoma of nose

C4A.39 Merkel cell carcinoma of other parts of face

C4A.4 Merkel cell carcinoma of scalp and neck

C4A.8 Merkel cell carcinoma of overlapping sites

C77.0 Secondary and unspecified malignant neoplasm of lymph nodes of head, face and neck

C7B.01 Secondary carcinoid tumors of distant lymph nodes

C7B.09 Secondary carcinoid tumors of other sites

C7B.1 Secondary Merkel cell carcinoma

C7B.8 Other secondary neuroendocrine tumors

C81.01 Nodular lymphocyte predominant Hodgkin lymphoma, lymph nodes of head, face, and neck

C81.11 Nodular sclerosis Hodgkin lymphoma, lymph nodes of head, face, and neck

C81.21 Mixed cellularity Hodgkin lymphoma, lymph nodes of head, face, and neck

C81.31 Lymphocyte depleted Hodgkin lymphoma, lymph nodes of head, face, and neck

C81.41 Lymphocyte-rich Hodgkin lymphoma, lymph nodes of head, face, and neck

C81.71 Other Hodgkin lymphoma, lymph nodes of head, face, and neck

C82.01 Follicular lymphoma grade I, lymph nodes of head, face, and neck

C82.11 Follicular lymphoma grade II, lymph nodes of head, face, and neck

C82.31 Follicular lymphoma grade IIIa, lymph nodes of head, face, and neck

C82.41 Follicular lymphoma grade IIIb, lymph nodes of head, face, and neck

C82.51 Diffuse follicle center lymphoma, lymph nodes of head, face, and neck

C82.61 Cutaneous follicle center lymphoma, lymph nodes of head, face, and neck

C82.81 Other types of follicular lymphoma, lymph nodes of head, face, and neck

C83.01 Small cell B-cell lymphoma, lymph nodes of head, face, and neck

C83.11 Mantle cell lymphoma, lymph nodes of head, face, and neck

C83.31 Diffuse large B-cell lymphoma, lymph nodes of head, face, and neck

C83.51 Lymphoblastic (diffuse) lymphoma, lymph nodes of head, face, and neck

C83.71 Burkitt lymphoma, lymph nodes of head, face, and neck

C83.81 Other non-follicular lymphoma, lymph nodes of head, face, and neck

C84.01 Mycosis fungoides, lymph nodes of head, face, and neck

C84.11 Sezary disease, lymph nodes of head, face, and neck

C84.41 Peripheral T-cell lymphoma, not classified, lymph nodes of head, face, and neck

C84.61 Anaplastic large cell lymphoma, ALK-positive, lymph nodes of head, face, and neck

C84.71 Anaplastic large cell lymphoma, ALK-negative, lymph nodes of head, face, and neck

C84.Z1 Other mature T/NK-cell lymphomas, lymph nodes of head, face, and neck

C85.21 Mediastinal (thymic) large B-cell lymphoma, lymph nodes of head, face, and neck

C85.81 Other specified types of non-Hodgkin lymphoma, lymph nodes of head, face, and neck

C86.0 Extranodal NK/T-cell lymphoma, nasal type

C88.4 Extranodal marginal zone B-cell lymphoma of mucosa-associated lymphoid tissue [MALT-lymphoma]

C91.40 Hairy cell leukemia not having achieved remission

C96.0 Multifocal and multisystemic (disseminated) Langerhans-cell histiocytosis

C96.21 Aggressive systemic mastocytosis

C96.22 Mast cell sarcoma

C96.29 Other malignant mast cell neoplasm

C96.A Histiocytic sarcoma

C96.Z Other specified malignant neoplasms of lymphoid, hematopoietic and related tissue

D48.7 Neoplasm of uncertain behavior of other specified sites

AMA: **38700** 2020,Dec,11; 2019,Feb,8; 2018,Jan,8; 2017,Jan,8; 2016,Jan,13; 2015,Jan,16

Relative Value Units/Medicare Edits

Non-Facility RVU	Work	PE	MP	Total
38700	12.81	8.77	1.83	23.41
Facility RVU	Work	PE	MP	Total
38700	12.81	8.77	1.83	23.41

	FUD	Status	MUE	Modifiers				IOM Reference
38700	90	A	1(2)	51	50	62*	80	None

* with documentation

Terms To Know

carcinoid tumor. Specific type of slow-growing neuroendocrine tumors. Carcinoid tumors occur most commonly in the hormone producing cells of the gastrointestinal tracts and can also occur in the pancreas, testes, ovaries, or lungs.

hyoid bone. Single, U-shaped bone palpable in the neck above the larynx and below the mandible (lower jaw) with various muscles attached but not articulating with any other bone.

Letterer-Siwe disease. Rare, inherited, and progressive form of Langerhans cell histiocytosis characterized by skin lesions, bleeding tendency, anemia, and enlarged liver and spleen.

lymphoma. Tumors occurring in the lymphoid tissues that are most commonly malignant.

38720

38720   Cervical lymphadenectomy (complete)

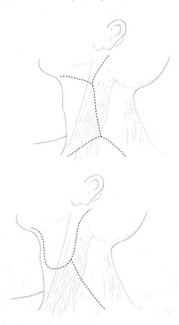

A variety of incisions may be used
for cervical lymphadenectomy

Explanation

The physician makes a large curved incision starting at the ear, going down the neck, and continuing to the chin. Incision may also be made starting at the original incision and continuing down the neck. The skin flaps are folded back and held in place with retractors. The tissue, lymph tissue, blood vessels, nerves, and muscles targeted for removal are dissected away and removed. The incision is closed with sutures.

Coding Tips

This is a unilateral procedure. If performed bilaterally, some payers require that the service be reported twice with modifier 50 appended to the second code while others require identification of the service only once with modifier 50 appended. Check with individual payers. Modifier 50 identifies a procedure performed identically on the opposite side of the body (mirror image). For suprahyoid lymphadenectomy, see 38700; for modified radical neck dissection, see 38724. If significant additional time and effort is documented, append modifier 22 and submit a cover letter and operative report.

ICD-10-CM Diagnostic Codes

C01	Malignant neoplasm of base of tongue
C02.0	Malignant neoplasm of dorsal surface of tongue
C02.1	Malignant neoplasm of border of tongue
C02.2	Malignant neoplasm of ventral surface of tongue
C02.4	Malignant neoplasm of lingual tonsil
C02.8	Malignant neoplasm of overlapping sites of tongue
C04.0	Malignant neoplasm of anterior floor of mouth
C04.1	Malignant neoplasm of lateral floor of mouth
C04.8	Malignant neoplasm of overlapping sites of floor of mouth
C05.0	Malignant neoplasm of hard palate
C05.1	Malignant neoplasm of soft palate
C05.2	Malignant neoplasm of uvula
C06.0	Malignant neoplasm of cheek mucosa
C06.1	Malignant neoplasm of vestibule of mouth
C06.2	Malignant neoplasm of retromolar area
C06.89	Malignant neoplasm of overlapping sites of other parts of mouth
C07	Malignant neoplasm of parotid gland
C08.0	Malignant neoplasm of submandibular gland
C08.1	Malignant neoplasm of sublingual gland
C12	Malignant neoplasm of pyriform sinus
C13.0	Malignant neoplasm of postcricoid region
C13.1	Malignant neoplasm of aryepiglottic fold, hypopharyngeal aspect
C13.2	Malignant neoplasm of posterior wall of hypopharynx
C13.8	Malignant neoplasm of overlapping sites of hypopharynx
C14.2	Malignant neoplasm of Waldeyer's ring
C14.8	Malignant neoplasm of overlapping sites of lip, oral cavity and pharynx
C15.3	Malignant neoplasm of upper third of esophagus
C15.4	Malignant neoplasm of middle third of esophagus
C15.8	Malignant neoplasm of overlapping sites of esophagus
C32.0	Malignant neoplasm of glottis
C32.1	Malignant neoplasm of supraglottis
C32.2	Malignant neoplasm of subglottis
C32.3	Malignant neoplasm of laryngeal cartilage
C32.8	Malignant neoplasm of overlapping sites of larynx
C33	Malignant neoplasm of trachea
C41.1	Malignant neoplasm of mandible
C43.4	Malignant melanoma of scalp and neck
C44.41	Basal cell carcinoma of skin of scalp and neck
C44.42	Squamous cell carcinoma of skin of scalp and neck
C44.49	Other specified malignant neoplasm of skin of scalp and neck
C4A.0	Merkel cell carcinoma of lip
C4A.111	Merkel cell carcinoma of right upper eyelid, including canthus ☑
C4A.112	Merkel cell carcinoma of right lower eyelid, including canthus ☑
C4A.121	Merkel cell carcinoma of left upper eyelid, including canthus ☑
C4A.122	Merkel cell carcinoma of left lower eyelid, including canthus ☑
C4A.21	Merkel cell carcinoma of right ear and external auricular canal ☑
C4A.22	Merkel cell carcinoma of left ear and external auricular canal ☑
C4A.31	Merkel cell carcinoma of nose
C4A.39	Merkel cell carcinoma of other parts of face
C4A.4	Merkel cell carcinoma of scalp and neck
C4A.8	Merkel cell carcinoma of overlapping sites
C73	Malignant neoplasm of thyroid gland
C75.0	Malignant neoplasm of parathyroid gland
C75.4	Malignant neoplasm of carotid body
C76.0	Malignant neoplasm of head, face and neck
C77.0	Secondary and unspecified malignant neoplasm of lymph nodes of head, face and neck
C7B.01	Secondary carcinoid tumors of distant lymph nodes
C7B.09	Secondary carcinoid tumors of other sites
C7B.1	Secondary Merkel cell carcinoma
C7B.8	Other secondary neuroendocrine tumors
D49.89	Neoplasm of unspecified behavior of other specified sites

Lymph Nodes

Relative Value Units/Medicare Edits

Non-Facility RVU	Work	PE	MP	Total
38720	21.95	13.56	3.53	39.04
Facility RVU	Work	PE	MP	Total
38720	21.95	13.56	3.53	39.04

	FUD	Status	MUE	Modifiers				IOM Reference
38720	90	A	1(2)	51	50	62*	80	None

* with documentation

Terms To Know

carcinoid tumor. Specific type of slow-growing neuroendocrine tumors. Carcinoid tumors occur most commonly in the hormone producing cells of the gastrointestinal tracts and can also occur in the pancreas, testes, ovaries, or lungs.

cervical. Relation to the cervical spine or to the cervix.

dissect. Cut apart or separate tissue for surgical purposes or for visual or microscopic study.

incision. Act of cutting into tissue or an organ.

lymphadenectomy. Dissection of lymph nodes free from the vessels and removal for examination by frozen section in a separate procedure to detect early-stage metastases.

malignant neoplasm. Any cancerous tumor or lesion exhibiting uncontrolled tissue growth that can progressively invade other parts of the body with its disease-generating cells.

Merkel cell carcinoma. Rare form of skin cancer that typically presents on the face, head, or neck as a flesh-colored or bluish-red lesion. This neoplasm is fast growing and can metastasize quickly to other areas of the body. Risk factors include older patients with weakened immune systems and/or long-term exposure to the sun.

38724

38724   Cervical lymphadenectomy (modified radical neck dissection)

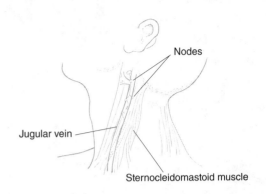

Explanation

The physician performs a cervical lymphadenectomy to preserve the spinal accessory nerve, jugular vein, and the sternocleidomastoid muscles. The physician makes a large curved incision starting at the ear, going down the neck, and continuing to the chin. Other incisions may be made down the neck from the original incision. Skin and tissue are retracted and the physician removes the lymph nodes. The incision is closed with sutures, including wound drains connected to suction. A tracheotomy may be performed.

Coding Tips

For suprahyoid lymphadenectomy, see 38700; complete cervical lymphadenectomy, see 38720. If significant additional time and effort is documented, append modifier 22 and submit a cover letter and operative report.

ICD-10-CM Diagnostic Codes

C01	Malignant neoplasm of base of tongue
C02.0	Malignant neoplasm of dorsal surface of tongue
C02.1	Malignant neoplasm of border of tongue
C02.2	Malignant neoplasm of ventral surface of tongue
C02.4	Malignant neoplasm of lingual tonsil
C02.8	Malignant neoplasm of overlapping sites of tongue
C04.0	Malignant neoplasm of anterior floor of mouth
C04.1	Malignant neoplasm of lateral floor of mouth
C04.8	Malignant neoplasm of overlapping sites of floor of mouth
C05.0	Malignant neoplasm of hard palate
C05.1	Malignant neoplasm of soft palate
C05.2	Malignant neoplasm of uvula
C06.0	Malignant neoplasm of cheek mucosa
C06.1	Malignant neoplasm of vestibule of mouth
C06.2	Malignant neoplasm of retromolar area
C06.89	Malignant neoplasm of overlapping sites of other parts of mouth
C07	Malignant neoplasm of parotid gland
C08.0	Malignant neoplasm of submandibular gland
C08.1	Malignant neoplasm of sublingual gland
C12	Malignant neoplasm of pyriform sinus
C13.0	Malignant neoplasm of postcricoid region
C13.1	Malignant neoplasm of aryepiglottic fold, hypopharyngeal aspect
C13.2	Malignant neoplasm of posterior wall of hypopharynx

Lymph Nodes

C13.8	Malignant neoplasm of overlapping sites of hypopharynx	
C14.2	Malignant neoplasm of Waldeyer's ring	
C14.8	Malignant neoplasm of overlapping sites of lip, oral cavity and pharynx	
C15.3	Malignant neoplasm of upper third of esophagus	
C15.4	Malignant neoplasm of middle third of esophagus	
C15.8	Malignant neoplasm of overlapping sites of esophagus	
C32.0	Malignant neoplasm of glottis	
C32.1	Malignant neoplasm of supraglottis	
C32.2	Malignant neoplasm of subglottis	
C32.3	Malignant neoplasm of laryngeal cartilage	
C32.8	Malignant neoplasm of overlapping sites of larynx	
C33	Malignant neoplasm of trachea	
C41.1	Malignant neoplasm of mandible	
C43.4	Malignant melanoma of scalp and neck	
C44.41	Basal cell carcinoma of skin of scalp and neck	
C44.42	Squamous cell carcinoma of skin of scalp and neck	
C44.49	Other specified malignant neoplasm of skin of scalp and neck	
C4A.0	Merkel cell carcinoma of lip	
C4A.111	Merkel cell carcinoma of right upper eyelid, including canthus ☑	
C4A.112	Merkel cell carcinoma of right lower eyelid, including canthus ☑	
C4A.21	Merkel cell carcinoma of right ear and external auricular canal ☑	
C4A.31	Merkel cell carcinoma of nose	
C4A.39	Merkel cell carcinoma of other parts of face	
C4A.4	Merkel cell carcinoma of scalp and neck	
C4A.8	Merkel cell carcinoma of overlapping sites	
C73	Malignant neoplasm of thyroid gland	
C75.0	Malignant neoplasm of parathyroid gland	
C75.4	Malignant neoplasm of carotid body	
C76.0	Malignant neoplasm of head, face and neck	
C77.0	Secondary and unspecified malignant neoplasm of lymph nodes of head, face and neck	
C7B.01	Secondary carcinoid tumors of distant lymph nodes	
C7B.09	Secondary carcinoid tumors of other sites	
C7B.1	Secondary Merkel cell carcinoma	
C7B.8	Other secondary neuroendocrine tumors	
D49.89	Neoplasm of unspecified behavior of other specified sites	

AMA: **38724** 2020,Dec,11; 2019,Mar,10; 2019,Feb,8; 2018,Jan,8; 2017,Jan,8; 2016,Jan,13; 2015,Jan,16

Relative Value Units/Medicare Edits

Non-Facility RVU	Work	PE	MP	Total
38724	23.95	14.74	3.47	42.16
Facility RVU	Work	PE	MP	Total
38724	23.95	14.74	3.47	42.16

	FUD	Status	MUE	Modifiers				IOM Reference
38724	90	A	1(2)	51	50	62*	80	None

* with documentation

38740-38745

38740 Axillary lymphadenectomy; superficial
38745   complete

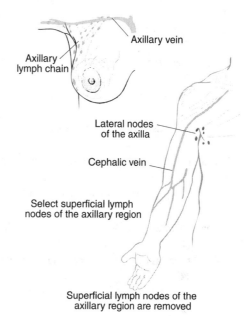

Select superficial lymph nodes of the axillary region

Superficial lymph nodes of the axillary region are removed

Explanation

The physician makes a diagonal incision across the lower axilla, exposing the axillary vein. The fatty tissue, lymph nodes, and vessels beneath the vein are dissected free. A drain is placed and connected to suction. The tissue and skin are closed with sutures. Report 38745 if a complete procedure is performed.

Coding Tips

For axillary lymphadenectomy with mastectomy, see 19302 or 19305–19307.

ICD-10-CM Diagnostic Codes

C40.01	Malignant neoplasm of scapula and long bones of right upper limb ☑	
C40.02	Malignant neoplasm of scapula and long bones of left upper limb ☑	
C40.11	Malignant neoplasm of short bones of right upper limb ☑	
C40.12	Malignant neoplasm of short bones of left upper limb ☑	
C46.3	Kaposi's sarcoma of lymph nodes	
C49.11	Malignant neoplasm of connective and soft tissue of right upper limb, including shoulder ☑	
C49.12	Malignant neoplasm of connective and soft tissue of left upper limb, including shoulder ☑	
C4A.52	Merkel cell carcinoma of skin of breast	
C4A.59	Merkel cell carcinoma of other part of trunk	
C4A.61	Merkel cell carcinoma of right upper limb, including shoulder ☑	
C4A.62	Merkel cell carcinoma of left upper limb, including shoulder ☑	
C4A.8	Merkel cell carcinoma of overlapping sites	
C50.111	Malignant neoplasm of central portion of right female breast ♀ ☑	
C50.112	Malignant neoplasm of central portion of left female breast ♀ ☑	
C50.121	Malignant neoplasm of central portion of right male breast ♂ ☑	
C50.122	Malignant neoplasm of central portion of left male breast ♂ ☑	

C50.211	Malignant neoplasm of upper-inner quadrant of right female breast ♀ ☑
C50.212	Malignant neoplasm of upper-inner quadrant of left female breast ♀ ☑
C50.221	Malignant neoplasm of upper-inner quadrant of right male breast ♂ ☑
C50.222	Malignant neoplasm of upper-inner quadrant of left male breast ♂ ☑
C50.311	Malignant neoplasm of lower-inner quadrant of right female breast ♀ ☑
C50.312	Malignant neoplasm of lower-inner quadrant of left female breast ♀ ☑
C50.321	Malignant neoplasm of lower-inner quadrant of right male breast ♂ ☑
C50.322	Malignant neoplasm of lower-inner quadrant of left male breast ♂ ☑
C50.411	Malignant neoplasm of upper-outer quadrant of right female breast ♀ ☑
C50.412	Malignant neoplasm of upper-outer quadrant of left female breast ♀ ☑
C50.421	Malignant neoplasm of upper-outer quadrant of right male breast ♂ ☑
C50.422	Malignant neoplasm of upper-outer quadrant of left male breast ♂ ☑
C50.511	Malignant neoplasm of lower-outer quadrant of right female breast ♀ ☑
C50.512	Malignant neoplasm of lower-outer quadrant of left female breast ♀ ☑
C50.521	Malignant neoplasm of lower-outer quadrant of right male breast ♂ ☑
C50.522	Malignant neoplasm of lower-outer quadrant of left male breast ♂ ☑
C50.611	Malignant neoplasm of axillary tail of right female breast ♀ ☑
C50.612	Malignant neoplasm of axillary tail of left female breast ♀ ☑
C50.621	Malignant neoplasm of axillary tail of right male breast ♂ ☑
C50.622	Malignant neoplasm of axillary tail of left male breast ♂ ☑
C50.811	Malignant neoplasm of overlapping sites of right female breast ♀ ☑
C50.812	Malignant neoplasm of overlapping sites of left female breast ♀ ☑
C50.821	Malignant neoplasm of overlapping sites of right male breast ♂ ☑
C50.822	Malignant neoplasm of overlapping sites of left male breast ♂ ☑
C76.1	Malignant neoplasm of thorax
C77.1	Secondary and unspecified malignant neoplasm of intrathoracic lymph nodes
C77.3	Secondary and unspecified malignant neoplasm of axilla and upper limb lymph nodes
C79.89	Secondary malignant neoplasm of other specified sites
C7B.01	Secondary carcinoid tumors of distant lymph nodes
C7B.09	Secondary carcinoid tumors of other sites
D05.01	Lobular carcinoma in situ of right breast ☑
D05.02	Lobular carcinoma in situ of left breast ☑
D05.11	Intraductal carcinoma in situ of right breast ☑
D05.12	Intraductal carcinoma in situ of left breast ☑
D05.81	Other specified type of carcinoma in situ of right breast ☑
D05.82	Other specified type of carcinoma in situ of left breast ☑
D19.7	Benign neoplasm of mesothelial tissue of other sites
D36.0	Benign neoplasm of lymph nodes
D36.7	Benign neoplasm of other specified sites
D48.7	Neoplasm of uncertain behavior of other specified sites
D49.3	Neoplasm of unspecified behavior of breast
N64.89	Other specified disorders of breast
R59.0	Localized enlarged lymph nodes
R59.1	Generalized enlarged lymph nodes

AMA: **38740** 2019,Feb,8; 2018,Jan,8; 2017,Jan,8; 2016,Jan,13; 2015,Jan,16
38745 2019,Feb,8

Relative Value Units/Medicare Edits

Non-Facility RVU	Work	PE	MP	Total
38740	10.7	7.43	2.54	20.67
38745	13.87	8.83	3.3	26.0
Facility RVU	**Work**	**PE**	**MP**	**Total**
38740	10.7	7.43	2.54	20.67
38745	13.87	8.83	3.3	26.0

	FUD	Status	MUE	Modifiers				IOM Reference
38740	90	A	1(2)	51	50	62*	80	None
38745	90	A	1(2)	51	50	62*	80	

* with documentation

Terms To Know

axillary. Area under the arm.

dissect. Cut apart or separate tissue for surgical purposes or for visual or microscopic study.

lymph nodes. Bean-shaped structures along the lymphatic vessels that intercept and destroy foreign materials in the tissue and bloodstream.

lymphadenectomy. Dissection of lymph nodes free from the vessels and removal for examination by frozen section in a separate procedure to detect early-stage metastases.

superficial. On the skin surface or near the surface of any involved structure or field of interest.

tissue. Group of similar cells with a similar function that form definite structures and organs. Tissue types include epithelial tissue, muscle tissue, connective tissue, and nervous tissue.

38746

+ **38746** Thoracic lymphadenectomy by thoracotomy, mediastinal and regional lymphadenectomy (List separately in addition to code for primary procedure)

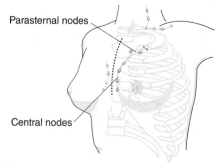

Parasternal nodes

Central nodes

Typical access incision for thoracic lymphadenectomy

Explanation

The physician performs a regional and mediastinal lymphadenectomy via an open approach. Using a scalpel, the surgeon makes a long incision around the side of the chest between two of the ribs. The incision is carried through all of the tissue layers into the chest cavity. Rib spreaders are inserted into the wound and the ribs are spread apart exposing the lung, the heart, and other structures. Alternately, the chest cavity can be opened and the operation performed through a vertical incision in the center of the chest through the sternum. The skin incision is carried down to the sternum bone and a saw is used to split the sternum. With the sternum split in half, the chest is entered by spreading the sternum apart with a set of rib spreaders. Lymph nodes near the lungs, around the heart, and behind the trachea are removed. The area is irrigated and the retractors are removed. If applicable, the sternotomy is repaired using wires to bring the two halves of the sternum together, and the operative wound is closed by sutures or staples.

Coding Tips

Report 38746 in addition to 21601, 31760–31766, 31786, 32096–32200, 32220–32320, 32440–32491, 32503–32505, 33025–33030, 33050–33130, 39200–39220, 39560–39561, 43101, 43112, 43117–43118, 43122–43123, 43351, 60270, or 60505. For this procedure, mediastinal lymph nodes include subcarinal, paraesophageal, and inferior pulmonary ligament on both sides. The right side also includes the paratracheal and the left side also includes the aortopulmonary window. For mediastinal and regional lymphadenectomy performed via thoracoscopy (VATS), see 32674.

ICD-10-CM Diagnostic Codes

C40.01	Malignant neoplasm of scapula and long bones of right upper limb ☑
C40.02	Malignant neoplasm of scapula and long bones of left upper limb ☑
C40.11	Malignant neoplasm of short bones of right upper limb ☑
C40.12	Malignant neoplasm of short bones of left upper limb ☑
C46.3	Kaposi's sarcoma of lymph nodes
C49.11	Malignant neoplasm of connective and soft tissue of right upper limb, including shoulder ☑
C49.12	Malignant neoplasm of connective and soft tissue of left upper limb, including shoulder ☑
C4A.52	Merkel cell carcinoma of skin of breast
C4A.59	Merkel cell carcinoma of other part of trunk

C4A.61	Merkel cell carcinoma of right upper limb, including shoulder ☑
C4A.62	Merkel cell carcinoma of left upper limb, including shoulder ☑
C4A.8	Merkel cell carcinoma of overlapping sites
C50.111	Malignant neoplasm of central portion of right female breast ♀ ☑
C50.112	Malignant neoplasm of central portion of left female breast ♀ ☑
C50.121	Malignant neoplasm of central portion of right male breast ♂ ☑
C50.122	Malignant neoplasm of central portion of left male breast ♂ ☑
C50.211	Malignant neoplasm of upper-inner quadrant of right female breast ♀ ☑
C50.212	Malignant neoplasm of upper-inner quadrant of left female breast ♀ ☑
C50.221	Malignant neoplasm of upper-inner quadrant of right male breast ♂ ☑
C50.222	Malignant neoplasm of upper-inner quadrant of left male breast ♂ ☑
C50.311	Malignant neoplasm of lower-inner quadrant of right female breast ♀ ☑
C50.312	Malignant neoplasm of lower-inner quadrant of left female breast ♀ ☑
C50.321	Malignant neoplasm of lower-inner quadrant of right male breast ♂ ☑
C50.322	Malignant neoplasm of lower-inner quadrant of left male breast ♂ ☑
C50.411	Malignant neoplasm of upper-outer quadrant of right female breast ♀ ☑
C50.412	Malignant neoplasm of upper-outer quadrant of left female breast ♀ ☑
C50.421	Malignant neoplasm of upper-outer quadrant of right male breast ♂ ☑
C50.422	Malignant neoplasm of upper-outer quadrant of left male breast ♂ ☑
C50.511	Malignant neoplasm of lower-outer quadrant of right female breast ♀ ☑
C50.512	Malignant neoplasm of lower-outer quadrant of left female breast ♀ ☑
C50.521	Malignant neoplasm of lower-outer quadrant of right male breast ♂ ☑
C50.522	Malignant neoplasm of lower-outer quadrant of left male breast ♂ ☑
C50.611	Malignant neoplasm of axillary tail of right female breast ♀ ☑
C50.612	Malignant neoplasm of axillary tail of left female breast ♀ ☑
C50.621	Malignant neoplasm of axillary tail of right male breast ♂ ☑
C50.622	Malignant neoplasm of axillary tail of left male breast ♂ ☑
C50.811	Malignant neoplasm of overlapping sites of right female breast ♀ ☑
C50.812	Malignant neoplasm of overlapping sites of left female breast ♀ ☑
C50.821	Malignant neoplasm of overlapping sites of right male breast ♂ ☑
C50.822	Malignant neoplasm of overlapping sites of left male breast ♂ ☑
C50.922	Malignant neoplasm of unspecified site of left male breast ♂ ☑
C76.1	Malignant neoplasm of thorax
C77.1	Secondary and unspecified malignant neoplasm of intrathoracic lymph nodes
C77.3	Secondary and unspecified malignant neoplasm of axilla and upper limb lymph nodes

C79.89	Secondary malignant neoplasm of other specified sites
C7B.01	Secondary carcinoid tumors of distant lymph nodes
C7B.09	Secondary carcinoid tumors of other sites
C80.2	Malignant neoplasm associated with transplanted organ
D05.01	Lobular carcinoma in situ of right breast ☑
D05.02	Lobular carcinoma in situ of left breast ☑
D05.11	Intraductal carcinoma in situ of right breast ☑
D05.12	Intraductal carcinoma in situ of left breast ☑
D05.81	Other specified type of carcinoma in situ of right breast ☑
D05.82	Other specified type of carcinoma in situ of left breast ☑
D19.7	Benign neoplasm of mesothelial tissue of other sites
D36.0	Benign neoplasm of lymph nodes
D36.7	Benign neoplasm of other specified sites
D48.7	Neoplasm of uncertain behavior of other specified sites
N64.89	Other specified disorders of breast
R59.0	Localized enlarged lymph nodes
R59.1	Generalized enlarged lymph nodes

AMA: 38746 2019,Feb,8; 2018,Jan,8; 2017,Jan,8; 2016,Jan,13; 2015,Jan,16

Relative Value Units/Medicare Edits

Non-Facility RVU	Work	PE	MP	Total
38746	4.12	1.21	0.95	6.28
Facility RVU	**Work**	**PE**	**MP**	**Total**
38746	4.12	1.21	0.95	6.28

	FUD	Status	MUE	Modifiers				IOM Reference
38746	N/A	A	1(2)	N/A	N/A	62*	80	None

* with documentation

Terms To Know

lymph nodes. Bean-shaped structures along the lymphatic vessels that intercept and destroy foreign materials in the tissue and bloodstream.

lymphadenectomy. Dissection of lymph nodes free from the vessels and removal for examination by frozen section in a separate procedure to detect early-stage metastases.

malignant. Any condition tending to progress toward death, specifically an invasive tumor with a loss of cellular differentiation that has the ability to spread or metastasize to other body areas.

mediastinum. Collection of organs and tissues that separate the pleural sacs. Located between the sternum and spine above the diaphragm, it contains the heart and great vessels, trachea and bronchi, esophagus, thymus, lymph nodes, and nerves.

retraction. Act of holding tissue or a structure back away from its normal position or the field of interest.

thoracic lymphadenectomy. Procedure to cut out the lymph nodes near the lungs, around the heart, and behind the trachea.

38747

+ **38747** Abdominal lymphadenectomy, regional, including celiac, gastric, portal, peripancreatic, with or without para-aortic and vena caval nodes (List separately in addition to code for primary procedure)

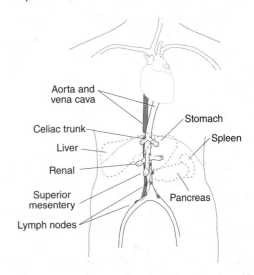

Explanation

The physician makes a midline abdominal incision. The abdominal contents are exposed, allowing the physician to locate the lymph nodes. Each lymph node grouping, with or without para-aortic and vena caval nodes, is dissected away from the surrounding tissue, nerves, and blood vessels, and removed. The incision is closed with sutures or staples.

Coding Tips

For regional thoracic lymphadenectomy, see 38746. For retroperitoneal transabdominal lymphadenectomy, see 38780.

ICD-10-CM Diagnostic Codes

C40.01	Malignant neoplasm of scapula and long bones of right upper limb ☑
C40.02	Malignant neoplasm of scapula and long bones of left upper limb ☑
C40.11	Malignant neoplasm of short bones of right upper limb ☑
C40.12	Malignant neoplasm of short bones of left upper limb ☑
C46.3	Kaposi's sarcoma of lymph nodes
C49.11	Malignant neoplasm of connective and soft tissue of right upper limb, including shoulder ☑
C49.12	Malignant neoplasm of connective and soft tissue of left upper limb, including shoulder ☑
C4A.52	Merkel cell carcinoma of skin of breast
C4A.59	Merkel cell carcinoma of other part of trunk
C4A.61	Merkel cell carcinoma of right upper limb, including shoulder ☑
C4A.62	Merkel cell carcinoma of left upper limb, including shoulder ☑
C4A.8	Merkel cell carcinoma of overlapping sites
C50.111	Malignant neoplasm of central portion of right female breast ♀ ☑
C50.112	Malignant neoplasm of central portion of left female breast ♀ ☑
C50.121	Malignant neoplasm of central portion of right male breast ♂ ☑
C50.122	Malignant neoplasm of central portion of left male breast ♂ ☑

C50.211	Malignant neoplasm of upper-inner quadrant of right female breast ♀ ☑
C50.212	Malignant neoplasm of upper-inner quadrant of left female breast ♀ ☑
C50.221	Malignant neoplasm of upper-inner quadrant of right male breast ♂ ☑
C50.222	Malignant neoplasm of upper-inner quadrant of left male breast ♂ ☑
C50.311	Malignant neoplasm of lower-inner quadrant of right female breast ♀ ☑
C50.312	Malignant neoplasm of lower-inner quadrant of left female breast ♀ ☑
C50.321	Malignant neoplasm of lower-inner quadrant of right male breast ♂ ☑
C50.322	Malignant neoplasm of lower-inner quadrant of left male breast ♂ ☑
C50.411	Malignant neoplasm of upper-outer quadrant of right female breast ♀ ☑
C50.412	Malignant neoplasm of upper-outer quadrant of left female breast ♀ ☑
C50.421	Malignant neoplasm of upper-outer quadrant of right male breast ♂ ☑
C50.422	Malignant neoplasm of upper-outer quadrant of left male breast ♂ ☑
C50.511	Malignant neoplasm of lower-outer quadrant of right female breast ♀ ☑
C50.512	Malignant neoplasm of lower-outer quadrant of left female breast ♀ ☑
C50.521	Malignant neoplasm of lower-outer quadrant of right male breast ♂ ☑
C50.522	Malignant neoplasm of lower-outer quadrant of left male breast ♂ ☑
C50.611	Malignant neoplasm of axillary tail of right female breast ♀ ☑
C50.612	Malignant neoplasm of axillary tail of left female breast ♀ ☑
C50.621	Malignant neoplasm of axillary tail of right male breast ♂ ☑
C50.622	Malignant neoplasm of axillary tail of left male breast ♂ ☑
C50.811	Malignant neoplasm of overlapping sites of right female breast ♀ ☑
C50.812	Malignant neoplasm of overlapping sites of left female breast ♀ ☑
C50.821	Malignant neoplasm of overlapping sites of right male breast ♂ ☑
C50.822	Malignant neoplasm of overlapping sites of left male breast ♂ ☑
C76.1	Malignant neoplasm of thorax
C77.1	Secondary and unspecified malignant neoplasm of intrathoracic lymph nodes
C77.2	Secondary and unspecified malignant neoplasm of intra-abdominal lymph nodes
C77.3	Secondary and unspecified malignant neoplasm of axilla and upper limb lymph nodes
C79.89	Secondary malignant neoplasm of other specified sites
C7B.01	Secondary carcinoid tumors of distant lymph nodes
C7B.09	Secondary carcinoid tumors of other sites
C80.2	Malignant neoplasm associated with transplanted organ
D05.01	Lobular carcinoma in situ of right breast ☑
D05.02	Lobular carcinoma in situ of left breast ☑

D05.11	Intraductal carcinoma in situ of right breast ☑
D05.12	Intraductal carcinoma in situ of left breast ☑
D05.81	Other specified type of carcinoma in situ of right breast ☑
D05.82	Other specified type of carcinoma in situ of left breast ☑
D19.7	Benign neoplasm of mesothelial tissue of other sites
D36.0	Benign neoplasm of lymph nodes
D36.7	Benign neoplasm of other specified sites
D48.7	Neoplasm of uncertain behavior of other specified sites
N64.89	Other specified disorders of breast
R59.0	Localized enlarged lymph nodes
R59.1	Generalized enlarged lymph nodes

AMA: **38747** 2020,Apr,10; 2019,Feb,8

Relative Value Units/Medicare Edits

Non-Facility RVU	Work	PE	MP	Total
38747	4.88	1.82	1.14	7.84
Facility RVU	**Work**	**PE**	**MP**	**Total**
38747	4.88	1.82	1.14	7.84

	FUD	Status	MUE	Modifiers				IOM Reference
38747	N/A	A	1(2)	N/A	N/A	62*	80	None

* with documentation

Terms To Know

dissection. (dis. apart; -section, act of cutting) Separating by cutting tissue or body structures apart.

Kaposi's sarcoma. Malignant neoplasm caused by vascular proliferation of cutaneous tumors characterized by channels lined with endothelial tissue containing vascular spaced.

lymph nodes. Bean-shaped structures along the lymphatic vessels that intercept and destroy foreign materials in the tissue and bloodstream.

lymphadenectomy. Dissection of lymph nodes free from the vessels and removal for examination by frozen section in a separate procedure to detect early-stage metastases.

Merkel cell carcinoma. Rare form of skin cancer that typically presents on the face, head, or neck as a flesh-colored or bluish-red lesion. This neoplasm is fast growing and can metastasize quickly to other areas of the body. Risk factors include older patients with weakened immune systems and/or long-term exposure to the sun.

Lymph Nodes

38760

38760 Inguinofemoral lymphadenectomy, superficial, including Cloquet's node (separate procedure)

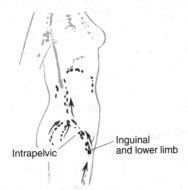

Superficial nodes of the inguinal region are removed along with certain pelvic nodes. Cloquet's node is of the deep inguinal group, but lies closest to the skin just under the inguinal ligament

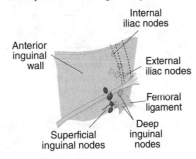

Explanation

The physician makes an incision across the groin area. The surrounding tissue, nerves, and blood vessels are dissected away, and the inguinal and femoral lymph nodes are visualized. The nodes are removed by group. The wound is closed with sutures or staples.

Coding Tips

This separate procedure, by definition, is usually a component of a more complex service and is not identified separately. When performed alone or with other unrelated procedures/services, it may be reported; if performed with other procedures/services, append modifier 59 or an X{EPSU} modifier. Code 38760 is a unilateral procedure. If performed bilaterally, some payers require that the service be reported twice with modifier 50 appended to the second code while others require identification of the service only once with modifier 50 appended. Check with individual payers. Modifier 50 identifies a procedure performed identically on the opposite side of the body (mirror image).

ICD-10-CM Diagnostic Codes

C19	Malignant neoplasm of rectosigmoid junction
C20	Malignant neoplasm of rectum
C46.3	Kaposi's sarcoma of lymph nodes
C4A.51	Merkel cell carcinoma of anal skin
C4A.59	Merkel cell carcinoma of other part of trunk
C4A.71	Merkel cell carcinoma of right lower limb, including hip ☑
C4A.72	Merkel cell carcinoma of left lower limb, including hip ☑
C4A.8	Merkel cell carcinoma of overlapping sites

C51.0	Malignant neoplasm of labium majus ♀
C51.1	Malignant neoplasm of labium minus ♀
C51.2	Malignant neoplasm of clitoris ♀
C52	Malignant neoplasm of vagina ♀
C53.0	Malignant neoplasm of endocervix ♀
C53.1	Malignant neoplasm of exocervix ♀
C53.8	Malignant neoplasm of overlapping sites of cervix uteri ♀
C54.0	Malignant neoplasm of isthmus uteri ♀
C54.1	Malignant neoplasm of endometrium ♀
C54.2	Malignant neoplasm of myometrium ♀
C54.3	Malignant neoplasm of fundus uteri ♀
C56.1	Malignant neoplasm of right ovary ♀ ☑
C56.2	Malignant neoplasm of left ovary ♀ ☑
C57.01	Malignant neoplasm of right fallopian tube ♀ ☑
C57.02	Malignant neoplasm of left fallopian tube ♀ ☑
C57.11	Malignant neoplasm of right broad ligament ♀ ☑
C57.12	Malignant neoplasm of left broad ligament ♀ ☑
C57.21	Malignant neoplasm of right round ligament ♀ ☑
C57.22	Malignant neoplasm of left round ligament ♀ ☑
C57.3	Malignant neoplasm of parametrium ♀
C57.7	Malignant neoplasm of other specified female genital organs ♀
C57.8	Malignant neoplasm of overlapping sites of female genital organs ♀
C60.0	Malignant neoplasm of prepuce ♂
C60.1	Malignant neoplasm of glans penis ♂
C60.2	Malignant neoplasm of body of penis ♂
C60.8	Malignant neoplasm of overlapping sites of penis ♂
C61	Malignant neoplasm of prostate ♂
C62.11	Malignant neoplasm of descended right testis ♂ ☑
C62.12	Malignant neoplasm of descended left testis ♂ ☑
C63.01	Malignant neoplasm of right epididymis ♂ ☑
C63.02	Malignant neoplasm of left epididymis ♂ ☑
C63.11	Malignant neoplasm of right spermatic cord ♂ ☑
C63.12	Malignant neoplasm of left spermatic cord ♂ ☑
C63.2	Malignant neoplasm of scrotum ♂
C63.7	Malignant neoplasm of other specified male genital organs ♂
C66.1	Malignant neoplasm of right ureter ☑
C66.2	Malignant neoplasm of left ureter ☑
C67.0	Malignant neoplasm of trigone of bladder
C67.1	Malignant neoplasm of dome of bladder
C67.2	Malignant neoplasm of lateral wall of bladder
C67.3	Malignant neoplasm of anterior wall of bladder
C67.4	Malignant neoplasm of posterior wall of bladder
C67.5	Malignant neoplasm of bladder neck
C67.6	Malignant neoplasm of ureteric orifice
C67.7	Malignant neoplasm of urachus
C67.8	Malignant neoplasm of overlapping sites of bladder
C68.0	Malignant neoplasm of urethra
C68.1	Malignant neoplasm of paraurethral glands
C77.4	Secondary and unspecified malignant neoplasm of inguinal and lower limb lymph nodes
C78.5	Secondary malignant neoplasm of large intestine and rectum
C7B.01	Secondary carcinoid tumors of distant lymph nodes

Lymph Nodes (side tab)

C7B.09	Secondary carcinoid tumors of other sites
C82.55	Diffuse follicle center lymphoma, lymph nodes of inguinal region and lower limb
C84.Z5	Other mature T/NK-cell lymphomas, lymph nodes of inguinal region and lower limb
C85.25	Mediastinal (thymic) large B-cell lymphoma, lymph nodes of inguinal region and lower limb
C85.85	Other specified types of non-Hodgkin lymphoma, lymph nodes of inguinal region and lower limb
D01.1	Carcinoma in situ of rectosigmoid junction
D01.2	Carcinoma in situ of rectum
D12.7	Benign neoplasm of rectosigmoid junction
D12.8	Benign neoplasm of rectum
D12.9	Benign neoplasm of anus and anal canal
D36.0	Benign neoplasm of lymph nodes
D37.5	Neoplasm of uncertain behavior of rectum
D3A.026	Benign carcinoid tumor of the rectum
R59.0	Localized enlarged lymph nodes
R59.1	Generalized enlarged lymph nodes

AMA: 38760 2019,Feb,8; 2018,Jan,8; 2017,Jan,8; 2016,Jan,13; 2015,Jan,16

Relative Value Units/Medicare Edits

Non-Facility RVU	Work	PE	MP	Total
38760	13.62	8.25	2.81	24.68
Facility RVU	**Work**	**PE**	**MP**	**Total**
38760	13.62	8.25	2.81	24.68

	FUD	Status	MUE	Modifiers				IOM Reference
38760	90	A	1(2)	51	50	62*	80	None

* with documentation

Terms To Know

Cloquet's node. Highest deep inguinofemoral lymph node.

femoral lymph node. Lymphatic, right lower extremity, left lower extremity.

inguinal. Within the groin region.

lymph nodes. Bean-shaped structures along the lymphatic vessels that intercept and destroy foreign materials in the tissue and bloodstream.

superficial. On the skin surface or near the surface of any involved structure or field of interest.

38765

38765	Inguinofemoral lymphadenectomy, superficial, in continuity with pelvic lymphadenectomy, including external iliac, hypogastric, and obturator nodes (separate procedure)

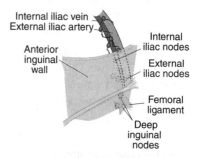

Internal iliac vein
External iliac artery
Internal iliac nodes
Anterior inguinal wall
External iliac nodes
Femoral ligament
Deep inguinal nodes

Nodes lying deep in the pelvic abdomen (internal iliac) are removed

Explanation

The physician makes an incision across the groin area. The surrounding tissue, nerves, and blood vessels are dissected away, and the inguinal and femoral lymph nodes are visualized. The nodes are removed by group. A pelvic lymphadenectomy is performed concurrently. The wound is closed with sutures or staples.

Coding Tips

This separate procedure by definition is usually a component of a more complex service and is not identified separately. When performed alone or with other unrelated procedures/services it may be reported. If performed with other procedures/services, list the code and append modifier 59 or an X{EPSU} modifier. This is a unilateral procedure. If performed bilaterally, some payers require that the service be reported twice with modifier 50 appended to the second code while others require identification of the service only once with modifier 50 appended. Check with individual payers. Modifier 50 identifies a procedure performed identically on the opposite side of the body (mirror image).

ICD-10-CM Diagnostic Codes

C19	Malignant neoplasm of rectosigmoid junction
C20	Malignant neoplasm of rectum
C4A.51	Merkel cell carcinoma of anal skin
C4A.59	Merkel cell carcinoma of other part of trunk
C4A.8	Merkel cell carcinoma of overlapping sites
C51.0	Malignant neoplasm of labium majus ♀
C51.1	Malignant neoplasm of labium minus ♀
C51.2	Malignant neoplasm of clitoris ♀
C53.0	Malignant neoplasm of endocervix ♀
C53.1	Malignant neoplasm of exocervix ♀
C53.8	Malignant neoplasm of overlapping sites of cervix uteri ♀
C54.0	Malignant neoplasm of isthmus uteri ♀
C54.1	Malignant neoplasm of endometrium ♀
C54.2	Malignant neoplasm of myometrium ♀
C54.3	Malignant neoplasm of fundus uteri ♀
C56.1	Malignant neoplasm of right ovary ♀ ☑
C56.2	Malignant neoplasm of left ovary ♀ ☑
C56.3	Malignant neoplasm of bilateral ovaries ♀ ☑

C57.01	Malignant neoplasm of right fallopian tube ♀ ☑
C57.02	Malignant neoplasm of left fallopian tube ♀ ☑
C57.11	Malignant neoplasm of right broad ligament ♀ ☑
C57.12	Malignant neoplasm of left broad ligament ♀ ☑
C57.21	Malignant neoplasm of right round ligament ♀ ☑
C57.22	Malignant neoplasm of left round ligament ♀ ☑
C57.3	Malignant neoplasm of parametrium ♀
C57.7	Malignant neoplasm of other specified female genital organs ♀
C57.8	Malignant neoplasm of overlapping sites of female genital organs ♀
C60.0	Malignant neoplasm of prepuce ♂
C60.1	Malignant neoplasm of glans penis ♂
C60.2	Malignant neoplasm of body of penis ♂
C60.8	Malignant neoplasm of overlapping sites of penis ♂
C61	Malignant neoplasm of prostate ♂
C62.11	Malignant neoplasm of descended right testis ♂ ☑
C62.12	Malignant neoplasm of descended left testis ♂ ☑
C63.01	Malignant neoplasm of right epididymis ♂ ☑
C63.02	Malignant neoplasm of left epididymis ♂ ☑
C63.11	Malignant neoplasm of right spermatic cord ♂ ☑
C63.12	Malignant neoplasm of left spermatic cord ♂ ☑
C63.2	Malignant neoplasm of scrotum ♂
C63.7	Malignant neoplasm of other specified male genital organs ♂
C66.1	Malignant neoplasm of right ureter ☑
C66.2	Malignant neoplasm of left ureter ☑
C67.0	Malignant neoplasm of trigone of bladder
C67.1	Malignant neoplasm of dome of bladder
C67.2	Malignant neoplasm of lateral wall of bladder
C67.3	Malignant neoplasm of anterior wall of bladder
C67.4	Malignant neoplasm of posterior wall of bladder
C67.5	Malignant neoplasm of bladder neck
C67.6	Malignant neoplasm of ureteric orifice
C67.7	Malignant neoplasm of urachus
C67.8	Malignant neoplasm of overlapping sites of bladder
C68.0	Malignant neoplasm of urethra
C68.1	Malignant neoplasm of paraurethral glands
C77.4	Secondary and unspecified malignant neoplasm of inguinal and lower limb lymph nodes
C78.5	Secondary malignant neoplasm of large intestine and rectum
C7B.09	Secondary carcinoid tumors of other sites
R59.0	Localized enlarged lymph nodes
R59.1	Generalized enlarged lymph nodes

AMA: 38765 2019,Feb,8; 2018,Jan,8; 2017,Jan,8; 2016,Jan,13; 2015,Jan,16

Relative Value Units/Medicare Edits

Non-Facility RVU	Work	PE	MP	Total
38765	21.91	12.09	4.36	38.36
Facility RVU	Work	PE	MP	Total
38765	21.91	12.09	4.36	38.36

	FUD	Status	MUE	Modifiers				IOM Reference
38765	90	A	1(2)	51	50	62*	80	None

* with documentation

Terms To Know

dissection. (dis. apart; -section, act of cutting) Separating by cutting tissue or body structures apart.

inguinal. Within the groin region.

lymph nodes. Bean-shaped structures along the lymphatic vessels that intercept and destroy foreign materials in the tissue and bloodstream.

lymphadenectomy. Dissection of lymph nodes free from the vessels and removal for examination by frozen section in a separate procedure to detect early-stage metastases.

malignant neoplasm. Any cancerous tumor or lesion exhibiting uncontrolled tissue growth that can progressively invade other parts of the body with its disease-generating cells.

superficial. On the skin surface or near the surface of any involved structure or field of interest.

38770

38770 Pelvic lymphadenectomy, including external iliac, hypogastric, and obturator nodes (separate procedure)

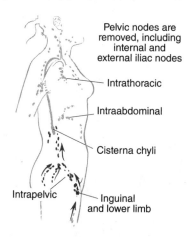

Pelvic nodes are removed, including internal and external iliac nodes

Intrathoracic

Intraabdominal

Cisterna chyli

Intrapelvic

Inguinal and lower limb

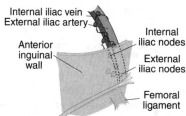

Internal iliac vein
External iliac artery

Anterior inguinal wall

Internal iliac nodes

External iliac nodes

Femoral ligament

Explanation

The physician makes a low abdominal vertical incision. The surrounding tissue, nerves, and blood vessels are dissected away, and the pelvic lymph nodes are visualized. The nodes are removed by group. The wound is closed with sutures or staples.

Coding Tips

This separate procedure, by definition, is usually a component of a more complex service and is not identified separately. When performed alone or with other unrelated procedures/services it may be reported. If performed with other procedures/services, list the code and append modifier 59 or an X{EPSU} modifier. This is a unilateral procedure. If performed bilaterally, some payers require that the service be reported twice with modifier 50 appended to the second code while others require identification of the service only once with modifier 50 appended. Check with individual payers. Modifier 50 identifies a procedure performed identically on the opposite side of the body (mirror image).

ICD-10-CM Diagnostic Codes

C51.0	Malignant neoplasm of labium majus ♀
C51.1	Malignant neoplasm of labium minus ♀
C51.2	Malignant neoplasm of clitoris ♀
C51.8	Malignant neoplasm of overlapping sites of vulva ♀
C52	Malignant neoplasm of vagina ♀
C53.0	Malignant neoplasm of endocervix ♀
C53.1	Malignant neoplasm of exocervix ♀
C53.8	Malignant neoplasm of overlapping sites of cervix uteri ♀
C54.0	Malignant neoplasm of isthmus uteri ♀
C54.1	Malignant neoplasm of endometrium ♀
C54.2	Malignant neoplasm of myometrium ♀
C54.3	Malignant neoplasm of fundus uteri ♀
C54.8	Malignant neoplasm of overlapping sites of corpus uteri ♀
C56.1	Malignant neoplasm of right ovary ♀ ☑
C56.2	Malignant neoplasm of left ovary ♀ ☑
C56.3	Malignant neoplasm of bilateral ovaries ♀ ☑
C57.01	Malignant neoplasm of right fallopian tube ♀ ☑
C57.02	Malignant neoplasm of left fallopian tube ♀ ☑
C57.11	Malignant neoplasm of right broad ligament ♀ ☑
C57.12	Malignant neoplasm of left broad ligament ♀ ☑
C57.21	Malignant neoplasm of right round ligament ♀ ☑
C57.22	Malignant neoplasm of left round ligament ♀ ☑
C57.3	Malignant neoplasm of parametrium ♀
C57.7	Malignant neoplasm of other specified female genital organs ♀
C57.8	Malignant neoplasm of overlapping sites of female genital organs ♀
C60.0	Malignant neoplasm of prepuce ♂
C60.1	Malignant neoplasm of glans penis ♂
C60.2	Malignant neoplasm of body of penis ♂
C60.8	Malignant neoplasm of overlapping sites of penis ♂
C61	Malignant neoplasm of prostate ♂
C62.11	Malignant neoplasm of descended right testis ♂ ☑
C62.12	Malignant neoplasm of descended left testis ♂ ☑
C63.01	Malignant neoplasm of right epididymis ♂ ☑
C63.02	Malignant neoplasm of left epididymis ♂ ☑
C63.11	Malignant neoplasm of right spermatic cord ♂ ☑
C63.12	Malignant neoplasm of left spermatic cord ♂ ☑
C63.2	Malignant neoplasm of scrotum ♂
C63.7	Malignant neoplasm of other specified male genital organs ♂
C63.8	Malignant neoplasm of overlapping sites of male genital organs ♂
C66.1	Malignant neoplasm of right ureter ☑
C66.2	Malignant neoplasm of left ureter ☑
C67.0	Malignant neoplasm of trigone of bladder
C67.1	Malignant neoplasm of dome of bladder
C67.2	Malignant neoplasm of lateral wall of bladder
C67.3	Malignant neoplasm of anterior wall of bladder
C67.4	Malignant neoplasm of posterior wall of bladder
C67.5	Malignant neoplasm of bladder neck
C67.6	Malignant neoplasm of ureteric orifice
C67.7	Malignant neoplasm of urachus
C67.8	Malignant neoplasm of overlapping sites of bladder
C68.0	Malignant neoplasm of urethra
C68.1	Malignant neoplasm of paraurethral glands
C77.5	Secondary and unspecified malignant neoplasm of intrapelvic lymph nodes
C7B.01	Secondary carcinoid tumors of distant lymph nodes
C7B.09	Secondary carcinoid tumors of other sites
D48.7	Neoplasm of uncertain behavior of other specified sites
D49.89	Neoplasm of unspecified behavior of other specified sites

AMA: **38770** 2019,Feb,8

Relative Value Units/Medicare Edits

Non-Facility RVU	Work	PE	MP	Total
38770	14.06	7.48	1.99	23.53
Facility RVU	Work	PE	MP	Total
38770	14.06	7.48	1.99	23.53

	FUD	Status	MUE	Modifiers				IOM Reference
38770	90	A	1(2)	51	50	62*	80	None

* with documentation

Terms To Know

broad ligament. Fold of peritoneum extending from the side of the uterus to the wall of the pelvis.

dissect. Cut apart or separate tissue for surgical purposes or for visual or microscopic study.

epididymis. Coiled tube on the back of the testis that is the site of sperm maturation and storage and where spermatozoa are propelled into the vas deferens toward the ejaculatory duct by contraction of smooth muscle.

lymph nodes. Bean-shaped structures along the lymphatic vessels that intercept and destroy foreign materials in the tissue and bloodstream.

lymphadenectomy. Dissection of lymph nodes free from the vessels and removal for examination by frozen section in a separate procedure to detect early-stage metastases.

malignant neoplasm. Any cancerous tumor or lesion exhibiting uncontrolled tissue growth that can progressively invade other parts of the body with its disease-generating cells.

round ligament. Ligament between the uterus and the pelvic wall.

38780

38780 Retroperitoneal transabdominal lymphadenectomy, extensive, including pelvic, aortic, and renal nodes (separate procedure)

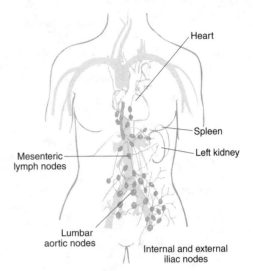

Extensive removal of lymph nodes of the retroperitoneal area

Explanation

The physician makes a large midline abdominal incision. The surrounding tissue, nerves, and blood vessels are dissected away, and the lymph nodes are visualized. The nodes are removed by group. Some surrounding tissues may also be removed. The wound is closed with sutures or staples.

Coding Tips

This separate procedure, by definition, is usually a component of a more complex service and is not identified separately. When performed alone or with other unrelated procedures/services it may be reported. If performed with other procedures/services, list the code and append modifier 59 or an X{EPSU} modifier. If significant additional time and effort is documented, append modifier 22 and submit a cover letter and operative report.

ICD-10-CM Diagnostic Codes

C17.0	Malignant neoplasm of duodenum
C18.5	Malignant neoplasm of splenic flexure
C20	Malignant neoplasm of rectum
C25.0	Malignant neoplasm of head of pancreas
C25.1	Malignant neoplasm of body of pancreas
C45.1	Mesothelioma of peritoneum
C48.0	Malignant neoplasm of retroperitoneum
C48.1	Malignant neoplasm of specified parts of peritoneum
C48.8	Malignant neoplasm of overlapping sites of retroperitoneum and peritoneum
C53.0	Malignant neoplasm of endocervix ♀
C53.1	Malignant neoplasm of exocervix ♀
C53.8	Malignant neoplasm of overlapping sites of cervix uteri ♀
C54.0	Malignant neoplasm of isthmus uteri ♀
C54.1	Malignant neoplasm of endometrium ♀
C54.2	Malignant neoplasm of myometrium ♀
C54.3	Malignant neoplasm of fundus uteri ♀
C54.8	Malignant neoplasm of overlapping sites of corpus uteri ♀

C56.1	Malignant neoplasm of right ovary ♀ ☑	
C56.2	Malignant neoplasm of left ovary ♀ ☑	
C56.3	Malignant neoplasm of bilateral ovaries ♀ ☑	
C57.01	Malignant neoplasm of right fallopian tube ♀ ☑	
C57.02	Malignant neoplasm of left fallopian tube ♀ ☑	
C57.11	Malignant neoplasm of right broad ligament ♀ ☑	
C57.12	Malignant neoplasm of left broad ligament ♀ ☑	
C57.21	Malignant neoplasm of right round ligament ♀ ☑	
C57.22	Malignant neoplasm of left round ligament ♀ ☑	
C57.3	Malignant neoplasm of parametrium ♀	
C61	Malignant neoplasm of prostate ♂	
C62.11	Malignant neoplasm of descended right testis ♂ ☑	
C62.12	Malignant neoplasm of descended left testis ♂ ☑	
C64.1	Malignant neoplasm of right kidney, except renal pelvis ☑	
C64.2	Malignant neoplasm of left kidney, except renal pelvis ☑	
C65.1	Malignant neoplasm of right renal pelvis ☑	
C65.2	Malignant neoplasm of left renal pelvis ☑	
C66.1	Malignant neoplasm of right ureter ☑	
C66.2	Malignant neoplasm of left ureter ☑	
C67.0	Malignant neoplasm of trigone of bladder	
C67.1	Malignant neoplasm of dome of bladder	
C67.2	Malignant neoplasm of lateral wall of bladder	
C67.3	Malignant neoplasm of anterior wall of bladder	
C67.4	Malignant neoplasm of posterior wall of bladder	
C67.5	Malignant neoplasm of bladder neck	
C67.6	Malignant neoplasm of ureteric orifice	
C67.8	Malignant neoplasm of overlapping sites of bladder	
C68.0	Malignant neoplasm of urethra	
C68.1	Malignant neoplasm of paraurethral glands	
C74.01	Malignant neoplasm of cortex of right adrenal gland ☑	
C74.02	Malignant neoplasm of cortex of left adrenal gland ☑	
C74.11	Malignant neoplasm of medulla of right adrenal gland ☑	
C74.12	Malignant neoplasm of medulla of left adrenal gland ☑	
C77.2	Secondary and unspecified malignant neoplasm of intra-abdominal lymph nodes	
C78.5	Secondary malignant neoplasm of large intestine and rectum	
C78.6	Secondary malignant neoplasm of retroperitoneum and peritoneum	
C78.7	Secondary malignant neoplasm of liver and intrahepatic bile duct	
C78.89	Secondary malignant neoplasm of other digestive organs	
C7A.093	Malignant carcinoid tumor of the kidney	
C7B.01	Secondary carcinoid tumors of distant lymph nodes	
C7B.04	Secondary carcinoid tumors of peritoneum	
C7B.09	Secondary carcinoid tumors of other sites	
C7B.1	Secondary Merkel cell carcinoma	
C7B.8	Other secondary neuroendocrine tumors	
D48.3	Neoplasm of uncertain behavior of retroperitoneum	
D48.7	Neoplasm of uncertain behavior of other specified sites	
D49.89	Neoplasm of unspecified behavior of other specified sites	

AMA: **38780** 2019,Feb,8

Relative Value Units/Medicare Edits

Non-Facility RVU	Work	PE	MP	Total
38780	17.7	9.79	2.91	30.4
Facility RVU	**Work**	**PE**	**MP**	**Total**
38780	17.7	9.79	2.91	30.4

	FUD	Status	MUE	Modifiers				IOM Reference
38780	90	A	1(2)	51	N/A	62*	80	None

* with documentation

Terms To Know

dissect. Cut apart or separate tissue for surgical purposes or for visual or microscopic study.

lymph nodes. Bean-shaped structures along the lymphatic vessels that intercept and destroy foreign materials in the tissue and bloodstream.

lymphadenectomy. Dissection of lymph nodes free from the vessels and removal for examination by frozen section in a separate procedure to detect early-stage metastases.

malignant. Any condition tending to progress toward death, specifically an invasive tumor with a loss of cellular differentiation that has the ability to spread or metastasize to other body areas.

retroperitoneal. Located behind the peritoneum, the membrane that lines the abdominopelvic walls and forms a covering for the internal organs.

suture. Numerous stitching techniques employed in wound closure.

tissue. Group of similar cells with a similar function that form definite structures and organs. Tissue types include epithelial tissue, muscle tissue, connective tissue, and nervous tissue.

38790

38790   Injection procedure; lymphangiography

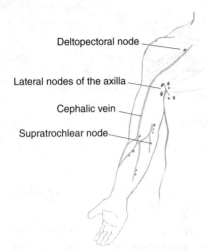

Deltopectoral node

Lateral nodes of the axilla

Cephalic vein

Supratrochlear node

The injection procedure is performed
to image lymph nodes of an extremity

Explanation

Vital blue dye is injected into the subcutaneous tissues for outlining of skin lymphatics. As soon as the lymphatic vessels are visualized by their blue color, the radiologist makes a small longitudinal incision over the area. Exposure of the lymph vessel is accomplished, the vessel is made taut, and it is cannulated with a 27 or 30 gauge needle with a fine catheter attached. A small amount of dye is injected to ensure correct placement, and the needle is advanced 2 to 3 mm into the vessel. The needle and catheter are secured. Dye is injected with a 10 cc syringe. X-rays are made and repeated 24 hours later. The physician removes the needle and closes the incision with sutures.

Coding Tips

Note that 38790 is a unilateral procedure. If performed bilaterally, some payers require that the service be reported twice with modifier 50 appended to the second code while others require identification of the service only once with modifier 50 appended. Check with individual payers. Modifier 50 identifies a procedure performed identically on the opposite side of the body (mirror image). For biopsy or excision of lymph nodes, see 38500–38542. Radiologic supervision and interpretation is reported with 75801–75807, when performed.

ICD-10-CM Diagnostic Codes

C81.04	Nodular lymphocyte predominant Hodgkin lymphoma, lymph nodes of axilla and upper limb
C81.08	Nodular lymphocyte predominant Hodgkin lymphoma, lymph nodes of multiple sites
C81.09	Nodular lymphocyte predominant Hodgkin lymphoma, extranodal and solid organ sites
C81.14	Nodular sclerosis Hodgkin lymphoma, lymph nodes of axilla and upper limb
C81.18	Nodular sclerosis Hodgkin lymphoma, lymph nodes of multiple sites
C81.19	Nodular sclerosis Hodgkin lymphoma, extranodal and solid organ sites
C81.24	Mixed cellularity Hodgkin lymphoma, lymph nodes of axilla and upper limb
C81.28	Mixed cellularity Hodgkin lymphoma, lymph nodes of multiple sites
C81.29	Mixed cellularity Hodgkin lymphoma, extranodal and solid organ sites
C81.38	Lymphocyte depleted Hodgkin lymphoma, lymph nodes of multiple sites
C81.39	Lymphocyte depleted Hodgkin lymphoma, extranodal and solid organ sites
C81.44	Lymphocyte-rich Hodgkin lymphoma, lymph nodes of axilla and upper limb
C81.48	Lymphocyte-rich Hodgkin lymphoma, lymph nodes of multiple sites
C81.74	Other Hodgkin lymphoma, lymph nodes of axilla and upper limb
C81.78	Other Hodgkin lymphoma, lymph nodes of multiple sites
C81.79	Other Hodgkin lymphoma, extranodal and solid organ sites
C82.04	Follicular lymphoma grade I, lymph nodes of axilla and upper limb
C82.08	Follicular lymphoma grade I, lymph nodes of multiple sites
C82.09	Follicular lymphoma grade I, extranodal and solid organ sites
C82.14	Follicular lymphoma grade II, lymph nodes of axilla and upper limb
C82.18	Follicular lymphoma grade II, lymph nodes of multiple sites
C82.19	Follicular lymphoma grade II, extranodal and solid organ sites
C82.34	Follicular lymphoma grade IIIa, lymph nodes of axilla and upper limb
C82.38	Follicular lymphoma grade IIIa, lymph nodes of multiple sites
C82.39	Follicular lymphoma grade IIIa, extranodal and solid organ sites
C82.44	Follicular lymphoma grade IIIb, lymph nodes of axilla and upper limb
C82.48	Follicular lymphoma grade IIIb, lymph nodes of multiple sites
C82.49	Follicular lymphoma grade IIIb, extranodal and solid organ sites
C82.54	Diffuse follicle center lymphoma, lymph nodes of axilla and upper limb
C82.58	Diffuse follicle center lymphoma, lymph nodes of multiple sites
C82.64	Cutaneous follicle center lymphoma, lymph nodes of axilla and upper limb
C82.69	Cutaneous follicle center lymphoma, extranodal and solid organ sites
C82.84	Other types of follicular lymphoma, lymph nodes of axilla and upper limb
C82.88	Other types of follicular lymphoma, lymph nodes of multiple sites
C83.04	Small cell B-cell lymphoma, lymph nodes of axilla and upper limb
C83.08	Small cell B-cell lymphoma, lymph nodes of multiple sites
C83.09	Small cell B-cell lymphoma, extranodal and solid organ sites
C83.14	Mantle cell lymphoma, lymph nodes of axilla and upper limb
C83.18	Mantle cell lymphoma, lymph nodes of multiple sites
C83.19	Mantle cell lymphoma, extranodal and solid organ sites
C83.34	Diffuse large B-cell lymphoma, lymph nodes of axilla and upper limb
C83.39	Diffuse large B-cell lymphoma, extranodal and solid organ sites
C83.54	Lymphoblastic (diffuse) lymphoma, lymph nodes of axilla and upper limb

C83.58	Lymphoblastic (diffuse) lymphoma, lymph nodes of multiple sites
C83.84	Other non-follicular lymphoma, lymph nodes of axilla and upper limb
C83.88	Other non-follicular lymphoma, lymph nodes of multiple sites
C83.89	Other non-follicular lymphoma, extranodal and solid organ sites
C84.14	Sezary disease, lymph nodes of axilla and upper limb
C84.18	Sezary disease, lymph nodes of multiple sites
C84.19	Sezary disease, extranodal and solid organ sites
C84.44	Peripheral T-cell lymphoma, not classified, lymph nodes of axilla and upper limb
C84.49	Peripheral T-cell lymphoma, not classified, extranodal and solid organ sites
C84.64	Anaplastic large cell lymphoma, ALK-positive, lymph nodes of axilla and upper limb
C84.68	Anaplastic large cell lymphoma, ALK-positive, lymph nodes of multiple sites
C84.74	Anaplastic large cell lymphoma, ALK-negative, lymph nodes of axilla and upper limb
C84.78	Anaplastic large cell lymphoma, ALK-negative, lymph nodes of multiple sites
C84.79	Anaplastic large cell lymphoma, ALK-negative, extranodal and solid organ sites
C84.Z4	Other mature T/NK-cell lymphomas, lymph nodes of axilla and upper limb
C84.Z8	Other mature T/NK-cell lymphomas, lymph nodes of multiple sites
C84.Z9	Other mature T/NK-cell lymphomas, extranodal and solid organ sites
C85.24	Mediastinal (thymic) large B-cell lymphoma, lymph nodes of axilla and upper limb
C85.28	Mediastinal (thymic) large B-cell lymphoma, lymph nodes of multiple sites
C85.29	Mediastinal (thymic) large B-cell lymphoma, extranodal and solid organ sites
C86.4	Blastic NK-cell lymphoma
C86.5	Angioimmunoblastic T-cell lymphoma
D36.0	Benign neoplasm of lymph nodes
R59.0	Localized enlarged lymph nodes
R59.1	Generalized enlarged lymph nodes

AMA: **38790** 2014,Jan,11

Relative Value Units/Medicare Edits

Non-Facility RVU	Work	PE	MP	Total
38790	1.29	0.88	0.21	2.38
Facility RVU	Work	PE	MP	Total
38790	1.29	0.88	0.21	2.38

	FUD	Status	MUE	Modifiers				IOM Reference
38790	0	A	1(2)	51	50	N/A	N/A	None

* with documentation

38792

| 38792 | Injection procedure; radioactive tracer for identification of sentinel node |

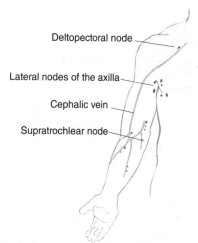

- Deltopectoral node
- Lateral nodes of the axilla
- Cephalic vein
- Supratrochlear node

A sentinel node is one in the cervical area that can be an indicator of a malignancy elsewhere in the body

Explanation

The physician injects radioactive material into the patient to identify the first lymph node to receive lymphatic drainage from a tumor (sentinel lymph node). This procedure is most commonly performed for breast cancer and melanoma. A radioactive tracer (radiotracer), such as radioactive technetium sulfur colloid, is injected around the tumor or, in cases of breast cancer, in periareolar or subareolar areas. Time is allowed for the tracer to flow to the sentinel lymph node. X-rays are taken and repeated 24 hours later.

Coding Tips

For biopsy or excision of sentinel nodes, see 38500–38542. When performed, intraoperative identification (e.g., mapping) of sentinel lymph nodes, including injection of non-radioactive dye, is reported with 38900. Nuclear medicine lymphatics and lymph gland imaging, when performed, is reported with 78195. For lymphangiography, see 38790.

ICD-10-CM Diagnostic Codes

C50.011	Malignant neoplasm of nipple and areola, right female breast ♀ ☑
C50.012	Malignant neoplasm of nipple and areola, left female breast ♀ ☑
C50.111	Malignant neoplasm of central portion of right female breast ♀ ☑
C50.112	Malignant neoplasm of central portion of left female breast ♀ ☑
C50.211	Malignant neoplasm of upper-inner quadrant of right female breast ♀ ☑
C50.212	Malignant neoplasm of upper-inner quadrant of left female breast ♀ ☑
C50.311	Malignant neoplasm of lower-inner quadrant of right female breast ♀ ☑
C50.312	Malignant neoplasm of lower-inner quadrant of left female breast ♀ ☑
C50.411	Malignant neoplasm of upper-outer quadrant of right female breast ♀ ☑
C50.412	Malignant neoplasm of upper-outer quadrant of left female breast ♀ ☑
C50.511	Malignant neoplasm of lower-outer quadrant of right female breast ♀ ☑

Lymph Nodes

C50.512	Malignant neoplasm of lower-outer quadrant of left female breast ♀ ☑	
C50.611	Malignant neoplasm of axillary tail of right female breast ♀ ☑	
C50.612	Malignant neoplasm of axillary tail of left female breast ♀ ☑	
C50.811	Malignant neoplasm of overlapping sites of right female breast ♀ ☑	
C50.812	Malignant neoplasm of overlapping sites of left female breast ♀ ☑	
C53.0	Malignant neoplasm of endocervix ♀	
C53.1	Malignant neoplasm of exocervix ♀	
C53.8	Malignant neoplasm of overlapping sites of cervix uteri ♀	
C62.01	Malignant neoplasm of undescended right testis ♂ ☑	
C62.02	Malignant neoplasm of undescended left testis ♂ ☑	
C62.11	Malignant neoplasm of descended right testis ♂ ☑	
C62.12	Malignant neoplasm of descended left testis ♂ ☑	
C73	Malignant neoplasm of thyroid gland	
C75.0	Malignant neoplasm of parathyroid gland	
C77.3	Secondary and unspecified malignant neoplasm of axilla and upper limb lymph nodes	
C7B.01	Secondary carcinoid tumors of distant lymph nodes	
C7B.09	Secondary carcinoid tumors of other sites	
C81.04	Nodular lymphocyte predominant Hodgkin lymphoma, lymph nodes of axilla and upper limb	
C81.14	Nodular sclerosis Hodgkin lymphoma, lymph nodes of axilla and upper limb	
C81.19	Nodular sclerosis Hodgkin lymphoma, extranodal and solid organ sites	
C81.24	Mixed cellularity Hodgkin lymphoma, lymph nodes of axilla and upper limb	
C81.29	Mixed cellularity Hodgkin lymphoma, extranodal and solid organ sites	
C81.34	Lymphocyte depleted Hodgkin lymphoma, lymph nodes of axilla and upper limb	
C81.39	Lymphocyte depleted Hodgkin lymphoma, extranodal and solid organ sites	
C81.74	Other Hodgkin lymphoma, lymph nodes of axilla and upper limb	
C82.54	Diffuse follicle center lymphoma, lymph nodes of axilla and upper limb	
C83.34	Diffuse large B-cell lymphoma, lymph nodes of axilla and upper limb	
C83.54	Lymphoblastic (diffuse) lymphoma, lymph nodes of axilla and upper limb	
C84.Z4	Other mature T/NK-cell lymphomas, lymph nodes of axilla and upper limb	
C85.24	Mediastinal (thymic) large B-cell lymphoma, lymph nodes of axilla and upper limb	
C85.84	Other specified types of non-Hodgkin lymphoma, lymph nodes of axilla and upper limb	
D18.1	Lymphangioma, any site	
R59.0	Localized enlarged lymph nodes	
R59.1	Generalized enlarged lymph nodes	

AMA: 38792 2019,Feb,8; 2018,Jan,8; 2017,Jan,8; 2016,Jan,13; 2015,Mar,5; 2015,Jan,16

Relative Value Units/Medicare Edits

Non-Facility RVU	Work	PE	MP	Total
38792	0.65	1.72	0.09	2.46
Facility RVU	Work	PE	MP	Total
38792	0.65	0.23	0.09	0.97

	FUD	Status	MUE	Modifiers				IOM Reference
38792	0	A	1(3)	51	50	N/A	N/A	None

* with documentation

Terms To Know

contrast material. Any internally administered substance that has a different opacity from soft tissue on radiography or computed tomograph; includes barium, used to opacify parts of the gastrointestinal tract; water-soluble iodinated compounds, used to opacify blood vessels or the genitourinary tract; may refer to air occurring naturally or introduced into the body; also, paramagnetic substances used in magnetic resonance imaging. Substances may also be documented as contrast agent or contrast medium.

injection. Forcing a liquid substance into a body part such as a joint or muscle.

lymph nodes. Bean-shaped structures along the lymphatic vessels that intercept and destroy foreign materials in the tissue and bloodstream.

malignant. Any condition tending to progress toward death, specifically an invasive tumor with a loss of cellular differentiation that has the ability to spread or metastasize to other body areas.

melanoma. Highly metastatic malignant neoplasm composed of melanocytes that occur most often on the skin from a preexisting mole or nevus but may also occur in the mouth, esophagus, anal canal, or vagina. Melanoma has four stages:

Stage 0: cells are found only in the outer layer of skin cells and have not invaded deeper tissues.

Stage I: Tumor is no more than 1 mm thick and the outer layer of skin may appear scraped or ulcerated; or the tumor is between 1 and 2 mm thick with no ulceration and no spread to nearby lymph nodes.

Stage II: Tumor is at least 1 mm thick with ulceration or the lesion is more than 2 mm thick without ulceration and no spread to lymph nodes.

Stage III: Cells have spread to one or more nearby lymph nodes or to tissues just outside the original lesion.

Stage IV: Malignant cells have spread to other organs, lymph nodes, or areas of the skin distant from the original tumor.

sentinel lymph node. First node to which lymph drainage and metastasis from a cancer can occur.

38900

+ **38900** Intraoperative identification (eg, mapping) of sentinel lymph node(s) includes injection of non-radioactive dye, when performed (List separately in addition to code for primary procedure)

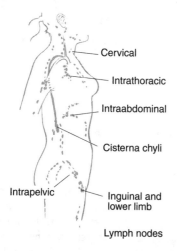

Lymph nodes

Explanation

Intraoperative mapping may be utilized during lymph node biopsy procedures. During the procedure, a nonradioactive dye such as methylene blue is injected into the area of focus. Following the path of the dye with the aid of fluorescence imaging, the first lymph node to receive lymphatic drainage from a tumor (sentinel lymph node) is identified and a separately reportable biopsy follows.

Coding Tips

Report 38900 in addition to 19302, 19307, 38500, 38510-38542, 38562, 38564, 38570-38572, 38740, or 38745, 38760-38780, 56630-56634, 56637, 56640. For injection of a radioactive tracer for identification of the sentinel node, see 38792.

ICD-10-CM Diagnostic Codes

C43.52	Malignant melanoma of skin of breast
C43.59	Malignant melanoma of other part of trunk
C43.61	Malignant melanoma of right upper limb, including shoulder ☑
C43.62	Malignant melanoma of left upper limb, including shoulder ☑
C50.111	Malignant neoplasm of central portion of right female breast ♀ ☑
C50.112	Malignant neoplasm of central portion of left female breast ♀ ☑
C50.121	Malignant neoplasm of central portion of right male breast ♂ ☑
C50.122	Malignant neoplasm of central portion of left male breast ♂ ☑
C50.211	Malignant neoplasm of upper-inner quadrant of right female breast ♀ ☑
C50.212	Malignant neoplasm of upper-inner quadrant of left female breast ♀ ☑
C50.221	Malignant neoplasm of upper-inner quadrant of right male breast ♂ ☑
C50.222	Malignant neoplasm of upper-inner quadrant of left male breast ♂ ☑
C50.311	Malignant neoplasm of lower-inner quadrant of right female breast ♀ ☑
C50.312	Malignant neoplasm of lower-inner quadrant of left female breast ♀ ☑
C50.321	Malignant neoplasm of lower-inner quadrant of right male breast ♂ ☑
C50.322	Malignant neoplasm of lower-inner quadrant of left male breast ♂ ☑
C50.411	Malignant neoplasm of upper-outer quadrant of right female breast ♀ ☑
C50.412	Malignant neoplasm of upper-outer quadrant of left female breast ♀ ☑
C50.511	Malignant neoplasm of lower-outer quadrant of right female breast ♀ ☑
C50.512	Malignant neoplasm of lower-outer quadrant of left female breast ♀ ☑
C50.521	Malignant neoplasm of lower-outer quadrant of right male breast ♂ ☑
C50.611	Malignant neoplasm of axillary tail of right female breast ♀ ☑
C50.621	Malignant neoplasm of axillary tail of right male breast ♂ ☑
C50.811	Malignant neoplasm of overlapping sites of right female breast ♀ ☑
C50.821	Malignant neoplasm of overlapping sites of right male breast ♂ ☑
C77.1	Secondary and unspecified malignant neoplasm of intrathoracic lymph nodes
C77.3	Secondary and unspecified malignant neoplasm of axilla and upper limb lymph nodes
D05.11	Intraductal carcinoma in situ of right breast ☑
D05.12	Intraductal carcinoma in situ of left breast ☑
D36.0	Benign neoplasm of lymph nodes

AMA: **38900** 2019,Feb,8; 2018,Jan,8; 2017,Jan,8; 2016,Jan,13; 2015,Mar,5

Relative Value Units/Medicare Edits

Non-Facility RVU	Work	PE	MP	Total
38900	2.5	0.96	0.59	4.05
Facility RVU	**Work**	**PE**	**MP**	**Total**
38900	2.5	0.96	0.59	4.05

	FUD	Status	MUE	Modifiers			IOM Reference
38900	N/A	A	1(3)	N/A	50	62*	80	None

* with documentation

Terms To Know

lymph nodes. Bean-shaped structures along the lymphatic vessels that intercept and destroy foreign materials in the tissue and bloodstream.

sentinel node biopsy. Tissue or fluid removed from the first lymph node from the breast for analysis of the cells and diagnosis.

39501

39501 Repair, laceration of diaphragm, any approach

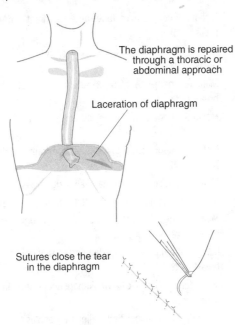

The diaphragm is repaired through a thoracic or abdominal approach

Laceration of diaphragm

Sutures close the tear in the diaphragm

Explanation

The physician makes an abdominal or chest incision and exposes a tear in the diaphragm. The tear is repaired with nonabsorbable sutures. Occasionally the tear may be so extensive that an artificial patch is used to repair defects or reinforce sutures. The incision is closed with sutures or staples, and a dressing is applied.

Coding Tips

When this procedure is performed with another separately identifiable procedure, the highest dollar value code is listed as the primary procedure, and subsequent procedures are appended with modifier 51. For transabdominal diaphragmatic (esophageal hiatal) hernia repair, see 43325. To report laparoscopic diaphragmatic (esophageal hiatal) hernia repairs and fundoplication, see codes 43280–43282.

ICD-10-CM Diagnostic Codes

S27.802A	Contusion of diaphragm, initial encounter
S27.803A	Laceration of diaphragm, initial encounter
S27.808A	Other injury of diaphragm, initial encounter

AMA: **39501** 2018,Jan,8; 2017,Jan,8; 2016,Jan,13; 2015,Jan,16

Relative Value Units/Medicare Edits

Non-Facility RVU	Work	PE	MP	Total
39501	13.98	8.05	3.16	25.19
Facility RVU	**Work**	**PE**	**MP**	**Total**
39501	13.98	8.05	3.16	25.19

	FUD	Status	MUE	Modifiers				IOM Reference
39501	90	A	1(3)	51	N/A	62*	80	None

* with documentation

39503

39503 Repair, neonatal diaphragmatic hernia, with or without chest tube insertion and with or without creation of ventral hernia

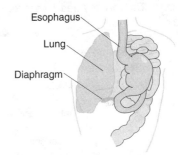

Esophagus

Lung

Diaphragm

A defect of the diaphragm can allow abdominal contents to herniate into the thoracic cavity

Explanation

The physician makes an incision across the abdomen. The herniated stomach is returned to its appropriate position in the abdomen, and the hernia sac is cut away and removed. The enlarged opening in the diaphragm through which the esophagus passes is narrowed by placing sutures in the two pillars connecting the spinal column and diaphragm. Reforming the stomach, cutting the vagus nerve or altering the size of the stomach-intestinal opening may be performed as well. Drains are placed, and the wound is sutured closed.

Coding Tips

Diaphragmatic or hiatus hernia in the newborn is a congenital anomaly in which the abdominal contents protrude into the thoracic cavity through a defect in the diaphragm. Severe cases are a medical emergency and must be repaired immediately after birth. For repair of a diaphragmatic hernia other than neonatal, see 39540–39541. For transthoracic diaphragmatic (esophageal hiatal) hernia repair, see 43334–43335. Report laparoscopic paraesophageal hernia repair with codes 43281–43282. Do not append modifier 63 to 39503 as the description or nature of the procedure includes infants up to 4 kg.

ICD-10-CM Diagnostic Codes

Q79.0	Congenital diaphragmatic hernia

AMA: **39503** 2018,Jan,8; 2017,Jan,8; 2016,Jan,13; 2015,Jan,16

Relative Value Units/Medicare Edits

Non-Facility RVU	Work	PE	MP	Total
39503	108.91	36.32	24.99	170.22
Facility RVU	**Work**	**PE**	**MP**	**Total**
39503	108.91	36.32	24.99	170.22

	FUD	Status	MUE	Modifiers				IOM Reference
39503	90	A	1(2)	51	N/A	62*	80	None

* with documentation

Terms To Know

congenital. Present at birth, occurring through heredity or an influence during gestation up to the moment of birth.

neonatal period. Period of an infant's life from birth to the age of 27 days, 23 hours, and 59 minutes.

Diaphragm

39540-39541

39540 Repair, diaphragmatic hernia (other than neonatal), traumatic; acute
39541   chronic

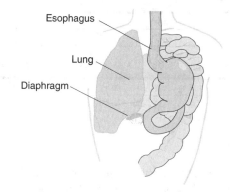

Explanation

A massive injury in the diaphragm is repaired, allowing organs to protrude into the chest cavity. The physician makes an incision into the chest or abdomen. The abdominal contents are drawn back into the abdomen, and the hole in the diaphragm is exposed. The opening is closed with sutures or by insertion of a patch. The tear is repaired with nonabsorbable sutures. The incision is closed with sutures or staples. Report 39541 if the hernia is chronic.

Coding Tips

Diaphragmatic hernias, also referred to as hiatus or sliding hiatal hernias, are caused by a defect in the diaphragm that allows abdominal contents to protrude above the diaphragm. They may be an acute, traumatic condition (39540) or a chronic condition (39541). To report transthoracic diaphragmatic (esophageal hiatal) hernia repair, see 43334–43335.

ICD-10-CM Diagnostic Codes

K44.0	Diaphragmatic hernia with obstruction, without gangrene
K44.1	Diaphragmatic hernia with gangrene
K44.9	Diaphragmatic hernia without obstruction or gangrene

AMA: 39540 2018,Jan,8; 2017,Jan,8; 2016,Jan,13; 2015,Jan,16 **39541** 2018,Jan,8; 2017,Jan,8; 2016,Jan,13; 2015,Jan,16

Relative Value Units/Medicare Edits

Non-Facility RVU	Work	PE	MP	Total
39540	14.57	7.55	3.31	25.43
39541	15.75	8.21	3.68	27.64
Facility RVU	**Work**	**PE**	**MP**	**Total**
39540	14.57	7.55	3.31	25.43
39541	15.75	8.21	3.68	27.64

	FUD	Status	MUE	Modifiers				IOM Reference
39540	90	A	1(2)	51	N/A	62*	80	None
39541	90	A	1(2)	51	N/A	62*	80	

* with documentation

39545

39545 Imbrication of diaphragm for eventration, transthoracic or transabdominal, paralytic or nonparalytic

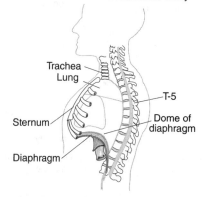

The diaphragm is the muscular wall separating the thorax from the abdominal cavity

Schematic showing diaphragm

Eventration is an abnormal elevation of the dome of the diaphragm

Explanation

The physician makes an incision across the chest or abdomen. The abdominal contents are drawn back into the abdomen, and the diaphragm is exposed. The connective tissue is used to stitch folds or tucks into the diaphragm to restore it to its original position. The incision is closed with sutures or staples.

Coding Tips

When 39545 is performed with another separately identifiable procedure, the highest dollar value code is listed as the primary procedure and subsequent procedures are appended with modifier 51. For repair of an acute, traumatic diaphragmatic hernia (other than neonatal), see 39540; chronic, see 39541.

ICD-10-CM Diagnostic Codes

J98.6	Disorders of diaphragm
Q79.1	Other congenital malformations of diaphragm

AMA: 39545 2018,Jan,8; 2017,Jan,8; 2016,Jan,13; 2015,Jan,16

Relative Value Units/Medicare Edits

Non-Facility RVU	Work	PE	MP	Total
39545	14.67	8.21	3.37	26.25
Facility RVU	**Work**	**PE**	**MP**	**Total**
39545	14.67	8.21	3.37	26.25

	FUD	Status	MUE	Modifiers				IOM Reference
39545	90	A	1(2)	51	N/A	62*	80	None

* with documentation

Terms To Know

imbricate. Process of building a surface of overlapping layers of apposing material, such as tissue, for closing a wound or other opening in a body part.

Diaphragm

39560-39561

39560   Resection, diaphragm; with simple repair (eg, primary suture)

39561   Resection, diaphragm; with complex repair (eg, prosthetic material, local muscle flap)

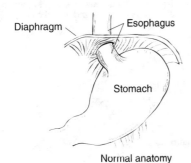

Diaphragm   Esophagus

Stomach

Normal anatomy

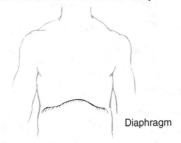

The diaphragm is the muscular wall separating the thorax from the abdominal cavity

Diaphragm

Explanation

Usually performed for tumors that have invaded the diaphragm, the surgeon removes part of the large muscle separating the chest and abdominal cavities. The patient is taken to the operating room and the chest is surgically opened using a midline incision. Occasionally, the xiphoid process is divided or removed to gain access. Retractors are placed to provide an optimal view of the subphrenic space. Using electrocautery, any affected tissue from the diaphragm is dissected and removed. The liver may be mobilized to provide better access to the surgical site. Once the tissue is removed, the diaphragm is repaired. Code 39560 involves using internal sutures. Code 39561 involves a complex repair using a muscle flap or synthetic material to correct the remaining large surgical defect. Hemostasis is confirmed and the operative wound is closed in layers.

Coding Tips

Any local muscle flap is included in the procedure and is not reported separately. For other open repairs of the diaphragm, see 39501–39541.

ICD-10-CM Diagnostic Codes

C49.3	Malignant neoplasm of connective and soft tissue of thorax
C79.89	Secondary malignant neoplasm of other specified sites
D21.3	Benign neoplasm of connective and other soft tissue of thorax
D48.1	Neoplasm of uncertain behavior of connective and other soft tissue
D49.2	Neoplasm of unspecified behavior of bone, soft tissue, and skin
J98.6	Disorders of diaphragm

AMA: **39560** 2018,Jan,8; 2017,Jan,8; 2016,Jan,13; 2015,Jan,16 **39561** 2018,Jan,8; 2017,Jan,8; 2016,Jan,13; 2015,Jan,16

Relative Value Units/Medicare Edits

Non-Facility RVU	Work	PE	MP	Total
39560	13.06	7.68	2.79	23.53
39561	19.99	12.05	4.56	36.6
Facility RVU	Work	PE	MP	Total
39560	13.06	7.68	2.79	23.53
39561	19.99	12.05	4.56	36.6

	FUD	Status	MUE	Modifiers			IOM Reference
39560	90	A	1(3)	51	N/A	62*	80	None
39561	90	A	1(3)	51	N/A	62*	80	

* with documentation

Terms To Know

abscess. Circumscribed collection of pus resulting from bacteria, frequently associated with swelling and other signs of inflammation.

absorbable sutures. Strands used for suture or repair of tissue prepared from collagen or a synthetic polymer and capable of being absorbed by tissue over time.

congenital. Present at birth, occurring through heredity or an influence during gestation up to the moment of birth.

diaphragm. Muscular wall separating the thorax and its structures from the abdomen.

electrocautery. Division or cutting of tissue using high-frequency electrical current to produce heat, which destroys cells.

mobilization. Therapy that consists of small passive movements, usually applied as a series of gentle stretches in a smooth, rhythmic fashion to the individual vertebrae. The movements are applied at various locations on each of the affected vertebrae, and at various angles, directed at relieving restriction in movement at any particular level of the spine. Mobilization stretches stiff joints to restore range. It also relieves pain. For example, it is especially effective with arthritic joints.

resection. Surgical removal of a part or all of an organ or body part.

wound repair. Surgical closure of a wound is divided into three categories: simple, intermediate, and complex. *simple repair:* Surgical closure of a superficial wound, requiring single layer suturing of the skin epidermis, dermis, or subcutaneous tissue. *intermediate repair:* Surgical closure of a wound requiring closure of one or more of the deeper subcutaneous tissue and non-muscle fascia layers in addition to suturing the skin; contaminated wounds with single layer closure that need extensive cleaning or foreign body removal. *complex repair:* Repair of wounds requiring more than layered closure (debridement, scar revision, stents, retention sutures).

42975

● **42975** Drug-induced sleep endoscopy, with dynamic evaluation of velum, pharynx, tongue base, and larynx for evaluation of sleep-disordered breathing, flexible, diagnostic

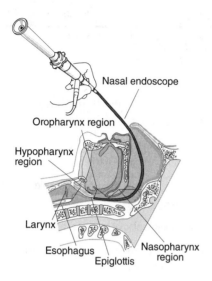

- Nasal endoscope
- Oropharynx region
- Hypopharynx region
- Larynx
- Esophagus
- Epiglottis
- Nasopharynx region

Explanation

The physician performs a diagnostic drug-induced sleep endoscopy (DISE) to evaluate the airway of a patient with obstructive sleep apnea (OSA). Also known as sleep nasoendoscopy (SNE), this procedure is typically performed in conjunction with an anesthesiologist. The patient is administered a sedative infusion, often propofol. The dose is carefully titrated in order to cause obstructive apnea but avoiding central apnea. The physician passes a fiberoptic nasopharyngoscope into the nasal cavity and performs a full examination to rule out any airway obstructions. The scope is advanced into the nasopharynx. The physician pauses at this point until the patient begins snoring, at which point the examination continues of the nasopharynx, velopharynx, and hypopharynx. The physician notes the degree of collapse using a standardized grading scale. Obstruction at the level of the palate (palate, tonsils, and lateral pharyngeal wall) and at the level of the hypopharynx (base of tongue, epiglottis, and lateral pharyngeal wall) is noted. The physician may advance the mandible 5 to 10 mm forward so that the action of a mandibular advancement device or a genioglossal advancement is reproduced. Insertion of a nasal trumpet or oral airway, or performance of a jaw thrust maneuver may also be a component of the evaluation.

Coding Tips

Do not report 42975 with 31231, unless performed for a condition other than a sleep-disordered breathing, and a separate endoscope is used. Do not report 42975 with 31575 or 92511.

ICD-10-CM Diagnostic Codes

G47.33   Obstructive sleep apnea (adult) (pediatric)

Relative Value Units/Medicare Edits

Non-Facility RVU	Work	PE	MP	Total
42975				
Facility RVU	**Work**	**PE**	**MP**	**Total**
42975				

	FUD	Status	MUE	Modifiers				IOM Reference
42975	N/A		-	N/A	N/A	N/A	N/A	None

* with documentation

Terms To Know

diagnostic procedures. Procedure performed on a patient to obtain information to assess the medical condition of the patient or to identify a disease and to determine the nature and severity of an illness or injury.

endoscopy. Visual inspection of the body using a fiberoptic scope.

OSAS. Obstructive sleep apnea syndrome. Headaches, high blood pressure, daytime sleepiness, and mental dullness usually associated with oxygen deprivation during sleep. Snoring is also common in OSAS. Confirmation of obstructive sleep apnea requires sleep testing.

sleep apnea. Intermittent cessation of breathing during sleep that may cause hypoxemia and pulmonary arterial hypertension.

Esophagus

43020

43020 Esophagotomy, cervical approach, with removal of foreign body

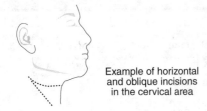

Example of horizontal and oblique incisions in the cervical area

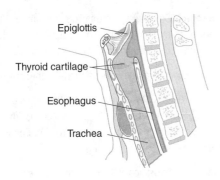

Epiglottis

Thyroid cartilage

Esophagus

Trachea

Explanation

The physician makes an incision in the esophagus to remove a foreign body from it. The physician makes a horizontal or oblique incision in the lateral neck and into the esophagus, using forceps to grasp and extract the foreign body. The incision is closed with sutured layers.

Coding Tips

For esophagotomy with removal of a foreign body via thoracic approach, see 43045. Esophagoscopy with removal of a foreign body is reported with 43215.

ICD-10-CM Diagnostic Codes

K22.2   Esophageal obstruction
S01.542A   Puncture wound with foreign body of oral cavity, initial encounter
S11.22XA   Laceration with foreign body of pharynx and cervical esophagus, initial encounter
S11.24XA   Puncture wound with foreign body of pharynx and cervical esophagus, initial encounter
T18.120A   Food in esophagus causing compression of trachea, initial encounter
T18.128A   Food in esophagus causing other injury, initial encounter
T18.190A   Other foreign object in esophagus causing compression of trachea, initial encounter
T18.198A   Other foreign object in esophagus causing other injury, initial encounter

AMA: 43020 2014,Jan,11

Relative Value Units/Medicare Edits

Non-Facility RVU	Work	PE	MP	Total
43020	8.23	6.45	1.99	16.67
Facility RVU	**Work**	**PE**	**MP**	**Total**
43020	8.23	6.45	1.99	16.67

	FUD	Status	MUE	Modifiers				IOM Reference
43020	90	A	1(2)	51	N/A	62*	80	None

* with documentation

Terms To Know

approach. Method or anatomical location used to gain access to a body organ or specific area for procedures.

epiglottis. Lid-like cartilaginous tissue that covers the entrance to the larynx and blocks food from entering the trachea.

esophagus. Muscular tube that carries swallowed liquids and foods from the pharynx to the stomach.

forceps. Tool used for grasping or compressing tissue.

foreign body. Any object or substance found in an organ and tissue that does not belong under normal circumstances.

incision. Act of cutting into tissue or an organ.

lateral. On/to the side.

stenosis. Narrowing or constriction of a passage.

stricture. Narrowing of an anatomical structure.

suture. Numerous stitching techniques employed in wound closure.

buried suture. Continuous or interrupted suture placed under the skin for a layered closure.

continuous suture. Running stitch with tension evenly distributed across a single strand to provide a leakproof closure line.

interrupted suture. Series of single stitches with tension isolated at each stitch, in which all stitches are not affected if one becomes loose, and the isolated sutures cannot act as a wick to transport an infection.

purse-string suture. Continuous suture placed around a tubular structure and tightened, to reduce or close the lumen.

retention suture. Secondary stitching that bridges the primary suture, providing support for the primary repair; a plastic or rubber bolster may be placed over the primary repair and under the retention sutures.

trachea. Tube descending from the larynx and branching into the right and left main bronchi.

Esophagus

43100-43101

43100 Excision of lesion, esophagus, with primary repair; cervical approach
43101 thoracic or abdominal approach

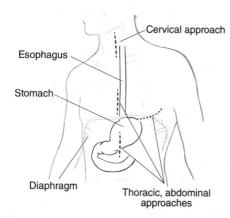

Cervical approach
Esophagus
Stomach
Diaphragm
Thoracic, abdominal approaches

Explanation

The physician removes a lesion in the esophagus. In 43100, the physician makes a horizontal or oblique incision of the lateral neck. Next, the physician makes an incision in the esophagus and excises the lesion. In 43101, for a thoracic approach, the physician incises and dissects the left posterior chest wall to access the esophagus. For an abdominal approach, the physician makes an upper midline abdominal incision to access the esophagus transhiatally. The physician excises the lesion. The remaining esophageal borders are sutured together. The incision is closed with sutured layers.

Coding Tips

For partial esophagectomy, see 43116–43123. For total or partial esophagectomy, without reconstruction (any approach), see 43124. If significant additional time and effort is documented, append modifier 22 and submit a cover letter and operative report.

ICD-10-CM Diagnostic Codes

C15.3	Malignant neoplasm of upper third of esophagus
C15.4	Malignant neoplasm of middle third of esophagus
C15.5	Malignant neoplasm of lower third of esophagus
C15.8	Malignant neoplasm of overlapping sites of esophagus
D00.1	Carcinoma in situ of esophagus
D13.0	Benign neoplasm of esophagus
K22.10	Ulcer of esophagus without bleeding
K22.11	Ulcer of esophagus with bleeding
K22.89	Other specified disease of esophagus
K23	Disorders of esophagus in diseases classified elsewhere
S27.818A	Other injury of esophagus (thoracic part), initial encounter
T28.1XXA	Burn of esophagus, initial encounter
T28.6XXA	Corrosion of esophagus, initial encounter

AMA: 43101 2018,Jan,8; 2017,Jan,8; 2016,Jan,13; 2015,Jan,16

Relative Value Units/Medicare Edits

Non-Facility RVU	Work	PE	MP	Total
43100	9.66	7.43	1.34	18.43
43101	17.07	8.55	3.93	29.55
Facility RVU	**Work**	**PE**	**MP**	**Total**
43100	9.66	7.43	1.34	18.43
43101	17.07	8.55	3.93	29.55

	FUD	Status	MUE	Modifiers			IOM Reference
43100	90	A	1(3)	51	N/A	62*	80	None
43101	90	A	1(3)	51	N/A	62*	80	

* with documentation

Terms To Know

approach. Method or anatomical location used to gain access to a body organ or specific area for procedures.

benign. Mild or nonmalignant in nature.

carcinoma in situ. Malignancy that arises from the cells of the vessel, gland, or organ of origin that remains confined to that site or has not invaded neighboring tissue.

dissection. Separating by cutting tissue or body structures apart.

excision. Surgical removal of an organ or tissue.

lesion. Area of damaged tissue that has lost continuity or function, due to disease or trauma. Lesions may be located on internal structures such as the brain, nerves, or kidneys, or visible on the skin.

malignant. Any condition tending to progress toward death, specifically an invasive tumor with a loss of cellular differentiation that has the ability to spread or metastasize to other body areas.

neoplasm. New abnormal growth, tumor.

repair. Surgical closure of a wound. The wound may be a result of injury/trauma or it may be a surgically created defect. Repairs are divided into three categories: simple, intermediate, and complex.

secondary. Second in order of occurrence or importance, or appearing during the course of another disease or condition.

43107

43107 Total or near total esophagectomy, without thoracotomy; with pharyngogastrostomy or cervical esophagogastrostomy, with or without pyloroplasty (transhiatal)

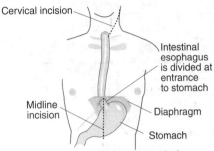

Cervical incision

Intestinal esophagus is divided at entrance to stomach

Midline incision

Diaphragm

Stomach

Esophagus is divided at the cervical level (shown) or at its origin in the pharynx

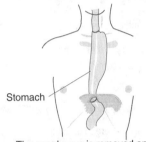

Stomach

The esophagus is removed and the stomach is pulled up and attached to the remaining esophagus or to the pharynx

Explanation

The physician removes most or all of the esophagus and attaches the stomach to the pharynx or cervical esophagus. The physician gains access to the esophagus through two incisions: an oblique cervical incision and a horizontal upper midline abdominal incision. The physician divides the esophagus at the cervical level (for an esophagogastrostomy) or at its origin at the pharynx (for a pharyngogastrostomy). The esophagus is removed through the abdominal incision and divided from the stomach. The stomach is pulled through the posterior mediastinum and anastomosed to the pharynx or the remaining cervical esophagus. If the stomach is used as the esophageal conduit, a pyloroplasty may be performed to open the pyloric sphincter. The incisions are repaired in sutured layers.

Coding Tips

If significant additional time and effort are documented, append modifier 22 and submit a cover letter and operative report. When this procedure is performed with colon interposition or small intestine reconstruction, including intestine mobilization, preparation, and anastomosis(es), see 43108.

ICD-10-CM Diagnostic Codes

C15.4	Malignant neoplasm of middle third of esophagus
C15.5	Malignant neoplasm of lower third of esophagus
C15.8	Malignant neoplasm of overlapping sites of esophagus
K22.0	Achalasia of cardia
K22.10	Ulcer of esophagus without bleeding
K22.11	Ulcer of esophagus with bleeding
K22.3	Perforation of esophagus
K22.710	Barrett's esophagus with low grade dysplasia
K22.711	Barrett's esophagus with high grade dysplasia

K22.89	Other specified disease of esophagus
K31.1	Adult hypertrophic pyloric stenosis △
Q39.3	Congenital stenosis and stricture of esophagus
Q39.5	Congenital dilatation of esophagus
Q39.6	Congenital diverticulum of esophagus
Q39.8	Other congenital malformations of esophagus
Q40.0	Congenital hypertrophic pyloric stenosis
S27.818A	Other injury of esophagus (thoracic part), initial encounter
T28.1XXA	Burn of esophagus, initial encounter
T28.6XXA	Corrosion of esophagus, initial encounter

AMA: **43107** 2014,Jan,11

Relative Value Units/Medicare Edits

Non-Facility RVU	Work	PE	MP	Total
43107	52.05	23.2	11.99	87.24
Facility RVU	Work	PE	MP	Total
43107	52.05	23.2	11.99	87.24

	FUD	Status	MUE	Modifiers				IOM Reference
43107	90	A	1(2)	51	N/A	62*	80	None

* with documentation

Terms To Know

anastomosis. Surgically created connection between ducts, blood vessels, or bowel segments to allow flow from one to the other.

esophagus. Muscular tube that carries swallowed liquids and foods from the pharynx to the stomach.

pharynx. Musculomembranous passage of the throat consisting of three regions: the nasopharynx is the passage at the back of the nostrils, above the level of the soft palate, and communicating with the eustachian tube.

pyloroplasty. Enlargement and reconstruction of the lower portion of the stomach opening into the duodenum performed after vagotomy to speed gastric emptying and treat duodenal ulcers.

sphincter. Ring-like band of muscle that surrounds a bodily opening, constricting and relaxing as required for normal physiological functioning.

thoracotomy. Surgical procedure for opening the chest wall in order to access the lungs, esophagus, trachea, aorta, heart, and diaphragm.

43108

43108 Total or near total esophagectomy, without thoracotomy; with colon interposition or small intestine reconstruction, including intestine mobilization, preparation and anastomosis(es)

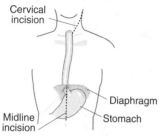

Esophagus is divided, at the cervical level (shown) or at its origin in the pharynx, and removed

Midline incision is made to access a section of colon or small bowel

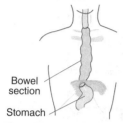

Resected bowel is attached to the stomach and to the remaining portion of esophagus or to the pharynx

Explanation

The physician removes most or all of the esophagus and uses a bowel or colon graft for reconstruction. The physician gains access to the esophagus through two incisions: an oblique cervical incision and a horizontal upper midline abdominal incision. The physician divides the esophagus at the cervical level (for an esophagogastrostomy) or at its origin at the pharynx (for a pharyngogastrostomy). The esophagus is removed through the abdominal incision and divided from the stomach. A portion of the colon or small bowel is excised and freed of attachments, taking care to preserve its major vascular supply. Gastrointestinal continuity is reestablished by securing the distal and proximal bowel margins. Finally, the excised portion of the colon or bowel is attached to the pharynx or cervical esophagus and the stomach. This anastomosis creates a usable esophagus. If the stomach is used as the esophageal conduit, a pyloroplasty may be performed to open the pyloric sphincter. The incisions are repaired in sutured layers.

Coding Tips

This procedure is performed without thoracotomy. When thoracotomy is performed, see 43113. For total or near total esophagectomy, without thoracotomy, with pharyngogastrostomy or cervical esophagogastrostomy, with or without pyloroplasty, see 43107; with thoracotomy, see 43112. For partial esophagectomy, see 43116–43123. For total or partial esophagectomy (any approach), without reconstruction, see 43124.

ICD-10-CM Diagnostic Codes

C15.4	Malignant neoplasm of middle third of esophagus
C15.5	Malignant neoplasm of lower third of esophagus
C15.8	Malignant neoplasm of overlapping sites of esophagus
K22.710	Barrett's esophagus with low grade dysplasia
K22.711	Barrett's esophagus with high grade dysplasia
K22.89	Other specified disease of esophagus
K23	Disorders of esophagus in diseases classified elsewhere
Q39.5	Congenital dilatation of esophagus
Q39.6	Congenital diverticulum of esophagus
Q39.8	Other congenital malformations of esophagus
S27.813A	Laceration of esophagus (thoracic part), initial encounter
S27.818A	Other injury of esophagus (thoracic part), initial encounter
T28.1XXA	Burn of esophagus, initial encounter
T28.6XXA	Corrosion of esophagus, initial encounter

AMA: 43108 2014,Jan,11

Relative Value Units/Medicare Edits

Non-Facility RVU	Work	PE	MP	Total
43108	82.87	28.24	19.02	130.13
Facility RVU	**Work**	**PE**	**MP**	**Total**
43108	82.87	28.24	19.02	130.13

	FUD	Status	MUE	Modifiers				IOM Reference
43108	90	A	1(2)	51	N/A	62*	80	None

* with documentation

Terms To Know

anastomosis. Surgically created connection between ducts, blood vessels, or bowel segments to allow flow from one to the other.

congenital. Present at birth, occurring through heredity or an influence during gestation up to the moment of birth.

distal. Located farther away from a specified reference point or the trunk.

diverticulum. Pouch or sac in the walls of an organ or canal.

esophagus. Muscular tube that carries swallowed liquids and foods from the pharynx to the stomach.

interposition. Placement between objects.

proximal. Located closest to a specified reference point, usually the midline or trunk.

reconstruction. Recreating, restoring, or rebuilding a body part or organ.

thoracotomy. Surgical procedure for opening the chest wall in order to access the lungs, esophagus, trachea, aorta, heart, and diaphragm.

Esophagus

43112

43112 Total or near total esophagectomy, with thoracotomy; with pharyngogastrostomy or cervical esophagogastrostomy, with or without pyloroplasty (ie, McKeown esophagectomy or tri-incisional esophagectomy)

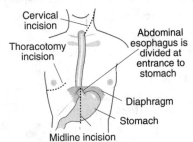

Esophagus is divided, either at the cervical level (shown) or at origin in the pharynx, and is discarded

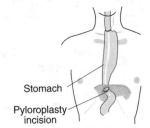

The esophagus is removed and the stomach is pulled up and attached to the remaining esophagus or to the pharynx

Explanation

The esophagus is removed through abdominal, chest, and neck incisions and replaced with stomach. The physician makes a midline abdominal incision. The stomach is dissected free of surrounding structures and the esophagus is mobilized as it passes through the diaphragm to the stomach. The physician makes an incision in the right chest between the ribs and exposes the esophagus. The esophagus is mobilized under direct vision in the chest from the diaphragm to the neck. A longitudinal incision is made in the left or right neck and the esophagus is identified and mobilized in the neck. The esophagus is divided at its junction with the stomach and in the neck and the esophagus is removed. The stomach is pulled through the middle of the chest into the neck and the stomach is connected to the stump of the esophagus in the neck. The incisions are closed. This procedure is also referred to as the McKeown procedure or the tri-incisional esophagectomy.

Coding Tips

This procedure is performed with thoracotomy. If the procedure is performed with colon interposition or small intestine reconstruction, including intestine mobilization, preparation, and anastomoses, see 43113. For total or near total esophagectomy, without thoracotomy, with pharyngogastrostomy or cervical esophagogastrostomy, with or without pyloroplasty, see 43107. For partial esophagectomy, see 43116–43123. For total or partial esophagectomy (any approach), without reconstruction, see 43124.

ICD-10-CM Diagnostic Codes

C15.4	Malignant neoplasm of middle third of esophagus
C15.5	Malignant neoplasm of lower third of esophagus
C15.8	Malignant neoplasm of overlapping sites of esophagus
C49.A1	Gastrointestinal stromal tumor of esophagus
K22.0	Achalasia of cardia
K22.10	Ulcer of esophagus without bleeding
K22.11	Ulcer of esophagus with bleeding
K22.3	Perforation of esophagus
K22.710	Barrett's esophagus with low grade dysplasia
K22.711	Barrett's esophagus with high grade dysplasia
K22.89	Other specified disease of esophagus
K23	Disorders of esophagus in diseases classified elsewhere
K31.1	Adult hypertrophic pyloric stenosis △
Q39.3	Congenital stenosis and stricture of esophagus
Q39.5	Congenital dilatation of esophagus
Q39.6	Congenital diverticulum of esophagus
Q39.8	Other congenital malformations of esophagus
Q40.0	Congenital hypertrophic pyloric stenosis
S27.812A	Contusion of esophagus (thoracic part), initial encounter
S27.813A	Laceration of esophagus (thoracic part), initial encounter
S27.818A	Other injury of esophagus (thoracic part), initial encounter
T28.1XXA	Burn of esophagus, initial encounter
T28.6XXA	Corrosion of esophagus, initial encounter

AMA: 43112 2018,Jul,7; 2018,Jan,8; 2017,Jan,8; 2016,Jan,13; 2015,Jan,16

Relative Value Units/Medicare Edits

Non-Facility RVU	Work	PE	MP	Total
43112	62.0	25.67	14.3	101.97
Facility RVU	**Work**	**PE**	**MP**	**Total**
43112	62.0	25.67	14.3	101.97

	FUD	Status	MUE	Modifiers				IOM Reference
43112	90	A	1(2)	51	N/A	62	80	None

* with documentation

Terms To Know

cervical. Relation to the cervical spine or to the cervix.

dissection. (dis. apart; -section, act of cutting) Separating by cutting tissue or body structures apart.

pyloroplasty. Enlargement and reconstruction of the lower portion of the stomach opening into the duodenum performed after vagotomy to speed gastric emptying and treat duodenal ulcers.

thoracotomy. Surgical procedure for opening the chest wall in order to access the lungs, esophagus, trachea, aorta, heart, and diaphragm.

43113

43113 Total or near total esophagectomy, with thoracotomy; with colon interposition or small intestine reconstruction, including intestine mobilization, preparation, and anastomosis(es)

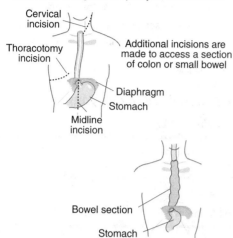

Esophagus is divided, either at the cervical level (shown) or at origin in the pharynx, and removed

Cervical incision

Thoracotomy incision

Additional incisions are made to access a section of colon or small bowel

Diaphragm

Stomach

Midline incision

Bowel section

Stomach

Resected bowel is attached to stomach and to remaining portion of esophagus or to the pharynx

Explanation

The physician removes the esophagus through abdominal, chest and neck incisions and replaces the esophagus with colon or small bowel. The physician makes a midline abdominal incision. The stomach is dissected free of surrounding structures and the esophagus is mobilized as it passes through the diagram to the stomach. The physician makes an incision in the right chest between the ribs and exposes the esophagus. The esophagus is mobilized under direct vision in the chest from the diaphragm to the neck. The esophagus is divided at its junction with the stomach and in the neck and the esophagus is removed. The physician selects an appropriate segment of colon or small bowel. The bowel is divided proximal and distal to this segment and the bowel ends are reapproximated. The selected segment of colon or small bowel is pulled through the middle section of the chest and connected to the stump of the esophagus in the neck and to the stomach in the abdomen. The incisions are closed.

Coding Tips

If significant additional time and effort are documented, append modifier 22 and submit a cover letter and operative report. For total or near total esophagectomy, without thoracotomy, with pharyngogastrostomy or cervical esophagogastrostomy, with or without pyloroplasty, see 43107; with colon interposition or small intestine reconstruction, including intestine mobilization, preparation, and anastomosis, see 43108. For partial esophagectomy, see 43116–43123. For total or partial esophagectomy (any approach), without reconstruction, see 43124.

ICD-10-CM Diagnostic Codes

C15.4	Malignant neoplasm of middle third of esophagus
C15.5	Malignant neoplasm of lower third of esophagus
C15.8	Malignant neoplasm of overlapping sites of esophagus
C49.A1	Gastrointestinal stromal tumor of esophagus
K22.710	Barrett's esophagus with low grade dysplasia
K22.711	Barrett's esophagus with high grade dysplasia
K22.89	Other specified disease of esophagus
K23	Disorders of esophagus in diseases classified elsewhere
Q39.5	Congenital dilatation of esophagus
Q39.6	Congenital diverticulum of esophagus
Q39.8	Other congenital malformations of esophagus
S27.812A	Contusion of esophagus (thoracic part), initial encounter
S27.813A	Laceration of esophagus (thoracic part), initial encounter
S27.818A	Other injury of esophagus (thoracic part), initial encounter
T28.1XXA	Burn of esophagus, initial encounter
T28.6XXA	Corrosion of esophagus, initial encounter

AMA: 43113 2014,Jan,11

Relative Value Units/Medicare Edits

Non-Facility RVU	Work	PE	MP	Total
43113	80.06	28.68	18.37	127.11
Facility RVU	**Work**	**PE**	**MP**	**Total**
43113	80.06	28.68	18.37	127.11

	FUD	Status	MUE	Modifiers				IOM Reference
43113	90	A	1(2)	51	N/A	62	80	None

* with documentation

Terms To Know

anastomosis. Surgically created connection between ducts, blood vessels, or bowel segments to allow flow from one to the other.

distal. Located farther away from a specified reference point or the trunk.

esophagus. Muscular tube that carries swallowed liquids and foods from the pharynx to the stomach.

interposition. Placement between objects.

proximal. Located closest to a specified reference point, usually the midline or trunk.

reconstruction. Recreating, restoring, or rebuilding a body part or organ.

thoracotomy. Surgical procedure for opening the chest wall in order to access the lungs, esophagus, trachea, aorta, heart, and diaphragm.

Esophagus

43116

43116 Partial esophagectomy, cervical, with free intestinal graft, including microvascular anastomosis, obtaining the graft and intestinal reconstruction

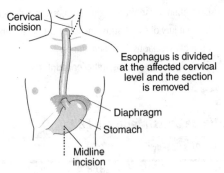

Cervical incision

Esophagus is divided at the affected cervical level and the section is removed

Diaphragm

Stomach

Midline incision

Midline incision is made to access a section of intestine

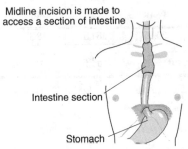

Intestine section

Stomach

Resected intestine is attached to the cervical esophagus; microvascular anastomosis is accomplished for blood supply

Explanation

The physician removes the affected portion of the esophagus and replaces it with a graft from the large or small intestine. The physician gains access to the esophagus through an oblique cervical incision. The physician resects the affected portion of the cervical esophagus. Next, the physician obtains a graft from the large or small intestine. To do this, the physician makes a midline abdominal incision and frees a portion of the large or small intestine of muscular and vascular attachments. The intestine is resected and interposed to reestablish gastrointestinal continuity in the cervical esophagus. Microsurgical techniques are used to create a new blood supply for the graft. The distal and proximal portions of the remaining intestine are reconnected (anastomosis).

Coding Tips

Do not report 43116 with 69990. Append modifier 52 to this code if intestinal or free jejunal graft with microvascular anastomosis is performed by another physician. Report 43496 for free jejunal transfer with microvascular anastomosis only.

ICD-10-CM Diagnostic Codes

C15.3	Malignant neoplasm of upper third of esophagus
C15.4	Malignant neoplasm of middle third of esophagus
C15.8	Malignant neoplasm of overlapping sites of esophagus
D00.1	Carcinoma in situ of esophagus
D13.0	Benign neoplasm of esophagus
K22.10	Ulcer of esophagus without bleeding
K22.11	Ulcer of esophagus with bleeding
K22.5	Diverticulum of esophagus, acquired
K22.70	Barrett's esophagus without dysplasia
K22.710	Barrett's esophagus with low grade dysplasia
K22.711	Barrett's esophagus with high grade dysplasia
K22.89	Other specified disease of esophagus
K23	Disorders of esophagus in diseases classified elsewhere
Q39.5	Congenital dilatation of esophagus
Q39.6	Congenital diverticulum of esophagus
Q39.8	Other congenital malformations of esophagus
T28.1XXA	Burn of esophagus, initial encounter
T28.6XXA	Corrosion of esophagus, initial encounter

AMA: **43116** 2016,Feb,12

Relative Value Units/Medicare Edits

Non-Facility RVU	Work	PE	MP	Total
43116	92.99	31.16	21.34	145.49
Facility RVU	**Work**	**PE**	**MP**	**Total**
43116	92.99	31.16	21.34	145.49

	FUD	Status	MUE	Modifiers				IOM Reference
43116	90	A	1(2)	51	N/A	62*	80	None

* with documentation

Terms To Know

anastomosis. Surgically created connection between ducts, blood vessels, or bowel segments to allow flow from one to the other.

cervical. Relation to the cervical spine or to the cervix.

graft. Tissue implant from another part of the body or another person.

interposition. Placement between objects.

reconstruction. Recreating, restoring, or rebuilding a body part or organ.

resection. Surgical removal of a part or all of an organ or body part.

Esophagus

43117

43117 Partial esophagectomy, distal two-thirds, with thoracotomy and separate abdominal incision, with or without proximal gastrectomy; with thoracic esophagogastrostomy, with or without pyloroplasty (Ivor Lewis)

The distal esophagus is removed, sometimes along with the upper part of the stomach

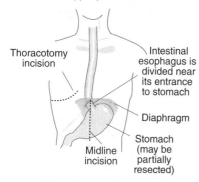

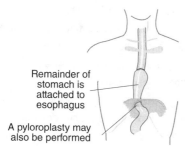

Remainder of stomach is attached to esophagus

A pyloroplasty may also be performed

Explanation

The physician removes the distal esophagus and possibly the proximal stomach through abdominal and chest incisions and replaces the esophagus with the remaining stomach. The physician makes a midline abdominal incision. The stomach is dissected free of surrounding structures and the esophagus is mobilized as it passes through the diaphragm to the stomach. The esophagus is divided at its connection to the stomach or the stomach may be divided near its middle portion. Next, a right chest incision is made between the ribs to expose the esophagus. The distal esophagus is mobilized under direct vision and divided above its diseased segment. The distal esophagus and attached proximal stomach are then removed. The remaining stomach is pulled up into the chest and connected to the stump of the proximal esophagus. Drains are placed into the chest near the new anastomosis and the incisions are closed.

Coding Tips

When this procedure is performed with colon interposition or small intestine reconstruction, including intestine mobilization, preparation, and anastomosis(es), see 43118. For partial esophagectomy, cervical, see 43116. For total or near total esophagectomy, without thoracotomy, with pharyngogastrostomy or cervical esophagogastrostomy, with or without pyloroplasty, see 43107; with colon interposition or small intestine reconstruction, including intestine mobilization, preparation, and anastomosis(es), see 43108.

ICD-10-CM Diagnostic Codes

C15.4	Malignant neoplasm of middle third of esophagus
C15.5	Malignant neoplasm of lower third of esophagus
C15.8	Malignant neoplasm of overlapping sites of esophagus
C16.0	Malignant neoplasm of cardia
C49.A1	Gastrointestinal stromal tumor of esophagus
C7A.092	Malignant carcinoid tumor of the stomach
D3A.092	Benign carcinoid tumor of the stomach
K22.10	Ulcer of esophagus without bleeding
K22.11	Ulcer of esophagus with bleeding
K22.5	Diverticulum of esophagus, acquired
K22.70	Barrett's esophagus without dysplasia
K22.710	Barrett's esophagus with low grade dysplasia
K22.711	Barrett's esophagus with high grade dysplasia
K22.89	Other specified disease of esophagus
K23	Disorders of esophagus in diseases classified elsewhere
K25.2	Acute gastric ulcer with both hemorrhage and perforation
K31.1	Adult hypertrophic pyloric stenosis ▲
Q39.5	Congenital dilatation of esophagus
Q39.6	Congenital diverticulum of esophagus
Q39.8	Other congenital malformations of esophagus
S27.812A	Contusion of esophagus (thoracic part), initial encounter
S27.813A	Laceration of esophagus (thoracic part), initial encounter
S27.818A	Other injury of esophagus (thoracic part), initial encounter
T28.1XXA	Burn of esophagus, initial encounter
T28.6XXA	Corrosion of esophagus, initial encounter

AMA: **43117** 2014,Jan,11

Relative Value Units/Medicare Edits

Non-Facility RVU	Work	PE	MP	Total
43117	57.5	24.41	13.4	95.31
Facility RVU	Work	PE	MP	Total
43117	57.5	24.41	13.4	95.31

	FUD	Status	MUE	Modifiers				IOM Reference
43117	90	A	1(2)	51	N/A	62	80	None

* with documentation

Terms To Know

anastomosis. Surgically created connection between ducts, blood vessels, or bowel segments to allow flow from one to the other.

distal. Located farther away from a specified reference point or the trunk.

pyloroplasty. Enlargement and reconstruction of the lower portion of the stomach opening into the duodenum performed after vagotomy to speed gastric emptying and treat duodenal ulcers.

Esophagus

43118

43118 Partial esophagectomy, distal two-thirds, with thoracotomy and separate abdominal incision, with or without proximal gastrectomy; with colon interposition or small intestine reconstruction, including intestine mobilization, preparation, and anastomosis(es)

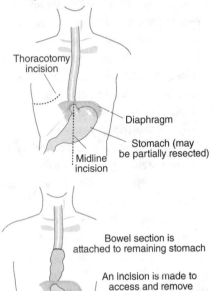

The distal esophagus is removed, sometimes along with the upper part of the stomach

Thoracotomy incision

Diaphragm

Stomach (may be partially resected)

Midline incision

Bowel section is attached to remaining stomach

An incision is made to access and remove bowel section to graft to the esophagus

Explanation

The physician removes the distal esophagus and possibly proximal stomach through abdominal and chest incisions and replaces the esophagus with colon or small bowel. The physician makes a midline abdominal incision. The stomach is dissected free of surrounding structures and the esophagus is mobilized as it passes through the diaphragm to the stomach. The esophagus is divided at its connection to the stomach or the stomach may be divided near its middle portion. An appropriate segment of colon or small bowel is selected and the bowel is divided proximal and distal to this segment and the bowel ends re-approximated. One end of the selected bowel segment is connected to the remaining stomach and the other end is placed through the diaphragm into the chest. A right chest incision is made between the ribs to expose the esophagus. The distal esophagus is mobilized under direct vision and divided above its diseased segment. The distal esophagus and attached proximal stomach are removed. The remaining end of the segment of colon or small bowel that has been attached to the stomach is pulled into the chest and connected to the stump of the proximal esophagus. Drains are placed into the chest near the new anastomosis and the incisions are closed.

Coding Tips

Partial esophagectomy procedures are defined by site. This code reports procedures on the distal (lower) two-thirds of the esophagus. The approach is considered inherent to the procedure and should not be reported separately. For partial esophagectomy of the cervical (proximal one-third) esophagus, see 43116. For partial esophagectomy, distal two-thirds, by thoracic approach with separate abdominal incision (Ivor Lewis procedure), see 43117; by thoracic approach only, see 43121; by thoracoabdominal or abdominal approach, see 43122.

ICD-10-CM Diagnostic Codes

C15.4	Malignant neoplasm of middle third of esophagus
C15.5	Malignant neoplasm of lower third of esophagus
C15.8	Malignant neoplasm of overlapping sites of esophagus
C16.0	Malignant neoplasm of cardia
C49.A1	Gastrointestinal stromal tumor of esophagus
C7A.092	Malignant carcinoid tumor of the stomach
D3A.092	Benign carcinoid tumor of the stomach
K22.10	Ulcer of esophagus without bleeding
K22.11	Ulcer of esophagus with bleeding
K22.5	Diverticulum of esophagus, acquired
K22.70	Barrett's esophagus without dysplasia
K22.710	Barrett's esophagus with low grade dysplasia
K22.711	Barrett's esophagus with high grade dysplasia
K22.89	Other specified disease of esophagus
K23	Disorders of esophagus in diseases classified elsewhere
K25.0	Acute gastric ulcer with hemorrhage
K25.2	Acute gastric ulcer with both hemorrhage and perforation
K25.3	Acute gastric ulcer without hemorrhage or perforation
K25.4	Chronic or unspecified gastric ulcer with hemorrhage
Q39.5	Congenital dilatation of esophagus
Q39.6	Congenital diverticulum of esophagus
Q39.8	Other congenital malformations of esophagus
S27.812A	Contusion of esophagus (thoracic part), initial encounter
S27.813A	Laceration of esophagus (thoracic part), initial encounter
S27.818A	Other injury of esophagus (thoracic part), initial encounter
T28.1XXA	Burn of esophagus, initial encounter
T28.6XXA	Corrosion of esophagus, initial encounter

AMA: **43118** 2014,Jan,11

Relative Value Units/Medicare Edits

Non-Facility RVU	Work	PE	MP	Total
43118	67.07	23.66	15.38	106.11
Facility RVU	**Work**	**PE**	**MP**	**Total**
43118	67.07	23.66	15.38	106.11

	FUD	Status	MUE	Modifiers				IOM Reference
43118	90	A	1(2)	51	N/A	62	80	None

* with documentation

Terms To Know

anastomosis. Surgically created connection between ducts, blood vessels, or bowel segments to allow flow from one to the other.

distal. Located farther away from a specified reference point or the trunk.

proximal. Located closest to a specified reference point, usually the midline or trunk.

43121

43121 Partial esophagectomy, distal two-thirds, with thoracotomy only, with or without proximal gastrectomy, with thoracic esophagogastrostomy, with or without pyloroplasty

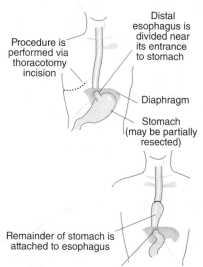

The distal esophagus is removed, sometimes along with the upper part of the stomach

Distal esophagus is divided near its entrance to stomach

Procedure is performed via thoracotomy incision

Diaphragm

Stomach (may be partially resected)

Remainder of stomach is attached to esophagus

A pyloroplasty may also be performed

Explanation

The physician removes the affected part of the esophagus and proximal stomach and reattaches the remaining stomach to the esophageal stump. The physician accesses the esophagus through a right posterolateral thoracotomy; no abdominal incision is made. The physician resects the affected portion of the distal esophagus and sometimes a portion of the proximal stomach. The resected area is removed. The stomach or gastric remnant is pulled into the thorax and sutured to the esophageal stump. If the stomach is used as the esophageal conduit, a pyloroplasty may be performed to open the pyloric sphincter. The incision is sutured in layers.

Coding Tips

For partial esophagectomy by thoracoabdominal or abdominal approach with esophagogastrostomy, with or without pyloroplasty, see 43122.

ICD-10-CM Diagnostic Codes

C15.4	Malignant neoplasm of middle third of esophagus
C15.5	Malignant neoplasm of lower third of esophagus
C15.8	Malignant neoplasm of overlapping sites of esophagus
C16.0	Malignant neoplasm of cardia
C49.A1	Gastrointestinal stromal tumor of esophagus
C7A.092	Malignant carcinoid tumor of the stomach
D3A.092	Benign carcinoid tumor of the stomach
K22.10	Ulcer of esophagus without bleeding
K22.11	Ulcer of esophagus with bleeding
K22.70	Barrett's esophagus without dysplasia
K22.710	Barrett's esophagus with low grade dysplasia
K22.711	Barrett's esophagus with high grade dysplasia
K22.89	Other specified disease of esophagus
K23	Disorders of esophagus in diseases classified elsewhere
K25.0	Acute gastric ulcer with hemorrhage
K25.2	Acute gastric ulcer with both hemorrhage and perforation
K25.3	Acute gastric ulcer without hemorrhage or perforation
K25.4	Chronic or unspecified gastric ulcer with hemorrhage
K31.1	Adult hypertrophic pyloric stenosis ▲
Q39.5	Congenital dilatation of esophagus
Q39.6	Congenital diverticulum of esophagus
Q39.8	Other congenital malformations of esophagus
S27.812A	Contusion of esophagus (thoracic part), initial encounter
S27.813A	Laceration of esophagus (thoracic part), initial encounter
S27.818A	Other injury of esophagus (thoracic part), initial encounter
T28.1XXA	Burn of esophagus, initial encounter
T28.6XXA	Corrosion of esophagus, initial encounter

AMA: **43121** 2014,Jan,11

Relative Value Units/Medicare Edits

Non-Facility RVU	Work	PE	MP	Total
43121	51.43	20.37	11.82	83.62
Facility RVU	**Work**	**PE**	**MP**	**Total**
43121	51.43	20.37	11.82	83.62

	FUD	Status	MUE	Modifiers				IOM Reference
43121	90	A	1(2)	51	N/A	62	80	None

* with documentation

Terms To Know

distal. Located farther away from a specified reference point or the trunk.

gastrectomy. Surgical excision of all or part of the stomach.

proximal. Located closest to a specified reference point, usually the midline or trunk.

pyloroplasty. Enlargement and reconstruction of the lower portion of the stomach opening into the duodenum performed after vagotomy to speed gastric emptying and treat duodenal ulcers.

thoracotomy. Surgical procedure for opening the chest wall in order to access the lungs, esophagus, trachea, aorta, heart, and diaphragm.

Esophagus

43122

43122 Partial esophagectomy, thoracoabdominal or abdominal approach, with or without proximal gastrectomy; with esophagogastrostomy, with or without pyloroplasty

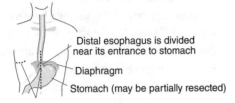

The distal esophagus is removed, sometimes along with the upper part of the stomach

Distal esophagus is divided near its entrance to stomach

Diaphragm

Stomach (may be partially resected)

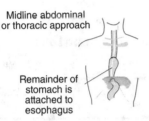

Midline abdominal or thoracic approach

Remainder of stomach is attached to esophagus

A pyloroplasty may also be performed

Explanation

The physician removes the distal esophagus and possibly proximal stomach through a combined abdominal and chest incision and replaces the esophagus with the remaining stomach. The physician makes a midline abdominal incision. The stomach is dissected free of surrounding structures and the esophagus is mobilized as it passes through the diaphragm to the stomach. The esophagus is divided proximally above the diseased area and distally at its junction with the stomach or the middle portion of the stomach may be divided. The distal esophagus and attached proximal stomach are removed. The remaining stomach is connected to the stump of the esophagus. The incision is closed.

Coding Tips

Proximal gastrectomy, esophagogastrostomy, pyloroplasty, and thoracoabdominal or abdominal approach are included in this procedure and are not reported separately. If this procedure is performed with colon interposition or small intestine reconstruction, including intestine mobilization, preparation, and anastomosis(es), see 43123.

ICD-10-CM Diagnostic Codes

C15.4	Malignant neoplasm of middle third of esophagus
C15.5	Malignant neoplasm of lower third of esophagus
C15.8	Malignant neoplasm of overlapping sites of esophagus
C16.0	Malignant neoplasm of cardia
C49.A1	Gastrointestinal stromal tumor of esophagus
C7A.092	Malignant carcinoid tumor of the stomach
D00.1	Carcinoma in situ of esophagus
D3A.092	Benign carcinoid tumor of the stomach
K21.9	Gastro-esophageal reflux disease without esophagitis
K22.10	Ulcer of esophagus without bleeding
K22.11	Ulcer of esophagus with bleeding
K22.70	Barrett's esophagus without dysplasia
K22.710	Barrett's esophagus with low grade dysplasia
K22.711	Barrett's esophagus with high grade dysplasia
K22.89	Other specified disease of esophagus
K23	Disorders of esophagus in diseases classified elsewhere
K25.0	Acute gastric ulcer with hemorrhage
K25.2	Acute gastric ulcer with both hemorrhage and perforation
K25.3	Acute gastric ulcer without hemorrhage or perforation
K25.4	Chronic or unspecified gastric ulcer with hemorrhage
K31.1	Adult hypertrophic pyloric stenosis 🅐
Q39.5	Congenital dilatation of esophagus
Q39.6	Congenital diverticulum of esophagus
Q39.8	Other congenital malformations of esophagus
S27.812A	Contusion of esophagus (thoracic part), initial encounter
S27.813A	Laceration of esophagus (thoracic part), initial encounter
S27.818A	Other injury of esophagus (thoracic part), initial encounter
T28.1XXA	Burn of esophagus, initial encounter
T28.6XXA	Corrosion of esophagus, initial encounter

AMA: **43122** 2014,Jan,11

Relative Value Units/Medicare Edits

Non-Facility RVU	Work	PE	MP	Total
43122	44.18	20.48	10.11	74.77
Facility RVU	**Work**	**PE**	**MP**	**Total**
43122	44.18	20.48	10.11	74.77

	FUD	Status	MUE	Modifiers				IOM Reference
43122	90	A	1(2)	51	N/A	62*	80	None

* with documentation

Terms To Know

approach. Method or anatomical location used to gain access to a body organ or specific area for procedures.

dissect. Cut apart or separate tissue for surgical purposes or for visual or microscopic study.

distal. Located farther away from a specified reference point or the trunk.

proximal. Located closest to a specified reference point, usually the midline or trunk.

Esophagus

43123

43123 Partial esophagectomy, thoracoabdominal or abdominal approach, with or without proximal gastrectomy; with colon interposition or small intestine reconstruction, including intestine mobilization, preparation, and anastomosis(es)

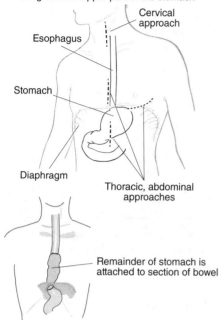

The diseased esophagus is removed, sometimes along with the upper part of the stomach

Cervical approach

Esophagus

Stomach

Diaphragm

Thoracic, abdominal approaches

Remainder of stomach is attached to section of bowel

A midline abdominal incision is made to access and remove bowel section to graft to the esophagus

Explanation

The physician removes the distal esophagus and possibly the proximal stomach through a combined abdominal and chest incision and replaces the esophagus with colon or small bowel. The physician makes a midline abdominal incision that may extend onto the chest between the ribs. The stomach is dissected free of surrounding structures and the esophagus is mobilized as it passes through the diaphragm to the stomach. The esophagus is divided proximally above the diseased area and distally at its junction with the stomach or the middle portion of the stomach may be divided. The distal esophagus and attached stomach are removed. An appropriate segment of colon or small bowel is selected. The bowel is divided proximal and distal to the segment and the bowel ends are re-approximated. The selected segment of bowel is connected proximally to the remaining esophageal stump and distally to the remaining stomach. The incision is closed.

Coding Tips

Proximal gastrectomy and thoracoabdominal or abdominal approach are included in this procedure and are not reported separately. When this procedure is performed without colon interposition or small intestine reconstruction, see 43122.

ICD-10-CM Diagnostic Codes

C15.4	Malignant neoplasm of middle third of esophagus
C15.5	Malignant neoplasm of lower third of esophagus
C15.8	Malignant neoplasm of overlapping sites of esophagus
C16.0	Malignant neoplasm of cardia
C16.1	Malignant neoplasm of fundus of stomach

C49.A1	Gastrointestinal stromal tumor of esophagus
C7A.092	Malignant carcinoid tumor of the stomach
D00.1	Carcinoma in situ of esophagus
D3A.092	Benign carcinoid tumor of the stomach
K21.9	Gastro-esophageal reflux disease without esophagitis
K22.10	Ulcer of esophagus without bleeding
K22.11	Ulcer of esophagus with bleeding
K22.70	Barrett's esophagus without dysplasia
K22.710	Barrett's esophagus with low grade dysplasia
K22.711	Barrett's esophagus with high grade dysplasia
K22.89	Other specified disease of esophagus
K23	Disorders of esophagus in diseases classified elsewhere
K25.0	Acute gastric ulcer with hemorrhage
K25.1	Acute gastric ulcer with perforation
K25.2	Acute gastric ulcer with both hemorrhage and perforation
K25.3	Acute gastric ulcer without hemorrhage or perforation
K25.4	Chronic or unspecified gastric ulcer with hemorrhage
Q39.5	Congenital dilatation of esophagus
Q39.6	Congenital diverticulum of esophagus
Q39.8	Other congenital malformations of esophagus
S27.812A	Contusion of esophagus (thoracic part), initial encounter
S27.813A	Laceration of esophagus (thoracic part), initial encounter
S27.818A	Other injury of esophagus (thoracic part), initial encounter
T28.1XXA	Burn of esophagus, initial encounter
T28.6XXA	Corrosion of esophagus, initial encounter

AMA: **43123** 2014,Jan,11

Relative Value Units/Medicare Edits

Non-Facility RVU	Work	PE	MP	Total
43123	83.12	29.57	19.08	131.77
Facility RVU	**Work**	**PE**	**MP**	**Total**
43123	83.12	29.57	19.08	131.77

	FUD	Status	MUE	Modifiers				IOM Reference
43123	90	A	1(2)	51	N/A	62*	80	None

* with documentation

Terms To Know

anastomosis. Surgically created connection between ducts, blood vessels, or bowel segments to allow flow from one to the other.

approach. Method or anatomical location used to gain access to a body organ or specific area for procedures.

gastrectomy. Surgical excision of all or part of the stomach.

interposition. Placement between objects.

proximal. Located closest to a specified reference point, usually the midline or trunk.

Esophagus

43124

43124 Total or partial esophagectomy, without reconstruction (any approach), with cervical esophagostomy

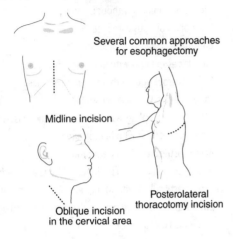

Several common approaches for esophagectomy

Midline incision

Oblique incision in the cervical area

Posterolateral thoracotomy incision

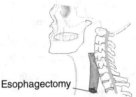

Esophagectomy

The esophagus is removed and the remaining stump is connected outside the body, creating a mucous fistula

Explanation

The physician removes the esophagus with no attempt to reconstruct the esophagus. The physician first creates a permanent tracheoplasty. The physician accesses the esophagus through an oblique cervical incision, a thoracotomy, and/or a midline abdominal incision and resects the affected portion of the esophagus. The esophageal stump is sutured to the cervical incision, creating a connection from the exterior of the neck to the esophageal lumen to provide drainage of saliva and mucus. The operative incisions are closed with sutured layers.

Coding Tips

The physician may use any method to accomplish the same result. The procedure is reported the same regardless of which method or technique is employed. If significant additional time and effort are documented, append modifier 22 and submit a cover letter and operative report.

ICD-10-CM Diagnostic Codes

C15.3	Malignant neoplasm of upper third of esophagus
C15.4	Malignant neoplasm of middle third of esophagus
C15.5	Malignant neoplasm of lower third of esophagus
C15.8	Malignant neoplasm of overlapping sites of esophagus
K22.10	Ulcer of esophagus without bleeding
K22.11	Ulcer of esophagus with bleeding
K22.3	Perforation of esophagus
K22.70	Barrett's esophagus without dysplasia
K22.710	Barrett's esophagus with low grade dysplasia
K22.711	Barrett's esophagus with high grade dysplasia
K22.89	Other specified disease of esophagus
K23	Disorders of esophagus in diseases classified elsewhere
Q39.3	Congenital stenosis and stricture of esophagus
Q39.5	Congenital dilatation of esophagus
Q39.6	Congenital diverticulum of esophagus
Q39.8	Other congenital malformations of esophagus
S11.25XA	Open bite of pharynx and cervical esophagus, initial encounter
S27.812A	Contusion of esophagus (thoracic part), initial encounter
S27.813A	Laceration of esophagus (thoracic part), initial encounter
S27.818A	Other injury of esophagus (thoracic part), initial encounter
T28.1XXA	Burn of esophagus, initial encounter
T28.6XXA	Corrosion of esophagus, initial encounter

AMA: **43124** 2018,Jan,8; 2017,Jan,8; 2016,Jan,13; 2015,Jan,16

Relative Value Units/Medicare Edits

Non-Facility RVU	Work	PE	MP	Total
43124	69.09	26.42	15.87	111.38
Facility RVU	**Work**	**PE**	**MP**	**Total**
43124	69.09	26.42	15.87	111.38

	FUD	Status	MUE	Modifiers				IOM Reference
43124	90	A	1(2)	51	N/A	62*	80	None

* with documentation

Terms To Know

approach. Method or anatomical location used to gain access to a body organ or specific area for procedures.

cervical. Relation to the cervical spine or to the cervix.

closure. Repairing an incision or wound by suture or other means.

esophagus. Muscular tube that carries swallowed liquids and foods from the pharynx to the stomach.

incision. Act of cutting into tissue or an organ.

lumen. Space inside an intestine, artery, vein, duct, or tube.

reconstruction. Recreating, restoring, or rebuilding a body part or organ.

thoracotomy. Surgical procedure for opening the chest wall in order to access the lungs, esophagus, trachea, aorta, heart, and diaphragm.

tracheoplasty. Plastic repair of the trachea, the tube descending from the larynx that branches into the right and left main bronchi.

43130-43135

43130 Diverticulectomy of hypopharynx or esophagus, with or without myotomy; cervical approach
43135 thoracic approach

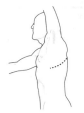

Example of posterolateral left thoracotomy incision

Example of oblique incision in the cervical area

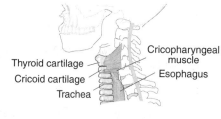

Thyroid cartilage
Cricoid cartilage
Trachea
Cricopharyngeal muscle
Esophagus

A diverticulum is removed from the hypopharynx or esophagus

Explanation

The physician removes a diverticulum from the hypopharynx or esophagus. A diverticulum is a pouch that occurs normally or because of a defect in the muscular membrane. In 43130 (cervical approach), the physician makes a lateral incision in the neck. In 43135 (thoracic approach), the physician incises and dissects the left posterior chest wall. The physician may dissect or incise the cricopharyngeus muscle to expose the diverticulum. If a myotomy is necessary, the physician makes a vertical incision through the cricopharyngeus muscle. The physician clamps the diverticulum and closes using sutures or staples. The incision is closed with sutured layers.

Coding Tips

The approach is considered inherent to the procedure and should not be reported separately. For excision of an esophageal lesion with primary repair via a thoracic or abdominal approach, see 43101. For endoscopic diverticulectomy of hypopharynx or cervical esophagus, see 43180.

ICD-10-CM Diagnostic Codes

K22.5   Diverticulum of esophagus, acquired
Q39.6   Congenital diverticulum of esophagus
Q39.8   Other congenital malformations of esophagus

AMA: **43130** 2018,Jan,8; 2017,Jan,8; 2016,Jan,13; 2015,Jan,16 **43135** 2018,Jan,8; 2017,Jan,8; 2016,Jan,13; 2015,Jan,16

Relative Value Units/Medicare Edits

Non-Facility RVU	Work	PE	MP	Total
43130	12.53	8.43	2.17	23.13
43135	26.17	10.91	6.0	43.08
Facility RVU	Work	PE	MP	Total
43130	12.53	8.43	2.17	23.13
43135	26.17	10.91	6.0	43.08

	FUD	Status	MUE	Modifiers				IOM Reference
43130	90	A	1(3)	51	N/A	62*	80	None
43135	90	A	1(3)	51	N/A	62*	80	

* with documentation

Terms To Know

anomaly. Irregularity in the structure or position of an organ or tissue.

approach. Method or anatomical location used to gain access to a body organ or specific area for procedures.

cervical. Relation to the cervical spine or to the cervix.

clamp. Tool used to grip, compress, join, or fasten body parts.

closure. Repairing an incision or wound by suture or other means.

congenital. Present at birth, occurring through heredity or an influence during gestation up to the moment of birth.

defect. Imperfection, flaw, or absence.

dissect. Cut apart or separate tissue for surgical purposes or for visual or microscopic study.

diverticulum. Pouch or sac in the walls of an organ or canal.

esophagus. Muscular tube that carries swallowed liquids and foods from the pharynx to the stomach.

excision. Surgical removal of an organ or tissue.

incision. Act of cutting into tissue or an organ.

myotomy. Surgical cutting of a muscle to gain access to underlying tissues or for therapeutic reasons.

pharynx. Musculomembranous passage of the throat consisting of three regions: the nasopharynx is the passage at the back of the nostrils, above the level of the soft palate, and communicating with the eustachian tube; the oropharynx is the region between the soft palate and the edge of the epiglottis; the hypopharynx is the region of the epiglottis to the juncture of the larynx and esophagus.

posterior. Located in the back part or caudal end of the body.

43180

43180 Esophagoscopy, rigid, transoral with diverticulectomy of hypopharynx or cervical esophagus (eg, Zenker's diverticulum), with cricopharyngeal myotomy, includes use of telescope or operating microscope and repair, when performed

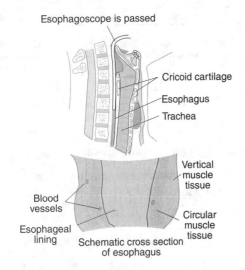

Esophagoscope is passed

Cricoid cartilage

Esophagus

Trachea

Vertical muscle tissue

Blood vessels

Esophageal lining

Circular muscle tissue

Schematic cross section of esophagus

Explanation

The physician examines the esophagus via a rigid esophagoscope inserted through the patient's mouth and into the esophagus under general anesthesia. The physician removes a diverticulum from the hypopharynx or esophagus. A diverticulum is a pouch that occurs normally or because of a defect in the muscular membrane of the upper esophagus. The physician may dissect or incise the cricopharyngeus muscle to expose the diverticulum. Cricopharyngeal myotomy is accomplished by making a vertical incision through the cricopharyngeus muscle. The physician clamps the diverticulum and closes using sutures or staples. The incision is closed with sutured layers.

Coding Tips

Esophagoscopy includes examination from the upper esophageal sphincter to and including the gastroesophageal junction, but may also include an examination of the proximal region of the stomach via retroflexion, if performed. Report the appropriate endoscopy for each anatomic site examined. Surgical endoscopy includes a diagnostic endoscopy; however, diagnostic endoscopy can be identified separately when performed at the same surgical session as an open procedure. For open diverticulectomy of the hypopharynx or esophagus, see 43130 or 43135. Use of an operating microscope is included in this procedure. Do not report 43180 with 43210 or 69990.

ICD-10-CM Diagnostic Codes

J39.2	Other diseases of pharynx
K22.5	Diverticulum of esophagus, acquired
K22.89	Other specified disease of esophagus
Q39.6	Congenital diverticulum of esophagus
Q39.8	Other congenital malformations of esophagus

AMA: 43180 2018,Jan,8; 2017,Jan,8; 2016,Jan,13; 2016,Feb,12; 2015,Nov,8

Relative Value Units/Medicare Edits

Non-Facility RVU	Work	PE	MP	Total
43180	9.03	5.59	1.29	15.91
Facility RVU	**Work**	**PE**	**MP**	**Total**
43180	9.03	5.59	1.29	15.91

	FUD	Status	MUE	Modifiers				IOM Reference
43180	90	A	1(2)	51	N/A	N/A	N/A	None

* with documentation

Terms To Know

defect. Imperfection, flaw, or absence.

dissect. Cut apart or separate tissue for surgical purposes or for visual or microscopic study.

diverticulum. Pouch or sac in the walls of an organ or canal.

esophagoscopy. Internal visual inspection of the esophagus through the use of an endoscope placed down the throat.

incise. To cut open or into.

myotomy. Surgical cutting of a muscle to gain access to underlying tissues or for therapeutic reasons.

operating microscope. Compound microscope with two or more lens systems or several grouped lenses in one unit that provides magnifying power to the surgeon up to 40X.

43191-43193

43191 Esophagoscopy, rigid, transoral; diagnostic, including collection of specimen(s) by brushing or washing when performed (separate procedure)
43192 with directed submucosal injection(s), any substance
43193 with biopsy, single or multiple

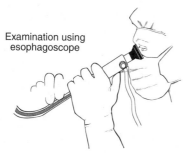

Examination using esophagoscope

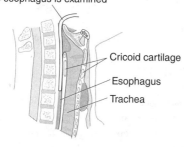

Esophagoscope is passed and the esophagus is examined

Cricoid cartilage
Esophagus
Trachea

Explanation

The physician views the esophagus via a rigid esophagoscope inserted through the patient's mouth and into the esophagus under general anesthesia. In 43191, a collection of cells may be taken by brushing or washing and/or aspirating the esophageal lining for specimens. In 43192, the physician injects any substance into a specific area through the scope. In 43193, biopsy forceps are used to obtain samples of the esophageal mucosa.

Coding Tips

Surgical endoscopy includes a diagnostic endoscopy; however, diagnostic endoscopy can be identified separately when performed at the same surgical session as an open procedure. Note that 43191, a separate procedure by definition, is usually a component of a more complex service and is not identified separately. When performed alone or with other unrelated procedures/services it may be reported. If performed alone, list the code; if performed with other procedures/services, list the code and append modifier 59 or an X{EPSU} modifier. Esophagoscopy includes examination from the upper esophageal sphincter to and including the gastroesophageal junction, but may also include an examination of the proximal region of the stomach via retroflexion, if performed. Report the appropriate endoscopy for each anatomic site examined. If a specimen is transported to an outside laboratory, report 99000 for handling or conveyance. For flexible transoral esophagoscopy, see 43200; with directed submucosal injection, any substance, see 43201; with biopsy, single or multiple, see 43202; with injection sclerosis of esophageal varices, see 43204; with injection of sclerosis via rigid transoral esophagoscopy, see 43499. For diagnostic transnasal esophagoscopy, diagnostic, see 43197; with biopsy, single or multiple, see 43198. Do not report 43191 with 43192–43198, 43210, or 43497. Do not report 43192 or 43193 with 43191, 43197, or 43198.

ICD-10-CM Diagnostic Codes

B37.81	Candidal esophagitis
C15.3	Malignant neoplasm of upper third of esophagus
C15.4	Malignant neoplasm of middle third of esophagus
C15.5	Malignant neoplasm of lower third of esophagus
C49.A1	Gastrointestinal stromal tumor of esophagus
D00.1	Carcinoma in situ of esophagus
D13.0	Benign neoplasm of esophagus
D49.0	Neoplasm of unspecified behavior of digestive system
I85.00	Esophageal varices without bleeding
I85.01	Esophageal varices with bleeding
I85.10	Secondary esophageal varices without bleeding
I85.11	Secondary esophageal varices with bleeding
K20.0	Eosinophilic esophagitis
K21.00	Gastro-esophageal reflux disease with esophagitis, without bleeding
K21.01	Gastro-esophageal reflux disease with esophagitis, with bleeding
K21.9	Gastro-esophageal reflux disease without esophagitis
K22.0	Achalasia of cardia
K22.10	Ulcer of esophagus without bleeding
K22.11	Ulcer of esophagus with bleeding
K22.2	Esophageal obstruction
K22.3	Perforation of esophagus
K22.4	Dyskinesia of esophagus
K22.5	Diverticulum of esophagus, acquired
K22.6	Gastro-esophageal laceration-hemorrhage syndrome
K22.70	Barrett's esophagus without dysplasia
K22.710	Barrett's esophagus with low grade dysplasia
K22.711	Barrett's esophagus with high grade dysplasia
K22.81	Esophageal polyp
K22.82	Esophagogastric junction polyp
K22.89	Other specified disease of esophagus
K23	Disorders of esophagus in diseases classified elsewhere
K30	Functional dyspepsia
K91.61	Intraoperative hemorrhage and hematoma of a digestive system organ or structure complicating a digestive system procedure
K91.62	Intraoperative hemorrhage and hematoma of a digestive system organ or structure complicating other procedure
K91.71	Accidental puncture and laceration of a digestive system organ or structure during a digestive system procedure
K91.72	Accidental puncture and laceration of a digestive system organ or structure during other procedure
K91.81	Other intraoperative complications of digestive system
K91.840	Postprocedural hemorrhage of a digestive system organ or structure following a digestive system procedure
K91.841	Postprocedural hemorrhage of a digestive system organ or structure following other procedure
K94.31	Esophagostomy hemorrhage
K94.32	Esophagostomy infection
K94.33	Esophagostomy malfunction
Q39.0	Atresia of esophagus without fistula
Q39.1	Atresia of esophagus with tracheo-esophageal fistula
Q39.2	Congenital tracheo-esophageal fistula without atresia

Esophagus

Q39.3	Congenital stenosis and stricture of esophagus
Q39.4	Esophageal web
Q39.5	Congenital dilatation of esophagus
Q39.6	Congenital diverticulum of esophagus
Q39.8	Other congenital malformations of esophagus
R13.0	Aphagia
R13.11	Dysphagia, oral phase
R13.12	Dysphagia, oropharyngeal phase
R13.13	Dysphagia, pharyngeal phase
R13.14	Dysphagia, pharyngoesophageal phase
S11.21XA	Laceration without foreign body of pharynx and cervical esophagus, initial encounter
S11.22XA	Laceration with foreign body of pharynx and cervical esophagus, initial encounter
S11.23XA	Puncture wound without foreign body of pharynx and cervical esophagus, initial encounter
S11.24XA	Puncture wound with foreign body of pharynx and cervical esophagus, initial encounter
S11.25XA	Open bite of pharynx and cervical esophagus, initial encounter
S27.812A	Contusion of esophagus (thoracic part), initial encounter
S27.813A	Laceration of esophagus (thoracic part), initial encounter
S27.818A	Other injury of esophagus (thoracic part), initial encounter
T85.511A	Breakdown (mechanical) of esophageal anti-reflux device, initial encounter
T85.521A	Displacement of esophageal anti-reflux device, initial encounter
T85.591A	Other mechanical complication of esophageal anti-reflux device, initial encounter
Z03.821	Encounter for observation for suspected ingested foreign body ruled out
Z48.815	Encounter for surgical aftercare following surgery on the digestive system

AMA: **43191** 2018,Jan,8; 2017,Jan,8; 2016,Jan,13; 2015,Nov,8; 2015,Jan,16 **43192** 2018,Jan,8; 2017,Jan,8; 2016,Jan,13; 2015,Jan,16 **43193** 2018,Jan,8; 2017,Jan,8; 2016,Jan,13; 2015,Jan,16

Relative Value Units/Medicare Edits

Non-Facility RVU	Work	PE	MP	Total
43191	2.49	1.65	0.36	4.5
43192	2.79	1.73	0.41	4.93
43193	2.79	1.72	0.39	4.9
Facility RVU	Work	PE	MP	Total
43191	2.49	1.65	0.36	4.5
43192	2.79	1.73	0.41	4.93
43193	2.79	1.72	0.39	4.9

	FUD	Status	MUE	Modifiers				IOM Reference
43191	0	A	1(3)	51	N/A	N/A	N/A	None
43192	0	A	1(3)	51	N/A	N/A	N/A	
43193	0	A	1(3)	51	N/A	N/A	N/A	
* with documentation								

43194

43194 Esophagoscopy, rigid, transoral; with removal of foreign body(s)

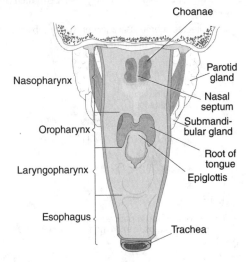

Esophageal anatomy

Explanation

The physician locates and removes a foreign body(s) from the esophagus via a rigid esophagoscope passed through the patient's mouth and into the esophagus. The foreign body is located. It may be suctioned or grasped with forceps and retracted through the scope. An alternative technique is to pass a balloon beyond the foreign body. The balloon is inflated and withdrawn, capturing the foreign body.

Coding Tips

Esophagoscopy includes examination from the upper esophageal sphincter to and including the gastroesophageal junction, but may also include an examination of the proximal region of the stomach via retroflexion, if performed. Report the appropriate endoscopy for each anatomic site examined. Surgical endoscopy includes a diagnostic endoscopy; however, diagnostic endoscopy can be identified separately when performed at the same surgical session as an open procedure. Report fluoroscopic guidance with 76000, when performed. Do not report 43194 with 43191, 43197, or 43198. For flexible transoral esophagoscopy with removal of a foreign body, see 43215.

ICD-10-CM Diagnostic Codes

S11.22XA	Laceration with foreign body of pharynx and cervical esophagus, initial encounter
S11.24XA	Puncture wound with foreign body of pharynx and cervical esophagus, initial encounter
T18.110A	Gastric contents in esophagus causing compression of trachea, initial encounter
T18.118A	Gastric contents in esophagus causing other injury, initial encounter
T18.120A	Food in esophagus causing compression of trachea, initial encounter
T18.128A	Food in esophagus causing other injury, initial encounter
T18.190A	Other foreign object in esophagus causing compression of trachea, initial encounter
T18.198A	Other foreign object in esophagus causing other injury, initial encounter

Esophagus

T85.511A	Breakdown (mechanical) of esophageal anti-reflux device, initial encounter
T85.521A	Displacement of esophageal anti-reflux device, initial encounter
T85.591A	Other mechanical complication of esophageal anti-reflux device, initial encounter
T85.598A	Other mechanical complication of other gastrointestinal prosthetic devices, implants and grafts, initial encounter

AMA: **43194** 2018,Jan,8; 2017,Jan,8; 2016,Jan,13; 2015,Jan,16

Relative Value Units/Medicare Edits

Non-Facility RVU	Work	PE	MP	Total
43194	3.51	1.55	0.53	5.59
Facility RVU	Work	PE	MP	Total
43194	3.51	1.55	0.53	5.59

	FUD	Status	MUE	Modifiers				IOM Reference
43194	0	A	1(3)	51	N/A	N/A	N/A	None

* with documentation

Terms To Know

balloon catheter. Any catheter equipped with an inflatable balloon at the end to hold it in place in a body cavity or to be used for dilation of a vessel lumen.

esophagoscopy. Internal visual inspection of the esophagus through the use of an endoscope placed down the throat.

esophagus. Muscular tube that carries swallowed liquids and foods from the pharynx to the stomach.

forceps. Tool used for grasping or compressing tissue.

foreign body. Any object or substance found in an organ and tissue that does not belong under normal circumstances.

suction. Vacuum evacuation of fluid or tissue.

43195-43196

| 43195 | Esophagoscopy, rigid, transoral; with balloon dilation (less than 30 mm diameter) |
| 43196 | with insertion of guide wire followed by dilation over guide wire |

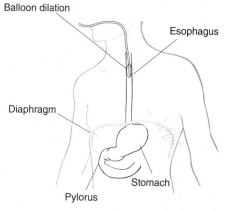

Rigid esophagoscopy with dilation

Explanation

The physician stretches esophageal tissue via a rigid esophagoscope passed through the patient's mouth and into the esophagus. A narrowing in the esophagus is expanded. In 43195, a balloon is advanced through the scope. After entering the obstructed region, the balloon is briefly inflated several times to achieve a satisfactory opening. In 43196, a guidewire is placed through the scope and the scope is removed. A dilator is passed over the guidewire. This process may be repeated several times using progressively larger dilators until the esophagus is opened satisfactorily.

Coding Tips

For esophageal dilation with balloon, 30 mm diameter or greater, see 43214 or 43233; without endoscopic visualization, see 43450 or 43453. For balloon dilation via flexible transoral esophagoscopy, less than 30 mm diameter, see 43220. Imaging guidance is reported with 74360, when performed. Do not report 43195–43196 with 43191 or 43197–43198.

ICD-10-CM Diagnostic Codes

C15.3	Malignant neoplasm of upper third of esophagus
C15.4	Malignant neoplasm of middle third of esophagus
C15.5	Malignant neoplasm of lower third of esophagus
C15.8	Malignant neoplasm of overlapping sites of esophagus
C49.A1	Gastrointestinal stromal tumor of esophagus
C78.89	Secondary malignant neoplasm of other digestive organs
D00.1	Carcinoma in situ of esophagus
D13.0	Benign neoplasm of esophagus
D37.8	Neoplasm of uncertain behavior of other specified digestive organs
D3A.098	Benign carcinoid tumors of other sites
K20.80	Other esophagitis without bleeding
K20.81	Other esophagitis with bleeding
K21.00	Gastro-esophageal reflux disease with esophagitis, without bleeding
K21.01	Gastro-esophageal reflux disease with esophagitis, with bleeding
K22.2	Esophageal obstruction
K22.89	Other specified disease of esophagus

Q39.0	Atresia of esophagus without fistula
Q39.1	Atresia of esophagus with tracheo-esophageal fistula
Q39.3	Congenital stenosis and stricture of esophagus
Q39.4	Esophageal web
Q39.8	Other congenital malformations of esophagus

AMA: 43195 2018,Jan,8; 2017,Jan,8; 2016,Jan,13; 2015,Jan,16 **43196** 2018,Jan,8; 2017,Jan,8; 2016,Jan,13; 2015,Jan,16

Relative Value Units/Medicare Edits

Non-Facility RVU	Work	PE	MP	Total
43195	3.07	1.83	0.43	5.33
43196	3.31	1.94	0.43	5.68
Facility RVU	**Work**	**PE**	**MP**	**Total**
43195	3.07	1.83	0.43	5.33
43196	3.31	1.94	0.43	5.68

	FUD	Status	MUE	Modifiers				IOM Reference
43195	0	A	1(3)	51	N/A	N/A	N/A	None
43196	0	A	1(3)	51	N/A	N/A	N/A	

* with documentation

Terms To Know

atresia. Congenital closure or absence of a tubular organ or an opening to the body surface.

balloon catheter. Any catheter equipped with an inflatable balloon at the end to hold it in place in a body cavity or to be used for dilation of a vessel lumen.

congenital. Present at birth, occurring through heredity or an influence during gestation up to the moment of birth.

diameter. Straight line connecting two opposite points on the surface of a lesion, spheric, or cylindric body.

dilation. Artificial increase in the diameter of an opening or lumen made by medication or by instrumentation.

dyskinesia. Impairment of voluntary movement.

esophagus. Muscular tube that carries swallowed liquids and foods from the pharynx to the stomach.

guidewire. Flexible metal instrument designed to lead another instrument in its proper course.

obstruction. Blockage that prevents normal function of the valve or structure.

stenosis. Narrowing or constriction of a passage.

stricture. Narrowing of an anatomical structure.

43197-43198

43197 Esophagoscopy, flexible, transnasal; diagnostic, including collection of specimen(s) by brushing or washing, when performed (separate procedure)

43198 with biopsy, single or multiple

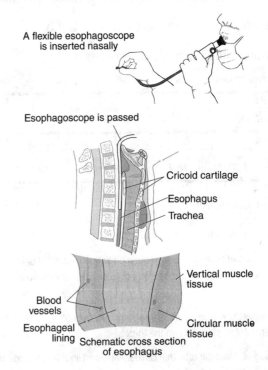

A flexible esophagoscope is inserted nasally

Esophagoscope is passed

Cricoid cartilage
Esophagus
Trachea

Vertical muscle tissue
Blood vessels
Circular muscle tissue
Esophageal lining   Schematic cross section of esophagus

Explanation

Transnasal flexible esophagoscopy is the safer, less-expensive, and more accurate technique as compared to conventional esophagoscopy. The physician examines the esophagus via a flexible esophagoscope inserted through one of the patient's nasal passages into the oropharynx and down into the esophagus. In 43197, a collection of specimen cells may be obtained by brushing or washing and/or aspirating the esophageal lining. In 43198, biopsy forceps are used to obtain samples of the esophageal mucosa.

Coding Tips

Do not report 43197 or 43198 with 31575, 43191–43196, 43200–43232, 43235–43259, 43266, 43270, 92511, 0652T-0654T, or each other. Additionally, do not report 43197 with 43497. For esophagoscopy performed transorally, see 43191 or 43200; with biopsy, see 43193 or 43202. Do not report 43197 or 43198 with 31231 unless a separate type of endoscope is used.

ICD-10-CM Diagnostic Codes

B37.81	Candidal esophagitis
C15.3	Malignant neoplasm of upper third of esophagus
C15.4	Malignant neoplasm of middle third of esophagus
C15.5	Malignant neoplasm of lower third of esophagus
C15.8	Malignant neoplasm of overlapping sites of esophagus
C49.A1	Gastrointestinal stromal tumor of esophagus
C78.89	Secondary malignant neoplasm of other digestive organs
D00.1	Carcinoma in situ of esophagus
D13.0	Benign neoplasm of esophagus
D37.8	Neoplasm of uncertain behavior of other specified digestive organs

Esophagus

I85.00	Esophageal varices without bleeding	
I85.01	Esophageal varices with bleeding	
I85.10	Secondary esophageal varices without bleeding	
I85.11	Secondary esophageal varices with bleeding	
K20.0	Eosinophilic esophagitis	
K20.80	Other esophagitis without bleeding	
K20.81	Other esophagitis with bleeding	
K21.00	Gastro-esophageal reflux disease with esophagitis, without bleeding	
K21.01	Gastro-esophageal reflux disease with esophagitis, with bleeding	
K21.9	Gastro-esophageal reflux disease without esophagitis	
K22.0	Achalasia of cardia	
K22.10	Ulcer of esophagus without bleeding	
K22.11	Ulcer of esophagus with bleeding	
K22.2	Esophageal obstruction	
K22.3	Perforation of esophagus	
K22.4	Dyskinesia of esophagus	
K22.5	Diverticulum of esophagus, acquired	
K22.6	Gastro-esophageal laceration-hemorrhage syndrome	
K22.70	Barrett's esophagus without dysplasia	
K22.710	Barrett's esophagus with low grade dysplasia	
K22.711	Barrett's esophagus with high grade dysplasia	
K22.81	Esophageal polyp	
K22.82	Esophagogastric junction polyp	
K22.89	Other specified disease of esophagus	
K23	Disorders of esophagus in diseases classified elsewhere	
K30	Functional dyspepsia	
K91.61	Intraoperative hemorrhage and hematoma of a digestive system organ or structure complicating a digestive system procedure	
K91.62	Intraoperative hemorrhage and hematoma of a digestive system organ or structure complicating other procedure	
K91.71	Accidental puncture and laceration of a digestive system organ or structure during a digestive system procedure	
K91.72	Accidental puncture and laceration of a digestive system organ or structure during other procedure	
K91.81	Other intraoperative complications of digestive system	
K91.840	Postprocedural hemorrhage of a digestive system organ or structure following a digestive system procedure	
K91.841	Postprocedural hemorrhage of a digestive system organ or structure following other procedure	
K91.870	Postprocedural hematoma of a digestive system organ or structure following a digestive system procedure	
K91.871	Postprocedural hematoma of a digestive system organ or structure following other procedure	
K91.872	Postprocedural seroma of a digestive system organ or structure following a digestive system procedure	
K91.873	Postprocedural seroma of a digestive system organ or structure following other procedure	
K94.31	Esophagostomy hemorrhage	
K94.32	Esophagostomy infection	
K94.33	Esophagostomy malfunction	
M35.08	Sjögren syndrome with gastrointestinal involvement	
Q39.0	Atresia of esophagus without fistula	
Q39.1	Atresia of esophagus with tracheo-esophageal fistula	

Q39.2	Congenital tracheo-esophageal fistula without atresia
Q39.3	Congenital stenosis and stricture of esophagus
Q39.4	Esophageal web
Q39.5	Congenital dilatation of esophagus
Q39.6	Congenital diverticulum of esophagus
Q39.8	Other congenital malformations of esophagus
Q40.1	Congenital hiatus hernia
Q40.8	Other specified congenital malformations of upper alimentary tract
R13.0	Aphagia
R13.11	Dysphagia, oral phase
R13.12	Dysphagia, oropharyngeal phase
R13.13	Dysphagia, pharyngeal phase
R13.14	Dysphagia, pharyngoesophageal phase
S11.21XA	Laceration without foreign body of pharynx and cervical esophagus, initial encounter
S11.22XA	Laceration with foreign body of pharynx and cervical esophagus, initial encounter
S11.23XA	Puncture wound without foreign body of pharynx and cervical esophagus, initial encounter
S11.24XA	Puncture wound with foreign body of pharynx and cervical esophagus, initial encounter
S11.25XA	Open bite of pharynx and cervical esophagus, initial encounter
S27.812A	Contusion of esophagus (thoracic part), initial encounter
S27.813A	Laceration of esophagus (thoracic part), initial encounter
T85.511A	Breakdown (mechanical) of esophageal anti-reflux device, initial encounter
T85.521A	Displacement of esophageal anti-reflux device, initial encounter
T85.591A	Other mechanical complication of esophageal anti-reflux device, initial encounter
T85.598A	Other mechanical complication of other gastrointestinal prosthetic devices, implants and grafts, initial encounter
Z03.821	Encounter for observation for suspected ingested foreign body ruled out

AMA: **43197** 2018,Jan,8; 2017,Jul,7; 2017,Jan,8; 2016,Sep,6; 2016,Jan,13; 2016,Dec,13; 2015,Nov,8; 2015,Jan,16 **43198** 2018,Jan,8; 2017,Jul,7; 2017,Jan,8; 2016,Sep,6; 2016,Jan,13; 2016,Dec,13; 2015,Jan,16

Relative Value Units/Medicare Edits

Non-Facility RVU	Work	PE	MP	Total
43197	1.52	4.07	0.23	5.82
43198	1.82	4.32	0.25	6.39
Facility RVU	Work	PE	MP	Total
43197	1.52	0.65	0.23	2.4
43198	1.82	0.79	0.25	2.86

	FUD	Status	MUE	Modifiers				IOM Reference
43197	0	A	1(3)	51	N/A	N/A	N/A	None
43198	0	A	1(3)	51	N/A	N/A	N/A	

* with documentation

Esophagus

43200-43202

43200   Esophagoscopy, flexible, transoral; diagnostic, including collection of specimen(s) by brushing or washing, when performed (separate procedure)

43201   with directed submucosal injection(s), any substance

43202   with biopsy, single or multiple

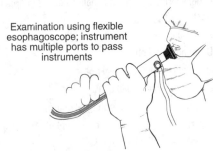

Examination using flexible esophagoscope; instrument has multiple ports to pass instruments

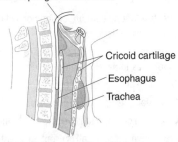

Esophagoscope is passed and the esophagus is examined

Cricoid cartilage
Esophagus
Trachea

Specimens may be obtained from the esophageal lining

Explanation

The physician views the esophagus via a flexible esophagoscope inserted through the patient's mouth and into the esophagus. In 43200, cells are collected for specimen by brushing or washing and/or aspirating the esophageal lining. In 43201, the physician injects any substance into a specific area through the scope while viewing the esophagus. In 43202, biopsy forceps are used to obtain samples of the esophageal mucosa.

Coding Tips

Note that 43200, a separate procedure by definition, is usually a component of a more complex service and is not identified separately. When performed alone or with other unrelated procedures/services, it may be reported. If performed alone, list the code; if performed with other procedures/services, list the code and append modifier 59 or an X{EPSU} modifier. Report the appropriate endoscopy for each anatomic site examined. Surgical endoscopy includes a diagnostic endoscopy; however, diagnostic endoscopy can be identified separately when performed at the same surgical session as an open procedure. If specimen is transported to an outside laboratory, report 99000 for handling or conveyance. For diagnostic esophagoscopy via rigid transoral, see 43191; flexible transnasal, see 43197. For injection sclerosis of esophageal varices via rigid transoral, see 43499; flexible transoral, see 43204. For directed submucosal injection via rigid transoral esophagoscopy, see 43192. For esophagoscopy with biopsy via rigid transoral, see 43193; flexible transnasal, see 43198. For diagnostic flexible esophagogastroduodenoscopy, see 43235. Do not report 43200–43202 with 43197–43198; 43200 with 43201–43232 or 43497; or 43201–43202 with 43200. Do not report 43201–43202 with 43211 or 43201 with 43204 or 43227 for the same lesion.

ICD-10-CM Diagnostic Codes

C15.3	Malignant neoplasm of upper third of esophagus
C15.4	Malignant neoplasm of middle third of esophagus
C15.5	Malignant neoplasm of lower third of esophagus
C15.8	Malignant neoplasm of overlapping sites of esophagus
C49.A1	Gastrointestinal stromal tumor of esophagus
D00.1	Carcinoma in situ of esophagus
D13.0	Benign neoplasm of esophagus
I85.00	Esophageal varices without bleeding
I85.01	Esophageal varices with bleeding
K21.00	Gastro-esophageal reflux disease with esophagitis, without bleeding
K21.01	Gastro-esophageal reflux disease with esophagitis, with bleeding
K21.9	Gastro-esophageal reflux disease without esophagitis
K22.0	Achalasia of cardia
K22.10	Ulcer of esophagus without bleeding
K22.11	Ulcer of esophagus with bleeding
K22.2	Esophageal obstruction
K22.3	Perforation of esophagus
K22.4	Dyskinesia of esophagus
K22.5	Diverticulum of esophagus, acquired
K22.6	Gastro-esophageal laceration-hemorrhage syndrome
K22.70	Barrett's esophagus without dysplasia
K22.710	Barrett's esophagus with low grade dysplasia
K22.711	Barrett's esophagus with high grade dysplasia
K22.89	Other specified disease of esophagus
K23	Disorders of esophagus in diseases classified elsewhere
M35.08	Sjögren syndrome with gastrointestinal involvement
Q39.5	Congenital dilatation of esophagus
Q39.6	Congenital diverticulum of esophagus
Q39.8	Other congenital malformations of esophagus
R07.0	Pain in throat
R12	Heartburn
R13.0	Aphagia
R13.11	Dysphagia, oral phase
R13.12	Dysphagia, oropharyngeal phase
R13.13	Dysphagia, pharyngeal phase
R13.14	Dysphagia, pharyngoesophageal phase
R13.19	Other dysphagia
S27.812A	Contusion of esophagus (thoracic part), initial encounter
S27.813A	Laceration of esophagus (thoracic part), initial encounter
S27.818A	Other injury of esophagus (thoracic part), initial encounter
Z03.821	Encounter for observation for suspected ingested foreign body ruled out

AMA: **43200** 2018,Jan,8; 2017,Jan,8; 2016,Jan,13; 2015,Nov,8; 2015,Jan,16 **43201** 2018,Jan,8; 2017,Jan,8; 2016,Jan,13; 2015,Jan,16 **43202** 2018,Jan,8; 2017,Jan,8; 2016,Jan,13; 2015,Jan,16

Relative Value Units/Medicare Edits

Non-Facility RVU	Work	PE	MP	Total
43200	1.42	6.21	0.21	7.84
43201	1.72	5.78	0.23	7.73
43202	1.72	8.94	0.22	10.88
Facility RVU	**Work**	**PE**	**MP**	**Total**
43200	1.42	0.92	0.21	2.55
43201	1.72	1.04	0.23	2.99
43202	1.72	1.05	0.22	2.99

	FUD	Status	MUE	Modifiers				IOM Reference
43200	0	A	1(3)	51	N/A	N/A	N/A	None
43201	0	A	1(2)	51	N/A	N/A	N/A	
43202	0	A	1(2)	51	N/A	N/A	N/A	

* with documentation

Terms To Know

achalasia. Failure of the smooth muscles within the gastrointestinal tract to relax at points of junction; most commonly referring to the esophagogastric sphincter's failure to relax when swallowing.

biopsy. Tissue or fluid removed for diagnostic purposes through analysis of the cells in the biopsy material.

diagnostic. Examination or procedure to which the patient is subjected, or which is performed on materials derived from a hospital outpatient, to obtain information to aid in the assessment of a medical condition or the identification of a disease. Among these examinations and tests are diagnostic laboratory services such as hematology and chemistry, diagnostic x-rays, isotope studies, EKGs, pulmonary function studies, thyroid function tests, psychological tests, and other tests given to determine the nature and severity of an ailment or injury.

dyskinesia of esophagus. Difficult or impaired voluntary muscle movement of the esophagus.

esophageal varices. Distended, tortuous varicose veins in the lower esophagus. Esophageal varices are frequently a cause of esophageal hemorrhaging and commonly a symptom of portal hypertension from chronic liver disease, especially alcoholic cirrhosis.

forceps. Tool used for grasping or compressing tissue.

injection. Forcing a liquid substance into a body part such as a joint or muscle.

malignant. Any condition tending to progress toward death, specifically an invasive tumor with a loss of cellular differentiation that has the ability to spread or metastasize to other body areas.

specimen. Tissue cells or sample of fluid taken for analysis, pathologic examination, and diagnosis.

therapeutic. Act meant to alleviate a medical or mental condition.

43204-43205

43204   Esophagoscopy, flexible, transoral; with injection sclerosis of esophageal varices

43205   with band ligation of esophageal varices

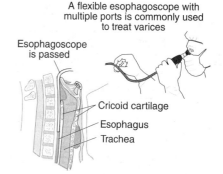

A flexible esophagoscope with multiple ports is commonly used to treat varices

Esophagoscope is passed

Cricoid cartilage
Esophagus
Trachea

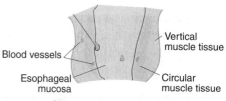

Vertical muscle tissue
Blood vessels
Esophageal mucosa
Circular muscle tissue

Schematic cross section of esophagus showing varices

Explanation

The physician passes a flexible esophagoscope through the patient's mouth and into the esophagus to identify and treat varices. Varices are dilated, enlarged, tortuous veins. In 43204, the physician passes a sclerotherapy needle through the scope and injects the varices with an agent that causes fibrosis (scarring). Over time, this results in obliteration of the varices. In 43205, the physician uses a suction tip to lift the varix and places a rubber band around the base of the varix.

Coding Tips

Report the appropriate endoscopy for each anatomic site examined. Surgical endoscopy includes a diagnostic endoscopy; however, diagnostic endoscopy can be identified separately when performed at the same surgical session as an open procedure. For injection sclerosis of esophageal varices, rigid transoral, see 43499. For control of nonvariceal bleeding via band ligation, see 43227. Do not report 43204–43205 with 43197–43198 or 43200. Do not report 43204 in addition to 43201 or 43204–43205 with 43227 for the same lesion.

ICD-10-CM Diagnostic Codes

I85.00	Esophageal varices without bleeding
I85.01	Esophageal varices with bleeding
I85.10	Secondary esophageal varices without bleeding
I85.11	Secondary esophageal varices with bleeding

AMA: 43204 2018,Jan,8; 2017,Jan,8; 2016,Jan,13; 2015,Jan,16 **43205** 2018,Jan,8; 2017,Jan,8; 2016,Jan,13; 2015,Jan,16

Esophagus

Relative Value Units/Medicare Edits

Non-Facility RVU	Work	PE	MP	Total
43204	2.33	1.35	0.25	3.93
43205	2.44	1.4	0.26	4.1
Facility RVU	Work	PE	MP	Total
43204	2.33	1.35	0.25	3.93
43205	2.44	1.4	0.26	4.1

	FUD	Status	MUE	Modifiers				IOM Reference
43204	0	A	1(2)	51	N/A	N/A	N/A	100-03,100.10
43205	0	A	1(2)	51	N/A	N/A	N/A	

* with documentation

Terms To Know

acute. Sudden, severe. Documentation and reporting of an acute condition is important to establishing medical necessity.

congenital. Present at birth, occurring through heredity or an influence during gestation up to the moment of birth.

dilation. Artificial increase in the diameter of an opening or lumen made by medication or by instrumentation.

esophageal varices. Distended, tortuous varicose veins in the lower esophagus. Esophageal varices are frequently a cause of esophageal hemorrhaging and commonly a symptom of portal hypertension from chronic liver disease, especially alcoholic cirrhosis.

esophagoscopy. Internal visual inspection of the esophagus through the use of an endoscope placed down the throat.

fibrosis. Formation of fibrous tissue as part of the restorative process.

ligation. Tying off a blood vessel or duct with a suture or a soft, thin wire.

obliterate. Get rid or do away with completely.

sclerotherapy. Injection of a chemical agent that will irritate, inflame, and cause fibrosis in a vein, eventually obliterating hemorrhoids or varicose veins.

43206

43206 Esophagoscopy, flexible, transoral; with optical endomicroscopy

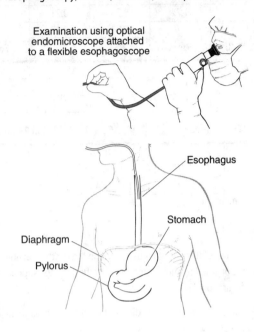

Examination using optical endomicroscope attached to a flexible esophagoscope

Esophagus

Stomach

Diaphragm

Pylorus

Explanation

The physician views the esophagus via a flexible esophagoscope inserted through the patient's mouth and into the esophagus. Any abnormalities of the mucosal lining of the esophagus can be seen using an endomicroscope that is attached to the esophagoscope. The endomicroscope uses laser light to magnify the cells of the mucosa in order to identify the histopathology in real time.

Coding Tips

Supplies used when providing this procedure may be reported with the appropriate HCPCS Level II code. Check with the specific payer to determine coverage. Do not report 43206 with 43197–43198, 43200, or 88375.

ICD-10-CM Diagnostic Codes

C15.3	Malignant neoplasm of upper third of esophagus
C15.4	Malignant neoplasm of middle third of esophagus
C15.5	Malignant neoplasm of lower third of esophagus
C15.8	Malignant neoplasm of overlapping sites of esophagus
C49.A1	Gastrointestinal stromal tumor of esophagus
D00.1	Carcinoma in situ of esophagus
D13.0	Benign neoplasm of esophagus
F45.8	Other somatoform disorders
I85.00	Esophageal varices without bleeding
I85.01	Esophageal varices with bleeding
K20.0	Eosinophilic esophagitis
K21.00	Gastro-esophageal reflux disease with esophagitis, without bleeding
K21.01	Gastro-esophageal reflux disease with esophagitis, with bleeding
K21.9	Gastro-esophageal reflux disease without esophagitis
K22.0	Achalasia of cardia
K22.10	Ulcer of esophagus without bleeding
K22.11	Ulcer of esophagus with bleeding
K22.2	Esophageal obstruction

Esophagus

K22.3	Perforation of esophagus
K22.4	Dyskinesia of esophagus
K22.5	Diverticulum of esophagus, acquired
K22.6	Gastro-esophageal laceration-hemorrhage syndrome
K22.70	Barrett's esophagus without dysplasia
K22.710	Barrett's esophagus with low grade dysplasia
K22.711	Barrett's esophagus with high grade dysplasia
K22.89	Other specified disease of esophagus
K23	Disorders of esophagus in diseases classified elsewhere
M35.08	Sjögren syndrome with gastrointestinal involvement
Q39.0	Atresia of esophagus without fistula
Q39.1	Atresia of esophagus with tracheo-esophageal fistula
Q39.3	Congenital stenosis and stricture of esophagus
Q39.5	Congenital dilatation of esophagus
Q39.6	Congenital diverticulum of esophagus
Q39.8	Other congenital malformations of esophagus
R13.0	Aphagia
R13.11	Dysphagia, oral phase
R13.12	Dysphagia, oropharyngeal phase
R13.13	Dysphagia, pharyngeal phase
R13.14	Dysphagia, pharyngoesophageal phase
R13.19	Other dysphagia

AMA: 43206 2018,Jan,8; 2017,Nov,10; 2017,Jan,8; 2016,Jan,13; 2015,Jan,16

Relative Value Units/Medicare Edits

Non-Facility RVU	Work	PE	MP	Total
43206	2.29	6.52	0.25	9.06
Facility RVU	**Work**	**PE**	**MP**	**Total**
43206	2.29	1.33	0.25	3.87

	FUD	Status	MUE	Modifiers				IOM Reference
43206	0	A	1(2)	51	N/A	N/A	N/A	None

* with documentation

43215

43215 Esophagoscopy, flexible, transoral; with removal of foreign body(s)

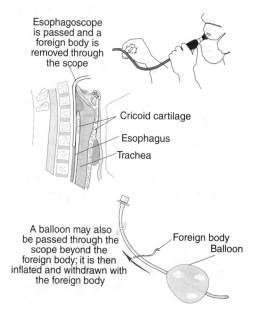

Esophagoscope is passed and a foreign body is removed through the scope

Cricoid cartilage
Esophagus
Trachea

A balloon may also be passed through the scope beyond the foreign body; it is then inflated and withdrawn with the foreign body

Foreign body
Balloon

Explanation

The physician passes a flexible esophagoscope through the patient's mouth and into the esophagus to locate and remove a foreign body(s). It may be suctioned or grasped with forceps and retracted through the scope. An alternative technique is to pass a balloon beyond the foreign body. When the balloon is inflated and withdrawn, the foreign body(s) is captured.

Coding Tips

Report the appropriate endoscopy for each anatomic site examined. Surgical endoscopy includes a diagnostic endoscopy; however, diagnostic endoscopy can be identified separately when performed at the same surgical session as an open procedure. For esophagoscopy with removal of a foreign body, rigid transoral, see 43194. For esophagogastroduodenoscopy, with removal of a foreign body, see 43247. Do not report 43215 with 43197, 43198, or 43200. Report 76000 for fluoroscopic guidance, when performed.

ICD-10-CM Diagnostic Codes

S11.22XA	Laceration with foreign body of pharynx and cervical esophagus, initial encounter
S11.24XA	Puncture wound with foreign body of pharynx and cervical esophagus, initial encounter
T18.110A	Gastric contents in esophagus causing compression of trachea, initial encounter
T18.118A	Gastric contents in esophagus causing other injury, initial encounter
T18.120A	Food in esophagus causing compression of trachea, initial encounter
T18.128A	Food in esophagus causing other injury, initial encounter
T18.190A	Other foreign object in esophagus causing compression of trachea, initial encounter
T18.198A	Other foreign object in esophagus causing other injury, initial encounter
T85.511A	Breakdown (mechanical) of esophageal anti-reflux device, initial encounter

Esophagus

T85.521A	Displacement of esophageal anti-reflux device, initial encounter
T85.591A	Other mechanical complication of esophageal anti-reflux device, initial encounter
T85.598A	Other mechanical complication of other gastrointestinal prosthetic devices, implants and grafts, initial encounter

AMA: 43215 2018,Jan,8; 2017,Jan,8; 2016,Jan,13; 2015,Jan,16

Relative Value Units/Medicare Edits

Non-Facility RVU	Work	PE	MP	Total
43215	2.44	9.3	0.34	12.08
Facility RVU	Work	PE	MP	Total
43215	2.44	1.33	0.34	4.11

	FUD	Status	MUE	Modifiers				IOM Reference
43215	0	A	1(3)	51	N/A	N/A	N/A	None

* with documentation

Terms To Know

balloon catheter. Any catheter equipped with an inflatable balloon at the end to hold it in place in a body cavity or to be used for dilation of a vessel lumen.

esophagus. Muscular tube that carries swallowed liquids and foods from the pharynx to the stomach.

forceps. Tool used for grasping or compressing tissue.

foreign body. Any object or substance found in an organ and tissue that does not belong under normal circumstances.

suction. Vacuum evacuation of fluid or tissue.

43216-43217

| 43216 | Esophagoscopy, flexible, transoral; with removal of tumor(s), polyp(s), or other lesion(s) by hot biopsy forceps |
| 43217 | with removal of tumor(s), polyp(s), or other lesion(s) by snare technique |

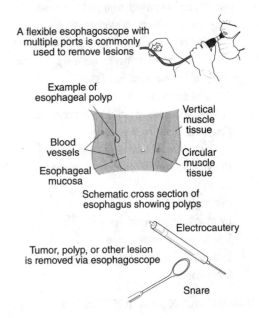

A flexible esophagoscope with multiple ports is commonly used to remove lesions

Example of esophageal polyp

Vertical muscle tissue

Blood vessels

Circular muscle tissue

Esophageal mucosa

Schematic cross section of esophagus showing polyps

Tumor, polyp, or other lesion is removed via esophagoscope

Electrocautery

Snare

Explanation

The physician uses an esophagoscope to remove tumors, polyps, or lesions from the esophagus. A flexible esophagoscope is passed through the patient's mouth and into the esophagus to locate the lesion. In 43216, the base of the lesion is electrocoagulated and severed using biopsy forceps. In 43217, a snare loop is placed around the base of the lesion and closed (the tissue is electrocoagulated and severed as the loop is closed). The severed tissue is withdrawn through the scope.

Coding Tips

Report the appropriate endoscopy for each anatomic site examined. Surgical endoscopy includes a diagnostic endoscopy; however, diagnostic endoscopy can be identified separately when performed at the same surgical session as an open procedure. If specimen is transported to an outside laboratory, report 99000 for handling or conveyance. For esophagoscopy with ablation of tumors, polyps, or lesions, see 43229. For esophagogastroduodenoscopy, with removal of tumors, polyps, or other lesions, by hot biopsy forceps, see 43250; by snare technique, see 43251; and with ablation of tumors, polyps, or lesions, see 43270. For esophagoscopy with endoscopic mucosal resection, see 43211. Do not report 43216 or 43217 with 43197, 43198, or 43200. Do not report 43217 in addition to 43211 when performed on the same lesion.

ICD-10-CM Diagnostic Codes

C15.3	Malignant neoplasm of upper third of esophagus
C15.4	Malignant neoplasm of middle third of esophagus
C15.5	Malignant neoplasm of lower third of esophagus
C15.8	Malignant neoplasm of overlapping sites of esophagus
D00.1	Carcinoma in situ of esophagus
D13.0	Benign neoplasm of esophagus
D37.8	Neoplasm of uncertain behavior of other specified digestive organs
K22.81	Esophageal polyp

K22.82	Esophagogastric junction polyp
K22.89	Other specified disease of esophagus
K23	Disorders of esophagus in diseases classified elsewhere

AMA: 43216 2018,Jan,8; 2017,Jan,8; 2016,Jan,13; 2015,Jan,16 **43217** 2020,May,13; 2018,Jan,8; 2017,Jan,8; 2016,Jan,13; 2015,Jan,16

Relative Value Units/Medicare Edits

Non-Facility RVU	Work	PE	MP	Total
43216	2.3	10.01	0.26	12.57
43217	2.8	9.72	0.3	12.82
Facility RVU	**Work**	**PE**	**MP**	**Total**
43216	2.3	1.33	0.26	3.89
43217	2.8	1.56	0.3	4.66

	FUD	Status	MUE	Modifiers				IOM Reference
43216	0	A	1(2)	51	N/A	N/A	N/A	None
43217	0	A	1(2)	51	N/A	N/A	N/A	

* with documentation

Terms To Know

carcinoma in situ. Malignancy that arises from the cells of the vessel, gland, or organ of origin that remains confined to that site or has not invaded neighboring tissue.

cauterize. Heat or chemicals used to burn or cut.

electrocautery. Division or cutting of tissue using high-frequency electrical current to produce heat, which destroys cells.

forceps. Tool used for grasping or compressing tissue.

hot biopsy. Using forceps technique, simultaneously excises and fulgurates polyps; avoids the bleeding associated with cold-forceps biopsy; and preserves the specimen for histologic examination (in contrast, a simple fulguration of the polyp destroys it).

lesion. Area of damaged tissue that has lost continuity or function, due to disease or trauma.

malignant neoplasm. Any cancerous tumor or lesion exhibiting uncontrolled tissue growth that can progressively invade other parts of the body with its disease-generating cells.

polyp. Small growth on a stalk-like attachment projecting from a mucous membrane.

snare. Wire used as a loop to excise a polyp or lesion.

technique. Manner of performance.

tumor. Pathological swelling or enlargement; a neoplastic growth of uncontrolled, abnormal multiplication of cells.

[43211]

| 43211 | Esophagoscopy, flexible, transoral; with endoscopic mucosal resection |

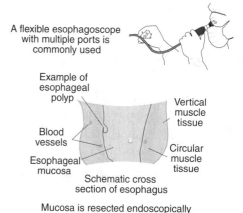

A flexible esophagoscope with multiple ports is commonly used

Example of esophageal polyp

Vertical muscle tissue

Blood vessels

Circular muscle tissue

Esophageal mucosa

Schematic cross section of esophagus

Mucosa is resected endoscopically

Explanation

The physician performs an endoscopic mucosal resection (EMR) to remove abnormal tissues from the esophagus. A flexible esophagoscope is passed through the patient's mouth and into the esophagus to locate the lesion in the inner lining of the esophagus. Saline or other solution is injected into the submucosa around the lesion to raise it from the surrounding deep muscle layer. Once the lesion is raised, it is removed using a snare, banding, or ligation and sent for pathology. The esophagoscope is removed.

Coding Tips

Do not report 43211 with 43197–43198 or 43200. Do not report 43211 in addition to 43201–43202 or 43217 when performed on the same lesion.

ICD-10-CM Diagnostic Codes

C15.3	Malignant neoplasm of upper third of esophagus
C15.4	Malignant neoplasm of middle third of esophagus
C15.5	Malignant neoplasm of lower third of esophagus
C15.8	Malignant neoplasm of overlapping sites of esophagus
C49.A1	Gastrointestinal stromal tumor of esophagus
C78.89	Secondary malignant neoplasm of other digestive organs
D00.1	Carcinoma in situ of esophagus
D13.0	Benign neoplasm of esophagus
I85.00	Esophageal varices without bleeding
I85.01	Esophageal varices with bleeding
K20.0	Eosinophilic esophagitis
K20.80	Other esophagitis without bleeding
K20.81	Other esophagitis with bleeding
K21.00	Gastro-esophageal reflux disease with esophagitis, without bleeding
K21.01	Gastro-esophageal reflux disease with esophagitis, with bleeding
K21.9	Gastro-esophageal reflux disease without esophagitis
K22.10	Ulcer of esophagus without bleeding
K22.11	Ulcer of esophagus with bleeding
K22.2	Esophageal obstruction
K22.3	Perforation of esophagus
K22.4	Dyskinesia of esophagus
K22.5	Diverticulum of esophagus, acquired
K22.6	Gastro-esophageal laceration-hemorrhage syndrome

Esophagus

K22.70	Barrett's esophagus without dysplasia
K22.710	Barrett's esophagus with low grade dysplasia
K22.711	Barrett's esophagus with high grade dysplasia
K22.89	Other specified disease of esophagus
Q39.1	Atresia of esophagus with tracheo-esophageal fistula
Q39.3	Congenital stenosis and stricture of esophagus

AMA: 43211 2019,Dec,14; 2018,Jan,8; 2017,Nov,10; 2017,Jan,8; 2016,Jan,13; 2015,Jan,16

Relative Value Units/Medicare Edits

Non-Facility RVU	Work	PE	MP	Total
43211	4.2	2.17	0.45	6.82
Facility RVU	**Work**	**PE**	**MP**	**Total**
43211	4.2	2.17	0.45	6.82

	FUD	Status	MUE	Modifiers			IOM Reference
43211	0	A	1(3)	51	N/A	N/A N/A	None

* with documentation

Terms To Know

esophagoscopy. Internal visual inspection of the esophagus through the use of an endoscope placed down the throat.

ligation. Tying off a blood vessel or duct with a suture or a soft, thin wire.

mucosa. Moist tissue lining the mouth (buccal mucosa), stomach (gastric mucosa), intestines, and respiratory tract.

resection. Surgical removal of a part or all of an organ or body part.

snare. Wire used as a loop to excise a polyp or lesion.

tissue. Group of similar cells with a similar function that form definite structures and organs. Tissue types include epithelial tissue, muscle tissue, connective tissue, and nervous tissue.

[43212]

43212   Esophagoscopy, flexible, transoral; with placement of endoscopic stent (includes pre- and post-dilation and guide wire passage, when performed)

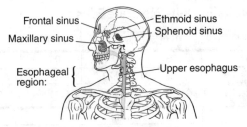

Endoscopically placed stent into esophagus

Explanation

A flexible esophagoscope is passed through the patient's mouth and the esophagus is examined. A guidewire is placed through the scope and the stent is advanced over the guidewire. The position of the stent is confirmed and the scope is withdrawn. This procedure usually follows dilation for an obstruction.

Coding Tips

Do not report 43212 with 43197–43198, 43200, 43220, 43226, or 43241. Report fluoroscopic guidance with 74360, when performed.

ICD-10-CM Diagnostic Codes

C15.3	Malignant neoplasm of upper third of esophagus
C15.4	Malignant neoplasm of middle third of esophagus
C15.5	Malignant neoplasm of lower third of esophagus
C15.8	Malignant neoplasm of overlapping sites of esophagus
C16.0	Malignant neoplasm of cardia
C49.A1	Gastrointestinal stromal tumor of esophagus
C78.89	Secondary malignant neoplasm of other digestive organs
C7A.098	Malignant carcinoid tumors of other sites
D00.1	Carcinoma in situ of esophagus
D13.0	Benign neoplasm of esophagus
D37.8	Neoplasm of uncertain behavior of other specified digestive organs
D3A.098	Benign carcinoid tumors of other sites
D49.0	Neoplasm of unspecified behavior of digestive system
K22.0	Achalasia of cardia
K22.2	Esophageal obstruction
K22.89	Other specified disease of esophagus
Q39.0	Atresia of esophagus without fistula
Q39.1	Atresia of esophagus with tracheo-esophageal fistula
Q39.3	Congenital stenosis and stricture of esophagus
Q39.4	Esophageal web
R13.11	Dysphagia, oral phase
R13.12	Dysphagia, oropharyngeal phase
R13.13	Dysphagia, pharyngeal phase
R13.14	Dysphagia, pharyngoesophageal phase

AMA: 43212 2018,Jan,8; 2017,Jan,8; 2016,Jan,13; 2015,Jan,16

Esophagus

Relative Value Units/Medicare Edits

Non-Facility RVU	Work	PE	MP	Total
43212	3.4	1.57	0.56	5.53
Facility RVU	Work	PE	MP	Total
43212	3.4	1.57	0.56	5.53

	FUD	Status	MUE	Modifiers				IOM Reference
43212	0	A	1(3)	51	N/A	N/A	N/A	None

* with documentation

Terms To Know

achalasia of cardia. Esophageal motility disorder that is caused by absence of the esophageal peristalsis and impaired relaxation of the lower esophageal sphincter. It is characterized by dysphagia, regurgitation, and heartburn.

atresia. Congenital closure or absence of a tubular organ or an opening to the body surface.

dysphagia. Difficulty and pain upon swallowing.

esophagoscopy. Internal visual inspection of the esophagus through the use of an endoscope placed down the throat.

guidewire. Flexible metal instrument designed to lead another instrument in its proper course.

obstruction. Blockage that prevents normal function of the valve or structure.

stent. Tube to provide support in a body cavity or lumen.

43220 [43214]

43220 Esophagoscopy, flexible, transoral; with transendoscopic balloon dilation (less than 30 mm diameter)

43214 Esophagoscopy, flexible, transoral; with dilation of esophagus with balloon (30 mm diameter or larger) (includes fluoroscopic guidance, when performed)

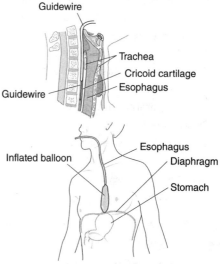

A guidewire is passed through the esophagoscope and a dilator is then passed over the guidewire

A balloon is delivered by scope into the esophagus where it is inflated, usually several times

Explanation

The physician passes a flexible esophagoscope through the patient's mouth and into the esophagus. A balloon is advanced through the scope to dilate the esophagus. After entering the obstructed region, the balloon is briefly inflated several times to stretch the esophageal tissue. Report 43220 when the balloon is dilated to a diameter of less than 30 mm and 43214 when the balloon is dilated to 30 mm or more.

Coding Tips

Report the appropriate endoscopy for each anatomic site examined. Surgical endoscopy includes a diagnostic endoscopy; however, diagnostic endoscopy can be identified separately when performed at the same surgical session as an open procedure. For esophagoscopy with balloon dilation, less than 30 mm, rigid transoral, see 43195. For dilation without endoscopic visualization, see 43450 or 43453. Do not report 43220 or 43214 with 43197–43198 or 43200. Do not report 43220 with 43212, 43226, or 43229. Do not report 43214 with 74360 or 76000. Fluoroscopic guidance is reported with 74360, when performed with 43220.

ICD-10-CM Diagnostic Codes

C15.3	Malignant neoplasm of upper third of esophagus
C15.4	Malignant neoplasm of middle third of esophagus
C15.5	Malignant neoplasm of lower third of esophagus
C15.8	Malignant neoplasm of overlapping sites of esophagus
C49.A1	Gastrointestinal stromal tumor of esophagus
C78.89	Secondary malignant neoplasm of other digestive organs
D00.1	Carcinoma in situ of esophagus
D13.0	Benign neoplasm of esophagus

Esophagus

D37.8	Neoplasm of uncertain behavior of other specified digestive organs
K20.80	Other esophagitis without bleeding
K20.81	Other esophagitis with bleeding
K21.00	Gastro-esophageal reflux disease with esophagitis, without bleeding
K21.01	Gastro-esophageal reflux disease with esophagitis, with bleeding
K22.2	Esophageal obstruction
K22.710	Barrett's esophagus with low grade dysplasia
K22.711	Barrett's esophagus with high grade dysplasia
K22.89	Other specified disease of esophagus
K23	Disorders of esophagus in diseases classified elsewhere
Q39.1	Atresia of esophagus with tracheo-esophageal fistula
Q39.3	Congenital stenosis and stricture of esophagus
Q39.4	Esophageal web
Q39.8	Other congenital malformations of esophagus
R13.11	Dysphagia, oral phase
R13.12	Dysphagia, oropharyngeal phase
R13.13	Dysphagia, pharyngeal phase
R13.14	Dysphagia, pharyngoesophageal phase
R13.19	Other dysphagia

AMA: 43214 2018,Jan,8; 2017,Jan,8; 2016,Jan,13; 2015,Jan,16 **43220** 2018,Jan,8; 2017,Jan,8; 2016,Jan,13; 2015,Jan,16

Relative Value Units/Medicare Edits

Non-Facility RVU	Work	PE	MP	Total
43220	2.0	27.96	0.26	30.22
43214	3.4	1.78	0.43	5.61
Facility RVU	**Work**	**PE**	**MP**	**Total**
43220	2.0	1.18	0.26	3.44
43214	3.4	1.78	0.43	5.61

	FUD	Status	MUE	Modifiers				IOM Reference
43220	0	A	1(3)	51	N/A	N/A	N/A	None
43214	0	A	1(3)	51	N/A	N/A	N/A	

* with documentation

[43213]

43213 Esophagoscopy, flexible, transoral; with dilation of esophagus, by balloon or dilator, retrograde (includes fluoroscopic guidance, when performed)

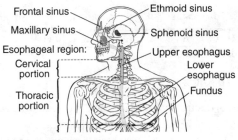

Retrograde balloon dilation is used to dilate the esophagus

Explanation

The physician stretches esophageal tissue in patients where routine esophageal dilation is not feasible. The physician passes a flexible esophagoscope through a patient's gastrostomy or jejunostomy. The scope is passed to the area of the stricture. A second flexible esophagoscope is inserted through the patient's mouth to the stricture. A guidewire is passed from either esophagoscope through the stricture. A balloon or dilators are passed over the guidewire through the scope. After entering the obstructed region, the balloon is briefly inflated several times or progressively larger dilators are passed in succession. Once the diameter of the stricture is acceptable, instruments are removed, the area is examined for perforation, and the scope is removed.

Coding Tips

Report transendoscopic balloon dilation of multiple strictures performed during the same operative session with 43213; append modifier 59 or an X{EPSU} modifier for each additional stricture dilated. Do not report 43213 with 43197–43198, 43200, 74360, or 76000.

ICD-10-CM Diagnostic Codes

C15.3	Malignant neoplasm of upper third of esophagus
C15.4	Malignant neoplasm of middle third of esophagus
C15.5	Malignant neoplasm of lower third of esophagus
C15.8	Malignant neoplasm of overlapping sites of esophagus
C49.A1	Gastrointestinal stromal tumor of esophagus
C78.89	Secondary malignant neoplasm of other digestive organs
D00.1	Carcinoma in situ of esophagus
D13.0	Benign neoplasm of esophagus
K20.80	Other esophagitis without bleeding
K20.81	Other esophagitis with bleeding
K21.00	Gastro-esophageal reflux disease with esophagitis, without bleeding
K21.01	Gastro-esophageal reflux disease with esophagitis, with bleeding
K22.2	Esophageal obstruction
K22.70	Barrett's esophagus without dysplasia
K22.710	Barrett's esophagus with low grade dysplasia
K22.711	Barrett's esophagus with high grade dysplasia
K22.89	Other specified disease of esophagus
Q39.0	Atresia of esophagus without fistula
Q39.1	Atresia of esophagus with tracheo-esophageal fistula

Q39.3	Congenital stenosis and stricture of esophagus
Q39.4	Esophageal web
Q39.5	Congenital dilatation of esophagus
Q39.6	Congenital diverticulum of esophagus
R13.0	Aphagia
R13.11	Dysphagia, oral phase
R13.12	Dysphagia, oropharyngeal phase
R13.13	Dysphagia, pharyngeal phase
R13.14	Dysphagia, pharyngoesophageal phase
R13.19	Other dysphagia

AMA: **43213** 2018,Jan,8; 2017,Jan,8; 2016,Jan,13; 2015,Jan,16

Relative Value Units/Medicare Edits

Non-Facility RVU	Work	PE	MP	Total
43213	4.63	33.35	0.68	38.66
Facility RVU	**Work**	**PE**	**MP**	**Total**
43213	4.63	2.24	0.68	7.55

	FUD	Status	MUE	Modifiers				IOM Reference
43213	0	A	1(2)	51	N/A	N/A	N/A	None

* with documentation

Terms To Know

balloon catheter. Any catheter equipped with an inflatable balloon at the end to hold it in place in a body cavity or to be used for dilation of a vessel lumen.

dilation. Artificial increase in the diameter of an opening or lumen made by medication or by instrumentation.

fluoroscopy. Radiology technique that allows visual examination of part of the body or a function of an organ using a device that projects an x-ray image on a fluorescent screen.

43226

43226 Esophagoscopy, flexible, transoral; with insertion of guide wire followed by passage of dilator(s) over guide wire

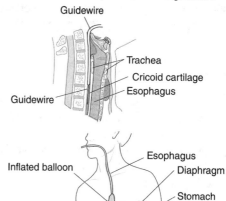

A guidewire is passed through the esophagoscope and a dilator is then passed over the guidewire

Guidewire
Trachea
Cricoid cartilage
Esophagus
Guidewire

Esophagus
Inflated balloon
Diaphragm
Stomach

Explanation

The physician passes a flexible esophagoscope through the patient's mouth and into the esophagus. A guidewire is placed through the scope. The scope is removed and a dilator is passed over the guidewire. This process is repeated several times using progressively larger dilators to stretch the esophageal tissue.

Coding Tips

For esophagoscopy, rigid transoral, with dilation over guidewire, see 43196. Fluoroscopic guidance is reported with 74360, when performed. Do not report 43226 with 43197–43198, 43200, 43212, or 43220. Do not report 43226 in addition to 43229 for the same lesion.

ICD-10-CM Diagnostic Codes

C15.3	Malignant neoplasm of upper third of esophagus
C15.4	Malignant neoplasm of middle third of esophagus
C15.5	Malignant neoplasm of lower third of esophagus
C15.8	Malignant neoplasm of overlapping sites of esophagus
C49.A1	Gastrointestinal stromal tumor of esophagus
D00.1	Carcinoma in situ of esophagus
D13.0	Benign neoplasm of esophagus
K22.2	Esophageal obstruction
K22.710	Barrett's esophagus with low grade dysplasia
K22.711	Barrett's esophagus with high grade dysplasia
K22.89	Other specified disease of esophagus
K23	Disorders of esophagus in diseases classified elsewhere
Q39.4	Esophageal web

AMA: **43226** 2018,Jan,8; 2017,Jan,8; 2016,Jan,13; 2015,Jan,16

Esophagus

Relative Value Units/Medicare Edits

Non-Facility RVU	Work	PE	MP	Total
43226	2.24	8.98	0.33	11.55
Facility RVU	Work	PE	MP	Total
43226	2.24	1.23	0.33	3.8

	FUD	Status	MUE	Modifiers				IOM Reference
43226	0	A	1(3)	51	N/A	N/A	N/A	None

* with documentation

Terms To Know

Barrett's esophagus. Complication of gastroesophageal reflux disease causing peptic ulcer and stricture in the lower part of the esophagus due to columnar epithelial cells from the lining of the stomach and intestine replacing the natural esophageal lining made of normal squamous cell epithelium. Barrett's esophagus is linked to an elevated risk of esophageal cancer, and is sometimes followed by esophageal adenocarcinoma.

dilation. Artificial increase in the diameter of an opening or lumen made by medication or by instrumentation.

esophagus. Muscular tube that carries swallowed liquids and foods from the pharynx to the stomach.

fluoroscopy. Radiology technique that allows visual examination of part of the body or a function of an organ using a device that projects an x-ray image on a fluorescent screen.

guidewire. Flexible metal instrument designed to lead another instrument in its proper course.

tissue. Group of similar cells with a similar function that form definite structures and organs. Tissue types include epithelial tissue, muscle tissue, connective tissue, and nervous tissue.

43227

43227   Esophagoscopy, flexible, transoral; with control of bleeding, any method

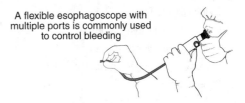

A flexible esophagoscope with multiple ports is commonly used to control bleeding

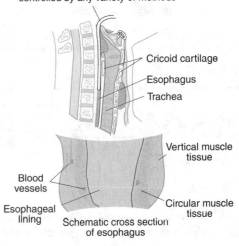

Esophagoscope is passed and bleeding is controlled by any variety of methods

Cricoid cartilage
Esophagus
Trachea
Vertical muscle tissue
Blood vessels
Circular muscle tissue
Esophageal lining

Schematic cross section of esophagus

Explanation

The physician passes a flexible esophagoscope through the patient's mouth and into the esophagus to identify the source of bleeding. Several endoscopic methods may be used to control bleeding, including the use of laser therapy, electrocoagulation, rubber band ligation, and the injection of the bleeding vessel with sclerosants, ethanol, or adrenaline.

Coding Tips

Surgical endoscopy includes a diagnostic endoscopy; however, diagnostic endoscopy can be identified separately when performed at the same surgical session as an open procedure. When endoscopic procedures are performed, report the appropriate endoscopy of each anatomic site examined. Do not report 43227 with 43197–43198 and 43200. Do not report 43227 in addition to 43201, 43204, or 43205 for the same lesion.

ICD-10-CM Diagnostic Codes

C15.3	Malignant neoplasm of upper third of esophagus
C15.4	Malignant neoplasm of middle third of esophagus
C15.5	Malignant neoplasm of lower third of esophagus
C15.8	Malignant neoplasm of overlapping sites of esophagus
C49.A1	Gastrointestinal stromal tumor of esophagus
D13.0	Benign neoplasm of esophagus
I85.01	Esophageal varices with bleeding
I85.11	Secondary esophageal varices with bleeding
K20.0	Eosinophilic esophagitis
K20.81	Other esophagitis with bleeding
K22.11	Ulcer of esophagus with bleeding
K22.3	Perforation of esophagus

K22.6	Gastro-esophageal laceration-hemorrhage syndrome
K22.70	Barrett's esophagus without dysplasia
K22.710	Barrett's esophagus with low grade dysplasia
K22.711	Barrett's esophagus with high grade dysplasia
K22.89	Other specified disease of esophagus
K23	Disorders of esophagus in diseases classified elsewhere
K91.840	Postprocedural hemorrhage of a digestive system organ or structure following a digestive system procedure
K91.841	Postprocedural hemorrhage of a digestive system organ or structure following other procedure
S27.812A	Contusion of esophagus (thoracic part), initial encounter
S27.813A	Laceration of esophagus (thoracic part), initial encounter
S27.818A	Other injury of esophagus (thoracic part), initial encounter
T85.838A	Hemorrhage due to other internal prosthetic devices, implants and grafts, initial encounter

AMA: **43227** 2018,Jan,8; 2017,Jan,8; 2016,Jan,13; 2015,Jan,16

Relative Value Units/Medicare Edits

Non-Facility RVU	Work	PE	MP	Total
43227	2.89	15.89	0.33	19.11
Facility RVU	**Work**	**PE**	**MP**	**Total**
43227	2.89	1.58	0.33	4.8

	FUD	Status	MUE	Modifiers				IOM Reference
43227	0	A	1(3)	51	N/A	N/A	N/A	None

* with documentation

Terms To Know

cautery. Destruction or burning of tissue by means of a hot instrument, an electric current, or a caustic chemical, such as silver nitrate.

electrosurgery. Use of electric currents to generate heat in performing surgery.

laser surgery. Use of concentrated, sharply defined light beams to cut, cauterize, coagulate, seal, or vaporize tissue.

ligation. Tying off a blood vessel or duct with a suture or a soft, thin wire.

perforation. Hole in an object, organ, or tissue, or the act of punching or boring holes through a part.

sclerotherapy. Injection of a chemical agent that will irritate, inflame, and cause fibrosis in a vein, eventually obliterating hemorrhoids or varicose veins.

ulcer. Open sore or excavating lesion of skin or the tissue on the surface of an organ from the sloughing of chronically inflamed and necrosing tissue.

varices. Enlarged, dilated, or twisted turning veins.

43229

43229   Esophagoscopy, flexible, transoral; with ablation of tumor(s), polyp(s), or other lesion(s) (includes pre- and post-dilation and guide wire passage, when performed)

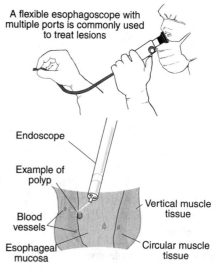

A flexible esophagoscope with multiple ports is commonly used to treat lesions

Endoscope

Example of polyp

Blood vessels

Esophageal mucosa

Vertical muscle tissue

Circular muscle tissue

Schematic cross section of esophagus showing laser ablation of polyp

Explanation

The physician removes tumors, polyps, or lesions from the esophagus by inserting a flexible esophagoscope through the patient's mouth and into the esophagus to locate the lesion. Laser therapy, electrocoagulation, or injection of toxic agents may be used to destroy the lesion.

Coding Tips

For photodynamic therapy of the esophagus, report 43229 in addition to 96570 and 96571, as appropriate. Do not report 43229 with 43197–43198 or 43200. Do not report 43229 in addition to 43220 or 43226 for the same lesion.

ICD-10-CM Diagnostic Codes

C15.3	Malignant neoplasm of upper third of esophagus
C15.4	Malignant neoplasm of middle third of esophagus
C15.5	Malignant neoplasm of lower third of esophagus
C15.8	Malignant neoplasm of overlapping sites of esophagus
C49.A1	Gastrointestinal stromal tumor of esophagus
C78.89	Secondary malignant neoplasm of other digestive organs
D00.1	Carcinoma in situ of esophagus
D13.0	Benign neoplasm of esophagus
D37.8	Neoplasm of uncertain behavior of other specified digestive organs
K22.710	Barrett's esophagus with low grade dysplasia
K22.711	Barrett's esophagus with high grade dysplasia
K22.81	Esophageal polyp
K22.82	Esophagogastric junction polyp
K22.89	Other specified disease of esophagus
K23	Disorders of esophagus in diseases classified elsewhere

AMA: **43229** 2018,Jan,8; 2017,Jan,8; 2016,Jan,13; 2015,Jan,16

Esophagus

Relative Value Units/Medicare Edits

Non-Facility RVU	Work	PE	MP	Total
43229	3.49	18.25	0.42	22.16
Facility RVU	Work	PE	MP	Total
43229	3.49	1.83	0.42	5.74

	FUD	Status	MUE	Modifiers				IOM Reference
43229	0	A	1(3)	51	N/A	N/A	N/A	None

* with documentation

Terms To Know

ablation. Removal or destruction of tissue by cutting, electrical energy, chemical substances, or excessive heat application.

Barrett's esophagus. Complication of gastroesophageal reflux disease causing peptic ulcer and stricture in the lower part of the esophagus due to columnar epithelial cells from the lining of the stomach and intestine replacing the natural esophageal lining made of normal squamous cell epithelium. Barrett's esophagus is linked to an elevated risk of esophageal cancer, and is sometimes followed by esophageal adenocarcinoma.

eosinophilic esophagitis. Disorder involving the accumulation of eosinophil in the tissues lining the esophagus, resulting in severe inflammation. Affecting the ability to swallow, it may result in malnutrition and possible failure to thrive in children.

guidewire. Flexible metal instrument designed to lead another instrument in its proper course.

laser surgery. Use of concentrated, sharply defined light beams to cut, cauterize, coagulate, seal, or vaporize tissue. The color and wavelength of the laser light is produced by its active medium, such as argon, CO_2, potassium titanyl phosphate (KTP), Krypton, and Nd:YAG, which determines the type of tissues it can best treat.

43231

43231   Esophagoscopy, flexible, transoral; with endoscopic ultrasound examination

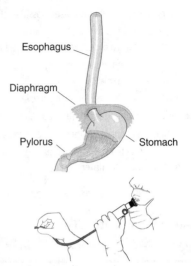

Esophagus
Diaphragm
Pylorus
Stomach

An endoscopic ultrasound is performed within the esophagus. An ultrasound device is passed through an endoscopic instrument. Readings of the esophagus and surrounding structures may be collected and interpreted

Explanation

The physician passes a flexible esophagoscope through the patient's mouth and into the esophagus to perform an endoscopic ultrasound examination. The esophagus is examined and the area of interest is identified. The esophagoscope is removed and replaced with an echoendoscope or an ultrasound probe is passed through the already placed esophagoscope. The echoendoscope or ultrasound probe is fitted with a water-filled balloon near the tip; the tip contains a transducer that picks up the ultrasound frequency and relays it to a processor, outside of the body. The water-filled tip is positioned in the esophagus, against the esophageal wall next to the area of interest. The area is scanned and an ultrasound image is projected through the processor to a monitor in real-time. When the ultrasound examination is complete, the echoendoscope or esophagoscope and ultrasound probe are removed.

Coding Tips

Report this service only once per session. Do not report 43231 with 43197–43198, 43200, 43232, or 76975.

ICD-10-CM Diagnostic Codes

C15.3	Malignant neoplasm of upper third of esophagus
C15.4	Malignant neoplasm of middle third of esophagus
C15.5	Malignant neoplasm of lower third of esophagus
C15.8	Malignant neoplasm of overlapping sites of esophagus
D00.1	Carcinoma in situ of esophagus
D13.0	Benign neoplasm of esophagus
I85.00	Esophageal varices without bleeding
I85.01	Esophageal varices with bleeding
K20.0	Eosinophilic esophagitis
K20.80	Other esophagitis without bleeding
K20.81	Other esophagitis with bleeding

K21.00	Gastro-esophageal reflux disease with esophagitis, without bleeding
K21.01	Gastro-esophageal reflux disease with esophagitis, with bleeding
K21.9	Gastro-esophageal reflux disease without esophagitis
K22.0	Achalasia of cardia
K22.10	Ulcer of esophagus without bleeding
K22.11	Ulcer of esophagus with bleeding
K22.2	Esophageal obstruction
K22.3	Perforation of esophagus
K22.4	Dyskinesia of esophagus
K22.5	Diverticulum of esophagus, acquired
K22.6	Gastro-esophageal laceration-hemorrhage syndrome
K22.70	Barrett's esophagus without dysplasia
K22.710	Barrett's esophagus with low grade dysplasia
K22.711	Barrett's esophagus with high grade dysplasia
K22.89	Other specified disease of esophagus
K23	Disorders of esophagus in diseases classified elsewhere
K92.0	Hematemesis
M35.08	Sjögren syndrome with gastrointestinal involvement
Q39.5	Congenital dilatation of esophagus
Q39.6	Congenital diverticulum of esophagus
Q39.8	Other congenital malformations of esophagus
R13.0	Aphagia
R13.11	Dysphagia, oral phase
R13.12	Dysphagia, oropharyngeal phase
R13.13	Dysphagia, pharyngeal phase
R13.14	Dysphagia, pharyngoesophageal phase
R13.19	Other dysphagia
S27.812A	Contusion of esophagus (thoracic part), initial encounter
S27.813A	Laceration of esophagus (thoracic part), initial encounter
S27.818A	Other injury of esophagus (thoracic part), initial encounter

AMA: 43231 2018,Jan,8; 2017,Jan,8; 2016,Jan,13; 2015,Jan,16

Relative Value Units/Medicare Edits

Non-Facility RVU	Work	PE	MP	Total
43231	2.8	1.55	0.28	4.63
Facility RVU	Work	PE	MP	Total
43231	2.8	1.55	0.28	4.63

	FUD	Status	MUE	Modifiers				IOM Reference
43231	0	A	1(2)	51	N/A	62	N/A	None

* with documentation

43232

43232 Esophagoscopy, flexible, transoral; with transendoscopic ultrasound-guided intramural or transmural fine needle aspiration/biopsy(s)

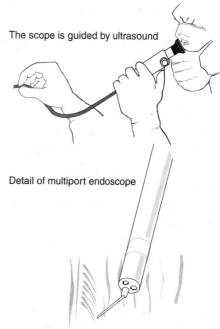

The scope is guided by ultrasound

Detail of multiport endoscope

A fine needle aspiration and/or biopsy is performed on the wall of the esophagus

Explanation

The physician views the esophagus and performs a transendoscopic ultrasound-guided intramural or transmural fine needle aspiration/biopsy. A flexible esophagoscope is passed through the patient's mouth and into the esophagus where the esophagus is examined and the area of interest is identified. The esophagoscope may be removed. A radial scanning echoendoscope is inserted and ultrasound scanning performed or an ultrasound probe is passed through the already placed esophagoscope. The site for a fine needle aspiration biopsy is determined. If a radial scanning echoendoscope is used it is removed and replaced with a curvilinear array echoendoscope. The echoendoscope or ultrasound probe is fitted with a water-filled balloon near the tip; the tip contains a transducer that picks up the ultrasound frequency and relays it to a processor outside of the body. The water-filled tip is positioned in the esophagus, against the esophageal wall next to the predetermined fine needle aspiration (FNA) biopsy site. The area is scanned and an ultrasound image is projected through the processor to a monitor in real-time. The FNA needle is passed through the scope to the biopsy site and the needle is inserted through the wall of the esophagus to the lesion or other structure, such as a lymph node, and a biopsy is taken. When the FNA is complete, the echoendoscope or esophagoscope and ultrasound probe is removed.

Coding Tips

Report this service only once per session. Do not report 43232 with 43197–43198, 43200, 43231, 76942, or 76975.

ICD-10-CM Diagnostic Codes

C15.3	Malignant neoplasm of upper third of esophagus
C15.4	Malignant neoplasm of middle third of esophagus
C15.5	Malignant neoplasm of lower third of esophagus

Esophagus

C15.8	Malignant neoplasm of overlapping sites of esophagus	
C49.A1	Gastrointestinal stromal tumor of esophagus	
D00.1	Carcinoma in situ of esophagus	
D13.0	Benign neoplasm of esophagus	
K20.80	Other esophagitis without bleeding	
K20.81	Other esophagitis with bleeding	
K21.00	Gastro-esophageal reflux disease with esophagitis, without bleeding	
K21.01	Gastro-esophageal reflux disease with esophagitis, with bleeding	
K22.0	Achalasia of cardia	
K22.10	Ulcer of esophagus without bleeding	
K22.11	Ulcer of esophagus with bleeding	
K22.5	Diverticulum of esophagus, acquired	
K22.70	Barrett's esophagus without dysplasia	
K22.710	Barrett's esophagus with low grade dysplasia	
K22.711	Barrett's esophagus with high grade dysplasia	
K22.89	Other specified disease of esophagus	
K23	Disorders of esophagus in diseases classified elsewhere	
K92.0	Hematemesis	
M35.08	Sjögren syndrome with gastrointestinal involvement	
R13.0	Aphagia	
R13.11	Dysphagia, oral phase	
R13.12	Dysphagia, oropharyngeal phase	
R13.13	Dysphagia, pharyngeal phase	
R13.14	Dysphagia, pharyngoesophageal phase	
R13.19	Other dysphagia	

AMA: 43232 2018,Jan,8; 2017,Jan,8; 2016,Jan,13; 2015,Jan,16

Relative Value Units/Medicare Edits

Non-Facility RVU	Work	PE	MP	Total
43232	3.59	1.83	0.37	5.79
Facility RVU	**Work**	**PE**	**MP**	**Total**
43232	3.59	1.83	0.37	5.79

	FUD	Status	MUE	Modifiers				IOM Reference
43232	0	A	1(2)	51	N/A	62	N/A	None

* with documentation

43235-43236

43235 Esophagogastroduodenoscopy, flexible, transoral; diagnostic, including collection of specimen(s) by brushing or washing, when performed (separate procedure)

43236 with directed submucosal injection(s), any substance

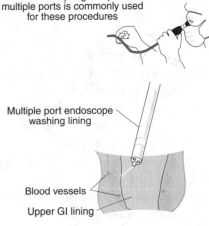

A flexible esophagoscope with multiple ports is commonly used for these procedures

Multiple port endoscope washing lining

Blood vessels

Upper GI lining

Schematic cross section of representative upper GI tract (distal stomach shown)

Explanation

The physician examines the upper gastrointestinal tract for diagnostic purposes. The physician passes an endoscope through the patient's mouth into the esophagus. The esophagus, stomach, duodenum, and sometimes the jejunum are viewed to determine if bleeding, tumors, erosions, ulcers, or other abnormalities are present. In 43235, specimens may be obtained by brushing or washing the esophageal lining with saline, followed by aspiration. Report 43236 if the physician injects any substance into the submucosa through the scope while viewing the upper gastrointestinal tract.

Coding Tips

Note that 43235, a separate procedure by definition, is usually a component of a more complex service and is not identified separately. When performed alone or with other unrelated procedures/services it may be reported. If performed alone, list the code; if performed with other procedures/services, list the code and append modifier 59 or an X{EPSU} modifier. Report the appropriate endoscopy for each anatomic site examined. Surgical endoscopy includes a diagnostic endoscopy; however, diagnostic endoscopy can be identified separately when performed at the same surgical session as an open procedure. For injection sclerosis of esophageal and/or gastric varices, see 43243. Supplies used when providing this procedure may be reported with the appropriate HCPCS Level II code. Check with the specific payer to determine coverage. Do not report 43235 with 43197–43198, 43210, 43236–43259, 43266, 43270, 43497, 44360–44361, 44363–44366, 44369–44370, 44372–44373, or 44376–44379. Do not report 43236 with 43197–43198, 43235, 44360–44361, 44363–44366, 44369–44370, 44372–44373, or 44376–44379. Do not report 43236 with 43243, 43254, or 43255 for the same lesion.

ICD-10-CM Diagnostic Codes

C15.3	Malignant neoplasm of upper third of esophagus
C15.4	Malignant neoplasm of middle third of esophagus
C15.5	Malignant neoplasm of lower third of esophagus
C16.0	Malignant neoplasm of cardia
C16.1	Malignant neoplasm of fundus of stomach

Esophagus

C16.2	Malignant neoplasm of body of stomach
C16.3	Malignant neoplasm of pyloric antrum
C16.4	Malignant neoplasm of pylorus
C17.1	Malignant neoplasm of jejunum
C49.A1	Gastrointestinal stromal tumor of esophagus
C49.A2	Gastrointestinal stromal tumor of stomach
C49.A3	Gastrointestinal stromal tumor of small intestine
C7A.010	Malignant carcinoid tumor of the duodenum
C7A.011	Malignant carcinoid tumor of the jejunum
C7A.092	Malignant carcinoid tumor of the stomach
D00.1	Carcinoma in situ of esophagus
D00.2	Carcinoma in situ of stomach
D13.0	Benign neoplasm of esophagus
D13.1	Benign neoplasm of stomach
D13.2	Benign neoplasm of duodenum
D13.39	Benign neoplasm of other parts of small intestine
D37.1	Neoplasm of uncertain behavior of stomach
D3A.010	Benign carcinoid tumor of the duodenum
D3A.011	Benign carcinoid tumor of the jejunum
D3A.092	Benign carcinoid tumor of the stomach
I85.01	Esophageal varices with bleeding
I85.11	Secondary esophageal varices with bleeding
K20.0	Eosinophilic esophagitis
K20.80	Other esophagitis without bleeding
K20.81	Other esophagitis with bleeding
K21.00	Gastro-esophageal reflux disease with esophagitis, without bleeding
K21.01	Gastro-esophageal reflux disease with esophagitis, with bleeding
K21.9	Gastro-esophageal reflux disease without esophagitis
K22.0	Achalasia of cardia
K22.10	Ulcer of esophagus without bleeding
K22.11	Ulcer of esophagus with bleeding
K22.2	Esophageal obstruction
K22.4	Dyskinesia of esophagus
K22.5	Diverticulum of esophagus, acquired
K22.6	Gastro-esophageal laceration-hemorrhage syndrome
K22.70	Barrett's esophagus without dysplasia
K22.710	Barrett's esophagus with low grade dysplasia
K22.711	Barrett's esophagus with high grade dysplasia
K22.81	Esophageal polyp
K22.82	Esophagogastric junction polyp
K22.89	Other specified disease of esophagus
K25.0	Acute gastric ulcer with hemorrhage
K25.1	Acute gastric ulcer with perforation
K25.2	Acute gastric ulcer with both hemorrhage and perforation
K25.3	Acute gastric ulcer without hemorrhage or perforation
K25.4	Chronic or unspecified gastric ulcer with hemorrhage
K25.5	Chronic or unspecified gastric ulcer with perforation
K25.6	Chronic or unspecified gastric ulcer with both hemorrhage and perforation
K25.7	Chronic gastric ulcer without hemorrhage or perforation
K26.0	Acute duodenal ulcer with hemorrhage
K26.1	Acute duodenal ulcer with perforation

K26.2	Acute duodenal ulcer with both hemorrhage and perforation
K26.3	Acute duodenal ulcer without hemorrhage or perforation
K26.4	Chronic or unspecified duodenal ulcer with hemorrhage
K26.5	Chronic or unspecified duodenal ulcer with perforation
K26.6	Chronic or unspecified duodenal ulcer with both hemorrhage and perforation
K26.7	Chronic duodenal ulcer without hemorrhage or perforation
K27.2	Acute peptic ulcer, site unspecified, with both hemorrhage and perforation
K27.6	Chronic or unspecified peptic ulcer, site unspecified, with both hemorrhage and perforation
K28.0	Acute gastrojejunal ulcer with hemorrhage
K28.1	Acute gastrojejunal ulcer with perforation
K28.2	Acute gastrojejunal ulcer with both hemorrhage and perforation
K28.3	Acute gastrojejunal ulcer without hemorrhage or perforation
K28.4	Chronic or unspecified gastrojejunal ulcer with hemorrhage
K28.7	Chronic gastrojejunal ulcer without hemorrhage or perforation
K29.01	Acute gastritis with bleeding
K29.21	Alcoholic gastritis with bleeding
K29.31	Chronic superficial gastritis with bleeding
K29.41	Chronic atrophic gastritis with bleeding
K29.80	Duodenitis without bleeding
K29.81	Duodenitis with bleeding
K30	Functional dyspepsia
K31.5	Obstruction of duodenum
K31.6	Fistula of stomach and duodenum
K31.7	Polyp of stomach and duodenum
K31.82	Dieulafoy lesion (hemorrhagic) of stomach and duodenum
K31.A11	Gastric intestinal metaplasia without dysplasia, involving the antrum
K31.A12	Gastric intestinal metaplasia without dysplasia, involving the body (corpus)
K31.A13	Gastric intestinal metaplasia without dysplasia, involving the fundus
K31.A21	Gastric intestinal metaplasia with low grade dysplasia
K31.A22	Gastric intestinal metaplasia with high grade dysplasia
K44.0	Diaphragmatic hernia with obstruction, without gangrene
K44.9	Diaphragmatic hernia without obstruction or gangrene
K50.00	Crohn's disease of small intestine without complications
K50.011	Crohn's disease of small intestine with rectal bleeding
K50.012	Crohn's disease of small intestine with intestinal obstruction
K50.013	Crohn's disease of small intestine with fistula
K50.014	Crohn's disease of small intestine with abscess
K50.814	Crohn's disease of both small and large intestine with abscess
K52.81	Eosinophilic gastritis or gastroenteritis
K52.89	Other specified noninfective gastroenteritis and colitis
K57.01	Diverticulitis of small intestine with perforation and abscess with bleeding
K90.0	Celiac disease
K92.0	Hematemesis
M35.08	Sjögren syndrome with gastrointestinal involvement
Q39.1	Atresia of esophagus with tracheo-esophageal fistula
Q39.2	Congenital tracheo-esophageal fistula without atresia
Q39.3	Congenital stenosis and stricture of esophagus

Esophagus

Q39.4	Esophageal web
Q39.5	Congenital dilatation of esophagus
Q39.6	Congenital diverticulum of esophagus
Q39.8	Other congenital malformations of esophagus
R13.11	Dysphagia, oral phase
R13.12	Dysphagia, oropharyngeal phase
R13.13	Dysphagia, pharyngeal phase
R13.14	Dysphagia, pharyngoesophageal phase
R62.7	Adult failure to thrive △
R63.0	Anorexia
R63.4	Abnormal weight loss
R63.6	Underweight

AMA: **43235** 2019,Oct,10; 2018,Jul,14; 2018,Jan,8; 2017,Jul,10; 2017,Jan,8; 2016,Jan,13; 2015,Nov,8; 2015,Jan,16 **43236** 2019,Oct,10; 2018,Jan,8; 2017,Jan,8; 2016,Jan,13; 2015,Jan,16

Relative Value Units/Medicare Edits

Non-Facility RVU	Work	PE	MP	Total
43235	2.09	6.59	0.25	8.93
43236	2.39	9.43	0.26	12.08
Facility RVU	**Work**	**PE**	**MP**	**Total**
43235	2.09	1.23	0.25	3.57
43236	2.39	1.37	0.26	4.02

	FUD	Status	MUE	Modifiers				IOM Reference
43235	0	A	1(3)	51	N/A	N/A	N/A	None
43236	0	A	1(2)	51	N/A	N/A	N/A	

* with documentation

Terms To Know

aspiration. Drawing fluid out by suction.

diagnostic. Examination or procedure to which the patient is subjected, or which is performed on materials derived from a hospital outpatient, to obtain information to aid in the assessment of a medical condition or the identification of a disease. Among these examinations and tests are diagnostic laboratory services such as hematology and chemistry, diagnostic x-rays, isotope studies, EKGs, pulmonary function studies, thyroid function tests, psychological tests, and other tests given to determine the nature and severity of an ailment or injury.

duodenum. First portion of the small intestine connected to the stomach at the pylorus and extending to the jejunum.

EGD. Esophagus, stomach, and duodenum.

esophagus. Muscular tube that carries swallowed liquids and foods from the pharynx to the stomach.

therapeutic. Act meant to alleviate a medical or mental condition.

tumor. Pathological swelling or enlargement; a neoplastic growth of uncontrolled, abnormal multiplication of cells.

ulcer. Open sore or excavating lesion of skin or the tissue on the surface of an organ from the sloughing of chronically inflamed and necrosing tissue.

43237-43238

43237 Esophagogastroduodenoscopy, flexible, transoral; with endoscopic ultrasound examination limited to the esophagus, stomach or duodenum, and adjacent structures

43238 with transendoscopic ultrasound-guided intramural or transmural fine needle aspiration/biopsy(s), (includes endoscopic ultrasound examination limited to the esophagus, stomach or duodenum, and adjacent structures)

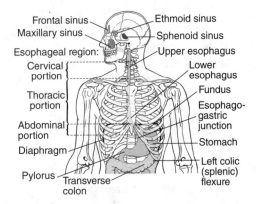

Transendoscopic ultrasound is utilized

Explanation

The physician performs an esophagogastroduodenoscopy (EGD) with a concomitant ultrasound examination for diagnostic purposes. The patient is prepped for an upper gastrointestinal exam and the scope is advanced through the mouth into the stomach and duodenum or jejunum. An examination is carried out to determine if any bleeding, tumors, erosions, ulcers, or other abnormalities are present. Report 43237 when the endoscope exam is followed by insertion of an echoendoscope for an ultrasound exam limited to the esophagus, stomach, duodenum, and adjacent structures. Report 43238 when the echoendoscope is inserted following the EGD examination and an ultrasound and transmural fine needle aspiration biopsy is performed. Using real-time ultrasonic imaging guidance, the physician inserts a 22-gauge needle through the scope to the biopsy site and tissue is removed. Several passes may be made for an adequate specimen before the scope is removed.

Coding Tips

Report the appropriate endoscopy for each anatomic site examined. Surgical endoscopy includes a diagnostic endoscopy; however, diagnostic endoscopy can be identified separately when performed at the same surgical session as an open procedure. These services should not be reported more than once per session. Do not report 43237–43238 with 43197–43198, 43235, 43242, 44360–44361, 44363–44366, 44369–44370, 44372–44373, 44376–44379, 76975, or each other. Do not report 43237 with 43253 and 43259 or 43238 with 76942.

ICD-10-CM Diagnostic Codes

C15.3	Malignant neoplasm of upper third of esophagus
C15.4	Malignant neoplasm of middle third of esophagus
C15.5	Malignant neoplasm of lower third of esophagus
C15.8	Malignant neoplasm of overlapping sites of esophagus
C49.A1	Gastrointestinal stromal tumor of esophagus
C49.A2	Gastrointestinal stromal tumor of stomach
C49.A3	Gastrointestinal stromal tumor of small intestine
D00.1	Carcinoma in situ of esophagus
D13.0	Benign neoplasm of esophagus

Esophagus

I85.00	Esophageal varices without bleeding
I85.01	Esophageal varices with bleeding
I85.11	Secondary esophageal varices with bleeding
K20.0	Eosinophilic esophagitis
K20.80	Other esophagitis without bleeding
K20.81	Other esophagitis with bleeding
K21.00	Gastro-esophageal reflux disease with esophagitis, without bleeding
K21.01	Gastro-esophageal reflux disease with esophagitis, with bleeding
K21.9	Gastro-esophageal reflux disease without esophagitis
K22.0	Achalasia of cardia
K22.10	Ulcer of esophagus without bleeding
K22.11	Ulcer of esophagus with bleeding
K22.2	Esophageal obstruction
K22.4	Dyskinesia of esophagus
K22.5	Diverticulum of esophagus, acquired
K22.6	Gastro-esophageal laceration-hemorrhage syndrome
K22.70	Barrett's esophagus without dysplasia
K22.710	Barrett's esophagus with low grade dysplasia
K22.711	Barrett's esophagus with high grade dysplasia
K22.89	Other specified disease of esophagus
K23	Disorders of esophagus in diseases classified elsewhere
K31.A11	Gastric intestinal metaplasia without dysplasia, involving the antrum
K31.A12	Gastric intestinal metaplasia without dysplasia, involving the body (corpus)
K31.A13	Gastric intestinal metaplasia without dysplasia, involving the fundus
K31.A21	Gastric intestinal metaplasia with low grade dysplasia
K31.A22	Gastric intestinal metaplasia with high grade dysplasia
K92.0	Hematemesis
M35.08	Sjögren syndrome with gastrointestinal involvement
Q39.0	Atresia of esophagus without fistula
Q39.1	Atresia of esophagus with tracheo-esophageal fistula
Q39.4	Esophageal web
Q39.5	Congenital dilatation of esophagus
Q39.6	Congenital diverticulum of esophagus
Q39.8	Other congenital malformations of esophagus
R07.0	Pain in throat
R13.0	Aphagia
R13.11	Dysphagia, oral phase
R13.12	Dysphagia, oropharyngeal phase
R13.13	Dysphagia, pharyngeal phase
R13.14	Dysphagia, pharyngoesophageal phase
R13.19	Other dysphagia
T18.120A	Food in esophagus causing compression of trachea, initial encounter
T18.128A	Food in esophagus causing other injury, initial encounter
T18.190A	Other foreign object in esophagus causing compression of trachea, initial encounter
T18.198A	Other foreign object in esophagus causing other injury, initial encounter
T18.8XXA	Foreign body in other parts of alimentary tract, initial encounter
T28.1XXA	Burn of esophagus, initial encounter

T28.6XXA	Corrosion of esophagus, initial encounter

AMA: **43237** 2019,Oct,10; 2018,Jan,8; 2017,Jan,8; 2016,Jan,13; 2016,Jan,11; 2015,Jan,16 **43238** 2019,Oct,10; 2018,Jan,8; 2017,Jan,8; 2016,Jan,13; 2015,Jan,16

Relative Value Units/Medicare Edits

Non-Facility RVU	Work	PE	MP	Total
43237	3.47	1.85	0.37	5.69
43238	4.16	2.15	0.45	6.76
Facility RVU	**Work**	**PE**	**MP**	**Total**
43237	3.47	1.85	0.37	5.69
43238	4.16	2.15	0.45	6.76

	FUD	Status	MUE	Modifiers				IOM Reference
43237	0	A	1(2)	51	N/A	N/A	N/A	None
43238	0	A	1(2)	51	N/A	N/A	N/A	

* with documentation

Terms To Know

EGD. Esophagus, stomach, and duodenum.

esophageal varices. Distended, tortuous varicose veins in the lower esophagus. Esophageal varices are frequently a cause of esophageal hemorrhaging and commonly a symptom of portal hypertension from chronic liver disease, especially alcoholic cirrhosis.

esophagitis. Inflammation of the esophagus.

fine needle aspiration biopsy. Insertion of a fine-gauge needle attached to a syringe into a tissue mass for the suctioned withdrawal of cells used for diagnostic study.

reflux esophagitis. Inflammation of the lower esophagus as a result of regurgitated gastric acid.

tissue. Group of similar cells with a similar function that form definite structures and organs. Tissue types include epithelial tissue, muscle tissue, connective tissue, and nervous tissue.

Esophagus

43239

43239 Esophagogastroduodenoscopy, flexible, transoral; with biopsy, single or multiple

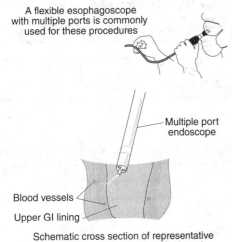

A flexible esophagoscope with multiple ports is commonly used for these procedures

Multiple port endoscope

Blood vessels

Upper GI lining

Schematic cross section of representative upper GI tract (distal stomach shown)

Explanation

The physician examines the upper gastrointestinal tract for diagnostic purposes. The physician passes an endoscope through the patient's mouth into the esophagus. The esophagus, stomach, duodenum, and sometimes the jejunum are viewed to determine if bleeding, tumors, erosions, ulcers, or other abnormalities are present. Single or multiple tissue samples from the upper gastrointestinal tract are obtained for biopsy specimens using biopsy forceps through the endoscope.

Coding Tips

Report the appropriate endoscopy for each anatomic site examined. Surgical endoscopy includes a diagnostic endoscopy; however, diagnostic endoscopy can be identified separately when performed at the same surgical session as an open procedure. Supplies used when providing this procedure may be reported with the appropriate HCPCS Level II code. Check with the specific payer to determine coverage. Do not report 43239 with 43197–43198, 43235, 44360–44361, 44363–44366, 44369–44370, 44372–44373, or 44376–44379. Do not report 43239 in addition to 43254 for the same lesion.

ICD-10-CM Diagnostic Codes

C15.3	Malignant neoplasm of upper third of esophagus
C15.4	Malignant neoplasm of middle third of esophagus
C15.5	Malignant neoplasm of lower third of esophagus
C16.0	Malignant neoplasm of cardia
C16.1	Malignant neoplasm of fundus of stomach
C16.2	Malignant neoplasm of body of stomach
C16.3	Malignant neoplasm of pyloric antrum
C16.4	Malignant neoplasm of pylorus
C17.0	Malignant neoplasm of duodenum
C17.1	Malignant neoplasm of jejunum
C49.A1	Gastrointestinal stromal tumor of esophagus
C49.A2	Gastrointestinal stromal tumor of stomach
C49.A3	Gastrointestinal stromal tumor of small intestine
C78.4	Secondary malignant neoplasm of small intestine
C78.89	Secondary malignant neoplasm of other digestive organs

C7A.010	Malignant carcinoid tumor of the duodenum
C7A.011	Malignant carcinoid tumor of the jejunum
C7A.092	Malignant carcinoid tumor of the stomach
D00.1	Carcinoma in situ of esophagus
D00.2	Carcinoma in situ of stomach
D13.0	Benign neoplasm of esophagus
D13.1	Benign neoplasm of stomach
D13.2	Benign neoplasm of duodenum
D37.1	Neoplasm of uncertain behavior of stomach
D37.2	Neoplasm of uncertain behavior of small intestine
D3A.010	Benign carcinoid tumor of the duodenum
D3A.011	Benign carcinoid tumor of the jejunum
D3A.092	Benign carcinoid tumor of the stomach
K20.0	Eosinophilic esophagitis
K20.80	Other esophagitis without bleeding
K20.81	Other esophagitis with bleeding
K21.00	Gastro-esophageal reflux disease with esophagitis, without bleeding
K21.01	Gastro-esophageal reflux disease with esophagitis, with bleeding
K22.0	Achalasia of cardia
K22.10	Ulcer of esophagus without bleeding
K22.11	Ulcer of esophagus with bleeding
K22.2	Esophageal obstruction
K22.4	Dyskinesia of esophagus
K22.5	Diverticulum of esophagus, acquired
K22.6	Gastro-esophageal laceration-hemorrhage syndrome
K22.70	Barrett's esophagus without dysplasia
K22.710	Barrett's esophagus with low grade dysplasia
K22.711	Barrett's esophagus with high grade dysplasia
K22.89	Other specified disease of esophagus
K25.0	Acute gastric ulcer with hemorrhage
K25.2	Acute gastric ulcer with both hemorrhage and perforation
K25.5	Chronic or unspecified gastric ulcer with perforation
K25.6	Chronic or unspecified gastric ulcer with both hemorrhage and perforation
K26.0	Acute duodenal ulcer with hemorrhage
K26.1	Acute duodenal ulcer with perforation
K26.3	Acute duodenal ulcer without hemorrhage or perforation
K26.4	Chronic or unspecified duodenal ulcer with hemorrhage
K26.6	Chronic or unspecified duodenal ulcer with both hemorrhage and perforation
K26.7	Chronic duodenal ulcer without hemorrhage or perforation
K27.5	Chronic or unspecified peptic ulcer, site unspecified, with perforation
K27.6	Chronic or unspecified peptic ulcer, site unspecified, with both hemorrhage and perforation
K28.0	Acute gastrojejunal ulcer with hemorrhage
K28.2	Acute gastrojejunal ulcer with both hemorrhage and perforation
K28.5	Chronic or unspecified gastrojejunal ulcer with perforation
K28.6	Chronic or unspecified gastrojejunal ulcer with both hemorrhage and perforation
K29.01	Acute gastritis with bleeding
K29.21	Alcoholic gastritis with bleeding
K29.31	Chronic superficial gastritis with bleeding

N Newborn: 0   **P** Pediatric: 0-17   **M** Maternity: 9-64   **A** Adult: 15-124   ♂ Male Only   ♀ Female Only   CPT © 2021 American Medical Association. All Rights Reserved.

Esophagus

K29.41	Chronic atrophic gastritis with bleeding
K29.61	Other gastritis with bleeding
K29.81	Duodenitis with bleeding
K31.4	Gastric diverticulum
K31.5	Obstruction of duodenum
K31.6	Fistula of stomach and duodenum
K31.7	Polyp of stomach and duodenum
K31.82	Dieulafoy lesion (hemorrhagic) of stomach and duodenum
K31.83	Achlorhydria
K31.A11	Gastric intestinal metaplasia without dysplasia, involving the antrum
K31.A12	Gastric intestinal metaplasia without dysplasia, involving the body (corpus)
K31.A13	Gastric intestinal metaplasia without dysplasia, involving the fundus
K31.A21	Gastric intestinal metaplasia with low grade dysplasia
K31.A22	Gastric intestinal metaplasia with high grade dysplasia
K50.011	Crohn's disease of small intestine with rectal bleeding
K50.012	Crohn's disease of small intestine with intestinal obstruction
K50.013	Crohn's disease of small intestine with fistula
K50.014	Crohn's disease of small intestine with abscess
K50.814	Crohn's disease of both small and large intestine with abscess
K52.81	Eosinophilic gastritis or gastroenteritis
K57.01	Diverticulitis of small intestine with perforation and abscess with bleeding
K92.0	Hematemesis
M35.08	Sjögren syndrome with gastrointestinal involvement
Q39.6	Congenital diverticulum of esophagus
R13.11	Dysphagia, oral phase
R13.14	Dysphagia, pharyngoesophageal phase

AMA: 43239 2020,Jan,12; 2019,Oct,10; 2018,Jul,14; 2018,Jan,8; 2017,Jan,8; 2016,Jan,13; 2015,Jan,16

Relative Value Units/Medicare Edits

Non-Facility RVU	Work	PE	MP	Total
43239	2.39	8.84	0.26	11.49
Facility RVU	**Work**	**PE**	**MP**	**Total**
43239	2.39	1.37	0.26	4.02

	FUD	Status	MUE	Modifiers				IOM Reference
43239	0	A	1(2)	51	N/A	N/A	N/A	None

* with documentation

Terms To Know

biopsy. Tissue or fluid removed for diagnostic purposes through analysis of the cells in the biopsy material.

forceps. Tool used for grasping or compressing tissue.

specimen. Tissue cells or sample of fluid taken for analysis, pathologic examination, and diagnosis.

tissue. Group of similar cells with a similar function that form definite structures and organs. Tissue types include epithelial tissue, muscle tissue, connective tissue, and nervous tissue.

43240

43240 Esophagogastroduodenoscopy, flexible, transoral; with transmural drainage of pseudocyst (includes placement of transmural drainage catheter[s]/stent[s], when performed, and endoscopic ultrasound, when performed)

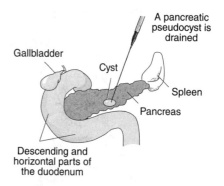

A pancreatic pseudocyst is drained

Gallbladder

Cyst

Spleen

Pancreas

Descending and horizontal parts of the duodenum

Explanation

The physician examines the upper gastrointestinal tract and performs transmural drainage of a pseudocyst. The physician passes an endoscope through the patient's mouth into the esophagus. The esophagus, stomach, duodenum, and sometimes the jejunum are examined. The site for drainage of the pseudocyst is identified. A needle is passed through the scope to the site and the needle is inserted through the small intestinal wall into the pancreatic pseudocyst. The pseudocyst is drained and the endoscope is removed.

Coding Tips

For open external drainage of a pseudocyst of the pancreas, see 48510. For pancreatic necrosectomy performed endoscopically, see 48999. This service should not be reported more than once per session. Do not report 43240 with 43197–43198, 43235, 43242, 43259, 43266, 44360–44361, 44363–44366, 44369–44370, 44372–44373, and 44376–44379 or with 43253 for the same lesion.

ICD-10-CM Diagnostic Codes

K86.2	Cyst of pancreas
K86.3	Pseudocyst of pancreas

AMA: 43240 2019,Oct,10; 2018,Jan,8; 2017,Jan,8; 2016,Jan,13; 2015,Jan,16

Relative Value Units/Medicare Edits

Non-Facility RVU	Work	PE	MP	Total
43240	7.15	3.48	0.76	11.39
Facility RVU	**Work**	**PE**	**MP**	**Total**
43240	7.15	3.48	0.76	11.39

	FUD	Status	MUE	Modifiers				IOM Reference
43240	0	A	1(2)	51	N/A	N/A	N/A	None

* with documentation

Esophagus

43241

43241 Esophagogastroduodenoscopy, flexible, transoral; with insertion of intraluminal tube or catheter

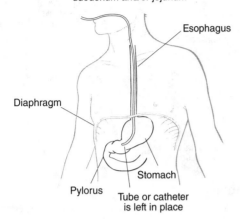

A tube or catheter is placed during a session in which the upper GI tract is scoped, including the esophagus, stomach, and either the duodenum and/or jejunum

Esophagus

Diaphragm

Stomach

Pylorus

Tube or catheter is left in place

Explanation

The physician examines the upper gastrointestinal tract and places a tube or catheter. The physician passes an endoscope through the patient's mouth into the esophagus. The esophagus, stomach, duodenum, and sometimes the jejunum are viewed. The physician places a tube or catheter through the endoscope. The endoscope is removed.

Coding Tips

Report the appropriate endoscopy for each anatomic site examined. Surgical endoscopy includes a diagnostic endoscopy; however, diagnostic endoscopy can be identified separately when performed at the same surgical session as an open procedure. For endoscopic naso- or orogastric tube placement, requiring a provider's skill and fluoroscopic guidance, see 43752; nonendoscopic enteric tube placement, see 44500 and 74340. For gastrostomy, with esophageal dilation and insertion of a permanent intraluminal tube, see 43510. Do not report 43241 with 43197–43198, 43212, 43235, 43266, 44360–44361, 44363–44366, 44369–44370, 44372–44373, or 44376–44379.

ICD-10-CM Diagnostic Codes

C15.3	Malignant neoplasm of upper third of esophagus
C15.4	Malignant neoplasm of middle third of esophagus
C15.5	Malignant neoplasm of lower third of esophagus
C16.0	Malignant neoplasm of cardia
C16.1	Malignant neoplasm of fundus of stomach
C16.2	Malignant neoplasm of body of stomach
C16.3	Malignant neoplasm of pyloric antrum
C16.4	Malignant neoplasm of pylorus
C17.0	Malignant neoplasm of duodenum
C17.1	Malignant neoplasm of jejunum
C49.A1	Gastrointestinal stromal tumor of esophagus
C49.A2	Gastrointestinal stromal tumor of stomach
C49.A3	Gastrointestinal stromal tumor of small intestine
C7A.010	Malignant carcinoid tumor of the duodenum
C7A.011	Malignant carcinoid tumor of the jejunum
C7A.092	Malignant carcinoid tumor of the stomach

D00.1	Carcinoma in situ of esophagus
D00.2	Carcinoma in situ of stomach
D13.1	Benign neoplasm of stomach
D3A.010	Benign carcinoid tumor of the duodenum
D3A.011	Benign carcinoid tumor of the jejunum
D3A.092	Benign carcinoid tumor of the stomach
K20.81	Other esophagitis with bleeding
K21.01	Gastro-esophageal reflux disease with esophagitis, with bleeding
K21.9	Gastro-esophageal reflux disease without esophagitis
K22.11	Ulcer of esophagus with bleeding
K22.2	Esophageal obstruction
K22.4	Dyskinesia of esophagus
K22.710	Barrett's esophagus with low grade dysplasia
K22.711	Barrett's esophagus with high grade dysplasia
K22.89	Other specified disease of esophagus
M35.08	Sjögren syndrome with gastrointestinal involvement
Q39.5	Congenital dilatation of esophagus
Q40.0	Congenital hypertrophic pyloric stenosis
Q40.2	Other specified congenital malformations of stomach
R13.0	Aphagia
R13.11	Dysphagia, oral phase
R13.12	Dysphagia, oropharyngeal phase
R13.13	Dysphagia, pharyngeal phase
R13.14	Dysphagia, pharyngoesophageal phase
T28.1XXA	Burn of esophagus, initial encounter
T28.6XXA	Corrosion of esophagus, initial encounter

AMA: **43241** 2019,Oct,10; 2018,Jan,8; 2017,Jan,8; 2016,Jan,13; 2015,Jan,16

Relative Value Units/Medicare Edits

Non-Facility RVU	Work	PE	MP	Total
43241	2.49	1.36	0.28	4.13
Facility RVU	**Work**	**PE**	**MP**	**Total**
43241	2.49	1.36	0.28	4.13

	FUD	Status	MUE	Modifiers				IOM Reference
43241	0	A	1(3)	51	N/A	N/A	N/A	None

* with documentation

Esophagus

43242

43242 Esophagogastroduodenoscopy, flexible, transoral; with transendoscopic ultrasound-guided intramural or transmural fine needle aspiration/biopsy(s) (includes endoscopic ultrasound examination of the esophagus, stomach, and either the duodenum or a surgically altered stomach where the jejunum is examined distal to the anastomosis)

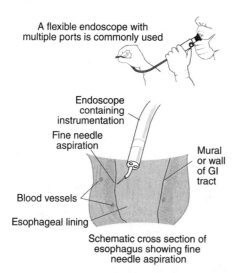

A flexible endoscope with multiple ports is commonly used

Endoscope containing instrumentation

Fine needle aspiration

Mural or wall of GI tract

Blood vessels

Esophageal lining

Schematic cross section of esophagus showing fine needle aspiration

An upper GI endoscopic session is performed with transendoscopic ultrasound-guided intramural or transmural fine needle aspiration and/or biopsy

Explanation

The physician examines the upper gastrointestinal tract and performs transendoscopic ultrasound-guided intramural or transmural fine needle aspiration/biopsy. The physician passes an endoscope through the patient's mouth into the esophagus. The esophagus, stomach, duodenum, and sometimes the jejunum are viewed. The endoscope may be removed. A radial scanning echoendoscope is inserted and ultrasound scanning is performed to examine the esophagus, stomach, and the duodenum and/or jejunum; or an ultrasound probe is passed through the already placed endoscope. The site for a fine needle aspiration biopsy is determined. If a radial scanning echoendoscope is used, it is removed and replaced with a curvilinear array echoendoscope. The echoendoscope or ultrasound probe is fitted with a water-filled balloon near the tip; the tip contains a transducer that picks up the ultrasound frequency and relays it to a processor outside of the body. The water-filled tip is positioned in the esophagus, stomach, or small intestine against the tissue wall next to the predetermined fine needle aspiration (FNA) biopsy site. The area is scanned and an ultrasound image is projected through the processor to a monitor in real-time. The needle is passed through the scope to the biopsy site and a biopsy is taken of the tissue or the needle is inserted through the wall of the esophagus, stomach, or small intestine and into a lesion or other structure, such as a lymph node. The area is biopsied. When the FNA/biopsy is complete, the instruments are removed.

Coding Tips

For transendoscopic ultrasound-guided transmural fine needle aspiration/biopsy limited to the esophagus, stomach, duodenum, or adjacent structures, see 43238. For interpretation of specimen, see 88172–88173. This service should not be reported more than once per session. Do not report 43242 with 43197–43198, 43235, 43237–43238, 43240, 43259–44361, 44363–44366, 44369–44370, 44372–44373, 44376–44379, 76942, or 76975.

ICD-10-CM Diagnostic Codes

C15.3	Malignant neoplasm of upper third of esophagus
C15.4	Malignant neoplasm of middle third of esophagus
C15.5	Malignant neoplasm of lower third of esophagus
C16.0	Malignant neoplasm of cardia
C16.1	Malignant neoplasm of fundus of stomach
C16.2	Malignant neoplasm of body of stomach
C16.3	Malignant neoplasm of pyloric antrum
C16.4	Malignant neoplasm of pylorus
C17.0	Malignant neoplasm of duodenum
C17.1	Malignant neoplasm of jejunum
C49.A1	Gastrointestinal stromal tumor of esophagus
C49.A2	Gastrointestinal stromal tumor of stomach
C49.A3	Gastrointestinal stromal tumor of small intestine
C7A.010	Malignant carcinoid tumor of the duodenum
C7A.011	Malignant carcinoid tumor of the jejunum
C7A.092	Malignant carcinoid tumor of the stomach
D00.1	Carcinoma in situ of esophagus
D00.2	Carcinoma in situ of stomach
D13.0	Benign neoplasm of esophagus
D13.1	Benign neoplasm of stomach
D13.2	Benign neoplasm of duodenum
D37.1	Neoplasm of uncertain behavior of stomach
D37.2	Neoplasm of uncertain behavior of small intestine
D3A.010	Benign carcinoid tumor of the duodenum
D3A.011	Benign carcinoid tumor of the jejunum
D3A.092	Benign carcinoid tumor of the stomach
K22.710	Barrett's esophagus with low grade dysplasia
K22.711	Barrett's esophagus with high grade dysplasia
K26.4	Chronic or unspecified duodenal ulcer with hemorrhage
K28.6	Chronic or unspecified gastrojejunal ulcer with both hemorrhage and perforation
K31.A11	Gastric intestinal metaplasia without dysplasia, involving the antrum
K31.A12	Gastric intestinal metaplasia without dysplasia, involving the body (corpus)
K31.A13	Gastric intestinal metaplasia without dysplasia, involving the fundus
K90.0	Celiac disease
K90.41	Non-celiac gluten sensitivity
R13.11	Dysphagia, oral phase
R13.12	Dysphagia, oropharyngeal phase

AMA: 43242 2019,Oct,10; 2018,Jan,8; 2017,Jan,8; 2016,Jan,13; 2015,Jan,16

Relative Value Units/Medicare Edits

Non-Facility RVU	Work	PE	MP	Total
43242	4.73	2.41	0.49	7.63
Facility RVU	Work	PE	MP	Total
43242	4.73	2.41	0.49	7.63

	FUD	Status	MUE	Modifiers				IOM Reference
43242	0	A	1(2)	51	N/A	N/A	N/A	None

* with documentation

Terms To Know

aspiration. Drawing fluid out by suction.

Barrett's esophagus. Complication of gastroesophageal reflux disease causing peptic ulcer and stricture in the lower part of the esophagus due to columnar epithelial cells from the lining of the stomach and intestine replacing the natural esophageal lining made of normal squamous cell epithelium. Barrett's esophagus is linked to an elevated risk of esophageal cancer, and is sometimes followed by esophageal adenocarcinoma.

biopsy. Tissue or fluid removed for diagnostic purposes.

carcinoid tumor. Specific type of slow-growing neuroendocrine tumors. Carcinoid tumors occur most commonly in the hormone producing cells of the gastrointestinal tracts and can also occur in the pancreas, testes, ovaries, or lungs.

real-time. Immediate imaging, with movement as it happens.

ultrasound. Imaging using ultra-high sound frequency bounced off body structures.

43243-43244

43243 Esophagogastroduodenoscopy, flexible, transoral; with injection sclerosis of esophageal/gastric varices
43244   with band ligation of esophageal/gastric varices

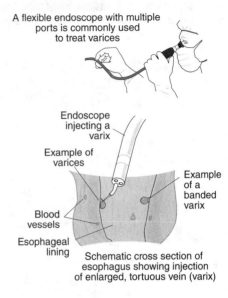

A flexible endoscope with multiple ports is commonly used to treat varices

Endoscope injecting a varix
Example of varices
Example of a banded varix
Blood vessels
Esophageal lining

Schematic cross section of esophagus showing injection of enlarged, tortuous vein (varix)

Explanation

The physician examines the upper gastrointestinal tract to identify and treat esophageal and/or gastric varices. Varices are dilated, enlarged, tortuous veins. The physician passes an endoscope through the patient's mouth into the esophagus. The esophagus, stomach, duodenum and sometimes the jejunum are viewed. The physician identifies the varices. In 43243, the physician passes a sclerotherapy needle through the scope, and injects the varices with an agent that causes fibrosis (scarring). The result is obliteration of the varices. In 43244, the physician uses a suction tip to lift the varix. The physician places a rubber band around the base of the varix.

Coding Tips

Report the appropriate endoscopy for each anatomic site examined. Surgical endoscopy includes a diagnostic endoscopy; however, diagnostic endoscopy can be identified separately when performed at the same surgical session as an open procedure. Report band ligation control of nonvariceal bleeding with 43255. For esophagoscopy, flexible, with injection sclerosis of esophageal varices, see 43204; with band ligation of esophageal varices, see 43205. Do not report 43243–43244 with 43197–43198, 43235, 44360–44361, 44363–44366, 44369–44370, 44372–44373, or 44376–44379. Do not report 43244 with 43255. Do not report 43243 in addition to 43236 or 43255 for the same lesion.

ICD-10-CM Diagnostic Codes

I85.00	Esophageal varices without bleeding
I85.01	Esophageal varices with bleeding
I85.10	Secondary esophageal varices without bleeding
I85.11	Secondary esophageal varices with bleeding
I86.4	Gastric varices
K22.2	Esophageal obstruction
K22.6	Gastro-esophageal laceration-hemorrhage syndrome
K23	Disorders of esophagus in diseases classified elsewhere
K31.82	Dieulafoy lesion (hemorrhagic) of stomach and duodenum
K76.6	Portal hypertension

K92.0	Hematemesis
K92.1	Melena
Q27.33	Arteriovenous malformation of digestive system vessel
Q27.8	Other specified congenital malformations of peripheral vascular system

AMA: **43243** 2019,Oct,10; 2018,Jan,8; 2017,Jan,8; 2016,Jan,13; 2015,Jan,16
43244 2019,Oct,10; 2018,Jan,8; 2017,Jan,8; 2016,Jan,13; 2015,Jan,16

Relative Value Units/Medicare Edits

Non-Facility RVU	Work	PE	MP	Total
43243	4.27	2.14	0.48	6.89
43244	4.4	2.26	0.46	7.12
Facility RVU	Work	PE	MP	Total
43243	4.27	2.14	0.48	6.89
43244	4.4	2.26	0.46	7.12

	FUD	Status	MUE	Modifiers				IOM Reference
43243	0	A	1(2)	51	N/A	N/A	N/A	None
43244	0	A	1(2)	51	N/A	N/A	N/A	

* with documentation

Terms To Know

esophageal varices. Distended, tortuous varicose veins in the lower esophagus. Esophageal varices are frequently a cause of esophageal hemorrhaging and commonly a symptom of portal hypertension from chronic liver disease, especially alcoholic cirrhosis.

fibrosis. Formation of fibrous tissue as part of the restorative process.

ligation. Tying off a blood vessel or duct with a suture or a soft, thin wire.

obliterate. Get rid or do away with completely.

sclerotherapy. Injection of a chemical agent that will irritate, inflame, and cause fibrosis in a vein, eventually obliterating hemorrhoids or varicose veins.

stenosis. Narrowing or constriction of a passage.

stricture. Narrowing of an anatomical structure.

43245

43245 Esophagogastroduodenoscopy, flexible, transoral; with dilation of gastric/duodenal stricture(s) (eg, balloon, bougie)

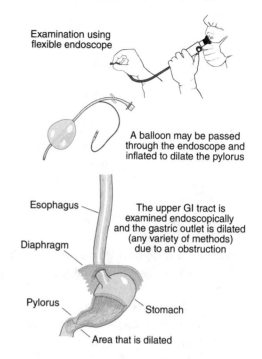

Explanation

The physician uses an endoscope to examine the upper gastrointestinal tract to locate an obstruction. The physician passes an endoscope through the patient's mouth into the esophagus. The esophagus, stomach, duodenum, and sometimes the jejunum are viewed. The gastric or duodenal stricture is located. The physician dilates it using various methods, such as a balloon or bougie. If balloon dilation is performed, the balloon is inflated briefly several times to enlarge the stricture. When the dilation is complete, the balloon and endoscope are removed.

Coding Tips

Report fluoroscopic guidance with 74360, when performed. Do not report 43245 with 43197–43198, 43235, 43266, 44360–44361, 44363–44366, 44369–44370, 44372–44373, or 44376–44379.

ICD-10-CM Diagnostic Codes

C16.2	Malignant neoplasm of body of stomach
C7A.092	Malignant carcinoid tumor of the stomach
D3A.092	Benign carcinoid tumor of the stomach
K25.0	Acute gastric ulcer with hemorrhage
K25.1	Acute gastric ulcer with perforation
K25.2	Acute gastric ulcer with both hemorrhage and perforation
K25.3	Acute gastric ulcer without hemorrhage or perforation
K25.4	Chronic or unspecified gastric ulcer with hemorrhage
K25.5	Chronic or unspecified gastric ulcer with perforation
K25.6	Chronic or unspecified gastric ulcer with both hemorrhage and perforation
K25.7	Chronic gastric ulcer without hemorrhage or perforation
K27.0	Acute peptic ulcer, site unspecified, with hemorrhage
K27.1	Acute peptic ulcer, site unspecified, with perforation

Esophagus

K27.2	Acute peptic ulcer, site unspecified, with both hemorrhage and perforation
K27.3	Acute peptic ulcer, site unspecified, without hemorrhage or perforation
K27.4	Chronic or unspecified peptic ulcer, site unspecified, with hemorrhage
K27.5	Chronic or unspecified peptic ulcer, site unspecified, with perforation
K27.6	Chronic or unspecified peptic ulcer, site unspecified, with both hemorrhage and perforation
K27.7	Chronic peptic ulcer, site unspecified, without hemorrhage or perforation
K31.1	Adult hypertrophic pyloric stenosis 🅐
K31.2	Hourglass stricture and stenosis of stomach
K31.3	Pylorospasm, not elsewhere classified
K31.4	Gastric diverticulum
K86.3	Pseudocyst of pancreas
Q40.0	Congenital hypertrophic pyloric stenosis
Q40.1	Congenital hiatus hernia
Q40.2	Other specified congenital malformations of stomach
Q40.8	Other specified congenital malformations of upper alimentary tract
Q43.8	Other specified congenital malformations of intestine
Q45.8	Other specified congenital malformations of digestive system
R10.0	Acute abdomen
R11.14	Bilious vomiting
R13.11	Dysphagia, oral phase
R13.12	Dysphagia, oropharyngeal phase
T18.2XXA	Foreign body in stomach, initial encounter

AMA: 43245 2019,Oct,10; 2018,Jan,8; 2017,Jan,8; 2016,Jan,13; 2015,Jan,16

Relative Value Units/Medicare Edits

Non-Facility RVU	Work	PE	MP	Total
43245	3.08	15.04	0.42	18.54
Facility RVU	Work	PE	MP	Total
43245	3.08	1.64	0.42	5.14

	FUD	Status	MUE	Modifiers				IOM Reference
43245	0	A	1(2)	51	N/A	N/A	N/A	None

* with documentation

Terms To Know

balloon catheter. Any catheter equipped with an inflatable balloon at the end to hold it in place in a body cavity or to be used for dilation of a vessel lumen.

bougie. Probe used to dilate or calibrate a body part.

stricture. Narrowing of an anatomical structure.

43246

43246 Esophagogastroduodenoscopy, flexible, transoral; with directed placement of percutaneous gastrostomy tube

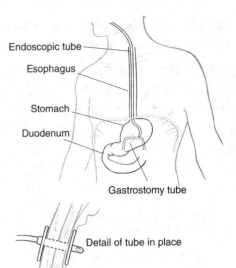

Endoscopic tube
Esophagus
Stomach
Duodenum
Gastrostomy tube
Detail of tube in place

Explanation

The physician uses an endoscope to examine the upper gastrointestinal tract to guide placement of a gastrostomy tube. The physician passes an endoscope through the patient's mouth into the esophagus. The esophagus, stomach, duodenum, and sometimes the jejunum are viewed. The endoscope is used to guide the placement of a percutaneous gastrostomy tube. The tube is inserted through an incision of the abdomen. When in place, the tube connects the gastric lumen with the exterior abdominal wall.

Coding Tips

Report the appropriate endoscopy for each anatomic site examined. Surgical endoscopy includes a diagnostic endoscopy; however, diagnostic endoscopy can be identified separately when performed at the same surgical session as an open procedure. For percutaneous placement of a gastrostomy tube, using fluoroscopy, see 49440. Replacement of a gastrostomy tube without the use of imaging or endoscopy is reported with 43762 or 43763. Do not report 43246 with 43197–43198, 43235, 44360–44366, 44369–44370, 44372, or 44376–44379.

ICD-10-CM Diagnostic Codes

C15.3	Malignant neoplasm of upper third of esophagus
C15.4	Malignant neoplasm of middle third of esophagus
C15.5	Malignant neoplasm of lower third of esophagus
C15.8	Malignant neoplasm of overlapping sites of esophagus
C16.2	Malignant neoplasm of body of stomach
C16.3	Malignant neoplasm of pyloric antrum
C16.4	Malignant neoplasm of pylorus
E41	Nutritional marasmus
E44.0	Moderate protein-calorie malnutrition
E44.1	Mild protein-calorie malnutrition
E45	Retarded development following protein-calorie malnutrition
E86.0	Dehydration
E86.1	Hypovolemia

F50.01	Anorexia nervosa, restricting type
F50.2	Bulimia nervosa
G12.21	Amyotrophic lateral sclerosis ▲
G12.24	Familial motor neuron disease
G20	Parkinson's disease
G35	Multiple sclerosis
G80.8	Other cerebral palsy
I69.291	Dysphagia following other nontraumatic intracranial hemorrhage
I69.391	Dysphagia following cerebral infarction
K22.2	Esophageal obstruction
K31.1	Adult hypertrophic pyloric stenosis ▲
K31.2	Hourglass stricture and stenosis of stomach
K31.3	Pylorospasm, not elsewhere classified
K31.4	Gastric diverticulum
K31.5	Obstruction of duodenum
K50.00	Crohn's disease of small intestine without complications
K50.018	Crohn's disease of small intestine with other complication
K86.3	Pseudocyst of pancreas
K91.89	Other postprocedural complications and disorders of digestive system
Q40.0	Congenital hypertrophic pyloric stenosis
Q40.2	Other specified congenital malformations of stomach
Q40.8	Other specified congenital malformations of upper alimentary tract
Q43.8	Other specified congenital malformations of intestine
Q45.8	Other specified congenital malformations of digestive system
R13.0	Aphagia
R13.11	Dysphagia, oral phase
R13.12	Dysphagia, oropharyngeal phase
R13.13	Dysphagia, pharyngeal phase
R13.14	Dysphagia, pharyngoesophageal phase
R13.19	Other dysphagia
R63.31	Pediatric feeding disorder, acute ℗
R63.32	Pediatric feeding disorder, chronic ℗
R63.4	Abnormal weight loss
T20.29XA	Burn of second degree of multiple sites of head, face, and neck, initial encounter
T20.39XA	Burn of third degree of multiple sites of head, face, and neck, initial encounter
T73.0XXA	Starvation, initial encounter

AMA: **43246** 2019,Oct,10; 2019,Feb,5; 2018,Jan,8; 2017,Jan,8; 2016,Jan,13; 2015,Jan,16

Relative Value Units/Medicare Edits

Non-Facility RVU	Work	PE	MP	Total
43246	3.56	1.78	0.49	5.83
Facility RVU	Work	PE	MP	Total
43246	3.56	1.78	0.49	5.83

	FUD	Status	MUE	Modifiers				IOM Reference
43246	0	A	1(2)	51	N/A	62	80*	None

* with documentation

43247

43247 Esophagogastroduodenoscopy, flexible, transoral; with removal of foreign body(s)

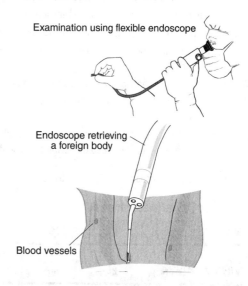

Examination using flexible endoscope

Endoscope retrieving a foreign body

Blood vessels

Explanation

The physician uses a flexible endoscope to examine the upper gastrointestinal tract to locate and remove a foreign body(s). The physician passes a flexible endoscope through the patient's mouth, down the esophagus, through the stomach, and into the duodenum; sometimes the jejunum is also examined. The foreign body(s) is located. It may be suctioned or grasped with forceps and retracted through the endoscope.

Coding Tips

Report the appropriate endoscopy for each anatomic site examined. Surgical endoscopy includes a diagnostic endoscopy; however, diagnostic endoscopy can be identified separately when performed at the same surgical session as an open procedure. Fluoroscopic guidance is reported with 76000, when performed. For esophagoscopy, flexible, with removal of a foreign body, see 43215. For gastrostomy, with exploration or removal of a foreign body, see 43500. Do not report 43247 with 43197–43198, 43235, 44360–44361, 44363–44366, 44369–44370, 44372–44373, or 44376–44379.

ICD-10-CM Diagnostic Codes

S11.22XA	Laceration with foreign body of pharynx and cervical esophagus, initial encounter
S11.24XA	Puncture wound with foreign body of pharynx and cervical esophagus, initial encounter
T17.220A	Food in pharynx causing asphyxiation, initial encounter
T17.228A	Food in pharynx causing other injury, initial encounter
T17.290A	Other foreign object in pharynx causing asphyxiation, initial encounter
T17.298A	Other foreign object in pharynx causing other injury, initial encounter
T18.110A	Gastric contents in esophagus causing compression of trachea, initial encounter
T18.118A	Gastric contents in esophagus causing other injury, initial encounter
T18.120A	Food in esophagus causing compression of trachea, initial encounter
T18.128A	Food in esophagus causing other injury, initial encounter

Esophagus

T18.190A	Other foreign object in esophagus causing compression of trachea, initial encounter
T18.198A	Other foreign object in esophagus causing other injury, initial encounter
T18.2XXA	Foreign body in stomach, initial encounter
T18.3XXA	Foreign body in small intestine, initial encounter
T18.8XXA	Foreign body in other parts of alimentary tract, initial encounter
T85.511A	Breakdown (mechanical) of esophageal anti-reflux device, initial encounter
T85.521A	Displacement of esophageal anti-reflux device, initial encounter
T85.591A	Other mechanical complication of esophageal anti-reflux device, initial encounter
T85.598A	Other mechanical complication of other gastrointestinal prosthetic devices, implants and grafts, initial encounter

AMA: 43247 2019,Oct,10; 2018,Jan,8; 2017,Jan,8; 2016,Jan,13; 2015,Jan,16

Relative Value Units/Medicare Edits

Non-Facility RVU	Work	PE	MP	Total
43247	3.11	8.12	0.37	11.6
Facility RVU	**Work**	**PE**	**MP**	**Total**
43247	3.11	1.67	0.37	5.15

	FUD	Status	MUE	Modifiers				IOM Reference
43247	0	A	1(2)	51	N/A	N/A	N/A	None

* with documentation

Terms To Know

complication. Condition arising after the beginning of observation and treatment that modifies the course of the patient's illness or the medical care required, or an undesired result or misadventure in medical care.

duodenum. First portion of the small intestine connected to the stomach at the pylorus and extending to the jejunum.

esophagoscopy. Internal visual inspection of the esophagus through the use of an endoscope placed down the throat.

forceps. Tool used for grasping or compressing tissue.

foreign body. Any object or substance found in an organ and tissue that does not belong under normal circumstances.

jejunum. Highly vascular upper two-fifths of the small intestine, extending from the duodenum to the ileum.

43248

43248 Esophagogastroduodenoscopy, flexible, transoral; with insertion of guide wire followed by passage of dilator(s) through esophagus over guide wire

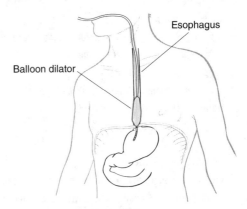

Balloon dilation of the esophagus

The esophagus is dilated during an endoscopic session of the upper GI tract, including the stomach and the duodenum and/or jejunum as appropriate

Explanation

The physician uses an endoscope to examine and dilate a portion of the upper gastrointestinal tract. The physician passes an endoscope through the patient's mouth into the esophagus. The esophagus, stomach, duodenum, and sometimes the jejunum are viewed. A guidewire is placed through the endoscope and the scope is removed. A dilator is passed into the esophagus over the guidewire. This may be repeated several times using progressively larger dilators.

Coding Tips

Report the appropriate endoscopy for each anatomic site examined. Surgical endoscopy includes a diagnostic endoscopy; however, diagnostic endoscopy can be identified separately when performed at the same surgical session as an open procedure. Fluoroscopic guidance is reported with 74360, when performed. Do not report 43248 with 43197–43198, 43235, 43266, 43270, 44360–44361, 44363–44366, 44369–44370, 44372–44373, or 44376–44379.

ICD-10-CM Diagnostic Codes

C15.3	Malignant neoplasm of upper third of esophagus
C15.4	Malignant neoplasm of middle third of esophagus
C15.5	Malignant neoplasm of lower third of esophagus
C15.8	Malignant neoplasm of overlapping sites of esophagus
C16.0	Malignant neoplasm of cardia
K20.0	Eosinophilic esophagitis
K20.80	Other esophagitis without bleeding
K20.81	Other esophagitis with bleeding
K21.00	Gastro-esophageal reflux disease with esophagitis, without bleeding
K21.01	Gastro-esophageal reflux disease with esophagitis, with bleeding
K21.9	Gastro-esophageal reflux disease without esophagitis
K22.2	Esophageal obstruction
K22.4	Dyskinesia of esophagus
K22.70	Barrett's esophagus without dysplasia
K22.710	Barrett's esophagus with low grade dysplasia

Esophagus

K22.711	Barrett's esophagus with high grade dysplasia
K22.89	Other specified disease of esophagus
K23	Disorders of esophagus in diseases classified elsewhere
Q39.3	Congenital stenosis and stricture of esophagus
Q39.4	Esophageal web
Q39.5	Congenital dilatation of esophagus
Q39.8	Other congenital malformations of esophagus
R13.0	Aphagia
R13.12	Dysphagia, oropharyngeal phase
R13.13	Dysphagia, pharyngeal phase
R13.14	Dysphagia, pharyngoesophageal phase

AMA: 43248 2019,Oct,10; 2018,Jan,8; 2017,Jul,10; 2017,Jan,8; 2016,Jan,13; 2015,Jan,16

Relative Value Units/Medicare Edits

Non-Facility RVU	Work	PE	MP	Total
43248	2.91	9.18	0.32	12.41
Facility RVU	**Work**	**PE**	**MP**	**Total**
43248	2.91	1.6	0.32	4.83

	FUD	Status	MUE	Modifiers			IOM Reference
43248	0	A	1(3)	51	N/A	N/A	N/A	None

* with documentation

Terms To Know

benign. Mild or nonmalignant in nature.

dilation. Artificial increase in the diameter of an opening or lumen made by medication or by instrumentation.

EGD. Esophagus, stomach, and duodenum.

eosinophilic esophagitis. Disorder involving the accumulation of eosinophil in the tissues lining the esophagus, resulting in severe inflammation. Affecting the ability to swallow, it may result in malnutrition and possible failure to thrive in children.

guidewire. Flexible metal instrument designed to lead another instrument in its proper course.

malignant. Any condition tending to progress toward death, specifically an invasive tumor with a loss of cellular differentiation that has the ability to spread or metastasize to other body areas.

stenosis. Narrowing or constriction of a passage.

stricture. Narrowing of an anatomical structure.

43249 [43233]

43249 Esophagogastroduodenoscopy, flexible, transoral; with transendoscopic balloon dilation of esophagus (less than 30 mm diameter)

43233 Esophagogastroduodenoscopy, flexible, transoral; with dilation of esophagus with balloon (30 mm diameter or larger) (includes fluoroscopic guidance, when performed)

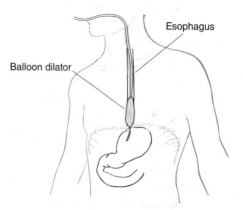

Balloon dilation of the esophagus

The esophagus is dilated during an endoscopic session of the upper GI tract

Explanation

The physician visualizes the esophagus, stomach, and proximal small bowel with an endoscope and dilates an esophageal stricture. The physician inserts the endoscope through the mouth into the esophagus. The endoscope is advanced under direct vision through the esophagus into the stomach. The stomach is visualized and the endoscope is advanced into and through the duodenum and into the proximal jejunum if possible. The endoscope is withdrawn. If an esophageal stricture is present, a balloon on a catheter is advanced through the endoscope and through the stricture. The balloon is inflated to correct volume, pressure, and duration according to the package insert. The endoscope is removed. Report 43249 if the balloon is dilated less than 30 mm and 43233 if the balloon is dilated 30 mm or more.

Coding Tips

Report 74360 for fluoroscopic guidance when performed with 43249. Do not report 43249 or 43233 with 43197–43198, 43235, 44360–44361, 44363–44366, 44369–44370, 44372–44373, or 44376–44379. Do not report 43249 with 43266 or 43270. Do not report 43233 with 74360 or 76000.

ICD-10-CM Diagnostic Codes

C15.3	Malignant neoplasm of upper third of esophagus
C15.4	Malignant neoplasm of middle third of esophagus
C15.5	Malignant neoplasm of lower third of esophagus
C15.8	Malignant neoplasm of overlapping sites of esophagus
C16.0	Malignant neoplasm of cardia
C16.1	Malignant neoplasm of fundus of stomach
C78.89	Secondary malignant neoplasm of other digestive organs
D00.1	Carcinoma in situ of esophagus
D13.0	Benign neoplasm of esophagus
D13.1	Benign neoplasm of stomach
D37.8	Neoplasm of uncertain behavior of other specified digestive organs

Esophagus

K20.0	Eosinophilic esophagitis
K20.80	Other esophagitis without bleeding
K20.81	Other esophagitis with bleeding
K21.00	Gastro-esophageal reflux disease with esophagitis, without bleeding
K21.01	Gastro-esophageal reflux disease with esophagitis, with bleeding
K21.9	Gastro-esophageal reflux disease without esophagitis
K22.0	Achalasia of cardia
K22.10	Ulcer of esophagus without bleeding
K22.2	Esophageal obstruction
K22.4	Dyskinesia of esophagus
K22.70	Barrett's esophagus without dysplasia
K22.710	Barrett's esophagus with low grade dysplasia
K22.711	Barrett's esophagus with high grade dysplasia
K22.89	Other specified disease of esophagus
K23	Disorders of esophagus in diseases classified elsewhere
Q39.0	Atresia of esophagus without fistula
Q39.3	Congenital stenosis and stricture of esophagus
Q39.4	Esophageal web
Q39.8	Other congenital malformations of esophagus
Q40.1	Congenital hiatus hernia
R13.0	Aphagia
R13.12	Dysphagia, oropharyngeal phase
R13.13	Dysphagia, pharyngeal phase
R13.14	Dysphagia, pharyngoesophageal phase
R13.19	Other dysphagia

AMA: 43233 2019,Oct,10; 2018,Jan,8; 2017,Jan,8; 2016,Jan,13; 2015,Jan,16
43249 2019,Oct,10; 2018,Jul,14; 2018,Jan,8; 2017,Jan,8; 2016,Jan,13; 2015,Jan,16

Relative Value Units/Medicare Edits

Non-Facility RVU	Work	PE	MP	Total
43249	2.67	31.47	0.31	34.45
43233	4.07	2.03	0.59	6.69
Facility RVU	**Work**	**PE**	**MP**	**Total**
43249	2.67	1.49	0.31	4.47
43233	4.07	2.03	0.59	6.69

	FUD	Status	MUE	Modifiers				IOM Reference
43249	0	A	1(3)	51	N/A	N/A	N/A	None
43233	0	A	1(3)	51	N/A	N/A	N/A	

* with documentation

43250-43251

43250	Esophagogastroduodenoscopy, flexible, transoral; with removal of tumor(s), polyp(s), or other lesion(s) by hot biopsy forceps
43251	with removal of tumor(s), polyp(s), or other lesion(s) by snare technique

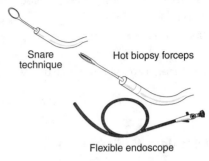

Snare technique   Hot biopsy forceps

Flexible endoscope

Lesions are removed endoscopically using any of a variety of techniques

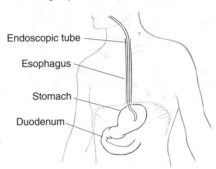

Endoscopic tube
Esophagus
Stomach
Duodenum

Explanation

The physician uses a flexible endoscope to examine the upper gastrointestinal tract and locate and remove tumors, polyps, or other lesions. The physician passes a flexible endoscope through the patient's mouth, down the esophagus, through the stomach, and into the duodenum; sometimes the jejunum is also examined to locate the lesion. Report 43250 when the base of the lesion is electrocoagulated and severed using biopsy forceps. Report 43251 when a snare loop is placed around the base of the lesion and closed (the tissue is electrocoagulated and severed as the loop is closed). The severed tissue is withdrawn through the endoscope. The endoscope is removed.

Coding Tips

Report the appropriate endoscopy for each anatomic site examined. Surgical endoscopy includes a diagnostic endoscopy; however, diagnostic endoscopy can be identified separately when performed at the same surgical session as an open procedure. If a specimen is transported to an outside laboratory, report 99000 for handling or conveyance. For esophagogastroduodenoscopy, with ablation of tumors, polyps, or other lesions, see 43270. For esophagoscopy, flexible, with removal of tumors, polyps, or lesions, by hot biopsy forceps, see 43216; by snare technique, see 43217; and for ablation by other methods, see 43229. For endoscopic mucosal resection, see 43254. Do not report 43250 or 43251 with 43197, 43198, 43235, 44360, 44361, 44363–44366, 44369, 44370, 44372, 44373, or 44376–44379. Do not report 43251 in addition to 43254 for the same lesion.

ICD-10-CM Diagnostic Codes

C15.3	Malignant neoplasm of upper third of esophagus
C15.4	Malignant neoplasm of middle third of esophagus
C15.5	Malignant neoplasm of lower third of esophagus

Esophagus

C15.8	Malignant neoplasm of overlapping sites of esophagus
C16.0	Malignant neoplasm of cardia
C16.1	Malignant neoplasm of fundus of stomach
C16.2	Malignant neoplasm of body of stomach
C16.3	Malignant neoplasm of pyloric antrum
C16.4	Malignant neoplasm of pylorus
C16.8	Malignant neoplasm of overlapping sites of stomach
C17.0	Malignant neoplasm of duodenum
C17.1	Malignant neoplasm of jejunum
C17.8	Malignant neoplasm of overlapping sites of small intestine
C49.A1	Gastrointestinal stromal tumor of esophagus
C49.A2	Gastrointestinal stromal tumor of stomach
C49.A3	Gastrointestinal stromal tumor of small intestine
C78.4	Secondary malignant neoplasm of small intestine
C79.89	Secondary malignant neoplasm of other specified sites
C7A.010	Malignant carcinoid tumor of the duodenum
C7A.011	Malignant carcinoid tumor of the jejunum
C7A.092	Malignant carcinoid tumor of the stomach
D00.1	Carcinoma in situ of esophagus
D00.2	Carcinoma in situ of stomach
D01.49	Carcinoma in situ of other parts of intestine
D13.0	Benign neoplasm of esophagus
D13.1	Benign neoplasm of stomach
D13.2	Benign neoplasm of duodenum
D13.39	Benign neoplasm of other parts of small intestine
D21.4	Benign neoplasm of connective and other soft tissue of abdomen
D37.1	Neoplasm of uncertain behavior of stomach
D37.2	Neoplasm of uncertain behavior of small intestine
D37.8	Neoplasm of uncertain behavior of other specified digestive organs
D3A.010	Benign carcinoid tumor of the duodenum
D3A.011	Benign carcinoid tumor of the jejunum
K20.80	Other esophagitis without bleeding
K20.81	Other esophagitis with bleeding
K21.00	Gastro-esophageal reflux disease with esophagitis, without bleeding
K21.01	Gastro-esophageal reflux disease with esophagitis, with bleeding
K21.9	Gastro-esophageal reflux disease without esophagitis
K22.81	Esophageal polyp
K22.82	Esophagogastric junction polyp
K22.89	Other specified disease of esophagus
K23	Disorders of esophagus in diseases classified elsewhere
K31.7	Polyp of stomach and duodenum
K31.811	Angiodysplasia of stomach and duodenum with bleeding
K31.819	Angiodysplasia of stomach and duodenum without bleeding
K31.82	Dieulafoy lesion (hemorrhagic) of stomach and duodenum
K31.89	Other diseases of stomach and duodenum
K92.81	Gastrointestinal mucositis (ulcerative)

AMA: 43250 2019,Oct,10; 2018,Jan,8; 2017,Jan,8; 2016,Jan,13; 2015,Jan,16
43251 2019,Oct,10; 2018,Jan,8; 2017,Jan,8; 2016,Jan,13; 2015,Jan,16

Relative Value Units/Medicare Edits

Non-Facility RVU	Work	PE	MP	Total
43250	2.97	10.44	0.43	13.84
43251	3.47	11.28	0.39	15.14
Facility RVU	Work	PE	MP	Total
43250	2.97	1.58	0.43	4.98
43251	3.47	1.84	0.39	5.7

	FUD	Status	MUE	Modifiers				IOM Reference
43250	0	A	1(2)	51	N/A	N/A	N/A	None
43251	0	A	1(2)	51	N/A	N/A	N/A	

* with documentation

Terms To Know

duodenum. First portion of the small intestine connected to the stomach at the pylorus and extending to the jejunum.

EGD. Esophagus, stomach, and duodenum.

esophagus. Muscular tube that carries swallowed liquids and foods from the pharynx to the stomach.

forceps. Tool used for grasping or compressing tissue.

hot biopsy. Using forceps technique, simultaneously excises and fulgurates polyps; avoids the bleeding associated with cold-forceps biopsy; and preserves the specimen for histologic examination (in contrast, a simple fulgeration of the polyp destroys it).

jejunum. Highly vascular upper two-fifths of the small intestine, extending from the duodenum to the ileum.

lesion. Area of damaged tissue that has lost continuity or function, due to disease or trauma.

polyp. Small growth on a stalk-like attachment projecting from a mucous membrane.

snare. Wire used as a loop to excise a polyp or lesion.

tumor. Pathological swelling or enlargement; a neoplastic growth of uncontrolled, abnormal multiplication of cells.

Esophagus

43252

43252 Esophagogastroduodenoscopy, flexible, transoral; with optical endomicroscopy

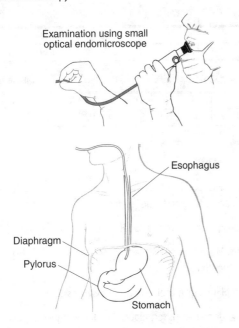

Examination using small optical endomicroscope

Esophagus

Diaphragm

Pylorus

Stomach

Explanation

The physician examines the upper gastrointestinal tract for diagnostic purposes. The physician passes an endoscope through the patient's mouth into the esophagus. The esophagus, stomach, duodenum, and sometimes the jejunum are viewed to determine if bleeding, tumors, erosions, ulcers, or other abnormalities are present. The physician views any abnormality of the mucosal lining using an endomicroscope that is attached to the esophagoscope. The endomicroscope uses laser light to magnify the cells of the mucosa in order to identify the histopathology in real time.

Coding Tips

For pathology of a biopsy specimen, see 88305. Do not report 43252 with 43197–43198, 43235, 44360–44361, 44363–44366, 44369–44370, 44372–44373, 44376–44379, or 88375.

ICD-10-CM Diagnostic Codes

C15.3	Malignant neoplasm of upper third of esophagus
C15.4	Malignant neoplasm of middle third of esophagus
C15.5	Malignant neoplasm of lower third of esophagus
C15.8	Malignant neoplasm of overlapping sites of esophagus
C16.0	Malignant neoplasm of cardia
C16.1	Malignant neoplasm of fundus of stomach
C16.2	Malignant neoplasm of body of stomach
C16.3	Malignant neoplasm of pyloric antrum
C16.4	Malignant neoplasm of pylorus
C17.0	Malignant neoplasm of duodenum
C17.1	Malignant neoplasm of jejunum
C49.A1	Gastrointestinal stromal tumor of esophagus
C49.A2	Gastrointestinal stromal tumor of stomach
C49.A3	Gastrointestinal stromal tumor of small intestine
C78.4	Secondary malignant neoplasm of small intestine
C7A.010	Malignant carcinoid tumor of the duodenum
C7A.011	Malignant carcinoid tumor of the jejunum
C7A.092	Malignant carcinoid tumor of the stomach
D00.1	Carcinoma in situ of esophagus
D00.2	Carcinoma in situ of stomach
D13.0	Benign neoplasm of esophagus
D13.1	Benign neoplasm of stomach
D13.2	Benign neoplasm of duodenum
D37.1	Neoplasm of uncertain behavior of stomach
D37.2	Neoplasm of uncertain behavior of small intestine
D3A.010	Benign carcinoid tumor of the duodenum
D3A.092	Benign carcinoid tumor of the stomach
I85.10	Secondary esophageal varices without bleeding
K20.0	Eosinophilic esophagitis
K20.80	Other esophagitis without bleeding
K20.81	Other esophagitis with bleeding
K21.00	Gastro-esophageal reflux disease with esophagitis, without bleeding
K21.01	Gastro-esophageal reflux disease with esophagitis, with bleeding
K21.9	Gastro-esophageal reflux disease without esophagitis
K22.0	Achalasia of cardia
K22.10	Ulcer of esophagus without bleeding
K22.11	Ulcer of esophagus with bleeding
K22.2	Esophageal obstruction
K22.4	Dyskinesia of esophagus
K22.5	Diverticulum of esophagus, acquired
K22.6	Gastro-esophageal laceration-hemorrhage syndrome
K22.70	Barrett's esophagus without dysplasia
K22.710	Barrett's esophagus with low grade dysplasia
K22.711	Barrett's esophagus with high grade dysplasia
K22.89	Other specified disease of esophagus
K23	Disorders of esophagus in diseases classified elsewhere
K25.0	Acute gastric ulcer with hemorrhage
K25.1	Acute gastric ulcer with perforation
K25.2	Acute gastric ulcer with both hemorrhage and perforation
K25.3	Acute gastric ulcer without hemorrhage or perforation
K25.4	Chronic or unspecified gastric ulcer with hemorrhage
K25.5	Chronic or unspecified gastric ulcer with perforation
K25.6	Chronic or unspecified gastric ulcer with both hemorrhage and perforation
K25.7	Chronic gastric ulcer without hemorrhage or perforation
K26.0	Acute duodenal ulcer with hemorrhage
K26.1	Acute duodenal ulcer with perforation
K26.2	Acute duodenal ulcer with both hemorrhage and perforation
K26.3	Acute duodenal ulcer without hemorrhage or perforation
K26.4	Chronic or unspecified duodenal ulcer with hemorrhage
K26.5	Chronic or unspecified duodenal ulcer with perforation
K26.6	Chronic or unspecified duodenal ulcer with both hemorrhage and perforation
K26.7	Chronic duodenal ulcer without hemorrhage or perforation
K27.2	Acute peptic ulcer, site unspecified, with both hemorrhage and perforation
K28.0	Acute gastrojejunal ulcer with hemorrhage
K28.1	Acute gastrojejunal ulcer with perforation

Esophagus

K28.2	Acute gastrojejunal ulcer with both hemorrhage and perforation
K28.4	Chronic or unspecified gastrojejunal ulcer with hemorrhage
K28.5	Chronic or unspecified gastrojejunal ulcer with perforation
K28.6	Chronic or unspecified gastrojejunal ulcer with both hemorrhage and perforation
K28.7	Chronic gastrojejunal ulcer without hemorrhage or perforation
K29.31	Chronic superficial gastritis with bleeding
K29.41	Chronic atrophic gastritis with bleeding
K29.61	Other gastritis with bleeding
K29.81	Duodenitis with bleeding
K31.4	Gastric diverticulum
K31.5	Obstruction of duodenum
K31.6	Fistula of stomach and duodenum
K31.7	Polyp of stomach and duodenum
K31.811	Angiodysplasia of stomach and duodenum with bleeding
K31.819	Angiodysplasia of stomach and duodenum without bleeding
K31.84	Gastroparesis
K31.89	Other diseases of stomach and duodenum
K31.A11	Gastric intestinal metaplasia without dysplasia, involving the antrum
K31.A12	Gastric intestinal metaplasia without dysplasia, involving the body (corpus)
K31.A13	Gastric intestinal metaplasia without dysplasia, involving the fundus
K31.A21	Gastric intestinal metaplasia with low grade dysplasia
K31.A22	Gastric intestinal metaplasia with high grade dysplasia
K90.0	Celiac disease
M35.08	Sjögren syndrome with gastrointestinal involvement
R13.14	Dysphagia, pharyngoesophageal phase

AMA: **43252** 2019,Oct,10; 2018,Jan,8; 2017,Jan,8; 2016,Jan,13; 2015,Jan,16

Relative Value Units/Medicare Edits

Non-Facility RVU	Work	PE	MP	Total
43252	2.96	6.86	0.34	10.16
Facility RVU	Work	PE	MP	Total
43252	2.96	1.6	0.34	4.9

	FUD	Status	MUE	Modifiers				IOM Reference
43252	0	A	1(2)	51	N/A	N/A	N/A	None

* with documentation

Terms To Know

duodenum. First portion of the small intestine connected to the stomach at the pylorus and extending to the jejunum.

endomicroscopy. Diagnostic technology that allows for the examination of tissue at the cellular level during endoscopy. The technology decreases the need for biopsy with histological examination for some types of lesions.

esophagus. Muscular tube that carries swallowed liquids and foods from the pharynx to the stomach.

jejunum. Highly vascular upper two-fifths of the small intestine, extending from the duodenum to the ileum.

43253

43253 Esophagogastroduodenoscopy, flexible, transoral; with transendoscopic ultrasound-guided transmural injection of diagnostic or therapeutic substance(s) (eg, anesthetic, neurolytic agent) or fiducial marker(s) (includes endoscopic ultrasound examination of the esophagus, stomach, and either the duodenum or a surgically altered stomach where the jejunum is examined distal to the anastomosis)

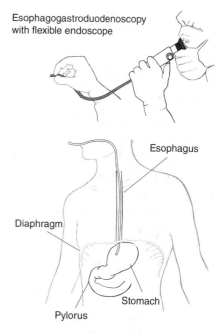

Esophagogastroduodenoscopy with flexible endoscope

Esophagus

Diaphragm

Pylorus

Stomach

Explanation

The physician examines the upper gastrointestinal tract and performs transendoscopic ultrasound-guided transmural injection. The physician passes an endoscope through the patient's mouth into the esophagus. The esophagus, stomach, duodenum, and sometimes the jejunum are viewed. The endoscope may be removed. A radial scanning echoendoscope is inserted and ultrasound scanning is performed to examine the esophagus, stomach, and the duodenum and/or jejunum or an ultrasound probe is passed through the already placed endoscope. The site for injection is determined. If a radial scanning echoendoscope is used, it is removed and replaced with a curvilinear array echoendoscope. The echoendoscope or ultrasound probe is fitted with a water-filled balloon near the tip; the tip contains a transducer that picks up the ultrasound frequency and relays it to a processor outside of the body. The water-filled tip is positioned in the esophagus, stomach, or small intestine against the tissue wall next to the injection site. The area is scanned and an ultrasound image is projected through the processor to a monitor in real-time. The needle is passed through the scope to the site and the injection of a diagnostic or therapeutic substance or fiducial marker is performed through the wall of the esophagus, stomach, or small intestine and into a lesion or other structure, such as a lymph node. When the injection is complete, the instruments are removed.

Coding Tips

Report this service only once per session. For transendoscopic ultrasound-guided transmural fine needle aspiration/biopsy, see 43238 and 43242. For interpretation of a specimen, see 88172–88173. Do not report 43253 with 43197–43198, 43235, 43237, 43259, 44360–44361, 44363–44366, 44369–44370, 44372–44373, 44376–44379, 76942, or 76975. Do not report 43253 in addition to 43240 for the same lesion.

Esophagus

ICD-10-CM Diagnostic Codes

C15.3	Malignant neoplasm of upper third of esophagus
C15.4	Malignant neoplasm of middle third of esophagus
C15.5	Malignant neoplasm of lower third of esophagus
C15.8	Malignant neoplasm of overlapping sites of esophagus
C16.0	Malignant neoplasm of cardia
C16.1	Malignant neoplasm of fundus of stomach
C16.2	Malignant neoplasm of body of stomach
C16.3	Malignant neoplasm of pyloric antrum
C16.4	Malignant neoplasm of pylorus
C16.8	Malignant neoplasm of overlapping sites of stomach
C17.0	Malignant neoplasm of duodenum
C17.1	Malignant neoplasm of jejunum
C17.8	Malignant neoplasm of overlapping sites of small intestine
C49.A1	Gastrointestinal stromal tumor of esophagus
C49.A2	Gastrointestinal stromal tumor of stomach
C49.A3	Gastrointestinal stromal tumor of small intestine
C78.4	Secondary malignant neoplasm of small intestine
C7A.010	Malignant carcinoid tumor of the duodenum
C7A.011	Malignant carcinoid tumor of the jejunum
C7A.092	Malignant carcinoid tumor of the stomach
D00.1	Carcinoma in situ of esophagus
D00.2	Carcinoma in situ of stomach
D13.0	Benign neoplasm of esophagus
D13.1	Benign neoplasm of stomach
D13.2	Benign neoplasm of duodenum
D13.39	Benign neoplasm of other parts of small intestine
D37.1	Neoplasm of uncertain behavior of stomach
D37.2	Neoplasm of uncertain behavior of small intestine
D3A.010	Benign carcinoid tumor of the duodenum
D3A.011	Benign carcinoid tumor of the jejunum
D3A.092	Benign carcinoid tumor of the stomach

AMA: **43253** 2019,Oct,10; 2018,Jan,8; 2018,Apr,10; 2017,Jan,8; 2016,Jan,13; 2015,Jan,16

Relative Value Units/Medicare Edits

Non-Facility RVU	Work	PE	MP	Total
43253	4.73	2.41	0.49	7.63
Facility RVU	**Work**	**PE**	**MP**	**Total**
43253	4.73	2.41	0.49	7.63

	FUD	Status	MUE	Modifiers				IOM Reference
43253	0	A	1(3)	51	N/A	N/A	N/A	None

* with documentation

43254

43254	Esophagogastroduodenoscopy, flexible, transoral; with endoscopic mucosal resection

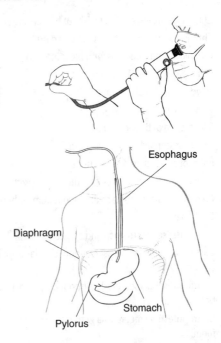

Explanation

The physician performs an endoscopic mucosal resection (EMR) to remove abnormal tissues from the upper gastrointestinal system. The physician passes an endoscope through the patient's mouth into the esophagus. The esophagus, stomach, duodenum, and sometimes the jejunum are viewed and the lesion in the inner lining of the upper gastrointestinal system is located. Saline or another solution is injected into the submucosa around the lesion to raise it from the surrounding deep muscle layer. Once the lesion is raised, it is removed using a snare, banding, or ligation and sent for pathology. The endoscope is removed.

Coding Tips

Biopsy of the same lesion is included in this procedure. Do not report 43254 with 43197–43198, 43235, 44360–44361, 44363–44366, 44369–44370, 44372–44373, or 44376–44379. Do not report 43254 in addition to 43236, 43239, or 43251 for the same lesion.

ICD-10-CM Diagnostic Codes

C15.3	Malignant neoplasm of upper third of esophagus
C15.4	Malignant neoplasm of middle third of esophagus
C15.5	Malignant neoplasm of lower third of esophagus
C15.8	Malignant neoplasm of overlapping sites of esophagus
C16.0	Malignant neoplasm of cardia
C16.1	Malignant neoplasm of fundus of stomach
C16.2	Malignant neoplasm of body of stomach
C16.3	Malignant neoplasm of pyloric antrum
C16.4	Malignant neoplasm of pylorus
C17.0	Malignant neoplasm of duodenum
C17.1	Malignant neoplasm of jejunum
C49.A1	Gastrointestinal stromal tumor of esophagus
C49.A2	Gastrointestinal stromal tumor of stomach
C49.A3	Gastrointestinal stromal tumor of small intestine

C78.89	Secondary malignant neoplasm of other digestive organs
C7A.010	Malignant carcinoid tumor of the duodenum
C7A.011	Malignant carcinoid tumor of the jejunum
C7A.092	Malignant carcinoid tumor of the stomach
D00.1	Carcinoma in situ of esophagus
D00.2	Carcinoma in situ of stomach
D13.0	Benign neoplasm of esophagus
D13.1	Benign neoplasm of stomach
D13.2	Benign neoplasm of duodenum
D13.39	Benign neoplasm of other parts of small intestine
D3A.092	Benign carcinoid tumor of the stomach
K20.80	Other esophagitis without bleeding
K20.81	Other esophagitis with bleeding
K21.00	Gastro-esophageal reflux disease with esophagitis, without bleeding
K21.01	Gastro-esophageal reflux disease with esophagitis, with bleeding
K22.710	Barrett's esophagus with low grade dysplasia
K22.711	Barrett's esophagus with high grade dysplasia
K22.89	Other specified disease of esophagus
K31.A11	Gastric intestinal metaplasia without dysplasia, involving the antrum
K31.A12	Gastric intestinal metaplasia without dysplasia, involving the body (corpus)
K31.A13	Gastric intestinal metaplasia without dysplasia, involving the fundus
K31.A21	Gastric intestinal metaplasia with low grade dysplasia
K31.A22	Gastric intestinal metaplasia with high grade dysplasia

AMA: **43254** 2019,Oct,10; 2019,Dec,14; 2018,Jan,8; 2017,Jan,8; 2016,Jan,13; 2015,Jan,16

Relative Value Units/Medicare Edits

Non-Facility RVU	Work	PE	MP	Total
43254	4.87	2.46	0.52	7.85
Facility RVU	**Work**	**PE**	**MP**	**Total**
43254	4.87	2.46	0.52	7.85

	FUD	Status	MUE	Modifiers				IOM Reference
43254	0	A	1(3)	51	N/A	N/A	N/A	None

* with documentation

Terms To Know

ligation. Tying off a blood vessel or duct with a suture or a soft, thin wire.

mucosa. Moist tissue lining the mouth (buccal mucosa), stomach (gastric mucosa), intestines, and respiratory tract.

resection. Surgical removal of a part or all of an organ or body part.

snare. Wire used as a loop to excise a polyp or lesion.

43255

43255	Esophagogastroduodenoscopy, flexible, transoral; with control of bleeding, any method

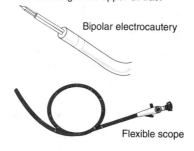

Any of a variety of methods, such as bipolar cautery, are used via a flexible scope to control bleeding in the upper GI tract

Bipolar electrocautery

Flexible scope

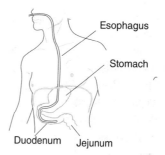

Esophagus

Stomach

Duodenum   Jejunum

Explanation

The physician uses an endoscope to access and control bleeding of the upper gastrointestinal tract. The physician passes an endoscope through the patient's mouth and into the esophagus. The esophagus, stomach, duodenum, and sometimes the jejunum are viewed. Control of bleeding may be achieved using several endoscopic methods including laser therapy, electrocoagulation, rubber band ligation, and injection of the bleeding vessel with sclerosants, ethanol, or adrenaline. The endoscope is removed.

Coding Tips

Report the appropriate endoscopy for each anatomic site examined. Surgical endoscopy includes a diagnostic endoscopy; however, diagnostic endoscopy can be identified separately when performed at the same surgical session as an open procedure. Do not report 43255 with 43197–43198, 43235, 44360–44361, 44363–44366, 44369–44370, 44372–44373, or 44376–44379. Do not report 43255 in addition to 43236 or 43243–43244 for the same lesion.

ICD-10-CM Diagnostic Codes

C15.5	Malignant neoplasm of lower third of esophagus
C16.1	Malignant neoplasm of fundus of stomach
C16.2	Malignant neoplasm of body of stomach
C16.3	Malignant neoplasm of pyloric antrum
C16.4	Malignant neoplasm of pylorus
C7A.092	Malignant carcinoid tumor of the stomach
D13.0	Benign neoplasm of esophagus
D13.1	Benign neoplasm of stomach
D13.2	Benign neoplasm of duodenum
D3A.010	Benign carcinoid tumor of the duodenum
D3A.011	Benign carcinoid tumor of the jejunum
D3A.092	Benign carcinoid tumor of the stomach

Esophagus

I85.01	Esophageal varices with bleeding	
K20.81	Other esophagitis with bleeding	
K22.11	Ulcer of esophagus with bleeding	
K22.6	Gastro-esophageal laceration-hemorrhage syndrome	
K22.70	Barrett's esophagus without dysplasia	
K22.710	Barrett's esophagus with low grade dysplasia	
K22.711	Barrett's esophagus with high grade dysplasia	
K22.89	Other specified disease of esophagus	
K25.0	Acute gastric ulcer with hemorrhage	
K25.2	Acute gastric ulcer with both hemorrhage and perforation	
K25.4	Chronic or unspecified gastric ulcer with hemorrhage	
K25.6	Chronic or unspecified gastric ulcer with both hemorrhage and perforation	
K27.0	Acute peptic ulcer, site unspecified, with hemorrhage	
K27.2	Acute peptic ulcer, site unspecified, with both hemorrhage and perforation	
K27.4	Chronic or unspecified peptic ulcer, site unspecified, with hemorrhage	
K27.6	Chronic or unspecified peptic ulcer, site unspecified, with both hemorrhage and perforation	
K29.31	Chronic superficial gastritis with bleeding	
K29.41	Chronic atrophic gastritis with bleeding	
K31.82	Dieulafoy lesion (hemorrhagic) of stomach and duodenum	
K55.21	Angiodysplasia of colon with hemorrhage	
K92.0	Hematemesis	

AMA: 43255 2019,Oct,10; 2018,Jan,8; 2017,Jan,8; 2016,Jan,13; 2015,Jan,16

Relative Value Units/Medicare Edits

Non-Facility RVU	Work	PE	MP	Total
43255	3.56	16.12	0.39	20.07
Facility RVU	Work	PE	MP	Total
43255	3.56	1.88	0.39	5.83

	FUD	Status	MUE	Modifiers				IOM Reference
43255	0	A	2(3)	51	N/A	N/A	N/A	None

* with documentation

[43266]

43266 Esophagogastroduodenoscopy, flexible, transoral; with placement of endoscopic stent (includes pre- and post-dilation and guide wire passage, when performed)

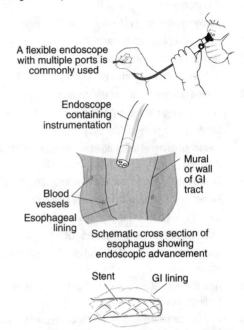

A flexible endoscope with multiple ports is commonly used

Endoscope containing instrumentation

Mural or wall of GI tract

Blood vessels

Esophageal lining

Schematic cross section of esophagus showing endoscopic advancement

Stent   GI lining

An upper GI endoscopic session is performed with endoscopic stent placement, including predilation before placement of the stent

Explanation

The physician uses an endoscope to examine the upper gastrointestinal tract and performs a stent placement. The physician passes an endoscope through the patient's mouth into the esophagus. The esophagus, stomach, duodenum, and sometimes the jejunum are viewed. The endoscope is placed at the site of an obstruction or stricture, the necessary stent length is determined, and predilation of the obstruction or stenosis may be performed. The stent (endoprosthesis) is introduced into the site of the obstruction. Using a commercial delivery system, a plastic covering over the stent is removed and the stent self-deploys, shoring-up the walls at a specific site in the esophagus or proximal small intestine. When necessary, a balloon catheter is placed into the stent and gently inflated to more fully deploy the stent. The delivery system and endoscope are removed.

Coding Tips

Report fluoroscopic guidance with 74360, when performed. Do not report 43266 with 43197–43198, 43235, 43240–43241, 43245, 43248–43249, 44360–44361, 44363–44366, 44369, 44370, 44372–44373, or 44376–44379.

ICD-10-CM Diagnostic Codes

C15.3	Malignant neoplasm of upper third of esophagus	
C15.4	Malignant neoplasm of middle third of esophagus	
C15.5	Malignant neoplasm of lower third of esophagus	
C15.8	Malignant neoplasm of overlapping sites of esophagus	
C16.0	Malignant neoplasm of cardia	
C16.1	Malignant neoplasm of fundus of stomach	
C16.2	Malignant neoplasm of body of stomach	
C16.3	Malignant neoplasm of pyloric antrum	
C16.4	Malignant neoplasm of pylorus	

Esophagus

C16.8	Malignant neoplasm of overlapping sites of stomach	
C17.0	Malignant neoplasm of duodenum	
C17.1	Malignant neoplasm of jejunum	
C17.8	Malignant neoplasm of overlapping sites of small intestine	
C49.A1	Gastrointestinal stromal tumor of esophagus	
C49.A2	Gastrointestinal stromal tumor of stomach	
C49.A3	Gastrointestinal stromal tumor of small intestine	
C78.4	Secondary malignant neoplasm of small intestine	
C78.89	Secondary malignant neoplasm of other digestive organs	
C7A.010	Malignant carcinoid tumor of the duodenum	
C7A.011	Malignant carcinoid tumor of the jejunum	
C7A.092	Malignant carcinoid tumor of the stomach	
D00.1	Carcinoma in situ of esophagus	
D00.2	Carcinoma in situ of stomach	
D13.0	Benign neoplasm of esophagus	
D13.1	Benign neoplasm of stomach	
D13.2	Benign neoplasm of duodenum	
D13.39	Benign neoplasm of other parts of small intestine	
D37.1	Neoplasm of uncertain behavior of stomach	
D37.2	Neoplasm of uncertain behavior of small intestine	
D3A.010	Benign carcinoid tumor of the duodenum	
D3A.011	Benign carcinoid tumor of the jejunum	
D3A.092	Benign carcinoid tumor of the stomach	
K22.0	Achalasia of cardia	
K22.2	Esophageal obstruction	
K22.4	Dyskinesia of esophagus	
K22.89	Other specified disease of esophagus	
K31.1	Adult hypertrophic pyloric stenosis 🅰	
K31.2	Hourglass stricture and stenosis of stomach	
K31.5	Obstruction of duodenum	
Q39.1	Atresia of esophagus with tracheo-esophageal fistula	
Q39.2	Congenital tracheo-esophageal fistula without atresia	
Q39.3	Congenital stenosis and stricture of esophagus	
Q39.4	Esophageal web	
Q39.5	Congenital dilatation of esophagus	
Q40.0	Congenital hypertrophic pyloric stenosis	

AMA: **43266** 2019,Oct,10; 2018,Jan,8; 2017,Jan,8; 2016,Jan,13; 2015,Jan,16

Relative Value Units/Medicare Edits

Non-Facility RVU	Work	PE	MP	Total
43266	3.92	1.93	0.48	6.33
Facility RVU	**Work**	**PE**	**MP**	**Total**
43266	3.92	1.93	0.48	6.33

	FUD	Status	MUE	Modifiers				IOM Reference
43266	0	A	1(3)	51	N/A	N/A	N/A	None

* with documentation

43257

43257 Esophagogastroduodenoscopy, flexible, transoral; with delivery of thermal energy to the muscle of lower esophageal sphincter and/or gastric cardia, for treatment of gastroesophageal reflux disease

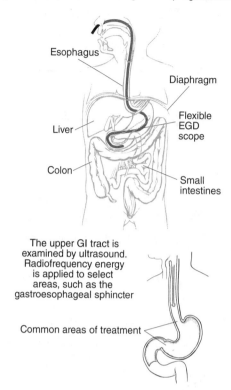

The upper GI tract is examined by ultrasound. Radiofrequency energy is applied to select areas, such as the gastroesophageal sphincter

Common areas of treatment

Explanation

The physician uses thermal energy to the muscle of the lower esophageal sphincter and/or gastric cardia to treat gastroesophageal reflux disease. The physician performs an esophagogastroduodenoscopy (EGD) with a concomitant ultrasound examination for diagnostic purposes. The patient is prepped for an upper gastrointestinal exam and the scope is advanced through the mouth into the stomach and duodenum or jejunum. An examination is carried out to determine if any bleeding, tumors, erosions, ulcers, or other abnormalities are present. Radiofrequency energy is applied through the scope equipment to apply heat to the muscle of the lower esophageal sphincter and/or the gastric cardia to treat gastroesophageal reflux disease (GERD). The heat is applied by electrodes placed in the esophageal tissue at multiple points above and below the squamocolumnar junction. Thermal lesions are created at the gastroesophageal junction that is thought to ablate the nerve pathways responsible for relaxing the sphincter and allowing reflux to occur. The thermal lesions are also thought to produce a "tightened" effect due to collagen contraction.

Coding Tips

Surgical endoscopy includes a diagnostic endoscopy; however, diagnostic endoscopy can be identified separately when performed at the same surgical session as an open procedure. For ablation of a metaplastic or dysplastic esophageal lesion (e.g., Barrett's esophagus), see 43229 or 43270. Do not report 43257 with 43197–43198, 43235, 44360–44361, 44363–44366, 44369–44370, 44372–44373, or 44376–44379.

ICD-10-CM Diagnostic Codes

K21.00	Gastro-esophageal reflux disease with esophagitis, without bleeding

Esophagus

| K21.01 | Gastro-esophageal reflux disease with esophagitis, with bleeding |
| K21.9 | Gastro-esophageal reflux disease without esophagitis |

AMA: **43257** 2019,Oct,10; 2018,Jan,8; 2017,Jan,8; 2016,Jan,13; 2015,Jan,16

Relative Value Units/Medicare Edits

Non-Facility RVU	Work	PE	MP	Total
43257	4.15	2.11	0.49	6.75
Facility RVU	**Work**	**PE**	**MP**	**Total**
43257	4.15	2.11	0.49	6.75

	FUD	Status	MUE	Modifiers			IOM Reference
43257	0	A	1(2)	51	N/A	N/A	N/A	None

* with documentation

Terms To Know

ablation. Removal or destruction of tissue by cutting, electrical energy, chemical substances, or excessive heat application.

cardia. Portion of the stomach next to and surrounding the cardiac esophageal opening.

duodenum. First portion of the small intestine connected to the stomach at the pylorus and extending to the jejunum.

erosion. Eating away or gradual breaking down of the surface of a structure.

esophagus. Muscular tube that carries swallowed liquids and foods from the pharynx to the stomach.

GERD. Gastroesophageal reflux disease. Disorder in which acidic gastric contents flow back into the esophagus as a chronic condition, causing pain, inflammation, and erosion of the esophagus.

hemorrhage. Internal or external bleeding with loss of significant amounts of blood.

jejunum. Highly vascular upper two-fifths of the small intestine, extending from the duodenum to the ileum.

radiofrequency ablation. To destroy by electromagnetic wave frequencies.

reflux esophagitis. Inflammation of the lower esophagus as a result of regurgitated gastric acid.

sphincter. Ring-like band of muscle that surrounds a bodily opening, constricting and relaxing as required for normal physiological functioning.

tissue. Group of similar cells with a similar function that form definite structures and organs. Tissue types include epithelial tissue, muscle tissue, connective tissue, and nervous tissue.

transverse. Crosswise at right angles to the long axis of a structure or part.

tumor. Pathological swelling or enlargement; a neoplastic growth of uncontrolled, abnormal multiplication of cells.

ulcer. Open sore or excavating lesion of skin or the tissue on the surface of an organ from the sloughing of chronically inflamed and necrosing tissue.

[43270]

| 43270 | Esophagogastroduodenoscopy, flexible, transoral; with ablation of tumor(s), polyp(s), or other lesion(s) (includes pre- and post-dilation and guide wire passage, when performed) |

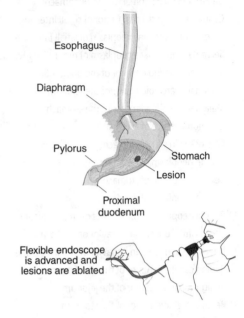

Flexible endoscope is advanced and lesions are ablated

Explanation

The physician uses an endoscope to locate and remove tumors, polyps, or lesions from the upper gastrointestinal tract. The physician passes an endoscope through the patient's mouth into the esophagus. The esophagus, stomach, duodenum, and sometimes the jejunum are viewed to locate the lesion. The lesion is destroyed using laser therapy, electrocoagulation, or injection of toxic agents. The endoscope is removed.

Coding Tips

For injection sclerosis of esophageal varices, flexible transoral, see 43204; esophagogastroduodenoscopy, flexible, transoral, see 43243. Report esophagoscopic photodynamic therapy with 43270 and 96570 or 96571 as appropriate. Do not report 43270 with 43197–43198, 43235, 44360–44361, 44363–44366, 44369–44370, 44372–44373, or 44376–44379. Do not report 43270 in addition to 43248–43249 for the same lesion.

ICD-10-CM Diagnostic Codes

C15.3	Malignant neoplasm of upper third of esophagus
C15.4	Malignant neoplasm of middle third of esophagus
C15.5	Malignant neoplasm of lower third of esophagus
C15.8	Malignant neoplasm of overlapping sites of esophagus
C16.0	Malignant neoplasm of cardia
C16.1	Malignant neoplasm of fundus of stomach
C16.2	Malignant neoplasm of body of stomach
C16.3	Malignant neoplasm of pyloric antrum
C16.4	Malignant neoplasm of pylorus
C16.8	Malignant neoplasm of overlapping sites of stomach
C17.0	Malignant neoplasm of duodenum
C49.A1	Gastrointestinal stromal tumor of esophagus
C49.A2	Gastrointestinal stromal tumor of stomach
C49.A3	Gastrointestinal stromal tumor of small intestine
C78.4	Secondary malignant neoplasm of small intestine

Esophagus

D00.1	Carcinoma in situ of esophagus	
D00.2	Carcinoma in situ of stomach	
D01.49	Carcinoma in situ of other parts of intestine	
D13.0	Benign neoplasm of esophagus	
D13.1	Benign neoplasm of stomach	
D13.2	Benign neoplasm of duodenum	
D37.1	Neoplasm of uncertain behavior of stomach	
D37.2	Neoplasm of uncertain behavior of small intestine	
D37.8	Neoplasm of uncertain behavior of other specified digestive organs	
D49.0	Neoplasm of unspecified behavior of digestive system	
K22.89	Other specified disease of esophagus	
R13.0	Aphagia	
R13.12	Dysphagia, oropharyngeal phase	
R13.13	Dysphagia, pharyngeal phase	
R13.14	Dysphagia, pharyngoesophageal phase	

AMA: 43270 2019,Oct,10; 2018,Jan,8; 2017,Jan,8; 2016,Jan,13; 2015,Jan,16

Relative Value Units/Medicare Edits

Non-Facility RVU	Work	PE	MP	Total
43270	4.01	18.21	0.44	22.66
Facility RVU	Work	PE	MP	Total
43270	4.01	2.08	0.44	6.53

	FUD	Status	MUE	Modifiers				IOM Reference
43270	0	A	1(3)	51	N/A	N/A	N/A	None

* with documentation

Terms To Know

ablation. Removal or destruction of tissue by cutting, electrical energy, chemical substances, or excessive heat application.

dilation. Artificial increase in the diameter of an opening or lumen made by medication or by instrumentation.

guidewire. Flexible metal instrument designed to lead another instrument in its proper course.

lesion. Area of damaged tissue that has lost continuity or function, due to disease or trauma.

polyp. Small growth on a stalk-like attachment projecting from a mucous membrane.

tumor. Pathological swelling or enlargement; a neoplastic growth of uncontrolled, abnormal multiplication of cells.

43259

43259 Esophagogastroduodenoscopy, flexible, transoral; with endoscopic ultrasound examination, including the esophagus, stomach, and either the duodenum or a surgically altered stomach where the jejunum is examined distal to the anastomosis

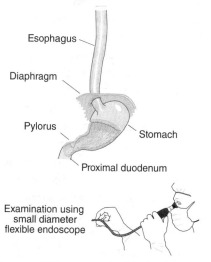

Esophagus
Diaphragm
Pylorus
Stomach
Proximal duodenum

Examination using small diameter flexible endoscope

The upper GI tract is examined. During the course of the exam, an endoscopic ultrasound device is fed through the endoscope and images viewed

Explanation

The physician uses an endoscope to examine the upper gastrointestinal tract and performs an endoscopic ultrasound examination of the esophagus, stomach, and the duodenum and/or jejunum. The physician passes an endoscope through the patient's mouth into the esophagus. The esophagus, stomach, duodenum, and sometimes the jejunum, are viewed. The endoscope may be removed and a radial scanning echoendoscope inserted or an ultrasound probe is passed through the already placed endoscope and an ultrasound examination is performed, including the esophagus, stomach, and the duodenum and/or jejunum. The echoendoscope or ultrasound probe is fitted with a water-filled balloon near the tip, which contains a transducer that picks up the ultrasound frequency and relays it to a processor outside of the body, where the internal images can be viewed on screen. When the ultrasound scanning is completed, the instruments are removed.

Coding Tips

Surgical endoscopy includes a diagnostic endoscopy; however, diagnostic endoscopy can be identified separately when performed at the same surgical session as an open procedure. When endoscopic procedures are performed, report the appropriate endoscopy of each anatomic site examined. For esophagogastroduodenoscopy, with removal of tumors, polyps, or lesions, by hot biopsy forceps, see 43250; by snare technique, see 43251; and for ablation by any other methods, see 43270. For esophagoscopy, flexible, transoral, with removal of tumors, polyps, or lesions, by hot biopsy forceps, see 43216; by snare technique, see 43217; and for ablation by any other method, see 43229. This service should only be reported once per session. Do not report 43259 with 43197–43198, 43235, 43237, 43240, 43242, 43253, 44360–44361, 44363–44366, 44369–44370, 44372–44373, 44376–44379, or 76975.

ICD-10-CM Diagnostic Codes

C15.3	Malignant neoplasm of upper third of esophagus
C15.4	Malignant neoplasm of middle third of esophagus

Esophagus

C15.5	Malignant neoplasm of lower third of esophagus
C15.8	Malignant neoplasm of overlapping sites of esophagus
C16.0	Malignant neoplasm of cardia
C16.1	Malignant neoplasm of fundus of stomach
C16.2	Malignant neoplasm of body of stomach
C16.3	Malignant neoplasm of pyloric antrum
C16.4	Malignant neoplasm of pylorus
C16.8	Malignant neoplasm of overlapping sites of stomach
C17.0	Malignant neoplasm of duodenum
C17.1	Malignant neoplasm of jejunum
C17.8	Malignant neoplasm of overlapping sites of small intestine
C49.A1	Gastrointestinal stromal tumor of esophagus
C49.A2	Gastrointestinal stromal tumor of stomach
C49.A3	Gastrointestinal stromal tumor of small intestine
C78.4	Secondary malignant neoplasm of small intestine
C78.89	Secondary malignant neoplasm of other digestive organs
C7A.010	Malignant carcinoid tumor of the duodenum
C7A.011	Malignant carcinoid tumor of the jejunum
C7A.092	Malignant carcinoid tumor of the stomach
D00.1	Carcinoma in situ of esophagus
D00.2	Carcinoma in situ of stomach
D13.0	Benign neoplasm of esophagus
D13.1	Benign neoplasm of stomach
D13.2	Benign neoplasm of duodenum
D13.39	Benign neoplasm of other parts of small intestine
D37.1	Neoplasm of uncertain behavior of stomach
D37.2	Neoplasm of uncertain behavior of small intestine
D3A.010	Benign carcinoid tumor of the duodenum
D3A.011	Benign carcinoid tumor of the jejunum
D3A.092	Benign carcinoid tumor of the stomach
I85.00	Esophageal varices without bleeding
I85.01	Esophageal varices with bleeding
I85.10	Secondary esophageal varices without bleeding
I85.11	Secondary esophageal varices with bleeding
K20.0	Eosinophilic esophagitis
K20.80	Other esophagitis without bleeding
K20.81	Other esophagitis with bleeding
K21.00	Gastro-esophageal reflux disease with esophagitis, without bleeding
K21.01	Gastro-esophageal reflux disease with esophagitis, with bleeding
K21.9	Gastro-esophageal reflux disease without esophagitis
K22.0	Achalasia of cardia
K22.10	Ulcer of esophagus without bleeding
K22.11	Ulcer of esophagus with bleeding
K22.2	Esophageal obstruction
K22.4	Dyskinesia of esophagus
K22.5	Diverticulum of esophagus, acquired
K22.6	Gastro-esophageal laceration-hemorrhage syndrome
K22.70	Barrett's esophagus without dysplasia
K22.710	Barrett's esophagus with low grade dysplasia
K22.711	Barrett's esophagus with high grade dysplasia
K22.89	Other specified disease of esophagus
K23	Disorders of esophagus in diseases classified elsewhere

K25.0	Acute gastric ulcer with hemorrhage
K25.2	Acute gastric ulcer with both hemorrhage and perforation
K25.3	Acute gastric ulcer without hemorrhage or perforation
K25.4	Chronic or unspecified gastric ulcer with hemorrhage
K25.6	Chronic or unspecified gastric ulcer with both hemorrhage and perforation
K25.7	Chronic gastric ulcer without hemorrhage or perforation
K26.0	Acute duodenal ulcer with hemorrhage
K26.1	Acute duodenal ulcer with perforation
K26.2	Acute duodenal ulcer with both hemorrhage and perforation
K28.0	Acute gastrojejunal ulcer with hemorrhage
K28.1	Acute gastrojejunal ulcer with perforation
K29.21	Alcoholic gastritis with bleeding
K29.31	Chronic superficial gastritis with bleeding
K29.41	Chronic atrophic gastritis with bleeding
K29.81	Duodenitis with bleeding
K31.5	Obstruction of duodenum
K31.6	Fistula of stomach and duodenum
K31.7	Polyp of stomach and duodenum
K31.A11	Gastric intestinal metaplasia without dysplasia, involving the antrum
K31.A12	Gastric intestinal metaplasia without dysplasia, involving the body (corpus)
K31.A13	Gastric intestinal metaplasia without dysplasia, involving the fundus
K31.A21	Gastric intestinal metaplasia with low grade dysplasia
K31.A22	Gastric intestinal metaplasia with high grade dysplasia
K50.011	Crohn's disease of small intestine with rectal bleeding
K50.012	Crohn's disease of small intestine with intestinal obstruction
K50.013	Crohn's disease of small intestine with fistula
K50.014	Crohn's disease of small intestine with abscess
K57.01	Diverticulitis of small intestine with perforation and abscess with bleeding
K90.0	Celiac disease
M35.08	Sjögren syndrome with gastrointestinal involvement
Q39.1	Atresia of esophagus with tracheo-esophageal fistula
Q39.2	Congenital tracheo-esophageal fistula without atresia
Q39.3	Congenital stenosis and stricture of esophagus
Q39.4	Esophageal web
Q39.6	Congenital diverticulum of esophagus

AMA: **43259** 2019,Oct,10; 2018,Jan,8; 2017,Jan,8; 2016,Jan,13; 2016,Jan,11; 2015,Jan,16

Relative Value Units/Medicare Edits

Non-Facility RVU	Work	PE	MP	Total
43259	4.04	2.1	0.43	6.57
Facility RVU	Work	PE	MP	Total
43259	4.04	2.1	0.43	6.57

	FUD	Status	MUE	Modifiers				IOM Reference
43259	0	A	1(2)	51	N/A	N/A	N/A	100-04,12,30.1

* with documentation

[43210]

43210 Esophagogastroduodenoscopy, flexible, transoral; with esophagogastric fundoplasty, partial or complete, includes duodenoscopy when performed

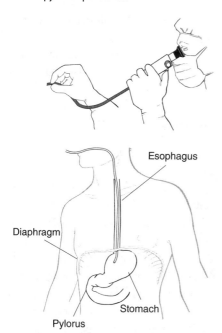

Esophagus

Diaphragm

Pylorus

Stomach

Esophagogastric fundoplasty is performed using an endomicroscope

Explanation

Esophagoscopy with esophagogastric fundoplasty involves an incisionless fundoplication technique; plication is the process of suturing one tissue to another, in this case part of the stomach around the esophagus. Fundoplication allows restoration of natural gastric and esophageal positioning resulting in the elimination of reflux and providing relief of gastroesophageal reflux disease (GERD) associated symptoms. By performing this procedure, the physician is able to treat the root cause of GERD by repairing an anatomic defect at the gastroesophageal valve. One procedure uses a proprietary device with a flexible video endoscope that provides visualization throughout the procedure. Another proprietary system combines a surgical stapler, ultrasonic sights to permit proper positioning, and a miniature video camera into a single device inserted through the patient's mouth to the gastrointestinal tract to perform esophagogastric fundoplication. The fundus of the stomach is wrapped around the lower end of the esophagus and secured. At the end of the procedure, the endoscope is removed.

Coding Tips

This code should be reported when a complete upper gastrointestinal endoscopy is performed in conjunction with a partial or complete fundoplasty of the esophagus and stomach. Report the appropriate endoscopy for each anatomic site examined. Surgical endoscopy includes a diagnostic endoscopy; however, diagnostic endoscopy can be identified separately when performed at the same surgical session as an open procedure. Do not report 43210 with 43180, 43191, 43197, 43200, or 43235.

ICD-10-CM Diagnostic Codes

K21.00	Gastro-esophageal reflux disease with esophagitis, without bleeding
K21.01	Gastro-esophageal reflux disease with esophagitis, with bleeding
K21.9	Gastro-esophageal reflux disease without esophagitis
K22.89	Other specified disease of esophagus
R13.11	Dysphagia, oral phase
R13.12	Dysphagia, oropharyngeal phase
R13.13	Dysphagia, pharyngeal phase
R13.14	Dysphagia, pharyngoesophageal phase
R13.19	Other dysphagia
R63.32	Pediatric feeding disorder, chronic 🅿
R63.39	Other feeding difficulties

AMA: 43210 2018,Jan,8; 2017,Jan,8; 2016,Jan,13; 2015,Nov,8

Relative Value Units/Medicare Edits

Non-Facility RVU	Work	PE	MP	Total
43210	7.75	3.59	1.25	12.59
Facility RVU	**Work**	**PE**	**MP**	**Total**
43210	7.75	3.59	1.25	12.59

	FUD	Status	MUE	Modifiers				IOM Reference
43210	0	A	1(2)	51	N/A	N/A	N/A	None

* with documentation

Terms To Know

esophagitis. Inflammation of the esophagus.

esophagoscopy. Internal visual inspection of the esophagus through the use of an endoscope placed down the throat.

GERD. Gastroesophageal reflux disease. Disorder in which acidic gastric contents flow back into the esophagus as a chronic condition, causing pain, inflammation, and erosion of the esophagus.

Nissen procedure (fundoplasty). Surgical repair technique that involves the fundus of the stomach being wrapped around the lower end of the esophagus to treat reflux esophagitis.

plication. Surgical technique involving folding, tucking, or pleating to reduce the size of a hollow structure or organ.

43260-43261

43260 Endoscopic retrograde cholangiopancreatography (ERCP); diagnostic, including collection of specimen(s) by brushing or washing, when performed (separate procedure)

43261 with biopsy, single or multiple

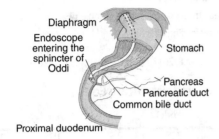

Diaphragm
Endoscope entering the sphincter of Oddi
Stomach
Pancreas
Pancreatic duct
Common bile duct
Proximal duodenum

An endoscope is fed through the stomach and into the duodenum. Usually a smaller subscope is fed up the sphincter of Oddi and into the ducts that drain the pancreas and the gallbladder (common bile)

Explanation

The physician performs an endoscopic retrograde cholangiopancreatography (ERCP) for diagnostic purposes. The physician passes the endoscope through the patient's oropharynx, esophagus, stomach, and into the small intestine. The ampulla of Vater is cannulated and filled with contrast. The common bile duct and the whole biliary tract, including the gallbladder, are visualized. Diagnostic brushing and washing may be performed in 43260. Report 43261 if a biopsy is performed.

Coding Tips

Note that 43260, a separate procedure by definition, is usually a component of a more complex service and is not identified separately. When performed alone or with other unrelated procedures/services it may be reported. If performed alone, list the code; if performed with other procedures/services, list the code and append modifier 59 or an X{EPSU} modifier. Report the appropriate endoscopy for each anatomic site examined. Surgical endoscopy includes a diagnostic endoscopy; however, diagnostic endoscopy can be identified separately when performed at the same surgical session as an open procedure. For endoluminal biopsy of the biliary tree, percutaneous, see 47543. Do not report 43260 with 43261–43265 or 43274–43278.

ICD-10-CM Diagnostic Codes

C22.1	Intrahepatic bile duct carcinoma
C23	Malignant neoplasm of gallbladder
C24.0	Malignant neoplasm of extrahepatic bile duct
C24.1	Malignant neoplasm of ampulla of Vater
C24.8	Malignant neoplasm of overlapping sites of biliary tract
C25.0	Malignant neoplasm of head of pancreas
C25.1	Malignant neoplasm of body of pancreas
C25.2	Malignant neoplasm of tail of pancreas
C25.3	Malignant neoplasm of pancreatic duct
C25.4	Malignant neoplasm of endocrine pancreas
C25.7	Malignant neoplasm of other parts of pancreas
C25.8	Malignant neoplasm of overlapping sites of pancreas
C78.7	Secondary malignant neoplasm of liver and intrahepatic bile duct
D01.5	Carcinoma in situ of liver, gallbladder and bile ducts

D13.5	Benign neoplasm of extrahepatic bile ducts
D37.6	Neoplasm of uncertain behavior of liver, gallbladder and bile ducts
E79.0	Hyperuricemia without signs of inflammatory arthritis and tophaceous disease
K56.3	Gallstone ileus
K80.00	Calculus of gallbladder with acute cholecystitis without obstruction
K80.01	Calculus of gallbladder with acute cholecystitis with obstruction
K80.10	Calculus of gallbladder with chronic cholecystitis without obstruction
K80.11	Calculus of gallbladder with chronic cholecystitis with obstruction
K80.12	Calculus of gallbladder with acute and chronic cholecystitis without obstruction
K80.13	Calculus of gallbladder with acute and chronic cholecystitis with obstruction
K80.18	Calculus of gallbladder with other cholecystitis without obstruction
K80.19	Calculus of gallbladder with other cholecystitis with obstruction
K80.20	Calculus of gallbladder without cholecystitis without obstruction
K80.21	Calculus of gallbladder without cholecystitis with obstruction
K80.32	Calculus of bile duct with acute cholangitis without obstruction
K80.33	Calculus of bile duct with acute cholangitis with obstruction
K80.34	Calculus of bile duct with chronic cholangitis without obstruction
K80.35	Calculus of bile duct with chronic cholangitis with obstruction
K80.36	Calculus of bile duct with acute and chronic cholangitis without obstruction
K80.37	Calculus of bile duct with acute and chronic cholangitis with obstruction
K80.42	Calculus of bile duct with acute cholecystitis without obstruction
K80.43	Calculus of bile duct with acute cholecystitis with obstruction
K80.44	Calculus of bile duct with chronic cholecystitis without obstruction
K80.45	Calculus of bile duct with chronic cholecystitis with obstruction
K80.46	Calculus of bile duct with acute and chronic cholecystitis without obstruction
K80.47	Calculus of bile duct with acute and chronic cholecystitis with obstruction
K80.50	Calculus of bile duct without cholangitis or cholecystitis without obstruction
K80.51	Calculus of bile duct without cholangitis or cholecystitis with obstruction
K80.62	Calculus of gallbladder and bile duct with acute cholecystitis without obstruction
K80.63	Calculus of gallbladder and bile duct with acute cholecystitis with obstruction
K80.64	Calculus of gallbladder and bile duct with chronic cholecystitis without obstruction
K80.65	Calculus of gallbladder and bile duct with chronic cholecystitis with obstruction
K80.66	Calculus of gallbladder and bile duct with acute and chronic cholecystitis without obstruction
K80.67	Calculus of gallbladder and bile duct with acute and chronic cholecystitis with obstruction
K80.70	Calculus of gallbladder and bile duct without cholecystitis without obstruction

Esophagus

K80.71	Calculus of gallbladder and bile duct without cholecystitis with obstruction
K80.80	Other cholelithiasis without obstruction
K80.81	Other cholelithiasis with obstruction
K81.0	Acute cholecystitis
K81.1	Chronic cholecystitis
K81.2	Acute cholecystitis with chronic cholecystitis
K82.0	Obstruction of gallbladder
K82.1	Hydrops of gallbladder
K82.2	Perforation of gallbladder
K82.3	Fistula of gallbladder
K82.4	Cholesterolosis of gallbladder
K82.8	Other specified diseases of gallbladder
K83.01	Primary sclerosing cholangitis
K83.09	Other cholangitis
K83.1	Obstruction of bile duct
K83.2	Perforation of bile duct
K83.3	Fistula of bile duct
K83.4	Spasm of sphincter of Oddi
K83.5	Biliary cyst
K83.8	Other specified diseases of biliary tract
K86.0	Alcohol-induced chronic pancreatitis
K86.1	Other chronic pancreatitis
K86.2	Cyst of pancreas
K86.3	Pseudocyst of pancreas
K86.81	Exocrine pancreatic insufficiency
K87	Disorders of gallbladder, biliary tract and pancreas in diseases classified elsewhere
K91.5	Postcholecystectomy syndrome
K91.86	Retained cholelithiasis following cholecystectomy
Q44.0	Agenesis, aplasia and hypoplasia of gallbladder
Q44.1	Other congenital malformations of gallbladder
Q44.4	Choledochal cyst
Q44.5	Other congenital malformations of bile ducts
Q45.0	Agenesis, aplasia and hypoplasia of pancreas
Q45.1	Annular pancreas
Q45.2	Congenital pancreatic cyst
Q45.3	Other congenital malformations of pancreas and pancreatic duct
R10.11	Right upper quadrant pain
R11.14	Bilious vomiting
R11.15	Cyclical vomiting syndrome unrelated to migraine

AMA: **43260** 2018,Jan,8; 2017,Jan,8; 2016,Jan,13; 2015,Jan,16; 2015,Dec,3
43261 2018,Jan,8; 2017,Jan,8; 2016,Jan,13; 2015,Jan,16; 2015,Dec,3

Relative Value Units/Medicare Edits

Non-Facility RVU	Work	PE	MP	Total
43260	5.85	2.9	0.63	9.38
43261	6.15	3.04	0.65	9.84
Facility RVU	**Work**	**PE**	**MP**	**Total**
43260	5.85	2.9	0.63	9.38
43261	6.15	3.04	0.65	9.84

	FUD	Status	MUE	Modifiers				IOM Reference
43260	0	A	1(3)	51	N/A	N/A	N/A	None
43261	0	A	1(2)	51	N/A	N/A	N/A	

* with documentation

Terms To Know

ampulla of Vater. Tubular structure with flask-like dilation where the common bile and pancreatic ducts join before emptying into the duodenum.

biopsy. Tissue or fluid removed for diagnostic purposes through analysis of the cells in the biopsy material.

contrast material. Any internally administered substance that has a different opacity from soft tissue on radiography or computed tomograph; includes barium, used to opacify parts of the gastrointestinal tract; water-soluble iodinated compounds, used to opacify blood vessels or the genitourinary tract; may refer to air occurring naturally or introduced into the body; also, paramagnetic substances used in magnetic resonance imaging. Substances may also be documented as contrast agent or contrast medium.

diagnostic. Examination or procedure to which the patient is subjected, or which is performed on materials derived from a hospital outpatient, to obtain information to aid in the assessment of a medical condition or the identification of a disease. Among these examinations and tests are diagnostic laboratory services such as hematology and chemistry, diagnostic x-rays, isotope studies, EKGs, pulmonary function studies, thyroid function tests, psychological tests, and other tests given to determine the nature and severity of an ailment or injury.

ERCP. Endoscopic retrograde cholangiopancreatography. Examination of the hepatobiliary system and gallbladder performed through a flexible fiberoptic endoscope.

esophagus. Muscular tube that carries swallowed liquids and foods from the pharynx to the stomach.

pharynx. Musculomembranous passage of the throat consisting of three regions: the nasopharynx is the passage at the back of the nostrils, above the level of the soft palate, and communicating with the eustachian tube.

specimen. Tissue cells or sample of fluid taken for analysis, pathologic examination, and diagnosis.

Esophagus

43262-43263

43262 Endoscopic retrograde cholangiopancreatography (ERCP); with sphincterotomy/papillotomy
43263   with pressure measurement of sphincter of Oddi

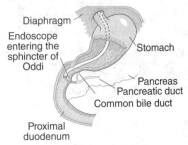

Diaphragm
Endoscope entering the sphincter of Oddi
Stomach
Pancreas
Pancreatic duct
Common bile duct
Proximal duodenum

An endoscope is fed through the stomach and into the duodenum. Usually a smaller subscope is fed up the sphincter of Oddi and into the ducts that drain the pancreas and the gallbladder (common bile)

Explanation

The physician performs an endoscopic retrograde cholangiopancreatography (ERCP). The physician passes the endoscope through the patient's oropharynx, esophagus, stomach, and into the small intestine. The ampulla of Vater is cannulated and filled with contrast. The common bile duct and the whole biliary tract, including the gallbladder, are visualized. In 43262, a sphincter/papillotomy is performed. The sphincter is cannulated using a sphincterotome. The sphincter is divided using electrocautery to control bleeding. In 43263, the physician performs an ERCP with sphincter of Oddi manometry for diagnostic purposes. A catheter is inserted into the bile duct and pancreatic ducts and connected to an external monitor to allow real time reading of the pressure of the muscle that controls the flow from the ducts to the duodenum.

Coding Tips

Report the appropriate endoscopy for each anatomic site examined. Surgical endoscopy includes a diagnostic endoscopy; however, diagnostic endoscopy can be identified separately when performed at the same surgical session as an open procedure. When 43262 is performed, it may be reported with 43261, 43263–43265, 43275, or 43278. Report 43263 only once per session. Do not report 43262–43263 with 43260 or 43262 with 43277. Do not report 43262 in addition to 43274 for stent placement or 43276 for stent exchange/replacement in the same location.

ICD-10-CM Diagnostic Codes

C22.1	Intrahepatic bile duct carcinoma
C23	Malignant neoplasm of gallbladder
C24.0	Malignant neoplasm of extrahepatic bile duct
C24.1	Malignant neoplasm of ampulla of Vater
C24.8	Malignant neoplasm of overlapping sites of biliary tract
C25.0	Malignant neoplasm of head of pancreas
C25.1	Malignant neoplasm of body of pancreas
C25.2	Malignant neoplasm of tail of pancreas
C25.3	Malignant neoplasm of pancreatic duct
C25.4	Malignant neoplasm of endocrine pancreas
C25.7	Malignant neoplasm of other parts of pancreas
C25.8	Malignant neoplasm of overlapping sites of pancreas

C78.7	Secondary malignant neoplasm of liver and intrahepatic bile duct
D01.5	Carcinoma in situ of liver, gallbladder and bile ducts
D13.5	Benign neoplasm of extrahepatic bile ducts
D37.6	Neoplasm of uncertain behavior of liver, gallbladder and bile ducts
E79.0	Hyperuricemia without signs of inflammatory arthritis and tophaceous disease
K56.3	Gallstone ileus
K80.00	Calculus of gallbladder with acute cholecystitis without obstruction
K80.01	Calculus of gallbladder with acute cholecystitis with obstruction
K80.10	Calculus of gallbladder with chronic cholecystitis without obstruction
K80.11	Calculus of gallbladder with chronic cholecystitis with obstruction
K80.12	Calculus of gallbladder with acute and chronic cholecystitis without obstruction
K80.13	Calculus of gallbladder with acute and chronic cholecystitis with obstruction
K80.18	Calculus of gallbladder with other cholecystitis without obstruction
K80.19	Calculus of gallbladder with other cholecystitis with obstruction
K80.20	Calculus of gallbladder without cholecystitis without obstruction
K80.21	Calculus of gallbladder without cholecystitis with obstruction
K80.32	Calculus of bile duct with acute cholangitis without obstruction
K80.33	Calculus of bile duct with acute cholangitis with obstruction
K80.34	Calculus of bile duct with chronic cholangitis without obstruction
K80.35	Calculus of bile duct with chronic cholangitis with obstruction
K80.36	Calculus of bile duct with acute and chronic cholangitis without obstruction
K80.37	Calculus of bile duct with acute and chronic cholangitis with obstruction
K80.42	Calculus of bile duct with acute cholecystitis without obstruction
K80.43	Calculus of bile duct with acute cholecystitis with obstruction
K80.44	Calculus of bile duct with chronic cholecystitis without obstruction
K80.45	Calculus of bile duct with chronic cholecystitis with obstruction
K80.46	Calculus of bile duct with acute and chronic cholecystitis without obstruction
K80.47	Calculus of bile duct with acute and chronic cholecystitis with obstruction
K80.50	Calculus of bile duct without cholangitis or cholecystitis without obstruction
K80.51	Calculus of bile duct without cholangitis or cholecystitis with obstruction
K80.62	Calculus of gallbladder and bile duct with acute cholecystitis without obstruction
K80.63	Calculus of gallbladder and bile duct with acute cholecystitis with obstruction
K80.64	Calculus of gallbladder and bile duct with chronic cholecystitis without obstruction
K80.65	Calculus of gallbladder and bile duct with chronic cholecystitis with obstruction
K80.66	Calculus of gallbladder and bile duct with acute and chronic cholecystitis without obstruction

Esophagus

K80.67	Calculus of gallbladder and bile duct with acute and chronic cholecystitis with obstruction
K80.70	Calculus of gallbladder and bile duct without cholecystitis without obstruction
K80.71	Calculus of gallbladder and bile duct without cholecystitis with obstruction
K80.80	Other cholelithiasis without obstruction
K80.81	Other cholelithiasis with obstruction
K81.0	Acute cholecystitis
K81.1	Chronic cholecystitis
K81.2	Acute cholecystitis with chronic cholecystitis
K82.0	Obstruction of gallbladder
K82.1	Hydrops of gallbladder
K82.2	Perforation of gallbladder
K82.3	Fistula of gallbladder
K82.4	Cholesterolosis of gallbladder
K82.8	Other specified diseases of gallbladder
K83.01	Primary sclerosing cholangitis
K83.09	Other cholangitis
K83.1	Obstruction of bile duct
K83.2	Perforation of bile duct
K83.3	Fistula of bile duct
K83.4	Spasm of sphincter of Oddi
K83.5	Biliary cyst
K83.8	Other specified diseases of biliary tract
K86.0	Alcohol-induced chronic pancreatitis
K86.1	Other chronic pancreatitis
K86.2	Cyst of pancreas
K86.3	Pseudocyst of pancreas
K86.81	Exocrine pancreatic insufficiency
K87	Disorders of gallbladder, biliary tract and pancreas in diseases classified elsewhere
K91.5	Postcholecystectomy syndrome
K91.86	Retained cholelithiasis following cholecystectomy
Q44.0	Agenesis, aplasia and hypoplasia of gallbladder
Q44.1	Other congenital malformations of gallbladder
Q44.4	Choledochal cyst
Q44.5	Other congenital malformations of bile ducts
Q45.0	Agenesis, aplasia and hypoplasia of pancreas
Q45.1	Annular pancreas
Q45.2	Congenital pancreatic cyst
Q45.3	Other congenital malformations of pancreas and pancreatic duct
R10.11	Right upper quadrant pain
R11.14	Bilious vomiting
R11.15	Cyclical vomiting syndrome unrelated to migraine

AMA: **43262** 2018,Jan,8; 2017,Jan,8; 2016,Jan,13; 2015,Jan,16; 2015,Dec,3
43263 2018,Jan,8; 2017,Jan,8; 2016,Jan,13; 2015,Jan,16

Relative Value Units/Medicare Edits

Non-Facility RVU	Work	PE	MP	Total
43262	6.5	3.19	0.7	10.39
43263	6.5	3.15	0.74	10.39
Facility RVU	Work	PE	MP	Total
43262	6.5	3.19	0.7	10.39
43263	6.5	3.15	0.74	10.39

	FUD	Status	MUE	Modifiers				IOM Reference
43262	0	A	2(2)	51	N/A	N/A	N/A	None
43263	0	A	1(2)	51	N/A	N/A	N/A	

* with documentation

Terms To Know

ampulla of Vater. Tubular structure with flask-like dilation where the common bile and pancreatic ducts join before emptying into the duodenum.

catheter. Flexible tube inserted into an area of the body for introducing or withdrawing fluid.

electrocautery. Division or cutting of tissue using high-frequency electrical current to produce heat, which destroys cells.

ERCP. Endoscopic retrograde cholangiopancreatography. Examination of the hepatobiliary system and gallbladder performed through a flexible fiberoptic endoscope.

manometry. Pressure measurement of liquids and gases along the esophagus.

sphincterotomy. Incision into the ring-like band of muscle that surrounds a bodily opening, constricting and relaxing as required for normal physiological functioning.

Esophagus

43264-43265

43264 Endoscopic retrograde cholangiopancreatography (ERCP); with removal of calculi/debris from biliary/pancreatic duct(s)

43265 with destruction of calculi, any method (eg, mechanical, electrohydraulic, lithotripsy)

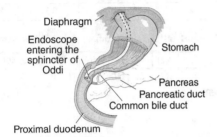

Diaphragm
Endoscope entering the sphincter of Oddi
Stomach
Pancreas
Pancreatic duct
Common bile duct
Proximal duodenum

An endoscope is fed through the stomach and into the duodenum. Usually a smaller subscope is fed up the sphincter of Oddi and into the ducts that drain the pancreas and the gallbladder (common bile)

Explanation

The physician performs an endoscopic retrograde cholangiopancreatography (ERCP) to destroy or remove calculi or debris. The physician passes the endoscope through the patient's oropharynx, esophagus, stomach, and into the small intestine. The ampulla of Vater is cannulated and filled with contrast. The common bile duct and the whole biliary tract, including the gallbladder, are visualized. Report 43264 if stones or debris are removed from biliary and/or pancreatic ducts. Report 43265 if stones are destroyed using any method and any remaining debris removed.

Coding Tips

Report the appropriate endoscopy for each anatomic site examined. Surgical endoscopy includes a diagnostic endoscopy; however, diagnostic endoscopy can be identified separately when performed at the same surgical session as an open procedure. For hepaticotomy or hepaticostomy with exploration, drainage, or removal of a calculus, see 47400. For choledochostomy, with exploration, drainage, or removal of a calculus, with or without cholecystotomy, without transduodenal sphincterotomy or sphincteroplasty, see 47420; with transduodenal sphincterotomy or sphincteroplasty, see 47425. For transduodenal sphincterotomy or sphincteroplasty, with or without transduodenal extraction of calculus, see 47460. For cholecystotomy with exploration, drainage, or removal of calculus, see 47480. For removal of a calculus or debris, percutaneously, see 47544. Do not report 43264–43265 with 43260 or each other. Do not report 43264 when no calculi or debris is found even with deployment of a balloon catheter.

ICD-10-CM Diagnostic Codes

K80.00	Calculus of gallbladder with acute cholecystitis without obstruction
K80.01	Calculus of gallbladder with acute cholecystitis with obstruction
K80.10	Calculus of gallbladder with chronic cholecystitis without obstruction
K80.11	Calculus of gallbladder with chronic cholecystitis with obstruction
K80.12	Calculus of gallbladder with acute and chronic cholecystitis without obstruction
K80.13	Calculus of gallbladder with acute and chronic cholecystitis with obstruction
K80.18	Calculus of gallbladder with other cholecystitis without obstruction
K80.19	Calculus of gallbladder with other cholecystitis with obstruction
K80.20	Calculus of gallbladder without cholecystitis without obstruction
K80.21	Calculus of gallbladder without cholecystitis with obstruction
K80.32	Calculus of bile duct with acute cholangitis without obstruction
K80.33	Calculus of bile duct with acute cholangitis with obstruction
K80.34	Calculus of bile duct with chronic cholangitis without obstruction
K80.35	Calculus of bile duct with chronic cholangitis with obstruction
K80.36	Calculus of bile duct with acute and chronic cholangitis without obstruction
K80.37	Calculus of bile duct with acute and chronic cholangitis with obstruction
K80.42	Calculus of bile duct with acute cholecystitis without obstruction
K80.43	Calculus of bile duct with acute cholecystitis with obstruction
K80.44	Calculus of bile duct with chronic cholecystitis without obstruction
K80.45	Calculus of bile duct with chronic cholecystitis with obstruction
K80.46	Calculus of bile duct with acute and chronic cholecystitis without obstruction
K80.47	Calculus of bile duct with acute and chronic cholecystitis with obstruction
K80.50	Calculus of bile duct without cholangitis or cholecystitis without obstruction
K80.51	Calculus of bile duct without cholangitis or cholecystitis with obstruction
K80.62	Calculus of gallbladder and bile duct with acute cholecystitis without obstruction
K80.63	Calculus of gallbladder and bile duct with acute cholecystitis with obstruction
K80.64	Calculus of gallbladder and bile duct with chronic cholecystitis without obstruction
K80.65	Calculus of gallbladder and bile duct with chronic cholecystitis with obstruction
K80.66	Calculus of gallbladder and bile duct with acute and chronic cholecystitis without obstruction
K80.67	Calculus of gallbladder and bile duct with acute and chronic cholecystitis with obstruction
K80.70	Calculus of gallbladder and bile duct without cholecystitis without obstruction
K80.71	Calculus of gallbladder and bile duct without cholecystitis with obstruction
K80.80	Other cholelithiasis without obstruction
K80.81	Other cholelithiasis with obstruction
K83.1	Obstruction of bile duct
K86.3	Pseudocyst of pancreas
K86.81	Exocrine pancreatic insufficiency
K87	Disorders of gallbladder, biliary tract and pancreas in diseases classified elsewhere
K91.86	Retained cholelithiasis following cholecystectomy

AMA: 43264 2018,Jan,8; 2017,Jan,8; 2016,Jan,13; 2015,Jan,16; 2015,Dec,3
43265 2018,Jan,8; 2017,Jan,8; 2016,Jan,13; 2015,Jan,16; 2015,Dec,3

Esophagus

Relative Value Units/Medicare Edits

Non-Facility RVU	Work	PE	MP	Total
43264	6.63	3.25	0.71	10.59
43265	7.93	3.83	0.85	12.61
Facility RVU	**Work**	**PE**	**MP**	**Total**
43264	6.63	3.25	0.71	10.59
43265	7.93	3.83	0.85	12.61

	FUD	Status	MUE	Modifiers				IOM Reference
43264	0	A	1(2)	51	N/A	N/A	N/A	None
43265	0	A	1(2)	51	N/A	N/A	N/A	

* with documentation

Terms To Know

ampulla of Vater. Tubular structure with flask-like dilation where the common bile and pancreatic ducts join before emptying into the duodenum.

calculus. Abnormal, stone-like concretion of calcium, cholesterol, mineral salts, or other substances that forms in any part of the body.

cannulation. Insertion of a flexible length of hollow tubing into a blood vessel, duct, or body cavity, usually for extracorporeal circulation or chemotherapy infusion to a particular region of the body.

contrast material. Any internally administered substance that has a different opacity from soft tissue on radiography or computed tomograph; includes barium, used to opacify parts of the gastrointestinal tract; water-soluble iodinated compounds, used to opacify blood vessels or the genitourinary tract; may refer to air occurring naturally or introduced into the body; also, paramagnetic substances used in magnetic resonance imaging. Substances may also be documented as contrast agent or contrast medium.

ERCP. Endoscopic retrograde cholangiopancreatography. Examination of the hepatobiliary system and gallbladder performed through a flexible fiberoptic endoscope.

lithotripsy. Destruction of calcified substances in the gallbladder or urinary system by smashing the concretion into small particles to be washed out. This may be done by surgical or noninvasive methods, such as ultrasound.

[43274]

43274 Endoscopic retrograde cholangiopancreatography (ERCP); with placement of endoscopic stent into biliary or pancreatic duct, including pre- and post-dilation and guide wire passage, when performed, including sphincterotomy, when performed, each stent

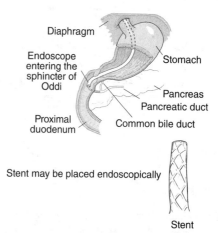

Stent may be placed endoscopically

Explanation

The physician performs an endoscopic retrograde cholangiopancreatography (ERCP) to insert a stent. The physician passes the endoscope through the patient's oropharynx, esophagus, stomach, and into the small intestine. The ampulla of Vater is cannulated and filled with contrast. The common bile duct and the whole biliary tract, including the gallbladder, are visualized. A sphincterotomy may be performed. A guidewire is threaded into the biliary or pancreatic duct. The stent is advanced over the guidewire and expanded in place. Balloon dilation may be performed to achieve desired outcome. The guidewire and surgical instruments are removed.

Coding Tips

This code is also used to report nasobiliary or nasopancreatic drainage tube insertion. For biliary stent placement, percutaneous, see 47538-47540. Do not report 43274 in addition to 43262 or 43275–43277 for stent insertion/replacement performed in the same duct.

ICD-10-CM Diagnostic Codes

C23	Malignant neoplasm of gallbladder
C24.0	Malignant neoplasm of extrahepatic bile duct
C24.1	Malignant neoplasm of ampulla of Vater
C24.8	Malignant neoplasm of overlapping sites of biliary tract
C78.7	Secondary malignant neoplasm of liver and intrahepatic bile duct
C78.89	Secondary malignant neoplasm of other digestive organs
C7A.098	Malignant carcinoid tumors of other sites
C7A.1	Malignant poorly differentiated neuroendocrine tumors
D01.5	Carcinoma in situ of liver, gallbladder and bile ducts
D01.7	Carcinoma in situ of other specified digestive organs
D13.5	Benign neoplasm of extrahepatic bile ducts
D13.6	Benign neoplasm of pancreas
D13.7	Benign neoplasm of endocrine pancreas
D37.6	Neoplasm of uncertain behavior of liver, gallbladder and bile ducts
K83.4	Spasm of sphincter of Oddi

Esophagus

Q44.2   Atresia of bile ducts

Q44.3   Congenital stenosis and stricture of bile ducts

AMA: 43274 2018,Jan,8; 2017,Jan,8; 2016,Jan,13; 2015,Jan,16

Relative Value Units/Medicare Edits

Non-Facility RVU	Work	PE	MP	Total
43274	8.48	4.07	0.92	13.47
Facility RVU	Work	PE	MP	Total
43274	8.48	4.07	0.92	13.47

	FUD	Status	MUE	Modifiers				IOM Reference
43274	0	A	2(3)	51	N/A	N/A	N/A	None

* with documentation

Terms To Know

dilation. Artificial increase in the diameter of an opening or lumen made by medication or by instrumentation.

ERCP. Endoscopic retrograde cholangiopancreatography. Examination of the hepatobiliary system and gallbladder performed through a flexible fiberoptic endoscope.

guidewire. Flexible metal instrument designed to lead another instrument in its proper course.

retrograde. Moving against the usual direction of flow.

sphincterotomy. Incision into the ring-like band of muscle that surrounds a bodily opening, constricting and relaxing as required for normal physiological functioning.

stent. Tube to provide support in a body cavity or lumen.

[43275]

43275   Endoscopic retrograde cholangiopancreatography (ERCP); with removal of foreign body(s) or stent(s) from biliary/pancreatic duct(s)

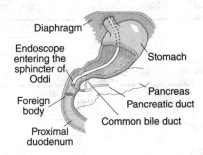

Foreign body or stent is retrieved endoscopically

Explanation

The physician performs an endoscopic retrograde cholangiopancreatography (ERCP) to remove a biliary stent or other foreign body. The physician passes the endoscope through the patient's oropharynx, esophagus, stomach, and into the small intestine. The ampulla of Vater is cannulated and filled with contrast. The common bile duct and the whole biliary tract, including the gallbladder, are visualized. A sphincterotomy may be performed. The previously placed stent or foreign body is located and removed using any method, including basket and snare techniques.

Coding Tips

For removal of biliary or pancreatic duct stents without ERCP, see 43247. For removal of a calculus or debris, percutaneously, see 47544. Report this code only one time per session regardless of the number of stents or foreign bodies removed. Do not report 43275 with 43260, 43274, or 43276.

ICD-10-CM Diagnostic Codes

T18.8XXA	Foreign body in other parts of alimentary tract, initial encounter
T81.514A	Adhesions due to foreign body accidentally left in body following endoscopic examination, initial encounter
T81.524A	Obstruction due to foreign body accidentally left in body following endoscopic examination, initial encounter
T81.594A	Other complications of foreign body accidentally left in body following endoscopic examination, initial encounter
T85.510A	Breakdown (mechanical) of bile duct prosthesis, initial encounter
T85.520A	Displacement of bile duct prosthesis, initial encounter
T85.590A	Other mechanical complication of bile duct prosthesis, initial encounter

AMA: 43275 2018,Jan,8; 2017,Jan,8; 2016,Jan,13; 2015,Jan,16

Relative Value Units/Medicare Edits

Non-Facility RVU	Work	PE	MP	Total
43275	6.86	3.35	0.74	10.95
Facility RVU	Work	PE	MP	Total
43275	6.86	3.35	0.74	10.95

	FUD	Status	MUE	Modifiers				IOM Reference
43275	0	A	1(3)	51	N/A	N/A	N/A	None

* with documentation

Esophagus

[43276]

43276 Endoscopic retrograde cholangiopancreatography (ERCP); with removal and exchange of stent(s), biliary or pancreatic duct, including pre- and post-dilation and guide wire passage, when performed, including sphincterotomy, when performed, each stent exchanged

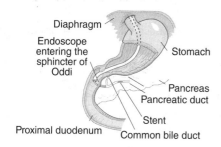

Diaphragm
Endoscope entering the sphincter of Oddi
Stomach
Pancreas
Pancreatic duct
Stent
Proximal duodenum
Common bile duct

An endoscope is fed through the stomach and into the duodenum. Usually a smaller subscope is fed up the sphincter of Oddi and into the ducts that drain the pancreas and the gallbladder (common bile)

Explanation

The physician performs an endoscopic retrograde cholangiopancreatography (ERCP) to exchange a biliary stent. The physician passes the endoscope through the patient's oropharynx, esophagus, stomach, and into the small intestine. The ampulla of Vater is cannulated and filled with contrast. The common bile duct and the whole biliary tract, including the gallbladder, are visualized. A sphincterotomy may be performed. The previously placed stent is located and removed using any method, including basket and snare techniques. A guidewire is threaded into the biliary or pancreatic duct. A new stent is advanced over the guidewire and expanded in place. Balloon dilation may be performed to achieve desired outcome. The guidewire and surgical instruments are removed.

Coding Tips

This procedure includes removal and replacement of one stent; append modifier 59 or an X{EPSU} modifier for additional stents performed during the same operative session. Do not report 43276 with 43260 or 43275. Do not report 43276 in addition to 43262 or 43274 when a stent is placed/exchanged in the same duct.

ICD-10-CM Diagnostic Codes

C23	Malignant neoplasm of gallbladder
C24.0	Malignant neoplasm of extrahepatic bile duct
C24.1	Malignant neoplasm of ampulla of Vater
C24.8	Malignant neoplasm of overlapping sites of biliary tract
C78.7	Secondary malignant neoplasm of liver and intrahepatic bile duct
C78.89	Secondary malignant neoplasm of other digestive organs
C7A.098	Malignant carcinoid tumors of other sites
C7A.1	Malignant poorly differentiated neuroendocrine tumors
D01.5	Carcinoma in situ of liver, gallbladder and bile ducts
D01.7	Carcinoma in situ of other specified digestive organs
D13.4	Benign neoplasm of liver
D13.5	Benign neoplasm of extrahepatic bile ducts
D13.6	Benign neoplasm of pancreas
D13.7	Benign neoplasm of endocrine pancreas

D37.6	Neoplasm of uncertain behavior of liver, gallbladder and bile ducts
K83.4	Spasm of sphincter of Oddi
Q44.2	Atresia of bile ducts
Q44.3	Congenital stenosis and stricture of bile ducts
T85.510A	Breakdown (mechanical) of bile duct prosthesis, initial encounter
T85.520A	Displacement of bile duct prosthesis, initial encounter
T85.590A	Other mechanical complication of bile duct prosthesis, initial encounter

AMA: 43276 2018,Jan,8; 2017,Jan,8; 2016,Jan,13; 2015,Jan,16

Relative Value Units/Medicare Edits

Non-Facility RVU	Work	PE	MP	Total
43276	8.84	4.24	0.94	14.02
Facility RVU	**Work**	**PE**	**MP**	**Total**
43276	8.84	4.24	0.94	14.02

	FUD	Status	MUE	Modifiers				IOM Reference
43276	0	A	2(3)	51	N/A	N/A	N/A	None

* with documentation

Terms To Know

balloon catheter. Any catheter equipped with an inflatable balloon at the end to hold it in place in a body cavity or to be used for dilation of a vessel lumen.

dilation. Artificial increase in the diameter of an opening or lumen made by medication or by instrumentation.

ERCP. Endoscopic retrograde cholangiopancreatography. Examination of the hepatobiliary system and gallbladder performed through a flexible fiberoptic endoscope.

guidewire. Flexible metal instrument designed to lead another instrument in its proper course.

sphincterotomy. Incision into the ring-like band of muscle that surrounds a bodily opening, constricting and relaxing as required for normal physiological functioning.

stent. Tube to provide support in a body cavity or lumen.

Esophagus

[43277]

43277 Endoscopic retrograde cholangiopancreatography (ERCP); with trans-endoscopic balloon dilation of biliary/pancreatic duct(s) or of ampulla (sphincteroplasty), including sphincterotomy, when performed, each duct

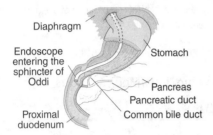

Explanation

The physician performs an endoscopic retrograde cholangiopancreatography (ERCP) to dilate a biliary duct or the ampulla of Vater. The physician passes the endoscope through the patient's oropharynx, esophagus, stomach, and into the small intestine. The ampulla is cannulated and filled with contrast. The common bile duct and the whole biliary tract, including the gallbladder, are visualized. A stricture or obstruction is visualized. A sphincterotomy may be performed to reach the area to be treated with the balloon dilator. Once the balloon is in place, it is expanded multiple times until the desired outcome is achieved. The endoscope and all surgical instruments are removed. Report 43277 for each biliary duct and ampulla dilated.

Coding Tips

Bilateral balloon dilation may be reported twice with modifier 59 or an X{EPSU} modifier appended to the subsequent procedure when performed. This code should not be reported for incidental dilation using a balloon for stone or debris removal, see 43264 and 43265. Report 43262 with modifier 59 or an X{EPSU} modifier for a sphincterotomy without sphincteroplasty performed on a separate pancreatic duct orifice during the same operative session. Append modifier 59 or an X{EPSU} modifier to this service code for each additional stricture dilated during the same operative session. For balloon dilation of the ampulla or biliary ducts, percutaneous, see 47542. Do not report 43277 in addition to 43260, 43262, or 43278 for the same lesion. Do not report 43277 in addition to 43274 or 43276 for dilation and stent placement/replacement procedures in the same duct.

ICD-10-CM Diagnostic Codes

C23	Malignant neoplasm of gallbladder
C24.0	Malignant neoplasm of extrahepatic bile duct
C24.1	Malignant neoplasm of ampulla of Vater
C24.8	Malignant neoplasm of overlapping sites of biliary tract
C78.7	Secondary malignant neoplasm of liver and intrahepatic bile duct
C78.89	Secondary malignant neoplasm of other digestive organs
C7A.098	Malignant carcinoid tumors of other sites
C7A.1	Malignant poorly differentiated neuroendocrine tumors
D01.5	Carcinoma in situ of liver, gallbladder and bile ducts
D01.7	Carcinoma in situ of other specified digestive organs
D13.6	Benign neoplasm of pancreas
D13.7	Benign neoplasm of endocrine pancreas
D37.6	Neoplasm of uncertain behavior of liver, gallbladder and bile ducts

K80.00	Calculus of gallbladder with acute cholecystitis without obstruction
K80.01	Calculus of gallbladder with acute cholecystitis with obstruction
K80.10	Calculus of gallbladder with chronic cholecystitis without obstruction
K80.11	Calculus of gallbladder with chronic cholecystitis with obstruction
K80.12	Calculus of gallbladder with acute and chronic cholecystitis without obstruction
K80.13	Calculus of gallbladder with acute and chronic cholecystitis with obstruction
K80.18	Calculus of gallbladder with other cholecystitis without obstruction
K80.19	Calculus of gallbladder with other cholecystitis with obstruction
K80.20	Calculus of gallbladder without cholecystitis without obstruction
K80.21	Calculus of gallbladder without cholecystitis with obstruction
K80.32	Calculus of bile duct with acute cholangitis without obstruction
K80.33	Calculus of bile duct with acute cholangitis with obstruction
K80.34	Calculus of bile duct with chronic cholangitis without obstruction
K80.35	Calculus of bile duct with chronic cholangitis with obstruction
K80.36	Calculus of bile duct with acute and chronic cholangitis without obstruction
K80.37	Calculus of bile duct with acute and chronic cholangitis with obstruction
K80.42	Calculus of bile duct with acute cholecystitis without obstruction
K80.43	Calculus of bile duct with acute cholecystitis with obstruction
K80.44	Calculus of bile duct with chronic cholecystitis without obstruction
K80.45	Calculus of bile duct with chronic cholecystitis with obstruction
K80.46	Calculus of bile duct with acute and chronic cholecystitis without obstruction
K80.47	Calculus of bile duct with acute and chronic cholecystitis with obstruction
K80.50	Calculus of bile duct without cholangitis or cholecystitis without obstruction
K80.51	Calculus of bile duct without cholangitis or cholecystitis with obstruction
K80.62	Calculus of gallbladder and bile duct with acute cholecystitis without obstruction
K80.63	Calculus of gallbladder and bile duct with acute cholecystitis with obstruction
K80.64	Calculus of gallbladder and bile duct with chronic cholecystitis without obstruction
K80.65	Calculus of gallbladder and bile duct with chronic cholecystitis with obstruction
K80.66	Calculus of gallbladder and bile duct with acute and chronic cholecystitis without obstruction
K80.67	Calculus of gallbladder and bile duct with acute and chronic cholecystitis with obstruction
K80.70	Calculus of gallbladder and bile duct without cholecystitis without obstruction
K80.71	Calculus of gallbladder and bile duct without cholecystitis with obstruction
K80.80	Other cholelithiasis without obstruction
K80.81	Other cholelithiasis with obstruction
K83.1	Obstruction of bile duct
K83.4	Spasm of sphincter of Oddi

Esophagus

Q44.2   Atresia of bile ducts

Q44.3   Congenital stenosis and stricture of bile ducts

AMA: **43277** 2018,Jan,8; 2017,Jan,8; 2016,Jan,13; 2015,Jan,16; 2015,Dec,3

Relative Value Units/Medicare Edits

Non-Facility RVU	Work	PE	MP	Total
43277	6.9	3.37	0.74	11.01
Facility RVU	**Work**	**PE**	**MP**	**Total**
43277	6.9	3.37	0.74	11.01

	FUD	Status	MUE	Modifiers				IOM Reference
43277	0	A	3(3)	51	N/A	N/A	N/A	None

* with documentation

Terms To Know

ampulla of Vater. Tubular structure with flask-like dilation where the common bile and pancreatic ducts join before emptying into the duodenum.

atresia. Congenital closure or absence of a tubular organ or an opening to the body surface.

balloon catheter. Any catheter equipped with an inflatable balloon at the end to hold it in place in a body cavity or to be used for dilation of a vessel lumen.

congenital. Present at birth, occurring through heredity or an influence during gestation up to the moment of birth.

retrograde. Moving against the usual direction of flow.

sphincteroplasty. Surgical repair done to correct, augment, or improve the muscular function of a sphincter, such as the anus or intestines.

sphincterotomy. Incision into the ring-like band of muscle that surrounds a bodily opening, constricting and relaxing as required for normal physiological functioning.

stricture. Narrowing of an anatomical structure.

[43278]

43278   Endoscopic retrograde cholangiopancreatography (ERCP); with ablation of tumor(s), polyp(s), or other lesion(s), including pre- and post-dilation and guide wire passage, when performed

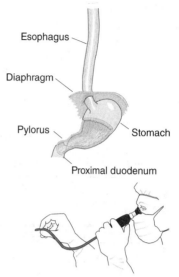

Flexible endoscope is used to ablate tumors, polyps, or other lesions

Explanation

The physician performs an endoscopic retrograde cholangiopancreatography (ERCP) to perform destruction of a tumor, polyp, or other lesion of the biliary system. The physician passes the endoscope through the patient's oropharynx, esophagus, stomach, and into the small intestine. The ampulla is cannulated and filled with contrast. The common bile duct and the whole biliary tract, including the gallbladder, are visualized to locate the lesion. The lesion is destroyed using laser therapy, electrocoagulation, or injection of toxic agents. The endoscope is removed.

Coding Tips

For ampullectomy, see 43254. Do not report 43278 with 43260 or in addition to 43277 for the same lesion.

ICD-10-CM Diagnostic Codes

C23	Malignant neoplasm of gallbladder
C24.0	Malignant neoplasm of extrahepatic bile duct
C24.1	Malignant neoplasm of ampulla of Vater
C24.8	Malignant neoplasm of overlapping sites of biliary tract
C25.4	Malignant neoplasm of endocrine pancreas
C78.7	Secondary malignant neoplasm of liver and intrahepatic bile duct
C78.89	Secondary malignant neoplasm of other digestive organs
D01.5	Carcinoma in situ of liver, gallbladder and bile ducts
D01.7	Carcinoma in situ of other specified digestive organs
D13.7	Benign neoplasm of endocrine pancreas
D37.6	Neoplasm of uncertain behavior of liver, gallbladder and bile ducts
D37.8	Neoplasm of uncertain behavior of other specified digestive organs
D49.0	Neoplasm of unspecified behavior of digestive system

Esophagus

K80.47	Calculus of bile duct with acute and chronic cholecystitis with obstruction
K80.50	Calculus of bile duct without cholangitis or cholecystitis without obstruction
K83.5	Biliary cyst
K86.2	Cyst of pancreas
K86.3	Pseudocyst of pancreas
Q45.1	Annular pancreas
Q45.2	Congenital pancreatic cyst

AMA: 43278 2018,Jan,8; 2017,Jan,8; 2016,Jan,13; 2015,Jan,16

Relative Value Units/Medicare Edits

Non-Facility RVU	Work	PE	MP	Total
43278	7.92	3.81	0.85	12.58
Facility RVU	**Work**	**PE**	**MP**	**Total**
43278	7.92	3.81	0.85	12.58

	FUD	Status	MUE	Modifiers				IOM Reference
43278	0	A	1(3)	51	N/A	N/A	N/A	None

* with documentation

Terms To Know

ablation. Removal or destruction of tissue by cutting, electrical energy, chemical substances, or excessive heat application.

cholesterolosis of gallbladder. Accumulation of cholesterol deposits within the tissues of the gallbladder.

contrast material. Any internally administered substance that has a different opacity from soft tissue on radiography or computed tomograph; includes barium, used to opacify parts of the gastrointestinal tract; water-soluble iodinated compounds, used to opacify blood vessels or the genitourinary tract; may refer to air occurring naturally or introduced into the body; also, paramagnetic substances used in magnetic resonance imaging. Substances may also be documented as contrast agent or contrast medium.

dilation. Artificial increase in the diameter of an opening or lumen made by medication or by instrumentation.

lesion. Area of damaged tissue that has lost continuity or function, due to disease or trauma.

polyp. Small growth on a stalk-like attachment projecting from a mucous membrane.

tumor. Pathological swelling or enlargement; a neoplastic growth of uncontrolled, abnormal multiplication of cells.

43273

+ **43273** Endoscopic cannulation of papilla with direct visualization of pancreatic/common bile duct(s) (List separately in addition to code(s) for primary procedure)

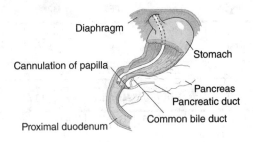

Explanation

At the same time as an endoscopic retrograde cholangiopancreatography (ERCP) with or without additional therapeutic or diagnostic procedures, the physician performs endoscopic cannulation of papilla with direct visualization of the pancreatic and/or common bile duct(s). A catheter or papillotome is inserted through the channel of the ERCP scope. With or without the use of a guidewire, the pancreatic and/or common bile duct are located and visually inspected.

Coding Tips

Report 43273 in addition to 43260–43265 or 43274–43278. Do not report this code more than once per procedure.

ICD-10-CM Diagnostic Codes

This/these CPT code(s) are add-on code(s). See the primary procedure code that this code is performed with for your ICD-10-CM code selections.

AMA: 43273 2018,Jan,8; 2017,Jan,8; 2016,Jan,13; 2015,Jan,16

Relative Value Units/Medicare Edits

Non-Facility RVU	Work	PE	MP	Total
43273	2.24	1.0	0.25	3.49
Facility RVU	**Work**	**PE**	**MP**	**Total**
43273	2.24	1.0	0.25	3.49

	FUD	Status	MUE	Modifiers				IOM Reference
43273	N/A	A	1(2)	N/A	N/A	N/A	80*	None

* with documentation

Terms To Know

ampulla of Vater. Tubular structure with flask-like dilation where the common bile and pancreatic ducts join before emptying into the duodenum.

cannulation. Insertion of a flexible length of hollow tubing into a blood vessel, duct, or body cavity, usually for extracorporeal circulation or chemotherapy infusion to a particular region of the body.

43279

43279 Laparoscopy, surgical, esophagomyotomy (Heller type), with fundoplasty, when performed

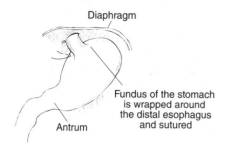

Diaphragm

Fundus of the stomach is wrapped around the distal esophagus and sutured

Antrum

Explanation

The physician performs laparoscopic esophagomyotomy (Heller myotomy), often for treatment of achalasia. Achalasia (a motility disorder of the esophagus) is caused by degeneration of the nerves in the esophageal wall and results in an absence of the typical wave-like motion of the esophagus and lack of relaxation of the lower esophagus. The physician makes several small incisions in the abdominal wall through which a video camera and laparoscopic instruments are inserted. An incision of the esophageal muscle is made using specialized laparoscopic instruments. To prevent reflux, a part of the upper stomach is then wrapped around the lower portion of the esophagus. Laparoscopic instruments are removed, and the small incisions are sutured. A swallowing study is typically obtained prior to discharge.

Coding Tips

A surgical laparoscopy always includes a diagnostic laparoscopy. Do not report 43279 with 43280. For an open approach, see 43330–43331.

ICD-10-CM Diagnostic Codes

C15.5	Malignant neoplasm of lower third of esophagus
C15.8	Malignant neoplasm of overlapping sites of esophagus
C16.0	Malignant neoplasm of cardia
K21.00	Gastro-esophageal reflux disease with esophagitis, without bleeding
K21.01	Gastro-esophageal reflux disease with esophagitis, with bleeding
K21.9	Gastro-esophageal reflux disease without esophagitis
K22.0	Achalasia of cardia
K22.10	Ulcer of esophagus without bleeding
K22.11	Ulcer of esophagus with bleeding
K22.2	Esophageal obstruction
K22.70	Barrett's esophagus without dysplasia
K22.710	Barrett's esophagus with low grade dysplasia
K22.711	Barrett's esophagus with high grade dysplasia
K22.89	Other specified disease of esophagus
Q39.0	Atresia of esophagus without fistula
Q39.1	Atresia of esophagus with tracheo-esophageal fistula
Q39.2	Congenital tracheo-esophageal fistula without atresia
Q39.3	Congenital stenosis and stricture of esophagus
Q39.4	Esophageal web
Q39.5	Congenital dilatation of esophagus
Q39.6	Congenital diverticulum of esophagus
Q39.8	Other congenital malformations of esophagus
R13.0	Aphagia
R13.11	Dysphagia, oral phase
R13.12	Dysphagia, oropharyngeal phase
R13.13	Dysphagia, pharyngeal phase
R13.14	Dysphagia, pharyngoesophageal phase
R13.19	Other dysphagia
R63.32	Pediatric feeding disorder, chronic 🅿
R63.39	Other feeding difficulties

AMA: **43279** 2018,Jan,8; 2017,Jan,8; 2017,Aug,6; 2016,Jan,13; 2015,Jan,16

Relative Value Units/Medicare Edits

Non-Facility RVU	Work	PE	MP	Total
43279	22.1	10.65	5.2	37.95
Facility RVU	**Work**	**PE**	**MP**	**Total**
43279	22.1	10.65	5.2	37.95

	FUD	Status	MUE	Modifiers				IOM Reference
43279	90	A	1(2)	51	N/A	62*	80	None

* with documentation

Terms To Know

achalasia. Failure of the smooth muscles within the gastrointestinal tract to relax at points of junction; most commonly referring to the esophagogastric sphincter's failure to relax when swallowing.

degeneration. Deterioration of an anatomic structure due to disease or other factors.

Heller myotomy. Longitudinal division of the distal esophageal muscle down to the submucosal layer. Cardia muscle fibers may also be divided. This procedure is used to treat achalasia.

laparoscopy. Direct visualization utilizing a thin, flexible, fiberoptic tube.

reflux. Return or backward flow.

Esophagus

43280

43280 Laparoscopy, surgical, esophagogastric fundoplasty (eg, Nissen, Toupet procedures)

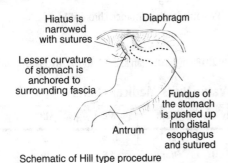

Hiatus is narrowed with sutures

Diaphragm

Lesser curvature of stomach is anchored to surrounding fascia

Fundus of the stomach is pushed up into distal esophagus and sutured

Antrum

Schematic of Hill type procedure

Explanation

The physician performs an esophagogastric fundoplasty using a laparoscope. With the patient under anesthesia, the physician places a trocar at the umbilicus into the abdomen and insufflates the abdominal cavity. The physician places a laparoscope through the umbilical incision and additional trocars are placed into the peritoneal space. Additional instruments are introduced through the trocars. The physician identifies the fundus and the esophagus and resects them. The fundus is wrapped around the lower end of the esophagus, which is rejoined to the stomach with sutures. The trocars are removed and the incisions are closed with sutures.

Coding Tips

Surgical laparoscopy always includes a diagnostic laparoscopy. For open esophagogastric fundoplasty (e.g., Nissen, Toupet procedure), see 43327–43328. For transoral esophagogastroduodenoscopy fundoplasty, partial or complete, see 43210. For augmentation of the esophageal sphincter with placement of a sphincter augmentation device, see 43284 and 43285. Do not report 43280 with 43279 or 43281-43282.

ICD-10-CM Diagnostic Codes

C15.4	Malignant neoplasm of middle third of esophagus
C15.5	Malignant neoplasm of lower third of esophagus
C15.8	Malignant neoplasm of overlapping sites of esophagus
C16.0	Malignant neoplasm of cardia
K21.00	Gastro-esophageal reflux disease with esophagitis, without bleeding
K21.01	Gastro-esophageal reflux disease with esophagitis, with bleeding
K21.9	Gastro-esophageal reflux disease without esophagitis
K22.0	Achalasia of cardia
K22.10	Ulcer of esophagus without bleeding
K22.11	Ulcer of esophagus with bleeding
K22.2	Esophageal obstruction
K22.70	Barrett's esophagus without dysplasia
K22.710	Barrett's esophagus with low grade dysplasia
K22.711	Barrett's esophagus with high grade dysplasia
Q39.0	Atresia of esophagus without fistula
Q39.1	Atresia of esophagus with tracheo-esophageal fistula
Q39.2	Congenital tracheo-esophageal fistula without atresia
Q39.3	Congenital stenosis and stricture of esophagus
Q39.4	Esophageal web
Q39.5	Congenital dilatation of esophagus
Q39.6	Congenital diverticulum of esophagus
Q39.8	Other congenital malformations of esophagus
R13.0	Aphagia
R13.11	Dysphagia, oral phase
R13.12	Dysphagia, oropharyngeal phase
R13.13	Dysphagia, pharyngeal phase
R13.14	Dysphagia, pharyngoesophageal phase
R13.19	Other dysphagia
R63.32	Pediatric feeding disorder, chronic 🅿
R63.39	Other feeding difficulties

AMA: 43280 2018,Jan,8; 2017,Jan,8; 2017,Aug,6; 2016,Jan,13; 2015,Nov,8; 2015,Jan,16

Relative Value Units/Medicare Edits

Non-Facility RVU	Work	PE	MP	Total
43280	18.1	9.46	4.33	31.89
Facility RVU	**Work**	**PE**	**MP**	**Total**
43280	18.1	9.46	4.33	31.89

	FUD	Status	MUE	Modifiers				IOM Reference
43280	90	A	1(2)	51	N/A	62*	80	None

* with documentation

Terms To Know

insufflation. Blowing air or gas into a body cavity.

laparoscopy. Direct visualization utilizing a thin, flexible, fiberoptic tube.

Nissen procedure (fundoplasty). Surgical repair technique that involves the fundus of the stomach being wrapped around the lower end of the esophagus to treat reflux esophagitis.

peritoneal. Space between the lining of the abdominal wall, or parietal peritoneum, and the surface layer of the abdominal organs, or visceral peritoneum. It contains a thin, watery fluid that keeps the peritoneal surfaces moist.

resect. Cutting out or removing a portion or all of a bone, organ, or other structure.

trocar. Cannula or a sharp pointed instrument used to puncture and aspirate fluid from cavities.

Esophagus

43281-43282

43281 Laparoscopy, surgical, repair of paraesophageal hernia, includes fundoplasty, when performed; without implantation of mesh
43282 with implantation of mesh

Diaphragm Esophagus

Stomach

Normal anatomy

Proximal part of stomach protrudes through gastroesophageal junction into mediastinum

Esophagus

Stomach

Paraesophageal hernia

Diaphragm

Gastroesophageal junction (remains in place)

Explanation

The physician repairs a paraesophageal hernia using a laparoscope and may also perform a fundoplasty when indicated. With the patient under anesthesia and in a supine position, the physician places laparoscopic ports in the upper abdomen, through which the appropriate surgical instruments are inserted. With the left lateral segment of the liver retracted, the hiatus is exposed. The physician reduces the herniated stomach into the abdomen and dissects the hernia sac and gastroesophageal fat pad using a combination of sharp and blunt dissection. If a fundoplasty is indicated, the physician identifies the fundus and the esophagus and resects them. The fundus is wrapped around the lower end of the esophagus, which is rejoined to the stomach with sutures. The instruments and trocars are removed and the incisions are closed with sutures. Report 43281 for a procedure performed without the implantation of mesh and 43282 for one requiring mesh implantation.

Coding Tips

Surgical laparoscopy always includes a diagnostic laparoscopy. These codes should not be reported with 43280, 43450, or 43453. For transthoracic diaphragmatic hernia repair, see 43334–43335; transabdominal paraesophageal hiatal hernia repair, see 43332–43333. For laparoscopic surgical esophagogastric fundoplasty (e.g., Nissen, Toupet procedure), see 43280.

ICD-10-CM Diagnostic Codes

K44.0	Diaphragmatic hernia with obstruction, without gangrene
K44.1	Diaphragmatic hernia with gangrene
K44.9	Diaphragmatic hernia without obstruction or gangrene
Q40.1	Congenital hiatus hernia
Q79.0	Congenital diaphragmatic hernia

AMA: 43281 2018,Sep,14; 2018,Nov,11; 2018,Jan,8; 2017,Jan,8; 2017,Aug,6; 2016,Jan,13; 2015,Jan,16 **43282** 2018,Jan,8; 2017,Jan,8; 2017,Aug,6; 2016,Jan,13; 2016,Aug,9; 2015,Jan,16

Relative Value Units/Medicare Edits

Non-Facility RVU	Work	PE	MP	Total
43281	26.6	12.53	6.38	45.51
43282	30.1	13.83	7.22	51.15
Facility RVU	Work	PE	MP	Total
43281	26.6	12.53	6.38	45.51
43282	30.1	13.83	7.22	51.15

	FUD	Status	MUE	Modifiers				IOM Reference
43281	90	A	1(2)	51	N/A	62*	80	None
43282	90	A	1(2)	51	N/A	62*	80	

* with documentation

Terms To Know

blunt dissection. Surgical technique used to expose an underlying area by separating along natural cleavage lines of tissue, without cutting.

hernia. Protrusion of a body structure through tissue.

implant. Material or device inserted or placed within the body for therapeutic, reconstructive, or diagnostic purposes.

laparoscopic. Minimally invasive procedure used for intraabdominal inspection; surgery that uses an endoscopic instrument inserted through small access incisions into the peritoneum for video-controlled imaging.

lateral. On/to the side.

mesh. Synthetic fabric used as a prosthetic patch in hernia repair.

trocar. Cannula or a sharp pointed instrument used to puncture and aspirate fluid from cavities.

Esophagus

43283

+ **43283** Laparoscopy, surgical, esophageal lengthening procedure (eg, Collis gastroplasty or wedge gastroplasty) (List separately in addition to code for primary procedure)

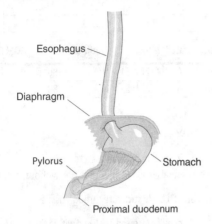

Esophagus

Diaphragm

Pylorus

Stomach

Proximal duodenum

Explanation

The physician performs a laparoscopic esophageal lengthening in order to extend a short esophagus prior to a separately reportable fundoplasty. This procedure is facilitated through a thoracoabdominal incision. With the patient under anesthesia, the physician places a trocar at the umbilicus into the abdomen and insufflates the abdominal cavity. The physician places a laparoscope through the umbilical incision and mobilizes the esophagus at the arch of the aorta. In the event that additional length is necessary, a gastric tube may be manipulated by separating the stomach with clamps and fixation of the proximal stomach that runs parallel with the lesser gastric curvature. A shortened esophagus may be due to damage caused by gastroesophageal reflux disease (GERD) thereby making fundoplasty difficult due to decreased tension necessary to reposition the GE junction. The trocars are removed and the incisions are closed with sutures.

Coding Tips

Report 43283 in addition to 43280–43282.

ICD-10-CM Diagnostic Codes

C15.4	Malignant neoplasm of middle third of esophagus
C15.5	Malignant neoplasm of lower third of esophagus
C15.8	Malignant neoplasm of overlapping sites of esophagus
C16.0	Malignant neoplasm of cardia
K20.80	Other esophagitis without bleeding
K20.81	Other esophagitis with bleeding
K21.00	Gastro-esophageal reflux disease with esophagitis, without bleeding
K21.01	Gastro-esophageal reflux disease with esophagitis, with bleeding
K21.9	Gastro-esophageal reflux disease without esophagitis
K22.0	Achalasia of cardia
K22.10	Ulcer of esophagus without bleeding
K22.11	Ulcer of esophagus with bleeding
K22.2	Esophageal obstruction
K22.70	Barrett's esophagus without dysplasia
K22.710	Barrett's esophagus with low grade dysplasia
K22.711	Barrett's esophagus with high grade dysplasia
K44.0	Diaphragmatic hernia with obstruction, without gangrene
K44.1	Diaphragmatic hernia with gangrene
K44.9	Diaphragmatic hernia without obstruction or gangrene
Q39.0	Atresia of esophagus without fistula
Q39.1	Atresia of esophagus with tracheo-esophageal fistula
Q39.2	Congenital tracheo-esophageal fistula without atresia
Q39.3	Congenital stenosis and stricture of esophagus
Q39.4	Esophageal web
Q39.5	Congenital dilatation of esophagus
Q39.6	Congenital diverticulum of esophagus
Q39.8	Other congenital malformations of esophagus
Q40.1	Congenital hiatus hernia
Q79.0	Congenital diaphragmatic hernia
R13.0	Aphagia
R13.11	Dysphagia, oral phase
R13.12	Dysphagia, oropharyngeal phase
R13.13	Dysphagia, pharyngeal phase
R13.14	Dysphagia, pharyngoesophageal phase
R13.19	Other dysphagia
R63.32	Pediatric feeding disorder, chronic 🅟
R63.39	Other feeding difficulties

AMA: **43283** 2018,Jan,8; 2017,Jan,8; 2016,Jan,13; 2015,Jan,16

Relative Value Units/Medicare Edits

Non-Facility RVU	Work	PE	MP	Total
43283	2.95	1.0	0.7	4.65
Facility RVU	**Work**	**PE**	**MP**	**Total**
43283	2.95	1.0	0.7	4.65

	FUD	Status	MUE	Modifiers				IOM Reference
43283	N/A	A	1(2)	N/A	N/A	62*	80	None

* with documentation

Esophagus

43286 Esophagectomy, total or near total, with laparoscopic mobilization of the abdominal and mediastinal esophagus and proximal gastrectomy, with laparoscopic pyloric drainage procedure if performed, with open cervical pharyngogastrostomy or esophagogastrostomy (ie, laparoscopic transhiatal esophagectomy)

43287 Esophagectomy, distal two-thirds, with laparoscopic mobilization of the abdominal and lower mediastinal esophagus and proximal gastrectomy, with laparoscopic pyloric drainage procedure if performed, with separate thoracoscopic mobilization of the middle and upper mediastinal esophagus and thoracic esophagogastrostomy (ie, laparoscopic thoracoscopic esophagectomy, Ivor Lewis esophagectomy)

43288 Esophagectomy, total or near total, with thoracoscopic mobilization of the upper, middle, and lower mediastinal esophagus, with separate laparoscopic proximal gastrectomy, with laparoscopic pyloric drainage procedure if performed, with open cervical pharyngogastrostomy or esophagogastrostomy (ie, thoracoscopic, laparoscopic and cervical incision esophagectomy, McKeown esophagectomy, tri-incisional esophagectomy)

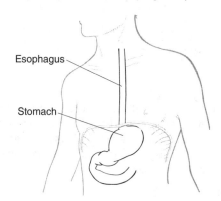

Esophagus

Stomach

Explanation

In laparoscopic or thoracoscopic esophagectomy, the physician partially or totally removes the esophagus, the upper stomach, and surrounding lymph nodes in patients diagnosed with esophageal cancer and/or Barrett's esophagus. In Barrett's esophagus, a complication resulting from chronic gastroesophageal reflux (GERD), the normal tissue lining the esophagus transforms into the tissue lining the intestine, which can develop into esophageal precancer or cancer. Laparoscopic/thoracoscopic esophagectomy is also used to treat patients who have damaged their esophagus by ingesting a caustic or burning substance or for patients with achalasia. In 43286, the physician removes all or most of the esophagus and attaches the stomach to the pharynx or cervical esophagus utilizing a combination of laparoscopic and open approaches. The physician gains access to the esophagus through an oblique cervical incision. Using a laparoscopic approach, the physician mobilizes portions of the esophagus and the proximal stomach. The esophagus is divided at the cervical level (for an esophagogastrostomy) or at its origin at the pharynx (for a pharyngogastrostomy). The esophagus is removed through the laparoscopic abdominal access site and is divided from the stomach. The stomach is anastomosed to the pharynx or the remaining cervical esophagus via the open cervical incision. The laparoscopic instruments are removed and all incisions are repaired in sutured layers. In 43287, the physician removes the distal two-thirds of the esophagus utilizing a combination of laparoscopic and thoracoscopic approaches. Also referred to as a laparoscopic/thoracoscopic Ivor Lewis esophagectomy, this procedure involves laparoscopic access to mobilize portions of the lower esophagus and stomach, to resect a portion of the proximal stomach and celiac axis lymph nodes, and to create a gastric

tube. Following removal of the abdominal trocars and closure of the trocar sites by layered suture, the patient is repositioned and the physician places appropriate trocars for separate thoracoscopic access to the chest. Via upper thoracoscopic technique, the physician mobilizes the middle and upper mediastinal esophagus. The esophagus is divided above the level of the azygos vein and the proximal esophageal margin is submitted for frozen-section pathological confirmation that no tumor remains. The distal esophagus and previously formed gastric conduit are brought into the chest. The thoracoscopic port is enlarged, the specimen is removed, and the gastric margin is evaluated by frozen-section pathology to confirm that it is tumor-free. The physician creates a side-to-side esophagogastric anastomosis. Chest tubes and drains are placed, trocars are removed, and trocar sites repaired with layered sutures. In 43288, the physician removes all or most of the esophagus utilizing a combination of laparoscopic, thoracoscopic, and open cervical approaches. The physician gains access to the esophagus through an oblique cervical incision. The esophagus is divided at the cervical level (for an esophagogastrostomy) or at its origin at the pharynx (for a pharyngogastrostomy). Using a laparoscopic approach, the physician mobilizes the stomach and performs a proximal gastrectomy. Utilizing a separate thoracoscopic approach, the physician mobilizes the upper, middle, and lower mediastinal esophagus and performs the appropriate resection. Anastomosis is performed via the open cervical incision. Laparoscopic pyloric drainage is included in all three techniques, when performed.

Coding Tips

Do not report 43287 or 43288 with 32551 when reporting a right tube thoracostomy.

ICD-10-CM Diagnostic Codes

C15.3	Malignant neoplasm of upper third of esophagus
C15.4	Malignant neoplasm of middle third of esophagus
C15.5	Malignant neoplasm of lower third of esophagus
C15.8	Malignant neoplasm of overlapping sites of esophagus
C16.0	Malignant neoplasm of cardia
C49.A1	Gastrointestinal stromal tumor of esophagus
C7A.092	Malignant carcinoid tumor of the stomach
C7A.094	Malignant carcinoid tumor of the foregut, unspecified
D3A.092	Benign carcinoid tumor of the stomach
D3A.094	Benign carcinoid tumor of the foregut, unspecified
K22.2	Esophageal obstruction
K22.3	Perforation of esophagus
K22.4	Dyskinesia of esophagus
K22.70	Barrett's esophagus without dysplasia
K22.710	Barrett's esophagus with low grade dysplasia
K22.711	Barrett's esophagus with high grade dysplasia
K22.89	Other specified disease of esophagus
K31.1	Adult hypertrophic pyloric stenosis ◩
Q39.1	Atresia of esophagus with tracheo-esophageal fistula
Q39.8	Other congenital malformations of esophagus
T28.1XXA	Burn of esophagus, initial encounter
T28.6XXA	Corrosion of esophagus, initial encounter

AMA: **43286** 2018,Jul,7 **43287** 2018,Jul,7 **43288** 2018,Jul,7

Esophagus

Relative Value Units/Medicare Edits

Non-Facility RVU	Work	PE	MP	Total
43286	55.0	25.45	13.0	93.45
43287	63.0	26.74	14.79	104.53
43288	66.42	28.37	15.27	110.06
Facility RVU	Work	PE	MP	Total
43286	55.0	25.45	13.0	93.45
43287	63.0	26.74	14.79	104.53
43288	66.42	28.37	15.27	110.06

	FUD	Status	MUE	Modifiers				IOM Reference
43286	90	A	1(2)	51	N/A	62*	80	None
43287	90	A	1(2)	51	N/A	62	80	
43288	90	A	1(2)	51	N/A	62	80	

* with documentation

Terms To Know

achalasia. Failure of the smooth muscles within the gastrointestinal tract to relax at points of junction; most commonly referring to the esophagogastric sphincter's failure to relax when swallowing.

distal. Located farther away from a specified reference point or the trunk.

gastrectomy. Surgical excision of all or part of the stomach.

proximal. Located closest to a specified reference point, usually the midline or trunk.

43300-43305

43300 Esophagoplasty (plastic repair or reconstruction), cervical approach; without repair of tracheoesophageal fistula
43305   with repair of tracheoesophageal fistula

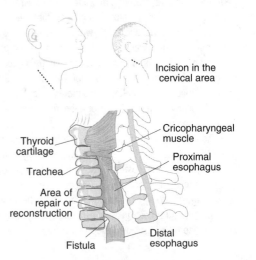

Incision in the cervical area

Thyroid cartilage

Cricopharyngeal muscle

Trachea

Proximal esophagus

Area of repair or reconstruction

Fistula

Distal esophagus

Example of esophageal atresia where the proximal esophagus fails to communicate with the lower portion; note that a fistula has developed from the trachea

Explanation

The physician repairs a defect in the esophagus using plastic repair or reconstruction. The physician makes a lateral neck incision to access the esophagus. The defect is identified and repaired. In 43305, the physician also transects the tracheoesophageal fistula. The physician closes the tracheal opening and repairs the esophagus. The incision is sutured in layers.

Coding Tips

If significant additional time and effort is documented, append modifier 22 and submit a cover letter and operative report. For esophagoplasty, thoracic approach, without repair of tracheoesophageal fistula, see 43310. For suture of an esophageal wound or injury, cervical approach, see 43410.

ICD-10-CM Diagnostic Codes

C15.3	Malignant neoplasm of upper third of esophagus
C15.4	Malignant neoplasm of middle third of esophagus
C15.5	Malignant neoplasm of lower third of esophagus
C15.8	Malignant neoplasm of overlapping sites of esophagus
D00.1	Carcinoma in situ of esophagus
D13.0	Benign neoplasm of esophagus
J95.04	Tracheo-esophageal fistula following tracheostomy
K22.10	Ulcer of esophagus without bleeding
K22.11	Ulcer of esophagus with bleeding
K22.2	Esophageal obstruction
K22.3	Perforation of esophagus
K22.4	Dyskinesia of esophagus
K22.5	Diverticulum of esophagus, acquired
K22.6	Gastro-esophageal laceration-hemorrhage syndrome
K22.70	Barrett's esophagus without dysplasia
K22.710	Barrett's esophagus with low grade dysplasia
K22.711	Barrett's esophagus with high grade dysplasia

Esophagus

N Newborn: 0   **P Pediatric: 0-17**   **M Maternity: 9-64**   **A Adult: 15-124**   ♂ **Male Only**   ♀ **Female Only**

Coding Companion for General Surgery/Gastroenterology

K22.89	Other specified disease of esophagus	
Q39.0	Atresia of esophagus without fistula	
Q39.1	Atresia of esophagus with tracheo-esophageal fistula	
Q39.2	Congenital tracheo-esophageal fistula without atresia	
Q39.3	Congenital stenosis and stricture of esophagus	
Q39.4	Esophageal web	
Q40.1	Congenital hiatus hernia	
Q40.8	Other specified congenital malformations of upper alimentary tract	
S27.813A	Laceration of esophagus (thoracic part), initial encounter	
S27.818A	Other injury of esophagus (thoracic part), initial encounter	
T18.190A	Other foreign object in esophagus causing compression of trachea, initial encounter	
T18.198A	Other foreign object in esophagus causing other injury, initial encounter	

AMA: **43300** 2014,Jan,11 **43305** 2014,Jan,11

Relative Value Units/Medicare Edits

Non-Facility RVU	Work	PE	MP	Total
43300	9.33	7.49	1.29	18.11
43305	18.1	11.15	2.71	31.96
Facility RVU	**Work**	**PE**	**MP**	**Total**
43300	9.33	7.49	1.29	18.11
43305	18.1	11.15	2.71	31.96

	FUD	Status	MUE	Modifiers				IOM Reference
43300	90	A	1(2)	51	N/A	62*	80	None
43305	90	A	1(2)	51	N/A	62*	80	

* with documentation

Terms To Know

approach. Method or anatomical location used to gain access to a body organ or specific area for procedures.

tracheoesophageal fistula. Abnormal opening between the trachea and the esophagus. There are three types of tracheoesophageal fistulas; congenital, formed from a previous tracheostomy, and fistula not caused by previous surgery.

43310-43312

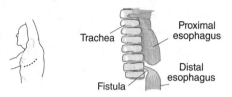

43310	Esophagoplasty (plastic repair or reconstruction), thoracic approach; without repair of tracheoesophageal fistula
43312	with repair of tracheoesophageal fistula

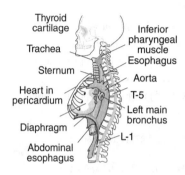

Detail of area of repair or reconstruction (atresia and fistula)

Explanation

The physician repairs a defect in the esophagus using plastic repair or reconstruction. The physician makes a thoracic incision to access the esophagus. In 43310, the defect is identified and repaired. In 43312, the physician also transects the tracheoesophageal fistula. The physician closes the tracheal opening and repairs the esophagus. The incision is sutured in layers.

Coding Tips

If significant additional time and effort are documented, append modifier 22 and submit a cover letter and operative report. For esophagoplasty, cervical approach, without repair of tracheoesophageal fistula, see 43300; with repair of tracheoesophageal fistula, see 43305. For suture of esophageal wound or injury, cervical approach, see 43410; transthoracic or transabdominal approach, see 43415.

ICD-10-CM Diagnostic Codes

C15.3	Malignant neoplasm of upper third of esophagus
C15.4	Malignant neoplasm of middle third of esophagus
C15.5	Malignant neoplasm of lower third of esophagus
C15.8	Malignant neoplasm of overlapping sites of esophagus
D00.1	Carcinoma in situ of esophagus
D13.0	Benign neoplasm of esophagus
J95.04	Tracheo-esophageal fistula following tracheostomy
K22.10	Ulcer of esophagus without bleeding
K22.11	Ulcer of esophagus with bleeding
K22.2	Esophageal obstruction
K22.3	Perforation of esophagus
K22.4	Dyskinesia of esophagus
K22.5	Diverticulum of esophagus, acquired
K22.6	Gastro-esophageal laceration-hemorrhage syndrome
K22.70	Barrett's esophagus without dysplasia

Esophagus

K22.710	Barrett's esophagus with low grade dysplasia	
K22.711	Barrett's esophagus with high grade dysplasia	
K22.89	Other specified disease of esophagus	
K44.0	Diaphragmatic hernia with obstruction, without gangrene	
K44.1	Diaphragmatic hernia with gangrene	
K44.9	Diaphragmatic hernia without obstruction or gangrene	
Q39.0	Atresia of esophagus without fistula	
Q39.1	Atresia of esophagus with tracheo-esophageal fistula	
Q39.2	Congenital tracheo-esophageal fistula without atresia	
Q39.3	Congenital stenosis and stricture of esophagus	
Q39.4	Esophageal web	
Q40.1	Congenital hiatus hernia	
Q40.8	Other specified congenital malformations of upper alimentary tract	
S27.813A	Laceration of esophagus (thoracic part), initial encounter	
S27.818A	Other injury of esophagus (thoracic part), initial encounter	
T18.190A	Other foreign object in esophagus causing compression of trachea, initial encounter	
T18.198A	Other foreign object in esophagus causing other injury, initial encounter	

AMA: **43310** 2014,Jan,11 **43312** 2014,Jan,11

Relative Value Units/Medicare Edits

Non-Facility RVU	Work	PE	MP	Total
43310	26.26	11.16	6.03	43.45
43312	29.25	10.58	6.7	46.53
Facility RVU	**Work**	**PE**	**MP**	**Total**
43310	26.26	11.16	6.03	43.45
43312	29.25	10.58	6.7	46.53

	FUD	Status	MUE	Modifiers				IOM Reference
43310	90	A	1(2)	51	N/A	62*	80	None
43312	90	A	1(2)	51	N/A	62*	80	

* with documentation

43313-43314

43313	Esophagoplasty for congenital defect (plastic repair or reconstruction), thoracic approach; without repair of congenital tracheoesophageal fistula
43314	with repair of congenital tracheoesophageal fistula

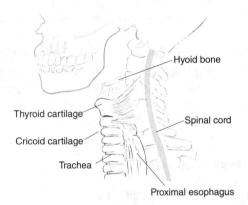

Explanation

There are multiple types of material and methods that may be used to repair the esophagus, including autologous grafts, nonautologous grafts, patches, and gastric tubes. In the case of an autologous graft, the graft or patch may be harvested from the patient's intestine or colon depending on the anatomy and vasculature. The patient is positioned for a right posterolateral incision at the sixth rib region. A muscle-sparing incision is made and an extrapleural approach is used to gain access to the esophageal anomaly. The anomalous part of the esophagus is opened longitudinally with significant margins above and below the affected area. The graft, patch, or tube is placed over the defect and sutured into place. Report 43314 when a transesophageal fistula is also present and repaired.

Coding Tips

If significant additional time and effort are documented, append modifier 22 and submit a cover letter and operative report. When these codes are performed with another separately identifiable procedure, the highest dollar value code is listed as the primary procedure and subsequent procedures are appended with modifier 51. For esophagoplasty, cervical approach, without repair of tracheoesophageal fistula, see 43300; with repair of tracheoesophageal fistula, see 43305; via thoracic approach, without repair of tracheoesophageal fistula, see 43310; with repair of tracheoesophageal fistula, see 43312. Do not append modifier 63 to these codes as the description or nature of the procedure includes infants up to 4 kg.

ICD-10-CM Diagnostic Codes

Q39.0	Atresia of esophagus without fistula
Q39.1	Atresia of esophagus with tracheo-esophageal fistula
Q39.2	Congenital tracheo-esophageal fistula without atresia
Q39.3	Congenital stenosis and stricture of esophagus
Q39.4	Esophageal web
Q39.5	Congenital dilatation of esophagus
Q39.6	Congenital diverticulum of esophagus
Q39.8	Other congenital malformations of esophagus
Q40.1	Congenital hiatus hernia
Q40.8	Other specified congenital malformations of upper alimentary tract

Relative Value Units/Medicare Edits

Non-Facility RVU	Work	PE	MP	Total
43313	48.45	20.46	11.12	80.03
43314	53.43	20.42	12.28	86.13
Facility RVU	**Work**	**PE**	**MP**	**Total**
43313	48.45	20.46	11.12	80.03
43314	53.43	20.42	12.28	86.13

	FUD	Status	MUE	Modifiers				IOM Reference
43313	90	A	1(2)	51	N/A	62*	80	None
43314	90	A	1(2)	51	N/A	62*	80	

* with documentation

Terms To Know

atresia. Congenital closure or absence of a tubular organ or an opening to the body surface.

autologous. Tissue, cells, or structure obtained from the same individual.

congenital. Present at birth, occurring through heredity or an influence during gestation up to the moment of birth.

dissect. Cut apart or separate tissue for surgical purposes or for visual or microscopic study.

esophagus. Muscular tube that carries swallowed liquids and foods from the pharynx to the stomach.

fistula. Abnormal tube-like passage between two body cavities or organs or from an organ to the outside surface.

graft. Tissue implant from another part of the body or another person.

harvest. Removal of cells or tissue from their native site to be used as a graft or transplant to another part of the donor's body or placed into another person.

hernia. Protrusion of a body structure through tissue.

stenosis. Narrowing or constriction of a passage.

43320

43320   Esophagogastrostomy (cardioplasty), with or without vagotomy and pyloroplasty, transabdominal or transthoracic approach

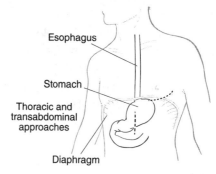

Esophagus

Stomach

Thoracic and transabdominal approaches

Diaphragm

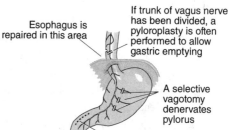

Esophagus is repaired in this area

If trunk of vagus nerve has been divided, a pyloroplasty is often performed to allow gastric emptying

A selective vagotomy denervates pylorus

Typical area of incision for pyloroplasty

Explanation

The physician performs a plastic repair of the lower esophagus where it joins the upper area (cardia) of the stomach. The physician may also transect the vagus nerve and/or enlarge the pylorus, the distal portion of the stomach. The physician accesses the esophagus through an upper abdominal or lateral thoracic incision. The diseased portion of the esophagus is resected. An anastomosis between the esophageal stump and the cardiac portion of the stomach is created. If the lesion is secondary to acid reflux, a vagotomy may be performed. The anterior and posterior trunks of the vagus nerve are transected to decrease acid production. If the gastric outlet area is decreased, a pyloroplasty may be performed to enlarge the pylorus. The incision is repaired in sutured layers.

Coding Tips

Vagotomy and pyloroplasty are included in this procedure, when performed, and should not be reported separately. For laparoscopic procedure, see 43280. For vagotomy including pyloroplasty, with or without gastrostomy, see 43640–43641. For pyloroplasty alone, see 43800; vagotomy alone, see 64755–64760.

ICD-10-CM Diagnostic Codes

C15.3	Malignant neoplasm of upper third of esophagus
C15.4	Malignant neoplasm of middle third of esophagus
C15.5	Malignant neoplasm of lower third of esophagus
C16.0	Malignant neoplasm of cardia
C7A.092	Malignant carcinoid tumor of the stomach
D00.1	Carcinoma in situ of esophagus
D00.2	Carcinoma in situ of stomach
I85.00	Esophageal varices without bleeding
I85.01	Esophageal varices with bleeding
I85.10	Secondary esophageal varices without bleeding
I85.11	Secondary esophageal varices with bleeding

Esophagus

K22.0	Achalasia of cardia
K22.10	Ulcer of esophagus without bleeding
K22.11	Ulcer of esophagus with bleeding
K22.2	Esophageal obstruction
K22.3	Perforation of esophagus
K22.70	Barrett's esophagus without dysplasia
K22.710	Barrett's esophagus with low grade dysplasia
K22.711	Barrett's esophagus with high grade dysplasia
Q39.0	Atresia of esophagus without fistula
Q39.1	Atresia of esophagus with tracheo-esophageal fistula
Q39.2	Congenital tracheo-esophageal fistula without atresia
Q39.3	Congenital stenosis and stricture of esophagus
Q39.4	Esophageal web
Q39.5	Congenital dilatation of esophagus
Q39.6	Congenital diverticulum of esophagus
Q39.8	Other congenital malformations of esophagus
S27.812A	Contusion of esophagus (thoracic part), initial encounter
S27.813A	Laceration of esophagus (thoracic part), initial encounter
S27.818A	Other injury of esophagus (thoracic part), initial encounter
T18.190A	Other foreign object in esophagus causing compression of trachea, initial encounter
T18.198A	Other foreign object in esophagus causing other injury, initial encounter

AMA: **43320** 2014,Jan,11

Relative Value Units/Medicare Edits

Non-Facility RVU	Work	PE	MP	Total
43320	23.31	12.35	5.69	41.35
Facility RVU	**Work**	**PE**	**MP**	**Total**
43320	23.31	12.35	5.69	41.35

	FUD	Status	MUE	Modifiers				IOM Reference
43320	90	A	1(2)	51	N/A	62*	80	None

* with documentation

Terms To Know

carcinoma in situ. Malignancy that arises from the cells of the vessel, gland, or organ of origin that remains confined to that site or has not invaded neighboring tissue.

pyloroplasty. Enlargement and reconstruction of the lower portion of the stomach opening into the duodenum performed after vagotomy to speed gastric emptying and treat duodenal ulcers.

stenosis. Narrowing or constriction of a passage.

vagotomy. Division of the vagus nerves, interrupting impulses resulting in lower gastric acid production and hastening gastric emptying.

43325

43325 Esophagogastric fundoplasty, with fundic patch (Thal-Nissen procedure)

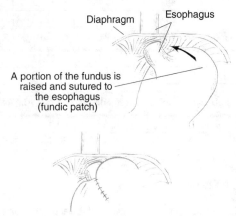

Diaphragm   Esophagus

A portion of the fundus is raised and sutured to the esophagus (fundic patch)

A Nissen type procedure is then typically performed

Explanation

The physician pulls up part of the gastric fundus to cover the affected distal esophagus. A bougie (dilating instrument) is placed in the distal esophagus to maintain the esophageal opening. The physician accesses the esophagus and stomach through a transverse abdominal incision. The physician picks up the stomach 1 cm below the gastroesophageal (GE) junction and attaches it 1 cm above the GE junction. This fundic patch is sutured to the esophagus. Next, a Nissen fundoplication is performed by wrapping the rest of the fundus around the esophagus and suturing it into place. The incision is sutured in layers.

Coding Tips

If significant additional time and effort are documented, append modifier 22 and submit a cover letter and operative report. For cricopharyngeal myotomy, see 43030. For esophagogastric fundoplasty, see 43327 and 43328. For laparoscopic esophagogastric fundoplasty (e.g., Nissen, Toupet procedure), see 43280.

ICD-10-CM Diagnostic Codes

K20.0	Eosinophilic esophagitis
K21.00	Gastro-esophageal reflux disease with esophagitis, without bleeding
K21.01	Gastro-esophageal reflux disease with esophagitis, with bleeding
K21.9	Gastro-esophageal reflux disease without esophagitis
K22.10	Ulcer of esophagus without bleeding
K22.11	Ulcer of esophagus with bleeding
K22.2	Esophageal obstruction
K22.70	Barrett's esophagus without dysplasia
K22.710	Barrett's esophagus with low grade dysplasia
K22.711	Barrett's esophagus with high grade dysplasia
K44.0	Diaphragmatic hernia with obstruction, without gangrene
K44.9	Diaphragmatic hernia without obstruction or gangrene
Q39.0	Atresia of esophagus without fistula
Q39.1	Atresia of esophagus with tracheo-esophageal fistula
Q39.2	Congenital tracheo-esophageal fistula without atresia
Q39.3	Congenital stenosis and stricture of esophagus
Q39.5	Congenital dilatation of esophagus

Esophagus

Q39.6   Congenital diverticulum of esophagus

Q39.8   Other congenital malformations of esophagus

AMA: 43325 2014,Jan,11

Relative Value Units/Medicare Edits

Non-Facility RVU	Work	PE	MP	Total
43325	22.6	12.09	5.53	40.22
Facility RVU	**Work**	**PE**	**MP**	**Total**
43325	22.6	12.09	5.53	40.22

	FUD	Status	MUE	Modifiers				IOM Reference
43325	90	A	1(2)	51	N/A	62*	80	None

* with documentation

Terms To Know

bougie. Probe used to dilate or calibrate a body part.

distal. Located farther away from a specified reference point or the trunk.

esophagus. Muscular tube that carries swallowed liquids and foods from the pharynx to the stomach.

Nissen procedure (fundoplasty). Surgical repair technique that involves the fundus of the stomach being wrapped around the lower end of the esophagus to treat reflux esophagitis.

transverse. Crosswise at right angles to the long axis of a structure or part.

43327-43328

43327	Esophagogastric fundoplasty partial or complete; laparotomy
43328	thoracotomy

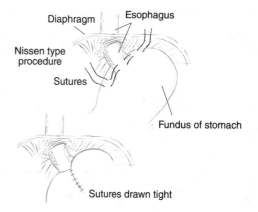

Explanation

The physician performs a partial or complete fundoplasty by an incision in the abdominal wall (43327) or an incision through the chest cavity (43328). Through this incision, the fundus of the stomach is wrapped around the lower 4 cm of the esophagus and sutured into position. This allows the sphincter at the distal end of the esophagus to pass through a small area within the stomach muscle, creating a new valve that prevents reflux.

Coding Tips

The Nissen fundoplasty is the most frequently performed with a 360-degree wrap of the stomach fundus around the gastroesophageal (GE) junction. A Toupet fundoplasty (modified Nissen) is a partial 270-degree wrap. For laparoscopic esophagogastric fundoplasty, see 43280. The Belsey IV is performed through a posterolateral thoracotomy, 240-degree wrap. The open Hill (median arcuate ligament repair) uses sutures to anchor the GE junction (posterior gastropexy). It does not use wrapping to accomplish the repair. If additional time and effort is documented, append modifier 22 and submit a cover letter and operative report. For transoral esophagogastroduodenoscopy fundoplasty, partial or complete, see 43210. For esophagogastric fundoplasty with a fundic patch (Thal-Nissen procedure), see 43325. For a cricopharyngeal myotomy, see 43030.

ICD-10-CM Diagnostic Codes

K20.0	Eosinophilic esophagitis
K21.00	Gastro-esophageal reflux disease with esophagitis, without bleeding
K21.01	Gastro-esophageal reflux disease with esophagitis, with bleeding
K21.9	Gastro-esophageal reflux disease without esophagitis
K22.10	Ulcer of esophagus without bleeding
K22.11	Ulcer of esophagus with bleeding
K22.2	Esophageal obstruction
K22.70	Barrett's esophagus without dysplasia
K22.710	Barrett's esophagus with low grade dysplasia
K22.711	Barrett's esophagus with high grade dysplasia
Q39.0	Atresia of esophagus without fistula
Q39.1	Atresia of esophagus with tracheo-esophageal fistula
Q39.2	Congenital tracheo-esophageal fistula without atresia
Q39.3	Congenital stenosis and stricture of esophagus
Q39.5	Congenital dilatation of esophagus

Q39.6   Congenital diverticulum of esophagus

Q39.8   Other congenital malformations of esophagus

AMA: **43327** 2018,Jan,8; 2017,Jan,8; 2016,Jan,13; 2015,Nov,8; 2015,Jan,16
43328 2018,Jan,8; 2017,Jan,8; 2016,Jan,13; 2015,Nov,8; 2015,Jan,16

Relative Value Units/Medicare Edits

Non-Facility RVU	Work	PE	MP	Total
43327	13.35	7.68	3.18	24.21
43328	19.91	8.5	4.56	32.97
Facility RVU	Work	PE	MP	Total
43327	13.35	7.68	3.18	24.21
43328	19.91	8.5	4.56	32.97

	FUD	Status	MUE	Modifiers				IOM Reference
43327	90	A	1(2)	51	N/A	62*	80	None
43328	90	A	1(2)	51	N/A	62*	80	

* with documentation

Terms To Know

distal. Located farther away from a specified reference point or the trunk.

esophagogastric fundoplasty. See Nissen procedure.

laparotomy. Incision through the flank or abdomen for therapeutic or diagnostic purposes.

Nissen procedure (fundoplasty). Surgical repair technique that involves the fundus of the stomach being wrapped around the lower end of the esophagus to treat reflux esophagitis.

reflux. Return or backward flow.

sphincter. Ring-like band of muscle that surrounds a bodily opening, constricting and relaxing as required for normal physiological functioning.

thoracotomy. Surgical procedure for opening the chest wall in order to access the lungs, esophagus, trachea, aorta, heart, and diaphragm.

43330-43331

43330   Esophagomyotomy (Heller type); abdominal approach

43331   thoracic approach

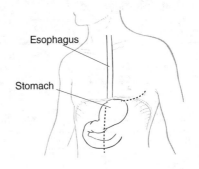

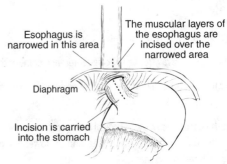

This relaxes the stricture in the esophagus

Explanation

The esophagus is repaired using a fundic flap. The physician accesses the esophagus through an upper abdominal or a thoracic incision. For an abdominal approach, report 43330. For a thoracic approach, report 43331. The physician makes an incision into the muscular layers of the distal esophagus and cardia of the stomach (myotomy), leaving a gastric fundic flap. The flap is pulled along the esophagus, and sutured onto the margins of the myotomy. Repair of a hiatal hernia is performed by restoring the herniated portion of the stomach back to the abdomen, then narrowing the hiatal opening of the diaphragm by suturing the left and right crura together. All incisions are sutured in layers.

Coding Tips

If significant additional time and effort are documented, append modifier 22 and submit a cover letter and operative report. Esophagomyotomy via laparoscopy, see 43279; via thoracoscopy, see 32665. For fundoplasty, see 43327–43328. For diverticulectomy of hypopharynx or esophagus, with or without myotomy, see 43130–43135.

ICD-10-CM Diagnostic Codes

C15.4	Malignant neoplasm of middle third of esophagus
C15.5	Malignant neoplasm of lower third of esophagus
C15.8	Malignant neoplasm of overlapping sites of esophagus
K21.00	Gastro-esophageal reflux disease with esophagitis, without bleeding
K21.01	Gastro-esophageal reflux disease with esophagitis, with bleeding
K21.9	Gastro-esophageal reflux disease without esophagitis
K22.0	Achalasia of cardia
K22.10	Ulcer of esophagus without bleeding
K22.11	Ulcer of esophagus with bleeding

Esophagus

K22.2	Esophageal obstruction
K22.3	Perforation of esophagus
K22.5	Diverticulum of esophagus, acquired
K22.70	Barrett's esophagus without dysplasia
K22.710	Barrett's esophagus with low grade dysplasia
K22.711	Barrett's esophagus with high grade dysplasia
K22.89	Other specified disease of esophagus
Q39.5	Congenital dilatation of esophagus
Q39.6	Congenital diverticulum of esophagus
Q39.8	Other congenital malformations of esophagus

AMA: **43330** 2018,Jan,8; 2017,Jan,8; 2016,Jan,13; 2015,Jan,16 **43331** 2018,Jan,8; 2017,Jan,8; 2016,Jan,13; 2015,Jan,16

Relative Value Units/Medicare Edits

Non-Facility RVU	Work	PE	MP	Total
43330	22.19	11.94	5.45	39.58
43331	23.06	10.92	5.29	39.27
Facility RVU	Work	PE	MP	Total
43330	22.19	11.94	5.45	39.58
43331	23.06	10.92	5.29	39.27

	FUD	Status	MUE	Modifiers				IOM Reference
43330	90	A	1(2)	51	N/A	62*	80	None
43331	90	A	1(2)	51	N/A	62*	80	

* with documentation

Terms To Know

achalasia. Failure of the smooth muscles within the gastrointestinal tract to relax at points of junction; most commonly referring to the esophagogastric sphincter's failure to relax when swallowing.

approach. Method or anatomical location used to gain access to a body organ or specific area for procedures.

diverticulum. Pouch or sac in the walls of an organ or canal.

fistula. Abnormal tube-like passage between two body cavities or organs or from an organ to the outside surface.

Heller myotomy. Longitudinal division of the distal esophageal muscle down to the submucosal layer. Cardia muscle fibers may also be divided. This procedure is used to treat achalasia.

stenosis. Narrowing or constriction of a passage.

43332-43333

43332 Repair, paraesophageal hiatal hernia (including fundoplication), via laparotomy, except neonatal; without implantation of mesh or other prosthesis

43333 with implantation of mesh or other prosthesis

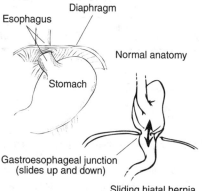

Explanation

The physician repairs a non-neonatal paraesophageal hiatal hernia via open approach in 43332. A paraesophageal hernia occurs when a portion of the stomach passes through the hiatus and rests in the chest next to the esophagus. The physician makes an incision into the abdomen, pulls the stomach back down into the correct position, and sutures it to the rectus sheath. The diaphragm is often secured with sutures and the hiatus is sutured along the gastroesophageal junction. Fundoplication is performed to prevent the stomach from moving out of position again. Report 43333 when mesh is sutured to the abdominal wall over the defect during the repair.

Coding Tips

For paraesophageal hiatal hernia repair via thoracotomy, see 43334–43335; via thoracoabdominal incision, see 43336–43337. For esophageal lengthening procedure (Collis gastroplasty) in addition to this procedure, see 43338. To report a neonatal diaphragmatic hernia repair, see 39503. If significant additional time and effort are documented, append modifier 22 and submit a cover letter and operative report.

ICD-10-CM Diagnostic Codes

K44.0	Diaphragmatic hernia with obstruction, without gangrene
K44.1	Diaphragmatic hernia with gangrene
K44.9	Diaphragmatic hernia without obstruction or gangrene
Q40.1	Congenital hiatus hernia
Q79.0	Congenital diaphragmatic hernia

AMA: **43332** 2018,Jan,8; 2017,Jan,8; 2016,Jan,13; 2015,Jan,16 **43333** 2018,Jan,8; 2017,Jan,8; 2016,Jan,13; 2015,Jan,16

Esophagus

Relative Value Units/Medicare Edits

Non-Facility RVU	Work	PE	MP	Total
43332	19.62	9.76	4.6	33.98
43333	21.46	10.67	5.11	37.24
Facility RVU	Work	PE	MP	Total
43332	19.62	9.76	4.6	33.98
43333	21.46	10.67	5.11	37.24

	FUD	Status	MUE	Modifiers				IOM Reference
43332	90	A	1(2)	51	N/A	62*	80	None
43333	90	A	1(2)	51	N/A	62*	80	

* with documentation

Terms To Know

acquired. Produced by outside influences and not by genetics or birth defect.

approach. Method or anatomical location used to gain access to a body organ or specific area for procedures. The approach is not coded separately although it may be a specified component of the procedure, such as laparoscopic versus incisional, or spinal procedures in which the amount of dissection required to expose the spine significantly alters with the site of approach.

congenital. Present at birth, occurring through heredity or an influence during gestation up to the moment of birth.

hiatal hernia. Protrusion of an abdominal organ, usually the stomach, through the esophageal opening within the diaphragm and occurring in two types: the sliding hiatal hernia and the paraesophageal hernia.

implant. Material or device inserted or placed within the body for therapeutic, reconstructive, or diagnostic purposes.

laparotomy. Incision through the flank or abdomen for therapeutic or diagnostic purposes.

mesh. Synthetic fabric used as a prosthetic patch in hernia repair.

prosthesis. Device that replaces all or part of an internal body organ or replaces all or part of the function of a permanently inoperative or malfunctioning internal body organ.

pyloroplasty. Enlargement and reconstruction of the lower portion of the stomach opening into the duodenum performed after vagotomy to speed gastric emptying and treat duodenal ulcers.

repair. Surgical closure of a wound. The wound may be a result of injury/trauma or it may be a surgically created defect. Repairs are divided into three categories: simple, intermediate, and complex.

43334-43335

43334   Repair, paraesophageal hiatal hernia (including fundoplication), via thoracotomy, except neonatal; without implantation of mesh or other prosthesis

43335   with implantation of mesh or other prosthesis

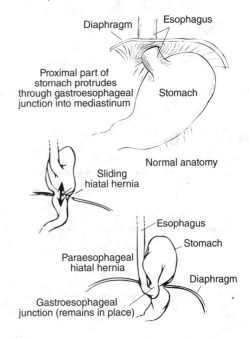

Explanation

The physician repairs a non-neonatal paraesophageal hiatal hernia via thoracotomy approach in 43334. A paraesophageal hernia occurs when a portion of the stomach passes through the hiatus and rests in the chest next to the esophagus. The physician makes the incision into the chest wall. The physician pulls the stomach back down into the abdomen and sutures it to the rectus sheath. The diaphragm is often secured with sutures and the hiatus is sutured along the gastroesophageal junction. Fundoplication is performed to prevent the stomach from moving out of position again. Report 43335 when mesh is sutured to the abdominal wall over the defect.

Coding Tips

For paraesophageal hiatal hernia repair via laparotomy, see 43332–43333; via thoracoabdominal incision, see 43336–43337. For esophageal lengthening procedure (Collis gastroplasty) in addition to this procedure, see 43338. To report a neonatal diaphragmatic hernia repair, see 39503. If significant additional time and effort are documented, append modifier 22 and submit a cover letter and operative report.

ICD-10-CM Diagnostic Codes

K44.0	Diaphragmatic hernia with obstruction, without gangrene
K44.1	Diaphragmatic hernia with gangrene
K44.9	Diaphragmatic hernia without obstruction or gangrene
Q40.1	Congenital hiatus hernia
Q79.0	Congenital diaphragmatic hernia

AMA: 43334 2018,Jan,8; 2017,Jan,8; 2016,Jan,13; 2015,Jan,16 **43335** 2018,Jan,8; 2017,Jan,8; 2016,Jan,13; 2015,Jan,16

Relative Value Units/Medicare Edits

Non-Facility RVU	Work	PE	MP	Total
43334	22.12	9.46	5.04	36.62
43335	23.97	9.67	5.51	39.15
Facility RVU	Work	PE	MP	Total
43334	22.12	9.46	5.04	36.62
43335	23.97	9.67	5.51	39.15

	FUD	Status	MUE	Modifiers				IOM Reference
43334	90	A	1(2)	51	N/A	62*	80	None
43335	90	A	1(2)	51	N/A	62*	80	

* with documentation

Terms To Know

approach. Method or anatomical location used to gain access to a body organ or specific area for procedures. The approach is not coded separately although it may be a specified component of the procedure, such as laparoscopic versus incisional, or spinal procedures in which the amount of dissection required to expose the spine significantly alters with the site of approach.

congenital. Present at birth, occurring through heredity or an influence during gestation up to the moment of birth.

gangrene. Death of tissue, usually resulting from a loss of vascular supply, followed by a bacterial attack or onset of disease.

hiatal hernia. Protrusion of an abdominal organ, usually the stomach, through the esophageal opening within the diaphragm and occurring in two types: the sliding hiatal hernia and the paraesophageal hernia.

implant. Material or device inserted or placed within the body for therapeutic, reconstructive, or diagnostic purposes.

mesh. Synthetic fabric used as a prosthetic patch in hernia repair.

neonatal period. Period of an infant's life from birth to the age of 27 days, 23 hours, and 59 minutes.

prosthesis. Device that replaces all or part of an internal body organ or replaces all or part of the function of a permanently inoperative or malfunctioning internal body organ.

thoracotomy. Surgical procedure for opening the chest wall in order to access the lungs, esophagus, trachea, aorta, heart, and diaphragm.

43336-43337

43336 Repair, paraesophageal hiatal hernia, (including fundoplication), via thoracoabdominal incision, except neonatal; without implantation of mesh or other prosthesis

43337 with implantation of mesh or other prosthesis

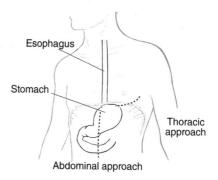

Esophagus
Stomach
Thoracic approach
Abdominal approach

Explanation

The physician repairs a non-neonatal paraesophageal hiatal hernia via thoracoabdominal incision in 43336. A paraesophageal hernia occurs when a portion of the stomach passes through the hiatus and rests in the chest next to the esophagus. The physician makes the incision into the chest wall and abdomen. The physician pulls the stomach back down into the abdomen and sutures it to the rectus sheath. The diaphragm is often secured with sutures and the hiatus is sutured along the gastroesophageal junction. Fundoplication is performed to prevent the stomach from moving out of position again. Report 43337 when mesh is sutured to the abdominal wall over the defect.

Coding Tips

For paraesophageal hiatal hernia repair via laparotomy, see 43332–43333; via thoracotomy, see 43334–43335. For esophageal lengthening procedure (Collis gastroplasty) in addition to this procedure, see 43338. To report a neonatal diaphragmatic hernia repair, see 39503. If significant additional time and effort are documented, append modifier 22 and submit a cover letter and operative report.

ICD-10-CM Diagnostic Codes

K44.0	Diaphragmatic hernia with obstruction, without gangrene
K44.1	Diaphragmatic hernia with gangrene
K44.9	Diaphragmatic hernia without obstruction or gangrene
Q40.1	Congenital hiatus hernia
Q79.0	Congenital diaphragmatic hernia

AMA: **43336** 2018,Jan,8; 2017,Jan,8; 2016,Jan,13; 2015,Jan,16 **43337** 2018,Jan,8; 2017,Jan,8; 2016,Jan,13; 2015,Jan,16

Relative Value Units/Medicare Edits

Non-Facility RVU	Work	PE	MP	Total
43336	25.81	10.79	5.94	42.54
43337	27.65	11.33	6.36	45.34
Facility RVU	Work	PE	MP	Total
43336	25.81	10.79	5.94	42.54
43337	27.65	11.33	6.36	45.34

	FUD	Status	MUE	Modifiers				IOM Reference
43336	90	A	1(2)	51	N/A	62*	80	None
43337	90	A	1(2)	51	N/A	62*	80	

* with documentation

Terms To Know

approach. Method or anatomical location used to gain access to a body organ or specific area for procedures. The approach is not coded separately although it may be a specified component of the procedure, such as laparoscopic versus incisional, or spinal procedures in which the amount of dissection required to expose the spine significantly alters with the site of approach.

hiatal hernia. Protrusion of an abdominal organ, usually the stomach, through the esophageal opening within the diaphragm and occurring in two types: the sliding hiatal hernia and the paraesophageal hernia.

incision. Act of cutting into tissue or an organ.

laparotomy. Incision through the flank or abdomen for therapeutic or diagnostic purposes.

mesh. Synthetic fabric used as a prosthetic patch in hernia repair.

neonatal period. Period of an infant's life from birth to the age of 27 days, 23 hours, and 59 minutes.

prosthesis. Device that replaces all or part of an internal body organ or replaces all or part of the function of a permanently inoperative or malfunctioning internal body organ.

repair. Surgical closure of a wound. The wound may be a result of injury/trauma or it may be a surgically created defect. Repairs are divided into three categories: simple, intermediate, and complex.

thoracotomy. Surgical procedure for opening the chest wall in order to access the lungs, esophagus, trachea, aorta, heart, and diaphragm.

vagotomy. Division of the vagus nerves, interrupting impulses resulting in lower gastric acid production and hastening gastric emptying.

43338

+ 43338 Esophageal lengthening procedure (eg, Collis gastroplasty or wedge gastroplasty) (List separately in addition to code for primary procedure)

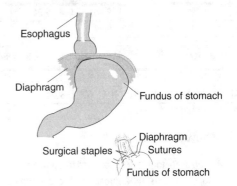

Collis procedure involves surgical staples along the stomach creating a longer esophagus

Explanation

In conjunction with a separately reportable fundoplasty procedure, the physician performs an esophageal lengthening procedure (also called a wedge gastroplasty) in order to extend a short esophagus. A bougie (dilating instrument) is passed through the esophagus into the stomach so that the bougie spans the gastroesophageal junction. The stomach is divided along the bougie with a gastric stapler, forming a gastric tube that effectively lengthens the esophagus.

Coding Tips

Report 43338 in addition to 43280 or 43327–43337.

ICD-10-CM Diagnostic Codes

This/these CPT code(s) are add-on code(s). See the primary procedure code that this code is performed with for your ICD-10-CM code selections.

AMA: **43338** 2018,Jan,8; 2017,Jan,8; 2016,Jan,13; 2015,Jan,16

Relative Value Units/Medicare Edits

Non-Facility RVU	Work	PE	MP	Total
43338	2.21	0.66	0.51	3.38
Facility RVU	Work	PE	MP	Total
43338	2.21	0.66	0.51	3.38

	FUD	Status	MUE	Modifiers				IOM Reference
43338	N/A	A	1(2)	N/A	N/A	62*	80	None

* with documentation

Terms To Know

bougie. Probe used to dilate or calibrate a body part.

Nissen procedure (fundoplasty). Surgical repair technique that involves the fundus of the stomach being wrapped around the lower end of the esophagus to treat reflux esophagitis.

Esophagus

43340-43341

43340 Esophagojejunostomy (without total gastrectomy); abdominal approach

43341   thoracic approach

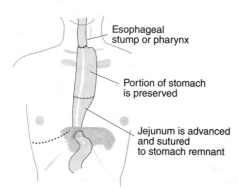

Esophageal stump or pharynx

Portion of stomach is preserved

Jejunum is advanced and sutured to stomach remnant

Explanation

The physician removes the affected esophagus and stomach, using the remaining stomach and jejunum to restore gastrointestinal continuity. The physician accesses the esophagus and stomach through an upper abdominal or a thoracic incision. For an abdominal approach, report 43340. For a thoracic approach, report 43341. The physician resects the affected part of the esophagus. The stomach is advanced through the hiatus and sutured to the esophageal remnant. The antral portion of the stomach is excised, and the proximal jejunum is sutured to the gastric remnant. The distal end of the duodenum is anastomosed to the jejunum; the proximal end of the duodenum is sutured closed to form a blind pouch. The incision is sutured in layers.

Coding Tips

For free jejunum transfer with microvascular anastomosis, see 43496. For total gastrectomy with formation of an intestinal pouch, any type, see 43622. For partial distal gastrectomy with gastroduodenostomy, see 43631; with gastrojejunostomy, see 43632.

ICD-10-CM Diagnostic Codes

C15.4	Malignant neoplasm of middle third of esophagus
C15.5	Malignant neoplasm of lower third of esophagus
C15.8	Malignant neoplasm of overlapping sites of esophagus
C16.0	Malignant neoplasm of cardia
C16.1	Malignant neoplasm of fundus of stomach
C16.2	Malignant neoplasm of body of stomach
C16.3	Malignant neoplasm of pyloric antrum
C16.4	Malignant neoplasm of pylorus
C16.8	Malignant neoplasm of overlapping sites of stomach
C7A.092	Malignant carcinoid tumor of the stomach
D13.0	Benign neoplasm of esophagus
D13.1	Benign neoplasm of stomach
D3A.092	Benign carcinoid tumor of the stomach
K20.0	Eosinophilic esophagitis
K21.00	Gastro-esophageal reflux disease with esophagitis, without bleeding
K21.01	Gastro-esophageal reflux disease with esophagitis, with bleeding
K25.4	Chronic or unspecified gastric ulcer with hemorrhage
K25.5	Chronic or unspecified gastric ulcer with perforation

AMA: **43340** 2014,Jan,11 **43341** 2014,Jan,11

Relative Value Units/Medicare Edits

Non-Facility RVU	Work	PE	MP	Total
43340	22.99	12.24	5.62	40.85
43341	24.23	11.26	5.56	41.05
Facility RVU	Work	PE	MP	Total
43340	22.99	12.24	5.62	40.85
43341	24.23	11.26	5.56	41.05

	FUD	Status	MUE	Modifiers				IOM Reference
43340	90	A	1(2)	51	N/A	62*	80	None
43341	90	A	1(2)	51	N/A	62*	80	

* with documentation

Terms To Know

anastomosis. Surgically created connection between ducts, blood vessels, or bowel segments to allow flow from one to the other.

approach. Method or anatomical location used to gain access to a body organ or specific area for procedures.

distal. Located farther away from a specified reference point or the trunk.

esophagus. Muscular tube that carries swallowed liquids and foods from the pharynx to the stomach.

jejunostomy. Permanent, surgical opening into the jejunum, the part of the small intestine between the duodenum and ileum, through the abdominal wall, often used for placing a feeding tube.

malignant. Any condition tending to progress toward death, specifically an invasive tumor with a loss of cellular differentiation that has the ability to spread or metastasize to other body areas.

proximal. Located closest to a specified reference point, usually the midline or trunk.

Esophagus

43351-43352

43351 Esophagostomy, fistulization of esophagus, external; thoracic approach
43352 cervical approach

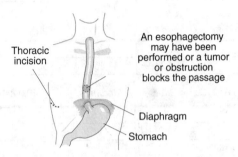

Thoracic incision

An esophagectomy may have been performed or a tumor or obstruction blocks the passage

Diaphragm

Stomach

Esophagus is incised and the upper portion is connected to the outside of the body, creating a fistula to drain mucous and saliva

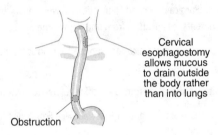

Cervical esophagostomy allows mucous to drain outside the body rather than into lungs

Obstruction

Explanation

The physician connects the esophagus to the exterior of the body, creating a fistula for drainage. In 43351, the physician uses a lateral thoracotomy to access the esophagus. In 43352, access is gained through a cervical incision. The physician makes an incision in the esophagus or the esophageal stump. The proximal limb of the esophagus is exteriorized and sutured into place, creating a connection from the exterior of the body to the esophageal lumen for mucus drainage. The incision is sutured in layers.

Coding Tips

For closure of an esophagostomy or fistula, cervical approach, see 43420; for transthoracic or transabdominal approach, see 43425.

ICD-10-CM Diagnostic Codes

C15.3	Malignant neoplasm of upper third of esophagus
C15.4	Malignant neoplasm of middle third of esophagus
C15.8	Malignant neoplasm of overlapping sites of esophagus
J86.0	Pyothorax with fistula
K22.0	Achalasia of cardia
K22.2	Esophageal obstruction
K22.3	Perforation of esophagus
K22.4	Dyskinesia of esophagus
K22.5	Diverticulum of esophagus, acquired
K22.6	Gastro-esophageal laceration-hemorrhage syndrome
K22.89	Other specified disease of esophagus
Q39.0	Atresia of esophagus without fistula
Q39.1	Atresia of esophagus with tracheo-esophageal fistula
S11.21XA	Laceration without foreign body of pharynx and cervical esophagus, initial encounter
S11.22XA	Laceration with foreign body of pharynx and cervical esophagus, initial encounter
S11.23XA	Puncture wound without foreign body of pharynx and cervical esophagus, initial encounter
S11.24XA	Puncture wound with foreign body of pharynx and cervical esophagus, initial encounter
S11.25XA	Open bite of pharynx and cervical esophagus, initial encounter
S27.813A	Laceration of esophagus (thoracic part), initial encounter
S27.818A	Other injury of esophagus (thoracic part), initial encounter
T28.1XXA	Burn of esophagus, initial encounter
T28.6XXA	Corrosion of esophagus, initial encounter

AMA: 43351 2014,Jan,11 **43352** 2014,Jan,11

Relative Value Units/Medicare Edits

Non-Facility RVU	Work	PE	MP	Total
43351	22.05	11.55	5.06	38.66
43352	17.81	9.4	4.1	31.31
Facility RVU	**Work**	**PE**	**MP**	**Total**
43351	22.05	11.55	5.06	38.66
43352	17.81	9.4	4.1	31.31

	FUD	Status	MUE	Modifiers				IOM Reference
43351	90	A	1(2)	51	N/A	62*	80	None
43352	90	A	1(2)	51	N/A	62*	80	

* with documentation

Terms To Know

approach. Method or anatomical location used to gain access to a body organ or specific area for procedures.

cervical. Relation to the cervical spine or to the cervix.

fistulization. Creation of a communication between two structures that were not previously connected.

lateral. On/to the side.

lumen. Space inside an intestine, artery, vein, duct, or tube.

proximal. Located closest to a specified reference point, usually the midline or trunk.

thoracotomy. Surgical procedure for opening the chest wall in order to access the lungs, esophagus, trachea, aorta, heart, and diaphragm.

Esophagus

43360-43361

43360 Gastrointestinal reconstruction for previous esophagectomy, for obstructing esophageal lesion or fistula, or for previous esophageal exclusion; with stomach, with or without pyloroplasty

43361 with colon interposition or small intestine reconstruction, including intestine mobilization, preparation, and anastomosis(es)

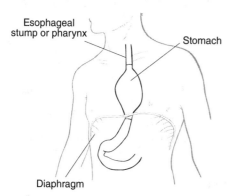

Esophageal stump or pharynx
Stomach
Diaphragm

A previous esophagectomy is reconstructed using the stomach to form a new esophageal passage

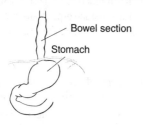

Bowel section
Stomach

Explanation

The physician repairs the esophagus and other gastronomic structures for a number of reasons. The physician uses a thoracoabdominal approach as a continuous incision or separate thoracic and abdominal incisions. The stomach is mobilized and repositioned in the chest in the original esophageal bed and sutured to the esophageal stump. The incision and esophageal stoma are closed. A jejunostomy tube is left in place. Report 43361 if performed with colon interposition or small bowel reconstruction, including bowel mobilization, preparation, and/or anastomosis.

Coding Tips

These codes report reconstruction of a previous esophagectomy only; with colon interposition or small intestine reconstruction, including intestine mobilization, preparation, and anastomosis(es), see 43361; for initial esophagectomy codes, see 43107–43124.

ICD-10-CM Diagnostic Codes

C15.3	Malignant neoplasm of upper third of esophagus
C15.4	Malignant neoplasm of middle third of esophagus
C15.5	Malignant neoplasm of lower third of esophagus
C15.8	Malignant neoplasm of overlapping sites of esophagus
K22.10	Ulcer of esophagus without bleeding
K22.11	Ulcer of esophagus with bleeding
K22.2	Esophageal obstruction
K22.70	Barrett's esophagus without dysplasia
K22.710	Barrett's esophagus with low grade dysplasia
K22.711	Barrett's esophagus with high grade dysplasia
K22.89	Other specified disease of esophagus

K23   Disorders of esophagus in diseases classified elsewhere

AMA: **43360** 2014,Jan,11 **43361** 2014,Jan,11

Relative Value Units/Medicare Edits

Non-Facility RVU	Work	PE	MP	Total
43360	40.11	16.56	9.21	65.88
43361	45.68	22.76	11.16	79.6
Facility RVU	**Work**	**PE**	**MP**	**Total**
43360	40.11	16.56	9.21	65.88
43361	45.68	22.76	11.16	79.6

	FUD	Status	MUE	Modifiers				IOM Reference
43360	90	A	1(2)	51	N/A	62*	80	None
43361	90	A	1(2)	51	N/A	62*	80	

* with documentation

Terms To Know

anastomosis. Surgically created connection between ducts, blood vessels, or bowel segments to allow flow from one to the other.

approach. Method or anatomical location used to gain access to a body organ or specific area for procedures.

fistula. Abnormal tube-like passage between two body cavities or organs or from an organ to the outside surface.

interposition. Placement between objects.

lesion. Area of damaged tissue that has lost continuity or function, due to disease or trauma.

pyloroplasty. Enlargement and reconstruction of the lower portion of the stomach opening into the duodenum performed after vagotomy to speed gastric emptying and treat duodenal ulcers.

reconstruction. Recreating, restoring, or rebuilding a body part or organ.

stoma. Opening created in the abdominal wall from an internal organ or structure for diversion of waste elimination, drainage, and access.

Esophagus

43405

43405   Ligation or stapling at gastroesophageal junction for pre-existing esophageal perforation

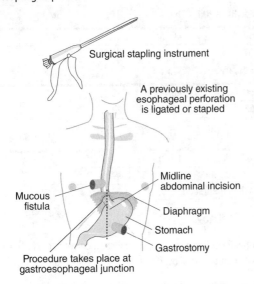

Surgical stapling instrument

A previously existing esophageal perforation is ligated or stapled

Mucous fistula

Midline abdominal incision

Diaphragm

Stomach

Gastrostomy

Procedure takes place at gastroesophageal junction

Explanation

The physician ligates or staples the esophagus to promote healing of a preexisting esophageal perforation. The physician makes a midline upper abdominal incision and retracts the soft tissues to expose the gastroesophageal junction. the physician staples or ligates the junction of the stomach and esophagus. A gastrostomy is created for feeding. The distal end of the esophagus may be exteriorized as a mucus fistula. The incision is sutured in layers.

Coding Tips

If significant additional time and effort are documented, append modifier 22 and submit a cover letter and operative report. For suture of an esophageal wound or injury, cervical approach, see 43410; for transthoracic or transabdominal approach, see 43415.

ICD-10-CM Diagnostic Codes

K22.3	Perforation of esophagus
K22.6	Gastro-esophageal laceration-hemorrhage syndrome
S27.813A	Laceration of esophagus (thoracic part), initial encounter
S27.818A	Other injury of esophagus (thoracic part), initial encounter

AMA: **43405** 2014,Jan,11

Relative Value Units/Medicare Edits

Non-Facility RVU	Work	PE	MP	Total
43405	24.73	12.31	5.68	42.72
Facility RVU	Work	PE	MP	Total
43405	24.73	12.31	5.68	42.72

	FUD	Status	MUE	Modifiers				IOM Reference
43405	90	A	1(2)	51	N/A	62*	80	None

* with documentation

43410-43415

43410   Suture of esophageal wound or injury; cervical approach
43415   transthoracic or transabdominal approach

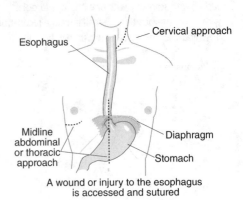

Esophagus

Cervical approach

Midline abdominal or thoracic approach

Diaphragm

Stomach

A wound or injury to the esophagus is accessed and sutured

Explanation

The physician sutures a wound or injury to the esophagus. The physician accesses the esophagus through a lateral neck, midline abdominal, or thoracic incision. For a cervical approach, report 43410. For a thoracic or transabdominal approach, report 43415. The physician exposes the affected segment of the esophagus, which is repaired by suturing. The incision is sutured in layers.

Coding Tips

If significant additional time and effort are documented, append modifier 22 and submit a cover letter and operative report. For ligation or stapling at the gastroesophageal junction for pre-existing esophageal perforation, see 43405. When 43410 or 43415 is performed with another separately identifiable procedure, the highest dollar value code is listed as the primary procedure, and subsequent procedures are appended with modifier 51. If the procedure is completed through an operating microscope, report 69990 in addition to the primary procedure. However, head gear (e.g., loupes or binoculars) is considered an integral part of this procedure.

ICD-10-CM Diagnostic Codes

K22.6	Gastro-esophageal laceration-hemorrhage syndrome
S11.21XA	Laceration without foreign body of pharynx and cervical esophagus, initial encounter
S11.22XA	Laceration with foreign body of pharynx and cervical esophagus, initial encounter
S11.23XA	Puncture wound without foreign body of pharynx and cervical esophagus, initial encounter
S11.24XA	Puncture wound with foreign body of pharynx and cervical esophagus, initial encounter
S11.25XA	Open bite of pharynx and cervical esophagus, initial encounter
S27.813A	Laceration of esophagus (thoracic part), initial encounter
S27.818A	Other injury of esophagus (thoracic part), initial encounter
T28.1XXA	Burn of esophagus, initial encounter
T28.6XXA	Corrosion of esophagus, initial encounter

AMA: **43410** 2018,Jan,8; 2017,Jan,8; 2016,Jan,13; 2015,Jan,16

N Newborn: 0   **P** Pediatric: 0-17   **M** Maternity: 9-64   **A** Adult: 15-124   ♂ Male Only   ♀ Female Only

Coding Companion for General Surgery/Gastroenterology

Esophagus

Relative Value Units/Medicare Edits

Non-Facility RVU	Work	PE	MP	Total
43410	16.41	11.2	2.26	29.87
43415	44.88	20.01	10.05	74.94
Facility RVU	Work	PE	MP	Total
43410	16.41	11.2	2.26	29.87
43415	44.88	20.01	10.05	74.94

	FUD	Status	MUE	Modifiers				IOM Reference
43410	90	A	1(3)	51	N/A	62*	80	None
43415	90	A	1(3)	51	N/A	62*	80	

* with documentation

Terms To Know

approach. Method or anatomical location used to gain access to a body organ or specific area for procedures. The approach is not coded separately although it may be a specified component of the procedure, such as laparoscopic versus incisional, or spinal procedures in which the amount of dissection required to expose the spine significantly alters with the site of approach.

diaphragm. Muscular wall separating the thorax and its structures from the abdomen.

esophagus. Muscular tube that carries swallowed liquids and foods from the pharynx to the stomach.

hemorrhage. Internal or external bleeding with loss of significant amounts of blood.

incision. Act of cutting into tissue or an organ.

puncture. Creating a hole.

43420-43425

43420	Closure of esophagostomy or fistula; cervical approach
43425	transthoracic or transabdominal approach

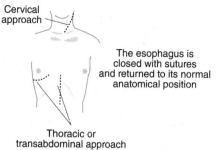

Cervical approach

The esophagus is closed with sutures and returned to its normal anatomical position

Thoracic or transabdominal approach

A surgically created esophageal fistula is repaired after it is no longer needed

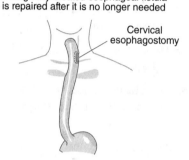

Cervical esophagostomy

Explanation

The physician closes an opening in the esophagus and returns it to its natural position. The physician accesses the defect through an oblique cervical incision along the border of the sternocleidomastoid muscle, a midline abdominal incision, or a thoracic incision. For a cervical approach, report 43420. For a thoracic or transabdominal approach, report 43425. The physician closes the opening with sutures and repositions the esophagus to its normal anatomical position. The incision is sutured in layers.

Coding Tips

For esophagostomy, fistulization of the esophagus, external, via a thoracic approach, see 43351; cervical approach, see 43352. The operative approach is considered inherent to the procedure and is not reported separately. To report transabdominal paraesophageal hiatal hernia repair, see codes 43332–43333; transthoracic diaphragmatic hernia repair, see 43334–43335.

ICD-10-CM Diagnostic Codes

K94.31	Esophagostomy hemorrhage
K94.32	Esophagostomy infection
K94.33	Esophagostomy malfunction
K94.39	Other complications of esophagostomy
Z43.4	Encounter for attention to other artificial openings of digestive tract

AMA: **43420** 2014,Jan,11 **43425** 2014,Jan,11

Esophagus

Relative Value Units/Medicare Edits

Non-Facility RVU	Work	PE	MP	Total
43420	16.78	10.46	2.3	29.54
43425	25.04	11.5	5.74	42.28
Facility RVU	Work	PE	MP	Total
43420	16.78	10.46	2.3	29.54
43425	25.04	11.5	5.74	42.28

	FUD	Status	MUE	Modifiers				IOM Reference
43420	90	A	1(3)	51	N/A	62*	80*	None
43425	90	A	1(3)	51	N/A	62*	80	

* with documentation

Terms To Know

fistula. Abnormal tube-like passage between two body cavities or organs or from an organ to the outside surface.

perforation. Hole in an object, organ, or tissue, or the act of punching or boring holes through a part.

sternocleidomastoid. Large superficial muscle that passes obliquely across the anterolateral neck, originating at the sternum and clavicle and inserting at the mastoid process of the temporal bone.

transabdominal. Across or through the belly or abdomen.

transthoracic. Across or through the chest.

43450-43453

43450   Dilation of esophagus, by unguided sound or bougie, single or multiple passes

43453   Dilation of esophagus, over guide wire

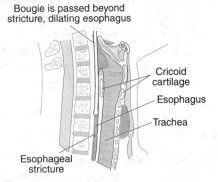

Bougie is passed beyond stricture, dilating esophagus

Cricoid cartilage

Esophagus

Trachea

Esophageal stricture

Explanation

In 43450, the physician dilates the esophagus using an unguided dilator. The physician passes a dilator into the patient's throat down into the esophagus until the end of the dilator passes the stricture. A stricture is a decrease in the esophagus opening as a result of cicatricial (scar) contraction or a deposit of abnormal tissue. The dilator is withdrawn after it passes the stricture. In 43453, the dilation is accomplished by passing dilators over a guidewire. The physician uses a fluoroscope to place a guidewire into the patient's throat, down the esophagus, and into the stomach. A series of dilators are passed over the guidewire and withdrawn. In both procedures, the process may be repeated several times to dilate the esophagus to an acceptable size.</p>

Coding Tips

If these procedures are performed with endoscopic visualization, dilation with balloon, less than 30 mm diameter, see 43195, 43220, and 43249; 30 mm diameter or larger, see 43214 or 43233; with balloon or dilators, see 43213; over guidewire, see 43226. For associated esophagogram, see 74220. Radiological supervision and interpretation is reported separately, see 74360.

ICD-10-CM Diagnostic Codes

K22.2   Esophageal obstruction

K23   Disorders of esophagus in diseases classified elsewhere

Q39.3   Congenital stenosis and stricture of esophagus

AMA: 43450 2018,Jan,8; 2017,Jul,10; 2017,Jan,8; 2016,Jan,13; 2015,Jan,16
43453 2018,Jan,8; 2017,Jan,8; 2016,Jan,13; 2015,Jan,16

Relative Value Units/Medicare Edits

Non-Facility RVU	Work	PE	MP	Total
43450	1.28	4.18	0.15	5.61
43453	1.41	25.1	0.16	26.67
Facility RVU	Work	PE	MP	Total
43450	1.28	0.88	0.15	2.31
43453	1.41	0.93	0.16	2.5

	FUD	Status	MUE	Modifiers				IOM Reference
43450	0	A	1(3)	51	N/A	N/A	N/A	None
43453	0	A	1(3)	51	N/A	N/A	N/A	

* with documentation

Coding Companion for General Surgery/Gastroenterology

Esophagus

43460

43460   Esophagogastric tamponade, with balloon (Sengstaken type)

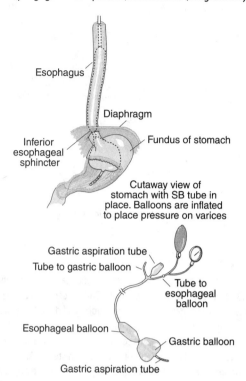

Esophagus

Diaphragm

Inferior esophageal sphincter

Fundus of stomach

Cutaway view of stomach with SB tube in place. Balloons are inflated to place pressure on varices

Gastric aspiration tube

Tube to gastric balloon

Tube to esophageal balloon

Esophageal balloon

Gastric balloon

Gastric aspiration tube

Explanation

The physician inserts a multilumen tube into the esophagus through which a balloon is passed for the tamponade of bleeding esophageal varices. The balloon is inflated to exert pressure on the varices to stop bleeding. The balloon is left inflated so coagulation can occur before the physician proceeds with definitive treatment.

Coding Tips

For esophagoscopy with injection sclerosis of esophageal varices, see 43204; with band ligation of esophageal varices, see 43205; for control of bleeding, any method, see 43227. For esophagogastroduodenoscopy, with injection sclerosis of gastric or esophageal varices, see 43243; with band ligation of esophageal and/or gastric varices, see 43244; with control of bleeding, any method, see 43255. Removal of foreign body by balloon catheter is reported with 43499 and 74235.

ICD-10-CM Diagnostic Codes

I85.01	Esophageal varices with bleeding
I85.11	Secondary esophageal varices with bleeding
I86.4	Gastric varices

AMA: 43460 2014,Jan,11

Relative Value Units/Medicare Edits

Non-Facility RVU	Work	PE	MP	Total
43460	3.79	1.97	0.42	6.18
Facility RVU	**Work**	**PE**	**MP**	**Total**
43460	3.79	1.97	0.42	6.18

	FUD	Status	MUE	Modifiers				IOM Reference
43460	0	A	1(3)	51	N/A	N/A	N/A	None

* with documentation

Terms To Know

acute. Sudden, severe. Documentation and reporting of an acute condition is important to establishing medical necessity.

balloon catheter. Any catheter equipped with an inflatable balloon at the end to hold it in place in a body cavity or to be used for dilation of a vessel lumen.

chronic. Persistent, continuing, or recurring.

esophagus. Muscular tube that carries swallowed liquids and foods from the pharynx to the stomach.

hemorrhage. Internal or external bleeding with loss of significant amounts of blood.

ligation. Tying off a blood vessel or duct with a suture or a soft, thin wire.

lumen. Space inside an intestine, artery, vein, duct, or tube.

tube. Long, hollow cylindrical instrument or body structure.

varices. Enlarged, dilated, or twisted turning veins.

43496

43496   Free jejunum transfer with microvascular anastomosis

Highly vascularized walls of jejunum

Vasa recta arteries

Free section of jejunum

Mesentery

The jejunum is the highly vascular, upper two-fifths of the small intestine; free transfers are often taken to graft other areas of the digestive tract, such as the esophagus

Explanation

The physician makes an abdominal incision to gain access to the omentum. The greater omentum is reflected to reveal the underlying small intestine. The jejunum is identified and removed. The remaining jejunum is reattached and the omentum is replaced. The free section of jejunum is transferred to another site with anastomosis of its vessels to another structure. Most commonly, the free transfer of a short segment of jejunum occurs between the pharynx and esophagus with microvascular anastomosis of jejunal vessels to the external carotid artery branches and the jugular vein. Portions of the pharynx and/or esophagus have already been resected with removal of cervical esophageal and hypopharyngeal carcinoma. Operative sites are sutured closed.

Coding Tips

Microvascular technique is included in 43496. Do not report 69990 in addition to 43496.

ICD-10-CM Diagnostic Codes

C14.2	Malignant neoplasm of Waldeyer's ring
C14.8	Malignant neoplasm of overlapping sites of lip, oral cavity and pharynx
C15.3	Malignant neoplasm of upper third of esophagus
C15.4	Malignant neoplasm of middle third of esophagus
C15.5	Malignant neoplasm of lower third of esophagus
C15.8	Malignant neoplasm of overlapping sites of esophagus
D00.1	Carcinoma in situ of esophagus

AMA: **43496** 2019,Dec,5; 2018,Jan,8; 2017,Jan,8; 2016,Jan,13; 2016,Feb,12; 2015,Jan,16

Relative Value Units/Medicare Edits

Non-Facility RVU	Work	PE	MP	Total
43496	0.0	0.0	0.0	0.0
Facility RVU	**Work**	**PE**	**MP**	**Total**
43496	0.0	0.0	0.0	0.0

	FUD	Status	MUE	Modifiers				IOM Reference
43496	90	C	1(3)	51	N/A	62*	80	None

* with documentation

43497

● 43497   Lower esophageal myotomy, transoral (ie, peroral endoscopic myotomy [POEM])

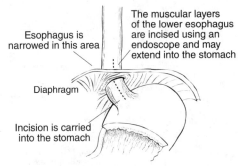

The muscular layers of the lower esophagus are incised using an endoscope and may extend into the stomach

Esophagus is narrowed in this area

Diaphragm

Incision is carried into the stomach

This relaxes the stricture in the esophagus

Explanation

The physician performs a transoral lower esophageal myotomy, also known as a peroral endoscopic myotomy or POEM. This procedure is often performed for the treatment of achalasia or spastic esophageal disorders (such as nutcracker esophagus or diffuse esophageal spasm) that have not responded to medical therapy. Prior to the procedure, an IV is inserted into a vein through which anesthesia, fluids, and antibiotics are administered. An arterial line is inserted for pressure monitoring during the procedure. The physician inserts an endoscope through the mouth and into the esophagus, observing the images on a monitor. The first incision is made into the internal lining of the esophagus, through which the endoscope is inserted. The muscle is exposed within the wall of the esophagus; the physician makes an incision (myotomy) in the inner muscle layer near the lower esophageal sphincter. Upon completion of the procedure, the physician repairs the esophageal incision using standard endoscopic clips. The patient is typically admitted for postoperative monitoring and administration of antibiotics.

Coding Tips

Do not report 43497 with 32665, 43191, 43197, 43200, or 43235.

ICD-10-CM Diagnostic Codes

K22.0	Achalasia of cardia
Q39.5	Congenital dilatation of esophagus

Relative Value Units/Medicare Edits

Non-Facility RVU	Work	PE	MP	Total
43497				
Facility RVU	**Work**	**PE**	**MP**	**Total**
43497				

	FUD	Status	MUE	Modifiers				IOM Reference
43497	N/A		-	N/A	N/A	N/A	N/A	None

* with documentation

Terms To Know

achalasia of cardia. Esophageal motility disorder that is caused by absence of the esophageal peristalsis and impaired relaxation of the lower esophageal sphincter. It is characterized by dysphagia, regurgitation, and heartburn.

Esophagus

43500-43510

43500 Gastrotomy; with exploration or foreign body removal
43501   with suture repair of bleeding ulcer
43502   with suture repair of pre-existing esophagogastric laceration (eg, Mallory-Weiss)
43510   with esophageal dilation and insertion of permanent intraluminal tube (eg, Celestin or Mousseaux-Barbin)

A Mallory-Weiss tear occurs after violent retching, usually near the junction

Esophagus
Diaphragm
Pylorus
Stomach
The stomach is incised and explored

Typical incision for gastrotomy

Explanation

The physician performs a gastrostomy and explores gastric area, removes a foreign body or corrects a mucosal defect. The physician makes a midline epigastric incision and retracts the skin and underlying tissues laterally. The stomach is incised and explored. In 43500, a foreign body is removed. In 43501, a bleeding ulcer is identified and bleeding is controlled with electrocautery or ligation of vessels, and the mucosa is drawn over the ulcer and sutured. In 43502, an esophagogastric laceration is identified and bleeding is controlled with electrocautery or ligation of vessels, and the mucosa is drawn over the defect and sutured. In 43510, the physician introduces dilators into the esophagus from the stomach to increase the diameter of the esophagus. When dilation is complete, a stent is placed and secured with sutures to maintain to patency. After exploration or repair, the stomach is sutured in layers, the soft tissues are returned to anatomical position, and the incision is sutured in layers.

Coding Tips

For esophagotomy, cervical approach, with removal of foreign body, see 43020; thoracic approach, see 43045. For dilation of the esophagus by balloon or dilator, retrograde, see 43213. For dilation of the esophagus with balloon (30 mm diameter or larger), see 43214 or 43233. For endoscopic dilation procedures, see 43213–43214, 43220–43226, 43233, 43245, 43248, and 43249.

ICD-10-CM Diagnostic Codes

A18.83	Tuberculosis of digestive tract organs, not elsewhere classified
C16.0	Malignant neoplasm of cardia
C16.1	Malignant neoplasm of fundus of stomach
C16.2	Malignant neoplasm of body of stomach
C16.3	Malignant neoplasm of pyloric antrum
C16.4	Malignant neoplasm of pylorus
C16.8	Malignant neoplasm of overlapping sites of stomach
D13.1	Benign neoplasm of stomach
D3A.092	Benign carcinoid tumor of the stomach
I86.4	Gastric varices
K22.6	Gastro-esophageal laceration-hemorrhage syndrome
K25.0	Acute gastric ulcer with hemorrhage
K25.2	Acute gastric ulcer with both hemorrhage and perforation
K25.3	Acute gastric ulcer without hemorrhage or perforation
K25.4	Chronic or unspecified gastric ulcer with hemorrhage
K25.5	Chronic or unspecified gastric ulcer with perforation
K25.6	Chronic or unspecified gastric ulcer with both hemorrhage and perforation
K25.7	Chronic gastric ulcer without hemorrhage or perforation
K29.41	Chronic atrophic gastritis with bleeding
K29.61	Other gastritis with bleeding
K31.2	Hourglass stricture and stenosis of stomach
K31.4	Gastric diverticulum
K31.6	Fistula of stomach and duodenum
K31.89	Other diseases of stomach and duodenum
Q40.0	Congenital hypertrophic pyloric stenosis
Q40.2	Other specified congenital malformations of stomach
S36.32XA	Contusion of stomach, initial encounter
S36.33XA	Laceration of stomach, initial encounter
S36.39XA	Other injury of stomach, initial encounter
T18.2XXA	Foreign body in stomach, initial encounter

AMA: **43500** 2014,Jan,11 **43501** 2014,Jan,11 **43502** 2014,Jan,11 **43510** 2014,Jan,11

Relative Value Units/Medicare Edits

Non-Facility RVU	Work	PE	MP	Total
43500	12.79	7.46	2.95	23.2
43501	22.6	11.94	5.3	39.84
43502	25.69	13.19	6.28	45.16
43510	15.14	9.27	3.72	28.13
Facility RVU	**Work**	**PE**	**MP**	**Total**
43500	12.79	7.46	2.95	23.2
43501	22.6	11.94	5.3	39.84
43502	25.69	13.19	6.28	45.16
43510	15.14	9.27	3.72	28.13

	FUD	Status	MUE	Modifiers				IOM Reference
43500	90	A	1(2)	51	N/A	62*	80	None
43501	90	A	1(3)	51	N/A	62*	80	
43502	90	A	1(2)	51	N/A	62*	80	
43510	90	A	1(2)	51	N/A	62*	80	

* with documentation

43520

43520 Pyloromyotomy, cutting of pyloric muscle (Fredet-Ramstedt type operation)

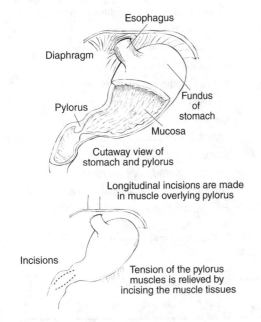

Esophagus

Diaphragm

Pylorus

Fundus of stomach

Mucosa

Cutaway view of stomach and pylorus

Longitudinal incisions are made in muscle overlying pylorus

Incisions

Tension of the pylorus muscles is relieved by incising the muscle tissues

Explanation

The physician incises the pyloric muscle. The physician makes a small subcostal incision over the pyloric olive. The peritoneum is incised, the tissues are retracted, and the pylorus is identified. The serosa is incised and the tension of the pyloric muscle is released with longitudinal incisions. The peritoneum is sutured closed and the operative site is sutured in layers.

Coding Tips

For vagotomy, including pyloroplasty, with or without gastrostomy, truncal or selective, see 43640; parietal cell, see 43641. For pyloroplasty, see 43800. Do not append modifier 63 to 43520 as the description or nature of the procedure includes infants up to 4 kg.

ICD-10-CM Diagnostic Codes

C16.3	Malignant neoplasm of pyloric antrum
C16.4	Malignant neoplasm of pylorus
C7A.092	Malignant carcinoid tumor of the stomach
K31.1	Adult hypertrophic pyloric stenosis 🅰
K31.3	Pylorospasm, not elsewhere classified
K31.811	Angiodysplasia of stomach and duodenum with bleeding
K31.819	Angiodysplasia of stomach and duodenum without bleeding
K31.89	Other diseases of stomach and duodenum
Q40.0	Congenital hypertrophic pyloric stenosis
R11.11	Vomiting without nausea
R11.12	Projectile vomiting

AMA: **43520** 2014,Jan,11

Relative Value Units/Medicare Edits

Non-Facility RVU	Work	PE	MP	Total
43520	11.29	6.51	2.48	20.28
Facility RVU	**Work**	**PE**	**MP**	**Total**
43520	11.29	6.51	2.48	20.28

	FUD	Status	MUE	Modifiers				IOM Reference
43520	90	A	1(2)	51	N/A	62*	80	None

* with documentation

Terms To Know

angiodysplasia. Vascular abnormalities, with or without bleeding.

closure. Repairing an incision or wound by suture or other means.

congenital. Present at birth, occurring through heredity or an influence during gestation up to the moment of birth.

diaphragm. Muscular wall separating the thorax and its structures from the abdomen.

duodenum. First portion of the small intestine connected to the stomach at the pylorus and extending to the jejunum.

hypertrophy. Overgrowth or enlargement of normal cells in tissue.

incision. Act of cutting into tissue or an organ.

malignant. Any condition tending to progress toward death, specifically an invasive tumor with a loss of cellular differentiation that has the ability to spread or metastasize to other body areas.

myotomy. Surgical cutting of a muscle to gain access to underlying tissues or for therapeutic reasons.

neoplasm. New abnormal growth, tumor.

peritoneum. Strong, continuous membrane that forms the lining of the abdominal and pelvic cavity. The parietal peritoneum, or outer layer, is attached to the abdominopelvic walls and the visceral peritoneum, or inner layer, surrounds the organs inside the abdominal cavity.

pylorus. Lower portion of the stomach, which opens into the duodenum.

release. Disconnection of a tendon or ligament.

retraction. Act of holding tissue or a structure back away from its normal position or the field of interest.

stenosis. Narrowing or constriction of a passage.

43605

43605 Biopsy of stomach, by laparotomy

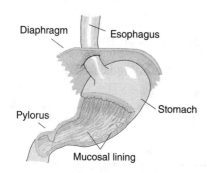

Biopsy specimens are collected from the stomach

Explanation

The physician obtains a biopsy of the stomach via open approach (laparotomy). The physician makes a midline abdominal incision. The peritoneum is incised and tissues are retracted to identify the anterior surface of the stomach. An incision is made in the stomach and the physician explores the mucosa to obtain biopsies. Once biopsies are acquired, the stomach incision is closed with sutures or staples. The peritoneum is sutured closed and the abdominal incision is closed using layered sutures.

Coding Tips

An excisional biopsy is not reported separately when a therapeutic excision is performed during the same surgical session. For esophagogastroduodenoscopy with biopsy of stomach, see 43239. Laparotomy, celiotomy (49000) is included in 43605 and should not be reported separately.

ICD-10-CM Diagnostic Codes

C16.0	Malignant neoplasm of cardia
C16.1	Malignant neoplasm of fundus of stomach
C16.2	Malignant neoplasm of body of stomach
C16.3	Malignant neoplasm of pyloric antrum
C16.4	Malignant neoplasm of pylorus
C16.8	Malignant neoplasm of overlapping sites of stomach
C49.A2	Gastrointestinal stromal tumor of stomach
C7A.092	Malignant carcinoid tumor of the stomach
D00.2	Carcinoma in situ of stomach
D13.1	Benign neoplasm of stomach
D37.1	Neoplasm of uncertain behavior of stomach
D49.0	Neoplasm of unspecified behavior of digestive system
K25.7	Chronic gastric ulcer without hemorrhage or perforation
K29.20	Alcoholic gastritis without bleeding
K29.21	Alcoholic gastritis with bleeding
K29.30	Chronic superficial gastritis without bleeding
K29.31	Chronic superficial gastritis with bleeding
K29.40	Chronic atrophic gastritis without bleeding
K29.41	Chronic atrophic gastritis with bleeding
K29.60	Other gastritis without bleeding
K29.61	Other gastritis with bleeding
K30	Functional dyspepsia
K31.7	Polyp of stomach and duodenum
K31.811	Angiodysplasia of stomach and duodenum with bleeding
K31.819	Angiodysplasia of stomach and duodenum without bleeding
K31.89	Other diseases of stomach and duodenum
K52.3	Indeterminate colitis
K52.81	Eosinophilic gastritis or gastroenteritis
K52.831	Collagenous colitis
K52.832	Lymphocytic colitis
K52.838	Other microscopic colitis
K92.0	Hematemesis
Q40.0	Congenital hypertrophic pyloric stenosis
Q40.2	Other specified congenital malformations of stomach

AMA: **43605** 2014,Jan,11

Relative Value Units/Medicare Edits

Non-Facility RVU	Work	PE	MP	Total
43605	13.72	7.86	3.2	24.78
Facility RVU	**Work**	**PE**	**MP**	**Total**
43605	13.72	7.86	3.2	24.78

	FUD	Status	MUE	Modifiers				IOM Reference
43605	90	A	1(2)	51	N/A	62*	80	None

* with documentation

Terms To Know

anterior. Situated in the front area or toward the belly surface of the body.

biopsy. Tissue or fluid removed for diagnostic purposes through analysis of the cells in the biopsy material.

laparotomy. Incision through the flank or abdomen for therapeutic or diagnostic purposes.

mucosa. Moist tissue lining the mouth (buccal mucosa), stomach (gastric mucosa), intestines, and respiratory tract.

peritoneum. Strong, continuous membrane that forms the lining of the abdominal and pelvic cavity. The parietal peritoneum, or outer layer, is attached to the abdominopelvic walls and the visceral peritoneum, or inner layer, surrounds the organs inside the abdominal cavity.

tissue. Group of similar cells with a similar function that form definite structures and organs. Tissue types include epithelial tissue, muscle tissue, connective tissue, and nervous tissue.

● **New** ▲ **Revised** + **Add On** ★ **Telemedicine** **AMA: CPT Assist** **[Resequenced]** ☑ **Laterality**

43610-43611

43610 Excision, local; ulcer or benign tumor of stomach
43611 malignant tumor of stomach

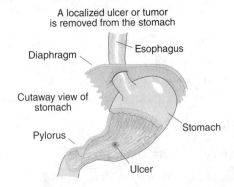

A localized ulcer or tumor
is removed from the stomach

Esophagus
Diaphragm
Cutaway view of
stomach
Stomach
Pylorus
Ulcer

Explanation

The physician performs a local excision of an ulcer or a benign tumor of the stomach. The physician makes a midline abdominal incision. Next, the stomach is dissected free of surrounding structures and the area of the tumor identified. The tumor is excised with a normal margin of stomach around the tumor. The defect created in the stomach is closed with sutures or a stapling device. The incision is closed. Report 43611 for local excision of a malignant tumor of the stomach.

Coding Tips

For gastrostomy with suture repair of a bleeding ulcer, see 43501. For esophagogastroduodenoscopy, with control of bleeding, any method, see 43255; removal or ablation of tumors, polyps, or lesions, see 43250–43251 or 43270.

ICD-10-CM Diagnostic Codes

C49.A2	Gastrointestinal stromal tumor of stomach
D13.1	Benign neoplasm of stomach
D3A.092	Benign carcinoid tumor of the stomach
K25.0	Acute gastric ulcer with hemorrhage
K25.1	Acute gastric ulcer with perforation
K25.2	Acute gastric ulcer with both hemorrhage and perforation
K25.3	Acute gastric ulcer without hemorrhage or perforation
K25.4	Chronic or unspecified gastric ulcer with hemorrhage
K25.5	Chronic or unspecified gastric ulcer with perforation
K25.6	Chronic or unspecified gastric ulcer with both hemorrhage and perforation
K25.7	Chronic gastric ulcer without hemorrhage or perforation
K27.0	Acute peptic ulcer, site unspecified, with hemorrhage
K27.1	Acute peptic ulcer, site unspecified, with perforation
K27.2	Acute peptic ulcer, site unspecified, with both hemorrhage and perforation
K27.3	Acute peptic ulcer, site unspecified, without hemorrhage or perforation
K27.4	Chronic or unspecified peptic ulcer, site unspecified, with hemorrhage
K27.5	Chronic or unspecified peptic ulcer, site unspecified, with perforation
K27.6	Chronic or unspecified peptic ulcer, site unspecified, with both hemorrhage and perforation
K27.7	Chronic peptic ulcer, site unspecified, without hemorrhage or perforation
K31.7	Polyp of stomach and duodenum

AMA: 43610 2014,Jan,11 **43611** 2014,Jan,11

Relative Value Units/Medicare Edits

Non-Facility RVU	Work	PE	MP	Total
43610	16.34	8.84	3.84	29.02
43611	20.38	10.99	4.78	36.15
Facility RVU	**Work**	**PE**	**MP**	**Total**
43610	16.34	8.84	3.84	29.02
43611	20.38	10.99	4.78	36.15

	FUD	Status	MUE	Modifiers				IOM Reference
43610	90	A	2(3)	51	N/A	62*	80	None
43611	90	A	2(3)	51	N/A	62*	80	

* with documentation

Terms To Know

benign. Mild or nonmalignant in nature.

malignant. Any condition tending to progress toward death, specifically an invasive tumor with a loss of cellular differentiation that has the ability to spread or metastasize to other body areas.

tumor. Pathological swelling or enlargement; a neoplastic growth of uncontrolled, abnormal multiplication of cells.

ulcer. Open sore or excavating lesion of skin or the tissue on the surface of an organ from the sloughing of chronically inflamed and necrosing tissue.

43620-43621

43620   Gastrectomy, total; with esophagoenterostomy
43621   with Roux-en-Y reconstruction

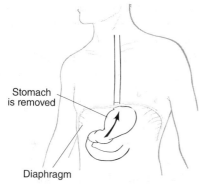

Stomach is removed

Diaphragm

The body of the stomach is removed. The remaining duodenum is mobilized upward and anastomosed to the distal esophagus

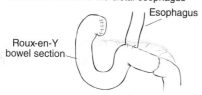

Esophagus

Roux-en-Y bowel section

Explanation

The physician removes the stomach and approximates a limb of small bowel to the esophagus by performing an esophagoenterostomy in 43620 or a Roux-en-Y esophagojejunostomy in 43621. The physician makes a midline abdominal incision. The stomach is dissected free of surrounding structures and its blood supply is divided. The stomach is divided at the gastroesophageal junction and at the gastroduodenal junction and removed. In 43620, the remaining duodenal end of the intestine is simply mobilized to the end of the esophagus and connected. In 43621, a measured limb of Roux, or limb of small intestine, is created by dividing the upper jejunum. The distal part of the now divided upper jejunum, the limb in continuity with the ileum, is brought up and anastomosed to the esophagus. The proximal end of the divided jejunum, the segment containing the duodenum, must be connected back into the limb of small bowel farther down from the esophageal anastomosis. This maintains continuity for the duodenal section, which was sealed upon removal of the stomach, but which is also receiving bile from the liver and gallbladder as well as pancreatic juice.

Coding Tips

For total gastrectomy with formation of an intestinal pouch, any type, see 43622. For partial distal gastrectomy, with gastroduodenostomy, see 43631; with gastrojejunostomy, see 43632; with Roux-en Y reconstruction, see 43633; with formation of a gastrointestinal pouch, see 43634.

ICD-10-CM Diagnostic Codes

C16.0	Malignant neoplasm of cardia
C16.1	Malignant neoplasm of fundus of stomach
C16.2	Malignant neoplasm of body of stomach
C16.3	Malignant neoplasm of pyloric antrum
C16.4	Malignant neoplasm of pylorus
C16.8	Malignant neoplasm of overlapping sites of stomach
C78.89	Secondary malignant neoplasm of other digestive organs

C7A.092	Malignant carcinoid tumor of the stomach
D13.1	Benign neoplasm of stomach
D37.1	Neoplasm of uncertain behavior of stomach
D3A.092	Benign carcinoid tumor of the stomach
D49.0	Neoplasm of unspecified behavior of digestive system
K25.0	Acute gastric ulcer with hemorrhage
K25.1	Acute gastric ulcer with perforation
K25.2	Acute gastric ulcer with both hemorrhage and perforation
K25.3	Acute gastric ulcer without hemorrhage or perforation
K25.4	Chronic or unspecified gastric ulcer with hemorrhage
K25.5	Chronic or unspecified gastric ulcer with perforation
K25.6	Chronic or unspecified gastric ulcer with both hemorrhage and perforation
K25.7	Chronic gastric ulcer without hemorrhage or perforation
K27.0	Acute peptic ulcer, site unspecified, with hemorrhage
K27.1	Acute peptic ulcer, site unspecified, with perforation
K27.2	Acute peptic ulcer, site unspecified, with both hemorrhage and perforation
K27.3	Acute peptic ulcer, site unspecified, without hemorrhage or perforation
K27.4	Chronic or unspecified peptic ulcer, site unspecified, with hemorrhage
K27.5	Chronic or unspecified peptic ulcer, site unspecified, with perforation
K27.6	Chronic or unspecified peptic ulcer, site unspecified, with both hemorrhage and perforation
K27.7	Chronic peptic ulcer, site unspecified, without hemorrhage or perforation
K31.7	Polyp of stomach and duodenum
S36.32XA	Contusion of stomach, initial encounter
S36.33XA	Laceration of stomach, initial encounter
S36.39XA	Other injury of stomach, initial encounter

AMA: **43620** 2014,Jan,11 **43621** 2014,Jan,11

Relative Value Units/Medicare Edits

Non-Facility RVU	Work	PE	MP	Total
43620	34.04	16.29	8.31	58.64
43621	39.53	18.14	9.4	67.07
Facility RVU	Work	PE	MP	Total
43620	34.04	16.29	8.31	58.64
43621	39.53	18.14	9.4	67.07

	FUD	Status	MUE	Modifiers				IOM Reference
43620	90	A	1(2)	51	N/A	62*	80	None
43621	90	A	1(2)	51	N/A	62*	80	

* with documentation

Stomach

43622

43622 Gastrectomy, total; with formation of intestinal pouch, any type

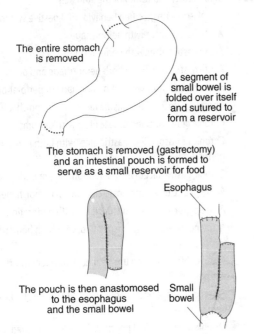

The entire stomach is removed

A segment of small bowel is folded over itself and sutured to form a reservoir

The stomach is removed (gastrectomy) and an intestinal pouch is formed to serve as a small reservoir for food

Esophagus

The pouch is then anastomosed to the esophagus and the small bowel

Small bowel

Explanation

The physician removes the stomach and forms a pouch of small bowel and approximates this to the esophagus. The physician makes a midline abdominal incision. Next, the stomach is dissected free of surrounding structures and its blood supply divided. The stomach is divided at the gastroesophageal junction and the gastroduodenal junction removed. The proximal jejunum is divided and the distal end of bowel is folded upon itself and approximated in such a way to form a pouch. The pouch is connected to the esophagus. The divided proximal jejunum is connected to the limb of small bowel distal to the esophageal anastomosis to restore intestinal continuity. The incisions are closed.

Coding Tips

For total gastrectomy with esophagoenterostomy, see 43620; with Roux-en-Y reconstruction, see 43621. For partial, distal gastrectomy with gastroduodenostomy, see 43631; with gastrojejunostomy, see 43632; with Roux-en-Y reconstruction, see 43633; with formation of an intestinal pouch, see 43634.

ICD-10-CM Diagnostic Codes

C16.0	Malignant neoplasm of cardia
C16.1	Malignant neoplasm of fundus of stomach
C16.2	Malignant neoplasm of body of stomach
C16.3	Malignant neoplasm of pyloric antrum
C16.4	Malignant neoplasm of pylorus
C16.8	Malignant neoplasm of overlapping sites of stomach
C78.89	Secondary malignant neoplasm of other digestive organs
C7A.092	Malignant carcinoid tumor of the stomach
D13.1	Benign neoplasm of stomach
D37.1	Neoplasm of uncertain behavior of stomach
D37.2	Neoplasm of uncertain behavior of small intestine
D3A.092	Benign carcinoid tumor of the stomach

K25.0	Acute gastric ulcer with hemorrhage
K25.1	Acute gastric ulcer with perforation
K25.2	Acute gastric ulcer with both hemorrhage and perforation
K25.3	Acute gastric ulcer without hemorrhage or perforation
K25.4	Chronic or unspecified gastric ulcer with hemorrhage
K25.5	Chronic or unspecified gastric ulcer with perforation
K25.6	Chronic or unspecified gastric ulcer with both hemorrhage and perforation
K25.7	Chronic gastric ulcer without hemorrhage or perforation
K27.0	Acute peptic ulcer, site unspecified, with hemorrhage
K27.1	Acute peptic ulcer, site unspecified, with perforation
K27.2	Acute peptic ulcer, site unspecified, with both hemorrhage and perforation
K27.3	Acute peptic ulcer, site unspecified, without hemorrhage or perforation
K27.4	Chronic or unspecified peptic ulcer, site unspecified, with hemorrhage
K27.5	Chronic or unspecified peptic ulcer, site unspecified, with perforation
K27.6	Chronic or unspecified peptic ulcer, site unspecified, with both hemorrhage and perforation
K27.7	Chronic peptic ulcer, site unspecified, without hemorrhage or perforation
K31.7	Polyp of stomach and duodenum
K56.0	Paralytic ileus
K56.1	Intussusception
K56.2	Volvulus
K56.51	Intestinal adhesions [bands], with partial obstruction
K56.52	Intestinal adhesions [bands] with complete obstruction
K56.690	Other partial intestinal obstruction
K56.691	Other complete intestinal obstruction
K91.31	Postprocedural partial intestinal obstruction
K91.32	Postprocedural complete intestinal obstruction
S36.32XA	Contusion of stomach, initial encounter
S36.33XA	Laceration of stomach, initial encounter
S36.39XA	Other injury of stomach, initial encounter

AMA: 43622 2014,Jan,11

Relative Value Units/Medicare Edits

Non-Facility RVU	Work	PE	MP	Total
43622	40.03	18.52	9.79	68.34
Facility RVU	**Work**	**PE**	**MP**	**Total**
43622	40.03	18.52	9.79	68.34

	FUD	Status	MUE	Modifiers				IOM Reference
43622	90	A	1(2)	51	N/A	62*	80	None

* with documentation

43631

43631 Gastrectomy, partial, distal; with gastroduodenostomy

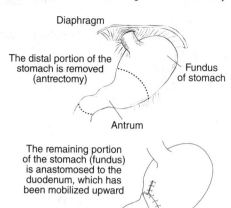

Diaphragm

The distal portion of the
stomach is removed
(antrectomy)

Fundus
of stomach

Antrum

The remaining portion
of the stomach (fundus)
is anastomosed to the
duodenum, which has
been mobilized upward

Duodenum

Explanation

The physician removes the distal stomach and approximates the proximal stomach to the duodenum. The physician makes a midline abdominal incision. The distal stomach (antrum) is dissected free from surrounding structures and the blood supply to the antrum is divided. Next, the gastroduodenal junction is divided and the stomach is divided in its middle portion removing the antrum. An anastomosis is made between the proximal stomach and the duodenum with staples or sutures. The incision is closed.

Coding Tips

For vagotomy performed with partial, distal gastrectomy, report 43635 in addition to this code. For total gastrectomy with esophagoenterostomy, see 43620; Roux-en-Y reconstruction, see 43621; with formation of an intestinal pouch, see 43622.

ICD-10-CM Diagnostic Codes

C16.0	Malignant neoplasm of cardia
C16.1	Malignant neoplasm of fundus of stomach
C16.2	Malignant neoplasm of body of stomach
C16.3	Malignant neoplasm of pyloric antrum
C16.4	Malignant neoplasm of pylorus
C16.8	Malignant neoplasm of overlapping sites of stomach
C7A.092	Malignant carcinoid tumor of the stomach
D13.1	Benign neoplasm of stomach
D37.1	Neoplasm of uncertain behavior of stomach
D3A.092	Benign carcinoid tumor of the stomach
K25.0	Acute gastric ulcer with hemorrhage
K25.1	Acute gastric ulcer with perforation
K25.2	Acute gastric ulcer with both hemorrhage and perforation
K25.4	Chronic or unspecified gastric ulcer with hemorrhage
K25.5	Chronic or unspecified gastric ulcer with perforation
K25.6	Chronic or unspecified gastric ulcer with both hemorrhage and perforation
K25.7	Chronic gastric ulcer without hemorrhage or perforation
K27.0	Acute peptic ulcer, site unspecified, with hemorrhage
K27.1	Acute peptic ulcer, site unspecified, with perforation
K27.2	Acute peptic ulcer, site unspecified, with both hemorrhage and perforation
K27.3	Acute peptic ulcer, site unspecified, without hemorrhage or perforation
K27.4	Chronic or unspecified peptic ulcer, site unspecified, with hemorrhage
K27.5	Chronic or unspecified peptic ulcer, site unspecified, with perforation
K27.6	Chronic or unspecified peptic ulcer, site unspecified, with both hemorrhage and perforation
K27.7	Chronic peptic ulcer, site unspecified, without hemorrhage or perforation
K31.1	Adult hypertrophic pyloric stenosis ▲
K31.2	Hourglass stricture and stenosis of stomach
K31.3	Pylorospasm, not elsewhere classified
K31.5	Obstruction of duodenum
K31.811	Angiodysplasia of stomach and duodenum with bleeding
K31.819	Angiodysplasia of stomach and duodenum without bleeding
K31.82	Dieulafoy lesion (hemorrhagic) of stomach and duodenum
K31.89	Other diseases of stomach and duodenum
K91.81	Other intraoperative complications of digestive system
S36.33XA	Laceration of stomach, initial encounter
S36.39XA	Other injury of stomach, initial encounter

AMA: 43631 2014,Jan,11

Relative Value Units/Medicare Edits

Non-Facility RVU	Work	PE	MP	Total
43631	24.51	12.57	5.79	42.87
Facility RVU	**Work**	**PE**	**MP**	**Total**
43631	24.51	12.57	5.79	42.87

	FUD	Status	MUE	Modifiers				IOM Reference
43631	90	A	1(2)	51	N/A	62*	80	None

* with documentation

43632

43632   Gastrectomy, partial, distal; with gastrojejunostomy

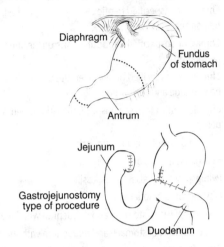

Diaphragm

Fundus of stomach

Antrum

Jejunum

Gastrojejunostomy type of procedure

Duodenum

The distal portion of the stomach (antrum) is surgically removed and the remainder is anastomosed to the jejunum

Explanation

The physician removes the distal stomach and approximates the proximal stomach to the jejunum. The physician makes a midline abdominal incision. The distal stomach (antrum) is dissected free from surrounding structures and the blood supply to the antrum is divided. Next, the gastroduodenal junction is divided and the stomach is divided in its middle portion removing the antrum. An anastomosis is made between the proximal stomach and the jejunum with staples or sutures. The incision is closed.

Coding Tips

For total gastrectomy with esophagoenterostomy, see 43620; Roux-en-Y reconstruction, see 43621; with formation of an intestinal pouch, see 43622. For partial, distal gastrectomy with gastroduodenostomy, see 43631; with Roux-en-Y reconstruction, see 43633; with formation of an intestinal pouch, see 43634.

ICD-10-CM Diagnostic Codes

C16.0	Malignant neoplasm of cardia
C16.1	Malignant neoplasm of fundus of stomach
C16.2	Malignant neoplasm of body of stomach
C16.3	Malignant neoplasm of pyloric antrum
C16.4	Malignant neoplasm of pylorus
C16.8	Malignant neoplasm of overlapping sites of stomach
C78.89	Secondary malignant neoplasm of other digestive organs
C7A.092	Malignant carcinoid tumor of the stomach
D13.1	Benign neoplasm of stomach
D37.1	Neoplasm of uncertain behavior of stomach
D3A.092	Benign carcinoid tumor of the stomach
K25.0	Acute gastric ulcer with hemorrhage
K25.1	Acute gastric ulcer with perforation
K25.2	Acute gastric ulcer with both hemorrhage and perforation
K25.4	Chronic or unspecified gastric ulcer with hemorrhage
K25.5	Chronic or unspecified gastric ulcer with perforation
K25.6	Chronic or unspecified gastric ulcer with both hemorrhage and perforation
K25.7	Chronic gastric ulcer without hemorrhage or perforation
K27.0	Acute peptic ulcer, site unspecified, with hemorrhage
K27.1	Acute peptic ulcer, site unspecified, with perforation
K27.2	Acute peptic ulcer, site unspecified, with both hemorrhage and perforation
K27.3	Acute peptic ulcer, site unspecified, without hemorrhage or perforation
K27.4	Chronic or unspecified peptic ulcer, site unspecified, with hemorrhage
K27.5	Chronic or unspecified peptic ulcer, site unspecified, with perforation
K27.6	Chronic or unspecified peptic ulcer, site unspecified, with both hemorrhage and perforation
K27.7	Chronic peptic ulcer, site unspecified, without hemorrhage or perforation
K31.1	Adult hypertrophic pyloric stenosis ◭
K31.2	Hourglass stricture and stenosis of stomach
K31.3	Pylorospasm, not elsewhere classified
K31.7	Polyp of stomach and duodenum
K31.811	Angiodysplasia of stomach and duodenum with bleeding
K31.819	Angiodysplasia of stomach and duodenum without bleeding
K31.82	Dieulafoy lesion (hemorrhagic) of stomach and duodenum
K31.84	Gastroparesis
K31.89	Other diseases of stomach and duodenum
K91.81	Other intraoperative complications of digestive system
S36.33XA	Laceration of stomach, initial encounter
S36.39XA	Other injury of stomach, initial encounter

AMA: 43632 2014,Jan,11

Relative Value Units/Medicare Edits

Non-Facility RVU	Work	PE	MP	Total
43632	35.14	16.5	8.32	59.96
Facility RVU	Work	PE	MP	Total
43632	35.14	16.5	8.32	59.96

	FUD	Status	MUE	Modifiers				IOM Reference
43632	90	A	1(2)	51	N/A	62*	80	None

* with documentation

43633

43633 Gastrectomy, partial, distal; with Roux-en-Y reconstruction

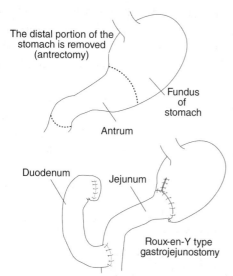

The distal portion of the
stomach is removed
(antrectomy)

Fundus
of
stomach

Antrum

Duodenum

Jejunum

Roux-en-Y type
gastrojejunostomy

The distal portion of the stomach (antrum) is
surgically removed and the remainder is
anastomosed, usually to the jejunum, and a
Roux-en-Y segment is fashioned from the duodenum

Explanation

The physician removes the distal stomach (antrum) and performs an anastomosis between the proximal stomach and a Roux-en-Y limb of jejunum. The physician makes a midline abdominal incision. Next, the distal stomach is dissected free of surrounding structures and the blood supply to the antrum is divided. The gastroduodenal junction and the middle portion of the stomach are divided and the antrum is removed. The vagus nerves, as they pass from the esophagus onto the stomach, are usually divided. The proximal jejunum is divided and the distal limb of jejunum is connected to the proximal stomach. The proximal jejunum is connected to the limb of jejunum distal to the gastrojejunostomy to restore intestinal continuity. The incisions are closed.

Coding Tips

For vagotomy performed with partial, distal gastrectomy, report 43635 in addition to this code. For total gastrectomy with esophagoenterostomy, see 43620; Roux-en-Y reconstruction, see 43621; with formation of an intestinal pouch, see 43622.

ICD-10-CM Diagnostic Codes

C16.0	Malignant neoplasm of cardia
C16.1	Malignant neoplasm of fundus of stomach
C16.2	Malignant neoplasm of body of stomach
C16.3	Malignant neoplasm of pyloric antrum
C16.4	Malignant neoplasm of pylorus
C16.8	Malignant neoplasm of overlapping sites of stomach
C78.89	Secondary malignant neoplasm of other digestive organs
C7A.092	Malignant carcinoid tumor of the stomach
D13.1	Benign neoplasm of stomach
D37.1	Neoplasm of uncertain behavior of stomach
D37.2	Neoplasm of uncertain behavior of small intestine
D3A.092	Benign carcinoid tumor of the stomach
K25.0	Acute gastric ulcer with hemorrhage
K25.1	Acute gastric ulcer with perforation
K25.2	Acute gastric ulcer with both hemorrhage and perforation
K25.3	Acute gastric ulcer without hemorrhage or perforation
K25.4	Chronic or unspecified gastric ulcer with hemorrhage
K25.5	Chronic or unspecified gastric ulcer with perforation
K25.6	Chronic or unspecified gastric ulcer with both hemorrhage and perforation
K25.7	Chronic gastric ulcer without hemorrhage or perforation
K27.0	Acute peptic ulcer, site unspecified, with hemorrhage
K27.1	Acute peptic ulcer, site unspecified, with perforation
K27.2	Acute peptic ulcer, site unspecified, with both hemorrhage and perforation
K27.3	Acute peptic ulcer, site unspecified, without hemorrhage or perforation
K27.4	Chronic or unspecified peptic ulcer, site unspecified, with hemorrhage
K27.5	Chronic or unspecified peptic ulcer, site unspecified, with perforation
K27.6	Chronic or unspecified peptic ulcer, site unspecified, with both hemorrhage and perforation
K27.7	Chronic peptic ulcer, site unspecified, without hemorrhage or perforation
K31.1	Adult hypertrophic pyloric stenosis ◣
K31.2	Hourglass stricture and stenosis of stomach
K31.3	Pylorospasm, not elsewhere classified
K31.7	Polyp of stomach and duodenum
S36.33XA	Laceration of stomach, initial encounter
S36.39XA	Other injury of stomach, initial encounter

AMA: 43633 2014,Jan,11

Relative Value Units/Medicare Edits

Non-Facility RVU	Work	PE	MP	Total
43633	33.14	15.74	7.86	56.74
Facility RVU	**Work**	**PE**	**MP**	**Total**
43633	33.14	15.74	7.86	56.74

	FUD	Status	MUE	Modifiers				IOM Reference
43633	90	A	1(2)	51	N/A	62*	80	None

* with documentation

Stomach

Stomach

43634

43634 Gastrectomy, partial, distal; with formation of intestinal pouch

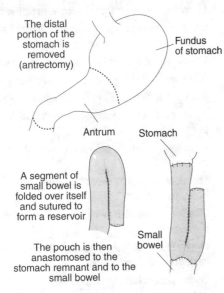

The distal portion of the stomach is removed (antrectomy)

Fundus of stomach

Antrum   Stomach

A segment of small bowel is folded over itself and sutured to form a reservoir

Small bowel

The pouch is then anastomosed to the stomach remnant and to the small bowel

The distal portion of the stomach is surgically removed and the remainder is anastomosed to the small bowel. An intestinal pouch is fashioned from bowel and sutured into place, forming a replacement for the removed antrum and pylorus

Explanation

The physician removes the distal stomach (antrum) and performs an anastomosis between the stomach and a pouch formed of jejunum. The physician makes a midline abdominal incision. The distal stomach is dissected free of surrounding structures and the blood supply to the antrum is divided. The gastroduodenal junction and the middle portion of the stomach are divided and the antrum is removed. The vagus nerves, as they pass from the esophagus onto the stomach, are usually divided. The proximal jejunum is divided and the distal end is folded upon itself and approximated in such a way to form a pouch. The pouch is connected to the proximal stomach and the proximal end of the divided jejunum is connected to the jejunal limb distal to the pouch anastomosis to establish intestinal continuity. The incision is closed.

Coding Tips

For a vagotomy performed with a partial, distal gastrectomy, report 43635 in addition to this code. For a total gastrectomy with an esophagoenterostomy, see 43620; Roux-en-Y reconstruction, see 43621; with formation of an intestinal pouch, see 43622.

ICD-10-CM Diagnostic Codes

C16.0	Malignant neoplasm of cardia
C16.1	Malignant neoplasm of fundus of stomach
C16.2	Malignant neoplasm of body of stomach
C16.3	Malignant neoplasm of pyloric antrum
C16.4	Malignant neoplasm of pylorus
C16.8	Malignant neoplasm of overlapping sites of stomach
C78.89	Secondary malignant neoplasm of other digestive organs
C7A.092	Malignant carcinoid tumor of the stomach
D13.1	Benign neoplasm of stomach
D37.1	Neoplasm of uncertain behavior of stomach
D3A.092	Benign carcinoid tumor of the stomach
K25.0	Acute gastric ulcer with hemorrhage
K25.1	Acute gastric ulcer with perforation
K25.2	Acute gastric ulcer with both hemorrhage and perforation
K25.3	Acute gastric ulcer without hemorrhage or perforation
K25.4	Chronic or unspecified gastric ulcer with hemorrhage
K25.5	Chronic or unspecified gastric ulcer with perforation
K25.6	Chronic or unspecified gastric ulcer with both hemorrhage and perforation
K25.7	Chronic gastric ulcer without hemorrhage or perforation
K27.0	Acute peptic ulcer, site unspecified, with hemorrhage
K27.1	Acute peptic ulcer, site unspecified, with perforation
K27.2	Acute peptic ulcer, site unspecified, with both hemorrhage and perforation
K27.3	Acute peptic ulcer, site unspecified, without hemorrhage or perforation
K27.4	Chronic or unspecified peptic ulcer, site unspecified, with hemorrhage
K27.5	Chronic or unspecified peptic ulcer, site unspecified, with perforation
K27.6	Chronic or unspecified peptic ulcer, site unspecified, with both hemorrhage and perforation
K27.7	Chronic peptic ulcer, site unspecified, without hemorrhage or perforation
K31.1	Adult hypertrophic pyloric stenosis △
K31.2	Hourglass stricture and stenosis of stomach
K31.3	Pylorospasm, not elsewhere classified
K31.7	Polyp of stomach and duodenum
S36.33XA	Laceration of stomach, initial encounter
S36.39XA	Other injury of stomach, initial encounter

AMA: **43634** 2014,Jan,11

Relative Value Units/Medicare Edits

Non-Facility RVU	Work	PE	MP	Total
43634	36.64	17.25	8.96	62.85
Facility RVU	**Work**	**PE**	**MP**	**Total**
43634	36.64	17.25	8.96	62.85

	FUD	Status	MUE	Modifiers				IOM Reference
43634	90	A	1(2)	51	N/A	62*	80	None

* with documentation

43635

+ **43635** Vagotomy when performed with partial distal gastrectomy (List separately in addition to code[s] for primary procedure)

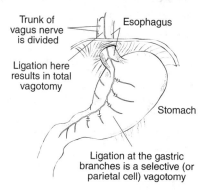

Trunk of vagus nerve is divided

Esophagus

Ligation here results in total vagotomy

Stomach

Ligation at the gastric branches is a selective (or parietal cell) vagotomy

Two main trunks of the vagus nerve run down the esophagus. They branch onto the stomach and govern gastric acid secretion

Explanation

The physician performs this with a separately reportable partial distal gastrectomy and repairs the stomach and severs vagus nerves. The physician uses a midline abdominal approach. The distal stomach (antrum) is dissected free and the blood supply to the antrum divided. The distal stomach is removed and the proximal stomach is sutured to the duodenum. Truncal vagotomy is performed by severing both right and left vagus nerves just below the diaphragm.

Coding Tips

Report 43635 in addition to 43631, 43632, 43633, and 43634.

ICD-10-CM Diagnostic Codes

C16.0	Malignant neoplasm of cardia
C16.1	Malignant neoplasm of fundus of stomach
C16.2	Malignant neoplasm of body of stomach
C16.3	Malignant neoplasm of pyloric antrum
C16.4	Malignant neoplasm of pylorus
C16.8	Malignant neoplasm of overlapping sites of stomach
C7A.092	Malignant carcinoid tumor of the stomach
D13.1	Benign neoplasm of stomach
D37.1	Neoplasm of uncertain behavior of stomach
D3A.092	Benign carcinoid tumor of the stomach
K25.0	Acute gastric ulcer with hemorrhage
K25.1	Acute gastric ulcer with perforation
K25.2	Acute gastric ulcer with both hemorrhage and perforation
K25.4	Chronic or unspecified gastric ulcer with hemorrhage
K25.5	Chronic or unspecified gastric ulcer with perforation
K25.6	Chronic or unspecified gastric ulcer with both hemorrhage and perforation
K25.7	Chronic gastric ulcer without hemorrhage or perforation
K27.0	Acute peptic ulcer, site unspecified, with hemorrhage
K27.1	Acute peptic ulcer, site unspecified, with perforation
K27.2	Acute peptic ulcer, site unspecified, with both hemorrhage and perforation
K27.3	Acute peptic ulcer, site unspecified, without hemorrhage or perforation
K27.4	Chronic or unspecified peptic ulcer, site unspecified, with hemorrhage
K27.5	Chronic or unspecified peptic ulcer, site unspecified, with perforation
K27.6	Chronic or unspecified peptic ulcer, site unspecified, with both hemorrhage and perforation
K27.7	Chronic peptic ulcer, site unspecified, without hemorrhage or perforation
K31.1	Adult hypertrophic pyloric stenosis ▲
K31.2	Hourglass stricture and stenosis of stomach
K31.3	Pylorospasm, not elsewhere classified
K31.5	Obstruction of duodenum
K31.811	Angiodysplasia of stomach and duodenum with bleeding
K31.819	Angiodysplasia of stomach and duodenum without bleeding
K31.82	Dieulafoy lesion (hemorrhagic) of stomach and duodenum
K31.89	Other diseases of stomach and duodenum
K91.81	Other intraoperative complications of digestive system
S36.33XA	Laceration of stomach, initial encounter
S36.39XA	Other injury of stomach, initial encounter

AMA: **43635** 2014,Jan,11

Relative Value Units/Medicare Edits

Non-Facility RVU	Work	PE	MP	Total
43635	2.06	0.76	0.48	3.3
Facility RVU	**Work**	**PE**	**MP**	**Total**
43635	2.06	0.76	0.48	3.3

	FUD	Status	MUE	Modifiers				IOM Reference
43635	N/A	A	1(2)	N/A	N/A	62*	80	None

* with documentation

Terms To Know

gastrectomy. Surgical excision of all or part of the stomach.

vagotomy. Division of the vagus nerves, interrupting impulses resulting in lower gastric acid production and hastening gastric emptying. Used in the treatment of chronic gastric, pyloric, and duodenal ulcers that can cause severe pain and difficulties in eating and sleeping.

43640-43641

43640 Vagotomy including pyloroplasty, with or without gastrostomy; truncal or selective

43641 parietal cell (highly selective)

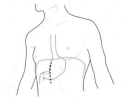

Upper abdominal midline incision

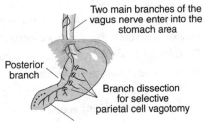

Two main branches of the vagus nerve enter into the stomach area

Posterior branch

Branch dissection for selective parietal cell vagotomy

A pyloroplasty is performed

A vagotomy and pyloroplasty are performed with or without construction of a gastrostomy

Explanation

The physician severs the vagus nerves and widens the pyloric canal, with or without making an incision in the stomach. The physician uses a midline upper abdominal incision to expose the muscular band surrounding the distal opening of the stomach. A longitudinal incision is made in the pylorus. The incision is closed with a single full thickness suture layer. The two branches of the vagus nerve are exposed and a truncal vagotomy is performed by severing both right and left vagus nerves. A gastrostomy may be created by inserting a tube from the stomach to the external surface of the abdominal wall. Report 43641 if performed with a parietal cell procedure.

Coding Tips

For partial, distal gastrectomy with gastroduodenostomy, see 43631; with gastrojejunostomy, see 43632; with Roux-en-Y reconstruction, see 43633; with formation of an intestinal pouch, see 43634. For pyloroplasty alone, see 43800. For vagotomy alone, see 64755–64760.

ICD-10-CM Diagnostic Codes

C16.4	Malignant neoplasm of pylorus
K25.0	Acute gastric ulcer with hemorrhage
K25.1	Acute gastric ulcer with perforation
K25.2	Acute gastric ulcer with both hemorrhage and perforation
K25.4	Chronic or unspecified gastric ulcer with hemorrhage
K25.5	Chronic or unspecified gastric ulcer with perforation
K25.6	Chronic or unspecified gastric ulcer with both hemorrhage and perforation
K25.7	Chronic gastric ulcer without hemorrhage or perforation
K26.0	Acute duodenal ulcer with hemorrhage
K26.1	Acute duodenal ulcer with perforation
K26.2	Acute duodenal ulcer with both hemorrhage and perforation
K26.3	Acute duodenal ulcer without hemorrhage or perforation
K26.4	Chronic or unspecified duodenal ulcer with hemorrhage
K26.5	Chronic or unspecified duodenal ulcer with perforation
K26.6	Chronic or unspecified duodenal ulcer with both hemorrhage and perforation
K26.7	Chronic duodenal ulcer without hemorrhage or perforation
K27.0	Acute peptic ulcer, site unspecified, with hemorrhage
K27.1	Acute peptic ulcer, site unspecified, with perforation
K27.2	Acute peptic ulcer, site unspecified, with both hemorrhage and perforation
K27.3	Acute peptic ulcer, site unspecified, without hemorrhage or perforation
K27.4	Chronic or unspecified peptic ulcer, site unspecified, with hemorrhage
K27.5	Chronic or unspecified peptic ulcer, site unspecified, with perforation
K27.6	Chronic or unspecified peptic ulcer, site unspecified, with both hemorrhage and perforation
K27.7	Chronic peptic ulcer, site unspecified, without hemorrhage or perforation
K30	Functional dyspepsia
K31.1	Adult hypertrophic pyloric stenosis 🅰
K31.89	Other diseases of stomach and duodenum

AMA: 43640 2014,Jan,11 **43641** 2014,Jan,11

Relative Value Units/Medicare Edits

Non-Facility RVU	Work	PE	MP	Total
43640	19.56	10.61	4.72	34.89
43641	19.81	11.01	4.84	35.66
Facility RVU	**Work**	**PE**	**MP**	**Total**
43640	19.56	10.61	4.72	34.89
43641	19.81	11.01	4.84	35.66

	FUD	Status	MUE	Modifiers				IOM Reference
43640	90	A	1(2)	51	N/A	62*	80	None
43641	90	A	1(2)	51	N/A	62*	80	

* with documentation

Terms To Know

gastrostomy. Temporary or permanent artificial opening made in the stomach for gastrointestinal decompression or to provide nutrition when not maintained by other methods.

pyloroplasty. Enlargement and reconstruction of the lower portion of the stomach opening into the duodenum performed after vagotomy to speed gastric emptying and treat duodenal ulcers.

vagotomy. Division of the vagus nerves, interrupting impulses resulting in lower gastric acid production and hastening gastric emptying.

43644

43644 Laparoscopy, surgical, gastric restrictive procedure; with gastric bypass and Roux-en-Y gastroenterostomy (roux limb 150 cm or less)

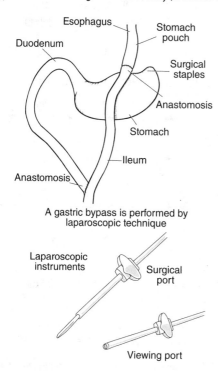

A gastric bypass is performed by laparoscopic technique

Laparoscopic instruments

Surgical port

Viewing port

Explanation

The physician performs a laparoscopic gastric bypass for morbid obesity by partitioning the stomach and performing a small bowel division with anastomosis to the proximal stomach (Roux-en-Y gastroenterostomy). This bypasses the majority of the stomach. The physician places a trocar though an incision above the umbilicus and insufflates the abdominal cavity. The laparoscope and additional trocars are placed through small portal incisions. The stomach is mobilized and the proximal stomach is divided with a stapling device along the lesser curvature, leaving only a small proximal pouch in continuity with the esophagus. A short limb of the proximal small bowel (150 cm or less) is divided and the distal end of the short intestinal limb is brought up and anastomosed to the proximal gastric pouch. The other end of the divided bowel is connected back into the small bowel distal to the short limb's gastric anastomosis to restore intestinal continuity. The instruments are removed.

Coding Tips

Surgical laparoscopy always includes diagnostic laparoscopy. Do not report 43644 with 43846 or 49320. Esophagogastroduodenoscopy (EGD) performed for a separate condition should be reported with modifier 59 or an X{EPSU} modifier. A gastric restrictive procedure with a roux limb greater than 150 cm is reported with 43645. For an open procedure, see 43846.

ICD-10-CM Diagnostic Codes

E27.8	Other specified disorders of adrenal gland
E35	Disorders of endocrine glands in diseases classified elsewhere
E66.01	Morbid (severe) obesity due to excess calories
E66.09	Other obesity due to excess calories
E66.1	Drug-induced obesity
E66.2	Morbid (severe) obesity with alveolar hypoventilation

E66.3	Overweight
E66.8	Other obesity
Z68.41	Body mass index [BMI] 40.0-44.9, adult Ⓐ
Z68.42	Body mass index [BMI] 45.0-49.9, adult Ⓐ
Z68.43	Body mass index [BMI] 50.0-59.9, adult Ⓐ
Z68.44	Body mass index [BMI] 60.0-69.9, adult Ⓐ
Z68.45	Body mass index [BMI] 70 or greater, adult Ⓐ

AMA: 43644 2014,Jan,11

Relative Value Units/Medicare Edits

Non-Facility RVU	Work	PE	MP	Total
43644	29.4	14.8	7.12	51.32
Facility RVU	**Work**	**PE**	**MP**	**Total**
43644	29.4	14.8	7.12	51.32

	FUD	Status	MUE	Modifiers				IOM Reference
43644	90	A	1(2)	51	N/A	62*	80	None

* with documentation

Terms To Know

BMI. Body mass index. Tool for calculating weight appropriateness in adults and may be a factor in determining medical necessity for bariatric procedures.

bypass. Auxiliary or diverted route to maintain continuous flow.

laparoscopy. Direct visualization of the peritoneal cavity, outer fallopian tubes, uterus, and ovaries utilizing a laparoscope, a thin, flexible fiberoptic tube.

morbid obesity. Accumulation of excess fat in the subcutaneous connective tissue with increased weight beyond the limits of skeletal requirements, defined as 125 percent or more over the ideal body weight. It is often associated with serious conditions that can become life threatening, such as diabetes, hypertension, and arteriosclerosis.

proximal. Located closest to a specified reference point, usually the midline or trunk.

Roux-en-Y anastomosis. Y-shaped attachment of the distal end of a divided small intestine segment to the stomach, esophagus, biliary tract, or other structure with anastomosis of the proximal end to the side of the small intestine further down for reflux-free drainage.

trocar. Cannula or a sharp pointed instrument used to puncture and aspirate fluid from cavities.

43645

43645   Laparoscopy, surgical, gastric restrictive procedure; with gastric bypass and small intestine reconstruction to limit absorption

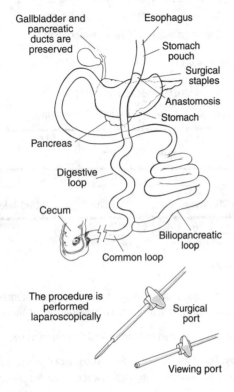

Gallbladder and pancreatic ducts are preserved

Esophagus

Stomach pouch

Surgical staples

Anastomosis

Stomach

Pancreas

Digestive loop

Cecum

Biliopancreatic loop

Common loop

The procedure is performed laparoscopically

Surgical port

Viewing port

Explanation

The physician performs a laparoscopic gastric bypass with small intestine reconstruction to limit absorption. This procedure is done to combine gastric restriction of intake with limited intestinal absorption. In one method used, the physician places a trocar though an incision above the umbilicus and insufflates the abdominal cavity. The laparoscope and additional trocars are placed through small portal incisions. The stomach is mobilized and the distal half is resected along a line from the lesser to greater curvature, leaving a "pouch" of stomach, which is connected directly to the final, distal section of small intestine. The bypassed duodenum, jejunum, and upper part of the divided ileum-the segment in connection with the gallbladder and pancreas, or the biliopancreatic loop-is anastomosed back to the common distal segment of the small intestine. This leaves a short common channel where food coming through the shortened alimentary tract combines with digestive juices from the much longer biliary tract before entering the colon. The instruments are removed.

Coding Tips

A surgical laparoscopy always includes a diagnostic laparoscopy. Do not report 43645 with 43847 or 49320. For open procedure, see 43847.

ICD-10-CM Diagnostic Codes

E27.8	Other specified disorders of adrenal gland
E35	Disorders of endocrine glands in diseases classified elsewhere
E66.01	Morbid (severe) obesity due to excess calories
E66.09	Other obesity due to excess calories
E66.1	Drug-induced obesity
E66.2	Morbid (severe) obesity with alveolar hypoventilation
E66.3	Overweight
E66.8	Other obesity
Z68.41	Body mass index [BMI] 40.0-44.9, adult △
Z68.42	Body mass index [BMI] 45.0-49.9, adult △
Z68.43	Body mass index [BMI] 50.0-59.9, adult △
Z68.44	Body mass index [BMI] 60.0-69.9, adult △
Z68.45	Body mass index [BMI] 70 or greater, adult △

AMA: **43645** 2018,Jan,8; 2017,Jan,8; 2016,Jan,13; 2015,Jan,16

Relative Value Units/Medicare Edits

Non-Facility RVU	Work	PE	MP	Total
43645	31.53	15.4	7.36	54.29
Facility RVU	**Work**	**PE**	**MP**	**Total**
43645	31.53	15.4	7.36	54.29

	FUD	Status	MUE	Modifiers				IOM Reference
43645	90	A	1(2)	51	N/A	62*	80	None

* with documentation

Terms To Know

anastomosis. Surgically created connection between ducts, blood vessels, or bowel segments to allow flow from one to the other.

BMI. Body mass index. Tool for calculating weight appropriateness in adults and may be a factor in determining medical necessity for bariatric procedures.

bypass. Auxiliary or diverted route to maintain continuous flow.

distal. Located farther away from a specified reference point or the trunk.

laparoscopy. Direct visualization of the peritoneal cavity, outer fallopian tubes, uterus, and ovaries utilizing a laparoscope, a thin, flexible fiberoptic tube.

morbid obesity. Accumulation of excess fat in the subcutaneous connective tissue with increased weight beyond the limits of skeletal requirements, defined as 125 percent or more over the ideal body weight. It is often associated with serious conditions that can become life threatening, such as diabetes, hypertension, and arteriosclerosis.

trocar. Cannula or a sharp pointed instrument used to puncture and aspirate fluid from cavities.

43647-43648

43647 Laparoscopy, surgical; implantation or replacement of gastric neurostimulator electrodes, antrum

43648 revision or removal of gastric neurostimulator electrodes, antrum

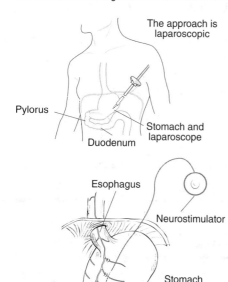

The approach is laparoscopic

Pylorus

Stomach and laparoscope

Duodenum

Esophagus

Neurostimulator

Stomach

Electrode

Explanation

The physician performs a laparoscopic placement of gastric neurostimulator electrodes. The physician makes an incision and places a trocar at the umbilicus to insufflate the abdomen. The laparoscope is placed through the umbilical port and additional trocars are placed into the abdominal cavity. The antrum of the stomach is identified and the physician secures two electrodes into the muscle of the pyloric antrum. The electrodes are connected to a neurostimulator that has been secured in a subcutaneous pocket in the abdomen in a separately reportable procedure. The physician removes the laparoscope and tools from the abdomen, which is deflated and repaired with sutures. Report 43647 if electrodes are placed or if existing electrodes are removed and replaced with new ones. Report 43648 for the revision or removal of the electrodes.

Coding Tips

If this procedure is performed with an open approach, see 43881–43882. For insertion of a gastric neurostimulator pulse generator, see 64590; revision or removal, see 64595. For electronic analysis and programming of gastric neurostimulator, see 95980–95982. For laparoscopic implantation, revision, or removal of gastric neurostimulator electrodes, lesser curvature (for morbid obesity), see 43659. Laparoscopic implantation, removal, replacement, or revision of vagus nerve blocking neurostimulator electrodes and/or pulse generator services are reported with 0312T-0317T.

ICD-10-CM Diagnostic Codes

E08.43	Diabetes mellitus due to underlying condition with diabetic autonomic (poly)neuropathy
E09.43	Drug or chemical induced diabetes mellitus with neurological complications with diabetic autonomic (poly)neuropathy
E10.43	Type 1 diabetes mellitus with diabetic autonomic (poly)neuropathy
E11.43	Type 2 diabetes mellitus with diabetic autonomic (poly)neuropathy
E66.01	Morbid (severe) obesity due to excess calories
E66.1	Drug-induced obesity
E66.2	Morbid (severe) obesity with alveolar hypoventilation
E66.3	Overweight
T85.518A	Breakdown (mechanical) of other gastrointestinal prosthetic devices, implants and grafts, initial encounter
T85.528A	Displacement of other gastrointestinal prosthetic devices, implants and grafts, initial encounter
T85.598A	Other mechanical complication of other gastrointestinal prosthetic devices, implants and grafts, initial encounter

AMA: **43647** 2019,Feb,6; 2018,Jan,8; 2017,Jan,8; 2016,Jan,13; 2015,Jan,16 **43648** 2019,Feb,6; 2018,Jan,8; 2017,Jan,8; 2016,Jan,13; 2015,Jan,16

Relative Value Units/Medicare Edits

Non-Facility RVU	Work	PE	MP	Total
43647	0.0	0.0	0.0	0.0
43648	0.0	0.0	0.0	0.0
Facility RVU	Work	PE	MP	Total
43647	0.0	0.0	0.0	0.0
43648	0.0	0.0	0.0	0.0

	FUD	Status	MUE	Modifiers				IOM Reference
43647	N/A	C	1(2)	51	N/A	62*	80	None
43648	N/A	C	1(2)	51	N/A	62*	80	

* with documentation

Terms To Know

antrum. Chamber or cavity, typically with a small opening.

diabetes mellitus. Endocrine disease manifested by high blood glucose levels and resulting in the inability to successfully metabolize carbohydrates, proteins, and fats, due to defects in insulin production and secretion, insulin action, or both.

gastroparesis. Delay in the emptying of food from the stomach into the small bowel due to a degree of paralysis in the muscles lining the stomach wall.

laparoscopy. Direct visualization utilizing a thin, flexible, fiberoptic tube.

morbid obesity. Accumulation of excess fat in the subcutaneous connective tissue with increased weight beyond the limits of skeletal requirements, defined as 125 percent or more over the ideal body weight. It is often associated with serious conditions that can become life threatening, such as diabetes, hypertension, and arteriosclerosis.

43651-43652

43651 Laparoscopy, surgical; transection of vagus nerves, truncal
43652 transection of vagus nerves, selective or highly selective

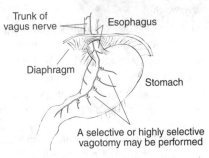

Trunk of vagus nerve
Esophagus
Diaphragm
Stomach

A selective or highly selective vagotomy may be performed

The vagus nerves are transected in a laparoscopic surgical session

Explanation

The physician performs laparoscopic truncal vagotomy. The physician places a trocar through an incision above the umbilicus and insufflates the abdominal cavity. The laparoscope is placed through the supraumbilical port and additional trocars are placed into the abdominal cavity. The fascial anterior to the esophagus is incised and the distal esophagus is mobilized. The anterior and posterior vagal nerve trunks are identified and divided. The physician removes a small segment of each nerve. In 43652, a selective or highly selective vagotomy is performed. The main nerve trunks are followed down onto the stomach and the branches from the nerves to the proximal half of the stomach are divided. The trocars are removed and the incisions are closed.

Coding Tips

Both truncal and selective vagotomies may require a drainage procedure, such as pyloroplasty to prevent gastric stasis. A pyloroplasty is accomplished by enlarging the pyloric opening between the stomach and duodenum. When a laparoscopic vagotomy is performed with a pyloroplasty, report the truncal vagotomy (43651) and the pyloroplasty code (43800) with modifier 51. Surgical laparoscopy always includes diagnostic laparoscopy. To report a diagnostic laparoscopy (peritoneoscopy) only, see 49320. For open vagotomy performed with partial distal gastrectomy, see 43635.

ICD-10-CM Diagnostic Codes

E16.4	Increased secretion of gastrin
K25.0	Acute gastric ulcer with hemorrhage
K25.1	Acute gastric ulcer with perforation
K25.2	Acute gastric ulcer with both hemorrhage and perforation
K25.3	Acute gastric ulcer without hemorrhage or perforation
K25.4	Chronic or unspecified gastric ulcer with hemorrhage
K25.5	Chronic or unspecified gastric ulcer with perforation
K25.6	Chronic or unspecified gastric ulcer with both hemorrhage and perforation
K25.7	Chronic gastric ulcer without hemorrhage or perforation
K26.0	Acute duodenal ulcer with hemorrhage
K26.1	Acute duodenal ulcer with perforation
K26.2	Acute duodenal ulcer with both hemorrhage and perforation
K26.3	Acute duodenal ulcer without hemorrhage or perforation
K26.4	Chronic or unspecified duodenal ulcer with hemorrhage
K26.5	Chronic or unspecified duodenal ulcer with perforation
K26.6	Chronic or unspecified duodenal ulcer with both hemorrhage and perforation
K26.7	Chronic duodenal ulcer without hemorrhage or perforation
K27.0	Acute peptic ulcer, site unspecified, with hemorrhage
K27.1	Acute peptic ulcer, site unspecified, with perforation
K27.2	Acute peptic ulcer, site unspecified, with both hemorrhage and perforation
K27.3	Acute peptic ulcer, site unspecified, without hemorrhage or perforation
K30	Functional dyspepsia
K31.1	Adult hypertrophic pyloric stenosis 🅰

AMA: 43651 2018,Jan,8; 2017,Jan,8; 2016,Jan,13; 2015,Jan,16 **43652** 2018,Jan,8; 2017,Jan,8; 2016,Jan,13; 2015,Jan,16

Relative Value Units/Medicare Edits

Non-Facility RVU	Work	PE	MP	Total
43651	10.13	6.84	2.47	19.44
43652	12.13	7.58	2.97	22.68
Facility RVU	**Work**	**PE**	**MP**	**Total**
43651	10.13	6.84	2.47	19.44
43652	12.13	7.58	2.97	22.68

	FUD	Status	MUE	Modifiers				IOM Reference
43651	90	A	1(2)	51	N/A	62*	80	None
43652	90	A	1(2)	51	N/A	62*	80	

* with documentation

Terms To Know

laparoscopy. Direct visualization of the peritoneal cavity, outer fallopian tubes, uterus, and ovaries utilizing a laparoscope, a thin, flexible fiberoptic tube.

transection. Transverse dissection; to cut across a long axis; cross section.

trocar. Cannula or a sharp pointed instrument used to puncture and aspirate fluid from cavities.

43653

43653 Laparoscopy, surgical; gastrostomy, without construction of gastric tube (eg, Stamm procedure) (separate procedure)

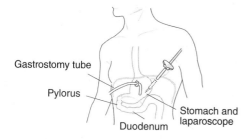

Gastrostomy tube
Pylorus
Stomach and laparoscope
Duodenum

A temporary gastrostomy tube is placed

Detail of tube in place

Explanation

Using a laparoscope, the physician constructs a temporary or permanent gastrostomy for feeding. With the patient under anesthesia, the physician places a trocar at the umbilicus into the abdomen and insufflates the abdominal cavity. The physician places a laparoscope through the umbilical incision. An additional trocar is inserted through the abdominal wall into the intra-abdominal cavity at a previously determined site where the gastrostomy will reside. The gastrostomy tube is pulled through the trocar from outside the abdomen into the intra-abdominal cavity. The physician identifies the stomach and introduces instruments to open the organ and create a viable receptacle for the tube. The tip of the gastrostomy tube is inserted into the stomach, and the tube is clamped off on the outside of the body and sutured into place on the stomach. Additional sutures are placed in the abdominal wall to hold the gastrostomy tube in place and to secure the tube. The trocars are removed and the incisions are closed with staples or sutures.

Coding Tips

Surgical laparoscopy always includes diagnostic laparoscopy. To report a diagnostic laparoscopy (peritoneoscopy) only, see 49320. This separate procedure by definition is usually a component of a more complex service and is not identified separately. When performed alone or with other unrelated procedures/services it may be reported. If performed alone, list the code; if performed with other procedures/services, list the code and append modifier 59 or an X{EPSU} modifier. For an open gastrostomy, see 43830–43832.

ICD-10-CM Diagnostic Codes

C10.0	Malignant neoplasm of vallecula
C10.1	Malignant neoplasm of anterior surface of epiglottis
C10.2	Malignant neoplasm of lateral wall of oropharynx
C10.3	Malignant neoplasm of posterior wall of oropharynx
C10.4	Malignant neoplasm of branchial cleft
C10.8	Malignant neoplasm of overlapping sites of oropharynx
C13.0	Malignant neoplasm of postcricoid region
C13.1	Malignant neoplasm of aryepiglottic fold, hypopharyngeal aspect
C13.2	Malignant neoplasm of posterior wall of hypopharynx
C13.8	Malignant neoplasm of overlapping sites of hypopharynx
C15.3	Malignant neoplasm of upper third of esophagus
C15.4	Malignant neoplasm of middle third of esophagus
C15.5	Malignant neoplasm of lower third of esophagus
C15.8	Malignant neoplasm of overlapping sites of esophagus
C16.0	Malignant neoplasm of cardia
C16.1	Malignant neoplasm of fundus of stomach
C16.2	Malignant neoplasm of body of stomach
C16.3	Malignant neoplasm of pyloric antrum
C16.4	Malignant neoplasm of pylorus
C16.8	Malignant neoplasm of overlapping sites of stomach
C76.0	Malignant neoplasm of head, face and neck
C78.89	Secondary malignant neoplasm of other digestive organs
C7A.092	Malignant carcinoid tumor of the stomach
D00.2	Carcinoma in situ of stomach
D13.1	Benign neoplasm of stomach
D3A.092	Benign carcinoid tumor of the stomach
E41	Nutritional marasmus
E44.0	Moderate protein-calorie malnutrition
E44.1	Mild protein-calorie malnutrition
E45	Retarded development following protein-calorie malnutrition
J95.04	Tracheo-esophageal fistula following tracheostomy
K22.0	Achalasia of cardia
K22.2	Esophageal obstruction
K22.3	Perforation of esophagus
K22.4	Dyskinesia of esophagus
K22.5	Diverticulum of esophagus, acquired
K22.89	Other specified disease of esophagus
K31.89	Other diseases of stomach and duodenum
Q39.0	Atresia of esophagus without fistula
Q39.1	Atresia of esophagus with tracheo-esophageal fistula
Q39.2	Congenital tracheo-esophageal fistula without atresia
Q39.3	Congenital stenosis and stricture of esophagus
Q39.4	Esophageal web
Q39.5	Congenital dilatation of esophagus
Q39.6	Congenital diverticulum of esophagus
Q39.8	Other congenital malformations of esophagus
Q40.0	Congenital hypertrophic pyloric stenosis
R13.11	Dysphagia, oral phase
R13.12	Dysphagia, oropharyngeal phase
R13.13	Dysphagia, pharyngeal phase
R13.14	Dysphagia, pharyngoesophageal phase
R62.7	Adult failure to thrive ▲
R63.0	Anorexia
R63.32	Pediatric feeding disorder, chronic ▣
R63.39	Other feeding difficulties
T73.0XXA	Starvation, initial encounter

AMA: 43653 2018,Jan,8; 2017,Jan,8; 2016,Jan,13; 2015,Jan,16

Relative Value Units/Medicare Edits

Non-Facility RVU	Work	PE	MP	Total
43653	8.48	6.62	2.03	17.13
Facility RVU	Work	PE	MP	Total
43653	8.48	6.62	2.03	17.13

	FUD	Status	MUE	Modifiers				IOM Reference
43653	90	A	1(2)	51	N/A	62*	80	None

* with documentation

Terms To Know

gastrostomy. Temporary or permanent artificial opening made in the stomach for gastrointestinal decompression or to provide nutrition when not maintained by other methods.

insufflation. Blowing air or gas into a body cavity.

intra. Within.

laparoscopy. Direct visualization utilizing a thin, flexible, fiberoptic tube.

separate procedures. Services commonly carried out as a fundamental part of a total service and, as such, do not usually warrant separate identification. These services are identified in CPT with the parenthetical phrase (separate procedure) at the end of the description and are payable only when performed alone.

trocar. Cannula or a sharp pointed instrument used to puncture and aspirate fluid from cavities.

43752

43752   Naso- or oro-gastric tube placement, requiring physician's skill and fluoroscopic guidance (includes fluoroscopy, image documentation and report)

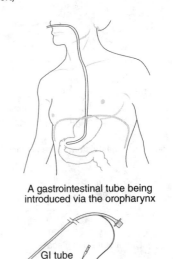

A gastrointestinal tube being introduced via the oropharynx

GI tube

A naso- or orogastric tube is placed by a physician

Explanation

The physician places a naso- or orogastric tube. The patient is placed in an upright position. The physician checks the nostrils for obstruction and selects the nostril for tube insertion. The physician may swab the nostril and spray the oropharynx with medication to numb the nasal passage and suppress the gag reflex. Next, the physician lubricates the tube, elevates the tip of the nose, and introduces the nasogastric tube into the nostril. The tube is advanced and the position of the tube is checked using fluoroscopy to ensure it is aligned to enter the oropharynx. As the patient swallows, the physician advances the tube through the pharynx, esophagus, and into the stomach. Air is injected into the tube (at the nose) while the physician listens with a stethoscope positioned at the stomach for the air to come out of the tube. Gastric contents are aspirated. These precautions are performed to ensure the tube is positioned in the stomach. The nasogastric tube is taped to the nostril. If the tube is fitted with a balloon (at the end of the tube in the stomach), it is inflated to hold the tube in place. This code includes the fluoroscopic guidance, image documentation, and report.

Coding Tips

Fluoroscopic guidance is included in 43752 and should not be reported separately. For enteric tube placement, see 44500 and 74340. For percutaneous placement of a gastrostomy tube, see 49440. Do not report 43752 with critical care codes 99291–99292, neonatal/pediatric intensive care codes 99468–99469 or 99471–99476, or low birth weight intensive care service codes 99478–99480.

ICD-10-CM Diagnostic Codes

C15.3	Malignant neoplasm of upper third of esophagus
C15.4	Malignant neoplasm of middle third of esophagus
C15.5	Malignant neoplasm of lower third of esophagus
C15.8	Malignant neoplasm of overlapping sites of esophagus
E03.5	Myxedema coma

E08.11	Diabetes mellitus due to underlying condition with ketoacidosis with coma
E08.641	Diabetes mellitus due to underlying condition with hypoglycemia with coma
E09.11	Drug or chemical induced diabetes mellitus with ketoacidosis with coma
E09.641	Drug or chemical induced diabetes mellitus with hypoglycemia with coma
E10.11	Type 1 diabetes mellitus with ketoacidosis with coma
E10.641	Type 1 diabetes mellitus with hypoglycemia with coma
E11.01	Type 2 diabetes mellitus with hyperosmolarity with coma
E11.641	Type 2 diabetes mellitus with hypoglycemia with coma
E13.11	Other specified diabetes mellitus with ketoacidosis with coma
E13.641	Other specified diabetes mellitus with hypoglycemia with coma
E40	Kwashiorkor
E41	Nutritional marasmus
E42	Marasmic kwashiorkor
F84.2	Rett's syndrome
G12.21	Amyotrophic lateral sclerosis △
G31.81	Alpers disease
G31.82	Leigh's disease
G93.1	Anoxic brain damage, not elsewhere classified
G93.82	Brain death
G94	Other disorders of brain in diseases classified elsewhere
I67.89	Other cerebrovascular disease
K21.00	Gastro-esophageal reflux disease with esophagitis, without bleeding
K21.01	Gastro-esophageal reflux disease with esophagitis, with bleeding
K22.10	Ulcer of esophagus without bleeding
K22.11	Ulcer of esophagus with bleeding
K22.89	Other specified disease of esophagus
R13.0	Aphagia
R13.11	Dysphagia, oral phase
R13.12	Dysphagia, oropharyngeal phase
R13.13	Dysphagia, pharyngeal phase
R13.14	Dysphagia, pharyngoesophageal phase
R13.19	Other dysphagia
R40.2111	Coma scale, eyes open, never, in the field [EMT or ambulance]
R40.2112	Coma scale, eyes open, never, at arrival to emergency department
R40.2113	Coma scale, eyes open, never, at hospital admission
R40.2114	Coma scale, eyes open, never, 24 hours or more after hospital admission
R40.2121	Coma scale, eyes open, to pain, in the field [EMT or ambulance]
R40.2122	Coma scale, eyes open, to pain, at arrival to emergency department
R40.2123	Coma scale, eyes open, to pain, at hospital admission
R40.2124	Coma scale, eyes open, to pain, 24 hours or more after hospital admission
R40.2211	Coma scale, best verbal response, none, in the field [EMT or ambulance]
R40.2212	Coma scale, best verbal response, none, at arrival to emergency department
R40.2213	Coma scale, best verbal response, none, at hospital admission
R40.2214	Coma scale, best verbal response, none, 24 hours or more after hospital admission
R40.2221	Coma scale, best verbal response, incomprehensible words, in the field [EMT or ambulance]
R40.2222	Coma scale, best verbal response, incomprehensible words, at arrival to emergency department
R40.2223	Coma scale, best verbal response, incomprehensible words, at hospital admission
R40.2224	Coma scale, best verbal response, incomprehensible words, 24 hours or more after hospital admission
R40.2311	Coma scale, best motor response, none, in the field [EMT or ambulance]
R40.2312	Coma scale, best motor response, none, at arrival to emergency department
R40.2313	Coma scale, best motor response, none, at hospital admission
R40.2314	Coma scale, best motor response, none, 24 hours or more after hospital admission
R40.2321	Coma scale, best motor response, extension, in the field [EMT or ambulance]
R40.2322	Coma scale, best motor response, extension, at arrival to emergency department
R40.2323	Coma scale, best motor response, extension, at hospital admission
R40.2324	Coma scale, best motor response, extension, 24 hours or more after hospital admission
R40.2341	Coma scale, best motor response, flexion withdrawal, in the field [EMT or ambulance]
R40.2342	Coma scale, best motor response, flexion withdrawal, at arrival to emergency department
R40.2343	Coma scale, best motor response, flexion withdrawal, at hospital admission
R40.2344	Coma scale, best motor response, flexion withdrawal, 24 hours or more after hospital admission
R62.51	Failure to thrive (child) ▣
R62.7	Adult failure to thrive △
R63.0	Anorexia
R63.32	Pediatric feeding disorder, chronic ▣
R63.39	Other feeding difficulties

AMA: **43752** 2019,Aug,8; 2018,Mar,11; 2018,Jan,8; 2017,Jan,8; 2016,Jan,13; 2015,Jan,16

Relative Value Units/Medicare Edits

Non-Facility RVU	Work	PE	MP	Total
43752	0.81	0.28	0.09	1.18
Facility RVU	Work	PE	MP	Total
43752	0.81	0.28	0.09	1.18

	FUD	Status	MUE	Modifiers				IOM Reference
43752	0	A	2(3)	N/A	N/A	N/A	N/A	None

* with documentation

43753-43755

43753 Gastric intubation and aspiration(s) therapeutic, necessitating physician's skill (eg, for gastrointestinal hemorrhage), including lavage if performed

43754 Gastric intubation and aspiration, diagnostic; single specimen (eg, acid analysis)

43755 collection of multiple fractional specimens with gastric stimulation, single or double lumen tube (gastric secretory study) (eg, histamine, insulin, pentagastrin, calcium, secretin), includes drug administration

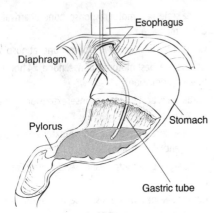

Esophagus

Diaphragm

Pylorus

Stomach

Gastric tube

The stomach contents are aspirated

Explanation

The physician performs therapeutic intubation and aspiration of the stomach (43753), often for indications such as poisoning or gastrointestinal hemorrhage. A gastric lavage (stomach pump) may also be performed. The physician inserts a Levin tube or other gastric lavage tube through the nose or mouth. The tube passes through the esophagus into the stomach. The stomach contents are removed by suction. The inside of the stomach may be rinsed with a salt water (saline) solution. If the intubation and aspiration are performed for diagnostic purposes (such as acid analysis) of a single specimen, report 43754. Report 43755 if the diagnostic procedure includes the collection of multiple specimens with gastric stimulation (gastric secretory study). The physician inserts a tube through the patient's nose or mouth and down into the stomach. Gastric contents are suctioned out for collection. Insulin, or another gastric secretion stimulant such as histamine, pentagastrin, calcium, or secretin, is given to the patient. Blood glucose is monitored while continued collection of gastric contents is done. Following sample collection, gastric contents undergo volume, pH, acid concentration, and volume measurements.

Coding Tips

For duodenal intubation and aspiration, diagnostic, including image guidance, see 43756–43757. For gastric acid analysis, see 82930. For naso- or orogastric tube placement by the physician, using fluoroscopic guidance, see 43752. Do not report 43753 with critical care codes 99291–99292, neonatal/pediatric intensive care codes 99468–99469 or 99471–99476, or low birth weight intensive care service codes 99477–99480.

ICD-10-CM Diagnostic Codes

I86.4	Gastric varices
K21.00	Gastro-esophageal reflux disease with esophagitis, without bleeding
K21.01	Gastro-esophageal reflux disease with esophagitis, with bleeding
K21.9	Gastro-esophageal reflux disease without esophagitis
K22.89	Other specified disease of esophagus
K25.0	Acute gastric ulcer with hemorrhage
K25.2	Acute gastric ulcer with both hemorrhage and perforation
K25.4	Chronic or unspecified gastric ulcer with hemorrhage
K28.0	Acute gastrojejunal ulcer with hemorrhage
K28.2	Acute gastrojejunal ulcer with both hemorrhage and perforation
K28.4	Chronic or unspecified gastrojejunal ulcer with hemorrhage
K28.6	Chronic or unspecified gastrojejunal ulcer with both hemorrhage and perforation
K29.01	Acute gastritis with bleeding
K29.21	Alcoholic gastritis with bleeding
K29.31	Chronic superficial gastritis with bleeding
K29.41	Chronic atrophic gastritis with bleeding
K29.61	Other gastritis with bleeding
K29.81	Duodenitis with bleeding
K30	Functional dyspepsia
K31.811	Angiodysplasia of stomach and duodenum with bleeding
K92.0	Hematemesis
T36.0X1A	Poisoning by penicillins, accidental (unintentional), initial encounter
T36.0X2A	Poisoning by penicillins, intentional self-harm, initial encounter
T36.0X4A	Poisoning by penicillins, undetermined, initial encounter
T36.4X1A	Poisoning by tetracyclines, accidental (unintentional), initial encounter
T36.7X4A	Poisoning by antifungal antibiotics, systemically used, undetermined, initial encounter
T36.8X1A	Poisoning by other systemic antibiotics, accidental (unintentional), initial encounter
T37.0X4A	Poisoning by sulfonamides, undetermined, initial encounter
T37.1X1A	Poisoning by antimycobacterial drugs, accidental (unintentional), initial encounter
T37.3X1A	Poisoning by other antiprotozoal drugs, accidental (unintentional), initial encounter
T37.3X2A	Poisoning by other antiprotozoal drugs, intentional self-harm, initial encounter
T37.5X1A	Poisoning by antiviral drugs, accidental (unintentional), initial encounter
T37.5X2A	Poisoning by antiviral drugs, intentional self-harm, initial encounter
T37.8X4A	Poisoning by other specified systemic anti-infectives and antiparasitics, undetermined, initial encounter
T38.1X4A	Poisoning by thyroid hormones and substitutes, undetermined, initial encounter
T38.2X1A	Poisoning by antithyroid drugs, accidental (unintentional), initial encounter
T38.3X1A	Poisoning by insulin and oral hypoglycemic [antidiabetic] drugs, accidental (unintentional), initial encounter
T38.3X2A	Poisoning by insulin and oral hypoglycemic [antidiabetic] drugs, intentional self-harm, initial encounter
T38.3X4A	Poisoning by insulin and oral hypoglycemic [antidiabetic] drugs, undetermined, initial encounter
T38.4X1A	Poisoning by oral contraceptives, accidental (unintentional), initial encounter
T38.5X1A	Poisoning by other estrogens and progestogens, accidental (unintentional), initial encounter

T38.5X4A	Poisoning by other estrogens and progestogens, undetermined, initial encounter
T38.7X1A	Poisoning by androgens and anabolic congeners, accidental (unintentional), initial encounter
T39.012A	Poisoning by aspirin, intentional self-harm, initial encounter
T39.014A	Poisoning by aspirin, undetermined, initial encounter
T40.0X2A	Poisoning by opium, intentional self-harm, initial encounter
T40.0X4A	Poisoning by opium, undetermined, initial encounter
T40.1X1A	Poisoning by heroin, accidental (unintentional), initial encounter
T40.2X2A	Poisoning by other opioids, intentional self-harm, initial encounter
T40.2X4A	Poisoning by other opioids, undetermined, initial encounter
T40.3X1A	Poisoning by methadone, accidental (unintentional), initial encounter
T40.3X2A	Poisoning by methadone, intentional self-harm, initial encounter
T40.412A	Poisoning by fentanyl or fentanyl analogs, intentional self-harm, initial encounter
T40.421A	Poisoning by tramadol, accidental (unintentional), initial encounter
T40.5X4A	Poisoning by cocaine, undetermined, initial encounter
T40.691A	Poisoning by other narcotics, accidental (unintentional), initial encounter
T40.711A	Poisoning by cannabis, accidental (unintentional), initial encounter
T40.712A	Poisoning by cannabis, intentional self-harm, initial encounter
T40.713A	Poisoning by cannabis, assault, initial encounter
T41.1X1A	Poisoning by intravenous anesthetics, accidental (unintentional), initial encounter
T41.1X4A	Poisoning by intravenous anesthetics, undetermined, initial encounter
T41.291A	Poisoning by other general anesthetics, accidental (unintentional), initial encounter
T41.5X4A	Poisoning by therapeutic gases, undetermined, initial encounter
T42.0X1A	Poisoning by hydantoin derivatives, accidental (unintentional), initial encounter
T42.3X1A	Poisoning by barbiturates, accidental (unintentional), initial encounter
T42.3X2A	Poisoning by barbiturates, intentional self-harm, initial encounter
T42.6X1A	Poisoning by other antiepileptic and sedative-hypnotic drugs, accidental (unintentional), initial encounter
T42.6X2A	Poisoning by other antiepileptic and sedative-hypnotic drugs, intentional self-harm, initial encounter
T42.8X4A	Poisoning by antiparkinsonism drugs and other central muscle-tone depressants, undetermined, initial encounter
T43.011A	Poisoning by tricyclic antidepressants, accidental (unintentional), initial encounter
T43.211A	Poisoning by selective serotonin and norepinephrine reuptake inhibitors, accidental (unintentional), initial encounter
T43.292A	Poisoning by other antidepressants, intentional self-harm, initial encounter
T43.294A	Poisoning by other antidepressants, undetermined, initial encounter
T43.4X4A	Poisoning by butyrophenone and thiothixene neuroleptics, undetermined, initial encounter
T43.611A	Poisoning by caffeine, accidental (unintentional), initial encounter
T43.624A	Poisoning by amphetamines, undetermined, initial encounter
T44.6X4A	Poisoning by alpha-adrenoreceptor antagonists, undetermined, initial encounter
T46.7X1A	Poisoning by peripheral vasodilators, accidental (unintentional), initial encounter
T47.2X1A	Poisoning by stimulant laxatives, accidental (unintentional), initial encounter
T47.2X2A	Poisoning by stimulant laxatives, intentional self-harm, initial encounter
T47.7X1A	Poisoning by emetics, accidental (unintentional), initial encounter
T48.5X4A	Poisoning by other anti-common-cold drugs, undetermined, initial encounter
T48.6X1A	Poisoning by antiasthmatics, accidental (unintentional), initial encounter
T51.0X1A	Toxic effect of ethanol, accidental (unintentional), initial encounter
T51.0X4A	Toxic effect of ethanol, undetermined, initial encounter
T51.1X2A	Toxic effect of methanol, intentional self-harm, initial encounter
T54.0X1A	Toxic effect of phenol and phenol homologues, accidental (unintentional), initial encounter
T54.0X2A	Toxic effect of phenol and phenol homologues, intentional self-harm, initial encounter

AMA: **43753** 2019,Aug,8; 2018,Jan,8; 2017,Jan,8; 2016,Jan,13; 2015,Jan,16 **43754** 2018,Jan,8; 2017,Jan,8; 2016,Jan,13; 2015,Jan,16 **43755** 2018,Jan,8; 2017,Jan,8; 2016,Jan,13; 2015,Jan,16

Relative Value Units/Medicare Edits

Non-Facility RVU	Work	PE	MP	Total
43753	0.45	0.11	0.09	0.65
43754	0.45	5.89	0.1	6.44
43755	0.94	4.82	0.1	5.86
Facility RVU	Work	PE	MP	Total
43753	0.45	0.11	0.09	0.65
43754	0.45	0.5	0.1	1.05
43755	0.94	0.69	0.1	1.73

	FUD	Status	MUE	Modifiers				IOM Reference
43753	0	A	1(3)	N/A	N/A	N/A	80	None
43754	0	A	1(3)	N/A	N/A	N/A	80	
43755	0	A	1(3)	N/A	N/A	N/A	80	

* with documentation

Terms To Know

aspiration. Drawing fluid out by suction.

hemorrhage. Internal or external bleeding with loss of significant amounts of blood.

intubation. Insertion of a tube into a hollow organ, canal, or cavity within the body.

lavage. Washing.

suction. Vacuum evacuation of fluid or tissue.

therapeutic. Act meant to alleviate a medical or mental condition.

43756-43757

43756 Duodenal intubation and aspiration, diagnostic, includes image guidance; single specimen (eg, bile study for crystals or afferent loop culture)

43757 collection of multiple fractional specimens with pancreatic or gallbladder stimulation, single or double lumen tube, includes drug administration

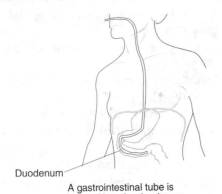

Duodenum

A gastrointestinal tube is advanced into the duodenum

Explanation

The physician performs diagnostic intubation and aspiration of the first portion of the small intestine (duodenum) using image guidance. A tube is inserted orally or nasally and positioned in the duodenum. In one method, the physician advances a double-lumen introducer tube containing an inflatable balloon through the esophagus. Upon reaching the stomach, the introducer tube is turned so that the balloon is positioned toward the greater curvature. As the physician inflates the balloon, it expands and conforms to the shape of the stomach. Once inflated, the distal end of the introducer tube abuts the pylorus. The physician inserts a duodenal catheter through the introducer tube into the duodenum. Following appropriate placement, the balloon is deflated and the introducer tube is removed, leaving the distal tip of the duodenal catheter within the duodenum. Report 43756 if the aspiration procedure is performed for a single specimen, such as an afferent loop culture or bile study for crystals. Report 43757 if multiple fractional specimens are collected and pancreatic or gallbladder stimulation occurs. Separately reportable chemical analysis procedures may follow. These codes include the administration of any drugs, although the drugs themselves are separately reportable.

Coding Tips

For gastric intubation and aspiration, therapeutic, including lavage, if performed, see 43753; diagnostic, see 43754–43755. To report chemical analysis procedures, see 89049–89240. For naso- or orogastric tube placement by the physician, using fluoroscopic guidance, see 43752.

ICD-10-CM Diagnostic Codes

K26.0	Acute duodenal ulcer with hemorrhage
K26.1	Acute duodenal ulcer with perforation
K26.2	Acute duodenal ulcer with both hemorrhage and perforation
K26.3	Acute duodenal ulcer without hemorrhage or perforation
K26.4	Chronic or unspecified duodenal ulcer with hemorrhage
K26.5	Chronic or unspecified duodenal ulcer with perforation
K26.6	Chronic or unspecified duodenal ulcer with both hemorrhage and perforation
K26.7	Chronic duodenal ulcer without hemorrhage or perforation
K80.00	Calculus of gallbladder with acute cholecystitis without obstruction
K80.01	Calculus of gallbladder with acute cholecystitis with obstruction
K80.10	Calculus of gallbladder with chronic cholecystitis without obstruction
K80.11	Calculus of gallbladder with chronic cholecystitis with obstruction
K80.12	Calculus of gallbladder with acute and chronic cholecystitis without obstruction
K80.13	Calculus of gallbladder with acute and chronic cholecystitis with obstruction
K80.18	Calculus of gallbladder with other cholecystitis without obstruction
K80.19	Calculus of gallbladder with other cholecystitis with obstruction
K80.32	Calculus of bile duct with acute cholangitis without obstruction
K80.33	Calculus of bile duct with acute cholangitis with obstruction
K80.34	Calculus of bile duct with chronic cholangitis without obstruction
K80.35	Calculus of bile duct with chronic cholangitis with obstruction
K80.36	Calculus of bile duct with acute and chronic cholangitis without obstruction
K80.37	Calculus of bile duct with acute and chronic cholangitis with obstruction
K80.42	Calculus of bile duct with acute cholecystitis without obstruction
K80.43	Calculus of bile duct with acute cholecystitis with obstruction
K80.44	Calculus of bile duct with chronic cholecystitis without obstruction
K80.45	Calculus of bile duct with chronic cholecystitis with obstruction
K80.46	Calculus of bile duct with acute and chronic cholecystitis without obstruction
K80.47	Calculus of bile duct with acute and chronic cholecystitis with obstruction
K80.62	Calculus of gallbladder and bile duct with acute cholecystitis without obstruction
K80.63	Calculus of gallbladder and bile duct with acute cholecystitis with obstruction
K80.64	Calculus of gallbladder and bile duct with chronic cholecystitis without obstruction
K80.65	Calculus of gallbladder and bile duct with chronic cholecystitis with obstruction
K80.66	Calculus of gallbladder and bile duct with acute and chronic cholecystitis without obstruction
K80.67	Calculus of gallbladder and bile duct with acute and chronic cholecystitis with obstruction
K80.81	Other cholelithiasis with obstruction
K81.0	Acute cholecystitis
K81.1	Chronic cholecystitis
K81.2	Acute cholecystitis with chronic cholecystitis
K83.01	Primary sclerosing cholangitis
K83.09	Other cholangitis
K85.00	Idiopathic acute pancreatitis without necrosis or infection
K85.01	Idiopathic acute pancreatitis with uninfected necrosis
K85.02	Idiopathic acute pancreatitis with infected necrosis
K85.10	Biliary acute pancreatitis without necrosis or infection
K85.11	Biliary acute pancreatitis with uninfected necrosis
K85.12	Biliary acute pancreatitis with infected necrosis
K85.22	Alcohol induced acute pancreatitis with infected necrosis

K85.31	Drug induced acute pancreatitis with uninfected necrosis	
R10.11	Right upper quadrant pain	

AMA: **43756** 2018,Jan,8; 2017,Jan,8; 2016,Jan,13; 2015,Jan,16 **43757** 2018,Jan,8; 2017,Jan,8; 2016,Jan,13; 2015,Jan,16

Relative Value Units/Medicare Edits

Non-Facility RVU	Work	PE	MP	Total
43756	0.77	7.5	0.09	8.36
43757	1.26	9.87	0.14	11.27
Facility RVU	Work	PE	MP	Total
43756	0.77	0.62	0.09	1.48
43757	1.26	0.83	0.14	2.23

	FUD	Status	MUE	Modifiers				IOM Reference
43756	0	A	1(2)	N/A	N/A	N/A	80	None
43757	0	A	1(2)	N/A	N/A	N/A	80	

* with documentation

Terms To Know

aspiration. Drawing fluid out by suction.

imaging. Radiologic means of producing pictures for clinical study of the internal structures and functions of the body, such as x-ray, ultrasound, magnetic resonance, or positron emission tomography.

intubation. Insertion of a tube into a hollow organ, canal, or cavity within the body.

specimen. Tissue cells or sample of fluid taken for analysis, pathologic examination, and diagnosis.

43761

43761	Repositioning of a naso- or oro-gastric feeding tube, through the duodenum for enteric nutrition

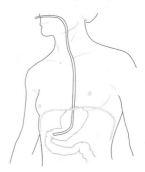

A gastrointestinal tube being introduced via the oropharynx

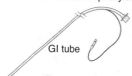

GI tube

A naso- or orogastric tube is placed by a physician

A previously placed naso- or orogastric feeding tube is repositioned through to the duodenum for enteric feeding

Explanation

The physician repositions a nasogastric or orogastric feeding tube through the duodenum for enteric nutrition. Under separately reportable fluoroscopic guidance, the physician passes the feeding tube through the stomach into the distal duodenum.

Coding Tips

Imaging guidance is reported separately with 76000, when performed. For percutaneous change of a gastrostomy tube, without imaging or endoscopic guidance, see 43762 and 43763; fluoroscopically guided replacement of a gastrostomy tube, see 49450. For endoscopic placement of a gastrostomy tube, see 43246. For open gastrostomy, without gastric tube construction, see 43830; open gastrostomy, neonatal, for feeding, see 43831; laparoscopic gastrostomy without gastric tube construction, see 43653. Do not report 43761 with 44500 or 49446.

ICD-10-CM Diagnostic Codes

Z43.4	Encounter for attention to other artificial openings of digestive tract
Z46.59	Encounter for fitting and adjustment of other gastrointestinal appliance and device

AMA: **43761** 2018,Jan,8; 2017,Jan,8; 2016,Jan,13; 2015,Jan,16

Relative Value Units/Medicare Edits

Non-Facility RVU	Work	PE	MP	Total
43761	2.01	1.32	0.3	3.63
Facility RVU	Work	PE	MP	Total
43761	2.01	0.73	0.3	3.04

	FUD	Status	MUE	Modifiers				IOM Reference
43761	0	A	2(3)	51	N/A	N/A	N/A	None

* with documentation

Terms To Know

distal. Located farther away from a specified reference point or the trunk.

enteral nutrition. Feeding of a nutrient mixture directly into or just proximal to the upper end of the small bowel via a tube or through an existing stoma. Patients are usually able to absorb the nutrients.

fluoroscopy. Radiology technique that allows visual examination of part of the body or a function of an organ using a device that projects an x-ray image on a fluorescent screen.

gastrostomy. Temporary or permanent artificial opening made in the stomach for gastrointestinal decompression or to provide nutrition when not maintained by other methods.

laparoscopy. Direct visualization utilizing a thin, flexible, fiberoptic tube.

nasogastric tube. Long, hollow, cylindrical catheter made of soft rubber or plastic that is inserted through the nose down into the stomach, and is used for feeding, instilling medication, or withdrawing gastric contents.

parenteral nutrition. Nutrients provided subcutaneously, intravenously, intramuscularly, or intradermally for patients during the postoperative period and in other conditions, such as shock, coma, and renal failure.

pylorus. Lower portion of the stomach, which opens into the duodenum.

reposition. Placement of an organ or structure into another position or return of an organ or structure to its original position.

43762-43763

43762 Replacement of gastrostomy tube, percutaneous, includes removal, when performed, without imaging or endoscopic guidance; not requiring revision of gastrostomy tract

43763 requiring revision of gastrostomy tract

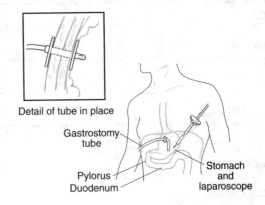

Detail of tube in place

Gastrostomy tube

Pylorus

Duodenum

Stomach and laparoscope

Gastrostomy tube is replaced

Explanation

In 43762, the physician replaces a gastrostomy tube via percutaneous approach that does not require revision (simple) of the gastrostomy tract. If the old gastrostomy tube has been placed endoscopically, the physician must remove it by snaring and pulling it out through the mouth. A new tube is placed percutaneously through the abdominal wall via the existing tract. In 43763, the replacement requires revision (complex). A small incision is made through the skin and fascia. A large bore needle with suture attached is passed through the incision into the lumen of the stomach. The needle is snared and the needle and suture are removed via the mouth. The gastrostomy tube is connected to the suture and passed through the mouth into the stomach and out the abdominal wall. The gastrostomy tube is sutured to the skin. No imaging or endoscopic guidance is utilized in either procedure.

Coding Tips

For percutaneous replacement of a gastrostomy tube using fluoroscopy, see 49450; endoscopic placement of a gastrostomy tube, see 43246. Surgical trays, A4550, are not separately reimbursed by Medicare; however, other third-party payers may cover them. Check with the specific payer to determine coverage.

ICD-10-CM Diagnostic Codes

K94.20	Gastrostomy complication, unspecified
K94.21	Gastrostomy hemorrhage
K94.22	Gastrostomy infection
K94.23	Gastrostomy malfunction
K94.29	Other complications of gastrostomy
Z43.1	Encounter for attention to gastrostomy
Z46.59	Encounter for fitting and adjustment of other gastrointestinal appliance and device
Z93.1	Gastrostomy status

AMA: **43762** 2019,Feb,5 **43763** 2019,Oct,10; 2019,Feb,5

Relative Value Units/Medicare Edits

Non-Facility RVU	Work	PE	MP	Total
43762	0.75	6.23	0.13	7.11
43763	1.41	9.02	0.25	10.68
Facility RVU	**Work**	**PE**	**MP**	**Total**
43762	0.75	0.23	0.13	1.11
43763	1.41	0.81	0.25	2.47

	FUD	Status	MUE	Modifiers				IOM Reference
43762	0	A	2(3)	51	N/A	N/A	N/A	None
43763	0	A	2(3)	51	N/A	N/A	N/A	

* with documentation

Terms To Know

endoscopy. Visual inspection of the body using a fiberoptic scope.

fascia. Fibrous sheet or band of tissue that envelops organs, muscles, and groupings of muscles.

gastrostomy. Temporary or permanent artificial opening made in the stomach for gastrointestinal decompression or to provide nutrition when not maintained by other methods.

imaging. Radiologic means of producing pictures for clinical study of the internal structures and functions of the body, such as x-ray, ultrasound, magnetic resonance, or positron emission tomography.

percutaneous approach. Method used to gain access to a body organ or specific area by puncture or minor incision through the skin or mucous membrane and/or any other body layers necessary to reach the procedure site.

43770

43770   Laparoscopy, surgical, gastric restrictive procedure; placement of adjustable gastric restrictive device (eg, gastric band and subcutaneous port components)

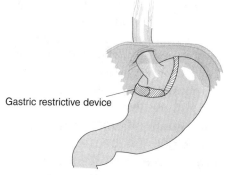

Gastric restrictive device

Gastric restrictive device is placed around the upper stomach and connected to an accessible port

Explanation

The physician performs a laparoscopic gastric restrictive procedure in which an adjustable gastric restrictive device, such as a gastric band with subcutaneous port components, is inserted. This is a gastric restrictive procedure for treatment of morbid obesity that does not permanently alter the gastrointestinal tract. The physician places a trocar though an incision, generally above the umbilicus, and insufflates the abdominal cavity. The laparoscope and additional trocars are placed through small portal incisions. The silicone gastric band is introduced into the peritoneal cavity via a trocar and is placed and secured around the upper stomach to form a smaller stomach pouch with a narrowed outlet. A small port, or reservoir, is placed under the skin at the time of surgery and connected to the silicone band by tubing to facilitate postoperative adjustments of the outlet size by the addition or removal of saline via the port. The instruments are removed and the incisions are closed.

Coding Tips

Surgical laparoscopy always includes diagnostic laparoscopy; the diagnostic laparoscopy should not be reported separately. Postoperative care following gastric restriction surgery using an adjustable gastric restrictive device includes subsequent device adjustments through the postoperative period and are not reported separately. Adjustment of a gastric restrictive device consists of modifying the device component diameter with aspiration of fluid or injection through a subcutaneous port. Placement of an individual component is reported by appending modifier 52 to this code.

ICD-10-CM Diagnostic Codes

E23.6	Other disorders of pituitary gland
E27.8	Other specified disorders of adrenal gland
E35	Disorders of endocrine glands in diseases classified elsewhere
E36.8	Other intraoperative complications of endocrine system
E66.01	Morbid (severe) obesity due to excess calories
E66.09	Other obesity due to excess calories
E66.1	Drug-induced obesity
E66.2	Morbid (severe) obesity with alveolar hypoventilation
E66.3	Overweight
E66.8	Other obesity
K91.1	Postgastric surgery syndromes

K95.01	Infection due to gastric band procedure
K95.09	Other complications of gastric band procedure
K95.81	Infection due to other bariatric procedure
K95.89	Other complications of other bariatric procedure
T85.518A	Breakdown (mechanical) of other gastrointestinal prosthetic devices, implants and grafts, initial encounter
T85.528A	Displacement of other gastrointestinal prosthetic devices, implants and grafts, initial encounter
T85.598A	Other mechanical complication of other gastrointestinal prosthetic devices, implants and grafts, initial encounter
Z46.51	Encounter for fitting and adjustment of gastric lap band
Z68.30	Body mass index [BMI] 30.0-30.9, adult 🅐
Z68.31	Body mass index [BMI] 31.0-31.9, adult 🅐
Z68.32	Body mass index [BMI] 32.0-32.9, adult 🅐
Z68.33	Body mass index [BMI] 33.0-33.9, adult 🅐
Z68.34	Body mass index [BMI] 34.0-34.9, adult 🅐
Z68.35	Body mass index [BMI] 35.0-35.9, adult 🅐
Z68.36	Body mass index [BMI] 36.0-36.9, adult 🅐
Z68.37	Body mass index [BMI] 37.0-37.9, adult 🅐
Z68.38	Body mass index [BMI] 38.0-38.9, adult 🅐
Z68.39	Body mass index [BMI] 39.0-39.9, adult 🅐
Z68.41	Body mass index [BMI] 40.0-44.9, adult 🅐
Z68.42	Body mass index [BMI] 45.0-49.9, adult 🅐
Z68.43	Body mass index [BMI] 50.0-59.9, adult 🅐
Z68.44	Body mass index [BMI] 60.0-69.9, adult 🅐
Z68.45	Body mass index [BMI] 70 or greater, adult 🅐

AMA: 43770 2018,Jan,8; 2017,Jan,8; 2016,Jan,13; 2015,Jan,16

Relative Value Units/Medicare Edits

Non-Facility RVU	Work	PE	MP	Total
43770	18.0	10.98	4.38	33.36
Facility RVU	Work	PE	MP	Total
43770	18.0	10.98	4.38	33.36

	FUD	Status	MUE	Modifiers				IOM Reference
43770	90	A	1(2)	51	N/A	62*	80	None

* with documentation

43771

43771 Laparoscopy, surgical, gastric restrictive procedure; revision of adjustable gastric restrictive device component only

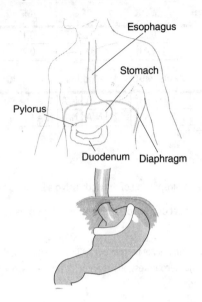

Explanation

The physician performs laparoscopic revision of an adjustable gastric restrictive device. This revision is most often performed for slippage of the device or for dilation of the gastric pouch. The physician places a trocar though an incision, generally above the umbilicus, and insufflates the abdominal cavity. The laparoscope and additional trocars are placed through small portal incisions. Saline is removed from the gastric restrictive device and the device is repositioned around the upper stomach. Saline is slowly reintroduced through the existing port to secure the device position. Once the device is in place, the instruments are removed and the incisions are closed. This code reports revision of the device component only.

Coding Tips

Surgical laparoscopy includes diagnostic laparoscopy. Restrictive device adjustments during the postoperative period are not separately reported. Code 43771 reports revision of the device component only. For removal of an adjustable gastric restrictive device, component only, report 43772; removal and replacement of an adjustable gastric restrictive device, component only, see 43773. For removal of an adjustable gastric restrictive device and subcutaneous port components, see 43774. To report the removal and replacement of both gastric band and subcutaneous port components, see 43659, unlisted laparoscopy procedure, stomach.

ICD-10-CM Diagnostic Codes

E23.6	Other disorders of pituitary gland
E27.8	Other specified disorders of adrenal gland
E35	Disorders of endocrine glands in diseases classified elsewhere
E36.8	Other intraoperative complications of endocrine system
E66.01	Morbid (severe) obesity due to excess calories
E66.09	Other obesity due to excess calories
E66.1	Drug-induced obesity
E66.2	Morbid (severe) obesity with alveolar hypoventilation
E66.3	Overweight
E66.8	Other obesity
K91.1	Postgastric surgery syndromes

K95.01	Infection due to gastric band procedure
K95.09	Other complications of gastric band procedure
K95.81	Infection due to other bariatric procedure
K95.89	Other complications of other bariatric procedure
T85.518A	Breakdown (mechanical) of other gastrointestinal prosthetic devices, implants and grafts, initial encounter
T85.528A	Displacement of other gastrointestinal prosthetic devices, implants and grafts, initial encounter
T85.598A	Other mechanical complication of other gastrointestinal prosthetic devices, implants and grafts, initial encounter
Z46.51	Encounter for fitting and adjustment of gastric lap band
Z68.30	Body mass index [BMI] 30.0-30.9, adult ◢
Z68.31	Body mass index [BMI] 31.0-31.9, adult ◢
Z68.32	Body mass index [BMI] 32.0-32.9, adult ◢
Z68.33	Body mass index [BMI] 33.0-33.9, adult ◢
Z68.34	Body mass index [BMI] 34.0-34.9, adult ◢
Z68.35	Body mass index [BMI] 35.0-35.9, adult ◢
Z68.36	Body mass index [BMI] 36.0-36.9, adult ◢
Z68.37	Body mass index [BMI] 37.0-37.9, adult ◢
Z68.38	Body mass index [BMI] 38.0-38.9, adult ◢
Z68.39	Body mass index [BMI] 39.0-39.9, adult ◢
Z68.41	Body mass index [BMI] 40.0-44.9, adult ◢
Z68.42	Body mass index [BMI] 45.0-49.9, adult ◢
Z68.43	Body mass index [BMI] 50.0-59.9, adult ◢
Z68.44	Body mass index [BMI] 60.0-69.9, adult ◢
Z68.45	Body mass index [BMI] 70 or greater, adult ◢

AMA: **43771** 2018,Jan,8; 2017,Jan,8; 2016,Jan,13; 2015,Jan,16

Relative Value Units/Medicare Edits

Non-Facility RVU	Work	PE	MP	Total
43771	20.79	12.04	5.08	37.91
Facility RVU	Work	PE	MP	Total
43771	20.79	12.04	5.08	37.91

	FUD	Status	MUE	Modifiers				IOM Reference
43771	90	A	1(2)	51	N/A	62*	80	None

* with documentation

43772-43773

43772 Laparoscopy, surgical, gastric restrictive procedure; removal of adjustable gastric restrictive device component only

43773   removal and replacement of adjustable gastric restrictive device component only

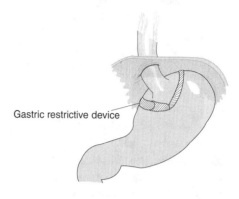

Gastric restrictive device

Explanation

The physician performs laparoscopic removal of an adjustable gastric restrictive device component. The physician places a trocar though an incision, generally above the umbilicus, and insufflates the abdominal cavity. The laparoscope and additional trocars are placed through small portal incisions. Saline is removed from the gastric restrictive device and the component is removed. Once the device component has been removed, the instruments are withdrawn and the incisions are closed. Report 43772 for removal of an adjustable gastric restrictive device component only. Report 43773 for removal and replacement of an adjustable gastric restrictive device component only.

Coding Tips

Laparoscopic placement of an adjustable gastric restrictive device is reported with 43770. For revision of the device component only, see 43771; removal of an adjustable gastric restrictive device, component only, see 43772; removal and replacement of an adjustable gastric restrictive device, component only, report 43773; removal of an adjustable gastric restrictive device and subcutaneous port components, see 43774. To report the removal and replacement of a gastric band and subcutaneous port components, see 43659.

ICD-10-CM Diagnostic Codes

E23.6	Other disorders of pituitary gland
E27.8	Other specified disorders of adrenal gland
E35	Disorders of endocrine glands in diseases classified elsewhere
E36.8	Other intraoperative complications of endocrine system
E66.01	Morbid (severe) obesity due to excess calories
E66.09	Other obesity due to excess calories
E66.1	Drug-induced obesity
E66.2	Morbid (severe) obesity with alveolar hypoventilation
E66.3	Overweight
E66.8	Other obesity
K91.1	Postgastric surgery syndromes
K95.01	Infection due to gastric band procedure
K95.09	Other complications of gastric band procedure
K95.81	Infection due to other bariatric procedure
K95.89	Other complications of other bariatric procedure
T85.518A	Breakdown (mechanical) of other gastrointestinal prosthetic devices, implants and grafts, initial encounter

T85.528A	Displacement of other gastrointestinal prosthetic devices, implants and grafts, initial encounter
T85.598A	Other mechanical complication of other gastrointestinal prosthetic devices, implants and grafts, initial encounter
Z46.51	Encounter for fitting and adjustment of gastric lap band
Z68.30	Body mass index [BMI] 30.0-30.9, adult 🄰
Z68.31	Body mass index [BMI] 31.0-31.9, adult 🄰
Z68.32	Body mass index [BMI] 32.0-32.9, adult 🄰
Z68.33	Body mass index [BMI] 33.0-33.9, adult 🄰
Z68.34	Body mass index [BMI] 34.0-34.9, adult 🄰
Z68.35	Body mass index [BMI] 35.0-35.9, adult 🄰
Z68.36	Body mass index [BMI] 36.0-36.9, adult 🄰
Z68.37	Body mass index [BMI] 37.0-37.9, adult 🄰
Z68.38	Body mass index [BMI] 38.0-38.9, adult 🄰
Z68.39	Body mass index [BMI] 39.0-39.9, adult 🄰
Z68.41	Body mass index [BMI] 40.0-44.9, adult 🄰
Z68.42	Body mass index [BMI] 45.0-49.9, adult 🄰
Z68.43	Body mass index [BMI] 50.0-59.9, adult 🄰
Z68.44	Body mass index [BMI] 60.0-69.9, adult 🄰
Z68.45	Body mass index [BMI] 70 or greater, adult 🄰

AMA: 43772 2018,Jan,8; 2017,Jan,8; 2016,Jan,13; 2015,Jan,16 **43773** 2018,Jan,8; 2017,Jan,8; 2016,Jan,13; 2015,Jan,16

Relative Value Units/Medicare Edits

Non-Facility RVU	Work	PE	MP	Total
43772	15.7	8.65	3.71	28.06
43773	20.79	12.04	5.08	37.91
Facility RVU	Work	PE	MP	Total
43772	15.7	8.65	3.71	28.06
43773	20.79	12.04	5.08	37.91

	FUD	Status	MUE	Modifiers				IOM Reference
43772	90	A	1(2)	51	N/A	62*	80	None
43773	90	A	1(2)	51	N/A	62*	80	

* with documentation

43774

43774 Laparoscopy, surgical, gastric restrictive procedure; removal of adjustable gastric restrictive device and subcutaneous port components

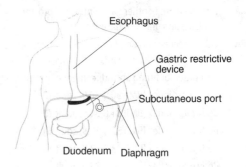

Explanation

The physician performs laparoscopic removal of an adjustable gastric restrictive device and subcutaneous port components. The physician places a trocar though an incision, generally above the umbilicus, and insufflates the abdominal cavity. The laparoscope and additional trocars are placed through small portal incisions. Saline is removed from the gastric device and the device is removed. Once the device has been removed, the subcutaneous port components are removed. The instruments are withdrawn and the incisions are closed.

Coding Tips

Laparoscopic placement of an adjustable gastric restrictive device is reported with 43770. Revision of an adjustable gastric restrictive device, component only, is reported with 43771. For removal of an adjustable gastric restrictive device, component only, see 43772; removal and replacement of an adjustable gastric restrictive device, component only, see 43773. For removal and replacement of both gastric band and subcutaneous port components, see 43659.

ICD-10-CM Diagnostic Codes

E23.6	Other disorders of pituitary gland
E27.8	Other specified disorders of adrenal gland
E35	Disorders of endocrine glands in diseases classified elsewhere
E36.8	Other intraoperative complications of endocrine system
E66.01	Morbid (severe) obesity due to excess calories
E66.09	Other obesity due to excess calories
E66.1	Drug-induced obesity
E66.2	Morbid (severe) obesity with alveolar hypoventilation
E66.3	Overweight
E66.8	Other obesity
K91.1	Postgastric surgery syndromes
K95.01	Infection due to gastric band procedure
K95.09	Other complications of gastric band procedure
K95.81	Infection due to other bariatric procedure
K95.89	Other complications of other bariatric procedure
T85.518A	Breakdown (mechanical) of other gastrointestinal prosthetic devices, implants and grafts, initial encounter
T85.528A	Displacement of other gastrointestinal prosthetic devices, implants and grafts, initial encounter

T85.598A	Other mechanical complication of other gastrointestinal prosthetic devices, implants and grafts, initial encounter
Z46.51	Encounter for fitting and adjustment of gastric lap band
Z68.30	Body mass index [BMI] 30.0-30.9, adult △
Z68.31	Body mass index [BMI] 31.0-31.9, adult △
Z68.32	Body mass index [BMI] 32.0-32.9, adult △
Z68.33	Body mass index [BMI] 33.0-33.9, adult △
Z68.34	Body mass index [BMI] 34.0-34.9, adult △
Z68.35	Body mass index [BMI] 35.0-35.9, adult △
Z68.36	Body mass index [BMI] 36.0-36.9, adult △
Z68.37	Body mass index [BMI] 37.0-37.9, adult △
Z68.38	Body mass index [BMI] 38.0-38.9, adult △
Z68.39	Body mass index [BMI] 39.0-39.9, adult △
Z68.41	Body mass index [BMI] 40.0-44.9, adult △
Z68.42	Body mass index [BMI] 45.0-49.9, adult △
Z68.43	Body mass index [BMI] 50.0-59.9, adult △
Z68.44	Body mass index [BMI] 60.0-69.9, adult △
Z68.45	Body mass index [BMI] 70 or greater, adult △

AMA: **43774** 2018,Jan,8; 2017,Jan,8; 2016,Jan,13; 2015,Jan,16

Relative Value Units/Medicare Edits

Non-Facility RVU	Work	PE	MP	Total
43774	15.76	8.85	3.82	28.43
Facility RVU	**Work**	**PE**	**MP**	**Total**
43774	15.76	8.85	3.82	28.43

	FUD	Status	MUE	Modifiers				IOM Reference
43774	90	A	1(2)	51	N/A	62*	80	None

* with documentation

43775

43775 Laparoscopy, surgical, gastric restrictive procedure; longitudinal gastrectomy (ie, sleeve gastrectomy)

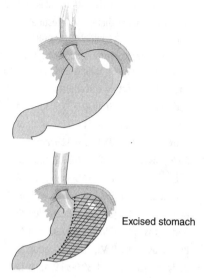

Excised stomach

The stomach is surgically restricted

Explanation

The physician performs a laparoscopic sleeve gastrectomy (LSG), a gastric restrictive procedure for the treatment of morbid obesity. Following appropriate anesthesia, the physician begins the longitudinal gastrectomy by placing a trocar though an incision, generally above the umbilicus, and insufflating the abdominal cavity. The laparoscope and additional trocars are placed through small portal incisions. The physician divides the greater curvature of the stomach from the left crus of the diaphragm to a point distal to the pylorus. The short gastric vessels are coagulated and gastric staplers are used. A gastric tube (sleeve) is formed and the remaining 80 percent of the stomach is excised. The instruments are removed and the incisions are closed.

Coding Tips

This code describes a laparoscopic gastric restrictive sleeve or longitudinal gastrectomy. For an open gastric restrictive procedure for morbid obesity, without gastric bypass, other than vertical-banded gastroplasty, see 43843. For laparoscopic implantation, removal, replacement, reprogramming, or revision of vagus nerve blocking neurostimulator electrodes and/or pulse generator, see 0312T-0317T.

ICD-10-CM Diagnostic Codes

E23.6	Other disorders of pituitary gland
E27.8	Other specified disorders of adrenal gland
E35	Disorders of endocrine glands in diseases classified elsewhere
E36.8	Other intraoperative complications of endocrine system
E66.01	Morbid (severe) obesity due to excess calories
E66.09	Other obesity due to excess calories
E66.1	Drug-induced obesity
E66.2	Morbid (severe) obesity with alveolar hypoventilation
E66.3	Overweight
E66.8	Other obesity
K91.1	Postgastric surgery syndromes

K95.01	Infection due to gastric band procedure
K95.09	Other complications of gastric band procedure
K95.81	Infection due to other bariatric procedure
K95.89	Other complications of other bariatric procedure
T85.518A	Breakdown (mechanical) of other gastrointestinal prosthetic devices, implants and grafts, initial encounter
T85.528A	Displacement of other gastrointestinal prosthetic devices, implants and grafts, initial encounter
T85.598A	Other mechanical complication of other gastrointestinal prosthetic devices, implants and grafts, initial encounter
Z46.51	Encounter for fitting and adjustment of gastric lap band
Z68.30	Body mass index [BMI] 30.0-30.9, adult ◭
Z68.31	Body mass index [BMI] 31.0-31.9, adult ◭
Z68.32	Body mass index [BMI] 32.0-32.9, adult ◭
Z68.33	Body mass index [BMI] 33.0-33.9, adult ◭
Z68.34	Body mass index [BMI] 34.0-34.9, adult ◭
Z68.35	Body mass index [BMI] 35.0-35.9, adult ◭
Z68.36	Body mass index [BMI] 36.0-36.9, adult ◭
Z68.37	Body mass index [BMI] 37.0-37.9, adult ◭
Z68.38	Body mass index [BMI] 38.0-38.9, adult ◭
Z68.39	Body mass index [BMI] 39.0-39.9, adult ◭
Z68.41	Body mass index [BMI] 40.0-44.9, adult ◭
Z68.42	Body mass index [BMI] 45.0-49.9, adult ◭
Z68.43	Body mass index [BMI] 50.0-59.9, adult ◭
Z68.44	Body mass index [BMI] 60.0-69.9, adult ◭
Z68.45	Body mass index [BMI] 70 or greater, adult ◭

AMA: **43775** 2019,Oct,10

Relative Value Units/Medicare Edits

Non-Facility RVU	Work	PE	MP	Total
43775	20.38	7.52	4.92	32.82
Facility RVU	**Work**	**PE**	**MP**	**Total**
43775	20.38	7.52	4.92	32.82

	FUD	Status	MUE	Modifiers				IOM Reference
43775	90	A	1(2)	51	N/A	62*	80	None

* with documentation

43800

43800 Pyloroplasty

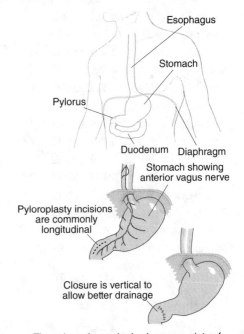

The pylorus is repaired using any variety of surgical pyloroplasty techniques

Explanation

The physician repairs the pylorus. The physician makes an upper abdominal incision through skin, fascia, and muscles to expose the pylorus, a muscular band surrounding the distal opening of the stomach. A longitudinal incision is made in the pylorus. The incision is closed with a single full thickness suture layer.

Coding Tips

When 43800 is performed with another separately identifiable procedure, the highest dollar value code is listed as the primary procedure and subsequent procedures are appended with modifier 51. For pyloroplasty and vagotomy, see 43640. Pyloromyotomy, cutting of pyloric muscles (Fredet-Ramstedt type operation), is reported with 43520.

ICD-10-CM Diagnostic Codes

C16.4	Malignant neoplasm of pylorus
K25.0	Acute gastric ulcer with hemorrhage
K25.1	Acute gastric ulcer with perforation
K25.2	Acute gastric ulcer with both hemorrhage and perforation
K25.3	Acute gastric ulcer without hemorrhage or perforation
K25.4	Chronic or unspecified gastric ulcer with hemorrhage
K25.5	Chronic or unspecified gastric ulcer with perforation
K25.6	Chronic or unspecified gastric ulcer with both hemorrhage and perforation
K25.7	Chronic gastric ulcer without hemorrhage or perforation
K26.0	Acute duodenal ulcer with hemorrhage
K26.1	Acute duodenal ulcer with perforation
K26.2	Acute duodenal ulcer with both hemorrhage and perforation
K26.3	Acute duodenal ulcer without hemorrhage or perforation
K26.4	Chronic or unspecified duodenal ulcer with hemorrhage

K26.5	Chronic or unspecified duodenal ulcer with perforation
K26.6	Chronic or unspecified duodenal ulcer with both hemorrhage and perforation
K26.7	Chronic duodenal ulcer without hemorrhage or perforation
K27.0	Acute peptic ulcer, site unspecified, with hemorrhage
K27.1	Acute peptic ulcer, site unspecified, with perforation
K27.2	Acute peptic ulcer, site unspecified, with both hemorrhage and perforation
K27.3	Acute peptic ulcer, site unspecified, without hemorrhage or perforation
K27.4	Chronic or unspecified peptic ulcer, site unspecified, with hemorrhage
K27.5	Chronic or unspecified peptic ulcer, site unspecified, with perforation
K27.6	Chronic or unspecified peptic ulcer, site unspecified, with both hemorrhage and perforation
K27.7	Chronic peptic ulcer, site unspecified, without hemorrhage or perforation
K30	Functional dyspepsia
K31.1	Adult hypertrophic pyloric stenosis ▲
K31.3	Pylorospasm, not elsewhere classified
K31.84	Gastroparesis
K31.89	Other diseases of stomach and duodenum
Q40.0	Congenital hypertrophic pyloric stenosis

AMA: 43800 2014,Jan,11

Relative Value Units/Medicare Edits

Non-Facility RVU	Work	PE	MP	Total
43800	15.43	8.42	3.7	27.55
Facility RVU	**Work**	**PE**	**MP**	**Total**
43800	15.43	8.42	3.7	27.55

	FUD	Status	MUE	Modifiers				IOM Reference
43800	90	A	1(2)	51	N/A	62*	80	None

* with documentation

Terms To Know

congenital. Present at birth, occurring through heredity or an influence during gestation up to the moment of birth.

fascia. Fibrous sheet or band of tissue that envelops organs, muscles, and groupings of muscles.

pylorus. Lower portion of the stomach, which opens into the duodenum.

stenosis. Narrowing or constriction of a passage.

43810

43810   Gastroduodenostomy

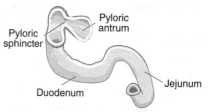

Cutaway view of the distal portion of the stomach and the duodenal tract

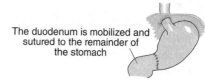

The duodenum is mobilized and sutured to the remainder of the stomach

A gastroduodenostomy is performed. The most distal part of the stomach, including the pylorus, is removed. The duodenum is pulled up and sutured to the stomach remnant

Explanation

The physician performs a gastroduodenostomy. The physician uses an upper midline epigastric incision through fascia and muscle. The distal end of the greater curvature of the stomach is removed. The duodenum is mobilized and connected to the greater curvature. The anastomosis is closed with interrupted stitches and the abdominal incision is closed.

Coding Tips

For partial, distal gastrectomy, with gastroduodenostomy, see 43631.

ICD-10-CM Diagnostic Codes

C16.0	Malignant neoplasm of cardia
C16.1	Malignant neoplasm of fundus of stomach
C16.2	Malignant neoplasm of body of stomach
C16.3	Malignant neoplasm of pyloric antrum
C16.4	Malignant neoplasm of pylorus
C16.8	Malignant neoplasm of overlapping sites of stomach
C17.0	Malignant neoplasm of duodenum
C78.4	Secondary malignant neoplasm of small intestine
C7A.010	Malignant carcinoid tumor of the duodenum
C7A.092	Malignant carcinoid tumor of the stomach
D37.1	Neoplasm of uncertain behavior of stomach
D3A.092	Benign carcinoid tumor of the stomach
K22.89	Other specified disease of esophagus
K25.0	Acute gastric ulcer with hemorrhage
K25.1	Acute gastric ulcer with perforation
K25.2	Acute gastric ulcer with both hemorrhage and perforation
K25.3	Acute gastric ulcer without hemorrhage or perforation
K25.4	Chronic or unspecified gastric ulcer with hemorrhage
K25.5	Chronic or unspecified gastric ulcer with perforation
K25.6	Chronic or unspecified gastric ulcer with both hemorrhage and perforation
K25.7	Chronic gastric ulcer without hemorrhage or perforation

K26.0	Acute duodenal ulcer with hemorrhage
K26.1	Acute duodenal ulcer with perforation
K26.2	Acute duodenal ulcer with both hemorrhage and perforation
K26.3	Acute duodenal ulcer without hemorrhage or perforation
K26.4	Chronic or unspecified duodenal ulcer with hemorrhage
K26.5	Chronic or unspecified duodenal ulcer with perforation
K26.6	Chronic or unspecified duodenal ulcer with both hemorrhage and perforation
K26.7	Chronic duodenal ulcer without hemorrhage or perforation
K27.0	Acute peptic ulcer, site unspecified, with hemorrhage
K27.1	Acute peptic ulcer, site unspecified, with perforation
K27.2	Acute peptic ulcer, site unspecified, with both hemorrhage and perforation
K27.3	Acute peptic ulcer, site unspecified, without hemorrhage or perforation
K27.4	Chronic or unspecified peptic ulcer, site unspecified, with hemorrhage
K27.5	Chronic or unspecified peptic ulcer, site unspecified, with perforation
K27.6	Chronic or unspecified peptic ulcer, site unspecified, with both hemorrhage and perforation
K27.7	Chronic peptic ulcer, site unspecified, without hemorrhage or perforation
K31.1	Adult hypertrophic pyloric stenosis 🅰
K31.3	Pylorospasm, not elsewhere classified
K31.89	Other diseases of stomach and duodenum
Q40.0	Congenital hypertrophic pyloric stenosis

AMA: **43810** 2014,Jan,11

Relative Value Units/Medicare Edits

Non-Facility RVU	Work	PE	MP	Total
43810	16.88	9.12	4.11	30.11
Facility RVU	Work	PE	MP	Total
43810	16.88	9.12	4.11	30.11

	FUD	Status	MUE	Modifiers				IOM Reference
43810	90	A	1(2)	51	N/A	62*	80	None

* with documentation

43820-43825

43820 Gastrojejunostomy; without vagotomy
43825   with vagotomy, any type

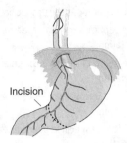

View of stomach showing anterior vagus nerve.
The distal part of the stomach is incised completely

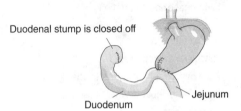

The stomach remnant is sutured directly to the jejunum

A gastrojejunostomy is performed with or without vagotomy. The distal portion of the stomach is incised and freed of the pylorus and duodenum. The duodenal stump is sutured closed. The stomach remnant is then anastomosed to the jejunum

Explanation

The physician performs a gastrojejunostomy to create a direct passage between the stomach and jejunum. The physician makes an upper abdominal incision to expose the stomach and small intestine. The distal portion of the stomach is resected and the jejunum is anastomosed to the gastric stump. The duodenal stump is closed. The vagal nerves are preserved. Report 43825 if a vagotomy is also performed.

Coding Tips

For partial, distal gastrectomy with gastrojejunostomy, see 43632.

ICD-10-CM Diagnostic Codes

C16.8	Malignant neoplasm of overlapping sites of stomach
C17.0	Malignant neoplasm of duodenum
C25.0	Malignant neoplasm of head of pancreas
C25.1	Malignant neoplasm of body of pancreas
C25.2	Malignant neoplasm of tail of pancreas
C25.3	Malignant neoplasm of pancreatic duct
C25.4	Malignant neoplasm of endocrine pancreas
C25.7	Malignant neoplasm of other parts of pancreas
C25.8	Malignant neoplasm of overlapping sites of pancreas
C78.4	Secondary malignant neoplasm of small intestine
C78.89	Secondary malignant neoplasm of other digestive organs
C7A.010	Malignant carcinoid tumor of the duodenum
C7A.092	Malignant carcinoid tumor of the stomach
D37.1	Neoplasm of uncertain behavior of stomach
K25.0	Acute gastric ulcer with hemorrhage

K25.1	Acute gastric ulcer with perforation
K25.2	Acute gastric ulcer with both hemorrhage and perforation
K25.3	Acute gastric ulcer without hemorrhage or perforation
K25.4	Chronic or unspecified gastric ulcer with hemorrhage
K25.5	Chronic or unspecified gastric ulcer with perforation
K25.6	Chronic or unspecified gastric ulcer with both hemorrhage and perforation
K25.7	Chronic gastric ulcer without hemorrhage or perforation
K26.0	Acute duodenal ulcer with hemorrhage
K26.1	Acute duodenal ulcer with perforation
K26.2	Acute duodenal ulcer with both hemorrhage and perforation
K26.3	Acute duodenal ulcer without hemorrhage or perforation
K26.4	Chronic or unspecified duodenal ulcer with hemorrhage
K26.5	Chronic or unspecified duodenal ulcer with perforation
K26.6	Chronic or unspecified duodenal ulcer with both hemorrhage and perforation
K26.7	Chronic duodenal ulcer without hemorrhage or perforation
K27.0	Acute peptic ulcer, site unspecified, with hemorrhage
K27.1	Acute peptic ulcer, site unspecified, with perforation
K27.2	Acute peptic ulcer, site unspecified, with both hemorrhage and perforation
K27.3	Acute peptic ulcer, site unspecified, without hemorrhage or perforation
K27.4	Chronic or unspecified peptic ulcer, site unspecified, with hemorrhage
K27.5	Chronic or unspecified peptic ulcer, site unspecified, with perforation
K27.6	Chronic or unspecified peptic ulcer, site unspecified, with both hemorrhage and perforation
K27.7	Chronic peptic ulcer, site unspecified, without hemorrhage or perforation
K28.0	Acute gastrojejunal ulcer with hemorrhage
K28.1	Acute gastrojejunal ulcer with perforation
K28.2	Acute gastrojejunal ulcer with both hemorrhage and perforation
K28.3	Acute gastrojejunal ulcer without hemorrhage or perforation
K28.4	Chronic or unspecified gastrojejunal ulcer with hemorrhage
K31.1	Adult hypertrophic pyloric stenosis △

AMA: 43820 2014,Jan,11 **43825** 2014,Jan,11

Relative Value Units/Medicare Edits

Non-Facility RVU	Work	PE	MP	Total
43820	22.53	11.87	5.32	39.72
43825	21.76	11.74	5.31	38.81
Facility RVU	Work	PE	MP	Total
43820	22.53	11.87	5.32	39.72
43825	21.76	11.74	5.31	38.81

	FUD	Status	MUE	Modifiers				IOM Reference
43820	90	A	1(2)	51	N/A	62*	80	None
43825	90	A	1(2)	51	N/A	62*	80	

* with documentation

43830-43831

43830   Gastrostomy, open; without construction of gastric tube (eg, Stamm procedure) (separate procedure)

43831   neonatal, for feeding

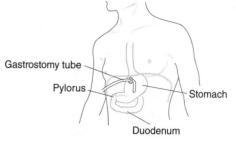

A temporary gastrostomy is usually performed as a surgical procedure. A tract is formed from the skin to the stomach. A large tube is inserted, usually for feeding purposes

Detail of tube in place

Explanation

The physician constructs a temporary or permanent gastrostomy for instillation of nutrients. After making a midline incision in the upper abdomen, the physician chooses a gastrostomy site on the middle anterior surface of the stomach. Stay sutures are placed and a small stab wound is made between purse string sutures. A gastrostomy tube is inserted and the purse string sutures are tied. The gastrostomy tube is withdrawn through a stab wound in the abdominal wall and stay sutures are placed in the posterior fascia. The abdominal incision is closed. Report 43831 if performed to facilitate feeding a neonate.

Coding Tips

Note that 43830 is a separate procedure by definition and is usually a component of a more complex service and is not identified separately. When performed alone or with other unrelated procedures/services it may be reported. If performed alone, list the code; if performed with other procedures/services, list the code and append modifier 59 or an X{EPSU} modifier. For partial, distal gastrectomy with gastrojejunostomy, see 43632. For percutaneous placement of a gastrostomy tube, see 43246. For percutaneous change of a gastrostomy tube, without imaging or endoscopic guidance, see 43762 and 43763; fluoroscopically guided replacement of a gastrostomy tube, see 49450. For repositioning of the gastric feeding tube through the duodenum for enteric nutrition, see 43761. For permanent gastrostomy with construction of a gastric tube, see 43832. Do not append modifier 63 to 43831 as the description or nature of the procedure includes infants up to 4 kg.

ICD-10-CM Diagnostic Codes

C15.3	Malignant neoplasm of upper third of esophagus
C15.4	Malignant neoplasm of middle third of esophagus
C15.5	Malignant neoplasm of lower third of esophagus
C15.8	Malignant neoplasm of overlapping sites of esophagus
C76.0	Malignant neoplasm of head, face and neck

E41	Nutritional marasmus
E44.0	Moderate protein-calorie malnutrition
E44.1	Mild protein-calorie malnutrition
E45	Retarded development following protein-calorie malnutrition
E86.0	Dehydration
E86.1	Hypovolemia
K22.2	Esophageal obstruction
K22.3	Perforation of esophagus
K22.4	Dyskinesia of esophagus
K22.89	Other specified disease of esophagus
K25.0	Acute gastric ulcer with hemorrhage
K25.1	Acute gastric ulcer with perforation
K25.2	Acute gastric ulcer with both hemorrhage and perforation
K25.3	Acute gastric ulcer without hemorrhage or perforation
K25.4	Chronic or unspecified gastric ulcer with hemorrhage
K25.5	Chronic or unspecified gastric ulcer with perforation
K25.6	Chronic or unspecified gastric ulcer with both hemorrhage and perforation
K25.7	Chronic gastric ulcer without hemorrhage or perforation
K26.0	Acute duodenal ulcer with hemorrhage
K26.1	Acute duodenal ulcer with perforation
K26.2	Acute duodenal ulcer with both hemorrhage and perforation
K26.3	Acute duodenal ulcer without hemorrhage or perforation
K26.4	Chronic or unspecified duodenal ulcer with hemorrhage
K26.5	Chronic or unspecified duodenal ulcer with perforation
K26.6	Chronic or unspecified duodenal ulcer with both hemorrhage and perforation
K26.7	Chronic duodenal ulcer without hemorrhage or perforation
K27.0	Acute peptic ulcer, site unspecified, with hemorrhage
K27.1	Acute peptic ulcer, site unspecified, with perforation
K27.2	Acute peptic ulcer, site unspecified, with both hemorrhage and perforation
K27.3	Acute peptic ulcer, site unspecified, without hemorrhage or perforation
K27.4	Chronic or unspecified peptic ulcer, site unspecified, with hemorrhage
K27.5	Chronic or unspecified peptic ulcer, site unspecified, with perforation
K31.7	Polyp of stomach and duodenum
K31.89	Other diseases of stomach and duodenum
Q39.5	Congenital dilatation of esophagus
Q40.0	Congenital hypertrophic pyloric stenosis
Q40.2	Other specified congenital malformations of stomach
R13.0	Aphagia
R13.11	Dysphagia, oral phase
R13.12	Dysphagia, oropharyngeal phase
R13.13	Dysphagia, pharyngeal phase
R13.14	Dysphagia, pharyngoesophageal phase
R13.19	Other dysphagia
R63.32	Pediatric feeding disorder, chronic 🄿
R63.39	Other feeding difficulties
T73.0XXA	Starvation, initial encounter

AMA: **43830** 2019,Feb,5; 2018,Jan,8; 2017,Jan,8; 2016,Jan,13; 2015,Jan,16
43831 2019,Feb,5; 2018,Jan,8; 2017,Jan,8; 2016,Jan,13; 2015,Jan,16

Relative Value Units/Medicare Edits

Non-Facility RVU	Work	PE	MP	Total
43830	10.85	7.44	2.54	20.83
43831	8.49	7.49	2.09	18.07
Facility RVU	**Work**	**PE**	**MP**	**Total**
43830	10.85	7.44	2.54	20.83
43831	8.49	7.49	2.09	18.07

	FUD	Status	MUE	Modifiers				IOM Reference
43830	90	A	1(2)	51	N/A	62*	80	None
43831	90	A	1(2)	51	N/A	62*	80	

* with documentation

Terms To Know

anterior. Situated in the front area or toward the belly surface of the body.

fascia. Fibrous sheet or band of tissue that envelops organs, muscles, and groupings of muscles.

gastrostomy. Temporary or permanent artificial opening made in the stomach for gastrointestinal decompression or to provide nutrition when not maintained by other methods.

posterior. Located in the back part or caudal end of the body.

separate procedures. Services commonly carried out as a fundamental part of a total service and, as such, do not usually warrant separate identification. These services are identified in CPT with the parenthetical phrase (separate procedure) at the end of the description and are payable only when performed alone.

43832

43832 Gastrostomy, open; with construction of gastric tube (eg, Janeway procedure)

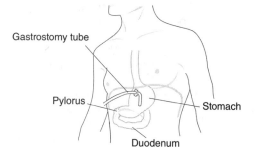

A permanent gastrostomy is performed as a surgical procedure. A mucosal-lined tract is formed from the skin to the stomach. A large tube is inserted and sutured to the skin

Explanation

The physician constructs a permanent gastrostomy for instillation of nutrients. After a small midline upper abdominal incision, the physician creates a flap with its base at the greater curvature of the stomach. The flap is converted into a tube by closure of the stomach incision. The tube is brought through the skin surface via a stab wound or tunnel. The end of the tube is everted slightly and sutured to the skin. The abdominal incision is closed with sutures.

Coding Tips

For percutaneous placement of a gastrostomy tube, see 43246. For change of a gastrostomy tube, see 43762 and 43763; repositioning, see 43761.

ICD-10-CM Diagnostic Codes

C13.2	Malignant neoplasm of posterior wall of hypopharynx
C13.8	Malignant neoplasm of overlapping sites of hypopharynx
C15.3	Malignant neoplasm of upper third of esophagus
C15.4	Malignant neoplasm of middle third of esophagus
C15.5	Malignant neoplasm of lower third of esophagus
C15.8	Malignant neoplasm of overlapping sites of esophagus
C16.0	Malignant neoplasm of cardia
C16.1	Malignant neoplasm of fundus of stomach
C16.2	Malignant neoplasm of body of stomach
C16.3	Malignant neoplasm of pyloric antrum
C16.4	Malignant neoplasm of pylorus
C76.0	Malignant neoplasm of head, face and neck
C7A.092	Malignant carcinoid tumor of the stomach
E41	Nutritional marasmus
E44.0	Moderate protein-calorie malnutrition
E44.1	Mild protein-calorie malnutrition
E45	Retarded development following protein-calorie malnutrition
E86.0	Dehydration
E86.1	Hypovolemia
F50.01	Anorexia nervosa, restricting type
F50.82	Avoidant/restrictive food intake disorder
G20	Parkinson's disease
G35	Multiple sclerosis
K22.2	Esophageal obstruction
K22.3	Perforation of esophagus
K22.4	Dyskinesia of esophagus
K22.89	Other specified disease of esophagus
K25.0	Acute gastric ulcer with hemorrhage
K25.1	Acute gastric ulcer with perforation
K25.2	Acute gastric ulcer with both hemorrhage and perforation
K25.3	Acute gastric ulcer without hemorrhage or perforation
K25.4	Chronic or unspecified gastric ulcer with hemorrhage
K25.5	Chronic or unspecified gastric ulcer with perforation
K25.6	Chronic or unspecified gastric ulcer with both hemorrhage and perforation
K25.7	Chronic gastric ulcer without hemorrhage or perforation
K26.0	Acute duodenal ulcer with hemorrhage
K26.1	Acute duodenal ulcer with perforation
K26.2	Acute duodenal ulcer with both hemorrhage and perforation
K26.3	Acute duodenal ulcer without hemorrhage or perforation
K26.4	Chronic or unspecified duodenal ulcer with hemorrhage
K26.5	Chronic or unspecified duodenal ulcer with perforation
K26.6	Chronic or unspecified duodenal ulcer with both hemorrhage and perforation
K26.7	Chronic duodenal ulcer without hemorrhage or perforation
K27.0	Acute peptic ulcer, site unspecified, with hemorrhage
K27.1	Acute peptic ulcer, site unspecified, with perforation
K27.2	Acute peptic ulcer, site unspecified, with both hemorrhage and perforation
K27.3	Acute peptic ulcer, site unspecified, without hemorrhage or perforation
K27.4	Chronic or unspecified peptic ulcer, site unspecified, with hemorrhage
K27.5	Chronic or unspecified peptic ulcer, site unspecified, with perforation
K31.89	Other diseases of stomach and duodenum
Q39.5	Congenital dilatation of esophagus
Q40.0	Congenital hypertrophic pyloric stenosis
Q40.2	Other specified congenital malformations of stomach
R13.0	Aphagia
R13.11	Dysphagia, oral phase
R13.12	Dysphagia, oropharyngeal phase
R13.13	Dysphagia, pharyngeal phase
R13.14	Dysphagia, pharyngoesophageal phase
R13.19	Other dysphagia
R63.32	Pediatric feeding disorder, chronic 🅿
R63.39	Other feeding difficulties
T73.0XXA	Starvation, initial encounter

AMA: **43832** 2018,Jan,8; 2017,Jan,8; 2016,Jan,13; 2015,Jan,16

Relative Value Units/Medicare Edits

Non-Facility RVU	Work	PE	MP	Total
43832	17.34	9.42	4.1	30.86
Facility RVU	Work	PE	MP	Total
43832	17.34	9.42	4.1	30.86

	FUD	Status	MUE	Modifiers				IOM Reference
43832	90	A	1(2)	51	N/A	62*	80	None

* with documentation

Terms To Know

dysphagia. Difficulty and pain upon swallowing.

flap. Mass of flesh and skin partially excised from its location but retaining its blood supply that is moved to another site to repair adjacent or distant defects.

gastrostomy. Temporary or permanent artificial opening made in the stomach for gastrointestinal decompression or to provide nutrition when not maintained by other methods.

incision. Act of cutting into tissue or an organ.

instillation. Administering a liquid slowly over time, drop by drop.

malignant neoplasm. Any cancerous tumor or lesion exhibiting uncontrolled tissue growth that can progressively invade other parts of the body with its disease-generating cells.

suture. Numerous stitching techniques employed in wound closure.

ulcer. Open sore or excavating lesion of skin or the tissue on the surface of an organ from the sloughing of chronically inflamed and necrosing tissue.

43840

43840   Gastrorrhaphy, suture of perforated duodenal or gastric ulcer, wound, or injury

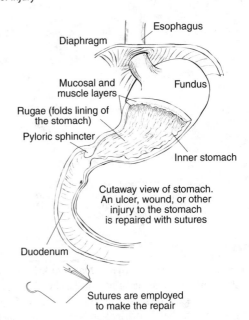

Cutaway view of stomach. An ulcer, wound, or other injury to the stomach is repaired with sutures

Sutures are employed to make the repair

Explanation

The physician repairs an ulcer, wound, or injury to the stomach or duodenum. The ulcer or wound is exposed by the physician via a midline upper abdominal incision or a transverse supraumbilical incision through skin, fascia, and muscle. The perforation is sutured closed and the peritoneal cavity is irrigated and suctioned to remove contamination. The abdominal fascia and peritoneum are closed in one layer. The skin and subcutaneous layers are closed.

Coding Tips

For gastrostomy with suture repair of a bleeding ulcer, see 43501; for pre-existing esophagogastric laceration (e.g., Mallory-Weiss), see 43502.

ICD-10-CM Diagnostic Codes

K25.1	Acute gastric ulcer with perforation
K25.2	Acute gastric ulcer with both hemorrhage and perforation
K25.5	Chronic or unspecified gastric ulcer with perforation
K25.6	Chronic or unspecified gastric ulcer with both hemorrhage and perforation
K26.1	Acute duodenal ulcer with perforation
K26.2	Acute duodenal ulcer with both hemorrhage and perforation
K26.5	Chronic or unspecified duodenal ulcer with perforation
K26.6	Chronic or unspecified duodenal ulcer with both hemorrhage and perforation
K27.0	Acute peptic ulcer, site unspecified, with hemorrhage
K27.1	Acute peptic ulcer, site unspecified, with perforation
K27.2	Acute peptic ulcer, site unspecified, with both hemorrhage and perforation
K27.5	Chronic or unspecified peptic ulcer, site unspecified, with perforation
K27.6	Chronic or unspecified peptic ulcer, site unspecified, with both hemorrhage and perforation
K28.1	Acute gastrojejunal ulcer with perforation

K28.5	Chronic or unspecified gastrojejunal ulcer with perforation
K28.6	Chronic or unspecified gastrojejunal ulcer with both hemorrhage and perforation
S36.33XA	Laceration of stomach, initial encounter
S36.39XA	Other injury of stomach, initial encounter
S36.410A	Primary blast injury of duodenum, initial encounter
S36.420A	Contusion of duodenum, initial encounter
S36.430A	Laceration of duodenum, initial encounter
S36.490A	Other injury of duodenum, initial encounter

AMA: 43840 2014,Jan,11

Relative Value Units/Medicare Edits

Non-Facility RVU	Work	PE	MP	Total
43840	22.83	11.96	5.38	40.17
Facility RVU	**Work**	**PE**	**MP**	**Total**
43840	22.83	11.96	5.38	40.17

	FUD	Status	MUE	Modifiers				IOM Reference
43840	90	A	2(3)	51	N/A	62*	80	None

* with documentation

Terms To Know

duodenum. First portion of the small intestine connected to the stomach at the pylorus and extending to the jejunum.

fascia. Fibrous sheet or band of tissue that envelops organs, muscles, and groupings of muscles.

gastrorrhaphy. Repair or suturing of a perforation of the stomach or duodenum.

irrigation. To wash out or cleanse a body cavity, wound, or tissue with water or other fluid.

perforation. Hole in an object, organ, or tissue, or the act of punching or boring holes through a part.

peritoneal cavity. Space between the lining of the abdominal wall, or parietal peritoneum, and the surface layer of the abdominal organs, or visceral peritoneum. It contains a thin, watery fluid that keeps the peritoneal surfaces moist.

transverse. Crosswise at right angles to the long axis of a structure or part.

ulcer. Open sore or excavating lesion of skin or the tissue on the surface of an organ from the sloughing of chronically inflamed and necrosing tissue.

43842-43843

| 43842 | Gastric restrictive procedure, without gastric bypass, for morbid obesity; vertical-banded gastroplasty |
| 43843 | other than vertical-banded gastroplasty |

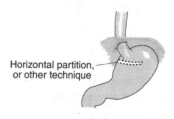

Explanation

The physician alters the stomach's size to help stem morbid obesity. The physician exposes the lesser curvature of the stomach via a midline abdominal incision through skin, fascia, and muscles. In 43842, a double row of staples is placed in the upper portion of the stomach to create a small stoma. A small strip of mesh or a Silastic ring is wrapped around the stoma and stapled to itself. Report 43843 if the technique used is other than the vertical-banded gastroplasty, and allows for staples restricting other parts of the stomach.

Coding Tips

For a gastric restrictive procedure with gastric bypass for morbid obesity, with short limb (less than 150 cm) Roux-en-Y gastroenterostomy, see 43846; with small intestine reconstruction to limit absorption, see 43847. For revision of a gastric restrictive procedure, see 43848.

ICD-10-CM Diagnostic Codes

E23.6	Other disorders of pituitary gland
E24.1	Nelson's syndrome
E27.8	Other specified disorders of adrenal gland
E35	Disorders of endocrine glands in diseases classified elsewhere
E66.01	Morbid (severe) obesity due to excess calories
E66.09	Other obesity due to excess calories
E66.1	Drug-induced obesity
E66.2	Morbid (severe) obesity with alveolar hypoventilation
E66.3	Overweight
E66.8	Other obesity

AMA: **43842** 2018,Jan,8; 2017,Jan,8; 2016,Jan,13; 2015,Jan,16 **43843** 2018,Jan,8; 2017,Jan,8; 2016,Jan,13; 2015,Jan,16

Relative Value Units/Medicare Edits

Non-Facility RVU	Work	PE	MP	Total
43842	21.03	10.98	1.67	33.68
43843	21.21	11.63	5.18	38.02
Facility RVU	Work	PE	MP	Total
43842	21.03	10.98	1.67	33.68
43843	21.21	11.63	5.18	38.02

	FUD	Status	MUE	Modifiers				IOM Reference
43842	90	N	0(3)	N/A	N/A	N/A	N/A	100-03,100.1
43843	90	A	1(2)	51	N/A	62	80	

* with documentation

Terms To Know

mesh. Synthetic fabric used as a prosthetic patch in hernia repair.

morbid obesity. Accumulation of excess fat in the subcutaneous connective tissue with increased weight beyond the limits of skeletal requirements, defined as 125 percent or more over the ideal body weight. It is often associated with serious conditions that can become life threatening, such as diabetes, hypertension, and arteriosclerosis.

pituitary gland. Hormone-controlling epithelial body located within the sella turcica at the base of the brain that secretes most of the body's hormones and regulates neurohormones received from the hypothalamus.

Roux-en-Y anastomosis. Y-shaped attachment of the distal end of a divided small intestine segment to the stomach, esophagus, biliary tract, or other structure with anastomosis of the proximal end to the side of the small intestine further down for reflux-free drainage.

stoma. Opening created in the abdominal wall from an internal organ or structure for diversion of waste elimination, drainage, and access.

43845

43845   Gastric restrictive procedure with partial gastrectomy, pylorus-preserving duodenoileostomy and ileoileostomy (50 to 100 cm common channel) to limit absorption (biliopancreatic diversion with duodenal switch)

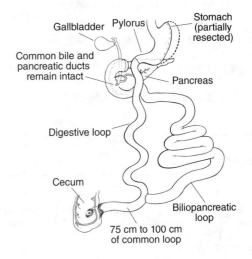

Explanation

A partial gastrectomy with pylorus-preserving duodenoileostomy and ileoileostomy is done to combine gastric restriction with limited intestinal absorption for weight loss. This procedure is called a biliopancreatic diversion with duodenal switch. The stomach is resected along the greater curvature, leaving the pyloric valve intact with the remaining stomach that maintains its functionality. A portion of the duodenum is also left within the food track to preserve the pylorus/duodenum pathway. The duodenum is divided near the pyloric valve. The small intestine is also divided. The distal end of the small intestine in continuity with the large intestine is brought up and anastomosed to the short duodenal segment on the stomach. The other end of the small intestine-the duodenal segment in connection with the gallbladder and pancreas, or the biliopancreatic loop-is attached to the newly anastomosed other limb further down near the large intestine. This forms a 75 cm to 100 cm "common loop" where the contents of both these segments channel together before dumping into the large intestine.

Coding Tips

Do not report 43845 with 43633, 43847, 44130, or 49000.

ICD-10-CM Diagnostic Codes

E23.6	Other disorders of pituitary gland
E27.8	Other specified disorders of adrenal gland
E35	Disorders of endocrine glands in diseases classified elsewhere
E66.01	Morbid (severe) obesity due to excess calories
E66.09	Other obesity due to excess calories
E66.1	Drug-induced obesity
E66.2	Morbid (severe) obesity with alveolar hypoventilation
E66.3	Overweight
E66.8	Other obesity
Z68.41	Body mass index [BMI] 40.0-44.9, adult 🄰
Z68.42	Body mass index [BMI] 45.0-49.9, adult 🄰
Z68.43	Body mass index [BMI] 50.0-59.9, adult 🄰
Z68.44	Body mass index [BMI] 60.0-69.9, adult 🄰

Z68.45   Body mass index [BMI] 70 or greater, adult ☒

AMA: **43845** 2018,Jan,8; 2017,Jan,8; 2016,Jan,13; 2015,Jan,16

Relative Value Units/Medicare Edits

Non-Facility RVU	Work	PE	MP	Total
43845	33.3	16.2	7.82	57.32
Facility RVU	**Work**	**PE**	**MP**	**Total**
43845	33.3	16.2	7.82	57.32

	FUD	Status	MUE	Modifiers				IOM Reference
43845	90	A	1(2)	51	N/A	62*	80	None

* with documentation

Terms To Know

anastomosis. Surgically created connection between ducts, blood vessels, or bowel segments to allow flow from one to the other.

BMI. Body mass index. Tool for calculating weight appropriateness in adults and may be a factor in determining medical necessity for bariatric procedures.

distal. Located farther away from a specified reference point or the trunk.

gastrectomy. Surgical excision of all or part of the stomach.

morbid obesity. Accumulation of excess fat in the subcutaneous connective tissue with increased weight beyond the limits of skeletal requirements, defined as 125 percent or more over the ideal body weight. It is often associated with serious conditions that can become life threatening, such as diabetes, hypertension, and arteriosclerosis.

43846-43847

43846   Gastric restrictive procedure, with gastric bypass for morbid obesity; with short limb (150 cm or less) Roux-en-Y gastroenterostomy
43847   with small intestine reconstruction to limit absorption

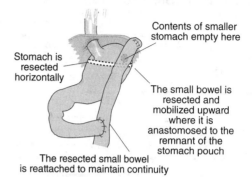

Contents of smaller stomach empty here

Stomach is resected horizontally

The small bowel is resected and mobilized upward where it is anastomosed to the remnant of the stomach pouch

The resected small bowel is reattached to maintain continuity

A gastric restrictive procedure with gastric bypass is performed

Explanation

The physician performs a gastric bypass for morbid obesity by partitioning the stomach and performing a small bowel division and anastomosis to the proximal stomach (Roux-en-Y gastrojejunostomy). This bypasses the majority of the stomach. The physician makes a midline abdominal incision. The stomach is mobilized and the proximal stomach is divided with a stapling device along the lesser curvature, leaving only a small proximal pouch in continuity with the esophagus. A short limb of the proximal small bowel (150 cm or less) is divided and the distal end of the short intestinal limb is brought up and anastomosed to the proximal gastric pouch. The other end of the divided bowel is connected back into the small bowel distal to the short limb's gastric anastomosis to restore intestinal continuity. The incision is closed. In 43847, the small intestine is reconstructed so that it is partially bypassed to limit the amount of area available for absorption of nutrients. The incision is closed.

Coding Tips

For roux limb greater than 150 cm, report 43847. For laparoscopic approach, see 43644–43645. For a gastric restrictive procedure, without gastric bypass for morbid obesity, vertical-banded gastroplasty, see 43842; other than vertical-banded gastroplasty, see 43843. For revision of a restrictive procedure, see 43848. For revision of a gastrojejunal anastomosis with reconstruction, with or without partial gastrectomy or intestine resection, without vagotomy, see 43860; with vagotomy, see 43865.

ICD-10-CM Diagnostic Codes

E23.6	Other disorders of pituitary gland
E27.8	Other specified disorders of adrenal gland
E35	Disorders of endocrine glands in diseases classified elsewhere
E66.01	Morbid (severe) obesity due to excess calories
E66.09	Other obesity due to excess calories
E66.1	Drug-induced obesity
E66.2	Morbid (severe) obesity with alveolar hypoventilation
E66.3	Overweight
E66.8	Other obesity
Z68.41	Body mass index [BMI] 40.0-44.9, adult ☒
Z68.42	Body mass index [BMI] 45.0-49.9, adult ☒
Z68.43	Body mass index [BMI] 50.0-59.9, adult ☒

Z68.44	Body mass index [BMI] 60.0-69.9, adult △	
Z68.45	Body mass index [BMI] 70 or greater, adult △	

AMA: **43846** 2018,Jan,8; 2017,Jan,8; 2016,Jan,13; 2015,Jan,16 **43847** 2018,Jan,8; 2017,Jan,8; 2016,Jan,13; 2015,Jan,16

Relative Value Units/Medicare Edits

Non-Facility RVU	Work	PE	MP	Total
43846	27.41	14.77	6.69	48.87
43847	30.28	15.82	7.41	53.51
Facility RVU	Work	PE	MP	Total
43846	27.41	14.77	6.69	48.87
43847	30.28	15.82	7.41	53.51

	FUD	Status	MUE	Modifiers				IOM Reference
43846	90	A	1(2)	51	N/A	62*	80	None
43847	90	A	1(2)	51	N/A	62*	80	

* with documentation

Terms To Know

morbid obesity. Accumulation of excess fat in the subcutaneous connective tissue with increased weight beyond the limits of skeletal requirements, defined as 125 percent or more over the ideal body weight. It is often associated with serious conditions that can become life threatening, such as diabetes, hypertension, and arteriosclerosis.

pituitary gland. Hormone-controlling epithelial body located within the sella turcica at the base of the brain that secretes most of the body's hormones and regulates neurohormones received from the hypothalamus.

proximal. Located closest to a specified reference point, usually the midline or trunk.

Roux-en-Y anastomosis. Y-shaped attachment of the distal end of a divided small intestine segment to the stomach, esophagus, biliary tract, or other structure with anastomosis of the proximal end to the side of the small intestine further down for reflux-free drainage.

43848

43848 Revision, open, of gastric restrictive procedure for morbid obesity, other than adjustable gastric restrictive device (separate procedure)

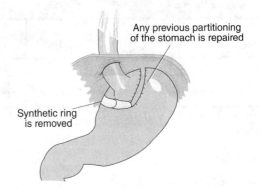

Any previous partitioning of the stomach is repaired

Synthetic ring is removed

Any type of previously performed gastric restrictive surgery for morbid obesity is revised

Explanation

The physician uses an open technique to revise a failed gastric restrictive procedure for morbid obesity. Indications for revision include stomal stenosis, stomal dilation, non-emptying gastric pouch, gastroesophageal reflux, staple dehiscence, intragastric foreign body, gastric fistula, gastroesophageal fistula, failure to maintain weight loss, breakdown of staple continuity, and restored gastric continuity. This code is not used to report revision of an adjustable gastric restrictive device. Revision techniques vary depending on the technique used in initial gastric restrictive procedure (i.e., gastroplasty, partial gastrectomy, gastric bypass) and the nature of the gastric restrictive failure. Types of revision include gastroplasty, conversion of a gastroplasty to a gastric bypass, and revision of a gastric bypass. The physician makes a midline abdominal incision. Next, the stomach and previous anastomoses are dissected free of surrounding structures. This can involve painstaking lysis of adhesions between the liver, stomach, distal esophagus, colon, and/or spleen. The physician performs the required revision. If a gastroplasty is performed, a double row of staples is placed in the upper portion of the stomach to create a small stoma. A small strip of mesh or a Silastic ring is wrapped around the stoma and stapled to itself. A partial gastrectomy involves resecting the stomach along the greater curvature and leaving the pyloric valve intact with the remaining stomach to maintain functionality. If a gastric bypass is performed, the stomach is partitioned, the small bowel divided, and the small bowel is reanastomosed to the proximal stomach.

Coding Tips

This separate procedure by definition is usually a component of a more complex service and is not identified separately. When performed alone or with other unrelated procedures/services it may be reported. If performed alone, list the code; if performed with other procedures/services, list the code and append modifier 59 or an X{EPSU} modifier. For laparoscopic adjustable gastric band procedures, see 43770–43775; open revision, removal, or removal with replacement of port components, see 43886–43888; removal of both gastric restrictive device and port components, see 43659. For open gastric restrictive procedure, without gastric bypass for morbid obesity, vertical-banded gastroplasty, see 43842; for other than vertical-banded gastroplasty, see 43843.

ICD-10-CM Diagnostic Codes

E23.6	Other disorders of pituitary gland
E27.8	Other specified disorders of adrenal gland

E35	Disorders of endocrine glands in diseases classified elsewhere
E66.01	Morbid (severe) obesity due to excess calories
E66.09	Other obesity due to excess calories
E66.1	Drug-induced obesity
E66.2	Morbid (severe) obesity with alveolar hypoventilation
E66.3	Overweight
E66.8	Other obesity
K91.1	Postgastric surgery syndromes
K91.89	Other postprocedural complications and disorders of digestive system
K95.01	Infection due to gastric band procedure
K95.09	Other complications of gastric band procedure
K95.81	Infection due to other bariatric procedure
K95.89	Other complications of other bariatric procedure
Z68.41	Body mass index [BMI] 40.0-44.9, adult ▲
Z68.42	Body mass index [BMI] 45.0-49.9, adult ▲
Z68.43	Body mass index [BMI] 50.0-59.9, adult ▲
Z68.44	Body mass index [BMI] 60.0-69.9, adult ▲
Z68.45	Body mass index [BMI] 70 or greater, adult ▲

AMA: **43848** 2018,Jan,8; 2017,Jan,8; 2016,Jan,13; 2015,Jan,16

Relative Value Units/Medicare Edits

Non-Facility RVU	Work	PE	MP	Total
43848	32.75	16.55	7.8	57.1
Facility RVU	**Work**	**PE**	**MP**	**Total**
43848	32.75	16.55	7.8	57.1

	FUD	Status	MUE	Modifiers				IOM Reference
43848	90	A	1(2)	51	N/A	62*	80	None

* with documentation

Terms To Know

anastomosis. Surgically created connection between ducts, blood vessels, or bowel segments to allow flow from one to the other.

morbid obesity. Accumulation of excess fat in the subcutaneous connective tissue with increased weight beyond the limits of skeletal requirements, defined as 125 percent or more over the ideal body weight. It is often associated with serious conditions that can become life threatening, such as diabetes, hypertension, and arteriosclerosis.

revision. Reordering or rearrangement of tissue to suit a particular need or function.

stoma. Opening created in the abdominal wall from an internal organ or structure for diversion of waste elimination, drainage, and access.

43860-43865

43860 Revision of gastrojejunal anastomosis (gastrojejunostomy) with reconstruction, with or without partial gastrectomy or intestine resection; without vagotomy

43865 with vagotomy

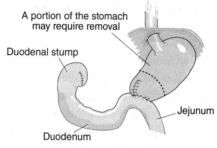

A portion of the stomach may require removal

Duodenal stump

Jejunum

Duodenum

A previous gastrojejunostomy is revised, with or without vagotomy

Any of a variety of revision techniques may be employed

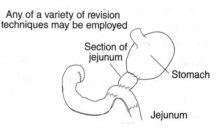

Section of jejunum

Stomach

Jejunum

Explanation

The physician revises an anastomoses between the stomach and the jejunum. The physician exposes the stomach and small intestine via a midline upper abdominal incision through skin, muscles, and fascia. About 8 cm to 10 cm of the jejunum limb is divided, reversed and connected to the distal end of the stomach. The short reversed segment is connected to the jejunum and the remnant of jejunum and duodenum are anastomosed to the long segment of jejunum. A partial gastrectomy or intestine resection may be performed. The abdominal incision is closed. Report 43865 if a vagotomy is performed in conjunction with this procedure.

Coding Tips

These codes report revision of a previously constructed gastrojejunostomy. For an initial gastroduodenostomy, see 43820; with vagotomy, any type, see 43825. For partial, distal gastrectomy, with gastroduodenostomy, see 43631; with vagotomy, see 43635.

ICD-10-CM Diagnostic Codes

C16.8	Malignant neoplasm of overlapping sites of stomach
C17.0	Malignant neoplasm of duodenum
C25.0	Malignant neoplasm of head of pancreas
C25.1	Malignant neoplasm of body of pancreas
C25.2	Malignant neoplasm of tail of pancreas
C25.3	Malignant neoplasm of pancreatic duct
C25.4	Malignant neoplasm of endocrine pancreas
C25.7	Malignant neoplasm of other parts of pancreas
C25.8	Malignant neoplasm of overlapping sites of pancreas
C78.4	Secondary malignant neoplasm of small intestine
C78.89	Secondary malignant neoplasm of other digestive organs
C7A.010	Malignant carcinoid tumor of the duodenum

C7A.092	Malignant carcinoid tumor of the stomach
D37.1	Neoplasm of uncertain behavior of stomach
K25.0	Acute gastric ulcer with hemorrhage
K25.1	Acute gastric ulcer with perforation
K25.2	Acute gastric ulcer with both hemorrhage and perforation
K25.3	Acute gastric ulcer without hemorrhage or perforation
K25.4	Chronic or unspecified gastric ulcer with hemorrhage
K25.5	Chronic or unspecified gastric ulcer with perforation
K25.6	Chronic or unspecified gastric ulcer with both hemorrhage and perforation
K25.7	Chronic gastric ulcer without hemorrhage or perforation
K26.0	Acute duodenal ulcer with hemorrhage
K26.1	Acute duodenal ulcer with perforation
K26.2	Acute duodenal ulcer with both hemorrhage and perforation
K26.3	Acute duodenal ulcer without hemorrhage or perforation
K26.4	Chronic or unspecified duodenal ulcer with hemorrhage
K26.5	Chronic or unspecified duodenal ulcer with perforation
K26.6	Chronic or unspecified duodenal ulcer with both hemorrhage and perforation
K26.7	Chronic duodenal ulcer without hemorrhage or perforation
K27.0	Acute peptic ulcer, site unspecified, with hemorrhage
K27.1	Acute peptic ulcer, site unspecified, with perforation
K27.2	Acute peptic ulcer, site unspecified, with both hemorrhage and perforation
K27.3	Acute peptic ulcer, site unspecified, without hemorrhage or perforation
K27.4	Chronic or unspecified peptic ulcer, site unspecified, with hemorrhage
K27.5	Chronic or unspecified peptic ulcer, site unspecified, with perforation
K27.6	Chronic or unspecified peptic ulcer, site unspecified, with both hemorrhage and perforation
K27.7	Chronic peptic ulcer, site unspecified, without hemorrhage or perforation
K28.0	Acute gastrojejunal ulcer with hemorrhage
K28.1	Acute gastrojejunal ulcer with perforation
K28.2	Acute gastrojejunal ulcer with both hemorrhage and perforation
K28.3	Acute gastrojejunal ulcer without hemorrhage or perforation
K28.4	Chronic or unspecified gastrojejunal ulcer with hemorrhage
K31.1	Adult hypertrophic pyloric stenosis A
K91.1	Postgastric surgery syndromes
K91.89	Other postprocedural complications and disorders of digestive system
K94.21	Gastrostomy hemorrhage
K94.22	Gastrostomy infection
K94.23	Gastrostomy malfunction
K94.29	Other complications of gastrostomy

AMA: 43860 2014,Jan,11 **43865** 2014,Jan,11

Relative Value Units/Medicare Edits

Non-Facility RVU	Work	PE	MP	Total
43860	27.89	13.94	6.44	48.27
43865	29.05	14.44	7.11	50.6
Facility RVU	**Work**	**PE**	**MP**	**Total**
43860	27.89	13.94	6.44	48.27
43865	29.05	14.44	7.11	50.6

	FUD	Status	MUE	Modifiers				IOM Reference
43860	90	A	1(2)	51	N/A	62*	80	None
43865	90	A	1(2)	51	N/A	62*	80	

* with documentation

Terms To Know

anastomosis. Surgically created connection between ducts, blood vessels, or bowel segments to allow flow from one to the other.

distal. Located farther away from a specified reference point or the trunk.

fascia. Fibrous sheet or band of tissue that envelops organs, muscles, and groupings of muscles.

gastrectomy. Surgical excision of all or part of the stomach.

gastrojejunostomy. Surgical creation of an opening from the stomach to the jejunum.

reconstruction. Recreating, restoring, or rebuilding a body part or organ.

resection. Surgical removal of a part or all of an organ or body part.

revision. Reordering or rearrangement of tissue to suit a particular need or function.

vagotomy. Division of the vagus nerves, interrupting impulses resulting in lower gastric acid production and hastening gastric emptying.

43870

43870 Closure of gastrostomy, surgical

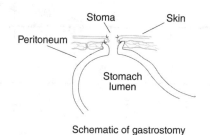

Schematic of gastrostomy

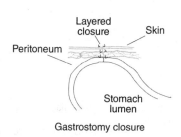

Gastrostomy closure

Explanation

The physician closes a gastrostomy no longer needed. The physician enters through a previous gastrostomy. The stomach is dissected free of the abdominal wall. The stomach gastrostomy site is closed with sutures. The abdominal incision is closed with layered sutures.

Coding Tips

For open gastrostomy, without gastric tube construction, see 43830; for neonatal for feeding, see 43831; for laparoscopic gastrostomy, see 43653. For permanent gastrostomy, with construction of a gastric tube, see 43832.

ICD-10-CM Diagnostic Codes

K94.21	Gastrostomy hemorrhage
K94.22	Gastrostomy infection
K94.23	Gastrostomy malfunction
K94.29	Other complications of gastrostomy
Z43.1	Encounter for attention to gastrostomy

AMA: 43870 2018,Jul,14

Relative Value Units/Medicare Edits

Non-Facility RVU	Work	PE	MP	Total
43870	11.44	6.99	2.59	21.02
Facility RVU	Work	PE	MP	Total
43870	11.44	6.99	2.59	21.02

	FUD	Status	MUE	Modifiers				IOM Reference
43870	90	A	1(2)	51	N/A	62*	80	None

* with documentation

43880

43880 Closure of gastrocolic fistula

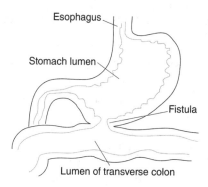

A fistula between the stomach and the colon is closed

Explanation

The physician closes a gastrocolic fistula. The physician exposes stomach and colon via a midline abdominal incision through skin, fascia, and muscle. The bowel is mobilized and the fistula is located. The stomach and intestinal tissue involving the fistula is resected en bloc with a margin of healthy adjacent tissue. The surgical defects of the stomach and intestine are repaired, the method depending on the extent of the defect. The abdominal incision is closed in layers.

Coding Tips

A fistula is an abnormal communication or passage between two structures. In order to select the correct procedure code, it is necessary to identify the structures the fistula connects. In this case, the fistula connects the stomach and the colon. For closure of an intestinal cutaneous fistula, see 44640; enteroenteric or enterocolic, see 44650; enterovesical, without intestinal or bladder resection, see 44660; with intestinal and/or bladder resection, see 44661; renocolic fistula, abdominal approach, see 50525; thoracic, see 50526; rectovesical fistula, see 45800; with colostomy, see 45805.

ICD-10-CM Diagnostic Codes

K31.6	Fistula of stomach and duodenum
Q40.2	Other specified congenital malformations of stomach

AMA: 43880 2014,Jan,11

Relative Value Units/Medicare Edits

Non-Facility RVU	Work	PE	MP	Total
43880	27.18	13.53	6.15	46.86
Facility RVU	Work	PE	MP	Total
43880	27.18	13.53	6.15	46.86

	FUD	Status	MUE	Modifiers				IOM Reference
43880	90	A	1(3)	51	N/A	62*	80	None

* with documentation

Stomach

43881-43882

43881 Implantation or replacement of gastric neurostimulator electrodes, antrum, open

43882 Revision or removal of gastric neurostimulator electrodes, antrum, open

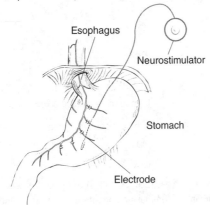

The procedure is performed via an open approach

Esophagus

Neurostimulator

Stomach

Electrode

Explanation

The physician performs placement of gastric neurostimulator electrodes in an open procedure. Through a laparotomy, the physician enters the abdominal cavity. The antrum of the stomach is identified and the physician secures two electrodes to the muscle of the pyloric antrum. The electrodes are connected to a neurostimulator that has been secured in a subcutaneous pocket in the abdomen in a separately reportable procedure. The physician closes the laparotomy with layered sutures. Report 43881 if electrodes are placed or if existing electrodes are removed and replaced with new ones. Report 43882 for the revision or removal of the electrodes.

Coding Tips

If this procedure is performed with a laparoscopic approach, see 43647–43648. For insertion or replacement of a gastric neurostimulator pulse generator, see 64590; for revision or removal, see 64595; electronic analysis, programming, and reprogramming, see 95980–95982. For open implantation, revision, or removal of gastric neurostimulator electrodes, lesser curvature (for morbid obesity), see 43999. Laparoscopic implantation, removal, replacement, reprogramming, or revision of vagus nerve blocking neurostimulator electrodes and/or pulse generator services are reported with 0312T-0317T.

ICD-10-CM Diagnostic Codes

E08.43	Diabetes mellitus due to underlying condition with diabetic autonomic (poly)neuropathy
E09.43	Drug or chemical induced diabetes mellitus with neurological complications with diabetic autonomic (poly)neuropathy
E10.43	Type 1 diabetes mellitus with diabetic autonomic (poly)neuropathy
E11.43	Type 2 diabetes mellitus with diabetic autonomic (poly)neuropathy
K31.84	Gastroparesis
T85.518A	Breakdown (mechanical) of other gastrointestinal prosthetic devices, implants and grafts, initial encounter
T85.528A	Displacement of other gastrointestinal prosthetic devices, implants and grafts, initial encounter
T85.598A	Other mechanical complication of other gastrointestinal prosthetic devices, implants and grafts, initial encounter

AMA: **43881** 2019,Feb,6; 2018,Jan,8; 2017,Jan,8; 2016,Jan,13; 2015,Jan,16
43882 2019,Feb,6; 2018,Jan,8; 2017,Jan,8; 2016,Jan,13; 2015,Jan,16

Relative Value Units/Medicare Edits

Non-Facility RVU	Work	PE	MP	Total
43881	0.0	0.0	0.0	0.0
43882	0.0	0.0	0.0	0.0
Facility RVU	**Work**	**PE**	**MP**	**Total**
43881	0.0	0.0	0.0	0.0
43882	0.0	0.0	0.0	0.0

	FUD	Status	MUE	Modifiers				IOM Reference
43881	N/A	C	1(3)	51	N/A	62*	80	None
43882	N/A	C	1(3)	51	N/A	62*	80	

* with documentation

Terms To Know

antrum. Chamber or cavity, typically with a small opening.

approach. Method or anatomical location used to gain access to a body organ or specific area for procedures.

diabetes mellitus. Endocrine disease manifested by high blood glucose levels and resulting in the inability to successfully metabolize carbohydrates, proteins, and fats, due to defects in insulin production and secretion, insulin action, or both.

gastroparesis. Delay in the emptying of food from the stomach into the small bowel due to a degree of paralysis in the muscles lining the stomach wall.

laparotomy. Incision through the flank or abdomen for therapeutic or diagnostic purposes.

morbid obesity. Accumulation of excess fat in the subcutaneous connective tissue with increased weight beyond the limits of skeletal requirements, defined as 125 percent or more over the ideal body weight. It is often associated with serious conditions that can become life threatening, such as diabetes, hypertension, and arteriosclerosis.

revision. Reordering or rearrangement of tissue to suit a particular need or function.

43886

43886   Gastric restrictive procedure, open; revision of subcutaneous port component only

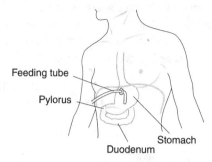

Feeding tube
Pylorus
Stomach
Duodenum

Gastric band is placed in laparoscopic approach

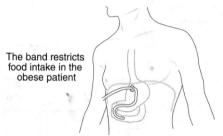

The band restricts food intake in the obese patient

A revision of subcutaneous port component

Explanation

The physician performs an open revision of the subcutaneous port component used in a gastric restrictive procedure for the treatment of morbid obesity. The subcutaneous port is the access point for infusing saline into the gastric band to adjust the band for optimal performance. The physician makes an incision through the old scar near the original port. Dissection is carried down to the port. The sutures adhering the port to the fascia may be removed so that necessary repairs and revisions can be made. The port is secured to the fascia with sutures. The incision is closed with sutures.

Coding Tips

Removal of subcutaneous port component only is reported with 43887; removal and replacement, see 43888; removal and replacement of both gastric band and subcutaneous port components, see 43659; via laparoscopic approach, see 43774.

ICD-10-CM Diagnostic Codes

E66.01	Morbid (severe) obesity due to excess calories
E66.09	Other obesity due to excess calories
E66.1	Drug-induced obesity
E66.2	Morbid (severe) obesity with alveolar hypoventilation
E66.3	Overweight
E66.8	Other obesity
K91.1	Postgastric surgery syndromes
K95.01	Infection due to gastric band procedure
K95.09	Other complications of gastric band procedure
K95.81	Infection due to other bariatric procedure
K95.89	Other complications of other bariatric procedure
T85.518A	Breakdown (mechanical) of other gastrointestinal prosthetic devices, implants and grafts, initial encounter
T85.528A	Displacement of other gastrointestinal prosthetic devices, implants and grafts, initial encounter
T85.598A	Other mechanical complication of other gastrointestinal prosthetic devices, implants and grafts, initial encounter
Z46.51	Encounter for fitting and adjustment of gastric lap band

AMA: 43886 2018,Jan,8; 2017,Jan,8; 2016,Jan,13; 2015,Jan,16

Relative Value Units/Medicare Edits

Non-Facility RVU	Work	PE	MP	Total
43886	4.64	5.14	1.14	10.92
Facility RVU	**Work**	**PE**	**MP**	**Total**
43886	4.64	5.14	1.14	10.92

	FUD	Status	MUE	Modifiers				IOM Reference
43886	90	A	1(2)	51	N/A	62*	80	None

* with documentation

Terms To Know

BMI. Body mass index. Tool for calculating weight appropriateness in adults and may be a factor in determining medical necessity for bariatric procedures.

deep fascia. Sheet of dense, fibrous tissue holding muscle groups together below the hypodermis layer or subcutaneous fat layer that lines the extremities and trunk.

dissection. (dis. apart; -section, act of cutting) Separating by cutting tissue or body structures apart.

incision. Act of cutting into tissue or an organ.

infusion. Introduction of a therapeutic fluid, other than blood, into the bloodstream.

revision. Reordering or rearrangement of tissue to suit a particular need or function.

subcutaneous. Below the skin.

suture. Numerous stitching techniques employed in wound closure.

Stomach

43887-43888

43887 Gastric restrictive procedure, open; removal of subcutaneous port component only
43888   removal and replacement of subcutaneous port component only

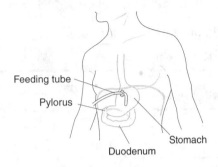

Feeding tube
Pylorus
Stomach
Duodenum

Gastric band is placed in laparoscopic approach

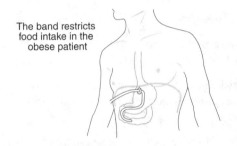

The band restricts food intake in the obese patient

Explanation

The physician performs an open removal or a removal and replacement of the subcutaneous port component used in a gastric restrictive procedure for the treatment of morbid obesity. The subcutaneous port is the access point for infusing saline into the gastric band to adjust the band for optimal performance. The physician makes an incision through the old scar near the original port. Dissection is carried down to the port and the sutures adhering the port to the fascia are removed. The physician severs the tubing connected to the port. In 43887, the subcutaneous port is removed. In 43888, the original subcutaneous port is removed and replaced with a new port to which the tubing is reattached. The replacement port is secured to the fascia with sutures. The incision is closed with sutures.

Coding Tips

Do not report 43888 with 43774 or 43887. For revision of the subcutaneous port component only, see 43886; via laparoscopy, see 43771. For removal only, see 43887; via laparoscopy, see 43772. For removal and replacement through a laparoscope, see 43773. For removal and replacement of the gastric band device and subcutaneous port components, see 43659.

ICD-10-CM Diagnostic Codes

E66.01	Morbid (severe) obesity due to excess calories
E66.09	Other obesity due to excess calories
E66.1	Drug-induced obesity
E66.2	Morbid (severe) obesity with alveolar hypoventilation
E66.3	Overweight
E66.8	Other obesity
K91.1	Postgastric surgery syndromes
K95.01	Infection due to gastric band procedure
K95.09	Other complications of gastric band procedure
K95.81	Infection due to other bariatric procedure
K95.89	Other complications of other bariatric procedure
T85.518A	Breakdown (mechanical) of other gastrointestinal prosthetic devices, implants and grafts, initial encounter
T85.528A	Displacement of other gastrointestinal prosthetic devices, implants and grafts, initial encounter
T85.598A	Other mechanical complication of other gastrointestinal prosthetic devices, implants and grafts, initial encounter
Z46.51	Encounter for fitting and adjustment of gastric lap band

AMA: **43887** 2018,Jan,8; 2017,Jan,8; 2016,Jan,13; 2015,Jan,16 **43888** 2018,Jan,8; 2017,Jan,8; 2016,Jan,13; 2015,Jan,16

Relative Value Units/Medicare Edits

Non-Facility RVU	Work	PE	MP	Total
43887	4.32	4.43	1.04	9.79
43888	6.44	5.8	1.58	13.82
Facility RVU	Work	PE	MP	Total
43887	4.32	4.43	1.04	9.79
43888	6.44	5.8	1.58	13.82

	FUD	Status	MUE	Modifiers				IOM Reference
43887	90	A	1(2)	51	N/A	62*	80	None
43888	90	A	1(2)	51	N/A	62*	80	

* with documentation

Terms To Know

BMI. Body mass index. Tool for calculating weight appropriateness in adults and may be a factor in determining medical necessity for bariatric procedures.

fascia. Fibrous sheet or band of tissue that envelops organs, muscles, and groupings of muscles.

incision. Act of cutting into tissue or an organ.

morbid obesity. Accumulation of excess fat in the subcutaneous connective tissue with increased weight beyond the limits of skeletal requirements, defined as 125 percent or more over the ideal body weight. It is often associated with serious conditions that can become life threatening, such as diabetes, hypertension, and arteriosclerosis.

suture. Numerous stitching techniques employed in wound closure.

buried suture. Continuous or interrupted suture placed under the skin for a layered closure.

continuous suture. Running stitch with tension evenly distributed across a single strand to provide a leakproof closure line.

interrupted suture. Series of single stitches with tension isolated at each stitch, in which all stitches are not affected if one becomes loose, and the isolated sutures cannot act as a wick to transport an infection.

purse-string suture. Continuous suture placed around a tubular structure and tightened, to reduce or close the lumen.

retention suture. Secondary stitching that bridges the primary suture, providing support for the primary repair; a plastic or rubber bolster may be placed over the primary repair and under the retention sutures.

44005

44005 Enterolysis (freeing of intestinal adhesion) (separate procedure)

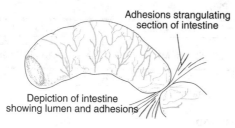

Adhesions strangulating section of intestine

Depiction of intestine showing lumen and adhesions

Explanation

The physician frees intestinal adhesions. The physician enters the abdomen through a midline abdominal incision. The bowel is freed from its attachments to itself, the abdominal wall and/or other abdominal organs. The abdominal incision is closed.

Coding Tips

This separate procedure, by definition, is usually a component of a more complex service and is not identified separately. When performed alone or with other unrelated procedures it may be reported. If performed alone, list the code; if performed with other procedures, list the code with modifier 59 or an X{EPSU} modifier. Do not report 44005 with 45136. For a laparoscopic approach, see 44180.

ICD-10-CM Diagnostic Codes

C17.0	Malignant neoplasm of duodenum
C17.1	Malignant neoplasm of jejunum
C17.2	Malignant neoplasm of ileum
C17.3	Meckel's diverticulum, malignant
C17.8	Malignant neoplasm of overlapping sites of small intestine
C18.0	Malignant neoplasm of cecum
C18.1	Malignant neoplasm of appendix
C18.2	Malignant neoplasm of ascending colon
C18.3	Malignant neoplasm of hepatic flexure
C18.4	Malignant neoplasm of transverse colon
C18.5	Malignant neoplasm of splenic flexure
C18.6	Malignant neoplasm of descending colon
C18.7	Malignant neoplasm of sigmoid colon
C19	Malignant neoplasm of rectosigmoid junction
C20	Malignant neoplasm of rectum
K31.5	Obstruction of duodenum
K31.6	Fistula of stomach and duodenum
K50.012	Crohn's disease of small intestine with intestinal obstruction
K50.112	Crohn's disease of large intestine with intestinal obstruction
K50.812	Crohn's disease of both small and large intestine with intestinal obstruction
K51.012	Ulcerative (chronic) pancolitis with intestinal obstruction
K51.312	Ulcerative (chronic) rectosigmoiditis with intestinal obstruction
K51.411	Inflammatory polyps of colon with rectal bleeding
K51.412	Inflammatory polyps of colon with intestinal obstruction
K51.413	Inflammatory polyps of colon with fistula
K51.414	Inflammatory polyps of colon with abscess
K51.512	Left sided colitis with intestinal obstruction

K51.812	Other ulcerative colitis with intestinal obstruction
K55.20	Angiodysplasia of colon without hemorrhage
K55.21	Angiodysplasia of colon with hemorrhage
K56.0	Paralytic ileus
K56.1	Intussusception
K56.2	Volvulus
K56.51	Intestinal adhesions [bands], with partial obstruction
K56.52	Intestinal adhesions [bands] with complete obstruction
K56.690	Other partial intestinal obstruction
K56.691	Other complete intestinal obstruction
K66.0	Peritoneal adhesions (postprocedural) (postinfection)
K91.31	Postprocedural partial intestinal obstruction
K91.32	Postprocedural complete intestinal obstruction
N73.6	Female pelvic peritoneal adhesions (postinfective) ♀
N80.5	Endometriosis of intestine ♀
N99.4	Postprocedural pelvic peritoneal adhesions
Q43.3	Congenital malformations of intestinal fixation

AMA: 44005 2018,Jan,8; 2018,Feb,11; 2017,Jan,8; 2016,Jan,13; 2015,Jan,16

Relative Value Units/Medicare Edits

Non-Facility RVU	Work	PE	MP	Total
44005	18.46	9.52	4.27	32.25
Facility RVU	**Work**	**PE**	**MP**	**Total**
44005	18.46	9.52	4.27	32.25

	FUD	Status	MUE	Modifiers				IOM Reference
44005	90	A	1(2)	51	N/A	62*	80	None

* with documentation

Terms To Know

intestinal or peritoneal adhesions with obstruction. Abnormal fibrous band growths joining separate tissues in the peritoneum or intestine, causing blockage.

laparoscopy. Direct visualization of the peritoneal cavity, outer fallopian tubes, uterus, and ovaries utilizing a laparoscope, a thin, flexible fiberoptic tube.

lysis. Destruction, breakdown, dissolution, or decomposition of cells or substances by a specific catalyzing agent.

44010

44010   Duodenotomy, for exploration, biopsy(s), or foreign body removal

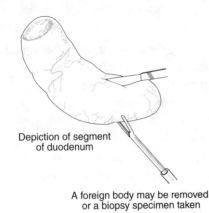

Depiction of segment
of duodenum

A foreign body may be removed
or a biopsy specimen taken

Explanation

The physician opens the duodenum, explores the segment, collects tissue samples for biopsy, or removes a foreign body. The physician exposes the proximal duodenum via a midline upper abdominal incision through skin, fascia, and muscles. The duodenum is incised in a longitudinal fashion and the area of concern is exposed. The physician may choose during exploration to excise tissues, biopsy, or remove foreign bodies. The duodenum is closed with transverse interrupted sutures. The abdominal incision is closed.

Coding Tips

For esophagogastroduodenoscopy, with biopsy, single or multiple, see 43239; with removal of foreign body, see 43247. For small intestinal endoscopy, with biopsy, single or multiple, see 44361; with removal of foreign body, see 44363. For biopsy of the intestine by capsule, tube or peroral (one or more specimens), see 44100. For small intestine enterotomy, other than duodenum, with biopsy or foreign body removal, see 44020. For colotomy, with biopsy or foreign body removal, see 44025.

ICD-10-CM Diagnostic Codes

B78.0	Intestinal strongyloidiasis
C17.0	Malignant neoplasm of duodenum
C7A.010	Malignant carcinoid tumor of the duodenum
D01.49	Carcinoma in situ of other parts of intestine
D13.2	Benign neoplasm of duodenum
D37.2	Neoplasm of uncertain behavior of small intestine
D3A.010	Benign carcinoid tumor of the duodenum
D49.0	Neoplasm of unspecified behavior of digestive system
K31.5	Obstruction of duodenum
K31.7	Polyp of stomach and duodenum
K31.811	Angiodysplasia of stomach and duodenum with bleeding
K31.819	Angiodysplasia of stomach and duodenum without bleeding
K31.82	Dieulafoy lesion (hemorrhagic) of stomach and duodenum
K31.89	Other diseases of stomach and duodenum
K90.0	Celiac disease
T18.3XXA	Foreign body in small intestine, initial encounter
T18.8XXA	Foreign body in other parts of alimentary tract, initial encounter

AMA: 44010 2014,Jan,11

Relative Value Units/Medicare Edits

Non-Facility RVU	Work	PE	MP	Total
44010	14.26	8.31	2.75	25.32
Facility RVU	Work	PE	MP	Total
44010	14.26	8.31	2.75	25.32

	FUD	Status	MUE	Modifiers				IOM Reference
44010	90	A	1(2)	51	N/A	62*	80	None

* with documentation

Terms To Know

biopsy. Tissue or fluid removed for diagnostic purposes through analysis of the cells in the biopsy material.

carcinoma in situ. Malignancy that arises from the cells of the vessel, gland, or organ of origin that remains confined to that site or has not invaded neighboring tissue.

duodenum. First portion of the small intestine connected to the stomach at the pylorus and extending to the jejunum.

fascia. Fibrous sheet or band of tissue that envelops organs, muscles, and groupings of muscles.

foreign body. Any object or substance found in an organ and tissue that does not belong under normal circumstances.

malignant. Any condition tending to progress toward death, specifically an invasive tumor with a loss of cellular differentiation that has the ability to spread or metastasize to other body areas.

neoplasm. New abnormal growth, tumor.

proximal. Located closest to a specified reference point, usually the midline or trunk.

skin. Outer protective covering of the body composed of the epidermis and dermis, situated above the subcutaneous tissues.

transverse. Crosswise at right angles to the long axis of a structure or part.

44015

+ **44015** Tube or needle catheter jejunostomy for enteral alimentation, intraoperative, any method (List separately in addition to primary procedure)

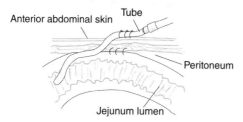

The tube is securely tacked to the inside of the abdominal wall

Explanation

The physician places a tube in the jejunum for feeding during a separately reportable operation. The physician makes an abdominal incision. A section of proximal jejunum is selected and a tube is placed in the jejunum and brought out through the abdominal wall. This segment of jejunum is securely tacked to the inside of the abdominal wall. The incision is closed.

Coding Tips

For laparoscopic jejunostomy for feeding, see 44186. For endoscopic placement of a percutaneous jejunostomy tube, see 44372.

ICD-10-CM Diagnostic Codes

This/these CPT code(s) are add-on code(s). See the primary procedure code that this code is performed with for your ICD-10-CM code selections.

AMA: **44015** 2018,Jan,8; 2017,Jan,8; 2016,Jan,13; 2015,Jan,16

Relative Value Units/Medicare Edits

Non-Facility RVU	Work	PE	MP	Total
44015	2.62	0.93	0.63	4.18
Facility RVU	**Work**	**PE**	**MP**	**Total**
44015	2.62	0.93	0.63	4.18

	FUD	Status	MUE	Modifiers				IOM Reference
44015	N/A	A	1(2)	N/A	N/A	62*	80	None

* with documentation

Terms To Know

hyperalimentation. Intake or ingestion of excessive amounts of food.

jejunostomy. Permanent, surgical opening into the jejunum, the part of the small intestine between the duodenum and ileum, through the abdominal wall, often used for placing a feeding tube.

peritoneum. Strong, continuous membrane that forms the lining of the abdominal and pelvic cavity. The parietal peritoneum, or outer layer, is attached to the abdominopelvic walls and the visceral peritoneum, or inner layer, surrounds the organs inside the abdominal cavity.

44020

44020 Enterotomy, small intestine, other than duodenum; for exploration, biopsy(s), or foreign body removal

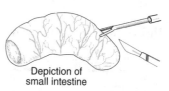

Depiction of small intestine

A foreign body may be removed or a biopsy specimen taken

Explanation

The physician makes an incision in the small intestine (enterotomy) for biopsy, exploration, or foreign body removal. The physician makes an abdominal incision. Next, the selected segment of small intestine is mobilized and incised to expose the area of interest. A biopsy is taken or a foreign body is removed. The enterotomy is closed with staples or sutures. The abdominal incision is closed.

Coding Tips

Enterotomy for decompression (e.g., Baker's tube) is reported with 44021. For esophagogastroduodenoscopy, with biopsy, single or multiple, see 43239; removal of foreign body, see 43247. For small intestinal endoscopy, with biopsy, single or multiple, see 44361; removal of foreign body, see 44363. Report biopsy of the intestine by capsule, tube, or peroral (one or more specimens) with 44100. For colotomy, with biopsy or foreign body removal, see 44025.

ICD-10-CM Diagnostic Codes

B78.0	Intestinal strongyloidiasis
C17.1	Malignant neoplasm of jejunum
C17.2	Malignant neoplasm of ileum
C78.4	Secondary malignant neoplasm of small intestine
C7A.011	Malignant carcinoid tumor of the jejunum
C7A.012	Malignant carcinoid tumor of the ileum
D01.49	Carcinoma in situ of other parts of intestine
D13.39	Benign neoplasm of other parts of small intestine
D37.2	Neoplasm of uncertain behavior of small intestine
D3A.011	Benign carcinoid tumor of the jejunum
D3A.012	Benign carcinoid tumor of the ileum
D49.0	Neoplasm of unspecified behavior of digestive system
K56.0	Paralytic ileus
K56.1	Intussusception
K56.2	Volvulus
K56.51	Intestinal adhesions [bands], with partial obstruction
K56.52	Intestinal adhesions [bands] with complete obstruction
K63.0	Abscess of intestine
K63.1	Perforation of intestine (nontraumatic)
K63.2	Fistula of intestine
K63.3	Ulcer of intestine
K63.4	Enteroptosis
K63.5	Polyp of colon
K63.81	Dieulafoy lesion of intestine

● **New**   ▲ **Revised**   + **Add On**   ★ **Telemedicine**   **AMA: CPT Assist**   **[Resequenced]**   ☑ **Laterality**

K63.89	Other specified diseases of intestine	
K90.0	Celiac disease	
T18.3XXA	Foreign body in small intestine, initial encounter	
T18.4XXA	Foreign body in colon, initial encounter	

AMA: **44020** 2014,Jan,11

Relative Value Units/Medicare Edits

Non-Facility RVU	Work	PE	MP	Total
44020	16.22	8.77	3.84	28.83
Facility RVU	Work	PE	MP	Total
44020	16.22	8.77	3.84	28.83

	FUD	Status	MUE	Modifiers				IOM Reference
44020	90	A	2(3)	51	N/A	62*	80	None

* with documentation

Terms To Know

biopsy. Tissue or fluid removed for diagnostic purposes through analysis of the cells in the biopsy material.

Dieulafoy lesion. Abnormally large submucosal artery protruding through a defect in the stomach mucosa or intestines that can cause massive and life-threatening hemorrhaging.

exploration. Examination for diagnostic purposes.

foreign body. Any object or substance found in an organ and tissue that does not belong under normal circumstances.

intussusception. Prolapse of one section of intestine into the lumen of an adjacent section of the bowel. This condition, which occurs mainly in children, causes pain, vomiting, and mucous passed from the rectum and requires surgical intervention.

jejunum. Highly vascular upper two-fifths of the small intestine, extending from the duodenum to the ileum.

volvulus. Twisting, knotting, or entanglement of the bowel on itself that may quickly compromise oxygen supply to the intestinal tissues. A volvulus usually occurs at the sigmoid and ileocecal areas of the intestines.

44021

44021	Enterotomy, small intestine, other than duodenum; for decompression (eg, Baker tube)

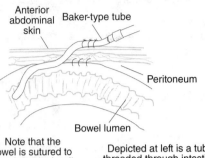

Note that the bowel is sutured to the abdominal wall

Depicted at left is a tube threaded through intestine for decompression

Explanation

The physician places a tube in the small bowel for decompression. The physician makes an abdominal incision. Next, the small bowel is dissected free of surrounding structures. The proximal small bowel is incised (enterotomy) and a tube is threaded through the small bowel. The proximal end of the tube is brought out through the abdominal wall. The bowel is tacked to the inside of the abdominal wall where the tube goes through. The abdominal incision is closed.

Coding Tips

For enterostomy or cecostomy tube (e.g., for decompression or feeding), see 44300. For small intestinal endoscopy, with placement of percutaneous jejunostomy tube, see 44372; with conversion of a gastrostomy tube to jejunostomy tube, percutaneous, see 44373.

ICD-10-CM Diagnostic Codes

C17.1	Malignant neoplasm of jejunum
C17.2	Malignant neoplasm of ileum
C7A.011	Malignant carcinoid tumor of the jejunum
C7A.012	Malignant carcinoid tumor of the ileum
K50.011	Crohn's disease of small intestine with rectal bleeding
K50.012	Crohn's disease of small intestine with intestinal obstruction
K50.013	Crohn's disease of small intestine with fistula
K50.014	Crohn's disease of small intestine with abscess
K51.013	Ulcerative (chronic) pancolitis with fistula
K56.0	Paralytic ileus
K56.1	Intussusception
K56.2	Volvulus
K56.49	Other impaction of intestine
K56.51	Intestinal adhesions [bands], with partial obstruction
K56.52	Intestinal adhesions [bands] with complete obstruction
K56.690	Other partial intestinal obstruction
K56.691	Other complete intestinal obstruction
K63.1	Perforation of intestine (nontraumatic)
K91.1	Postgastric surgery syndromes
K91.31	Postprocedural partial intestinal obstruction
K91.32	Postprocedural complete intestinal obstruction
Q43.0	Meckel's diverticulum (displaced) (hypertrophic)
Q43.1	Hirschsprung's disease

Intestines

Q43.2	Other congenital functional disorders of colon		
Q43.3	Congenital malformations of intestinal fixation		

AMA: 44021 2014,Jan,11

Relative Value Units/Medicare Edits

Non-Facility RVU	Work	PE	MP	Total
44021	16.31	8.71	3.78	28.8
Facility RVU	Work	PE	MP	Total
44021	16.31	8.71	3.78	28.8

	FUD	Status	MUE	Modifiers				IOM Reference
44021	90	A	1(3)	51	N/A	62*	80	None

* with documentation

Terms To Know

decompression. Release of pressure.

dissect. Cut apart or separate tissue for surgical purposes or for visual or microscopic study.

ileum. Lower portion of the small intestine, from the jejunum to the cecum.

intestinal or peritoneal adhesions with obstruction. Abnormal fibrous band growths joining separate tissues in the peritoneum or intestine, causing blockage.

jejunum. Highly vascular upper two-fifths of the small intestine, extending from the duodenum to the ileum.

proximal. Located closest to a specified reference point, usually the midline or trunk.

44025

44025	Colotomy, for exploration, biopsy(s), or foreign body removal

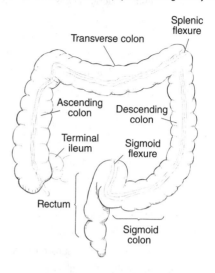

Explanation

The physician makes an incision in the colon (colotomy) through which the colon is explored for biopsy or foreign body removal. The physician makes an abdominal incision. Next, the selected segment of colon is mobilized and a colotomy is made in the area of interest. The colon is explored and a biopsy performed or foreign body removed. The colotomy is closed with staples or sutures. The abdominal incision is closed.

Coding Tips

For proctosigmoidoscopy with biopsy, see 45305; foreign body removal, see 45307. Sigmoidoscopy with biopsy is reported with 45331; removal of foreign body, see 45332. To report colonoscopy with biopsy, see 45380; removal of foreign body, see 45379.

ICD-10-CM Diagnostic Codes

C18.3	Malignant neoplasm of hepatic flexure
C18.4	Malignant neoplasm of transverse colon
C18.6	Malignant neoplasm of descending colon
C78.5	Secondary malignant neoplasm of large intestine and rectum
C7A.023	Malignant carcinoid tumor of the transverse colon
C7A.024	Malignant carcinoid tumor of the descending colon
D12.2	Benign neoplasm of ascending colon
D12.3	Benign neoplasm of transverse colon
D12.4	Benign neoplasm of descending colon
D12.5	Benign neoplasm of sigmoid colon
D3A.023	Benign carcinoid tumor of the transverse colon
D3A.024	Benign carcinoid tumor of the descending colon
D3A.025	Benign carcinoid tumor of the sigmoid colon
K51.00	Ulcerative (chronic) pancolitis without complications
K51.011	Ulcerative (chronic) pancolitis with rectal bleeding
K51.012	Ulcerative (chronic) pancolitis with intestinal obstruction
K51.013	Ulcerative (chronic) pancolitis with fistula
K51.014	Ulcerative (chronic) pancolitis with abscess
K51.018	Ulcerative (chronic) pancolitis with other complication
K51.30	Ulcerative (chronic) rectosigmoiditis without complications

K51.311	Ulcerative (chronic) rectosigmoiditis with rectal bleeding
K51.312	Ulcerative (chronic) rectosigmoiditis with intestinal obstruction
K51.313	Ulcerative (chronic) rectosigmoiditis with fistula
K51.314	Ulcerative (chronic) rectosigmoiditis with abscess
K51.318	Ulcerative (chronic) rectosigmoiditis with other complication
K51.40	Inflammatory polyps of colon without complications
K51.411	Inflammatory polyps of colon with rectal bleeding
K51.412	Inflammatory polyps of colon with intestinal obstruction
K51.413	Inflammatory polyps of colon with fistula
K51.414	Inflammatory polyps of colon with abscess
K51.418	Inflammatory polyps of colon with other complication
K51.50	Left sided colitis without complications
K51.511	Left sided colitis with rectal bleeding
K51.512	Left sided colitis with intestinal obstruction
K51.513	Left sided colitis with fistula
K51.514	Left sided colitis with abscess
K51.518	Left sided colitis with other complication
K51.812	Other ulcerative colitis with intestinal obstruction
K51.813	Other ulcerative colitis with fistula
K51.814	Other ulcerative colitis with abscess
K52.82	Eosinophilic colitis
K55.031	Focal (segmental) acute (reversible) ischemia of large intestine
K55.032	Diffuse acute (reversible) ischemia of large intestine
K55.041	Focal (segmental) acute infarction of large intestine
K55.042	Diffuse acute infarction of large intestine
K55.1	Chronic vascular disorders of intestine
K55.20	Angiodysplasia of colon without hemorrhage
K55.21	Angiodysplasia of colon with hemorrhage
K55.8	Other vascular disorders of intestine
K56.51	Intestinal adhesions [bands], with partial obstruction
K56.52	Intestinal adhesions [bands] with complete obstruction
K56.690	Other partial intestinal obstruction
K56.691	Other complete intestinal obstruction
K57.20	Diverticulitis of large intestine with perforation and abscess without bleeding
K57.21	Diverticulitis of large intestine with perforation and abscess with bleeding
K57.30	Diverticulosis of large intestine without perforation or abscess without bleeding
K57.31	Diverticulosis of large intestine without perforation or abscess with bleeding
K57.32	Diverticulitis of large intestine without perforation or abscess without bleeding
K57.33	Diverticulitis of large intestine without perforation or abscess with bleeding
K63.2	Fistula of intestine
K63.4	Enteroptosis
K63.5	Polyp of colon
K63.81	Dieulafoy lesion of intestine
K91.31	Postprocedural partial intestinal obstruction
K91.32	Postprocedural complete intestinal obstruction
T18.4XXA	Foreign body in colon, initial encounter

AMA: **44025** 2014,Jan,11

Relative Value Units/Medicare Edits

Non-Facility RVU	Work	PE	MP	Total
44025	16.51	8.77	3.61	28.89
Facility RVU	**Work**	**PE**	**MP**	**Total**
44025	16.51	8.77	3.61	28.89

	FUD	Status	MUE	Modifiers				IOM Reference
44025	90	A	1(3)	51	N/A	62*	80	None

* with documentation

Terms To Know

angiodysplasia. Vascular abnormalities, with or without bleeding.

biopsy. Tissue or fluid removed for diagnostic purposes through analysis of the cells in the biopsy material.

colitis. Inflammation of the colon, caused by an infection or external influences such as laxatives, radiation, or antibiotics.

ulcerative colitis. Chronic recurrent inflammation of the large intestine (colon) causing mucosal and submucosal ulceration of unknown cause, and leading to symptoms of abdominal pain, diarrhea with passage of non-fecal discharges, and rectal bleeding.

44050-44055

44050 Reduction of volvulus, intussusception, internal hernia, by laparotomy
44055 Correction of malrotation by lysis of duodenal bands and/or reduction of midgut volvulus (eg, Ladd procedure)

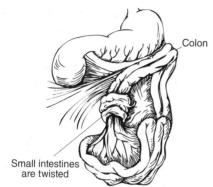

Colon

Small intestines are twisted

These conditions often arise during fetal development and intervention will be early in life.

Volvulus is the twisting of a bowel segment and intussusception is the prolapse of one segment of bowel into another; both can cause obstructions

Explanation

The physician reduces a volvulus, intussusception, or internal hernia through an abdominal incision. The physician makes an abdominal incision. Next, the abdomen is explored and the twisted segment of bowel (volvulus), telescoped segment of bowel (intussusception), or internal hernia is manually reduced. The bowel is inspected to ensure viability. The incision is closed. Report 44055 if the problem is corrected by lysis of duodenal bands or reduction of midgut volvulus.

Coding Tips

Proctosigmoidoscopy with decompression of volvulus is reported with 45321. To report flexible sigmoidoscopy with decompression of volvulus, any method, see 45337. Do not append modifier 63 to 44055 as the description or nature of the procedure includes infants less than 4 kg.

ICD-10-CM Diagnostic Codes

K42.0	Umbilical hernia with obstruction, without gangrene
K42.1	Umbilical hernia with gangrene
K42.9	Umbilical hernia without obstruction or gangrene
K43.0	Incisional hernia with obstruction, without gangrene
K43.1	Incisional hernia with gangrene
K43.2	Incisional hernia without obstruction or gangrene
K43.3	Parastomal hernia with obstruction, without gangrene
K43.4	Parastomal hernia with gangrene
K43.5	Parastomal hernia without obstruction or gangrene
K45.0	Other specified abdominal hernia with obstruction, without gangrene
K45.1	Other specified abdominal hernia with gangrene
K45.8	Other specified abdominal hernia without obstruction or gangrene
K56.0	Paralytic ileus
K56.1	Intussusception
K56.2	Volvulus
K56.51	Intestinal adhesions [bands], with partial obstruction
K56.52	Intestinal adhesions [bands] with complete obstruction
K56.690	Other partial intestinal obstruction
K56.691	Other complete intestinal obstruction
K57.00	Diverticulitis of small intestine with perforation and abscess without bleeding
K57.01	Diverticulitis of small intestine with perforation and abscess with bleeding
K57.10	Diverticulosis of small intestine without perforation or abscess without bleeding
K57.11	Diverticulosis of small intestine without perforation or abscess with bleeding
K57.12	Diverticulitis of small intestine without perforation or abscess without bleeding
K57.13	Diverticulitis of small intestine without perforation or abscess with bleeding
K57.20	Diverticulitis of large intestine with perforation and abscess without bleeding
K57.21	Diverticulitis of large intestine with perforation and abscess with bleeding
K57.30	Diverticulosis of large intestine without perforation or abscess without bleeding
K57.31	Diverticulosis of large intestine without perforation or abscess with bleeding
K57.32	Diverticulitis of large intestine without perforation or abscess without bleeding
K57.33	Diverticulitis of large intestine without perforation or abscess with bleeding
K63.5	Polyp of colon
K63.89	Other specified diseases of intestine
K91.31	Postprocedural partial intestinal obstruction
K91.32	Postprocedural complete intestinal obstruction
Q43.2	Other congenital functional disorders of colon
Q43.3	Congenital malformations of intestinal fixation
Q43.8	Other specified congenital malformations of intestine

AMA: **44050** 2014,Jan,11 **44055** 2014,Jan,11

Relative Value Units/Medicare Edits

Non-Facility RVU	Work	PE	MP	Total
44050	15.52	8.5	3.63	27.65
44055	25.63	12.35	5.98	43.96
Facility RVU	**Work**	**PE**	**MP**	**Total**
44050	15.52	8.5	3.63	27.65
44055	25.63	12.35	5.98	43.96

	FUD	Status	MUE	Modifiers				IOM Reference
44050	90	A	1(2)	51	N/A	62*	80	None
44055	90	A	1(2)	51	N/A	62*	80	

* with documentation

44100

44100 Biopsy of intestine by capsule, tube, peroral (1 or more specimens)

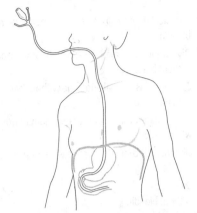

A biopsy capsule is delivered orally by tube through to the duodenum, jejunum, or small intestine. The capsule blade is activated, a biopsy specimen is collected, and the tube is withdrawn

Explanation

The physician performs a peroral biopsy of the small intestine with a capsule. The physician places a biopsy capsule attached to a tube through the mouth and directs it into the small intestine usually with fluoroscopy. The capsule blade is fired by placing suction on the tube and a biopsy obtained. The tube and capsule are withdrawn.

Coding Tips

For biopsy of the stomach by laparotomy, see 43605. Exploration, biopsy, or foreign body removal, by duodenotomy, see 44010; by enterotomy, small intestine, other than duodenum, see 44020; by colotomy, see 44025.

ICD-10-CM Diagnostic Codes

C17.0	Malignant neoplasm of duodenum
C17.1	Malignant neoplasm of jejunum
C17.2	Malignant neoplasm of ileum
C17.8	Malignant neoplasm of overlapping sites of small intestine
C78.4	Secondary malignant neoplasm of small intestine
C7A.010	Malignant carcinoid tumor of the duodenum
C7A.011	Malignant carcinoid tumor of the jejunum
C7A.012	Malignant carcinoid tumor of the ileum
D13.2	Benign neoplasm of duodenum
D13.39	Benign neoplasm of other parts of small intestine
D37.2	Neoplasm of uncertain behavior of small intestine
D3A.010	Benign carcinoid tumor of the duodenum
D3A.011	Benign carcinoid tumor of the jejunum
D3A.012	Benign carcinoid tumor of the ileum
K50.00	Crohn's disease of small intestine without complications
K50.011	Crohn's disease of small intestine with rectal bleeding
K50.012	Crohn's disease of small intestine with intestinal obstruction
K50.013	Crohn's disease of small intestine with fistula
K50.014	Crohn's disease of small intestine with abscess
K50.811	Crohn's disease of both small and large intestine with rectal bleeding
K50.812	Crohn's disease of both small and large intestine with intestinal obstruction
K50.813	Crohn's disease of both small and large intestine with fistula
K50.814	Crohn's disease of both small and large intestine with abscess
K55.011	Focal (segmental) acute (reversible) ischemia of small intestine
K55.012	Diffuse acute (reversible) ischemia of small intestine
K55.021	Focal (segmental) acute infarction of small intestine
K55.022	Diffuse acute infarction of small intestine
K55.1	Chronic vascular disorders of intestine
K56.51	Intestinal adhesions [bands], with partial obstruction
K56.52	Intestinal adhesions [bands] with complete obstruction
K57.00	Diverticulitis of small intestine with perforation and abscess without bleeding
K57.01	Diverticulitis of small intestine with perforation and abscess with bleeding
K57.11	Diverticulosis of small intestine without perforation or abscess with bleeding
K57.12	Diverticulitis of small intestine without perforation or abscess without bleeding
K57.13	Diverticulitis of small intestine without perforation or abscess with bleeding
K63.81	Dieulafoy lesion of intestine
K90.0	Celiac disease
K91.31	Postprocedural partial intestinal obstruction
K91.32	Postprocedural complete intestinal obstruction
K92.1	Melena
Q41.0	Congenital absence, atresia and stenosis of duodenum
Q41.1	Congenital absence, atresia and stenosis of jejunum
Q41.2	Congenital absence, atresia and stenosis of ileum
Q41.8	Congenital absence, atresia and stenosis of other specified parts of small intestine
Q43.1	Hirschsprung's disease
Q43.2	Other congenital functional disorders of colon
R19.5	Other fecal abnormalities
R62.7	Adult failure to thrive ▲
R63.4	Abnormal weight loss
R63.6	Underweight

AMA: **44100** 2014,Jan,11

Relative Value Units/Medicare Edits

Non-Facility RVU	Work	PE	MP	Total
44100	2.01	0.89	0.21	3.11
Facility RVU	**Work**	**PE**	**MP**	**Total**
44100	2.01	0.89	0.21	3.11

	FUD	Status	MUE	Modifiers				IOM Reference
44100	0	A	1(2)	51	N/A	N/A	N/A	None

* with documentation

44110-44111

44110 Excision of 1 or more lesions of small or large intestine not requiring anastomosis, exteriorization, or fistulization; single enterotomy
44111 multiple enterotomies

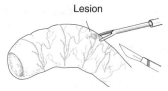

Lesion

Depiction of intestine
showing lesion removal

One or more bowel lesions are excised without
anastomosis, exteriorization, or fistulization

Explanation

The physician removes one or more lesions in the small or large intestine through an incision in the colon (colotomy) or small intestine (enterotomy) without bowel resection. The physician makes an abdominal incision. Next, the segment of small intestine or colon containing the lesions is mobilized. An incision is made in the small intestine or colon and the lesions are removed. The enterotomy or colotomy is closed with staples or sutures. The abdominal incision is closed. Report 44111 when multiple enterotomies are performed.

Coding Tips

If significant additional time and effort is documented, append modifier 22 and submit a cover letter and operative report. When these codes are performed with another separately identifiable procedure, the highest dollar value code is listed as the primary procedure and subsequent procedures are appended with modifier 51. Excision of the stomach for ulcer or benign tumor, see 43610; malignant, see 43611.

ICD-10-CM Diagnostic Codes

C17.1	Malignant neoplasm of jejunum
C17.2	Malignant neoplasm of ileum
C17.3	Meckel's diverticulum, malignant
C18.0	Malignant neoplasm of cecum
C18.1	Malignant neoplasm of appendix
C18.2	Malignant neoplasm of ascending colon
C18.3	Malignant neoplasm of hepatic flexure
C18.4	Malignant neoplasm of transverse colon
C18.5	Malignant neoplasm of splenic flexure
C18.6	Malignant neoplasm of descending colon
C18.7	Malignant neoplasm of sigmoid colon
C18.8	Malignant neoplasm of overlapping sites of colon
C49.A3	Gastrointestinal stromal tumor of small intestine
C49.A4	Gastrointestinal stromal tumor of large intestine
C7A.010	Malignant carcinoid tumor of the duodenum
C7A.011	Malignant carcinoid tumor of the jejunum
C7A.012	Malignant carcinoid tumor of the ileum
C7A.021	Malignant carcinoid tumor of the cecum
C7A.023	Malignant carcinoid tumor of the transverse colon
C7A.024	Malignant carcinoid tumor of the descending colon
C7A.025	Malignant carcinoid tumor of the sigmoid colon
D01.0	Carcinoma in situ of colon
D01.1	Carcinoma in situ of rectosigmoid junction
D01.2	Carcinoma in situ of rectum
D12.0	Benign neoplasm of cecum
D12.1	Benign neoplasm of appendix
D12.2	Benign neoplasm of ascending colon
D12.3	Benign neoplasm of transverse colon
D12.4	Benign neoplasm of descending colon
D12.5	Benign neoplasm of sigmoid colon
D13.2	Benign neoplasm of duodenum
D37.2	Neoplasm of uncertain behavior of small intestine
D37.3	Neoplasm of uncertain behavior of appendix
D37.4	Neoplasm of uncertain behavior of colon
D37.5	Neoplasm of uncertain behavior of rectum
D3A.010	Benign carcinoid tumor of the duodenum
D3A.011	Benign carcinoid tumor of the jejunum
D3A.012	Benign carcinoid tumor of the ileum
D3A.021	Benign carcinoid tumor of the cecum
D3A.022	Benign carcinoid tumor of the ascending colon
D3A.023	Benign carcinoid tumor of the transverse colon
D3A.024	Benign carcinoid tumor of the descending colon
D3A.025	Benign carcinoid tumor of the sigmoid colon
K56.51	Intestinal adhesions [bands], with partial obstruction
K56.52	Intestinal adhesions [bands] with complete obstruction
K63.5	Polyp of colon
N80.5	Endometriosis of intestine ♀
Q43.1	Hirschsprung's disease
Q43.2	Other congenital functional disorders of colon

AMA: **44110** 2014,Jan,11 **44111** 2014,Jan,11

Relative Value Units/Medicare Edits

Non-Facility RVU	Work	PE	MP	Total
44110	14.04	8.1	2.88	25.02
44111	16.52	8.98	3.27	28.77
Facility RVU	Work	PE	MP	Total
44110	14.04	8.1	2.88	25.02
44111	16.52	8.98	3.27	28.77

	FUD	Status	MUE	Modifiers				IOM Reference
44110	90	A	1(2)	51	N/A	62*	80	None
44111	90	A	1(2)	51	N/A	62*	80	

* with documentation

44120-44125

44120   Enterectomy, resection of small intestine; single resection and anastomosis

+   44121   each additional resection and anastomosis (List separately in addition to code for primary procedure)

   44125   with enterostomy

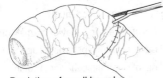

Depiction of small bowel
showing end-to-end anastomosis

Detail of enterostomy
at skin surface

A section of small bowel is removed and
continuity restored by anastomosis. An enterostomy
may be performed after the resection

Explanation

In 44120, the physician resects a single segment of small intestine and performs an anastomosis between the remaining bowel ends. The physician makes an abdominal incision. Next, the selected segment of small bowel is isolated and divided proximally and distally to the remaining bowel and removed. The remaining bowel ends are reapproximated using staples or sutures. The incision is closed. Report 44121 for each additional resection and anastomosis; enterostomy performed with this procedure is reported with 44125.

Coding Tips

Report 44121 in addition to 44120. If significant additional time and effort is documented, append modifier 22 and submit a cover letter and operative report.

ICD-10-CM Diagnostic Codes

C17.0	Malignant neoplasm of duodenum
C17.1	Malignant neoplasm of jejunum
C17.2	Malignant neoplasm of ileum
C17.3	Meckel's diverticulum, malignant
C49.A3	Gastrointestinal stromal tumor of small intestine
C78.4	Secondary malignant neoplasm of small intestine
C7A.010	Malignant carcinoid tumor of the duodenum
C7A.011	Malignant carcinoid tumor of the jejunum
C7A.012	Malignant carcinoid tumor of the ileum
D13.2	Benign neoplasm of duodenum
D13.39	Benign neoplasm of other parts of small intestine
D37.2	Neoplasm of uncertain behavior of small intestine
D3A.010	Benign carcinoid tumor of the duodenum
D3A.011	Benign carcinoid tumor of the jejunum
D3A.012	Benign carcinoid tumor of the ileum
D49.0	Neoplasm of unspecified behavior of digestive system
K26.0	Acute duodenal ulcer with hemorrhage
K26.1	Acute duodenal ulcer with perforation
K26.2	Acute duodenal ulcer with both hemorrhage and perforation
K26.3	Acute duodenal ulcer without hemorrhage or perforation
K26.4	Chronic or unspecified duodenal ulcer with hemorrhage
K26.5	Chronic or unspecified duodenal ulcer with perforation
K26.6	Chronic or unspecified duodenal ulcer with both hemorrhage and perforation
K26.7	Chronic duodenal ulcer without hemorrhage or perforation
K31.5	Obstruction of duodenum
K31.6	Fistula of stomach and duodenum
K31.811	Angiodysplasia of stomach and duodenum with bleeding
K31.819	Angiodysplasia of stomach and duodenum without bleeding
K31.82	Dieulafoy lesion (hemorrhagic) of stomach and duodenum
K43.0	Incisional hernia with obstruction, without gangrene
K43.1	Incisional hernia with gangrene
K45.1	Other specified abdominal hernia with gangrene
K50.011	Crohn's disease of small intestine with rectal bleeding
K50.012	Crohn's disease of small intestine with intestinal obstruction
K50.013	Crohn's disease of small intestine with fistula
K50.014	Crohn's disease of small intestine with abscess
K50.018	Crohn's disease of small intestine with other complication
K50.812	Crohn's disease of both small and large intestine with intestinal obstruction
K50.813	Crohn's disease of both small and large intestine with fistula
K50.814	Crohn's disease of both small and large intestine with abscess
K55.011	Focal (segmental) acute (reversible) ischemia of small intestine
K55.012	Diffuse acute (reversible) ischemia of small intestine
K55.021	Focal (segmental) acute infarction of small intestine
K55.022	Diffuse acute infarction of small intestine
K55.1	Chronic vascular disorders of intestine
K56.0	Paralytic ileus
K56.1	Intussusception
K56.2	Volvulus
K56.51	Intestinal adhesions [bands], with partial obstruction
K56.52	Intestinal adhesions [bands] with complete obstruction
K56.690	Other partial intestinal obstruction
K56.691	Other complete intestinal obstruction
K57.00	Diverticulitis of small intestine with perforation and abscess without bleeding
K57.01	Diverticulitis of small intestine with perforation and abscess with bleeding
K57.10	Diverticulosis of small intestine without perforation or abscess without bleeding
K57.11	Diverticulosis of small intestine without perforation or abscess with bleeding
K57.12	Diverticulitis of small intestine without perforation or abscess without bleeding
K57.13	Diverticulitis of small intestine without perforation or abscess with bleeding
K57.40	Diverticulitis of both small and large intestine with perforation and abscess without bleeding
K57.41	Diverticulitis of both small and large intestine with perforation and abscess with bleeding
K57.50	Diverticulosis of both small and large intestine without perforation or abscess without bleeding
K57.51	Diverticulosis of both small and large intestine without perforation or abscess with bleeding
K57.52	Diverticulitis of both small and large intestine without perforation or abscess without bleeding

Intestines

K57.53	Diverticulitis of both small and large intestine without perforation or abscess with bleeding
K63.0	Abscess of intestine
K63.1	Perforation of intestine (nontraumatic)
K63.2	Fistula of intestine
K63.3	Ulcer of intestine
K91.31	Postprocedural partial intestinal obstruction
K91.32	Postprocedural complete intestinal obstruction
K91.71	Accidental puncture and laceration of a digestive system organ or structure during a digestive system procedure
K91.72	Accidental puncture and laceration of a digestive system organ or structure during other procedure
K91.81	Other intraoperative complications of digestive system
K91.89	Other postprocedural complications and disorders of digestive system
N80.5	Endometriosis of intestine ♀
Q41.0	Congenital absence, atresia and stenosis of duodenum
Q41.1	Congenital absence, atresia and stenosis of jejunum
Q41.2	Congenital absence, atresia and stenosis of ileum
Q41.8	Congenital absence, atresia and stenosis of other specified parts of small intestine
Q43.0	Meckel's diverticulum (displaced) (hypertrophic)
Q43.3	Congenital malformations of intestinal fixation
S36.430A	Laceration of duodenum, initial encounter
S36.438A	Laceration of other part of small intestine, initial encounter

AMA: **44120** 2018,Nov,11; 2018,Jan,8; 2017,Jan,8; 2016,Jan,13; 2015,Jan,16

Relative Value Units/Medicare Edits

Non-Facility RVU	Work	PE	MP	Total
44120	20.82	10.44	4.79	36.05
44121	4.44	1.66	1.0	7.1
44125	20.03	10.27	4.43	34.73
Facility RVU	**Work**	**PE**	**MP**	**Total**
44120	20.82	10.44	4.79	36.05
44121	4.44	1.66	1.0	7.1
44125	20.03	10.27	4.43	34.73

	FUD	Status	MUE	Modifiers				IOM Reference
44120	90	A	1(2)	51	N/A	62*	80	None
44121	N/A	A	2(3)	N/A	N/A	62*	80	
44125	90	A	1(2)	51	N/A	62*	80	

* with documentation

44126-44128

44126 Enterectomy, resection of small intestine for congenital atresia, single resection and anastomosis of proximal segment of intestine; without tapering

44127 with tapering

+ 44128 Enterectomy, resection of small intestine for congenital atresia, single resection and anastomosis of proximal segment of intestine; each additional resection and anastomosis (List separately in addition to code for primary procedure)

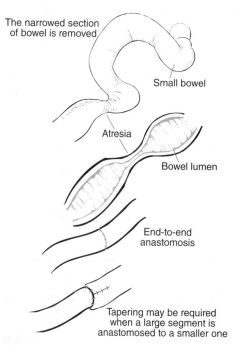

The narrowed section of bowel is removed

Small bowel

Atresia

Bowel lumen

End-to-end anastomosis

Tapering may be required when a large segment is anastomosed to a smaller one

Explanation

The physician resects a segment of small intestine and may perform tapering to fit the area of anastomosis. The physician makes an abdominal incision. The selected segment of small intestine is isolated and divided proximally and distally to the remaining bowel and removed. An end-to-end anastomosis of the proximal rectum to the distal anal canal is performed. The remaining bowel ends are reapproximated using staples or sutures. The incision is closed. Report 44126 for a single resection and anastomosis. Report 44127 when tapering (gradually narrowing toward one end) of the bowel is performed with the resection and anastomosis. Report 44128 for each additional resection and anastomosis beyond the first one.

Coding Tips

Report 44128 in addition to 44126–44127. If significant additional time and effort is documented, append modifier 22 and submit a cover letter and operative report. For enterectomy, resection, and anastomosis of the small intestine, single resection, see 44120; each additional resection and anastomosis, see 44121; with enterostomy, see 44125. Do not append modifier 63 to these codes as the description or nature of the procedure includes infants up to 4 kg.

ICD-10-CM Diagnostic Codes

Q41.0	Congenital absence, atresia and stenosis of duodenum
Q41.1	Congenital absence, atresia and stenosis of jejunum
Q41.2	Congenital absence, atresia and stenosis of ileum

Q41.8   Congenital absence, atresia and stenosis of other specified parts of small intestine

AMA: **44126** 2014,Jan,11 **44127** 2014,Jan,11 **44128** 2014,Jan,11

Relative Value Units/Medicare Edits

Non-Facility RVU	Work	PE	MP	Total
44126	42.23	20.43	10.33	72.99
44127	49.3	22.95	12.06	84.31
44128	4.44	1.65	1.1	7.19
Facility RVU	Work	PE	MP	Total
44126	42.23	20.43	10.33	72.99
44127	49.3	22.95	12.06	84.31
44128	4.44	1.65	1.1	7.19

	FUD	Status	MUE	Modifiers				IOM Reference
44126	90	A	1(2)	51	N/A	62*	80	None
44127	90	A	1(2)	51	N/A	62*	80	
44128	N/A	A	2(3)	N/A	N/A	62*	80	

* with documentation

Terms To Know

anastomosis. Surgically created connection between ducts, blood vessels, or bowel segments to allow flow from one to the other.

atresia. Congenital closure or absence of a tubular organ or an opening to the body surface.

congenital. Present at birth, occurring through heredity or an influence during gestation up to the moment of birth.

distal. Located farther away from a specified reference point or the trunk.

proximal. Located closest to a specified reference point, usually the midline or trunk.

resection. Surgical removal of a part or all of an organ or body part.

segment. Group of related data elements in a transaction.

stenosis. Narrowing or constriction of a passage.

44130

44130	Enteroenterostomy, anastomosis of intestine, with or without cutaneous enterostomy (separate procedure)

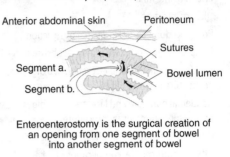

Enteroenterostomy is the surgical creation of an opening from one segment of bowel into another segment of bowel

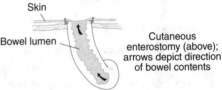

Cutaneous enterostomy (above); arrows depict direction of bowel contents

Explanation

The physician performs a small bowel anastomosis and may bring one end of small bowel through the abdominal wall onto the skin as a stoma. The physician makes an abdominal incision. A segment of small bowel may be resected. Next, a small bowel anastomosis is performed with staples or sutures. An end or loop of small bowel may be brought through a separate incision in the abdominal wall onto the skin as a stoma. The initial incision is closed.

Coding Tips

This separate procedure by definition is usually a component of a more complex service and is not identified separately. When performed alone or with other unrelated procedures/services it may be reported. If performed alone, list the code; if performed with other procedures/services, list the code and append modifier 59 or an X{EPSU} modifier. For enterectomy resection of the small intestine, with enterostomy, see 44125.

ICD-10-CM Diagnostic Codes

C17.0	Malignant neoplasm of duodenum
C17.1	Malignant neoplasm of jejunum
C17.2	Malignant neoplasm of ileum
C17.3	Meckel's diverticulum, malignant
C17.8	Malignant neoplasm of overlapping sites of small intestine
C49.A3	Gastrointestinal stromal tumor of small intestine
C78.4	Secondary malignant neoplasm of small intestine
C7A.010	Malignant carcinoid tumor of the duodenum
C7A.011	Malignant carcinoid tumor of the jejunum
C7A.012	Malignant carcinoid tumor of the ileum
D01.49	Carcinoma in situ of other parts of intestine
D13.2	Benign neoplasm of duodenum
D13.39	Benign neoplasm of other parts of small intestine
D37.2	Neoplasm of uncertain behavior of small intestine
D3A.010	Benign carcinoid tumor of the duodenum
D3A.011	Benign carcinoid tumor of the jejunum
D3A.012	Benign carcinoid tumor of the ileum
D49.0	Neoplasm of unspecified behavior of digestive system

K31.5	Obstruction of duodenum
K31.6	Fistula of stomach and duodenum
K31.7	Polyp of stomach and duodenum
K31.811	Angiodysplasia of stomach and duodenum with bleeding
K31.82	Dieulafoy lesion (hemorrhagic) of stomach and duodenum
K31.89	Other diseases of stomach and duodenum
K50.011	Crohn's disease of small intestine with rectal bleeding
K50.012	Crohn's disease of small intestine with intestinal obstruction
K50.013	Crohn's disease of small intestine with fistula
K50.014	Crohn's disease of small intestine with abscess
K50.018	Crohn's disease of small intestine with other complication
K50.812	Crohn's disease of both small and large intestine with intestinal obstruction
K50.813	Crohn's disease of both small and large intestine with fistula
K50.814	Crohn's disease of both small and large intestine with abscess
K55.011	Focal (segmental) acute (reversible) ischemia of small intestine
K55.012	Diffuse acute (reversible) ischemia of small intestine
K55.021	Focal (segmental) acute infarction of small intestine
K55.022	Diffuse acute infarction of small intestine
K55.1	Chronic vascular disorders of intestine
K55.8	Other vascular disorders of intestine
K56.0	Paralytic ileus
K56.1	Intussusception
K56.2	Volvulus
K56.49	Other impaction of intestine
K56.51	Intestinal adhesions [bands], with partial obstruction
K56.52	Intestinal adhesions [bands] with complete obstruction
K56.690	Other partial intestinal obstruction
K56.691	Other complete intestinal obstruction
K57.00	Diverticulitis of small intestine with perforation and abscess without bleeding
K57.01	Diverticulitis of small intestine with perforation and abscess with bleeding
K57.10	Diverticulosis of small intestine without perforation or abscess without bleeding
K57.11	Diverticulosis of small intestine without perforation or abscess with bleeding
K57.12	Diverticulitis of small intestine without perforation or abscess without bleeding
K57.13	Diverticulitis of small intestine without perforation or abscess with bleeding
K57.40	Diverticulitis of both small and large intestine with perforation and abscess without bleeding
K57.41	Diverticulitis of both small and large intestine with perforation and abscess with bleeding
K57.50	Diverticulosis of both small and large intestine without perforation or abscess without bleeding
K57.51	Diverticulosis of both small and large intestine without perforation or abscess with bleeding
K57.52	Diverticulitis of both small and large intestine without perforation or abscess without bleeding
K57.53	Diverticulitis of both small and large intestine without perforation or abscess with bleeding
K63.0	Abscess of intestine
K63.1	Perforation of intestine (nontraumatic)
K63.2	Fistula of intestine
K63.3	Ulcer of intestine
K63.4	Enteroptosis
K63.81	Dieulafoy lesion of intestine
K63.89	Other specified diseases of intestine
K91.31	Postprocedural partial intestinal obstruction
K91.32	Postprocedural complete intestinal obstruction
K91.71	Accidental puncture and laceration of a digestive system organ or structure during a digestive system procedure
K91.72	Accidental puncture and laceration of a digestive system organ or structure during other procedure
K91.81	Other intraoperative complications of digestive system
K91.89	Other postprocedural complications and disorders of digestive system
K92.89	Other specified diseases of the digestive system
N80.5	Endometriosis of intestine ♀
Q43.0	Meckel's diverticulum (displaced) (hypertrophic)
Q43.3	Congenital malformations of intestinal fixation
Q43.8	Other specified congenital malformations of intestine
S36.410A	Primary blast injury of duodenum, initial encounter
S36.418A	Primary blast injury of other part of small intestine, initial encounter
S36.430A	Laceration of duodenum, initial encounter
S36.438A	Laceration of other part of small intestine, initial encounter
S36.490A	Other injury of duodenum, initial encounter
S36.498A	Other injury of other part of small intestine, initial encounter

AMA: **44130** 2014,Jan,11

Relative Value Units/Medicare Edits

Non-Facility RVU	Work	PE	MP	Total
44130	22.11	11.68	5.01	38.8
Facility RVU	**Work**	**PE**	**MP**	**Total**
44130	22.11	11.68	5.01	38.8

	FUD	Status	MUE	Modifiers				IOM Reference
44130	90	A	2(3)	51	N/A	62*	80	None

* with documentation

44132-44133

44132 Donor enterectomy (including cold preservation), open; from cadaver donor

44133 partial, from living donor

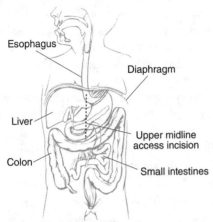

A section of the gut is harvested in an open procedure from a cadaver donor or a living donor

Explanation

The physician performs an open donor enterectomy from a cadaver donor in 44132 and an open partial enterectomy from a living donor in 44133. With the cadaver or living donor supine on the operating room table, the physician performs a midline abdominal incision. Tissue is incised and muscles are separated down to the level of the small intestine. In 44132, the small intestine can be mobilized and excised from the cadaver, as needed. In 44133, only a portion of the small intestine can be excised from the living donor and the bowel ends are anastomosed to restore continuity. Any bleeding is controlled, the area is irrigated, and the incision is closed with layered sutures. The acquired intestine is preserved for transplantation into the recipient, who may be hundreds of miles away. The organ remains under refrigeration, specially packed in a sealable container with some preserving solution and kept on ice in a suitable carrier.

Coding Tips

For intestinal allotransplantation, see 44135–44136. For backbench intestinal graft preparation or reconstruction, see 44715, 44720, and 44721.

ICD-10-CM Diagnostic Codes

Z52.89   Donor of other specified organs or tissues

AMA: **44132** 2014,Jan,11 **44133** 2014,Jan,11

Relative Value Units/Medicare Edits

Non-Facility RVU	Work	PE	MP	Total
44132	0.0	0.0	0.0	0.0
44133	0.0	0.0	0.0	0.0
Facility RVU	Work	PE	MP	Total
44132	0.0	0.0	0.0	0.0
44133	0.0	0.0	0.0	0.0

	FUD	Status	MUE	Modifiers				IOM Reference
44132	N/A	R	1(2)	N/A	N/A	N/A	80*	None
44133	N/A	R	1(2)	N/A	N/A	N/A	80*	

* with documentation

Terms To Know

allograft. Graft from one individual to another of the same species.

anastomosis. Surgically created connection between ducts, blood vessels, or bowel segments to allow flow from one to the other.

donor. Person from whom tissues or organs are removed for transplantation.

excision. Surgical removal of an organ or tissue.

harvest. Removal of cells or tissue from their native site to be used as a graft or transplant to another part of the donor's body or placed into another person.

incision. Act of cutting into tissue or an organ.

irrigation. To wash out or cleanse a body cavity, wound, or tissue with water or other fluid.

peritoneum. Strong, continuous membrane that forms the lining of the abdominal and pelvic cavity. The parietal peritoneum, or outer layer, is attached to the abdominopelvic walls and the visceral peritoneum, or inner layer, surrounds the organs inside the abdominal cavity.

skin. Outer protective covering of the body composed of the epidermis and dermis, situated above the subcutaneous tissues.

small intestine. First portion of intestine connecting to the pylorus at the proximal end and consisting of the duodenum, jejunum, and ileum.

supine. Lying on the back.

suture. Numerous stitching techniques employed in wound closure.

buried suture. Continuous or interrupted suture placed under the skin for a layered closure.

continuous suture. Running stitch with tension evenly distributed across a single strand to provide a leakproof closure line.

interrupted suture. Series of single stitches with tension isolated at each stitch, in which all stitches are not affected if one becomes loose, and the isolated sutures cannot act as a wick to transport an infection.

purse-string suture. Continuous suture placed around a tubular structure and tightened, to reduce or close the lumen.

retention suture. Secondary stitching that bridges the primary suture, providing support for the primary repair; a plastic or rubber bolster may be placed over the primary repair and under the retention sutures.

44135-44136

44135 Intestinal allotransplantation; from cadaver donor
44136   from living donor

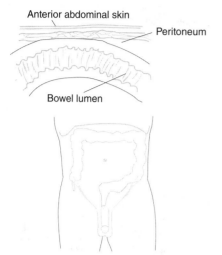

Anterior abdominal skin

Peritoneum

Bowel lumen

An intestinal transplantation is performed

Explanation

The physician performs an intestinal allotransplantation. The patient is placed supine on the operating room table. After adequate preparation, the physician performs a midline abdominal incision, tissue is incised, and muscles are separated down to the level of the small intestine. The area of small intestine to be transplanted is located. An incision is made through the intestine, the area is examined, and the free intestinal edges are debrided or excised in order to accept the intestinal transplant. The previously excised small intestinal allograft, from a cadaver (44135) or partially excised small intestinal allograft, from a living donor (44136) are removed from the maintenance solution, and irrigated. The allograft is sized and is anastomosed first to one free end of the patient's small intestine and then the opposite end of the patient's small intestine. Any bleeding is controlled, the area is irrigated, and the small bowel is anatomically positioned in the abdominal cavity. The wound is closed with layered sutures over a drain. A dressing is applied.

Coding Tips

An intestinal allograft is frequently performed at the same operative session as a liver transplant or multivisceral grafts. For donor enterectomy, see 44132–44133.

ICD-10-CM Diagnostic Codes

C17.0	Malignant neoplasm of duodenum
C17.1	Malignant neoplasm of jejunum
C17.2	Malignant neoplasm of ileum
C17.3	Meckel's diverticulum, malignant
C17.8	Malignant neoplasm of overlapping sites of small intestine
C78.4	Secondary malignant neoplasm of small intestine
C7A.010	Malignant carcinoid tumor of the duodenum
C7A.011	Malignant carcinoid tumor of the jejunum
C7A.012	Malignant carcinoid tumor of the ileum
K31.5	Obstruction of duodenum
K31.6	Fistula of stomach and duodenum
K31.811	Angiodysplasia of stomach and duodenum with bleeding
K31.819	Angiodysplasia of stomach and duodenum without bleeding

K31.82	Dieulafoy lesion (hemorrhagic) of stomach and duodenum
K31.89	Other diseases of stomach and duodenum
K50.00	Crohn's disease of small intestine without complications
K50.011	Crohn's disease of small intestine with rectal bleeding
K50.012	Crohn's disease of small intestine with intestinal obstruction
K50.013	Crohn's disease of small intestine with fistula
K50.014	Crohn's disease of small intestine with abscess
K50.018	Crohn's disease of small intestine with other complication
K50.112	Crohn's disease of large intestine with intestinal obstruction
K50.812	Crohn's disease of both small and large intestine with intestinal obstruction
K50.813	Crohn's disease of both small and large intestine with fistula
K50.814	Crohn's disease of both small and large intestine with abscess
K51.00	Ulcerative (chronic) pancolitis without complications
K51.011	Ulcerative (chronic) pancolitis with rectal bleeding
K51.012	Ulcerative (chronic) pancolitis with intestinal obstruction
K51.212	Ulcerative (chronic) proctitis with intestinal obstruction
K51.312	Ulcerative (chronic) rectosigmoiditis with intestinal obstruction
K51.412	Inflammatory polyps of colon with intestinal obstruction
K51.512	Left sided colitis with intestinal obstruction
K51.80	Other ulcerative colitis without complications
K51.811	Other ulcerative colitis with rectal bleeding
K51.812	Other ulcerative colitis with intestinal obstruction
K51.813	Other ulcerative colitis with fistula
K51.814	Other ulcerative colitis with abscess
K51.818	Other ulcerative colitis with other complication
K52.3	Indeterminate colitis
K52.831	Collagenous colitis
K52.832	Lymphocytic colitis
K55.1	Chronic vascular disorders of intestine
K55.21	Angiodysplasia of colon with hemorrhage
K55.8	Other vascular disorders of intestine
K56.0	Paralytic ileus
K56.1	Intussusception
K56.2	Volvulus
K56.51	Intestinal adhesions [bands], with partial obstruction
K56.52	Intestinal adhesions [bands] with complete obstruction
K56.690	Other partial intestinal obstruction
K56.691	Other complete intestinal obstruction
K57.00	Diverticulitis of small intestine with perforation and abscess without bleeding
K57.01	Diverticulitis of small intestine with perforation and abscess with bleeding
K57.11	Diverticulosis of small intestine without perforation or abscess with bleeding
K57.12	Diverticulitis of small intestine without perforation or abscess without bleeding
K57.13	Diverticulitis of small intestine without perforation or abscess with bleeding
K57.40	Diverticulitis of both small and large intestine with perforation and abscess without bleeding
K57.41	Diverticulitis of both small and large intestine with perforation and abscess with bleeding

K57.51	Diverticulosis of both small and large intestine without perforation or abscess with bleeding
K57.52	Diverticulitis of both small and large intestine without perforation or abscess without bleeding
K57.53	Diverticulitis of both small and large intestine without perforation or abscess with bleeding
K63.0	Abscess of intestine
K63.1	Perforation of intestine (nontraumatic)
K63.2	Fistula of intestine
K63.3	Ulcer of intestine
K63.4	Enteroptosis
K91.31	Postprocedural partial intestinal obstruction
K91.32	Postprocedural complete intestinal obstruction
N80.5	Endometriosis of intestine ♀
Q41.0	Congenital absence, atresia and stenosis of duodenum
Q41.1	Congenital absence, atresia and stenosis of jejunum
Q41.2	Congenital absence, atresia and stenosis of ileum
Q41.8	Congenital absence, atresia and stenosis of other specified parts of small intestine
Q43.0	Meckel's diverticulum (displaced) (hypertrophic)
Q43.1	Hirschsprung's disease
Q43.3	Congenital malformations of intestinal fixation
Q43.8	Other specified congenital malformations of intestine
S36.410A	Primary blast injury of duodenum, initial encounter
S36.418A	Primary blast injury of other part of small intestine, initial encounter
S36.430A	Laceration of duodenum, initial encounter
S36.438A	Laceration of other part of small intestine, initial encounter

AMA: **44135** 2014,Jan,11 **44136** 2014,Jan,11

Relative Value Units/Medicare Edits

Non-Facility RVU	Work	PE	MP	Total
44135	0.0	0.0	0.0	0.0
44136	0.0	0.0	0.0	0.0
Facility RVU	**Work**	**PE**	**MP**	**Total**
44135	0.0	0.0	0.0	0.0
44136	0.0	0.0	0.0	0.0

	FUD	Status	MUE	Modifiers				IOM Reference
44135	N/A	R	1(2)	N/A	N/A	N/A	80*	None
44136	N/A	R	1(2)	N/A	N/A	N/A	80*	

* with documentation

44137

44137 Removal of transplanted intestinal allograft, complete

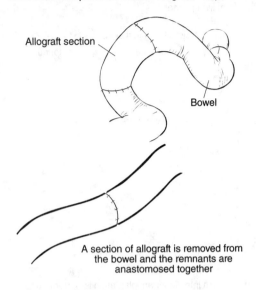

Allograft section

Bowel

A section of allograft is removed from the bowel and the remnants are anastomosed together

Explanation

The physician removes a previously transplanted intestinal allograft due to complications such as infection or rejection. The physician makes an abdominal incision. The intestinal allograft is isolated and resected at sites distal and proximal to the anastomosis sites of the previously placed intestinal graft. The distal and proximal ends of the remaining intestine are reapproximated using staples or sutures. The incision is closed.

Coding Tips

For partial removal of a transplant allograft, see 44120, 44121, or 44140.

ICD-10-CM Diagnostic Codes

T86.850	Intestine transplant rejection
T86.851	Intestine transplant failure
T86.852	Intestine transplant infection
T86.858	Other complications of intestine transplant
Z94.82	Intestine transplant status

AMA: **44137** 2014,Jan,11

Relative Value Units/Medicare Edits

Non-Facility RVU	Work	PE	MP	Total
44137	0.0	0.0	0.0	0.0
Facility RVU	**Work**	**PE**	**MP**	**Total**
44137	0.0	0.0	0.0	0.0

	FUD	Status	MUE	Modifiers				IOM Reference
44137	N/A	C	1(2)	51	N/A	62*	80	None

* with documentation

44139

+ **44139** Mobilization (take-down) of splenic flexure performed in conjunction with partial colectomy (List separately in addition to primary procedure)

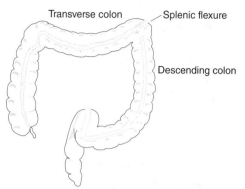

Transverse colon — Splenic flexure

Descending colon

The splenic flexure of the colon is attached to the posterior and lateral walls of the intestinal cavity. The attachments are released and the colon mobilized to allow for anastomosis after a partial colectomy

Explanation

The physician mobilizes the splenic flexure in conjunction with a partial colon resection. The physician makes an abdominal incision. The attachments between the splenic flexure of the colon and the lateral abdominal wall and spleen are dissected free and taken down to mobilize the colon. This is done to mobilize adequate length of colon in conjunction with a partial colon resection. At the completion of the procedure the abdominal incision is closed.

Coding Tips

Report 44139 in addition to 44140–44147. Splenic flexure mobilization performed in addition to a colectomy is reported separately.

ICD-10-CM Diagnostic Codes

This/these CPT code(s) are add-on code(s). See the primary procedure code that this code is performed with for your ICD-10-CM code selections.

AMA: **44139** 2014,Jan,11

Relative Value Units/Medicare Edits

Non-Facility RVU	Work	PE	MP	Total
44139	2.23	0.83	0.48	3.54
Facility RVU	Work	PE	MP	Total
44139	2.23	0.83	0.48	3.54

	FUD	Status	MUE	Modifiers				IOM Reference
44139	N/A	A	1(2)	N/A	N/A	62*	80	None

* with documentation

44140

44140 Colectomy, partial; with anastomosis

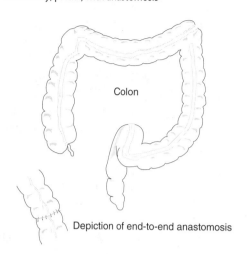

Colon

Depiction of end-to-end anastomosis

Explanation

The physician resects a segment of colon and performs an anastomosis between the remaining ends of colon. The physician makes an abdominal incision. Next, the selected segment of colon is isolated and divided proximally and distally to the remaining colon and removed. The remaining ends of colon are reapproximated with staples or sutures. The incision is closed.

Coding Tips

Mobilization (take-down) of splenic flexure and intraoperative colonic lavage performed in conjunction with partial colectomy are reported separately, see 44139 and 44701, respectively. For laparoscopic approach, see 44204.

ICD-10-CM Diagnostic Codes

C18.0	Malignant neoplasm of cecum
C18.2	Malignant neoplasm of ascending colon
C18.3	Malignant neoplasm of hepatic flexure
C18.4	Malignant neoplasm of transverse colon
C18.5	Malignant neoplasm of splenic flexure
C18.6	Malignant neoplasm of descending colon
C18.7	Malignant neoplasm of sigmoid colon
C18.8	Malignant neoplasm of overlapping sites of colon
C19	Malignant neoplasm of rectosigmoid junction
C49.A4	Gastrointestinal stromal tumor of large intestine
C78.5	Secondary malignant neoplasm of large intestine and rectum
C7A.021	Malignant carcinoid tumor of the cecum
C7A.022	Malignant carcinoid tumor of the ascending colon
C7A.023	Malignant carcinoid tumor of the transverse colon
C7A.024	Malignant carcinoid tumor of the descending colon
C7A.025	Malignant carcinoid tumor of the sigmoid colon
D01.0	Carcinoma in situ of colon
D01.1	Carcinoma in situ of rectosigmoid junction
D12.0	Benign neoplasm of cecum
D12.1	Benign neoplasm of appendix
D12.2	Benign neoplasm of ascending colon
D12.3	Benign neoplasm of transverse colon
D12.4	Benign neoplasm of descending colon

D12.5	Benign neoplasm of sigmoid colon
D12.7	Benign neoplasm of rectosigmoid junction
D37.3	Neoplasm of uncertain behavior of appendix
D37.4	Neoplasm of uncertain behavior of colon
D3A.022	Benign carcinoid tumor of the ascending colon
D3A.023	Benign carcinoid tumor of the transverse colon
D3A.024	Benign carcinoid tumor of the descending colon
D3A.025	Benign carcinoid tumor of the sigmoid colon
D49.0	Neoplasm of unspecified behavior of digestive system
K50.111	Crohn's disease of large intestine with rectal bleeding
K50.112	Crohn's disease of large intestine with intestinal obstruction
K50.113	Crohn's disease of large intestine with fistula
K50.114	Crohn's disease of large intestine with abscess
K50.118	Crohn's disease of large intestine with other complication
K50.811	Crohn's disease of both small and large intestine with rectal bleeding
K50.812	Crohn's disease of both small and large intestine with intestinal obstruction
K50.813	Crohn's disease of both small and large intestine with fistula
K50.814	Crohn's disease of both small and large intestine with abscess
K50.818	Crohn's disease of both small and large intestine with other complication
K51.011	Ulcerative (chronic) pancolitis with rectal bleeding
K51.012	Ulcerative (chronic) pancolitis with intestinal obstruction
K51.013	Ulcerative (chronic) pancolitis with fistula
K51.014	Ulcerative (chronic) pancolitis with abscess
K51.018	Ulcerative (chronic) pancolitis with other complication
K51.311	Ulcerative (chronic) rectosigmoiditis with rectal bleeding
K51.312	Ulcerative (chronic) rectosigmoiditis with intestinal obstruction
K51.313	Ulcerative (chronic) rectosigmoiditis with fistula
K51.314	Ulcerative (chronic) rectosigmoiditis with abscess
K51.318	Ulcerative (chronic) rectosigmoiditis with other complication
K51.411	Inflammatory polyps of colon with rectal bleeding
K51.412	Inflammatory polyps of colon with intestinal obstruction
K51.413	Inflammatory polyps of colon with fistula
K51.414	Inflammatory polyps of colon with abscess
K51.418	Inflammatory polyps of colon with other complication
K51.511	Left sided colitis with rectal bleeding
K51.512	Left sided colitis with intestinal obstruction
K51.513	Left sided colitis with fistula
K51.514	Left sided colitis with abscess
K51.518	Left sided colitis with other complication
K55.041	Focal (segmental) acute infarction of large intestine
K55.042	Diffuse acute infarction of large intestine
K55.1	Chronic vascular disorders of intestine
K55.20	Angiodysplasia of colon without hemorrhage
K55.21	Angiodysplasia of colon with hemorrhage
K56.0	Paralytic ileus
K56.1	Intussusception
K56.2	Volvulus
K56.51	Intestinal adhesions [bands], with partial obstruction
K56.52	Intestinal adhesions [bands] with complete obstruction

K57.20	Diverticulitis of large intestine with perforation and abscess without bleeding
K57.21	Diverticulitis of large intestine with perforation and abscess with bleeding
K57.31	Diverticulosis of large intestine without perforation or abscess with bleeding
K57.33	Diverticulitis of large intestine without perforation or abscess with bleeding
K57.40	Diverticulitis of both small and large intestine with perforation and abscess without bleeding
K57.41	Diverticulitis of both small and large intestine with perforation and abscess with bleeding
K59.31	Toxic megacolon
K59.81	Ogilvie syndrome
K63.0	Abscess of intestine
K63.1	Perforation of intestine (nontraumatic)
K63.2	Fistula of intestine
K63.3	Ulcer of intestine
K63.4	Enteroptosis
K63.5	Polyp of colon
N32.1	Vesicointestinal fistula
Q42.8	Congenital absence, atresia and stenosis of other parts of large intestine
Q43.1	Hirschsprung's disease
Q43.2	Other congenital functional disorders of colon
Q43.3	Congenital malformations of intestinal fixation
Q43.4	Duplication of intestine
S36.530A	Laceration of ascending [right] colon, initial encounter
S36.531A	Laceration of transverse colon, initial encounter
S36.532A	Laceration of descending [left] colon, initial encounter
S36.533A	Laceration of sigmoid colon, initial encounter
S36.538A	Laceration of other part of colon, initial encounter

AMA: 44140 2020,Apr,10; 2018,Jan,8; 2017,Jan,8; 2016,Jan,13; 2015,Jan,16

Relative Value Units/Medicare Edits

Non-Facility RVU	Work	PE	MP	Total
44140	22.59	11.88	5.11	39.58
Facility RVU	**Work**	**PE**	**MP**	**Total**
44140	22.59	11.88	5.11	39.58

	FUD	Status	MUE	Modifiers				IOM Reference
44140	90	A	2(3)	51	N/A	62*	80	None

* with documentation

44141-44143

44141 Colectomy, partial; with skin level cecostomy or colostomy
44143 with end colostomy and closure of distal segment (Hartmann type procedure)

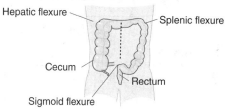

The colon showing a midline

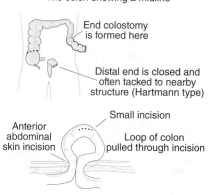

End colostomy is formed here

Distal end is closed and often tacked to nearby structure (Hartmann type)

Small incision

Anterior abdominal skin incision

Loop of colon pulled through incision

Explanation

The physician resects a segment of colon and brings the proximal end of colon through the abdominal wall onto the skin as a colostomy. The physician makes an abdominal incision. The selected segment of colon is isolated and divided proximally and distally to the remaining colon and removed. The proximal end of colon is brought through a separate incision on the abdominal wall and onto the skin as a colostomy. In 44141, the remaining bowel ends may be reapproximated and a loop of colon proximal to the anastomosis brought through a separate incision on the abdominal wall onto the skin as a loop colostomy. In 44143, the distal end of colon is closed with staples or sutures and left in the abdomen. The initial incision is closed.

Coding Tips

Mobilization (take-down) of splenic flexure performed in conjunction with partial colectomy is reported separately, see 44139. For colectomy, partial, with anastomosis, see 44140; with end colostomy and closure of distal segment (Hartmann type procedure), see 44143; with abdominal and transanal approach, see 44147. For laparoscopic approach, see 44206.

ICD-10-CM Diagnostic Codes

C18.0	Malignant neoplasm of cecum
C18.1	Malignant neoplasm of appendix
C18.2	Malignant neoplasm of ascending colon
C18.3	Malignant neoplasm of hepatic flexure
C18.4	Malignant neoplasm of transverse colon
C18.5	Malignant neoplasm of splenic flexure
C18.6	Malignant neoplasm of descending colon
C18.7	Malignant neoplasm of sigmoid colon
C18.8	Malignant neoplasm of overlapping sites of colon
C19	Malignant neoplasm of rectosigmoid junction
C49.A4	Gastrointestinal stromal tumor of large intestine
C78.5	Secondary malignant neoplasm of large intestine and rectum
C7A.021	Malignant carcinoid tumor of the cecum
C7A.022	Malignant carcinoid tumor of the ascending colon
C7A.023	Malignant carcinoid tumor of the transverse colon
C7A.024	Malignant carcinoid tumor of the descending colon
C7A.025	Malignant carcinoid tumor of the sigmoid colon
D01.0	Carcinoma in situ of colon
D01.1	Carcinoma in situ of rectosigmoid junction
D12.0	Benign neoplasm of cecum
D12.1	Benign neoplasm of appendix
D12.2	Benign neoplasm of ascending colon
D12.3	Benign neoplasm of transverse colon
D12.4	Benign neoplasm of descending colon
D12.5	Benign neoplasm of sigmoid colon
D12.7	Benign neoplasm of rectosigmoid junction
D37.4	Neoplasm of uncertain behavior of colon
D3A.021	Benign carcinoid tumor of the cecum
D3A.022	Benign carcinoid tumor of the ascending colon
D3A.023	Benign carcinoid tumor of the transverse colon
D3A.024	Benign carcinoid tumor of the descending colon
D3A.025	Benign carcinoid tumor of the sigmoid colon
K50.111	Crohn's disease of large intestine with rectal bleeding
K50.112	Crohn's disease of large intestine with intestinal obstruction
K50.113	Crohn's disease of large intestine with fistula
K50.114	Crohn's disease of large intestine with abscess
K50.118	Crohn's disease of large intestine with other complication
K50.811	Crohn's disease of both small and large intestine with rectal bleeding
K50.812	Crohn's disease of both small and large intestine with intestinal obstruction
K50.813	Crohn's disease of both small and large intestine with fistula
K50.814	Crohn's disease of both small and large intestine with abscess
K50.818	Crohn's disease of both small and large intestine with other complication
K51.011	Ulcerative (chronic) pancolitis with rectal bleeding
K51.012	Ulcerative (chronic) pancolitis with intestinal obstruction
K51.013	Ulcerative (chronic) pancolitis with fistula
K51.014	Ulcerative (chronic) pancolitis with abscess
K51.018	Ulcerative (chronic) pancolitis with other complication
K51.311	Ulcerative (chronic) rectosigmoiditis with rectal bleeding
K51.312	Ulcerative (chronic) rectosigmoiditis with intestinal obstruction
K51.313	Ulcerative (chronic) rectosigmoiditis with fistula
K51.314	Ulcerative (chronic) rectosigmoiditis with abscess
K51.318	Ulcerative (chronic) rectosigmoiditis with other complication
K51.411	Inflammatory polyps of colon with rectal bleeding
K51.412	Inflammatory polyps of colon with intestinal obstruction
K51.413	Inflammatory polyps of colon with fistula
K51.414	Inflammatory polyps of colon with abscess
K51.418	Inflammatory polyps of colon with other complication
K51.511	Left sided colitis with rectal bleeding
K51.512	Left sided colitis with intestinal obstruction
K51.513	Left sided colitis with fistula
K51.514	Left sided colitis with abscess

K51.518	Left sided colitis with other complication
K51.811	Other ulcerative colitis with rectal bleeding
K51.812	Other ulcerative colitis with intestinal obstruction
K55.041	Focal (segmental) acute infarction of large intestine
K55.042	Diffuse acute infarction of large intestine
K55.1	Chronic vascular disorders of intestine
K55.20	Angiodysplasia of colon without hemorrhage
K55.21	Angiodysplasia of colon with hemorrhage
K56.0	Paralytic ileus
K56.1	Intussusception
K56.2	Volvulus
K56.51	Intestinal adhesions [bands], with partial obstruction
K56.52	Intestinal adhesions [bands] with complete obstruction
K57.20	Diverticulitis of large intestine with perforation and abscess without bleeding
K57.21	Diverticulitis of large intestine with perforation and abscess with bleeding
K57.31	Diverticulosis of large intestine without perforation or abscess with bleeding
K57.33	Diverticulitis of large intestine without perforation or abscess with bleeding
K57.40	Diverticulitis of both small and large intestine with perforation and abscess without bleeding
K57.41	Diverticulitis of both small and large intestine with perforation and abscess with bleeding
K59.31	Toxic megacolon
K59.81	Ogilvie syndrome
K63.0	Abscess of intestine
K63.1	Perforation of intestine (nontraumatic)
K63.2	Fistula of intestine
K63.3	Ulcer of intestine
K63.4	Enteroptosis
K63.5	Polyp of colon
N32.1	Vesicointestinal fistula
Q42.8	Congenital absence, atresia and stenosis of other parts of large intestine
Q43.1	Hirschsprung's disease
Q43.2	Other congenital functional disorders of colon
Q43.3	Congenital malformations of intestinal fixation
Q43.4	Duplication of intestine
S36.530A	Laceration of ascending [right] colon, initial encounter
S36.531A	Laceration of transverse colon, initial encounter
S36.532A	Laceration of descending [left] colon, initial encounter
S36.533A	Laceration of sigmoid colon, initial encounter
S36.538A	Laceration of other part of colon, initial encounter

AMA: 44141 2018,Jan,8; 2017,Jan,8; 2016,Jan,13; 2015,Jan,16 **44143** 2018,Jan,8; 2017,Jan,8; 2016,Jan,13; 2015,Jan,16

Relative Value Units/Medicare Edits

Non-Facility RVU	Work	PE	MP	Total
44141	29.91	17.07	6.76	53.74
44143	27.79	14.94	6.28	49.01
Facility RVU	Work	PE	MP	Total
44141	29.91	17.07	6.76	53.74
44143	27.79	14.94	6.28	49.01

	FUD	Status	MUE	Modifiers				IOM Reference
44141	90	A	1(3)	51	N/A	62*	80	None
44143	90	A	1(2)	51	N/A	62*	80	

* with documentation

Terms To Know

carcinoid tumor. Specific type of slow-growing neuroendocrine tumors. Carcinoid tumors occur most commonly in the hormone producing cells of the gastrointestinal tracts and can also occur in the pancreas, testes, ovaries, or lungs.

Crohn's disease. Chronic inflammation of the gastrointestinal tract characterized by chronic granulomatous disease, most commonly affecting the intestines and the terminal ileum.

enteroptosis. Condition in which the intestines are abnormally positioned downward in the abdominal cavity and often associated with displacement of other internal organs.

Hirschsprung's disease. Congenital enlargement or dilation of the colon, with the absence of nerve cells in a segment of colon distally that causes the inability to defecate.

Ogilvie's syndrome. Colonic obstruction with symptoms of persistent contraction of intestinal musculature, caused by a defect in the sympathetic nerve supply.

44144

44144 Colectomy, partial; with resection, with colostomy or ileostomy and creation of mucofistula

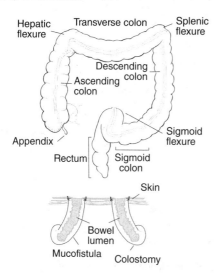

Explanation

The physician resects a segment of colon. The proximal and distal ends of colon are brought through the abdominal wall onto the skin as a colostomy and mucus fistula. The physician makes an abdominal incision. Next, the selected segment of colon is isolated and divided proximally and distally to the remaining colon and removed. The proximal end of colon or terminal ileum and the distal end of colon are brought through separate incisions on the abdominal wall onto the skin as an ileostomy or colostomy and mucus fistula. The initial abdominal incision is closed.

Coding Tips

Mobilization (take-down) of splenic flexure performed in conjunction with partial colectomy is reported separately, see 44139. For colectomy, partial, with coloproctostomy (low pelvic anastomosis), with colostomy, see 44146; with abdominal and transanal approach, see 44147.

ICD-10-CM Diagnostic Codes

C18.0	Malignant neoplasm of cecum
C18.2	Malignant neoplasm of ascending colon
C18.3	Malignant neoplasm of hepatic flexure
C18.4	Malignant neoplasm of transverse colon
C18.5	Malignant neoplasm of splenic flexure
C18.6	Malignant neoplasm of descending colon
C18.7	Malignant neoplasm of sigmoid colon
C18.8	Malignant neoplasm of overlapping sites of colon
C19	Malignant neoplasm of rectosigmoid junction
C49.A4	Gastrointestinal stromal tumor of large intestine
C78.5	Secondary malignant neoplasm of large intestine and rectum
C7A.021	Malignant carcinoid tumor of the cecum
C7A.022	Malignant carcinoid tumor of the ascending colon
C7A.023	Malignant carcinoid tumor of the transverse colon
C7A.024	Malignant carcinoid tumor of the descending colon
C7A.025	Malignant carcinoid tumor of the sigmoid colon
D01.0	Carcinoma in situ of colon
D01.1	Carcinoma in situ of rectosigmoid junction

D12.0	Benign neoplasm of cecum
D12.1	Benign neoplasm of appendix
D12.2	Benign neoplasm of ascending colon
D12.3	Benign neoplasm of transverse colon
D12.4	Benign neoplasm of descending colon
D12.5	Benign neoplasm of sigmoid colon
D12.7	Benign neoplasm of rectosigmoid junction
D37.3	Neoplasm of uncertain behavior of appendix
D37.4	Neoplasm of uncertain behavior of colon
D3A.022	Benign carcinoid tumor of the ascending colon
D3A.023	Benign carcinoid tumor of the transverse colon
D3A.024	Benign carcinoid tumor of the descending colon
D3A.025	Benign carcinoid tumor of the sigmoid colon
D49.0	Neoplasm of unspecified behavior of digestive system
K50.111	Crohn's disease of large intestine with rectal bleeding
K50.112	Crohn's disease of large intestine with intestinal obstruction
K50.113	Crohn's disease of large intestine with fistula
K50.114	Crohn's disease of large intestine with abscess
K50.811	Crohn's disease of both small and large intestine with rectal bleeding
K50.812	Crohn's disease of both small and large intestine with intestinal obstruction
K50.813	Crohn's disease of both small and large intestine with fistula
K50.814	Crohn's disease of both small and large intestine with abscess
K50.818	Crohn's disease of both small and large intestine with other complication
K51.011	Ulcerative (chronic) pancolitis with rectal bleeding
K51.012	Ulcerative (chronic) pancolitis with intestinal obstruction
K51.013	Ulcerative (chronic) pancolitis with fistula
K51.014	Ulcerative (chronic) pancolitis with abscess
K51.311	Ulcerative (chronic) rectosigmoiditis with rectal bleeding
K51.312	Ulcerative (chronic) rectosigmoiditis with intestinal obstruction
K51.313	Ulcerative (chronic) rectosigmoiditis with fistula
K51.314	Ulcerative (chronic) rectosigmoiditis with abscess
K51.318	Ulcerative (chronic) rectosigmoiditis with other complication
K51.411	Inflammatory polyps of colon with rectal bleeding
K51.412	Inflammatory polyps of colon with intestinal obstruction
K51.413	Inflammatory polyps of colon with fistula
K51.414	Inflammatory polyps of colon with abscess
K51.511	Left sided colitis with rectal bleeding
K51.512	Left sided colitis with intestinal obstruction
K51.513	Left sided colitis with fistula
K51.514	Left sided colitis with abscess
K55.041	Focal (segmental) acute infarction of large intestine
K55.042	Diffuse acute infarction of large intestine
K55.1	Chronic vascular disorders of intestine
K55.20	Angiodysplasia of colon without hemorrhage
K55.21	Angiodysplasia of colon with hemorrhage
K55.31	Stage 1 necrotizing enterocolitis
K55.32	Stage 2 necrotizing enterocolitis
K55.33	Stage 3 necrotizing enterocolitis
K56.0	Paralytic ileus
K56.1	Intussusception

K56.2	Volvulus	
K56.51	Intestinal adhesions [bands], with partial obstruction	
K56.52	Intestinal adhesions [bands] with complete obstruction	
K56.690	Other partial intestinal obstruction	
K56.691	Other complete intestinal obstruction	
K57.20	Diverticulitis of large intestine with perforation and abscess without bleeding	
K57.21	Diverticulitis of large intestine with perforation and abscess with bleeding	
K57.31	Diverticulosis of large intestine without perforation or abscess with bleeding	
K57.33	Diverticulitis of large intestine without perforation or abscess with bleeding	
K57.40	Diverticulitis of both small and large intestine with perforation and abscess without bleeding	
K57.41	Diverticulitis of both small and large intestine with perforation and abscess with bleeding	
K59.31	Toxic megacolon	
K59.81	Ogilvie syndrome	
K63.1	Perforation of intestine (nontraumatic)	
K63.2	Fistula of intestine	
K63.3	Ulcer of intestine	
K63.4	Enteroptosis	
K63.5	Polyp of colon	
K91.31	Postprocedural partial intestinal obstruction	
K91.32	Postprocedural complete intestinal obstruction	
N32.1	Vesicointestinal fistula	
P76.8	Other specified intestinal obstruction of newborn ℕ	
P77.1	Stage 1 necrotizing enterocolitis in newborn ℕ	
P77.2	Stage 2 necrotizing enterocolitis in newborn ℕ	
P77.3	Stage 3 necrotizing enterocolitis in newborn ℕ	
Q42.8	Congenital absence, atresia and stenosis of other parts of large intestine	
Q43.1	Hirschsprung's disease	
Q43.2	Other congenital functional disorders of colon	
Q43.3	Congenital malformations of intestinal fixation	
Q43.4	Duplication of intestine	
S36.530A	Laceration of ascending [right] colon, initial encounter	
S36.531A	Laceration of transverse colon, initial encounter	
S36.532A	Laceration of descending [left] colon, initial encounter	
S36.533A	Laceration of sigmoid colon, initial encounter	

AMA: 44144 2018,Jan,8; 2017,Jan,8; 2016,Jan,13; 2015,Jan,16

Relative Value Units/Medicare Edits

Non-Facility RVU	Work	PE	MP	Total
44144	29.91	15.5	6.65	52.06
Facility RVU	**Work**	**PE**	**MP**	**Total**
44144	29.91	15.5	6.65	52.06

	FUD	Status	MUE	Modifiers				IOM Reference
44144	90	A	1(3)	51	N/A	62*	80	None

* with documentation

44145-44146

44145   Colectomy, partial; with coloproctostomy (low pelvic anastomosis)
44146   with coloproctostomy (low pelvic anastomosis), with colostomy

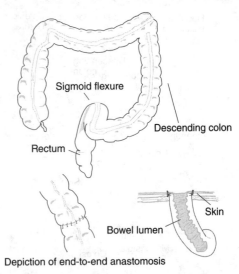

Depiction of end-to-end anastomosis

The descending colon, sigmoid, and rectum is the site of partial colectomy with coloproctostomy

Explanation

The physician resects a segment of distal colon or rectum and performs a low colorectal anastomosis in the pelvis. The physician makes an abdominal incision. The distal colon and rectum are mobilized, and the selected segment divided proximally and distally to the remaining colon. In 44145, an anastomosis is created between the proximal colon and remaining rectum in the pelvis with staples or sutures. In 44146, the distal colon and rectum are mobilized, and the selected segment of diseased colon and/or rectal tissue is removed. The new ends are brought together, and an anastomosis is done between the colon and the rectum low in the pelvis with staples or sutures (coloproctostomy). A loop of colon above the newly sutured anastomosis is brought out through a separate incision in the abdominal wall and fixed there so the colon will empty through this artificial opening in the skin as a colostomy, usually temporary, to divert the fecal stream while the anastomosis heals. The incision is closed.

Coding Tips

Mobilization (take-down) of splenic flexure and intraoperative colonic lavage performed in conjunction with partial colectomy is reported separately, see 44139 and 44701. For colectomy, partial, with skin level cecostomy or colostomy, see 44141; with end colostomy and closure of distal segment (Hartmann type procedure), see 44143; with coloproctostomy (low pelvic anastomosis, with colostomy), see 44146; with abdominal and transanal approach, see 44147; laparoscopic approach, see 44207. For colectomy, partial, with coloproctostomy (low pelvic anastomosis), see 44145; with abdominal and transanal approach, see 44147; laparoscopic approach, see 44208.

ICD-10-CM Diagnostic Codes

C18.0	Malignant neoplasm of cecum
C18.2	Malignant neoplasm of ascending colon
C18.3	Malignant neoplasm of hepatic flexure
C18.4	Malignant neoplasm of transverse colon
C18.5	Malignant neoplasm of splenic flexure
C18.6	Malignant neoplasm of descending colon

C18.7	Malignant neoplasm of sigmoid colon
C18.8	Malignant neoplasm of overlapping sites of colon
C19	Malignant neoplasm of rectosigmoid junction
C49.A4	Gastrointestinal stromal tumor of large intestine
C78.5	Secondary malignant neoplasm of large intestine and rectum
C7A.021	Malignant carcinoid tumor of the cecum
C7A.024	Malignant carcinoid tumor of the descending colon
C7A.025	Malignant carcinoid tumor of the sigmoid colon
D01.1	Carcinoma in situ of rectosigmoid junction
D12.0	Benign neoplasm of cecum
D12.1	Benign neoplasm of appendix
D12.4	Benign neoplasm of descending colon
D12.5	Benign neoplasm of sigmoid colon
D12.7	Benign neoplasm of rectosigmoid junction
D37.3	Neoplasm of uncertain behavior of appendix
D3A.024	Benign carcinoid tumor of the descending colon
D3A.025	Benign carcinoid tumor of the sigmoid colon
D49.0	Neoplasm of unspecified behavior of digestive system
K50.111	Crohn's disease of large intestine with rectal bleeding
K50.112	Crohn's disease of large intestine with intestinal obstruction
K50.113	Crohn's disease of large intestine with fistula
K50.114	Crohn's disease of large intestine with abscess
K50.118	Crohn's disease of large intestine with other complication
K50.811	Crohn's disease of both small and large intestine with rectal bleeding
K50.812	Crohn's disease of both small and large intestine with intestinal obstruction
K50.813	Crohn's disease of both small and large intestine with fistula
K50.814	Crohn's disease of both small and large intestine with abscess
K50.818	Crohn's disease of both small and large intestine with other complication
K51.011	Ulcerative (chronic) pancolitis with rectal bleeding
K51.012	Ulcerative (chronic) pancolitis with intestinal obstruction
K51.013	Ulcerative (chronic) pancolitis with fistula
K51.014	Ulcerative (chronic) pancolitis with abscess
K51.018	Ulcerative (chronic) pancolitis with other complication
K51.311	Ulcerative (chronic) rectosigmoiditis with rectal bleeding
K51.312	Ulcerative (chronic) rectosigmoiditis with intestinal obstruction
K51.313	Ulcerative (chronic) rectosigmoiditis with fistula
K51.314	Ulcerative (chronic) rectosigmoiditis with abscess
K51.318	Ulcerative (chronic) rectosigmoiditis with other complication
K51.411	Inflammatory polyps of colon with rectal bleeding
K51.412	Inflammatory polyps of colon with intestinal obstruction
K51.413	Inflammatory polyps of colon with fistula
K51.414	Inflammatory polyps of colon with abscess
K51.418	Inflammatory polyps of colon with other complication
K51.511	Left sided colitis with rectal bleeding
K51.512	Left sided colitis with intestinal obstruction
K51.513	Left sided colitis with fistula
K51.514	Left sided colitis with abscess
K51.518	Left sided colitis with other complication
K55.021	Focal (segmental) acute infarction of small intestine
K55.022	Diffuse acute infarction of small intestine

K55.031	Focal (segmental) acute (reversible) ischemia of large intestine
K55.032	Diffuse acute (reversible) ischemia of large intestine
K55.041	Focal (segmental) acute infarction of large intestine
K55.042	Diffuse acute infarction of large intestine
K55.1	Chronic vascular disorders of intestine
K55.20	Angiodysplasia of colon without hemorrhage
K55.21	Angiodysplasia of colon with hemorrhage
K55.31	Stage 1 necrotizing enterocolitis
K55.32	Stage 2 necrotizing enterocolitis
K55.33	Stage 3 necrotizing enterocolitis
K56.0	Paralytic ileus
K56.1	Intussusception
K56.2	Volvulus
K56.51	Intestinal adhesions [bands], with partial obstruction
K56.52	Intestinal adhesions [bands] with complete obstruction
K56.690	Other partial intestinal obstruction
K56.691	Other complete intestinal obstruction
K57.20	Diverticulitis of large intestine with perforation and abscess without bleeding
K57.21	Diverticulitis of large intestine with perforation and abscess with bleeding
K57.33	Diverticulitis of large intestine without perforation or abscess with bleeding
K57.40	Diverticulitis of both small and large intestine with perforation and abscess without bleeding
K57.41	Diverticulitis of both small and large intestine with perforation and abscess with bleeding
K57.52	Diverticulitis of both small and large intestine without perforation or abscess without bleeding
K57.53	Diverticulitis of both small and large intestine without perforation or abscess with bleeding
K59.31	Toxic megacolon
K59.81	Ogilvie syndrome
K63.0	Abscess of intestine
K63.1	Perforation of intestine (nontraumatic)
K63.2	Fistula of intestine
K63.3	Ulcer of intestine
K63.4	Enteroptosis
K63.5	Polyp of colon
K91.31	Postprocedural partial intestinal obstruction
K91.32	Postprocedural complete intestinal obstruction
N32.1	Vesicointestinal fistula
Q42.8	Congenital absence, atresia and stenosis of other parts of large intestine
Q43.1	Hirschsprung's disease
Q43.2	Other congenital functional disorders of colon
Q43.3	Congenital malformations of intestinal fixation
Q43.4	Duplication of intestine
S36.530A	Laceration of ascending [right] colon, initial encounter
S36.531A	Laceration of transverse colon, initial encounter
S36.532A	Laceration of descending [left] colon, initial encounter
S36.533A	Laceration of sigmoid colon, initial encounter
S36.538A	Laceration of other part of colon, initial encounter

AMA: 44146 2018,Jun,11; 2018,Jan,8; 2017,Jan,8; 2016,Jan,13; 2015,Jan,16

Relative Value Units/Medicare Edits

Non-Facility RVU	Work	PE	MP	Total
44145	28.58	14.05	5.87	48.5
44146	35.3	19.42	7.24	61.96
Facility RVU	**Work**	**PE**	**MP**	**Total**
44145	28.58	14.05	5.87	48.5
44146	35.3	19.42	7.24	61.96

	FUD	Status	MUE	Modifiers				IOM Reference
44145	90	A	1(2)	51	N/A	62*	80	None
44146	90	A	1(2)	51	N/A	62*	80	

* with documentation

Terms To Know

anastomosis. Surgically created connection between ducts, blood vessels, or bowel segments to allow flow from one to the other.

Crohn's disease. Chronic inflammation of the gastrointestinal tract characterized by chronic granulomatous disease, most commonly affecting the intestines and the terminal ileum.

megacolon. Enlargement or dilation of the large intestines or the colon.

Ogilvie's syndrome. Colonic obstruction with symptoms of persistent contraction of intestinal musculature, caused by a defect in the sympathetic nerve supply.

pancolitis. Severe form of ulcerative colitis, where inflammation affects the entire colon. May be caused by infection or external influences such as laxatives, radiation, or antibiotics.

volvulus. Twisting, knotting, or entanglement of the bowel on itself that may quickly compromise oxygen supply to the intestinal tissues. A volvulus usually occurs at the sigmoid and ileocecal areas of the intestines.

44147

44147   Colectomy, partial; abdominal and transanal approach

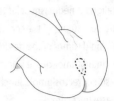

Transanal phase of surgery involves a deep incision to free the anus from its muscle attachments

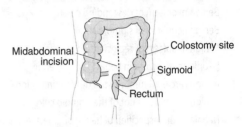

A portion of the distal colon is resected

Explanation

The physician removes a segment of colon through a combined abdominal and transanal approach and reapproximates the remaining ends of the colon. The physician makes an abdominal incision. The distal colon and rectum are mobilized also by using a transanal approach. The segment of the colon to be eliminated is divided at the appropriate distal and proximal points and the remaining ends are anastomosed. The abdominal and transanal incisions are closed.

Coding Tips

Mobilization (take-down) of splenic flexure performed in conjunction with partial colectomy is reported separately, see 44139. For colectomy, partial, with skin level cecostomy or colostomy, see 44141; with end colostomy and closure of distal segment (Hartmann type procedure), see 44143; with coloproctostomy (low pelvic anastomosis), see 44145; with coloproctostomy (low pelvic anastomosis with colostomy), see 44146. For colectomy, partial, with removal of terminal ileum and ileocolostomy, see 44160.

ICD-10-CM Diagnostic Codes

C18.0	Malignant neoplasm of cecum
C18.1	Malignant neoplasm of appendix
C18.6	Malignant neoplasm of descending colon
C18.7	Malignant neoplasm of sigmoid colon
C18.8	Malignant neoplasm of overlapping sites of colon
C19	Malignant neoplasm of rectosigmoid junction
C49.A4	Gastrointestinal stromal tumor of large intestine
C78.5	Secondary malignant neoplasm of large intestine and rectum
C7A.021	Malignant carcinoid tumor of the cecum
C7A.024	Malignant carcinoid tumor of the descending colon
C7A.025	Malignant carcinoid tumor of the sigmoid colon
D01.1	Carcinoma in situ of rectosigmoid junction
D12.4	Benign neoplasm of descending colon
D12.5	Benign neoplasm of sigmoid colon
D12.7	Benign neoplasm of rectosigmoid junction
D3A.021	Benign carcinoid tumor of the cecum

D3A.024	Benign carcinoid tumor of the descending colon
D3A.025	Benign carcinoid tumor of the sigmoid colon
D49.0	Neoplasm of unspecified behavior of digestive system
K50.111	Crohn's disease of large intestine with rectal bleeding
K50.112	Crohn's disease of large intestine with intestinal obstruction
K50.113	Crohn's disease of large intestine with fistula
K50.114	Crohn's disease of large intestine with abscess
K50.812	Crohn's disease of both small and large intestine with intestinal obstruction
K50.813	Crohn's disease of both small and large intestine with fistula
K50.814	Crohn's disease of both small and large intestine with abscess
K51.011	Ulcerative (chronic) pancolitis with rectal bleeding
K51.012	Ulcerative (chronic) pancolitis with intestinal obstruction
K51.013	Ulcerative (chronic) pancolitis with fistula
K51.014	Ulcerative (chronic) pancolitis with abscess
K51.212	Ulcerative (chronic) proctitis with intestinal obstruction
K51.213	Ulcerative (chronic) proctitis with fistula
K51.312	Ulcerative (chronic) rectosigmoiditis with intestinal obstruction
K51.313	Ulcerative (chronic) rectosigmoiditis with fistula
K51.314	Ulcerative (chronic) rectosigmoiditis with abscess
K51.411	Inflammatory polyps of colon with rectal bleeding
K51.412	Inflammatory polyps of colon with intestinal obstruction
K51.413	Inflammatory polyps of colon with fistula
K51.414	Inflammatory polyps of colon with abscess
K51.512	Left sided colitis with intestinal obstruction
K51.513	Left sided colitis with fistula
K51.514	Left sided colitis with abscess
K52.82	Eosinophilic colitis
K55.041	Focal (segmental) acute infarction of large intestine
K55.042	Diffuse acute infarction of large intestine
K55.1	Chronic vascular disorders of intestine
K55.21	Angiodysplasia of colon with hemorrhage
K56.0	Paralytic ileus
K56.1	Intussusception
K56.2	Volvulus
K57.20	Diverticulitis of large intestine with perforation and abscess without bleeding
K57.21	Diverticulitis of large intestine with perforation and abscess with bleeding
K57.33	Diverticulitis of large intestine without perforation or abscess with bleeding
K57.40	Diverticulitis of both small and large intestine with perforation and abscess without bleeding
K57.41	Diverticulitis of both small and large intestine with perforation and abscess with bleeding
K57.51	Diverticulosis of both small and large intestine without perforation or abscess with bleeding
K59.31	Toxic megacolon
K59.81	Ogilvie syndrome
K63.1	Perforation of intestine (nontraumatic)
K63.2	Fistula of intestine
K63.3	Ulcer of intestine
K63.4	Enteroptosis

Q42.8	Congenital absence, atresia and stenosis of other parts of large intestine
Q43.1	Hirschsprung's disease
Q43.2	Other congenital functional disorders of colon
Q43.3	Congenital malformations of intestinal fixation
Q43.8	Other specified congenital malformations of intestine
S36.530A	Laceration of ascending [right] colon, initial encounter
S36.531A	Laceration of transverse colon, initial encounter
S36.532A	Laceration of descending [left] colon, initial encounter
S36.533A	Laceration of sigmoid colon, initial encounter

AMA: **44147** 2018,Jan,8; 2017,Jan,8; 2016,Jan,13; 2015,Jan,16

Relative Value Units/Medicare Edits

Non-Facility RVU	Work	PE	MP	Total
44147	33.69	15.97	7.26	56.92
Facility RVU	Work	PE	MP	Total
44147	33.69	15.97	7.26	56.92

	FUD	Status	MUE	Modifiers				IOM Reference
44147	90	A	1(3)	51	N/A	62*	80	None

* with documentation

Terms To Know

Crohn's disease. Chronic inflammation of the gastrointestinal tract characterized by chronic granulomatous disease, most commonly affecting the intestines and the terminal ileum.

diverticulosis. Saclike pouches of the mucous membrane lining the intestine, herniating through the muscular wall of the colon, and occurring without inflammation.

pancolitis. Severe form of ulcerative colitis, where inflammation affects the entire colon. May be caused by infection or external influences such as laxatives, radiation, or antibiotics.

Intestines

44150-44151

44150 Colectomy, total, abdominal, without proctectomy; with ileostomy or ileoproctostomy

44151 with continent ileostomy

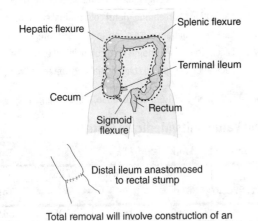

Hepatic flexure

Splenic flexure

Terminal ileum

Cecum

Rectum

Sigmoid flexure

Distal ileum anastomosed to rectal stump

Total removal will involve construction of an end ileostomy or an ileoproctostomy

Explanation

The physician removes the entire colon. In 44150, an ileostomy or an anastomosis between the ileum and rectum is performed. The physician makes an abdominal incision. The entire colon is mobilized and the colorectal junction and terminal ileum are divided. The colon is removed. The terminal ileum is approximated to the rectum or brought out through a separate incision on the abdominal wall onto the skin as an ileostomy. In 44151, a reservoir of distal ileum (Kock pouch) is created. The reservoir is brought out through the abdominal wall as a continent stoma. The physician makes an abdominal incision. Next, the colon is mobilized. The colorectal junction and terminal ileum are divided and the colon removed. The distal ileum is folded upon itself and approximated to form a pouch and valve. The distal end of the pouch is brought through a separate incision on the abdominal wall onto the skin as a continent ileostomy. The initial incision is closed.

Coding Tips

Intraoperative colonic lavage performed with 44150 is reported separately, see 44701. For colectomy, total, abdominal, with proctectomy, with ileostomy, see 44155; and with continent ileostomy, see 44156; with ileoanal anastomosis, loop ileostomy and rectal mucosectomy, when performed, see 44157; with ileoanal anastomosis, creation of ileal reservoir (S or J), loop ileostomy and rectal mucosectomy, when performed, see 44158. For laparoscopic approach, see 44210.

ICD-10-CM Diagnostic Codes

C18.0	Malignant neoplasm of cecum
C18.1	Malignant neoplasm of appendix
C18.2	Malignant neoplasm of ascending colon
C18.3	Malignant neoplasm of hepatic flexure
C18.4	Malignant neoplasm of transverse colon
C18.5	Malignant neoplasm of splenic flexure
C18.6	Malignant neoplasm of descending colon
C18.7	Malignant neoplasm of sigmoid colon
C18.8	Malignant neoplasm of overlapping sites of colon
C19	Malignant neoplasm of rectosigmoid junction
C49.A4	Gastrointestinal stromal tumor of large intestine
C78.5	Secondary malignant neoplasm of large intestine and rectum
C7A.021	Malignant carcinoid tumor of the cecum
C7A.022	Malignant carcinoid tumor of the ascending colon
C7A.023	Malignant carcinoid tumor of the transverse colon
C7A.024	Malignant carcinoid tumor of the descending colon
C7A.025	Malignant carcinoid tumor of the sigmoid colon
D01.0	Carcinoma in situ of colon
D01.1	Carcinoma in situ of rectosigmoid junction
D12.0	Benign neoplasm of cecum
D12.1	Benign neoplasm of appendix
D12.2	Benign neoplasm of ascending colon
D12.3	Benign neoplasm of transverse colon
D12.4	Benign neoplasm of descending colon
D12.5	Benign neoplasm of sigmoid colon
D12.7	Benign neoplasm of rectosigmoid junction
D37.3	Neoplasm of uncertain behavior of appendix
D37.4	Neoplasm of uncertain behavior of colon
D3A.021	Benign carcinoid tumor of the cecum
D3A.022	Benign carcinoid tumor of the ascending colon
D3A.023	Benign carcinoid tumor of the transverse colon
D3A.024	Benign carcinoid tumor of the descending colon
D3A.025	Benign carcinoid tumor of the sigmoid colon
D49.0	Neoplasm of unspecified behavior of digestive system
K50.111	Crohn's disease of large intestine with rectal bleeding
K50.112	Crohn's disease of large intestine with intestinal obstruction
K50.113	Crohn's disease of large intestine with fistula
K50.114	Crohn's disease of large intestine with abscess
K50.812	Crohn's disease of both small and large intestine with intestinal obstruction
K50.813	Crohn's disease of both small and large intestine with fistula
K50.814	Crohn's disease of both small and large intestine with abscess
K51.011	Ulcerative (chronic) pancolitis with rectal bleeding
K51.012	Ulcerative (chronic) pancolitis with intestinal obstruction
K51.013	Ulcerative (chronic) pancolitis with fistula
K51.014	Ulcerative (chronic) pancolitis with abscess
K51.312	Ulcerative (chronic) rectosigmoiditis with intestinal obstruction
K51.313	Ulcerative (chronic) rectosigmoiditis with fistula
K51.411	Inflammatory polyps of colon with rectal bleeding
K51.412	Inflammatory polyps of colon with intestinal obstruction
K51.413	Inflammatory polyps of colon with fistula
K51.414	Inflammatory polyps of colon with abscess
K51.511	Left sided colitis with rectal bleeding
K51.512	Left sided colitis with intestinal obstruction
K51.513	Left sided colitis with fistula
K51.514	Left sided colitis with abscess
K52.82	Eosinophilic colitis
K55.041	Focal (segmental) acute infarction of large intestine
K55.042	Diffuse acute infarction of large intestine
K55.1	Chronic vascular disorders of intestine
K55.21	Angiodysplasia of colon with hemorrhage
K55.32	Stage 2 necrotizing enterocolitis
K55.33	Stage 3 necrotizing enterocolitis
K56.2	Volvulus

Intestines

K56.52	Intestinal adhesions [bands] with complete obstruction
K57.20	Diverticulitis of large intestine with perforation and abscess without bleeding
K57.21	Diverticulitis of large intestine with perforation and abscess with bleeding
K57.33	Diverticulitis of large intestine without perforation or abscess with bleeding
K57.40	Diverticulitis of both small and large intestine with perforation and abscess without bleeding
K57.41	Diverticulitis of both small and large intestine with perforation and abscess with bleeding
K57.51	Diverticulosis of both small and large intestine without perforation or abscess with bleeding
K59.31	Toxic megacolon
K59.81	Ogilvie syndrome
K63.1	Perforation of intestine (nontraumatic)
K63.2	Fistula of intestine
K63.3	Ulcer of intestine
K63.4	Enteroptosis
P77.1	Stage 1 necrotizing enterocolitis in newborn N
P77.2	Stage 2 necrotizing enterocolitis in newborn N
P77.3	Stage 3 necrotizing enterocolitis in newborn N
P78.0	Perinatal intestinal perforation N
Q43.1	Hirschsprung's disease
Q43.2	Other congenital functional disorders of colon
S36.530A	Laceration of ascending [right] colon, initial encounter
S36.531A	Laceration of transverse colon, initial encounter
S36.532A	Laceration of descending [left] colon, initial encounter
S36.533A	Laceration of sigmoid colon, initial encounter

AMA: **44150** 2014,Jan,11 **44151** 2014,Jan,11

Relative Value Units/Medicare Edits

Non-Facility RVU	Work	PE	MP	Total
44150	30.18	18.21	6.42	54.81
44151	34.92	20.46	8.54	63.92
Facility RVU	Work	PE	MP	Total
44150	30.18	18.21	6.42	54.81
44151	34.92	20.46	8.54	63.92

	FUD	Status	MUE	Modifiers				IOM Reference
44150	90	A	1(2)	51	N/A	62*	80	None
44151	90	A	1(2)	51	N/A	62*	80	

* with documentation

44155-44156

44155   Colectomy, total, abdominal, with proctectomy; with ileostomy
44156   with continent ileostomy

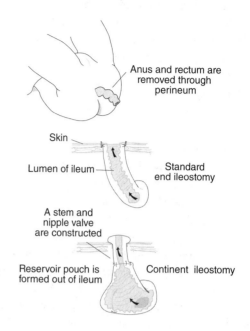

Anus and rectum are removed through perineum

Skin

Lumen of ileum

Standard end ileostomy

A stem and nipple valve are constructed

Reservoir pouch is formed out of ileum

Continent ileostomy

Explanation

The physician removes the entire colon and rectum and brings the terminal ileum or a pouch created from the terminal ileum out through the abdominal wall onto the skin as an ileostomy. The physician makes an abdominal incision. Next, the entire colon and rectum are mobilized, the proximal rectum and distal ileum are divided, and the colon and proximal rectum are removed. The distal rectum is mobilized and removed through a perineal approach. In 44155, the terminal ileum is brought out through a separate incision on the abdominal wall onto the skin as an ileostomy. In 44156, the terminal ileum is folded upon itself and approximated to form a pouch with a valve. The end of the pouch is brought out through a separate abdominal incision onto the skin as a continent ileostomy. Abdominal and perineal incisions are closed.

Coding Tips

For laparoscopic approach, see 44212.

ICD-10-CM Diagnostic Codes

C18.0	Malignant neoplasm of cecum
C18.1	Malignant neoplasm of appendix
C18.2	Malignant neoplasm of ascending colon
C18.3	Malignant neoplasm of hepatic flexure
C18.4	Malignant neoplasm of transverse colon
C18.5	Malignant neoplasm of splenic flexure
C18.6	Malignant neoplasm of descending colon
C18.7	Malignant neoplasm of sigmoid colon
C18.8	Malignant neoplasm of overlapping sites of colon
C19	Malignant neoplasm of rectosigmoid junction
C49.A4	Gastrointestinal stromal tumor of large intestine
C78.5	Secondary malignant neoplasm of large intestine and rectum
C7A.021	Malignant carcinoid tumor of the cecum
C7A.024	Malignant carcinoid tumor of the descending colon
C7A.025	Malignant carcinoid tumor of the sigmoid colon

D01.1	Carcinoma in situ of rectosigmoid junction
D01.2	Carcinoma in situ of rectum
D12.0	Benign neoplasm of cecum
D12.1	Benign neoplasm of appendix
D12.4	Benign neoplasm of descending colon
D12.5	Benign neoplasm of sigmoid colon
D12.7	Benign neoplasm of rectosigmoid junction
D12.8	Benign neoplasm of rectum
D37.3	Neoplasm of uncertain behavior of appendix
D37.5	Neoplasm of uncertain behavior of rectum
D3A.021	Benign carcinoid tumor of the cecum
D3A.024	Benign carcinoid tumor of the descending colon
D3A.025	Benign carcinoid tumor of the sigmoid colon
D49.0	Neoplasm of unspecified behavior of digestive system
K50.111	Crohn's disease of large intestine with rectal bleeding
K50.112	Crohn's disease of large intestine with intestinal obstruction
K50.113	Crohn's disease of large intestine with fistula
K50.114	Crohn's disease of large intestine with abscess
K50.118	Crohn's disease of large intestine with other complication
K50.812	Crohn's disease of both small and large intestine with intestinal obstruction
K50.813	Crohn's disease of both small and large intestine with fistula
K50.814	Crohn's disease of both small and large intestine with abscess
K51.011	Ulcerative (chronic) pancolitis with rectal bleeding
K51.012	Ulcerative (chronic) pancolitis with intestinal obstruction
K51.013	Ulcerative (chronic) pancolitis with fistula
K51.014	Ulcerative (chronic) pancolitis with abscess
K51.211	Ulcerative (chronic) proctitis with rectal bleeding
K51.212	Ulcerative (chronic) proctitis with intestinal obstruction
K51.213	Ulcerative (chronic) proctitis with fistula
K51.214	Ulcerative (chronic) proctitis with abscess
K51.312	Ulcerative (chronic) rectosigmoiditis with intestinal obstruction
K51.313	Ulcerative (chronic) rectosigmoiditis with fistula
K51.314	Ulcerative (chronic) rectosigmoiditis with abscess
K51.411	Inflammatory polyps of colon with rectal bleeding
K51.412	Inflammatory polyps of colon with intestinal obstruction
K51.413	Inflammatory polyps of colon with fistula
K51.414	Inflammatory polyps of colon with abscess
K51.511	Left sided colitis with rectal bleeding
K51.512	Left sided colitis with intestinal obstruction
K51.513	Left sided colitis with fistula
K51.514	Left sided colitis with abscess
K52.82	Eosinophilic colitis
K55.041	Focal (segmental) acute infarction of large intestine
K55.042	Diffuse acute infarction of large intestine
K55.1	Chronic vascular disorders of intestine
K55.21	Angiodysplasia of colon with hemorrhage
K55.31	Stage 1 necrotizing enterocolitis
K55.32	Stage 2 necrotizing enterocolitis
K55.33	Stage 3 necrotizing enterocolitis
K55.8	Other vascular disorders of intestine
K56.2	Volvulus

K57.20	Diverticulitis of large intestine with perforation and abscess without bleeding
K57.21	Diverticulitis of large intestine with perforation and abscess with bleeding
K57.33	Diverticulitis of large intestine without perforation or abscess with bleeding
K57.40	Diverticulitis of both small and large intestine with perforation and abscess without bleeding
K57.41	Diverticulitis of both small and large intestine with perforation and abscess with bleeding
K57.51	Diverticulosis of both small and large intestine without perforation or abscess with bleeding
K59.31	Toxic megacolon
K59.81	Ogilvie syndrome
K63.1	Perforation of intestine (nontraumatic)
K63.2	Fistula of intestine
K63.3	Ulcer of intestine
K63.4	Enteroptosis
P77.1	Stage 1 necrotizing enterocolitis in newborn 🅽
P77.2	Stage 2 necrotizing enterocolitis in newborn 🅽
P77.3	Stage 3 necrotizing enterocolitis in newborn 🅽
P78.0	Perinatal intestinal perforation 🅽
Q42.8	Congenital absence, atresia and stenosis of other parts of large intestine
Q43.1	Hirschsprung's disease
Q43.2	Other congenital functional disorders of colon
S36.530A	Laceration of ascending [right] colon, initial encounter
S36.531A	Laceration of transverse colon, initial encounter
S36.532A	Laceration of descending [left] colon, initial encounter
S36.533A	Laceration of sigmoid colon, initial encounter

AMA: 44155 2014,Jan,11 **44156** 2014,Jan,11

Relative Value Units/Medicare Edits

Non-Facility RVU	Work	PE	MP	Total
44155	34.42	19.69	6.74	60.85
44156	37.42	21.86	9.13	68.41
Facility RVU	Work	PE	MP	Total
44155	34.42	19.69	6.74	60.85
44156	37.42	21.86	9.13	68.41

	FUD	Status	MUE	Modifiers				IOM Reference
44155	90	A	1(2)	51	N/A	62*	80	None
44156	90	A	1(2)	51	N/A	62*	80	

* with documentation

44157-44158

44157 Colectomy, total, abdominal, with proctectomy; with ileoanal anastomosis, includes loop ileostomy, and rectal mucosectomy, when performed

44158 with ileoanal anastomosis, creation of ileal reservoir (S or J), includes loop ileostomy, and rectal mucosectomy, when performed

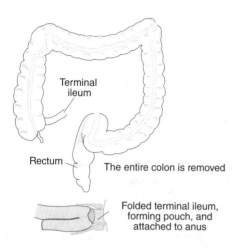

Terminal ileum

Rectum

The entire colon is removed

Folded terminal ileum, forming pouch, and attached to anus

A loop colostomy may also be created above this site to eliminate waste during the healing period

Explanation

The physician removes the entire colon and rectum, strips the mucosa from the distal rectum, and performs an anastomosis between the terminal ileum and anus. The physician makes an abdominal incision. Next, the colon and rectum are mobilized. The mucosa of the distal rectum is stripped from a perineal approach. In 44157, the terminal ileum and rectum are divided and the colon is removed. The terminal ileum is pulled through the remaining muscular cuff of the rectum and approximated to the anus with sutures. A loop of ileum may be brought out through the abdominal wall onto the skin as an ileostomy proximal to the anastomosis. In 44158, the terminal ileum is folded upon itself and approximated in order to form a pouch. The pouch is pulled through the remaining muscular tube of the rectum and approximated to the anus with sutures. A loop of ileum may be brought out through a separate incision on the abdominal wall onto the skin as an ileostomy proximal to the anastomosis.

Coding Tips

For colectomy, partial, with anastomosis, see 44140; with skin level cecostomy or colostomy, see 44141; with end colostomy and closure of distal segment (Hartmann type procedure), see 44143; with coloproctostomy (low pelvic anastomosis), see 44145; with coloproctostomy (low pelvic anastomosis), with colostomy, see 44146; with abdominal and transanal approach, see 44147; laparoscopic approach, see 44211.

ICD-10-CM Diagnostic Codes

C18.0	Malignant neoplasm of cecum
C18.1	Malignant neoplasm of appendix
C18.2	Malignant neoplasm of ascending colon
C18.3	Malignant neoplasm of hepatic flexure
C18.4	Malignant neoplasm of transverse colon
C18.5	Malignant neoplasm of splenic flexure
C18.6	Malignant neoplasm of descending colon
C18.7	Malignant neoplasm of sigmoid colon
C18.8	Malignant neoplasm of overlapping sites of colon
C19	Malignant neoplasm of rectosigmoid junction
C20	Malignant neoplasm of rectum
C49.A4	Gastrointestinal stromal tumor of large intestine
C78.5	Secondary malignant neoplasm of large intestine and rectum
C7A.021	Malignant carcinoid tumor of the cecum
C7A.024	Malignant carcinoid tumor of the descending colon
C7A.025	Malignant carcinoid tumor of the sigmoid colon
D01.1	Carcinoma in situ of rectosigmoid junction
D01.2	Carcinoma in situ of rectum
D12.0	Benign neoplasm of cecum
D12.1	Benign neoplasm of appendix
D12.4	Benign neoplasm of descending colon
D12.5	Benign neoplasm of sigmoid colon
D12.7	Benign neoplasm of rectosigmoid junction
D12.8	Benign neoplasm of rectum
D37.3	Neoplasm of uncertain behavior of appendix
D37.5	Neoplasm of uncertain behavior of rectum
D3A.021	Benign carcinoid tumor of the cecum
D3A.024	Benign carcinoid tumor of the descending colon
D3A.025	Benign carcinoid tumor of the sigmoid colon
D49.0	Neoplasm of unspecified behavior of digestive system
K50.111	Crohn's disease of large intestine with rectal bleeding
K50.112	Crohn's disease of large intestine with intestinal obstruction
K50.113	Crohn's disease of large intestine with fistula
K50.114	Crohn's disease of large intestine with abscess
K50.118	Crohn's disease of large intestine with other complication
K50.812	Crohn's disease of both small and large intestine with intestinal obstruction
K50.813	Crohn's disease of both small and large intestine with fistula
K50.814	Crohn's disease of both small and large intestine with abscess
K51.011	Ulcerative (chronic) pancolitis with rectal bleeding
K51.012	Ulcerative (chronic) pancolitis with intestinal obstruction
K51.013	Ulcerative (chronic) pancolitis with fistula
K51.014	Ulcerative (chronic) pancolitis with abscess
K51.211	Ulcerative (chronic) proctitis with rectal bleeding
K51.212	Ulcerative (chronic) proctitis with intestinal obstruction
K51.213	Ulcerative (chronic) proctitis with fistula
K51.214	Ulcerative (chronic) proctitis with abscess
K51.312	Ulcerative (chronic) rectosigmoiditis with intestinal obstruction
K51.313	Ulcerative (chronic) rectosigmoiditis with fistula
K51.314	Ulcerative (chronic) rectosigmoiditis with abscess
K51.411	Inflammatory polyps of colon with rectal bleeding
K51.412	Inflammatory polyps of colon with intestinal obstruction
K51.413	Inflammatory polyps of colon with fistula
K51.414	Inflammatory polyps of colon with abscess
K51.511	Left sided colitis with rectal bleeding
K51.512	Left sided colitis with intestinal obstruction
K51.513	Left sided colitis with fistula

K51.514	Left sided colitis with abscess
K52.82	Eosinophilic colitis
K55.041	Focal (segmental) acute infarction of large intestine
K55.042	Diffuse acute infarction of large intestine
K55.1	Chronic vascular disorders of intestine
K55.21	Angiodysplasia of colon with hemorrhage
K55.8	Other vascular disorders of intestine
K56.2	Volvulus
K57.20	Diverticulitis of large intestine with perforation and abscess without bleeding
K57.21	Diverticulitis of large intestine with perforation and abscess with bleeding
K57.33	Diverticulitis of large intestine without perforation or abscess with bleeding
K57.40	Diverticulitis of both small and large intestine with perforation and abscess without bleeding
K57.41	Diverticulitis of both small and large intestine with perforation and abscess with bleeding
K57.51	Diverticulosis of both small and large intestine without perforation or abscess with bleeding
K59.31	Toxic megacolon
K59.81	Ogilvie syndrome
K63.1	Perforation of intestine (nontraumatic)
K63.2	Fistula of intestine
K63.3	Ulcer of intestine
K63.4	Enteroptosis
P77.1	Stage 1 necrotizing enterocolitis in newborn ℕ
P77.2	Stage 2 necrotizing enterocolitis in newborn ℕ
P77.3	Stage 3 necrotizing enterocolitis in newborn ℕ
P78.0	Perinatal intestinal perforation ℕ
Q43.1	Hirschsprung's disease
Q43.2	Other congenital functional disorders of colon
S36.530A	Laceration of ascending [right] colon, initial encounter
S36.531A	Laceration of transverse colon, initial encounter
S36.532A	Laceration of descending [left] colon, initial encounter
S36.533A	Laceration of sigmoid colon, initial encounter
S36.62XA	Contusion of rectum, initial encounter
S36.63XA	Laceration of rectum, initial encounter

AMA: 44157 2014,Jan,11 **44158** 2014,Jan,11

Relative Value Units/Medicare Edits

Non-Facility RVU	Work	PE	MP	Total
44157	35.7	20.44	8.74	64.88
44158	36.7	20.81	8.96	66.47
Facility RVU	**Work**	**PE**	**MP**	**Total**
44157	35.7	20.44	8.74	64.88
44158	36.7	20.81	8.96	66.47

	FUD	Status	MUE	Modifiers				IOM Reference
44157	90	A	1(2)	51	N/A	62*	80	None
44158	90	A	1(2)	51	N/A	62*	80	

* with documentation

44160

44160   Colectomy, partial, with removal of terminal ileum with ileocolostomy

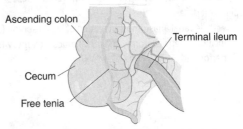

Ascending colon
Terminal ileum
Cecum
Free tenia

Detail of the juncture of the ileum and the colon

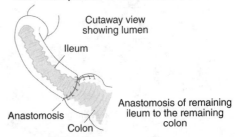

Cutaway view showing lumen
Ileum
Anastomosis
Colon
Anastomosis of remaining ileum to the remaining colon

Explanation

The physician makes an abdominal incision and removes a segment of the colon and terminal ileum and performs an anastomosis between the remaining ileum and colon. The physician makes an abdominal incision. Next, the selected segment of colon and terminal ileum are isolated and divided proximal and distal to the remaining bowel and removed. An anastomosis is created between the distal ileum and remaining colon with staples or sutures. The incision is closed.

Coding Tips

For colectomy, partial, with anastomosis, see 44140; with skin level cecostomy or colostomy, see 44141; with end colostomy and closure of distal segment (Hartmann type procedure), see 44143; with coloproctostomy (low pelvic anastomosis), see 44145; with coloproctostomy (low pelvic anastomosis), with colostomy, see 44146; with abdominal and transanal approach, see 44147.

ICD-10-CM Diagnostic Codes

C17.2	Malignant neoplasm of ileum
C17.3	Meckel's diverticulum, malignant
C18.0	Malignant neoplasm of cecum
C18.1	Malignant neoplasm of appendix
C18.2	Malignant neoplasm of ascending colon
C18.3	Malignant neoplasm of hepatic flexure
C18.4	Malignant neoplasm of transverse colon
C18.5	Malignant neoplasm of splenic flexure
C18.6	Malignant neoplasm of descending colon
C18.7	Malignant neoplasm of sigmoid colon
C18.8	Malignant neoplasm of overlapping sites of colon
C19	Malignant neoplasm of rectosigmoid junction
C49.A4	Gastrointestinal stromal tumor of large intestine
C78.5	Secondary malignant neoplasm of large intestine and rectum
C7A.012	Malignant carcinoid tumor of the ileum
C7A.021	Malignant carcinoid tumor of the cecum
C7A.022	Malignant carcinoid tumor of the ascending colon

C7A.023	Malignant carcinoid tumor of the transverse colon	
C7A.024	Malignant carcinoid tumor of the descending colon	
C7A.025	Malignant carcinoid tumor of the sigmoid colon	
D01.0	Carcinoma in situ of colon	
D01.1	Carcinoma in situ of rectosigmoid junction	
D12.0	Benign neoplasm of cecum	
D12.1	Benign neoplasm of appendix	
D12.2	Benign neoplasm of ascending colon	
D12.3	Benign neoplasm of transverse colon	
D12.4	Benign neoplasm of descending colon	
D12.5	Benign neoplasm of sigmoid colon	
D12.7	Benign neoplasm of rectosigmoid junction	
D13.39	Benign neoplasm of other parts of small intestine	
D37.3	Neoplasm of uncertain behavior of appendix	
D37.4	Neoplasm of uncertain behavior of colon	
D3A.021	Benign carcinoid tumor of the cecum	
D3A.022	Benign carcinoid tumor of the ascending colon	
D3A.023	Benign carcinoid tumor of the transverse colon	
D3A.024	Benign carcinoid tumor of the descending colon	
D3A.025	Benign carcinoid tumor of the sigmoid colon	
D49.0	Neoplasm of unspecified behavior of digestive system	
K50.111	Crohn's disease of large intestine with rectal bleeding	
K50.112	Crohn's disease of large intestine with intestinal obstruction	
K50.113	Crohn's disease of large intestine with fistula	
K50.114	Crohn's disease of large intestine with abscess	
K50.118	Crohn's disease of large intestine with other complication	
K50.812	Crohn's disease of both small and large intestine with intestinal obstruction	
K50.813	Crohn's disease of both small and large intestine with fistula	
K50.814	Crohn's disease of both small and large intestine with abscess	
K51.011	Ulcerative (chronic) pancolitis with rectal bleeding	
K51.012	Ulcerative (chronic) pancolitis with intestinal obstruction	
K51.013	Ulcerative (chronic) pancolitis with fistula	
K51.014	Ulcerative (chronic) pancolitis with abscess	
K51.311	Ulcerative (chronic) rectosigmoiditis with rectal bleeding	
K51.312	Ulcerative (chronic) rectosigmoiditis with intestinal obstruction	
K51.313	Ulcerative (chronic) rectosigmoiditis with fistula	
K51.314	Ulcerative (chronic) rectosigmoiditis with abscess	
K51.411	Inflammatory polyps of colon with rectal bleeding	
K51.412	Inflammatory polyps of colon with intestinal obstruction	
K51.413	Inflammatory polyps of colon with fistula	
K51.414	Inflammatory polyps of colon with abscess	
K51.511	Left sided colitis with rectal bleeding	
K51.512	Left sided colitis with intestinal obstruction	
K51.513	Left sided colitis with fistula	
K51.514	Left sided colitis with abscess	
K52.82	Eosinophilic colitis	
K55.041	Focal (segmental) acute infarction of large intestine	
K55.042	Diffuse acute infarction of large intestine	
K55.1	Chronic vascular disorders of intestine	
K55.21	Angiodysplasia of colon with hemorrhage	
K55.8	Other vascular disorders of intestine	
K56.0	Paralytic ileus	
K56.1	Intussusception	
K56.2	Volvulus	
K56.51	Intestinal adhesions [bands], with partial obstruction	
K56.52	Intestinal adhesions [bands] with complete obstruction	
K56.690	Other partial intestinal obstruction	
K56.691	Other complete intestinal obstruction	
K57.20	Diverticulitis of large intestine with perforation and abscess without bleeding	
K57.21	Diverticulitis of large intestine with perforation and abscess with bleeding	
K57.33	Diverticulitis of large intestine without perforation or abscess with bleeding	
K57.40	Diverticulitis of both small and large intestine with perforation and abscess without bleeding	
K57.41	Diverticulitis of both small and large intestine with perforation and abscess with bleeding	
K57.51	Diverticulosis of both small and large intestine without perforation or abscess with bleeding	
K59.31	Toxic megacolon	
K59.81	Ogilvie syndrome	
K63.1	Perforation of intestine (nontraumatic)	
K63.2	Fistula of intestine	
K63.3	Ulcer of intestine	
K63.4	Enteroptosis	
P77.1	Stage 1 necrotizing enterocolitis in newborn N	
P77.2	Stage 2 necrotizing enterocolitis in newborn N	
P77.3	Stage 3 necrotizing enterocolitis in newborn N	
P78.0	Perinatal intestinal perforation N	
Q43.1	Hirschsprung's disease	
Q43.2	Other congenital functional disorders of colon	
S36.530A	Laceration of ascending [right] colon, initial encounter	
S36.531A	Laceration of transverse colon, initial encounter	
S36.532A	Laceration of descending [left] colon, initial encounter	
S36.533A	Laceration of sigmoid colon, initial encounter	

AMA: 44160 2018,Jan,8; 2017,Jan,8; 2016,Jan,13; 2015,Jan,16

Relative Value Units/Medicare Edits

Non-Facility RVU	Work	PE	MP	Total
44160	20.89	11.07	4.59	36.55
Facility RVU	**Work**	**PE**	**MP**	**Total**
44160	20.89	11.07	4.59	36.55

	FUD	Status	MUE	Modifiers				IOM Reference
44160	90	A	1(2)	51	N/A	62*	80	None

* with documentation

44180

44180 Laparoscopy, surgical, enterolysis (freeing of intestinal adhesion) (separate procedure)

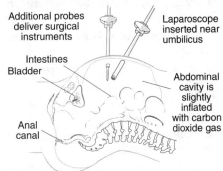

Intestinal adhesions are removed laparoscopically after the abdominal cavity has been insufflated

Additional probes deliver surgical instruments

Laparoscope inserted near umbilicus

Intestines
Bladder

Abdominal cavity is slightly inflated with carbon dioxide gas

Anal canal

Explanation

The physician performs laparoscopic enterolysis to free intestinal adhesions. With the patient under anesthesia, the physician places a trocar at the umbilicus into the abdominal or retroperitoneal space and insufflates the abdominal cavity. The physician places a laparoscope through the umbilical incision and additional trocars are placed into the abdomen. Intestinal adhesions are identified and instruments are passed through to dissect and remove the adhesions. The trocars are removed and the incisions are closed with sutures.

Coding Tips

This separate procedure by definition is usually a component of a more complex service and is not identified separately. When performed with other unrelated procedures, list the code and append modifier 59 or an X{EPSU} modifier. Surgical laparoscopy always includes diagnostic laparoscopy.

ICD-10-CM Diagnostic Codes

K31.5	Obstruction of duodenum
K50.012	Crohn's disease of small intestine with intestinal obstruction
K50.112	Crohn's disease of large intestine with intestinal obstruction
K50.812	Crohn's disease of both small and large intestine with intestinal obstruction
K51.012	Ulcerative (chronic) pancolitis with intestinal obstruction
K51.312	Ulcerative (chronic) rectosigmoiditis with intestinal obstruction
K51.412	Inflammatory polyps of colon with intestinal obstruction
K51.512	Left sided colitis with intestinal obstruction
K51.812	Other ulcerative colitis with intestinal obstruction
K56.51	Intestinal adhesions [bands], with partial obstruction
K56.52	Intestinal adhesions [bands] with complete obstruction
K56.690	Other partial intestinal obstruction
K56.691	Other complete intestinal obstruction
K66.0	Peritoneal adhesions (postprocedural) (postinfection)
K91.31	Postprocedural partial intestinal obstruction
K91.32	Postprocedural complete intestinal obstruction
Q43.3	Congenital malformations of intestinal fixation
R10.31	Right lower quadrant pain
R10.32	Left lower quadrant pain
R10.33	Periumbilical pain
R10.84	Generalized abdominal pain
R19.01	Right upper quadrant abdominal swelling, mass and lump
R19.02	Left upper quadrant abdominal swelling, mass and lump
R19.03	Right lower quadrant abdominal swelling, mass and lump
R19.04	Left lower quadrant abdominal swelling, mass and lump
R19.05	Periumbilic swelling, mass or lump
R19.06	Epigastric swelling, mass or lump
R19.07	Generalized intra-abdominal and pelvic swelling, mass and lump
R19.09	Other intra-abdominal and pelvic swelling, mass and lump

AMA: **44180** 2018,Jan,8; 2018,Feb,11; 2017,Jan,8; 2016,Jan,13; 2015,Jan,16

Relative Value Units/Medicare Edits

Non-Facility RVU	Work	PE	MP	Total
44180	15.27	8.35	3.55	27.17
Facility RVU	**Work**	**PE**	**MP**	**Total**
44180	15.27	8.35	3.55	27.17

	FUD	Status	MUE	Modifiers				IOM Reference
44180	90	A	1(2)	51	N/A	62*	80	None

* with documentation

Terms To Know

adhesion. Abnormal fibrous connection between two structures, soft tissue or bony structures, that may occur as the result of surgery, infection, or trauma.

enterolysis. Division of intestinal adhesions.

retroperitoneal. Located behind the peritoneum, the membrane that lines the abdominopelvic walls and forms a covering for the internal organs.

trocar. Cannula or a sharp pointed instrument used to puncture and aspirate fluid from cavities.

44186-44187

44186 Laparoscopy, surgical; jejunostomy (eg, for decompression or feeding)
44187 ileostomy or jejunostomy, non-tube

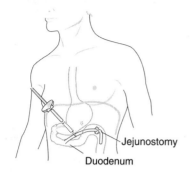

Jejunostomy
Duodenum

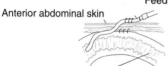

Feeding tube
Anterior abdominal skin
Bowel lumen

A route from the bowel to
the skin surface is established

Explanation

In 44186, the physician constructs a jejunostomy using a laparoscope. With the patient under anesthesia, the physician makes small incisions into the abdomen, places one trocar at the umbilicus into the abdomen, and insufflates the abdominal cavity. The physician places a laparoscope through one of the incisions with additional instruments introduced through the trocars. The tube is placed into the jejunostomy with the other end sutured to the skin at the exit point. The trocars are removed and the incisions are closed with sutures. In 44187, the physician constructs a non-tube ileostomy or jejunostomy using a laparoscope. With the patient under general anesthesia, the physician places a trocar at the umbilicus into the abdomen and insufflates the abdominal cavity. The physician places a laparoscope through the umbilical incision. Additional trocars are placed through which the specialized surgical instruments are inserted. Next, the selected segment of jejunum or ileum is isolated. A loop or end of the selected segment of bowel is located and grasped. The skin and fat are excised, the fascia is opened, and the loop is exteriorized through a previously defined ileostomy or jejunostomy site. The laparoscope is removed, the ports are closed with incisions, and the stoma is matured.

Coding Tips

Surgical laparoscopy always includes diagnostic laparoscopy. For open non-tube ileostomy or jejunostomy, see 44310.

ICD-10-CM Diagnostic Codes

C15.3	Malignant neoplasm of upper third of esophagus
C15.4	Malignant neoplasm of middle third of esophagus
C15.5	Malignant neoplasm of lower third of esophagus
C15.8	Malignant neoplasm of overlapping sites of esophagus
C16.0	Malignant neoplasm of cardia
C16.1	Malignant neoplasm of fundus of stomach
C16.2	Malignant neoplasm of body of stomach
C16.3	Malignant neoplasm of pyloric antrum
C16.4	Malignant neoplasm of pylorus
C16.8	Malignant neoplasm of overlapping sites of stomach
C17.0	Malignant neoplasm of duodenum
C25.0	Malignant neoplasm of head of pancreas
C25.1	Malignant neoplasm of body of pancreas
C25.2	Malignant neoplasm of tail of pancreas
C25.3	Malignant neoplasm of pancreatic duct
C25.4	Malignant neoplasm of endocrine pancreas
C25.7	Malignant neoplasm of other parts of pancreas
C25.8	Malignant neoplasm of overlapping sites of pancreas
C76.0	Malignant neoplasm of head, face and neck
C78.4	Secondary malignant neoplasm of small intestine
C78.89	Secondary malignant neoplasm of other digestive organs
C7A.010	Malignant carcinoid tumor of the duodenum
C7A.092	Malignant carcinoid tumor of the stomach
D00.2	Carcinoma in situ of stomach
E41	Nutritional marasmus
E44.0	Moderate protein-calorie malnutrition
E44.1	Mild protein-calorie malnutrition
E45	Retarded development following protein-calorie malnutrition
E86.0	Dehydration
E86.1	Hypovolemia
I69.091	Dysphagia following nontraumatic subarachnoid hemorrhage
I69.191	Dysphagia following nontraumatic intracerebral hemorrhage
I69.291	Dysphagia following other nontraumatic intracranial hemorrhage
I69.391	Dysphagia following cerebral infarction
K20.80	Other esophagitis without bleeding
K20.81	Other esophagitis with bleeding
K21.00	Gastro-esophageal reflux disease with esophagitis, without bleeding
K21.01	Gastro-esophageal reflux disease with esophagitis, with bleeding
K22.2	Esophageal obstruction
K22.3	Perforation of esophagus
K22.4	Dyskinesia of esophagus
K25.0	Acute gastric ulcer with hemorrhage
K25.1	Acute gastric ulcer with perforation
K25.2	Acute gastric ulcer with both hemorrhage and perforation
K25.4	Chronic or unspecified gastric ulcer with hemorrhage
K25.5	Chronic or unspecified gastric ulcer with perforation
K25.6	Chronic or unspecified gastric ulcer with both hemorrhage and perforation
K26.0	Acute duodenal ulcer with hemorrhage
K26.2	Acute duodenal ulcer with both hemorrhage and perforation
K26.5	Chronic or unspecified duodenal ulcer with perforation
K26.6	Chronic or unspecified duodenal ulcer with both hemorrhage and perforation
K26.7	Chronic duodenal ulcer without hemorrhage or perforation
K28.0	Acute gastrojejunal ulcer with hemorrhage
K28.1	Acute gastrojejunal ulcer with perforation
K28.2	Acute gastrojejunal ulcer with both hemorrhage and perforation
K28.4	Chronic or unspecified gastrojejunal ulcer with hemorrhage
K28.5	Chronic or unspecified gastrojejunal ulcer with perforation
K28.6	Chronic or unspecified gastrojejunal ulcer with both hemorrhage and perforation
K28.7	Chronic gastrojejunal ulcer without hemorrhage or perforation

K86.0	Alcohol-induced chronic pancreatitis
K86.1	Other chronic pancreatitis
K86.2	Cyst of pancreas
K86.3	Pseudocyst of pancreas
K91.1	Postgastric surgery syndromes
K91.2	Postsurgical malabsorption, not elsewhere classified
K91.89	Other postprocedural complications and disorders of digestive system
Q39.5	Congenital dilatation of esophagus
Q40.2	Other specified congenital malformations of stomach
Q41.0	Congenital absence, atresia and stenosis of duodenum
R13.0	Aphagia
R13.11	Dysphagia, oral phase
R13.12	Dysphagia, oropharyngeal phase
R13.13	Dysphagia, pharyngeal phase
R13.14	Dysphagia, pharyngoesophageal phase
R62.7	Adult failure to thrive 🅰
R63.0	Anorexia
R63.32	Pediatric feeding disorder, chronic 🅿
R63.39	Other feeding difficulties
S36.430A	Laceration of duodenum, initial encounter
S36.438A	Laceration of other part of small intestine, initial encounter
S36.490A	Other injury of duodenum, initial encounter
S36.498A	Other injury of other part of small intestine, initial encounter
T73.0XXA	Starvation, initial encounter

AMA: 44186 2018,Jan,8; 2017,Jan,8; 2016,Jan,13; 2015,Jan,16 **44187** 2019,Sep,10; 2018,Jan,8; 2017,Jan,8; 2016,Jan,13; 2015,Jan,16

Relative Value Units/Medicare Edits

Non-Facility RVU	Work	PE	MP	Total
44186	10.38	6.44	2.46	19.28
44187	17.4	11.59	3.27	32.26
Facility RVU	Work	PE	MP	Total
44186	10.38	6.44	2.46	19.28
44187	17.4	11.59	3.27	32.26

	FUD	Status	MUE	Modifiers				IOM Reference
44186	90	A	1(2)	51	N/A	62*	80	None
44187	90	A	1(3)	51	N/A	62*	80	

* with documentation

44188

44188 Laparoscopy, surgical, colostomy or skin level cecostomy

A colostomy or skin level cecostomy is performed

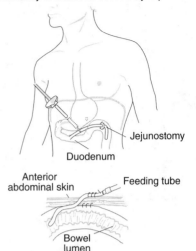

Explanation

The physician constructs a colostomy or skin level cecostomy using a laparoscope. With the patient under general anesthesia, the physician places a trocar at the umbilicus into the abdomen and insufflates the abdominal cavity. The physician places a laparoscope through the umbilical incision. Additional trocars are placed, through which the specialized surgical instruments are inserted. The selected segment of colon or cecum is isolated. The physician brings a loop, end of colon, or cecum onto the skin as a stoma (colostomy or cecostomy) through a small incision in the abdominal wall. The laparoscope is removed, the ports are closed with incisions, and the stoma is matured.

Coding Tips

Surgical laparoscopy always includes diagnostic laparoscopy. Do not report this code with 44970. For open approach, see 44320.

ICD-10-CM Diagnostic Codes

C18.0	Malignant neoplasm of cecum
C18.3	Malignant neoplasm of hepatic flexure
C18.4	Malignant neoplasm of transverse colon
C18.6	Malignant neoplasm of descending colon
C18.7	Malignant neoplasm of sigmoid colon
C19	Malignant neoplasm of rectosigmoid junction
C20	Malignant neoplasm of rectum
C21.1	Malignant neoplasm of anal canal
C21.2	Malignant neoplasm of cloacogenic zone
C21.8	Malignant neoplasm of overlapping sites of rectum, anus and anal canal
C78.5	Secondary malignant neoplasm of large intestine and rectum
C7A.020	Malignant carcinoid tumor of the appendix
C7A.021	Malignant carcinoid tumor of the cecum
C7A.022	Malignant carcinoid tumor of the ascending colon
C7A.023	Malignant carcinoid tumor of the transverse colon
C7A.024	Malignant carcinoid tumor of the descending colon

C7A.025	Malignant carcinoid tumor of the sigmoid colon	
C7A.026	Malignant carcinoid tumor of the rectum	
D01.0	Carcinoma in situ of colon	
D01.1	Carcinoma in situ of rectosigmoid junction	
D01.2	Carcinoma in situ of rectum	
D01.7	Carcinoma in situ of other specified digestive organs	
D12.0	Benign neoplasm of cecum	
D12.1	Benign neoplasm of appendix	
D12.2	Benign neoplasm of ascending colon	
D12.3	Benign neoplasm of transverse colon	
D12.4	Benign neoplasm of descending colon	
D12.5	Benign neoplasm of sigmoid colon	
D37.4	Neoplasm of uncertain behavior of colon	
D37.5	Neoplasm of uncertain behavior of rectum	
D3A.020	Benign carcinoid tumor of the appendix	
D3A.021	Benign carcinoid tumor of the cecum	
D3A.022	Benign carcinoid tumor of the ascending colon	
D3A.023	Benign carcinoid tumor of the transverse colon	
D3A.024	Benign carcinoid tumor of the descending colon	
D3A.025	Benign carcinoid tumor of the sigmoid colon	
D3A.026	Benign carcinoid tumor of the rectum	
D49.0	Neoplasm of unspecified behavior of digestive system	
K50.111	Crohn's disease of large intestine with rectal bleeding	
K50.112	Crohn's disease of large intestine with intestinal obstruction	
K50.113	Crohn's disease of large intestine with fistula	
K50.114	Crohn's disease of large intestine with abscess	
K50.118	Crohn's disease of large intestine with other complication	
K50.80	Crohn's disease of both small and large intestine without complications	
K50.811	Crohn's disease of both small and large intestine with rectal bleeding	
K50.813	Crohn's disease of both small and large intestine with fistula	
K50.814	Crohn's disease of both small and large intestine with abscess	
K51.011	Ulcerative (chronic) pancolitis with rectal bleeding	
K51.012	Ulcerative (chronic) pancolitis with intestinal obstruction	
K51.014	Ulcerative (chronic) pancolitis with abscess	
K51.211	Ulcerative (chronic) proctitis with rectal bleeding	
K51.212	Ulcerative (chronic) proctitis with intestinal obstruction	
K51.213	Ulcerative (chronic) proctitis with fistula	
K51.214	Ulcerative (chronic) proctitis with abscess	
K51.311	Ulcerative (chronic) rectosigmoiditis with rectal bleeding	
K51.313	Ulcerative (chronic) rectosigmoiditis with fistula	
K51.314	Ulcerative (chronic) rectosigmoiditis with abscess	
K51.412	Inflammatory polyps of colon with intestinal obstruction	
K51.413	Inflammatory polyps of colon with fistula	
K51.512	Left sided colitis with intestinal obstruction	
K51.513	Left sided colitis with fistula	
K51.514	Left sided colitis with abscess	
K52.82	Eosinophilic colitis	
K55.021	Focal (segmental) acute infarction of small intestine	
K55.022	Diffuse acute infarction of small intestine	
K56.2	Volvulus	
K56.51	Intestinal adhesions [bands], with partial obstruction	

K56.52	Intestinal adhesions [bands] with complete obstruction
K56.690	Other partial intestinal obstruction
K56.691	Other complete intestinal obstruction
K57.20	Diverticulitis of large intestine with perforation and abscess without bleeding
K57.31	Diverticulosis of large intestine without perforation or abscess with bleeding
K57.33	Diverticulitis of large intestine without perforation or abscess with bleeding
K57.41	Diverticulitis of both small and large intestine with perforation and abscess with bleeding
K57.53	Diverticulitis of both small and large intestine without perforation or abscess with bleeding
K59.81	Ogilvie syndrome
K60.3	Anal fistula
K60.4	Rectal fistula
K60.5	Anorectal fistula
K61.1	Rectal abscess
K62.5	Hemorrhage of anus and rectum
K62.6	Ulcer of anus and rectum
K62.7	Radiation proctitis
K63.0	Abscess of intestine
K63.1	Perforation of intestine (nontraumatic)
K63.2	Fistula of intestine
K63.3	Ulcer of intestine
N32.1	Vesicointestinal fistula
N82.3	Fistula of vagina to large intestine ♀
Q42.0	Congenital absence, atresia and stenosis of rectum with fistula
Q42.2	Congenital absence, atresia and stenosis of anus with fistula
Q43.1	Hirschsprung's disease
Q43.8	Other specified congenital malformations of intestine
Q64.73	Congenital urethrorectal fistula
R15.9	Full incontinence of feces

AMA: **44188** 2018,Jan,8; 2017,Jan,8; 2016,Jan,13; 2015,Jan,16

Relative Value Units/Medicare Edits

Non-Facility RVU	Work	PE	MP	Total
44188	19.35	12.54	4.06	35.95
Facility RVU	Work	PE	MP	Total
44188	19.35	12.54	4.06	35.95

	FUD	Status	MUE	Modifiers				IOM Reference
44188	90	A	1(3)	51	N/A	62*	80	None

* with documentation

Terms To Know

colostomy. Artificial surgical opening anywhere along the length of the colon to the skin surface for the diversion of feces.

stoma. Opening created in the abdominal wall from an internal organ or structure for diversion of waste elimination, drainage, and access.

44202-44203

44202 Laparoscopy, surgical; enterectomy, resection of small intestine, single resection and anastomosis

+ 44203 each additional small intestine resection and anastomosis (List separately in addition to code for primary procedure)

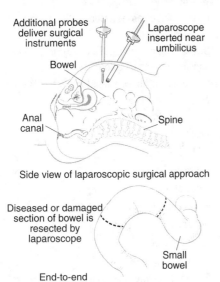

Additional probes deliver surgical instruments

Laparoscope inserted near umbilicus

Bowel

Anal canal

Spine

Side view of laparoscopic surgical approach

Diseased or damaged section of bowel is resected by laparoscope

Small bowel

End-to-end anastomosis

Explanation

The physician performs a laparoscopic single resection and anastomosis of the small intestine. With the patient under general anesthesia, a urinary catheter is inserted and the patient is placed in a supine or Trendelenburg position on the operating table. Carbon dioxide gas is used to insufflate the abdomen through a laparoscopic port placed through the umbilicus. The laparoscope is positioned in the abdominal cavity and a diagnostic laparoscopy is performed. The remaining laparoscopic ports are placed under direct vision. The transverse colon is located and maintained in upward traction. The ligament of Treitz is identified and the small intestine is run. The targeted section of small intestine is marked and suspended with traction sutures through the mesentery. The peritoneum overlying the mesentery is scored and the segment of small intestine marked for resection is devascularized. The bowel is divided proximal and distal to the segment with a stapler. The segment is brought out through an enlarged trocar site. The divided bowel ends are anastomosed with staples and inspected. The mesentery is closed with interrupted sutures. The trocars and laparoscope are removed and the incisions are closed with sutures. Report 44203 for each additional small intestine resection and anastomosis beyond the first.

Coding Tips

Report 44203 in addition to 44202. Surgical laparoscopy always includes diagnostic laparoscopy. For an open approach, see 44120–44121.

ICD-10-CM Diagnostic Codes

C17.0	Malignant neoplasm of duodenum
C17.1	Malignant neoplasm of jejunum
C17.2	Malignant neoplasm of ileum
C17.3	Meckel's diverticulum, malignant
C49.A3	Gastrointestinal stromal tumor of small intestine
C78.4	Secondary malignant neoplasm of small intestine
C7A.010	Malignant carcinoid tumor of the duodenum
C7A.011	Malignant carcinoid tumor of the jejunum
C7A.012	Malignant carcinoid tumor of the ileum
D01.7	Carcinoma in situ of other specified digestive organs
D13.2	Benign neoplasm of duodenum
D13.39	Benign neoplasm of other parts of small intestine
D37.2	Neoplasm of uncertain behavior of small intestine
D3A.010	Benign carcinoid tumor of the duodenum
D3A.011	Benign carcinoid tumor of the jejunum
D3A.012	Benign carcinoid tumor of the ileum
K26.0	Acute duodenal ulcer with hemorrhage
K26.1	Acute duodenal ulcer with perforation
K26.2	Acute duodenal ulcer with both hemorrhage and perforation
K26.3	Acute duodenal ulcer without hemorrhage or perforation
K26.4	Chronic or unspecified duodenal ulcer with hemorrhage
K26.5	Chronic or unspecified duodenal ulcer with perforation
K26.6	Chronic or unspecified duodenal ulcer with both hemorrhage and perforation
K26.7	Chronic duodenal ulcer without hemorrhage or perforation
K31.5	Obstruction of duodenum
K31.6	Fistula of stomach and duodenum
K31.811	Angiodysplasia of stomach and duodenum with bleeding
K31.819	Angiodysplasia of stomach and duodenum without bleeding
K31.82	Dieulafoy lesion (hemorrhagic) of stomach and duodenum
K31.89	Other diseases of stomach and duodenum
K43.0	Incisional hernia with obstruction, without gangrene
K43.1	Incisional hernia with gangrene
K50.011	Crohn's disease of small intestine with rectal bleeding
K50.012	Crohn's disease of small intestine with intestinal obstruction
K50.013	Crohn's disease of small intestine with fistula
K50.014	Crohn's disease of small intestine with abscess
K50.812	Crohn's disease of both small and large intestine with intestinal obstruction
K50.813	Crohn's disease of both small and large intestine with fistula
K50.814	Crohn's disease of both small and large intestine with abscess
K55.021	Focal (segmental) acute infarction of small intestine
K55.022	Diffuse acute infarction of small intestine
K55.1	Chronic vascular disorders of intestine
K56.0	Paralytic ileus
K56.1	Intussusception
K56.2	Volvulus
K56.51	Intestinal adhesions [bands], with partial obstruction
K56.52	Intestinal adhesions [bands] with complete obstruction
K57.00	Diverticulitis of small intestine with perforation and abscess without bleeding
K57.01	Diverticulitis of small intestine with perforation and abscess with bleeding
K57.10	Diverticulosis of small intestine without perforation or abscess without bleeding
K57.11	Diverticulosis of small intestine without perforation or abscess with bleeding
K57.12	Diverticulitis of small intestine without perforation or abscess without bleeding

Intestines

K57.13	Diverticulitis of small intestine without perforation or abscess with bleeding
K57.40	Diverticulitis of both small and large intestine with perforation and abscess without bleeding
K57.41	Diverticulitis of both small and large intestine with perforation and abscess with bleeding
K57.50	Diverticulosis of both small and large intestine without perforation or abscess without bleeding
K57.51	Diverticulosis of both small and large intestine without perforation or abscess with bleeding
K57.52	Diverticulitis of both small and large intestine without perforation or abscess without bleeding
K57.53	Diverticulitis of both small and large intestine without perforation or abscess with bleeding
K63.0	Abscess of intestine
K63.1	Perforation of intestine (nontraumatic)
K63.2	Fistula of intestine
K63.3	Ulcer of intestine
K91.31	Postprocedural partial intestinal obstruction
K91.32	Postprocedural complete intestinal obstruction
K91.71	Accidental puncture and laceration of a digestive system organ or structure during a digestive system procedure
K91.72	Accidental puncture and laceration of a digestive system organ or structure during other procedure
N80.5	Endometriosis of intestine ♀
Q41.0	Congenital absence, atresia and stenosis of duodenum
Q41.1	Congenital absence, atresia and stenosis of jejunum
Q41.2	Congenital absence, atresia and stenosis of ileum
Q43.0	Meckel's diverticulum (displaced) (hypertrophic)
Q43.3	Congenital malformations of intestinal fixation
S36.410A	Primary blast injury of duodenum, initial encounter
S36.418A	Primary blast injury of other part of small intestine, initial encounter
S36.430A	Laceration of duodenum, initial encounter
S36.438A	Laceration of other part of small intestine, initial encounter

AMA: **44202** 2020,Jul,13; 2018,Jan,8; 2017,Jan,8; 2016,Jan,13; 2015,Jan,16
44203 2018,Jan,8; 2017,Jan,8; 2016,Jan,13; 2015,Jan,16

Relative Value Units/Medicare Edits

Non-Facility RVU	Work	PE	MP	Total
44202	23.39	12.17	5.3	40.86
44203	4.44	1.63	0.98	7.05
Facility RVU	Work	PE	MP	Total
44202	23.39	12.17	5.3	40.86
44203	4.44	1.63	0.98	7.05

	FUD	Status	MUE	Modifiers				IOM Reference
44202	90	A	1(2)	51	N/A	62*	80	None
44203	N/A	A	2(3)	N/A	N/A	62*	80	
* with documentation								

44204

44204 Laparoscopy, surgical; colectomy, partial, with anastomosis

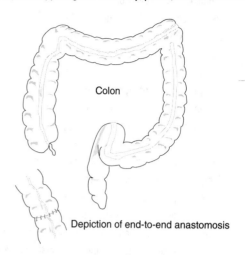

Colon

Depiction of end-to-end anastomosis

The colon is surgically accessed and a section is removed. The two ends are anastomosed together

Explanation

With the patient under general anesthesia, a urinary catheter is inserted and the patient is placed supine or in a Trendelenburg position on the operating table. Carbon dioxide gas is used to insufflate the abdomen through a laparoscopic port placed through the umbilicus. The laparoscope is positioned in the abdominal cavity and a diagnostic laparoscopy is performed. The remaining laparoscopic ports are placed under direct vision. The physician incises peritoneum along both sides to mobilize the colon. The greater omentum and colon are separated by incision to mobilize the hepatic and splenic flexures. The colon is mobilized centrally onto its mesentery and the mesenteric vessels are divided intracorporeally using titanium clips. The colon is divided with an endoscopic stapler, and the specimen is removed through an enlarged trocar site. If the procedure is being performed for malignancy, a wound protector is used. The divided bowel ends are anastomosed and inspected. The abdomen is deflated. The laparoscope and trocar incisions are closed.

Coding Tips

For open approach, see 44140. Surgical laparoscopy always includes diagnostic laparoscopy. For mobilization (takedown) of splenic flexure performed with this code, see 44213.

ICD-10-CM Diagnostic Codes

C18.2	Malignant neoplasm of ascending colon
C18.3	Malignant neoplasm of hepatic flexure
C18.4	Malignant neoplasm of transverse colon
C18.5	Malignant neoplasm of splenic flexure
C18.6	Malignant neoplasm of descending colon
C18.7	Malignant neoplasm of sigmoid colon
C19	Malignant neoplasm of rectosigmoid junction
C49.A4	Gastrointestinal stromal tumor of large intestine
C78.5	Secondary malignant neoplasm of large intestine and rectum
C7A.021	Malignant carcinoid tumor of the cecum
C7A.022	Malignant carcinoid tumor of the ascending colon
C7A.023	Malignant carcinoid tumor of the transverse colon
C7A.024	Malignant carcinoid tumor of the descending colon

C7A.025	Malignant carcinoid tumor of the sigmoid colon
D01.0	Carcinoma in situ of colon
D01.1	Carcinoma in situ of rectosigmoid junction
D12.0	Benign neoplasm of cecum
D12.1	Benign neoplasm of appendix
D12.2	Benign neoplasm of ascending colon
D12.3	Benign neoplasm of transverse colon
D12.4	Benign neoplasm of descending colon
D12.5	Benign neoplasm of sigmoid colon
D12.7	Benign neoplasm of rectosigmoid junction
D37.3	Neoplasm of uncertain behavior of appendix
D37.4	Neoplasm of uncertain behavior of colon
D3A.022	Benign carcinoid tumor of the ascending colon
D3A.023	Benign carcinoid tumor of the transverse colon
D3A.024	Benign carcinoid tumor of the descending colon
D3A.025	Benign carcinoid tumor of the sigmoid colon
D49.0	Neoplasm of unspecified behavior of digestive system
K50.111	Crohn's disease of large intestine with rectal bleeding
K50.112	Crohn's disease of large intestine with intestinal obstruction
K50.113	Crohn's disease of large intestine with fistula
K50.114	Crohn's disease of large intestine with abscess
K50.811	Crohn's disease of both small and large intestine with rectal bleeding
K50.812	Crohn's disease of both small and large intestine with intestinal obstruction
K50.813	Crohn's disease of both small and large intestine with fistula
K50.814	Crohn's disease of both small and large intestine with abscess
K51.011	Ulcerative (chronic) pancolitis with rectal bleeding
K51.012	Ulcerative (chronic) pancolitis with intestinal obstruction
K51.013	Ulcerative (chronic) pancolitis with fistula
K51.014	Ulcerative (chronic) pancolitis with abscess
K51.311	Ulcerative (chronic) rectosigmoiditis with rectal bleeding
K51.312	Ulcerative (chronic) rectosigmoiditis with intestinal obstruction
K51.313	Ulcerative (chronic) rectosigmoiditis with fistula
K51.314	Ulcerative (chronic) rectosigmoiditis with abscess
K51.411	Inflammatory polyps of colon with rectal bleeding
K51.412	Inflammatory polyps of colon with intestinal obstruction
K51.413	Inflammatory polyps of colon with fistula
K51.414	Inflammatory polyps of colon with abscess
K51.511	Left sided colitis with rectal bleeding
K51.512	Left sided colitis with intestinal obstruction
K51.513	Left sided colitis with fistula
K51.514	Left sided colitis with abscess
K55.041	Focal (segmental) acute infarction of large intestine
K55.042	Diffuse acute infarction of large intestine
K55.1	Chronic vascular disorders of intestine
K55.20	Angiodysplasia of colon without hemorrhage
K55.21	Angiodysplasia of colon with hemorrhage
K56.0	Paralytic ileus
K56.1	Intussusception
K56.2	Volvulus
K56.51	Intestinal adhesions [bands], with partial obstruction
K56.52	Intestinal adhesions [bands] with complete obstruction

K57.20	Diverticulitis of large intestine with perforation and abscess without bleeding
K57.21	Diverticulitis of large intestine with perforation and abscess with bleeding
K57.31	Diverticulosis of large intestine without perforation or abscess with bleeding
K57.32	Diverticulitis of large intestine without perforation or abscess without bleeding
K57.33	Diverticulitis of large intestine without perforation or abscess with bleeding
K57.40	Diverticulitis of both small and large intestine with perforation and abscess without bleeding
K57.41	Diverticulitis of both small and large intestine with perforation and abscess with bleeding
K59.31	Toxic megacolon
K59.81	Ogilvie syndrome
K63.0	Abscess of intestine
K63.1	Perforation of intestine (nontraumatic)
K63.2	Fistula of intestine
K63.3	Ulcer of intestine
K63.4	Enteroptosis
K63.5	Polyp of colon
N32.1	Vesicointestinal fistula
P77.1	Stage 1 necrotizing enterocolitis in newborn N
P77.2	Stage 2 necrotizing enterocolitis in newborn N
P77.3	Stage 3 necrotizing enterocolitis in newborn N
Q42.8	Congenital absence, atresia and stenosis of other parts of large intestine
Q43.1	Hirschsprung's disease
Q43.2	Other congenital functional disorders of colon
Q43.3	Congenital malformations of intestinal fixation
Q43.4	Duplication of intestine
S36.530A	Laceration of ascending [right] colon, initial encounter
S36.531A	Laceration of transverse colon, initial encounter
S36.532A	Laceration of descending [left] colon, initial encounter
S36.533A	Laceration of sigmoid colon, initial encounter
S36.538A	Laceration of other part of colon, initial encounter

AMA: **44204** 2018,Jan,8; 2017,Jan,8; 2017,Dec,14; 2016,Jan,13; 2015,Jan,16

Relative Value Units/Medicare Edits

Non-Facility RVU	Work	PE	MP	Total
44204	26.42	13.23	5.5	45.15
Facility RVU	**Work**	**PE**	**MP**	**Total**
44204	26.42	13.23	5.5	45.15

	FUD	Status	MUE	Modifiers				IOM Reference
44204	90	A	2(3)	51	N/A	62*	80	None

* with documentation

44205

44205 Laparoscopy, surgical; colectomy, partial, with removal of terminal ileum with ileocolostomy

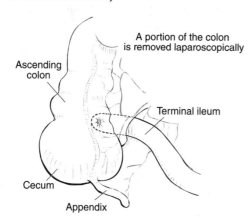

A portion of the colon is removed laparoscopically

Ascending colon

Terminal ileum

Cecum

Appendix

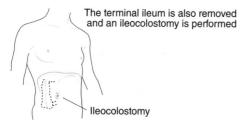

The terminal ileum is also removed and an ileocolostomy is performed

Ileocolostomy

Explanation

With the patient under general anesthesia, a urinary catheter is inserted and the patient is placed supine or in a Trendelenburg position on the operating table. Carbon dioxide gas is used to insufflate the abdomen through a laparoscopic port placed through the umbilicus. The laparoscope is positioned in the abdominal cavity and a diagnostic laparoscopy is performed. The remaining laparoscopic ports are placed under direct vision. The physician incises peritoneum along both sides to mobilize the colon. The greater omentum and colon are separated by incision to mobilize the hepatic and splenic flexures. The colon is mobilized centrally onto its mesentery and the mesenteric vessels are divided intracorporeally using titanium clips. The colon is divided with an endoscopic stapler and the specimen is removed through an enlarged trocar site. If the procedure is being performed for malignancy, a wound protector is used. The selected segment of colon and terminal ileum are isolated and divided proximal and distal to the remaining bowel and removed. An anastomosis is created between the distal ileum and remaining colon. The abdomen is deflated and the laparoscope and trocar incisions are closed.

Coding Tips

For open approach, see 44160. Surgical laparoscopy always includes diagnostic laparoscopy. For mobilization (takedown) of splenic flexure performed with this code, see 44213.

ICD-10-CM Diagnostic Codes

C17.2	Malignant neoplasm of ileum
C17.3	Meckel's diverticulum, malignant
C18.0	Malignant neoplasm of cecum
C18.2	Malignant neoplasm of ascending colon
C18.3	Malignant neoplasm of hepatic flexure
C18.4	Malignant neoplasm of transverse colon
C18.5	Malignant neoplasm of splenic flexure
C18.6	Malignant neoplasm of descending colon
C18.7	Malignant neoplasm of sigmoid colon
C18.8	Malignant neoplasm of overlapping sites of colon
C19	Malignant neoplasm of rectosigmoid junction
C49.A4	Gastrointestinal stromal tumor of large intestine
C78.5	Secondary malignant neoplasm of large intestine and rectum
C7A.012	Malignant carcinoid tumor of the ileum
C7A.021	Malignant carcinoid tumor of the cecum
C7A.022	Malignant carcinoid tumor of the ascending colon
C7A.023	Malignant carcinoid tumor of the transverse colon
C7A.024	Malignant carcinoid tumor of the descending colon
C7A.025	Malignant carcinoid tumor of the sigmoid colon
D01.0	Carcinoma in situ of colon
D01.1	Carcinoma in situ of rectosigmoid junction
D12.0	Benign neoplasm of cecum
D12.1	Benign neoplasm of appendix
D12.2	Benign neoplasm of ascending colon
D12.3	Benign neoplasm of transverse colon
D12.4	Benign neoplasm of descending colon
D12.5	Benign neoplasm of sigmoid colon
D12.7	Benign neoplasm of rectosigmoid junction
D13.39	Benign neoplasm of other parts of small intestine
D37.3	Neoplasm of uncertain behavior of appendix
D37.4	Neoplasm of uncertain behavior of colon
D3A.021	Benign carcinoid tumor of the cecum
D3A.022	Benign carcinoid tumor of the ascending colon
D3A.023	Benign carcinoid tumor of the transverse colon
D3A.024	Benign carcinoid tumor of the descending colon
D3A.025	Benign carcinoid tumor of the sigmoid colon
D49.0	Neoplasm of unspecified behavior of digestive system
K50.111	Crohn's disease of large intestine with rectal bleeding
K50.112	Crohn's disease of large intestine with intestinal obstruction
K50.113	Crohn's disease of large intestine with fistula
K50.114	Crohn's disease of large intestine with abscess
K50.118	Crohn's disease of large intestine with other complication
K50.812	Crohn's disease of both small and large intestine with intestinal obstruction
K50.813	Crohn's disease of both small and large intestine with fistula
K50.814	Crohn's disease of both small and large intestine with abscess
K51.011	Ulcerative (chronic) pancolitis with rectal bleeding
K51.012	Ulcerative (chronic) pancolitis with intestinal obstruction
K51.013	Ulcerative (chronic) pancolitis with fistula
K51.014	Ulcerative (chronic) pancolitis with abscess
K51.411	Inflammatory polyps of colon with rectal bleeding
K51.412	Inflammatory polyps of colon with intestinal obstruction
K51.413	Inflammatory polyps of colon with fistula
K51.414	Inflammatory polyps of colon with abscess
K51.511	Left sided colitis with rectal bleeding
K51.512	Left sided colitis with intestinal obstruction
K51.513	Left sided colitis with fistula
K51.514	Left sided colitis with abscess
K55.041	Focal (segmental) acute infarction of large intestine
K55.042	Diffuse acute infarction of large intestine

K55.1	Chronic vascular disorders of intestine
K55.21	Angiodysplasia of colon with hemorrhage
K55.8	Other vascular disorders of intestine
K56.0	Paralytic ileus
K56.1	Intussusception
K56.2	Volvulus
K56.51	Intestinal adhesions [bands], with partial obstruction
K56.52	Intestinal adhesions [bands] with complete obstruction
K57.20	Diverticulitis of large intestine with perforation and abscess without bleeding
K57.21	Diverticulitis of large intestine with perforation and abscess with bleeding
K57.33	Diverticulitis of large intestine without perforation or abscess with bleeding
K57.40	Diverticulitis of both small and large intestine with perforation and abscess without bleeding
K57.41	Diverticulitis of both small and large intestine with perforation and abscess with bleeding
K57.51	Diverticulosis of both small and large intestine without perforation or abscess with bleeding
K59.31	Toxic megacolon
K59.81	Ogilvie syndrome
K63.1	Perforation of intestine (nontraumatic)
K63.2	Fistula of intestine
K63.3	Ulcer of intestine
K63.4	Enteroptosis
P77.1	Stage 1 necrotizing enterocolitis in newborn ☒
P77.2	Stage 2 necrotizing enterocolitis in newborn ☒
P77.3	Stage 3 necrotizing enterocolitis in newborn ☒
P78.0	Perinatal intestinal perforation ☒
Q43.1	Hirschsprung's disease
Q43.2	Other congenital functional disorders of colon
S36.530A	Laceration of ascending [right] colon, initial encounter
S36.531A	Laceration of transverse colon, initial encounter
S36.532A	Laceration of descending [left] colon, initial encounter
S36.533A	Laceration of sigmoid colon, initial encounter

AMA: 44205 2018,Jan,8; 2017,Jan,8; 2016,Jan,13; 2015,Jan,16

Relative Value Units/Medicare Edits

Non-Facility RVU	Work	PE	MP	Total
44205	22.95	11.62	4.64	39.21
Facility RVU	**Work**	**PE**	**MP**	**Total**
44205	22.95	11.62	4.64	39.21

	FUD	Status	MUE	Modifiers				IOM Reference
44205	90	A	1(2)	51	N/A	62*	80	None

* with documentation

44206-44207

44206 Laparoscopy, surgical; colectomy, partial, with end colostomy and closure of distal segment (Hartmann type procedure)

44207 colectomy, partial, with anastomosis, with coloproctostomy (low pelvic anastomosis)

A portion of the colon is removed laparoscopically

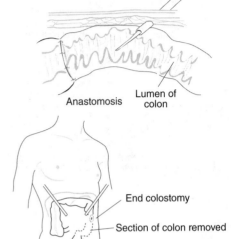

Explanation

The physician performs a laparoscopic partial colectomy with end colostomy and closure of the distal segment (Hartmann type) in 44206 and with anastomosis and coloproctostomy in 44207. With the patient under general anesthesia, a urinary catheter is inserted and the patient is positioned supine. Carbon dioxide gas is used to insufflate the abdomen through a laparoscopic port placed through the umbilicus. A 10 to 12 mm cannula is used to facilitate insertion of the laparoscope into the abdominal cavity. Cannulae are inserted in the right middle quadrant, the suprapubic area, and in the left middle quadrant to allow instrument access to the surgical site. The laparoscope is placed through the left cannula for mobilization of the colon. The physician dissects along the peritoneum to mobilize the colon. Once mobilized, the laparoscope is placed in the suprapubic cannula and the omentum is dissected using electrocautery and vascular clips. A 4 to 6 cm transverse incision is made at the appropriate cannula site depending on the portion of the resection. The colon is exteriorized and the distal segment is resected. In 44206, the new proximal end of the colon is brought through an opening made in the abdominal wall and anastomosed so as to exit onto the skin for a colostomy and the remaining distal end is closed off. In 44207, after the distal segment of diseased colon and/or rectal tissue is resected, the new ends are brought together and an anastomosis is done between the colon and the rectum low in the pelvis with staples or sutures (coloproctostomy). The abdominal cavity is inspected through the laparoscope for hemostasis and irrigated. The instruments are removed and the remaining abdominal wounds are closed.

Coding Tips

For open approach, see 44143 and 44145. Surgical laparoscopy always includes diagnostic laparoscopy. For mobilization (takedown) of splenic flexure performed with this code, see 44213.

ICD-10-CM Diagnostic Codes

C18.6	Malignant neoplasm of descending colon
C18.7	Malignant neoplasm of sigmoid colon

C18.8	Malignant neoplasm of overlapping sites of colon
C19	Malignant neoplasm of rectosigmoid junction
C49.A4	Gastrointestinal stromal tumor of large intestine
C78.5	Secondary malignant neoplasm of large intestine and rectum
C7A.024	Malignant carcinoid tumor of the descending colon
C7A.025	Malignant carcinoid tumor of the sigmoid colon
D01.1	Carcinoma in situ of rectosigmoid junction
D12.4	Benign neoplasm of descending colon
D12.5	Benign neoplasm of sigmoid colon
D12.7	Benign neoplasm of rectosigmoid junction
D3A.024	Benign carcinoid tumor of the descending colon
D3A.025	Benign carcinoid tumor of the sigmoid colon
D49.0	Neoplasm of unspecified behavior of digestive system
K50.111	Crohn's disease of large intestine with rectal bleeding
K50.112	Crohn's disease of large intestine with intestinal obstruction
K50.113	Crohn's disease of large intestine with fistula
K50.114	Crohn's disease of large intestine with abscess
K50.118	Crohn's disease of large intestine with other complication
K50.811	Crohn's disease of both small and large intestine with rectal bleeding
K50.812	Crohn's disease of both small and large intestine with intestinal obstruction
K50.813	Crohn's disease of both small and large intestine with fistula
K50.814	Crohn's disease of both small and large intestine with abscess
K50.818	Crohn's disease of both small and large intestine with other complication
K51.011	Ulcerative (chronic) pancolitis with rectal bleeding
K51.012	Ulcerative (chronic) pancolitis with intestinal obstruction
K51.013	Ulcerative (chronic) pancolitis with fistula
K51.014	Ulcerative (chronic) pancolitis with abscess
K51.018	Ulcerative (chronic) pancolitis with other complication
K51.212	Ulcerative (chronic) proctitis with intestinal obstruction
K51.213	Ulcerative (chronic) proctitis with fistula
K51.214	Ulcerative (chronic) proctitis with abscess
K51.311	Ulcerative (chronic) rectosigmoiditis with rectal bleeding
K51.312	Ulcerative (chronic) rectosigmoiditis with intestinal obstruction
K51.313	Ulcerative (chronic) rectosigmoiditis with fistula
K51.314	Ulcerative (chronic) rectosigmoiditis with abscess
K51.318	Ulcerative (chronic) rectosigmoiditis with other complication
K51.411	Inflammatory polyps of colon with rectal bleeding
K51.412	Inflammatory polyps of colon with intestinal obstruction
K51.413	Inflammatory polyps of colon with fistula
K51.414	Inflammatory polyps of colon with abscess
K51.418	Inflammatory polyps of colon with other complication
K51.511	Left sided colitis with rectal bleeding
K51.512	Left sided colitis with intestinal obstruction
K51.513	Left sided colitis with fistula
K51.514	Left sided colitis with abscess
K51.518	Left sided colitis with other complication
K55.041	Focal (segmental) acute infarction of large intestine
K55.042	Diffuse acute infarction of large intestine
K55.1	Chronic vascular disorders of intestine
K55.20	Angiodysplasia of colon without hemorrhage
K55.21	Angiodysplasia of colon with hemorrhage
K55.31	Stage 1 necrotizing enterocolitis
K55.32	Stage 2 necrotizing enterocolitis
K55.33	Stage 3 necrotizing enterocolitis
K56.0	Paralytic ileus
K56.1	Intussusception
K56.2	Volvulus
K56.51	Intestinal adhesions [bands], with partial obstruction
K56.52	Intestinal adhesions [bands] with complete obstruction
K56.690	Other partial intestinal obstruction
K56.691	Other complete intestinal obstruction
K57.20	Diverticulitis of large intestine with perforation and abscess without bleeding
K57.21	Diverticulitis of large intestine with perforation and abscess with bleeding
K57.31	Diverticulosis of large intestine without perforation or abscess with bleeding
K57.32	Diverticulitis of large intestine without perforation or abscess without bleeding
K57.33	Diverticulitis of large intestine without perforation or abscess with bleeding
K57.40	Diverticulitis of both small and large intestine with perforation and abscess without bleeding
K57.41	Diverticulitis of both small and large intestine with perforation and abscess with bleeding
K59.31	Toxic megacolon
K59.81	Ogilvie syndrome
K63.0	Abscess of intestine
K63.1	Perforation of intestine (nontraumatic)
K63.2	Fistula of intestine
K63.3	Ulcer of intestine
K63.4	Enteroptosis
K63.5	Polyp of colon
K91.31	Postprocedural partial intestinal obstruction
K91.32	Postprocedural complete intestinal obstruction
N32.1	Vesicointestinal fistula
Q42.8	Congenital absence, atresia and stenosis of other parts of large intestine
Q43.1	Hirschsprung's disease
Q43.2	Other congenital functional disorders of colon
Q43.3	Congenital malformations of intestinal fixation
Q43.4	Duplication of intestine
S36.530A	Laceration of ascending [right] colon, initial encounter
S36.531A	Laceration of transverse colon, initial encounter
S36.532A	Laceration of descending [left] colon, initial encounter
S36.533A	Laceration of sigmoid colon, initial encounter
S36.538A	Laceration of other part of colon, initial encounter

AMA: 44206 2018,Jan,8; 2017,Jan,8; 2016,Jan,13; 2015,Jan,16 **44207** 2018,Jan,8; 2017,Jan,8; 2016,Jan,13; 2015,Jan,16

Relative Value Units/Medicare Edits

Non-Facility RVU	Work	PE	MP	Total
44206	29.79	15.32	6.27	51.38
44207	31.92	15.07	6.16	53.15
Facility RVU	Work	PE	MP	Total
44206	29.79	15.32	6.27	51.38
44207	31.92	15.07	6.16	53.15

	FUD	Status	MUE	Modifiers				IOM Reference
44206	90	A	1(2)	51	N/A	62*	80	None
44207	90	A	1(2)	51	N/A	62*	80	

* with documentation

Terms To Know

anastomosis. Surgically created connection between ducts, blood vessels, or bowel segments to allow flow from one to the other.

colectomy. Excision of a segment or all of the colon.

colostomy. Artificial surgical opening anywhere along the length of the colon to the skin surface for the diversion of feces.

distal. Located farther away from a specified reference point or the trunk.

Hartmann procedure. The lower part of the sigmoid colon and/or the upper part of the rectum is excised. The descending colon is manipulated and sutured to the skin to create a colostomy. The proximal end of the descending colon is oversewn and a pouch is formed.

insufflation. Blowing air or gas into a body cavity.

laparoscopy. Direct visualization of the peritoneal cavity, outer fallopian tubes, uterus, and ovaries utilizing a laparoscope, a thin, flexible fiberoptic tube.

44208

44208 Laparoscopy, surgical; colectomy, partial, with anastomosis, with coloproctostomy (low pelvic anastomosis) with colostomy

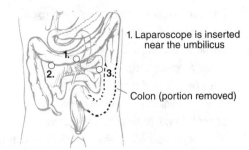

1. Laparoscope is inserted near the umbilicus

Colon (portion removed)

2. and 3. Ports for trocars and surgical instruments

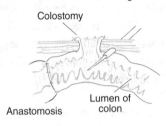

Colostomy

Anastomosis

Lumen of colon

Explanation

The physician performs a laparoscopic partial colectomy with anastomosis and coloproctostomy, with a colostomy. With the patient under general anesthesia, a urinary catheter is inserted and the patient is positioned supine. Carbon dioxide gas is used to insufflate the abdomen through a laparoscopic port placed through the umbilicus. A 10 12 mm cannula is used to facilitate insertion of the laparoscope into the abdominal cavity. Cannulae are inserted in the right middle quadrant, the suprapubic area, and in the left middle quadrant to allow instrument access to the surgical site. The laparoscope is placed through the left cannula for mobilization of the colon. The physician dissects along the peritoneum to mobilize the colon. Once mobilized, the laparoscope is placed in the suprapubic cannula and the omentum is dissected using electrocautery and vascular clips. A 4 to 6 cm transverse incision is made at the appropriate cannula site depending on the portion of the resection. The distal segment of diseased colon and/or rectal tissue is resected and the new ends are brought together and an anastomosis is done between the colon and the rectum low in the pelvis with staples or sutures (coloproctostomy). A loop of colon above the newly sutured anastomosis is brought out through a separate incision in the abdominal wall and fixed there so the colon will empty through this artificial opening in the skin as a colostomy, usually temporary, to divert the fecal stream while the anastomosis heals.

Coding Tips

For open approach, see 44146. Surgical laparoscopy always includes diagnostic laparoscopy. For mobilization (takedown) of splenic flexure performed with this code, see 44213.

ICD-10-CM Diagnostic Codes

C18.6	Malignant neoplasm of descending colon
C18.7	Malignant neoplasm of sigmoid colon
C18.8	Malignant neoplasm of overlapping sites of colon
C19	Malignant neoplasm of rectosigmoid junction
C20	Malignant neoplasm of rectum
C49.A4	Gastrointestinal stromal tumor of large intestine
C78.5	Secondary malignant neoplasm of large intestine and rectum

C7A.024	Malignant carcinoid tumor of the descending colon	
C7A.025	Malignant carcinoid tumor of the sigmoid colon	
C7A.026	Malignant carcinoid tumor of the rectum	
D01.1	Carcinoma in situ of rectosigmoid junction	
D01.2	Carcinoma in situ of rectum	
D12.4	Benign neoplasm of descending colon	
D12.5	Benign neoplasm of sigmoid colon	
D12.7	Benign neoplasm of rectosigmoid junction	
D3A.024	Benign carcinoid tumor of the descending colon	
D3A.025	Benign carcinoid tumor of the sigmoid colon	
D3A.026	Benign carcinoid tumor of the rectum	
D49.0	Neoplasm of unspecified behavior of digestive system	

K50.111 Crohn's disease of large intestine with rectal bleeding
K50.112 Crohn's disease of large intestine with intestinal obstruction
K50.113 Crohn's disease of large intestine with fistula
K50.114 Crohn's disease of large intestine with abscess
K50.118 Crohn's disease of large intestine with other complication
K50.811 Crohn's disease of both small and large intestine with rectal bleeding
K50.812 Crohn's disease of both small and large intestine with intestinal obstruction
K50.813 Crohn's disease of both small and large intestine with fistula
K50.818 Crohn's disease of both small and large intestine with other complication
K51.011 Ulcerative (chronic) pancolitis with rectal bleeding
K51.012 Ulcerative (chronic) pancolitis with intestinal obstruction
K51.013 Ulcerative (chronic) pancolitis with fistula
K51.014 Ulcerative (chronic) pancolitis with abscess
K51.018 Ulcerative (chronic) pancolitis with other complication
K51.212 Ulcerative (chronic) proctitis with intestinal obstruction
K51.213 Ulcerative (chronic) proctitis with fistula
K51.214 Ulcerative (chronic) proctitis with abscess
K51.311 Ulcerative (chronic) rectosigmoiditis with rectal bleeding
K51.312 Ulcerative (chronic) rectosigmoiditis with intestinal obstruction
K51.313 Ulcerative (chronic) rectosigmoiditis with fistula
K51.314 Ulcerative (chronic) rectosigmoiditis with abscess
K51.411 Inflammatory polyps of colon with rectal bleeding
K51.412 Inflammatory polyps of colon with intestinal obstruction
K51.413 Inflammatory polyps of colon with fistula
K51.414 Inflammatory polyps of colon with abscess
K51.511 Left sided colitis with rectal bleeding
K51.512 Left sided colitis with intestinal obstruction
K51.513 Left sided colitis with fistula
K55.041 Focal (segmental) acute infarction of large intestine
K55.042 Diffuse acute infarction of large intestine
K55.1 Chronic vascular disorders of intestine
K55.20 Angiodysplasia of colon without hemorrhage
K55.21 Angiodysplasia of colon with hemorrhage
K55.31 Stage 1 necrotizing enterocolitis
K55.32 Stage 2 necrotizing enterocolitis
K55.33 Stage 3 necrotizing enterocolitis
K56.0 Paralytic ileus
K56.1 Intussusception

K56.2 Volvulus
K56.51 Intestinal adhesions [bands], with partial obstruction
K56.52 Intestinal adhesions [bands] with complete obstruction
K57.20 Diverticulitis of large intestine with perforation and abscess without bleeding
K57.21 Diverticulitis of large intestine with perforation and abscess with bleeding
K57.31 Diverticulosis of large intestine without perforation or abscess with bleeding
K57.33 Diverticulitis of large intestine without perforation or abscess with bleeding
K57.40 Diverticulitis of both small and large intestine with perforation and abscess without bleeding
K57.41 Diverticulitis of both small and large intestine with perforation and abscess with bleeding
K59.31 Toxic megacolon
K59.81 Ogilvie syndrome
K63.0 Abscess of intestine
K63.1 Perforation of intestine (nontraumatic)
K63.2 Fistula of intestine
K63.3 Ulcer of intestine
K63.4 Enteroptosis
K63.5 Polyp of colon
N32.1 Vesicointestinal fistula
P76.8 Other specified intestinal obstruction of newborn 🆕
P77.1 Stage 1 necrotizing enterocolitis in newborn 🆕
P77.2 Stage 2 necrotizing enterocolitis in newborn 🆕
P77.3 Stage 3 necrotizing enterocolitis in newborn 🆕
P78.0 Perinatal intestinal perforation 🆕
Q42.8 Congenital absence, atresia and stenosis of other parts of large intestine
Q43.1 Hirschsprung's disease
Q43.2 Other congenital functional disorders of colon
Q43.3 Congenital malformations of intestinal fixation
Q43.4 Duplication of intestine
S36.532A Laceration of descending [left] colon, initial encounter
S36.533A Laceration of sigmoid colon, initial encounter

AMA: **44208** 2018,Jan,8; 2017,Jan,8; 2016,Jan,13; 2015,Jan,16

Relative Value Units/Medicare Edits

Non-Facility RVU	Work	PE	MP	Total
44208	33.99	17.48	6.44	57.91
Facility RVU	**Work**	**PE**	**MP**	**Total**
44208	33.99	17.48	6.44	57.91

	FUD	Status	MUE	Modifiers				IOM Reference
44208	90	A	1(2)	51	N/A	62*	80	None

* with documentation

44210

44210 Laparoscopy, surgical; colectomy, total, abdominal, without proctectomy, with ileostomy or ileoproctostomy

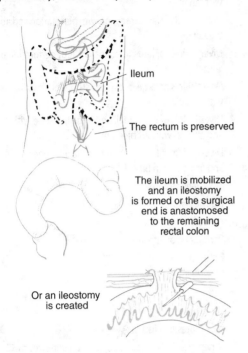

Ileum

The rectum is preserved

The ileum is mobilized and an ileostomy is formed or the surgical end is anastomosed to the remaining rectal colon

Or an ileostomy is created

Explanation

The physician performs a laparoscopic total colectomy with ileostomy or ileoproctostomy. With the patient under general anesthesia, a urinary catheter is inserted and the patient is positioned supine. Carbon dioxide gas is used to insufflate the abdomen through a laparoscopic port placed through the umbilicus. A 10 to 12 mm cannula is used to facilitate insertion of the laparoscope into the abdominal cavity. Cannulae are inserted in the right middle quadrant, the suprapubic area, and in the left middle quadrant to allow instrument access to the surgical site. The laparoscope is placed through the left cannula for mobilization of the colon. The physician dissects along the peritoneum to mobilize the colon. Once mobilized, the laparoscope is placed in the suprapubic cannula and the omentum is dissected using electrocautery and vascular clips. A 4 to 6 cm transverse incision is made at the appropriate cannula site depending on the portion of the resection. After the colon has been mobilized, the colorectal junction and the terminal ileum are divided. The whole colon is removed. The terminal ileum is approximated to the rectum and the ends anastomosed together or it is brought out through a separate incision on the abdominal wall and sutured as an ileostomy artificial opening onto the skin.

Coding Tips

Surgical laparoscopy always includes diagnostic laparoscopy. For open approach, see 44150.

ICD-10-CM Diagnostic Codes

C18.0	Malignant neoplasm of cecum
C18.1	Malignant neoplasm of appendix
C18.2	Malignant neoplasm of ascending colon
C18.3	Malignant neoplasm of hepatic flexure
C18.4	Malignant neoplasm of transverse colon
C18.5	Malignant neoplasm of splenic flexure
C18.6	Malignant neoplasm of descending colon
C18.7	Malignant neoplasm of sigmoid colon
C18.8	Malignant neoplasm of overlapping sites of colon
C19	Malignant neoplasm of rectosigmoid junction
C49.A4	Gastrointestinal stromal tumor of large intestine
C78.5	Secondary malignant neoplasm of large intestine and rectum
C7A.021	Malignant carcinoid tumor of the cecum
C7A.022	Malignant carcinoid tumor of the ascending colon
C7A.023	Malignant carcinoid tumor of the transverse colon
C7A.024	Malignant carcinoid tumor of the descending colon
C7A.025	Malignant carcinoid tumor of the sigmoid colon
D01.0	Carcinoma in situ of colon
D01.1	Carcinoma in situ of rectosigmoid junction
D12.0	Benign neoplasm of cecum
D12.1	Benign neoplasm of appendix
D12.2	Benign neoplasm of ascending colon
D12.3	Benign neoplasm of transverse colon
D12.4	Benign neoplasm of descending colon
D12.5	Benign neoplasm of sigmoid colon
D12.7	Benign neoplasm of rectosigmoid junction
D37.3	Neoplasm of uncertain behavior of appendix
D37.4	Neoplasm of uncertain behavior of colon
D3A.021	Benign carcinoid tumor of the cecum
D3A.022	Benign carcinoid tumor of the ascending colon
D3A.023	Benign carcinoid tumor of the transverse colon
D3A.024	Benign carcinoid tumor of the descending colon
D3A.025	Benign carcinoid tumor of the sigmoid colon
D49.0	Neoplasm of unspecified behavior of digestive system
K50.111	Crohn's disease of large intestine with rectal bleeding
K50.112	Crohn's disease of large intestine with intestinal obstruction
K50.113	Crohn's disease of large intestine with fistula
K50.114	Crohn's disease of large intestine with abscess
K50.118	Crohn's disease of large intestine with other complication
K50.812	Crohn's disease of both small and large intestine with intestinal obstruction
K50.813	Crohn's disease of both small and large intestine with fistula
K50.814	Crohn's disease of both small and large intestine with abscess
K51.011	Ulcerative (chronic) pancolitis with rectal bleeding
K51.012	Ulcerative (chronic) pancolitis with intestinal obstruction
K51.013	Ulcerative (chronic) pancolitis with fistula
K51.014	Ulcerative (chronic) pancolitis with abscess
K51.312	Ulcerative (chronic) rectosigmoiditis with intestinal obstruction
K51.313	Ulcerative (chronic) rectosigmoiditis with fistula
K51.411	Inflammatory polyps of colon with rectal bleeding
K51.412	Inflammatory polyps of colon with intestinal obstruction
K51.413	Inflammatory polyps of colon with fistula
K51.414	Inflammatory polyps of colon with abscess
K51.511	Left sided colitis with rectal bleeding
K51.512	Left sided colitis with intestinal obstruction
K51.513	Left sided colitis with fistula
K51.514	Left sided colitis with abscess
K55.041	Focal (segmental) acute infarction of large intestine
K55.042	Diffuse acute infarction of large intestine
K55.1	Chronic vascular disorders of intestine

N Newborn: 0   **P** Pediatric: 0-17   **M** Maternity: 9-64   **A** Adult: 15-124   ♂ Male Only   ♀ Female Only   CPT © 2021 American Medical Association. All Rights Reserved.

Coding Companion for General Surgery/Gastroenterology

Intestines

K55.21	Angiodysplasia of colon with hemorrhage
K55.8	Other vascular disorders of intestine
K56.2	Volvulus
K57.20	Diverticulitis of large intestine with perforation and abscess without bleeding
K57.21	Diverticulitis of large intestine with perforation and abscess with bleeding
K57.33	Diverticulitis of large intestine without perforation or abscess with bleeding
K57.40	Diverticulitis of both small and large intestine with perforation and abscess without bleeding
K57.41	Diverticulitis of both small and large intestine with perforation and abscess with bleeding
K57.51	Diverticulosis of both small and large intestine without perforation or abscess with bleeding
K59.31	Toxic megacolon
K59.81	Ogilvie syndrome
K63.1	Perforation of intestine (nontraumatic)
K63.2	Fistula of intestine
K63.3	Ulcer of intestine
K63.4	Enteroptosis
P77.1	Stage 1 necrotizing enterocolitis in newborn N
P77.2	Stage 2 necrotizing enterocolitis in newborn N
P77.3	Stage 3 necrotizing enterocolitis in newborn N
P78.0	Perinatal intestinal perforation N
Q43.1	Hirschsprung's disease
Q43.2	Other congenital functional disorders of colon
S36.530A	Laceration of ascending [right] colon, initial encounter
S36.531A	Laceration of transverse colon, initial encounter
S36.532A	Laceration of descending [left] colon, initial encounter
S36.533A	Laceration of sigmoid colon, initial encounter

AMA: **44210** 2018,Jan,8; 2017,Jan,8; 2016,Jan,13; 2015,Jan,16

Relative Value Units/Medicare Edits

Non-Facility RVU	Work	PE	MP	Total
44210	30.09	16.44	5.27	51.8
Facility RVU	**Work**	**PE**	**MP**	**Total**
44210	30.09	16.44	5.27	51.8

	FUD	Status	MUE	Modifiers				IOM Reference
44210	90	A	1(2)	51	N/A	62*	80	None

* with documentation

44211

44211 Laparoscopy, surgical; colectomy, total, abdominal, with proctectomy, with ileoanal anastomosis, creation of ileal reservoir (S or J), with loop ileostomy, includes rectal mucosectomy, when performed

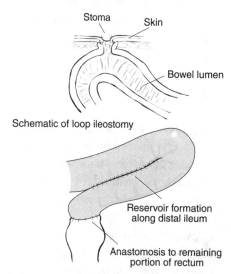

Schematic of loop ileostomy

The distal ileum is mobilized and a reservoir is formed to store waste. The distal end is anastomosed to the remnant of the rectum. A loop enterostomy is performed to eliminate waste during the healing period

Explanation

The physician performs a laparoscopic total colectomy with proctectomy with ileoanal anastomosis and creation of an ileal reservoir, with loop ileostomy, with or without rectal mucosectomy. With the patient under general anesthesia, a urinary catheter is inserted and the patient is positioned supine. Carbon dioxide gas is used to insufflate the abdomen through a laparoscopic port placed through the umbilicus. A 10 to 12 mm cannula is used to facilitate insertion of the laparoscope into the abdominal cavity. Cannulae are inserted in the right middle quadrant, the suprapubic area, and in the left middle quadrant to allow instrument access to the surgical site. The laparoscope is placed through the left cannula for mobilization of the colon. The physician dissects along the peritoneum to mobilize the colon. Once mobilized, the laparoscope is placed in the suprapubic cannula and the omentum is dissected using electrocautery and vascular clips. A 4 to 6 cm transverse incision is made at the appropriate cannula site depending on the portion of the resection. After the colon and rectum have been mobilized, they are removed. The mucosa of the remaining distal rectum may be stripped. The terminal ileum is folded upon itself and approximated in order to form a pouch and the terminal ileum is pulled through the remaining muscular tube of the rectum and approximated to the anus with sutures. A loop of ileum above the newly sutured ileoanal anastomosis is brought out through a separate incision in the abdominal wall and fixed there so the ileum will empty through this artificial opening in the skin as an ileostomy, usually temporary, to divert the fecal stream while the anastomosis heals.

Coding Tips

Surgical laparoscopy always includes diagnostic laparoscopy. For open approach, see 44157–44158.

ICD-10-CM Diagnostic Codes

| C18.0 | Malignant neoplasm of cecum |
| C18.1 | Malignant neoplasm of appendix |

C18.2	Malignant neoplasm of ascending colon
C18.3	Malignant neoplasm of hepatic flexure
C18.4	Malignant neoplasm of transverse colon
C18.5	Malignant neoplasm of splenic flexure
C18.6	Malignant neoplasm of descending colon
C18.7	Malignant neoplasm of sigmoid colon
C19	Malignant neoplasm of rectosigmoid junction
C20	Malignant neoplasm of rectum
C49.A4	Gastrointestinal stromal tumor of large intestine
C7A.021	Malignant carcinoid tumor of the cecum
C7A.022	Malignant carcinoid tumor of the ascending colon
C7A.023	Malignant carcinoid tumor of the transverse colon
C7A.024	Malignant carcinoid tumor of the descending colon
C7A.025	Malignant carcinoid tumor of the sigmoid colon
C7A.026	Malignant carcinoid tumor of the rectum
D01.0	Carcinoma in situ of colon
D01.1	Carcinoma in situ of rectosigmoid junction
D01.2	Carcinoma in situ of rectum
D12.0	Benign neoplasm of cecum
D12.2	Benign neoplasm of ascending colon
D12.3	Benign neoplasm of transverse colon
D12.4	Benign neoplasm of descending colon
D12.5	Benign neoplasm of sigmoid colon
D12.7	Benign neoplasm of rectosigmoid junction
D12.8	Benign neoplasm of rectum
D37.3	Neoplasm of uncertain behavior of appendix
D37.4	Neoplasm of uncertain behavior of colon
D3A.021	Benign carcinoid tumor of the cecum
D3A.022	Benign carcinoid tumor of the ascending colon
D3A.023	Benign carcinoid tumor of the transverse colon
D3A.024	Benign carcinoid tumor of the descending colon
D3A.025	Benign carcinoid tumor of the sigmoid colon
D3A.026	Benign carcinoid tumor of the rectum
K50.111	Crohn's disease of large intestine with rectal bleeding
K50.112	Crohn's disease of large intestine with intestinal obstruction
K50.113	Crohn's disease of large intestine with fistula
K50.114	Crohn's disease of large intestine with abscess
K50.812	Crohn's disease of both small and large intestine with intestinal obstruction
K50.813	Crohn's disease of both small and large intestine with fistula
K50.814	Crohn's disease of both small and large intestine with abscess
K51.011	Ulcerative (chronic) pancolitis with rectal bleeding
K51.012	Ulcerative (chronic) pancolitis with intestinal obstruction
K51.013	Ulcerative (chronic) pancolitis with fistula
K51.014	Ulcerative (chronic) pancolitis with abscess
K51.312	Ulcerative (chronic) rectosigmoiditis with intestinal obstruction
K51.313	Ulcerative (chronic) rectosigmoiditis with fistula
K51.411	Inflammatory polyps of colon with rectal bleeding
K51.412	Inflammatory polyps of colon with intestinal obstruction
K51.413	Inflammatory polyps of colon with fistula
K51.414	Inflammatory polyps of colon with abscess
K51.511	Left sided colitis with rectal bleeding
K51.512	Left sided colitis with intestinal obstruction
K51.513	Left sided colitis with fistula
K51.514	Left sided colitis with abscess
K55.041	Focal (segmental) acute infarction of large intestine
K55.042	Diffuse acute infarction of large intestine
K55.1	Chronic vascular disorders of intestine
K55.21	Angiodysplasia of colon with hemorrhage
K55.8	Other vascular disorders of intestine
K56.2	Volvulus
K57.20	Diverticulitis of large intestine with perforation and abscess without bleeding
K57.21	Diverticulitis of large intestine with perforation and abscess with bleeding
K57.33	Diverticulitis of large intestine without perforation or abscess with bleeding
K57.40	Diverticulitis of both small and large intestine with perforation and abscess without bleeding
K59.31	Toxic megacolon
K59.81	Ogilvie syndrome
K63.1	Perforation of intestine (nontraumatic)
K63.2	Fistula of intestine
K63.3	Ulcer of intestine
K63.4	Enteroptosis
P77.1	Stage 1 necrotizing enterocolitis in newborn N
P77.2	Stage 2 necrotizing enterocolitis in newborn N
P77.3	Stage 3 necrotizing enterocolitis in newborn N
P78.0	Perinatal intestinal perforation N
Q43.1	Hirschsprung's disease
S36.530A	Laceration of ascending [right] colon, initial encounter
S36.531A	Laceration of transverse colon, initial encounter
S36.532A	Laceration of descending [left] colon, initial encounter
S36.533A	Laceration of sigmoid colon, initial encounter

AMA: **44211** 2018,Jan,8; 2017,Jan,8; 2016,Jan,13; 2015,Jan,16

Relative Value Units/Medicare Edits

Non-Facility RVU	Work	PE	MP	Total
44211	37.08	19.85	4.73	61.66
Facility RVU	**Work**	**PE**	**MP**	**Total**
44211	37.08	19.85	4.73	61.66

	FUD	Status	MUE	Modifiers				IOM Reference
44211	90	A	1(2)	51	N/A	62*	80	None

* with documentation

44212

44212 Laparoscopy, surgical; colectomy, total, abdominal, with proctectomy, with ileostomy

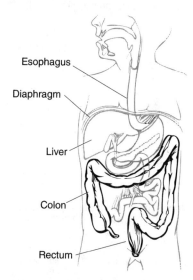

The entire colon and rectum (dark) are removed

Explanation

The physician performs a laparoscopic total colectomy with proctectomy, with ileostomy. With the patient under general anesthesia, a urinary catheter is inserted and the patient is positioned supine. Carbon dioxide gas is used to insufflate the abdomen through a laparoscopic port placed through the umbilicus. A 10 to 12 mm cannula is used to facilitate insertion of the laparoscope into the abdominal cavity. Cannulae are inserted in the right middle quadrant, the suprapubic area, and in the left middle quadrant to allow instrument access to the surgical site. The laparoscope is placed through the left cannula for mobilization of the colon. The physician dissects along the peritoneum to mobilize the colon. Once mobilized, the laparoscope is placed in the suprapubic cannula and the omentum is dissected using electrocautery and vascular clips. A 4 to 6 cm transverse incision is made at the appropriate cannula site depending on the portion of the resection. After the colon and rectum have been mobilized, they are removed. The terminal ileum is brought out through a separate incision on the abdominal wall and sutured as an ileostomy artificial opening onto the skin.

Coding Tips

Surgical laparoscopy always includes diagnostic laparoscopy. For open approach, see 44155.

ICD-10-CM Diagnostic Codes

C18.0	Malignant neoplasm of cecum
C18.1	Malignant neoplasm of appendix
C18.2	Malignant neoplasm of ascending colon
C18.3	Malignant neoplasm of hepatic flexure
C18.4	Malignant neoplasm of transverse colon
C18.5	Malignant neoplasm of splenic flexure
C18.6	Malignant neoplasm of descending colon
C18.7	Malignant neoplasm of sigmoid colon
C18.8	Malignant neoplasm of overlapping sites of colon
C19	Malignant neoplasm of rectosigmoid junction
C20	Malignant neoplasm of rectum
C49.A4	Gastrointestinal stromal tumor of large intestine
C78.5	Secondary malignant neoplasm of large intestine and rectum
C7A.021	Malignant carcinoid tumor of the cecum
C7A.022	Malignant carcinoid tumor of the ascending colon
C7A.023	Malignant carcinoid tumor of the transverse colon
C7A.024	Malignant carcinoid tumor of the descending colon
C7A.025	Malignant carcinoid tumor of the sigmoid colon
D01.0	Carcinoma in situ of colon
D01.1	Carcinoma in situ of rectosigmoid junction
D01.2	Carcinoma in situ of rectum
D12.0	Benign neoplasm of cecum
D12.1	Benign neoplasm of appendix
D12.2	Benign neoplasm of ascending colon
D12.3	Benign neoplasm of transverse colon
D12.4	Benign neoplasm of descending colon
D12.5	Benign neoplasm of sigmoid colon
D12.7	Benign neoplasm of rectosigmoid junction
D12.8	Benign neoplasm of rectum
D37.3	Neoplasm of uncertain behavior of appendix
D37.4	Neoplasm of uncertain behavior of colon
D3A.021	Benign carcinoid tumor of the cecum
D3A.022	Benign carcinoid tumor of the ascending colon
D3A.023	Benign carcinoid tumor of the transverse colon
D3A.024	Benign carcinoid tumor of the descending colon
D3A.025	Benign carcinoid tumor of the sigmoid colon
D3A.026	Benign carcinoid tumor of the rectum
D49.0	Neoplasm of unspecified behavior of digestive system
K50.111	Crohn's disease of large intestine with rectal bleeding
K50.112	Crohn's disease of large intestine with intestinal obstruction
K50.113	Crohn's disease of large intestine with fistula
K50.114	Crohn's disease of large intestine with abscess
K50.118	Crohn's disease of large intestine with other complication
K50.812	Crohn's disease of both small and large intestine with intestinal obstruction
K50.813	Crohn's disease of both small and large intestine with fistula
K50.814	Crohn's disease of both small and large intestine with abscess
K51.011	Ulcerative (chronic) pancolitis with rectal bleeding
K51.012	Ulcerative (chronic) pancolitis with intestinal obstruction
K51.013	Ulcerative (chronic) pancolitis with fistula
K51.014	Ulcerative (chronic) pancolitis with abscess
K51.312	Ulcerative (chronic) rectosigmoiditis with intestinal obstruction
K51.313	Ulcerative (chronic) rectosigmoiditis with fistula
K51.314	Ulcerative (chronic) rectosigmoiditis with abscess
K51.411	Inflammatory polyps of colon with rectal bleeding
K51.412	Inflammatory polyps of colon with intestinal obstruction
K51.413	Inflammatory polyps of colon with fistula
K51.414	Inflammatory polyps of colon with abscess
K51.512	Left sided colitis with intestinal obstruction
K51.513	Left sided colitis with fistula
K55.041	Focal (segmental) acute infarction of large intestine
K55.042	Diffuse acute infarction of large intestine
K55.1	Chronic vascular disorders of intestine
K55.21	Angiodysplasia of colon with hemorrhage

Labels on figure: Esophagus, Diaphragm, Liver, Colon, Rectum

K55.8	Other vascular disorders of intestine
K56.2	Volvulus
K57.20	Diverticulitis of large intestine with perforation and abscess without bleeding
K57.21	Diverticulitis of large intestine with perforation and abscess with bleeding
K57.33	Diverticulitis of large intestine without perforation or abscess with bleeding
K57.40	Diverticulitis of both small and large intestine with perforation and abscess without bleeding
K57.41	Diverticulitis of both small and large intestine with perforation and abscess with bleeding
K57.51	Diverticulosis of both small and large intestine without perforation or abscess with bleeding
K59.31	Toxic megacolon
K59.81	Ogilvie syndrome
K63.1	Perforation of intestine (nontraumatic)
K63.2	Fistula of intestine
K63.3	Ulcer of intestine
K63.4	Enteroptosis
P77.1	Stage 1 necrotizing enterocolitis in newborn N
P77.2	Stage 2 necrotizing enterocolitis in newborn N
P77.3	Stage 3 necrotizing enterocolitis in newborn N
P78.0	Perinatal intestinal perforation N
Q42.8	Congenital absence, atresia and stenosis of other parts of large intestine
Q43.1	Hirschsprung's disease
Q43.2	Other congenital functional disorders of colon
S36.530A	Laceration of ascending [right] colon, initial encounter
S36.531A	Laceration of transverse colon, initial encounter
S36.532A	Laceration of descending [left] colon, initial encounter
S36.533A	Laceration of sigmoid colon, initial encounter

AMA: **44212** 2018,Jan,8; 2017,Jan,8; 2016,Jan,13; 2015,Jan,16

Relative Value Units/Medicare Edits

Non-Facility RVU	Work	PE	MP	Total
44212	34.58	19.14	5.81	59.53
Facility RVU	**Work**	**PE**	**MP**	**Total**
44212	34.58	19.14	5.81	59.53

	FUD	Status	MUE	Modifiers				IOM Reference
44212	90	A	1(2)	51	N/A	62*	80	None

* with documentation

44213

+ **44213** Laparoscopy, surgical, mobilization (take-down) of splenic flexure performed in conjunction with partial colectomy (List separately in addition to primary procedure)

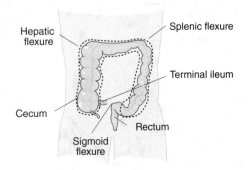

Mobilization of splenic flexure is performed laparoscopically in conjunction with partial colectomy

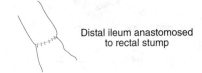

Distal ileum anastomosed to rectal stump

Explanation

The physician mobilizes the splenic flexure via a laparoscopic approach in conjunction with a separately reportable partial colon resection. With the patient under general anesthesia, a urinary catheter is inserted and the patient is placed supine or in a Trendelenburg position on the operating table. A 15-mmHg carbon dioxide pneumoperitoneum is established with a laparoscopic port placed through the umbilicus using a direct open technique. The laparoscope is positioned in the abdominal cavity and a diagnostic laparoscopy is performed. The remaining laparoscopic ports are placed under direct vision. The attachments between the splenic flexure of the colon and the lateral abdominal wall and spleen are dissected free and taken down in order to mobilize an adequate length of colon in conjunction with a partial colon resection. At the completion of the procedure, the abdomen is deflated and the laparoscope and trocar incisions are closed.

Coding Tips

Report 44213 in addition to 44204–44208. Surgical laparoscopy always includes diagnostic laparoscopy. For an open approach, see 44139.

ICD-10-CM Diagnostic Codes

This/these CPT code(s) are add-on code(s). See the primary procedure code that this code is performed with for your ICD-10-CM code selections.

AMA: **44213** 2018,Jan,8; 2017,Jan,8; 2016,Jan,13; 2015,Jan,16

Relative Value Units/Medicare Edits

Non-Facility RVU	Work	PE	MP	Total
44213	3.5	1.29	0.69	5.48
Facility RVU	**Work**	**PE**	**MP**	**Total**
44213	3.5	1.29	0.69	5.48

	FUD	Status	MUE	Modifiers				IOM Reference
44213	N/A	A	1(2)	N/A	N/A	62*	80	None

* with documentation

44227

44227 Laparoscopy, surgical, closure of enterostomy, large or small intestine, with resection and anastomosis

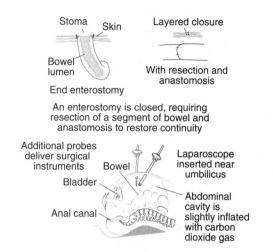

Stoma / Skin
Bowel lumen
End enterostomy

Layered closure
With resection and anastomosis

An enterostomy is closed, requiring resection of a segment of bowel and anastomosis to restore continuity

Additional probes deliver surgical instruments
Bowel
Bladder
Anal canal
Laparoscope inserted near umbilicus
Abdominal cavity is slightly inflated with carbon dioxide gas

Explanation

The physician takes down (closes) a previously created enterostomy (stoma) of the large or small intestine using a laparoscope. With the patient under general anesthesia, the physician places a trocar at the umbilicus into the abdomen and insufflates the abdominal cavity. The physician places a laparoscope through the umbilical incision. Additional trocars are placed, through which the specialized surgical instruments are inserted. The stoma is mobilized and taken down from the abdominal wall. The stoma is resected and the bowel ends are reapproximated with staples or sutures. The laparoscope is removed, the ports are closed with incisions, and the stoma is matured.

Coding Tips

To indicate that this is a staged or related procedure performed during the postoperative period by the same physician, append modifier 58. Surgical laparoscopy always includes diagnostic laparoscopy. For open approach, see codes 44620–44626.

ICD-10-CM Diagnostic Codes

K56.51	Intestinal adhesions [bands], with partial obstruction
K56.52	Intestinal adhesions [bands] with complete obstruction
K91.89	Other postprocedural complications and disorders of digestive system
K94.01	Colostomy hemorrhage
K94.02	Colostomy infection
K94.03	Colostomy malfunction
K94.09	Other complications of colostomy
K94.11	Enterostomy hemorrhage
K94.12	Enterostomy infection
K94.13	Enterostomy malfunction
K94.19	Other complications of enterostomy
Z43.2	Encounter for attention to ileostomy
Z43.3	Encounter for attention to colostomy
Z43.4	Encounter for attention to other artificial openings of digestive tract
Z93.2	Ileostomy status
Z93.3	Colostomy status
Z93.4	Other artificial openings of gastrointestinal tract status
Z93.8	Other artificial opening status

AMA: **44227** 2018,Jan,8; 2017,Jan,8; 2016,Jan,13; 2015,Jan,16

Relative Value Units/Medicare Edits

Non-Facility RVU	Work	PE	MP	Total
44227	28.62	14.16	6.12	48.9
Facility RVU	**Work**	**PE**	**MP**	**Total**
44227	28.62	14.16	6.12	48.9

	FUD	Status	MUE	Modifiers			IOM Reference
44227	90	A	1(3)	51	N/A	62* 80	None

* with documentation

Terms To Know

anastomosis. Surgically created connection between ducts, blood vessels, or bowel segments to allow flow from one to the other.

colostomy. Artificial surgical opening anywhere along the length of the colon to the skin surface for the diversion of feces.

complication. Condition arising after the beginning of observation and treatment that modifies the course of the patient's illness or the medical care required, or an undesired result or misadventure in medical care.

enterostomy. Surgically created opening into the intestine through the abdominal wall.

insufflation. Blowing air or gas into a body cavity.

laparoscopy. Direct visualization of the peritoneal cavity, outer fallopian tubes, uterus, and ovaries utilizing a laparoscope, a thin, flexible fiberoptic tube.

resection. Surgical removal of a part or all of an organ or body part.

trocar. Cannula or a sharp pointed instrument used to puncture and aspirate fluid from cavities.

44300

44300 Placement, enterostomy or cecostomy, tube open (eg, for feeding or decompression) (separate procedure)

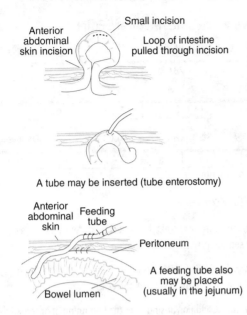

Anterior abdominal skin incision

Small incision

Loop of intestine pulled through incision

A tube may be inserted (tube enterostomy)

Anterior abdominal skin

Feeding tube

Peritoneum

A feeding tube also may be placed (usually in the jejunum)

Bowel lumen

Explanation

The physician places a tube in the small bowel for feeding or into the cecum for decompression via an open approach. The physician makes an abdominal incision. Next, a segment of proximal small bowel or the cecum is isolated. A tube is placed into the small bowel or cecum and brought out through the abdominal wall. The incision is closed.

Coding Tips

This separate procedure, by definition, is usually a component of a more complex service and is not identified separately. When performed alone or with other unrelated procedures/services it may be reported. If performed alone, list the code; if performed with other procedures/services, list the code and append modifier 59 or an X{EPSU} modifier. Do not report 44300 with 44701 when a colon cannulation is performed for an intraoperative colonic lavage. Report percutaneous placement of a duodenostomy, jejunostomy, gastrojejunostomy, cecostomy, or other colonic tube including fluoroscopic imaging guidance with 49441-49442.

ICD-10-CM Diagnostic Codes

C15.3	Malignant neoplasm of upper third of esophagus
C15.4	Malignant neoplasm of middle third of esophagus
C15.5	Malignant neoplasm of lower third of esophagus
C16.0	Malignant neoplasm of cardia
C16.1	Malignant neoplasm of fundus of stomach
C16.2	Malignant neoplasm of body of stomach
C16.3	Malignant neoplasm of pyloric antrum
C16.4	Malignant neoplasm of pylorus
C17.0	Malignant neoplasm of duodenum
C25.0	Malignant neoplasm of head of pancreas
C25.1	Malignant neoplasm of body of pancreas
C25.2	Malignant neoplasm of tail of pancreas
C25.3	Malignant neoplasm of pancreatic duct
C25.4	Malignant neoplasm of endocrine pancreas
C25.7	Malignant neoplasm of other parts of pancreas
C78.4	Secondary malignant neoplasm of small intestine
C7A.010	Malignant carcinoid tumor of the duodenum
C7A.092	Malignant carcinoid tumor of the stomach
D00.2	Carcinoma in situ of stomach
E41	Nutritional marasmus
E44.0	Moderate protein-calorie malnutrition
E44.1	Mild protein-calorie malnutrition
E84.19	Cystic fibrosis with other intestinal manifestations
E86.0	Dehydration
E86.1	Hypovolemia
F50.01	Anorexia nervosa, restricting type
F50.81	Binge eating disorder
F50.89	Other specified eating disorder
G82.21	Paraplegia, complete
G82.22	Paraplegia, incomplete
G82.51	Quadriplegia, C1-C4 complete
G82.53	Quadriplegia, C5-C7 complete
G82.54	Quadriplegia, C5-C7 incomplete
I69.091	Dysphagia following nontraumatic subarachnoid hemorrhage
I69.191	Dysphagia following nontraumatic intracerebral hemorrhage
I69.391	Dysphagia following cerebral infarction
I69.891	Dysphagia following other cerebrovascular disease
K22.0	Achalasia of cardia
K22.10	Ulcer of esophagus without bleeding
K22.11	Ulcer of esophagus with bleeding
K22.2	Esophageal obstruction
K22.3	Perforation of esophagus
K22.4	Dyskinesia of esophagus
K22.6	Gastro-esophageal laceration-hemorrhage syndrome
K22.70	Barrett's esophagus without dysplasia
K22.710	Barrett's esophagus with low grade dysplasia
K22.89	Other specified disease of esophagus
K25.0	Acute gastric ulcer with hemorrhage
K25.1	Acute gastric ulcer with perforation
K25.5	Chronic or unspecified gastric ulcer with perforation
K25.6	Chronic or unspecified gastric ulcer with both hemorrhage and perforation
K25.7	Chronic gastric ulcer without hemorrhage or perforation
K26.0	Acute duodenal ulcer with hemorrhage
K26.2	Acute duodenal ulcer with both hemorrhage and perforation
K26.3	Acute duodenal ulcer without hemorrhage or perforation
K26.5	Chronic or unspecified duodenal ulcer with perforation
K26.7	Chronic duodenal ulcer without hemorrhage or perforation
K28.0	Acute gastrojejunal ulcer with hemorrhage
K28.2	Acute gastrojejunal ulcer with both hemorrhage and perforation
K28.4	Chronic or unspecified gastrojejunal ulcer with hemorrhage
K28.5	Chronic or unspecified gastrojejunal ulcer with perforation
K31.1	Adult hypertrophic pyloric stenosis △
K31.2	Hourglass stricture and stenosis of stomach
K31.5	Obstruction of duodenum
K31.6	Fistula of stomach and duodenum
K31.811	Angiodysplasia of stomach and duodenum with bleeding

Intestines

K31.84	Gastroparesis
K86.0	Alcohol-induced chronic pancreatitis
K86.1	Other chronic pancreatitis
K86.2	Cyst of pancreas
K86.3	Pseudocyst of pancreas
K86.81	Exocrine pancreatic insufficiency
K91.1	Postgastric surgery syndromes
K91.2	Postsurgical malabsorption, not elsewhere classified
Q41.0	Congenital absence, atresia and stenosis of duodenum
T28.0XXA	Burn of mouth and pharynx, initial encounter
T28.1XXA	Burn of esophagus, initial encounter
T28.5XXA	Corrosion of mouth and pharynx, initial encounter
T28.7XXA	Corrosion of other parts of alimentary tract, initial encounter
T73.0XXA	Starvation, initial encounter

AMA: 44300 2018,Jan,8; 2017,Jan,8; 2016,Jan,13; 2015,Jan,16

Relative Value Units/Medicare Edits

Non-Facility RVU	Work	PE	MP	Total
44300	13.75	7.89	3.24	24.88
Facility RVU	Work	PE	MP	Total
44300	13.75	7.89	3.24	24.88

	FUD	Status	MUE	Modifiers				IOM Reference
44300	90	A	1(3)	51	N/A	62*	80	None

* with documentation

Terms To Know

approach. Method or anatomical location used to gain access to a body organ or specific area for procedures.

decompression. Release of pressure.

enterostomy. Surgically created opening into the intestine through the abdominal wall.

proximal. Located closest to a specified reference point, usually the midline or trunk.

44310

44310 Ileostomy or jejunostomy, non-tube

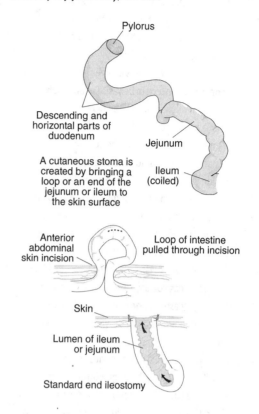

Explanation

The physician brings a loop or end of jejunum or ileum through the abdominal wall onto the skin as a stoma. The physician makes an abdominal incision. Next, the selected segment of jejunum or ileum is isolated. A loop or end of the selected segment of bowel is secured through a separate incision on the abdominal wall onto the skin as a stoma. The initial incision is closed. This stoma is created for purposes other than enteral feeding.

Coding Tips

Do not report 44310 with 44144, 44150–44151, 44155–44156, 45113, 45119, or 45136. For a laparoscopic approach, see 44187.

ICD-10-CM Diagnostic Codes

C18.0	Malignant neoplasm of cecum
C18.2	Malignant neoplasm of ascending colon
C18.3	Malignant neoplasm of hepatic flexure
C18.4	Malignant neoplasm of transverse colon
C18.5	Malignant neoplasm of splenic flexure
C18.6	Malignant neoplasm of descending colon
C7A.020	Malignant carcinoid tumor of the appendix
C7A.021	Malignant carcinoid tumor of the cecum
C7A.022	Malignant carcinoid tumor of the ascending colon
C7A.023	Malignant carcinoid tumor of the transverse colon
C7A.024	Malignant carcinoid tumor of the descending colon
C7A.025	Malignant carcinoid tumor of the sigmoid colon
D01.2	Carcinoma in situ of rectum
D12.0	Benign neoplasm of cecum

D12.1	Benign neoplasm of appendix
D12.2	Benign neoplasm of ascending colon
D12.3	Benign neoplasm of transverse colon
D12.4	Benign neoplasm of descending colon
D12.5	Benign neoplasm of sigmoid colon
D12.7	Benign neoplasm of rectosigmoid junction
D12.8	Benign neoplasm of rectum
D12.9	Benign neoplasm of anus and anal canal
D37.3	Neoplasm of uncertain behavior of appendix
D37.4	Neoplasm of uncertain behavior of colon
D37.5	Neoplasm of uncertain behavior of rectum
D3A.020	Benign carcinoid tumor of the appendix
D3A.021	Benign carcinoid tumor of the cecum
D3A.022	Benign carcinoid tumor of the ascending colon
D3A.023	Benign carcinoid tumor of the transverse colon
D3A.024	Benign carcinoid tumor of the descending colon
D3A.025	Benign carcinoid tumor of the sigmoid colon
D3A.026	Benign carcinoid tumor of the rectum
K50.112	Crohn's disease of large intestine with intestinal obstruction
K50.113	Crohn's disease of large intestine with fistula
K50.114	Crohn's disease of large intestine with abscess
K51.211	Ulcerative (chronic) proctitis with rectal bleeding
K51.213	Ulcerative (chronic) proctitis with fistula
K51.214	Ulcerative (chronic) proctitis with abscess
K51.311	Ulcerative (chronic) rectosigmoiditis with rectal bleeding
K51.312	Ulcerative (chronic) rectosigmoiditis with intestinal obstruction
K51.314	Ulcerative (chronic) rectosigmoiditis with abscess
K51.411	Inflammatory polyps of colon with rectal bleeding
K51.413	Inflammatory polyps of colon with fistula
K51.414	Inflammatory polyps of colon with abscess
K51.511	Left sided colitis with rectal bleeding
K51.512	Left sided colitis with intestinal obstruction
K51.513	Left sided colitis with fistula
K51.514	Left sided colitis with abscess
K51.811	Other ulcerative colitis with rectal bleeding
K51.812	Other ulcerative colitis with intestinal obstruction
K51.813	Other ulcerative colitis with fistula
K55.021	Focal (segmental) acute infarction of small intestine
K55.022	Diffuse acute infarction of small intestine
K55.1	Chronic vascular disorders of intestine
K55.20	Angiodysplasia of colon without hemorrhage
K55.21	Angiodysplasia of colon with hemorrhage
K56.0	Paralytic ileus
K56.2	Volvulus
K57.20	Diverticulitis of large intestine with perforation and abscess without bleeding
K57.21	Diverticulitis of large intestine with perforation and abscess with bleeding
K57.31	Diverticulosis of large intestine without perforation or abscess with bleeding
K57.33	Diverticulitis of large intestine without perforation or abscess with bleeding
K57.40	Diverticulitis of both small and large intestine with perforation and abscess without bleeding
K57.41	Diverticulitis of both small and large intestine with perforation and abscess with bleeding
K59.2	Neurogenic bowel, not elsewhere classified
K59.31	Toxic megacolon
K59.81	Ogilvie syndrome
K63.1	Perforation of intestine (nontraumatic)
K63.3	Ulcer of intestine
P77.1	Stage 1 necrotizing enterocolitis in newborn 🅽
P77.2	Stage 2 necrotizing enterocolitis in newborn 🅽
P77.3	Stage 3 necrotizing enterocolitis in newborn 🅽
P78.0	Perinatal intestinal perforation 🅽
Q42.0	Congenital absence, atresia and stenosis of rectum with fistula
Q42.1	Congenital absence, atresia and stenosis of rectum without fistula
Q42.2	Congenital absence, atresia and stenosis of anus with fistula
Q43.1	Hirschsprung's disease
Q43.2	Other congenital functional disorders of colon
Q43.3	Congenital malformations of intestinal fixation
Q43.8	Other specified congenital malformations of intestine
Q45.8	Other specified congenital malformations of digestive system

AMA: **44310** 2018,Jan,8; 2017,Jan,8; 2016,Jan,13; 2015,Jan,16

Relative Value Units/Medicare Edits

Non-Facility RVU	Work	PE	MP	Total
44310	17.59	9.36	3.61	30.56
Facility RVU	**Work**	**PE**	**MP**	**Total**
44310	17.59	9.36	3.61	30.56

	FUD	Status	MUE	Modifiers				IOM Reference
44310	90	A	2(3)	51	N/A	62*	80	None

* with documentation

Terms To Know

ileostomy. Artificial surgical opening that brings the end of the ileum out through the abdominal wall to the skin surface for the diversion of feces through a stoma.

jejunostomy. Permanent, surgical opening into the jejunum, the part of the small intestine between the duodenum and ileum, through the abdominal wall, often used for placing a feeding tube.

Ogilvie's syndrome. Colonic obstruction with symptoms of persistent contraction of intestinal musculature, caused by a defect in the sympathetic nerve supply.

stoma. Opening created in the abdominal wall from an internal organ or structure for diversion of waste elimination, drainage, and access.

44312-44314

44312 Revision of ileostomy; simple (release of superficial scar) (separate procedure)

44314 complicated (reconstruction in-depth) (separate procedure)

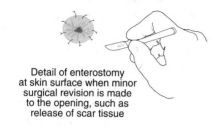

Detail of enterostomy at skin surface when minor surgical revision is made to the opening, such as release of scar tissue

In a complicated revision, the site of the ileostomy may be moved

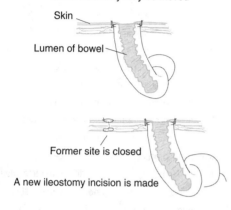

Skin

Lumen of bowel

Former site is closed

A new ileostomy incision is made

Explanation

In 44312, the physician revises an ileostomy through an incision around the stoma with release of scar tissue. The physician makes and incision around the ileostomy site. Next, the stoma is dissected free of the surrounding abdominal wall and constricting scar tissue is released. The stoma is reapproximated to the skin or the distal end of the stoma may be transected. Additional ileum may be pulled through the abdominal wall and approximated to the skin as a revised ileostomy. In 44314, the physician revises an ileostomy by forming a new stoma site. The physician makes an abdominal incision and the previous ileostomy is completely taken down. The distal ileum is brought through a new incision on the abdominal wall onto the skin as an ileostomy at a new site. The initial incision and former stoma site are closed.

Coding Tips

These separate procedures by definition are usually a component of a more complex service and are not identified separately. When performed alone or with other unrelated procedures/services they may be reported. If performed with other procedures, list the code and append modifier 59 or an X{EPSU} modifier.

ICD-10-CM Diagnostic Codes

K56.51	Intestinal adhesions [bands], with partial obstruction
K56.52	Intestinal adhesions [bands] with complete obstruction
K91.89	Other postprocedural complications and disorders of digestive system
K94.11	Enterostomy hemorrhage
K94.12	Enterostomy infection
K94.13	Enterostomy malfunction
K94.19	Other complications of enterostomy

Z43.2	Encounter for attention to ileostomy
Z46.89	Encounter for fitting and adjustment of other specified devices

AMA: 44312 2014,Jan,11 **44314** 2014,Jan,11

Relative Value Units/Medicare Edits

Non-Facility RVU	Work	PE	MP	Total
44312	9.43	6.24	1.89	17.56
44314	16.74	9.55	3.27	29.56
Facility RVU	**Work**	**PE**	**MP**	**Total**
44312	9.43	6.24	1.89	17.56
44314	16.74	9.55	3.27	29.56

	FUD	Status	MUE		Modifiers			IOM Reference
44312	90	A	1(2)	51	N/A	N/A	80*	None
44314	90	A	1(2)	51	N/A	62*	80	

* with documentation

Terms To Know

adhesion. Abnormal fibrous connection between two structures, soft tissue or bony structures, that may occur as the result of surgery, infection, or trauma.

dissect. Cut apart or separate tissue for surgical purposes or for visual or microscopic study.

distal. Located farther away from a specified reference point or the trunk.

ileostomy. Artificial surgical opening that brings the end of the ileum out through the abdominal wall to the skin surface for the diversion of feces through a stoma.

infection. Presence of microorganisms in body tissues that may result in cellular damage.

intestinal or peritoneal adhesions with obstruction. Abnormal fibrous band growths joining separate tissues in the peritoneum or intestine, causing blockage.

reconstruction. Recreating, restoring, or rebuilding a body part or organ.

release. Disconnection of a tendon or ligament.

revision. Reordering or rearrangement of tissue to suit a particular need or function.

scar tissue. Fibrous connective tissue that forms around a wounded area or injury, composed mainly of fibroblasts or collagenous fibers.

stoma. Opening created in the abdominal wall from an internal organ or structure for diversion of waste elimination, drainage, and access.

superficial. On the skin surface or near the surface of any involved structure or field of interest.

transection. Transverse dissection; to cut across a long axis; cross section.

44316

44316 Continent ileostomy (Kock procedure) (separate procedure)

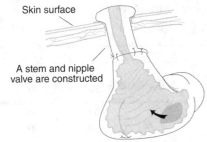

Skin surface

A stem and nipple valve are constructed

Reservoir pouch is formed out of ileum

Explanation

The physician forms a reservoir of distal ileum (Kock pouch) and brings it through the abdominal wall onto the skin as a continent ileostomy. The physician makes an abdominal incision. Next, the distal ileum is folded upon itself and approximated in such a way to form a pouch with a valve. The end of the pouch is brought through a separate incision on the abdominal wall onto the skin as a continent ileostomy. The initial incision is closed.

Coding Tips

This separate procedure by definition is usually a component of a more complex service and is not identified separately. When performed alone or with other unrelated procedures/services it may be reported. If performed alone, list the code; if performed with other procedures/services, list the code and append modifier 59 or an X{EPSU} modifier. For total abdominal colectomy with proctectomy, with continent ileostomy, see 44156. For revision of ileostomy, simple, see 44312; complicated, see 44314. For diagnostic endoscopic evaluation of small intestinal pouch (fiberoptic evaluation), see 44385.

ICD-10-CM Diagnostic Codes

C18.0	Malignant neoplasm of cecum
C18.2	Malignant neoplasm of ascending colon
C18.3	Malignant neoplasm of hepatic flexure
C18.4	Malignant neoplasm of transverse colon
C18.5	Malignant neoplasm of splenic flexure
C18.6	Malignant neoplasm of descending colon
C18.8	Malignant neoplasm of overlapping sites of colon
C19	Malignant neoplasm of rectosigmoid junction
C78.5	Secondary malignant neoplasm of large intestine and rectum
C7A.020	Malignant carcinoid tumor of the appendix
C7A.021	Malignant carcinoid tumor of the cecum
C7A.022	Malignant carcinoid tumor of the ascending colon
C7A.023	Malignant carcinoid tumor of the transverse colon
C7A.024	Malignant carcinoid tumor of the descending colon
C7A.025	Malignant carcinoid tumor of the sigmoid colon
D01.0	Carcinoma in situ of colon
D01.1	Carcinoma in situ of rectosigmoid junction
D01.2	Carcinoma in situ of rectum
D12.0	Benign neoplasm of cecum
D12.1	Benign neoplasm of appendix
D12.2	Benign neoplasm of ascending colon
D12.3	Benign neoplasm of transverse colon
D12.4	Benign neoplasm of descending colon
D12.5	Benign neoplasm of sigmoid colon
D12.7	Benign neoplasm of rectosigmoid junction
D12.8	Benign neoplasm of rectum
D37.3	Neoplasm of uncertain behavior of appendix
D37.4	Neoplasm of uncertain behavior of colon
D37.5	Neoplasm of uncertain behavior of rectum
D3A.020	Benign carcinoid tumor of the appendix
D3A.021	Benign carcinoid tumor of the cecum
D3A.022	Benign carcinoid tumor of the ascending colon
D3A.023	Benign carcinoid tumor of the transverse colon
D3A.024	Benign carcinoid tumor of the descending colon
D3A.025	Benign carcinoid tumor of the sigmoid colon
D3A.026	Benign carcinoid tumor of the rectum
D49.0	Neoplasm of unspecified behavior of digestive system
K51.011	Ulcerative (chronic) pancolitis with rectal bleeding
K51.012	Ulcerative (chronic) pancolitis with intestinal obstruction
K51.013	Ulcerative (chronic) pancolitis with fistula
K51.014	Ulcerative (chronic) pancolitis with abscess
K51.211	Ulcerative (chronic) proctitis with rectal bleeding
K51.212	Ulcerative (chronic) proctitis with intestinal obstruction
K51.213	Ulcerative (chronic) proctitis with fistula
K51.214	Ulcerative (chronic) proctitis with abscess
K51.311	Ulcerative (chronic) rectosigmoiditis with rectal bleeding
K51.312	Ulcerative (chronic) rectosigmoiditis with intestinal obstruction
K51.313	Ulcerative (chronic) rectosigmoiditis with fistula
K51.314	Ulcerative (chronic) rectosigmoiditis with abscess
K51.411	Inflammatory polyps of colon with rectal bleeding
K51.412	Inflammatory polyps of colon with intestinal obstruction
K51.413	Inflammatory polyps of colon with fistula
K51.414	Inflammatory polyps of colon with abscess
K51.511	Left sided colitis with rectal bleeding
K51.512	Left sided colitis with intestinal obstruction
K51.513	Left sided colitis with fistula
K51.514	Left sided colitis with abscess
K55.021	Focal (segmental) acute infarction of small intestine
K55.022	Diffuse acute infarction of small intestine
K55.1	Chronic vascular disorders of intestine
K55.8	Other vascular disorders of intestine
K57.20	Diverticulitis of large intestine with perforation and abscess without bleeding
K57.21	Diverticulitis of large intestine with perforation and abscess with bleeding
K57.33	Diverticulitis of large intestine without perforation or abscess with bleeding
K57.40	Diverticulitis of both small and large intestine with perforation and abscess without bleeding
K57.41	Diverticulitis of both small and large intestine with perforation and abscess with bleeding
K57.51	Diverticulosis of both small and large intestine without perforation or abscess with bleeding
K59.81	Ogilvie syndrome
K63.1	Perforation of intestine (nontraumatic)

K63.3	Ulcer of intestine		
K63.4	Enteroptosis		
K94.11	Enterostomy hemorrhage		
K94.12	Enterostomy infection		
K94.19	Other complications of enterostomy		
P77.1	Stage 1 necrotizing enterocolitis in newborn N		
P77.2	Stage 2 necrotizing enterocolitis in newborn N		
P77.3	Stage 3 necrotizing enterocolitis in newborn N		
P78.0	Perinatal intestinal perforation N		
S36.530A	Laceration of ascending [right] colon, initial encounter		
S36.531A	Laceration of transverse colon, initial encounter		
S36.532A	Laceration of descending [left] colon, initial encounter		
S36.533A	Laceration of sigmoid colon, initial encounter		

AMA: 44316 2014,Jan,11

Relative Value Units/Medicare Edits

Non-Facility RVU	Work	PE	MP	Total
44316	23.59	12.52	5.77	41.88
Facility RVU	**Work**	**PE**	**MP**	**Total**
44316	23.59	12.52	5.77	41.88

	FUD	Status	MUE	Modifiers				IOM Reference
44316	90	A	1(2)	51	N/A	62*	80	None

* with documentation

Terms To Know

distal. Located farther away from a specified reference point or the trunk.

ileostomy. Artificial surgical opening that brings the end of the ileum out through the abdominal wall to the skin surface for the diversion of feces through a stoma.

Kock procedure. Surgical procedure in which the physician forms a reservoir of distal ileum (Kock pouch) and brings it through the abdominal wall onto the skin as a continent ileostomy.

44320-44322

44320	Colostomy or skin level cecostomy;
44322	with multiple biopsies (eg, for congenital megacolon) (separate procedure)

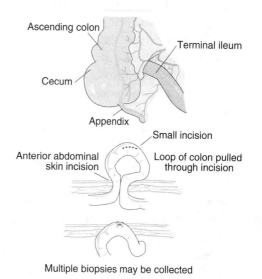

Multiple biopsies may be collected

Explanation

The physician performs a colostomy or skin level cecostomy. An abdominal incision is made and the peritoneum is entered, followed by a thorough exploratory exam of abdominal organs and tissues, including lysis of any adhesions. The small bowel is mobilized and isolated out of the way. The distal bowel is measured for the appropriate length for pouch creation. A proximal point from the distal end is separated from its blood supply to be made into a pouch nipple valve. The pouch is fashioned into the right configuration and secured in place. The nipple valve component is intussuscepted and secured in place. The pouch end of colon (or cecum) is brought out through a separate incision on the abdominal wall onto the skin as a stoma (cecostomy or colostomy) and secured in place with a pouch nipple to mucocutaneous tissue anastomosis. The abdomen is irrigated, a final inspection is made, and a closed-system suction drain may be placed. The abdominal wall skin is closed and dressed and a pouch intubation catheter is placed into the nipple valve and pouch. Report 44322 when multiple biopsies are obtained during the procedure.

Coding Tips

Note that 44322, a separate procedure by definition, is usually a component of a more complex service and is not identified separately. When performed alone or with other unrelated procedures, it may be reported. If performed with other procedures, list the code and append modifier 59 or an X{EPSU} modifier. Do not report 44320 with 44141, 44144, 44146, 44605, 45110, 45119, 45126, 45563, 45805, 45825, 50810, 51597, 57307, or 58240. For a laparoscopic approach, see 44188.

ICD-10-CM Diagnostic Codes

C18.0	Malignant neoplasm of cecum
C18.3	Malignant neoplasm of hepatic flexure
C18.6	Malignant neoplasm of descending colon
C18.7	Malignant neoplasm of sigmoid colon
C19	Malignant neoplasm of rectosigmoid junction
C78.5	Secondary malignant neoplasm of large intestine and rectum
C7A.021	Malignant carcinoid tumor of the cecum

C7A.022	Malignant carcinoid tumor of the ascending colon
C7A.023	Malignant carcinoid tumor of the transverse colon
C7A.024	Malignant carcinoid tumor of the descending colon
C7A.025	Malignant carcinoid tumor of the sigmoid colon
D01.0	Carcinoma in situ of colon
D01.1	Carcinoma in situ of rectosigmoid junction
D12.0	Benign neoplasm of cecum
D12.1	Benign neoplasm of appendix
D12.2	Benign neoplasm of ascending colon
D12.3	Benign neoplasm of transverse colon
D12.4	Benign neoplasm of descending colon
D12.5	Benign neoplasm of sigmoid colon
D37.3	Neoplasm of uncertain behavior of appendix
D37.4	Neoplasm of uncertain behavior of colon
D3A.022	Benign carcinoid tumor of the ascending colon
D3A.023	Benign carcinoid tumor of the transverse colon
D3A.024	Benign carcinoid tumor of the descending colon
D3A.025	Benign carcinoid tumor of the sigmoid colon
D49.0	Neoplasm of unspecified behavior of digestive system
K50.111	Crohn's disease of large intestine with rectal bleeding
K50.112	Crohn's disease of large intestine with intestinal obstruction
K50.113	Crohn's disease of large intestine with fistula
K50.114	Crohn's disease of large intestine with abscess
K50.811	Crohn's disease of both small and large intestine with rectal bleeding
K50.812	Crohn's disease of both small and large intestine with intestinal obstruction
K50.813	Crohn's disease of both small and large intestine with fistula
K50.814	Crohn's disease of both small and large intestine with abscess
K51.011	Ulcerative (chronic) pancolitis with rectal bleeding
K51.012	Ulcerative (chronic) pancolitis with intestinal obstruction
K51.013	Ulcerative (chronic) pancolitis with fistula
K51.014	Ulcerative (chronic) pancolitis with abscess
K51.311	Ulcerative (chronic) rectosigmoiditis with rectal bleeding
K51.312	Ulcerative (chronic) rectosigmoiditis with intestinal obstruction
K51.313	Ulcerative (chronic) rectosigmoiditis with fistula
K51.314	Ulcerative (chronic) rectosigmoiditis with abscess
K51.411	Inflammatory polyps of colon with rectal bleeding
K51.412	Inflammatory polyps of colon with intestinal obstruction
K51.413	Inflammatory polyps of colon with fistula
K51.414	Inflammatory polyps of colon with abscess
K51.511	Left sided colitis with rectal bleeding
K51.512	Left sided colitis with intestinal obstruction
K51.513	Left sided colitis with fistula
K51.514	Left sided colitis with abscess
K55.041	Focal (segmental) acute infarction of large intestine
K55.042	Diffuse acute infarction of large intestine
K55.20	Angiodysplasia of colon without hemorrhage
K55.21	Angiodysplasia of colon with hemorrhage
K56.0	Paralytic ileus
K56.2	Volvulus
K56.51	Intestinal adhesions [bands], with partial obstruction
K56.52	Intestinal adhesions [bands] with complete obstruction

K57.20	Diverticulitis of large intestine with perforation and abscess without bleeding
K57.21	Diverticulitis of large intestine with perforation and abscess with bleeding
K57.31	Diverticulosis of large intestine without perforation or abscess with bleeding
K57.33	Diverticulitis of large intestine without perforation or abscess with bleeding
K57.40	Diverticulitis of both small and large intestine with perforation and abscess without bleeding
K57.41	Diverticulitis of both small and large intestine with perforation and abscess with bleeding
K59.31	Toxic megacolon
K59.81	Ogilvie syndrome
K63.0	Abscess of intestine
K63.1	Perforation of intestine (nontraumatic)
K63.2	Fistula of intestine
K63.3	Ulcer of intestine
K63.4	Enteroptosis
K63.5	Polyp of colon
K91.31	Postprocedural partial intestinal obstruction
K91.32	Postprocedural complete intestinal obstruction
N32.1	Vesicointestinal fistula
Q43.1	Hirschsprung's disease
Q43.2	Other congenital functional disorders of colon
Q43.3	Congenital malformations of intestinal fixation
S36.530A	Laceration of ascending [right] colon, initial encounter
S36.531A	Laceration of transverse colon, initial encounter
S36.532A	Laceration of descending [left] colon, initial encounter
S36.533A	Laceration of sigmoid colon, initial encounter
S36.538A	Laceration of other part of colon, initial encounter

AMA: **44320** 2018,Jan,8; 2017,Jan,8; 2016,Jan,13; 2015,Jan,16

Relative Value Units/Medicare Edits

Non-Facility RVU	Work	PE	MP	Total
44320	19.91	11.13	4.33	35.37
44322	13.32	13.51	3.27	30.1
Facility RVU	Work	PE	MP	Total
44320	19.91	11.13	4.33	35.37
44322	13.32	13.51	3.27	30.1

	FUD	Status	MUE	Modifiers				IOM Reference
44320	90	A	1(2)	51	N/A	62*	80	None
44322	90	A	1(2)	51	N/A	62*	80	

* with documentation

44340-44346

44340 Revision of colostomy; simple (release of superficial scar) (separate procedure)
44345 complicated (reconstruction in-depth) (separate procedure)
44346 with repair of paracolostomy hernia (separate procedure)

Detail of colostomy at skin surface. A minor revision is made to the opening

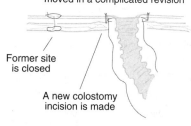
The site of the colostomy is often moved in a complicated revision

Former site is closed

A new colostomy incision is made

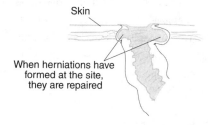
Skin

When herniations have formed at the site, they are repaired

Explanation

The physician revises a colostomy through an incision around the stoma site. In 44340, a release of scar tissue is performed. The physician makes an incision around the stoma site. The stoma is dissected free of the surrounding abdominal wall and constricting scar tissue is released. The stoma is reapproximated to the skin or the distal stoma is transected and additional colon pulled through the abdominal wall and approximated to the skin as a revised colostomy. In 44345, a new stoma site is formed. The previous colostomy is completely taken down. The distal end of colon is brought through a separate incision on the abdominal wall onto the skin at a new site as a revised colostomy. The initial incision and previous stoma site are closed. In 44346, the physician repairs a paracolostomy hernia. The previous colostomy site is taken down. The hernia at the former colostomy site is repaired. The end of colon is brought through a separate incision on the abdominal wall at a new site and onto the skin as a revised colostomy. The initial incision and previous stoma site are closed.

Coding Tips

These separate procedures by definition are usually a component of a more complex service and are not identified separately. When performed alone or with other unrelated procedures/services it may be reported. If performed alone, list the code; if performed with other procedures/services, list the code and append modifier 59 or an X{EPSU} modifier.

ICD-10-CM Diagnostic Codes

K43.3 Parastomal hernia with obstruction, without gangrene
K43.4 Parastomal hernia with gangrene
K43.5 Parastomal hernia without obstruction or gangrene
K91.89 Other postprocedural complications and disorders of digestive system

K94.01 Colostomy hemorrhage
K94.02 Colostomy infection
K94.03 Colostomy malfunction
K94.09 Other complications of colostomy
T81.31XA Disruption of external operation (surgical) wound, not elsewhere classified, initial encounter
Z43.3 Encounter for attention to colostomy

AMA: **44346** 2018,Jan,8; 2017,Jan,8; 2016,Jan,13; 2015,Jan,16

Relative Value Units/Medicare Edits

Non-Facility RVU	Work	PE	MP	Total
44340	9.28	7.16	1.94	18.38
44345	17.22	10.09	3.57	30.88
44346	19.63	11.03	4.18	34.84
Facility RVU	Work	PE	MP	Total
44340	9.28	7.16	1.94	18.38
44345	17.22	10.09	3.57	30.88
44346	19.63	11.03	4.18	34.84

	FUD	Status	MUE	Modifiers			IOM Reference
44340	90	A	1(2)	51	N/A	62*	N/A	None
44345	90	A	1(2)	51	N/A	62*	80	
44346	90	A	1(2)	51	N/A	62*	80	

* with documentation

Terms To Know

colostomy. Artificial surgical opening anywhere along the length of the colon to the skin surface for the diversion of feces.

complication. Condition arising after the beginning of observation and treatment that modifies the course of the patient's illness or the medical care required, or an undesired result or misadventure in medical care.

dissection. Separating by cutting tissue or body structures apart.

infection. Presence of microorganisms in body tissues that may result in cellular damage.

intestinal or peritoneal adhesions with obstruction. Abnormal fibrous band growths joining separate tissues in the peritoneum or intestine, causing blockage.

revision. Reordering or rearrangement of tissue to suit a particular need or function.

stoma. Opening created in the abdominal wall from an internal organ or structure for diversion of waste elimination, drainage, and access.

transection. Transverse dissection; to cut across a long axis; cross section.

Intestines

44360-44361

44360 Small intestinal endoscopy, enteroscopy beyond second portion of duodenum, not including ileum; diagnostic, including collection of specimen(s) by brushing or washing, when performed (separate procedure)

44361 with biopsy, single or multiple

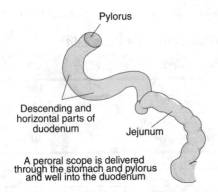

Pylorus

Descending and horizontal parts of duodenum

Jejunum

A peroral scope is delivered through the stomach and pylorus and well into the duodenum

Specimens are collected by brushing, washing, or biopsy

Explanation

The physician performs endoscopy of the proximal small bowel and may obtain brushings or washings. The physician places an endoscope through the mouth and advances it into the small intestine beyond the second portion of the duodenum, but not including the ileum. An abdominal incision may be made to mobilize the small bowel and assist in running the bowel over the endoscope. The lumen of the small bowel is examined and brushings or washings may be obtained of suspicious areas. The endoscope is withdrawn at the completion of the procedure. If an incision was made, it is closed. Report 44361 when biopsies are obtained.

Coding Tips

Note that 44360, a separate procedure by definition, and is usually a component of a more complex service and is not identified separately. When performed alone or with other unrelated procedures/services it may be reported. If performed alone, list the code; if performed with other procedures/services, list the code and append modifier 59 or an X{EPSU} modifier. Report the appropriate endoscopy for each anatomic site examined. Surgical endoscopy includes diagnostic endoscopy; however, diagnostic endoscopy can be identified separately when performed at the same surgical session as an open procedure. Bleeding that occurs as the result of an endoscopic procedure, and controlled during the same operative session, is not reported separately. Do not report 44360 or 44361 with 43233, 43235–43259, 43266, 43270, or 44376–44379.

ICD-10-CM Diagnostic Codes

A04.0	Enteropathogenic Escherichia coli infection
A04.1	Enterotoxigenic Escherichia coli infection
A04.2	Enteroinvasive Escherichia coli infection
A04.3	Enterohemorrhagic Escherichia coli infection
A04.4	Other intestinal Escherichia coli infections
C17.0	Malignant neoplasm of duodenum
C17.1	Malignant neoplasm of jejunum
C17.3	Meckel's diverticulum, malignant
C49.A3	Gastrointestinal stromal tumor of small intestine
C7A.010	Malignant carcinoid tumor of the duodenum
C7A.011	Malignant carcinoid tumor of the jejunum
C88.3	Immunoproliferative small intestinal disease
D13.2	Benign neoplasm of duodenum
D13.39	Benign neoplasm of other parts of small intestine
D3A.010	Benign carcinoid tumor of the duodenum
D3A.011	Benign carcinoid tumor of the jejunum
D52.0	Dietary folate deficiency anemia
K26.0	Acute duodenal ulcer with hemorrhage
K26.1	Acute duodenal ulcer with perforation
K26.2	Acute duodenal ulcer with both hemorrhage and perforation
K26.3	Acute duodenal ulcer without hemorrhage or perforation
K26.4	Chronic or unspecified duodenal ulcer with hemorrhage
K26.5	Chronic or unspecified duodenal ulcer with perforation
K26.6	Chronic or unspecified duodenal ulcer with both hemorrhage and perforation
K26.7	Chronic duodenal ulcer without hemorrhage or perforation
K28.0	Acute gastrojejunal ulcer with hemorrhage
K28.1	Acute gastrojejunal ulcer with perforation
K28.2	Acute gastrojejunal ulcer with both hemorrhage and perforation
K28.3	Acute gastrojejunal ulcer without hemorrhage or perforation
K28.4	Chronic or unspecified gastrojejunal ulcer with hemorrhage
K28.5	Chronic or unspecified gastrojejunal ulcer with perforation
K28.6	Chronic or unspecified gastrojejunal ulcer with both hemorrhage and perforation
K29.80	Duodenitis without bleeding
K29.81	Duodenitis with bleeding
K31.5	Obstruction of duodenum
K31.82	Dieulafoy lesion (hemorrhagic) of stomach and duodenum
K50.011	Crohn's disease of small intestine with rectal bleeding
K50.012	Crohn's disease of small intestine with intestinal obstruction
K50.013	Crohn's disease of small intestine with fistula
K50.014	Crohn's disease of small intestine with abscess
K50.80	Crohn's disease of both small and large intestine without complications
K50.811	Crohn's disease of both small and large intestine with rectal bleeding
K50.812	Crohn's disease of both small and large intestine with intestinal obstruction
K50.813	Crohn's disease of both small and large intestine with fistula
K50.814	Crohn's disease of both small and large intestine with abscess
K50.818	Crohn's disease of both small and large intestine with other complication
K52.0	Gastroenteritis and colitis due to radiation
K52.1	Toxic gastroenteritis and colitis
K52.21	Food protein-induced enterocolitis syndrome
K52.22	Food protein-induced enteropathy
K52.29	Other allergic and dietetic gastroenteritis and colitis
K52.3	Indeterminate colitis
K52.81	Eosinophilic gastritis or gastroenteritis
K52.831	Collagenous colitis
K52.832	Lymphocytic colitis
K52.838	Other microscopic colitis
K52.89	Other specified noninfective gastroenteritis and colitis
K55.021	Focal (segmental) acute infarction of small intestine

K55.022	Diffuse acute infarction of small intestine
K55.1	Chronic vascular disorders of intestine
K55.8	Other vascular disorders of intestine
K57.00	Diverticulitis of small intestine with perforation and abscess without bleeding
K57.01	Diverticulitis of small intestine with perforation and abscess with bleeding
K57.11	Diverticulosis of small intestine without perforation or abscess with bleeding
K57.12	Diverticulitis of small intestine without perforation or abscess without bleeding
K57.13	Diverticulitis of small intestine without perforation or abscess with bleeding
K57.40	Diverticulitis of both small and large intestine with perforation and abscess without bleeding
K57.41	Diverticulitis of both small and large intestine with perforation and abscess with bleeding
K57.51	Diverticulosis of both small and large intestine without perforation or abscess with bleeding
K57.53	Diverticulitis of both small and large intestine without perforation or abscess with bleeding
K58.0	Irritable bowel syndrome with diarrhea
K58.1	Irritable bowel syndrome with constipation
K58.2	Mixed irritable bowel syndrome
K58.8	Other irritable bowel syndrome
K58.9	Irritable bowel syndrome without diarrhea
K59.1	Functional diarrhea
K63.3	Ulcer of intestine
K63.81	Dieulafoy lesion of intestine
K90.0	Celiac disease
K90.1	Tropical sprue
K90.81	Whipple's disease
K90.89	Other intestinal malabsorption
K92.0	Hematemesis
K92.1	Melena
M35.08	Sjögren syndrome with gastrointestinal involvement
N82.2	Fistula of vagina to small intestine ♀
Q43.0	Meckel's diverticulum (displaced) (hypertrophic)
R62.7	Adult failure to thrive Ⓐ
R63.4	Abnormal weight loss
R63.6	Underweight

AMA: **44360** 2019,Oct,10; 2018,Jan,8; 2017,Jan,8; 2016,Jan,13; 2015,Jan,16
44361 2019,Oct,10

Relative Value Units/Medicare Edits

Non-Facility RVU	Work	PE	MP	Total
44360	2.49	1.42	0.26	4.17
44361	2.77	1.55	0.3	4.62
Facility RVU	**Work**	**PE**	**MP**	**Total**
44360	2.49	1.42	0.26	4.17
44361	2.77	1.55	0.3	4.62

	FUD	Status	MUE	Modifiers				IOM Reference
44360	0	A	1(3)	51	N/A	N/A	N/A	None
44361	0	A	1(2)	51	N/A	N/A	N/A	

* with documentation

Terms To Know

carcinoid tumor. Specific type of slow-growing neuroendocrine tumors. Carcinoid tumors occur most commonly in the hormone producing cells of the gastrointestinal tracts and can also occur in the pancreas, testes, ovaries, or lungs.

duodenum. First portion of the small intestine connected to the stomach at the pylorus and extending to the jejunum.

hemorrhage. Internal or external bleeding with loss of significant amounts of blood.

ileum. Lower portion of the small intestine, from the jejunum to the cecum.

Meckel's diverticulum. Congenital, abnormal remnant of embryonic digestive system development that leaves a sacculation or outpouching from the wall of the small intestine near the terminal part of the ileum made of acid-secreting tissue as in the stomach.

44363

44363   Small intestinal endoscopy, enteroscopy beyond second portion of duodenum, not including ileum; with removal of foreign body(s)

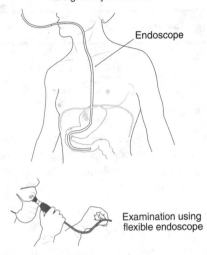

An endoscope is delivered through the stomach and pylorus and well into the duodenum and a foreign body is removed

Endoscope

Examination using flexible endoscope

Explanation

The physician performs endoscopy of the proximal small bowel and removes a foreign body(s). The physician places an endoscope through the mouth and advances it into the small intestine beyond the second portion of the duodenum, but not including the ileum. An abdominal incision may be made to mobilize the small bowel and assist in running the bowel over the endoscope. The bowel lumen is examined and the foreign body(s) located. A snare or forceps is advanced through the endoscope and the foreign body(s) grasped and removed. The endoscope is withdrawn at the completion of the procedure. If an incision was made, it is closed.

Coding Tips

Report the appropriate endoscopy for each anatomic site examined. Surgical endoscopy includes diagnostic endoscopy; however, diagnostic endoscopy can be identified separately when performed at the same surgical session as an open procedure. For esophagogastroduodenoscopy, with removal of a foreign body, see 43247. Bleeding that occurs as the result of an endoscopic procedure, and controlled during the same operative session, is not reported separately. Do not report 44363 with 43233, 43235–43259, 43266, 43270, or 44376–44379.

ICD-10-CM Diagnostic Codes

T18.3XXA   Foreign body in small intestine, initial encounter
T18.8XXA   Foreign body in other parts of alimentary tract, initial encounter

AMA: 44363 2019,Oct,10

Relative Value Units/Medicare Edits

Non-Facility RVU	Work	PE	MP	Total
44363	3.39	1.8	0.38	5.57
Facility RVU	Work	PE	MP	Total
44363	3.39	1.8	0.38	5.57

	FUD	Status	MUE	Modifiers				IOM Reference
44363	0	A	1(3)	51	N/A	N/A	80*	None

* with documentation

Terms To Know

closure. Repairing an incision or wound by suture or other means.

duodenum. First portion of the small intestine connected to the stomach at the pylorus and extending to the jejunum.

endoscopy. Visual inspection of the body using a fiberoptic scope.

forceps. Tool used for grasping or compressing tissue.

foreign body. Any object or substance found in an organ and tissue that does not belong under normal circumstances.

ileum. Lower portion of the small intestine, from the jejunum to the cecum.

incision. Act of cutting into tissue or an organ.

jejunum. Highly vascular upper two-fifths of the small intestine, extending from the duodenum to the ileum.

lumen. Space inside an intestine, artery, vein, duct, or tube.

proximal. Located closest to a specified reference point, usually the midline or trunk.

small intestine. First portion of intestine connecting to the pylorus at the proximal end and consisting of the duodenum, jejunum, and ileum.

snare. Wire used as a loop to excise a polyp or lesion.

44364-44365

44364 Small intestinal endoscopy, enteroscopy beyond second portion of duodenum, not including ileum; with removal of tumor(s), polyp(s), or other lesion(s) by snare technique

44365 with removal of tumor(s), polyp(s), or other lesion(s) by hot biopsy forceps or bipolar cautery

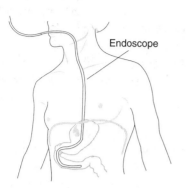

An endoscope is delivered through the stomach and pylorus and well into the duodenum. Tumors, polyps, or other lesions are removed

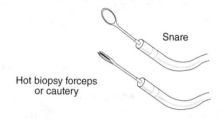

Explanation

The physician performs endoscopy of the proximal small bowel and removes a tumor or polyp by snare technique. The physician places an endoscope through the mouth and advances it into the small intestine. An abdominal incision may be made to mobilize the small bowel and assist in running the bowel over the endoscope. The bowel lumen is examined and the polyp or tumor is located and removed with a snare placed through the endoscope. The endoscope is withdrawn at the completion of the procedure. If an incision was made it is closed. Report 44365 when hot biopsy forceps or cautery is used to remove the tumor or polyp.

Coding Tips

Report the appropriate endoscopy for each anatomic site examined. Surgical endoscopy includes diagnostic endoscopy; however, diagnostic endoscopy can be identified separately when performed at the same surgical session as an open procedure. Bleeding that occurs as the result of an endoscopic procedure, and controlled during the same operative session, is not reported separately. Do not report 44364–44365 with 43233, 43235–43259, 43266, 43270, or 44376–44379.

ICD-10-CM Diagnostic Codes

C17.0	Malignant neoplasm of duodenum
C17.1	Malignant neoplasm of jejunum
C17.8	Malignant neoplasm of overlapping sites of small intestine
C49.A3	Gastrointestinal stromal tumor of small intestine
C78.4	Secondary malignant neoplasm of small intestine
C7A.010	Malignant carcinoid tumor of the duodenum
C7A.011	Malignant carcinoid tumor of the jejunum

D01.49	Carcinoma in situ of other parts of intestine
D13.2	Benign neoplasm of duodenum
D13.39	Benign neoplasm of other parts of small intestine
D37.2	Neoplasm of uncertain behavior of small intestine
D3A.010	Benign carcinoid tumor of the duodenum
D3A.011	Benign carcinoid tumor of the jejunum
D49.0	Neoplasm of unspecified behavior of digestive system
K26.0	Acute duodenal ulcer with hemorrhage
K26.1	Acute duodenal ulcer with perforation
K26.2	Acute duodenal ulcer with both hemorrhage and perforation
K26.3	Acute duodenal ulcer without hemorrhage or perforation
K26.4	Chronic or unspecified duodenal ulcer with hemorrhage
K26.5	Chronic or unspecified duodenal ulcer with perforation
K26.6	Chronic or unspecified duodenal ulcer with both hemorrhage and perforation
K26.7	Chronic duodenal ulcer without hemorrhage or perforation
K28.0	Acute gastrojejunal ulcer with hemorrhage
K28.1	Acute gastrojejunal ulcer with perforation
K28.2	Acute gastrojejunal ulcer with both hemorrhage and perforation
K28.3	Acute gastrojejunal ulcer without hemorrhage or perforation
K28.4	Chronic or unspecified gastrojejunal ulcer with hemorrhage
K28.5	Chronic or unspecified gastrojejunal ulcer with perforation
K28.6	Chronic or unspecified gastrojejunal ulcer with both hemorrhage and perforation
K28.7	Chronic gastrojejunal ulcer without hemorrhage or perforation
K31.89	Other diseases of stomach and duodenum
K92.89	Other specified diseases of the digestive system

AMA: **44364** 2019,Oct,10 **44365** 2019,Oct,10

Relative Value Units/Medicare Edits

Non-Facility RVU	Work	PE	MP	Total
44364	3.63	1.92	0.39	5.94
44365	3.21	1.74	0.34	5.29
Facility RVU	**Work**	**PE**	**MP**	**Total**
44364	3.63	1.92	0.39	5.94
44365	3.21	1.74	0.34	5.29

	FUD	Status	MUE	Modifiers				IOM Reference
44364	0	A	1(2)	51	N/A	N/A	80*	None
44365	0	A	1(2)	51	N/A	N/A	80*	

* with documentation

44366

44366 Small intestinal endoscopy, enteroscopy beyond second portion of duodenum, not including ileum; with control of bleeding (eg, injection, bipolar cautery, unipolar cautery, laser, heater probe, stapler, plasma coagulator)

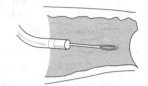

Bleeding may be controlled by any method, such as electrocautery

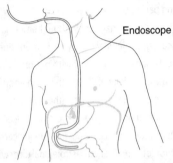

Endoscope

An endoscope is delivered into the upper small bowel and delivered well into the duodenum where bleeding is controlled by any of a variety of methods

Explanation

The physician performs endoscopy of the proximal small bowel and controls an area of bleeding. The physician places an endoscope through the mouth and advances it into the small intestine. An abdominal incision may be made to mobilize the small bowel and assist in running the bowel over the endoscope. The bowel lumen is examined and the area of bleeding is identified and controlled. The endoscope is withdrawn at the completion of the procedure. If an incision was made, it is closed.

Coding Tips

Report the appropriate endoscopy for each anatomic site examined. Surgical endoscopy includes diagnostic endoscopy; however, diagnostic endoscopy can be identified separately when performed at the same surgical session as an open procedure. Bleeding that occurs as the result of an endoscopic procedure, and controlled during the same operative session, is not reported separately. For esophagogastroduodenoscopy, with control of bleeding, see 43255. For colonoscopy, with control of bleeding, see 45382. Do not report 44366 with 43233, 43235–43259, 43266, 43270, 44376–44379.

ICD-10-CM Diagnostic Codes

C17.0	Malignant neoplasm of duodenum
C17.1	Malignant neoplasm of jejunum
C17.8	Malignant neoplasm of overlapping sites of small intestine
C78.4	Secondary malignant neoplasm of small intestine
C7A.010	Malignant carcinoid tumor of the duodenum
C7A.011	Malignant carcinoid tumor of the jejunum
D01.49	Carcinoma in situ of other parts of intestine
D13.2	Benign neoplasm of duodenum
D13.39	Benign neoplasm of other parts of small intestine
D37.2	Neoplasm of uncertain behavior of small intestine

D3A.010	Benign carcinoid tumor of the duodenum
D3A.011	Benign carcinoid tumor of the jejunum
D49.0	Neoplasm of unspecified behavior of digestive system
K26.0	Acute duodenal ulcer with hemorrhage
K26.1	Acute duodenal ulcer with perforation
K26.2	Acute duodenal ulcer with both hemorrhage and perforation
K26.4	Chronic or unspecified duodenal ulcer with hemorrhage
K26.6	Chronic or unspecified duodenal ulcer with both hemorrhage and perforation
K28.0	Acute gastrojejunal ulcer with hemorrhage
K28.2	Acute gastrojejunal ulcer with both hemorrhage and perforation
K28.4	Chronic or unspecified gastrojejunal ulcer with hemorrhage
K28.6	Chronic or unspecified gastrojejunal ulcer with both hemorrhage and perforation
K29.81	Duodenitis with bleeding
K31.82	Dieulafoy lesion (hemorrhagic) of stomach and duodenum
K31.89	Other diseases of stomach and duodenum
K50.011	Crohn's disease of small intestine with rectal bleeding
K50.811	Crohn's disease of both small and large intestine with rectal bleeding
K63.81	Dieulafoy lesion of intestine
K91.89	Other postprocedural complications and disorders of digestive system

AMA: **44366** 2019,Oct,10; 2018,Jan,8; 2017,Jan,8; 2016,Jan,13; 2015,Jan,16

Relative Value Units/Medicare Edits

Non-Facility RVU	Work	PE	MP	Total
44366	4.3	2.22	0.45	6.97
Facility RVU	**Work**	**PE**	**MP**	**Total**
44366	4.3	2.22	0.45	6.97

	FUD	Status	MUE	Modifiers				IOM Reference
44366	0	A	1(3)	51	N/A	N/A	N/A	None

* with documentation

Terms To Know

cautery. Destruction or burning of tissue by means of a hot instrument, an electric current, or a caustic chemical, such as silver nitrate.

duodenum. First portion of the small intestine connected to the stomach at the pylorus and extending to the jejunum.

endoscopy. Visual inspection of the body using a fiberoptic scope.

hemorrhage. Internal or external bleeding with loss of significant amounts of blood.

Coding Companion for General Surgery/Gastroenterology

Intestines

44369

44369 Small intestinal endoscopy, enteroscopy beyond second portion of duodenum, not including ileum; with ablation of tumor(s), polyp(s), or other lesion(s) not amenable to removal by hot biopsy forceps, bipolar cautery or snare technique

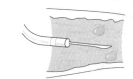

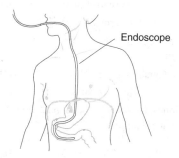

An endoscope is delivered into the upper small bowel and delivered well into the duodenum where tumors, polyps, or other lesions are removed

Endoscope

Explanation

The physician performs endoscopy of the proximal small bowel and ablates a tumor or polyp or other lesion. The physician places an endoscope through the mouth and advances it into the small intestine. An abdominal incision may be made to mobilize the small bowel and assist in running the bowel over the endoscope. The bowel lumen is examined and the tumor, polyp, or other lesion is identified and ablated. The endoscope is withdrawn at the completion of the procedure. If an incision was made it is closed.

Coding Tips

Report the appropriate endoscopy for each anatomic site examined. Surgical endoscopy includes diagnostic endoscopy; however, diagnostic endoscopy can be identified separately when performed at the same surgical session as an open procedure. For removal of tumors, polyps, or lesions, by snare technique, see 44364; by hot biopsy forceps or bipolar cautery, see 44365. For esophagogastroduodenoscopy, with removal of tumors, polyps, or lesions, by hot biopsy forceps or bipolar cautery, see 43250; by snare technique, see 43251; and ablation, see 43270. For colonoscopy, with removal of tumors, polyps, or lesions, by hot biopsy forceps or bipolar cautery, see 45384; by snare technique, see 45385; with ablation by other method, see 45388. Bleeding that occurs as the result of an endoscopic procedure, and controlled during the same operative session, is not reported separately. Do not report 44369 with 43233, 43235–43259, 43266, 43270, or 44376–44379.

ICD-10-CM Diagnostic Codes

C17.0	Malignant neoplasm of duodenum
C17.1	Malignant neoplasm of jejunum
C17.8	Malignant neoplasm of overlapping sites of small intestine
C49.A3	Gastrointestinal stromal tumor of small intestine
C78.4	Secondary malignant neoplasm of small intestine
C7A.010	Malignant carcinoid tumor of the duodenum
C7A.011	Malignant carcinoid tumor of the jejunum

D01.49	Carcinoma in situ of other parts of intestine
D13.2	Benign neoplasm of duodenum
D13.39	Benign neoplasm of other parts of small intestine
D37.2	Neoplasm of uncertain behavior of small intestine
D3A.010	Benign carcinoid tumor of the duodenum
D3A.011	Benign carcinoid tumor of the jejunum
D49.0	Neoplasm of unspecified behavior of digestive system
K28.1	Acute gastrojejunal ulcer with perforation
K28.2	Acute gastrojejunal ulcer with both hemorrhage and perforation
K28.3	Acute gastrojejunal ulcer without hemorrhage or perforation
K31.89	Other diseases of stomach and duodenum
K92.89	Other specified diseases of the digestive system

AMA: 44369 2019,Oct,10

Relative Value Units/Medicare Edits

Non-Facility RVU	Work	PE	MP	Total
44369	4.41	2.27	0.46	7.14
Facility RVU	**Work**	**PE**	**MP**	**Total**
44369	4.41	2.27	0.46	7.14

	FUD	Status	MUE	Modifiers				IOM Reference
44369	0	A	1(2)	51	N/A	N/A	80*	None

* with documentation

Terms To Know

ablation. Removal or destruction of a body part or tissue or its function. Ablation may be performed by surgical means, hormones, drugs, radiofrequency, heat, chemical application, or other methods.

cauterize. Heat or chemicals used to burn or cut.

duodenum. First portion of the small intestine connected to the stomach at the pylorus and extending to the jejunum.

endoscopy. Visual inspection of the body using a fiberoptic scope.

jejunum. Highly vascular upper two-fifths of the small intestine, extending from the duodenum to the ileum.

lumen. Space inside an intestine, artery, vein, duct, or tube.

neoplasm. New abnormal growth, tumor.

polyp. Small growth on a stalk-like attachment projecting from a mucous membrane.

44370

44370 Small intestinal endoscopy, enteroscopy beyond second portion of duodenum, not including ileum; with transendoscopic stent placement (includes predilation)

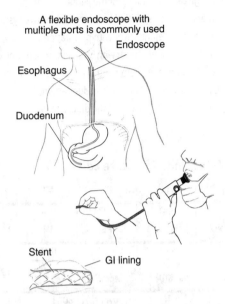

A flexible endoscope with multiple ports is commonly used

Endoscope

Esophagus

Duodenum

Stent — GI lining

An upper GI endoscopic session is performed beyond the duodenum with transendoscopic stent placement, including predilation

Explanation

The physician uses an endoscope to examine the proximal small intestine and performs a transendoscopic placement of a stent in the small intestine. The physician places an endoscope through the mouth and advances it into the small intestine. The lumen of the entire small intestine is visualized. The endoscope is placed at the site of an obstruction or stricture, the necessary stent length is determined and predilation of the obstruction or stenosis may be performed. The stent (endoprosthesis) is introduced into the site of the obstruction. Using a commercial delivery system, a plastic covering over the stent is removed and the stent self-deploys, shoring-up the walls at a specific site in the small intestine beyond the second portion of duodenum, not including the ileum. When necessary, a balloon catheter is placed into the stent and gently inflated to more fully deploy the stent. The delivery system and endoscope are removed.

Coding Tips

For endoscopic stent placement through an esophagogastroduodenoscopy, see 43266. Bleeding that occurs as the result of an endoscopic procedure, and controlled during the same operative session, is not reported separately. Do not report 44370 with 43233, 43235–43259, 43266, 43270, or 44376–44379.

ICD-10-CM Diagnostic Codes

C17.0	Malignant neoplasm of duodenum
C17.1	Malignant neoplasm of jejunum
C17.8	Malignant neoplasm of overlapping sites of small intestine
C78.4	Secondary malignant neoplasm of small intestine
C7A.010	Malignant carcinoid tumor of the duodenum
C7A.011	Malignant carcinoid tumor of the jejunum
D01.49	Carcinoma in situ of other parts of intestine
D13.2	Benign neoplasm of duodenum
D13.39	Benign neoplasm of other parts of small intestine
D37.2	Neoplasm of uncertain behavior of small intestine
D3A.010	Benign carcinoid tumor of the duodenum
D3A.011	Benign carcinoid tumor of the jejunum
D49.0	Neoplasm of unspecified behavior of digestive system
K31.5	Obstruction of duodenum
K50.012	Crohn's disease of small intestine with intestinal obstruction
K50.112	Crohn's disease of large intestine with intestinal obstruction
K50.812	Crohn's disease of both small and large intestine with intestinal obstruction
K56.51	Intestinal adhesions [bands], with partial obstruction
K56.52	Intestinal adhesions [bands] with complete obstruction
K56.690	Other partial intestinal obstruction
K56.691	Other complete intestinal obstruction
K91.31	Postprocedural partial intestinal obstruction
K91.32	Postprocedural complete intestinal obstruction
K91.89	Other postprocedural complications and disorders of digestive system
Q41.0	Congenital absence, atresia and stenosis of duodenum
Q41.1	Congenital absence, atresia and stenosis of jejunum
Q41.8	Congenital absence, atresia and stenosis of other specified parts of small intestine

AMA: **44370** 2019,Oct,10; 2018,Jan,8; 2017,Jan,8; 2016,Jan,13; 2015,Jan,16

Relative Value Units/Medicare Edits

Non-Facility RVU	Work	PE	MP	Total
44370	4.69	2.55	0.49	7.73
Facility RVU	**Work**	**PE**	**MP**	**Total**
44370	4.69	2.55	0.49	7.73

	FUD	Status	MUE	Modifiers				IOM Reference
44370	0	A	1(2)	51	N/A	N/A	80*	None

* with documentation

Terms To Know

atresia. Congenital closure or absence of a tubular organ or an opening to the body surface.

endoprosthesis. Intravascular device in the form of a hollow stent placed within a duct or artery to provide passage through an obstructed area, such as in a bile duct, or to act as a replacement for damaged arterial walls, as in treating an aneurysm.

stent. Tube to provide support in a body cavity or lumen.

44372-44373

44372 Small intestinal endoscopy, enteroscopy beyond second portion of duodenum, not including ileum; with placement of percutaneous jejunostomy tube

44373 with conversion of percutaneous gastrostomy tube to percutaneous jejunostomy tube

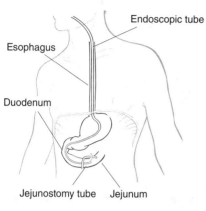

Esophagus

Endoscopic tube

Duodenum

Jejunostomy tube   Jejunum

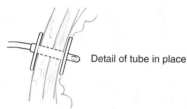

Detail of tube in place

Explanation

The physician performs endoscopy of the proximal small bowel and places a percutaneous jejunostomy tube. The physician places an endoscope into the mouth and advances it into the small intestine. The bowel lumen is visualized and transilluminated through the abdominal skin. A needle is placed through the skin into the lumen of the jejunum under visualization of the endoscope. A wire is threaded through the needle into the bowel lumen. The needle is removed. A jejunostomy tube is placed over the wire, through the skin, into the jejunum, and secured into place. In 44373, a jejunostomy tube is advanced through the previously placed gastrostomy tube. The tube is grasped with a snare or forceps placed through the endoscope and advanced with the endoscope into the proximal jejunum. The endoscope is withdrawn.

Coding Tips

Surgical endoscopy includes diagnostic endoscopy; however, diagnostic endoscopy can be identified separately when performed at the same surgical session as an open procedure. Bleeding that occurs as the result of an endoscopic procedure, and controlled during the same operative session, is not reported separately. Do not report 44372–44373 with 43233, 43235–43259, 43266, 43270, or 44376–44379.

ICD-10-CM Diagnostic Codes

C15.3	Malignant neoplasm of upper third of esophagus
C15.4	Malignant neoplasm of middle third of esophagus
C15.5	Malignant neoplasm of lower third of esophagus
C15.8	Malignant neoplasm of overlapping sites of esophagus
C16.0	Malignant neoplasm of cardia
C16.1	Malignant neoplasm of fundus of stomach
C16.2	Malignant neoplasm of body of stomach
C16.3	Malignant neoplasm of pyloric antrum
C16.4	Malignant neoplasm of pylorus
C16.8	Malignant neoplasm of overlapping sites of stomach
C17.0	Malignant neoplasm of duodenum
C76.0	Malignant neoplasm of head, face and neck
C78.4	Secondary malignant neoplasm of small intestine
C78.89	Secondary malignant neoplasm of other digestive organs
C7A.010	Malignant carcinoid tumor of the duodenum
C7A.092	Malignant carcinoid tumor of the stomach
D00.2	Carcinoma in situ of stomach
E41	Nutritional marasmus
E44.0	Moderate protein-calorie malnutrition
E44.1	Mild protein-calorie malnutrition
E86.0	Dehydration
E86.1	Hypovolemia
I69.091	Dysphagia following nontraumatic subarachnoid hemorrhage
I69.191	Dysphagia following nontraumatic intracerebral hemorrhage
I69.291	Dysphagia following other nontraumatic intracranial hemorrhage
I69.391	Dysphagia following cerebral infarction
I69.891	Dysphagia following other cerebrovascular disease
K22.0	Achalasia of cardia
K22.10	Ulcer of esophagus without bleeding
K22.11	Ulcer of esophagus with bleeding
K22.2	Esophageal obstruction
K22.3	Perforation of esophagus
K22.4	Dyskinesia of esophagus
K25.0	Acute gastric ulcer with hemorrhage
K25.1	Acute gastric ulcer with perforation
K25.2	Acute gastric ulcer with both hemorrhage and perforation
K25.3	Acute gastric ulcer without hemorrhage or perforation
K25.7	Chronic gastric ulcer without hemorrhage or perforation
K26.0	Acute duodenal ulcer with hemorrhage
K26.1	Acute duodenal ulcer with perforation
K26.2	Acute duodenal ulcer with both hemorrhage and perforation
K26.3	Acute duodenal ulcer without hemorrhage or perforation
K26.4	Chronic or unspecified duodenal ulcer with hemorrhage
K26.5	Chronic or unspecified duodenal ulcer with perforation
K28.0	Acute gastrojejunal ulcer with hemorrhage
K28.1	Acute gastrojejunal ulcer with perforation
K28.2	Acute gastrojejunal ulcer with both hemorrhage and perforation
K28.6	Chronic or unspecified gastrojejunal ulcer with both hemorrhage and perforation
K28.7	Chronic gastrojejunal ulcer without hemorrhage or perforation
K31.1	Adult hypertrophic pyloric stenosis ▲
K31.6	Fistula of stomach and duodenum
K31.89	Other diseases of stomach and duodenum
K86.0	Alcohol-induced chronic pancreatitis
K86.1	Other chronic pancreatitis
K86.2	Cyst of pancreas
K86.3	Pseudocyst of pancreas
K86.81	Exocrine pancreatic insufficiency
K86.89	Other specified diseases of pancreas
K91.1	Postgastric surgery syndromes

Intestines

K94.21	Gastrostomy hemorrhage
K94.22	Gastrostomy infection
K94.23	Gastrostomy malfunction
K94.29	Other complications of gastrostomy
Q40.2	Other specified congenital malformations of stomach
Q41.0	Congenital absence, atresia and stenosis of duodenum
R13.0	Aphagia
R13.11	Dysphagia, oral phase
R13.12	Dysphagia, oropharyngeal phase
R13.13	Dysphagia, pharyngeal phase
R13.14	Dysphagia, pharyngoesophageal phase
R13.19	Other dysphagia
R62.7	Adult failure to thrive △
R63.0	Anorexia
R63.32	Pediatric feeding disorder, chronic 🅿
R63.39	Other feeding difficulties

AMA: 44372 2019,Oct,10; 2018,Jan,8; 2017,Jan,8; 2016,Jan,13; 2015,Jan,16
44373 2019,Oct,10; 2018,Jan,8; 2017,Jan,8; 2016,Jan,13; 2015,Jan,16

Relative Value Units/Medicare Edits

Non-Facility RVU	Work	PE	MP	Total
44372	4.3	2.14	0.52	6.96
44373	3.39	1.77	0.43	5.59
Facility RVU	Work	PE	MP	Total
44372	4.3	2.14	0.52	6.96
44373	3.39	1.77	0.43	5.59

	FUD	Status	MUE	Modifiers				IOM Reference
44372	0	A	1(2)	51	N/A	N/A	N/A	None
44373	0	A	1(2)	51	N/A	N/A	N/A	

* with documentation

44376-44377

44376 Small intestinal endoscopy, enteroscopy beyond second portion of duodenum, including ileum; diagnostic, with or without collection of specimen(s) by brushing or washing (separate procedure)

44377   with biopsy, single or multiple

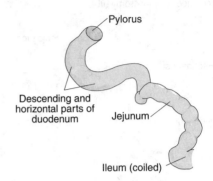

Explanation

The physician performs endoscopy of the small bowel and may obtain brushings or washings. The physician places the endoscope into the mouth and advances it into the small intestine. An abdominal incision may be made to mobilize the small bowel and assist in running the bowel over the endoscope. The lumen of the small bowel is visualized and brushings or washings may be obtained. The endoscope is withdrawn at the completion of the procedure. If an incision was made, it is closed. Report 44377 when biopsies are obtained.

Coding Tips

Note that 44376, a separate procedure by definition, is usually a component of a more complex service and is not identified separately. When performed alone or with other unrelated procedures/services it may be reported. If performed alone, list the code; if performed with other procedures/services, list the code and append modifier 59 or an X{EPSU} modifier. Surgical endoscopy includes diagnostic endoscopy; however, diagnostic endoscopy can be identified separately when performed at the same surgical session as an open procedure. For esophagogastroduodenoscopy (EGD), see 43210, 43233, 43235–43259, 43266, and 43270. Bleeding that occurs as the result of an endoscopic procedure, and controlled during the same operative session, is not reported separately. Do not report 44376–44377 with 43233, 43235-43259, 43266, 43270, 44360–44361, 44363–44366, 44369–44370, or 44372–44373.

ICD-10-CM Diagnostic Codes

B77.0	Ascariasis with intestinal complications
B78.0	Intestinal strongyloidiasis
B79	Trichuriasis
B96.81	Helicobacter pylori [H. pylori] as the cause of diseases classified elsewhere
C17.0	Malignant neoplasm of duodenum
C17.1	Malignant neoplasm of jejunum
C17.2	Malignant neoplasm of ileum
C17.3	Meckel's diverticulum, malignant
C7A.010	Malignant carcinoid tumor of the duodenum
C7A.011	Malignant carcinoid tumor of the jejunum
C7A.012	Malignant carcinoid tumor of the ileum
C88.3	Immunoproliferative small intestinal disease

D13.2	Benign neoplasm of duodenum
D3A.010	Benign carcinoid tumor of the duodenum
D3A.011	Benign carcinoid tumor of the jejunum
D3A.012	Benign carcinoid tumor of the ileum
K26.0	Acute duodenal ulcer with hemorrhage
K26.1	Acute duodenal ulcer with perforation
K26.2	Acute duodenal ulcer with both hemorrhage and perforation
K26.3	Acute duodenal ulcer without hemorrhage or perforation
K26.4	Chronic or unspecified duodenal ulcer with hemorrhage
K26.7	Chronic duodenal ulcer without hemorrhage or perforation
K28.0	Acute gastrojejunal ulcer with hemorrhage
K28.1	Acute gastrojejunal ulcer with perforation
K28.2	Acute gastrojejunal ulcer with both hemorrhage and perforation
K28.4	Chronic or unspecified gastrojejunal ulcer with hemorrhage
K28.5	Chronic or unspecified gastrojejunal ulcer with perforation
K28.6	Chronic or unspecified gastrojejunal ulcer with both hemorrhage and perforation
K28.7	Chronic gastrojejunal ulcer without hemorrhage or perforation
K29.80	Duodenitis without bleeding
K29.81	Duodenitis with bleeding
K31.5	Obstruction of duodenum
K31.82	Dieulafoy lesion (hemorrhagic) of stomach and duodenum
K50.011	Crohn's disease of small intestine with rectal bleeding
K50.012	Crohn's disease of small intestine with intestinal obstruction
K50.013	Crohn's disease of small intestine with fistula
K50.014	Crohn's disease of small intestine with abscess
K50.811	Crohn's disease of both small and large intestine with rectal bleeding
K50.812	Crohn's disease of both small and large intestine with intestinal obstruction
K50.813	Crohn's disease of both small and large intestine with fistula
K50.814	Crohn's disease of both small and large intestine with abscess
K52.0	Gastroenteritis and colitis due to radiation
K52.1	Toxic gastroenteritis and colitis
K52.21	Food protein-induced enterocolitis syndrome
K52.22	Food protein-induced enteropathy
K52.29	Other allergic and dietetic gastroenteritis and colitis
K52.3	Indeterminate colitis
K52.81	Eosinophilic gastritis or gastroenteritis
K52.831	Collagenous colitis
K52.832	Lymphocytic colitis
K55.1	Chronic vascular disorders of intestine
K56.51	Intestinal adhesions [bands], with partial obstruction
K56.52	Intestinal adhesions [bands] with complete obstruction
K57.00	Diverticulitis of small intestine with perforation and abscess without bleeding
K57.01	Diverticulitis of small intestine with perforation and abscess with bleeding
K57.11	Diverticulosis of small intestine without perforation or abscess with bleeding
K57.12	Diverticulitis of small intestine without perforation or abscess without bleeding
K57.13	Diverticulitis of small intestine without perforation or abscess with bleeding

K57.40	Diverticulitis of both small and large intestine with perforation and abscess without bleeding
K57.41	Diverticulitis of both small and large intestine with perforation and abscess with bleeding
K57.51	Diverticulosis of both small and large intestine without perforation or abscess with bleeding
K57.53	Diverticulitis of both small and large intestine without perforation or abscess with bleeding
K58.0	Irritable bowel syndrome with diarrhea
K58.9	Irritable bowel syndrome without diarrhea
K59.1	Functional diarrhea
K63.3	Ulcer of intestine
K63.81	Dieulafoy lesion of intestine
K90.0	Celiac disease
K90.1	Tropical sprue
K90.41	Non-celiac gluten sensitivity
K90.81	Whipple's disease
K92.0	Hematemesis
K92.1	Melena
M35.08	Sjögren syndrome with gastrointestinal involvement
N82.2	Fistula of vagina to small intestine ♀
Q43.0	Meckel's diverticulum (displaced) (hypertrophic)
R62.7	Adult failure to thrive ▲
R63.4	Abnormal weight loss
R63.6	Underweight

AMA: **44376** 2018,Jan,8; 2017,Jan,8; 2016,Jan,13; 2015,Jan,16 **44377** 2018,Jan,8; 2017,Jan,8; 2016,Jan,13; 2015,Jan,16

Relative Value Units/Medicare Edits

Non-Facility RVU	Work	PE	MP	Total
44376	5.15	2.57	0.53	8.25
44377	5.42	2.68	0.59	8.69
Facility RVU	Work	PE	MP	Total
44376	5.15	2.57	0.53	8.25
44377	5.42	2.68	0.59	8.69

	FUD	Status	MUE	Modifiers				IOM Reference
44376	0	A	1(3)	51	N/A	N/A	80*	None
44377	0	A	1(2)	51	N/A	N/A	80*	

* with documentation

44378

44378 Small intestinal endoscopy, enteroscopy beyond second portion of duodenum, including ileum; with control of bleeding (eg, injection, bipolar cautery, unipolar cautery, laser, heater probe, stapler, plasma coagulator)

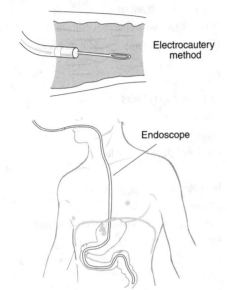

Bleeding is controlled by any of a variety of methods

Explanation

The physician performs endoscopy of the small intestine, which may include the ileum, and controls an area of bleeding. The physician places the endoscope into the mouth and advances it into the small intestine. The lumen of the small intestine is visualized and any area of bleeding is controlled using various methods, such as cautery, injection, or laser. In some cases, a separately reportable abdominal incision is made to mobilize the small intestine and assist in running the intestine over the endoscope. The endoscope is withdrawn at the completion of the procedure.

Coding Tips

Report the appropriate endoscopy for each anatomic site examined. Surgical endoscopy includes diagnostic endoscopy; however, diagnostic endoscopy can be identified separately when performed at the same surgical session as an open procedure. For a small intestinal endoscopy, not including the ileum, with control of bleeding, any method, see 44366. For esophagogastroduodenoscopy (EGD), see 43210, 43233, 43235–43259, 43266, and 43270. Bleeding that occurs as the result of an endoscopic procedure, and is controlled during the same operative session, is not reported separately. Do not report 44378 with 43233, 43235-43259, 43266, 43270, 44360–44361, 44363–44366, 44369–44370, or 44372–44373.

ICD-10-CM Diagnostic Codes

C17.0	Malignant neoplasm of duodenum
C17.1	Malignant neoplasm of jejunum
C17.2	Malignant neoplasm of ileum
C17.8	Malignant neoplasm of overlapping sites of small intestine
C78.4	Secondary malignant neoplasm of small intestine
C7A.010	Malignant carcinoid tumor of the duodenum
C7A.011	Malignant carcinoid tumor of the jejunum
C7A.012	Malignant carcinoid tumor of the ileum
D01.49	Carcinoma in situ of other parts of intestine
D13.2	Benign neoplasm of duodenum
D13.39	Benign neoplasm of other parts of small intestine
D37.2	Neoplasm of uncertain behavior of small intestine
D3A.010	Benign carcinoid tumor of the duodenum
D3A.011	Benign carcinoid tumor of the jejunum
D3A.012	Benign carcinoid tumor of the ileum
K26.0	Acute duodenal ulcer with hemorrhage
K26.2	Acute duodenal ulcer with both hemorrhage and perforation
K26.4	Chronic or unspecified duodenal ulcer with hemorrhage
K26.6	Chronic or unspecified duodenal ulcer with both hemorrhage and perforation
K28.0	Acute gastrojejunal ulcer with hemorrhage
K28.2	Acute gastrojejunal ulcer with both hemorrhage and perforation
K28.4	Chronic or unspecified gastrojejunal ulcer with hemorrhage
K28.6	Chronic or unspecified gastrojejunal ulcer with both hemorrhage and perforation
K28.7	Chronic gastrojejunal ulcer without hemorrhage or perforation
K29.81	Duodenitis with bleeding
K31.82	Dieulafoy lesion (hemorrhagic) of stomach and duodenum
K31.89	Other diseases of stomach and duodenum
K50.011	Crohn's disease of small intestine with rectal bleeding
K50.811	Crohn's disease of both small and large intestine with rectal bleeding
K63.3	Ulcer of intestine
K63.81	Dieulafoy lesion of intestine
K91.89	Other postprocedural complications and disorders of digestive system
K92.89	Other specified diseases of the digestive system
Q27.33	Arteriovenous malformation of digestive system vessel

AMA: 44378 2018,Jan,8; 2017,Jan,8; 2016,Jan,13; 2015,Jan,16

Relative Value Units/Medicare Edits

Non-Facility RVU	Work	PE	MP	Total
44378	7.02	3.42	0.74	11.18
Facility RVU	**Work**	**PE**	**MP**	**Total**
44378	7.02	3.42	0.74	11.18

	FUD	Status	MUE	Modifiers				IOM Reference
44378	0	A	1(3)	51	N/A	N/A	80*	None

* with documentation

44379

44379 Small intestinal endoscopy, enteroscopy beyond second portion of duodenum, including ileum; with transendoscopic stent placement (includes predilation)

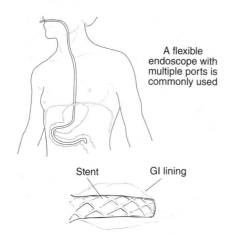

A flexible endoscope with multiple ports is commonly used

Stent   GI lining

An upper GI endoscopic session is performed beyond the duodenum with transendoscopic stent placement, including predilation

Explanation

The physician uses an endoscope to examine the small intestine and performs transendoscopic placement of a stent in the small intestine. The physician performs endoscopy of the small bowel and places a transendoscopic stent. The physician places an endoscope into the mouth and advances it into the small intestine. The lumen of the small intestine is visualized. The endoscope is placed at the site of an obstruction or stricture and the necessary stent length is determined. The stent (endoprosthesis) is introduced into the site of the obstruction. Using a commercial delivery system, a plastic covering over the stent is removed and the stent self-deploys, shoring-up the walls at a specific site in the small intestine beyond the second portion of the duodenum, including the ileum. When necessary, a balloon catheter is placed into the stent and gently inflated to more fully deploy the stent. The delivery system and endoscope are removed.

Coding Tips

For transendoscopic stent placement not including the ileum, see 44370; through stoma via ileoscopy, see 44384. For esophagogastroduodenoscopy (EGD), see 43210, 43233, 43235–43259, 43266, and 43270. Bleeding that occurs as the result of an endoscopic procedure, and is controlled during the same operative session, is not reported separately. Do not report 44379 with 43233, 43235-43259, 43266, 43270, 44360–44361, 44363–44366, 44369–44370, or 44372–44373.

ICD-10-CM Diagnostic Codes

C17.0	Malignant neoplasm of duodenum
C17.1	Malignant neoplasm of jejunum
C17.2	Malignant neoplasm of ileum
C17.3	Meckel's diverticulum, malignant
C17.8	Malignant neoplasm of overlapping sites of small intestine
C78.4	Secondary malignant neoplasm of small intestine
C7A.010	Malignant carcinoid tumor of the duodenum
C7A.011	Malignant carcinoid tumor of the jejunum
C7A.012	Malignant carcinoid tumor of the ileum
D13.2	Benign neoplasm of duodenum
D13.39	Benign neoplasm of other parts of small intestine
D37.2	Neoplasm of uncertain behavior of small intestine
D3A.010	Benign carcinoid tumor of the duodenum
D3A.011	Benign carcinoid tumor of the jejunum
D3A.012	Benign carcinoid tumor of the ileum
K31.5	Obstruction of duodenum
K50.011	Crohn's disease of small intestine with rectal bleeding
K50.012	Crohn's disease of small intestine with intestinal obstruction
K50.013	Crohn's disease of small intestine with fistula
K50.014	Crohn's disease of small intestine with abscess
K50.112	Crohn's disease of large intestine with intestinal obstruction
K50.811	Crohn's disease of both small and large intestine with rectal bleeding
K50.812	Crohn's disease of both small and large intestine with intestinal obstruction
K50.813	Crohn's disease of both small and large intestine with fistula
K50.814	Crohn's disease of both small and large intestine with abscess
K50.818	Crohn's disease of both small and large intestine with other complication
K56.51	Intestinal adhesions [bands], with partial obstruction
K56.52	Intestinal adhesions [bands] with complete obstruction
K56.690	Other partial intestinal obstruction
K56.691	Other complete intestinal obstruction
K91.31	Postprocedural partial intestinal obstruction
K91.32	Postprocedural complete intestinal obstruction
K91.89	Other postprocedural complications and disorders of digestive system
Q41.0	Congenital absence, atresia and stenosis of duodenum
Q41.1	Congenital absence, atresia and stenosis of jejunum
Q41.2	Congenital absence, atresia and stenosis of ileum
Q41.8	Congenital absence, atresia and stenosis of other specified parts of small intestine

AMA: **44379** 2018,Jan,8; 2017,Jan,8; 2016,Jan,13; 2015,Jan,16

Relative Value Units/Medicare Edits

Non-Facility RVU	Work	PE	MP	Total
44379	7.36	3.74	0.78	11.88
Facility RVU	**Work**	**PE**	**MP**	**Total**
44379	7.36	3.74	0.78	11.88

	FUD	Status	MUE	Modifiers				IOM Reference
44379	0	A	1(2)	51	N/A	N/A	80*	None

* with documentation

44380, 44382

44380 Ileoscopy, through stoma; diagnostic, including collection of specimen(s) by brushing or washing, when performed (separate procedure)

44382   with biopsy, single or multiple

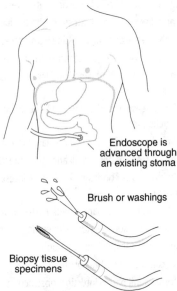

Specimens are collected by brushing, washing, or biopsy

Endoscope is advanced through an existing stoma

Brush or washings

Biopsy tissue specimens

Explanation

An ileostomy is an artificial opening (called a stoma) created in the abdomen. The physician performs endoscopy through an ileostomy and may obtain brushings or washings (44380) or biopsies (44382). The physician places the endoscope into the ileostomy and advances the endoscope into the small intestine. The lumen of the ileum, the last part of the small intestine, is visualized and brushings, washings, or biopsies may be obtained. The endoscope is withdrawn at the completion of the procedure.

Coding Tips

Note that 44380, a separate procedure by definition, is usually a component of a more complex service and is not identified separately. When performed alone or with other unrelated procedures it may be reported. If performed alone, list the code; if performed with other procedures/services, list the code and append modifier 59 or an X{EPSU} modifier. Report the appropriate endoscopy for each anatomic site examined. Surgical endoscopy includes diagnostic endoscopy; however, diagnostic endoscopy can be identified separately when performed at the same surgical session as an open procedure. For diagnostic endoscopic evaluation of the small intestinal pouch, with or without brushing or washing, see 44385; with biopsy, single or multiple, see 44386. For colonoscopy through stoma, with or without brushing or washing, see 44388; with biopsy, single or multiple, see 44389. Bleeding that occurs as the result of an endoscopic procedure, and controlled during the same operative session, is not reported separately. Do not report 44380 with 44381, 44382, or 44384. Do not report 44382 with 44380.

ICD-10-CM Diagnostic Codes

B78.0	Intestinal strongyloidiasis
B79	Trichuriasis
C17.2	Malignant neoplasm of ileum
C17.3	Meckel's diverticulum, malignant
C17.8	Malignant neoplasm of overlapping sites of small intestine
C49.A3	Gastrointestinal stromal tumor of small intestine
C7A.012	Malignant carcinoid tumor of the ileum
C88.3	Immunoproliferative small intestinal disease
D13.39	Benign neoplasm of other parts of small intestine
D3A.012	Benign carcinoid tumor of the ileum
K50.011	Crohn's disease of small intestine with rectal bleeding
K50.012	Crohn's disease of small intestine with intestinal obstruction
K50.013	Crohn's disease of small intestine with fistula
K50.014	Crohn's disease of small intestine with abscess
K50.018	Crohn's disease of small intestine with other complication
K50.811	Crohn's disease of both small and large intestine with rectal bleeding
K50.812	Crohn's disease of both small and large intestine with intestinal obstruction
K50.813	Crohn's disease of both small and large intestine with fistula
K50.814	Crohn's disease of both small and large intestine with abscess
K50.818	Crohn's disease of both small and large intestine with other complication
K52.0	Gastroenteritis and colitis due to radiation
K52.1	Toxic gastroenteritis and colitis
K52.89	Other specified noninfective gastroenteritis and colitis
K55.021	Focal (segmental) acute infarction of small intestine
K55.022	Diffuse acute infarction of small intestine
K55.1	Chronic vascular disorders of intestine
K55.8	Other vascular disorders of intestine
K56.49	Other impaction of intestine
K56.51	Intestinal adhesions [bands], with partial obstruction
K56.52	Intestinal adhesions [bands] with complete obstruction
K56.690	Other partial intestinal obstruction
K56.691	Other complete intestinal obstruction
K57.00	Diverticulitis of small intestine with perforation and abscess without bleeding
K57.01	Diverticulitis of small intestine with perforation and abscess with bleeding
K57.10	Diverticulosis of small intestine without perforation or abscess without bleeding
K57.11	Diverticulosis of small intestine without perforation or abscess with bleeding
K57.12	Diverticulitis of small intestine without perforation or abscess without bleeding
K57.13	Diverticulitis of small intestine without perforation or abscess with bleeding
K57.40	Diverticulitis of both small and large intestine with perforation and abscess without bleeding
K57.41	Diverticulitis of both small and large intestine with perforation and abscess with bleeding
K57.50	Diverticulosis of both small and large intestine without perforation or abscess without bleeding
K57.51	Diverticulosis of both small and large intestine without perforation or abscess with bleeding
K57.52	Diverticulitis of both small and large intestine without perforation or abscess without bleeding
K57.53	Diverticulitis of both small and large intestine without perforation or abscess with bleeding

Intestines

K58.0	Irritable bowel syndrome with diarrhea	
K58.1	Irritable bowel syndrome with constipation	
K58.2	Mixed irritable bowel syndrome	
K58.9	Irritable bowel syndrome without diarrhea	
K59.1	Functional diarrhea	
K59.81	Ogilvie syndrome	
K63.1	Perforation of intestine (nontraumatic)	
K63.3	Ulcer of intestine	
K63.81	Dieulafoy lesion of intestine	
K90.0	Celiac disease	
K90.1	Tropical sprue	
K90.41	Non-celiac gluten sensitivity	
K90.81	Whipple's disease	
K90.89	Other intestinal malabsorption	
K92.0	Hematemesis	
K92.1	Melena	
M35.08	Sjögren syndrome with gastrointestinal involvement	
N82.2	Fistula of vagina to small intestine ♀	
N82.4	Other female intestinal-genital tract fistulae ♀	
Q41.2	Congenital absence, atresia and stenosis of ileum	
Q43.0	Meckel's diverticulum (displaced) (hypertrophic)	
R62.7	Adult failure to thrive △	
R63.4	Abnormal weight loss	
R63.6	Underweight	
Z11.0	Encounter for screening for intestinal infectious diseases	
Z12.13	Encounter for screening for malignant neoplasm of small intestine	

AMA: 44380 2018,Jan,8; 2017,Jan,8; 2016,Jan,13; 2015,Jan,16 **44382** 2018,Jan,8; 2017,Jan,8; 2016,Jan,13; 2015,Jan,16

Relative Value Units/Medicare Edits

Non-Facility RVU	Work	PE	MP	Total
44380	0.87	4.95	0.1	5.92
44382	1.17	7.87	0.14	9.18
Facility RVU	Work	PE	MP	Total
44380	0.87	0.67	0.1	1.64
44382	1.17	0.83	0.14	2.14

	FUD	Status	MUE	Modifiers				IOM Reference
44380	0	A	1(3)	51	N/A	N/A	N/A	None
44382	0	A	1(2)	51	N/A	N/A	N/A	

* with documentation

[44381]

44381   Ileoscopy, through stoma; with transendoscopic balloon dilation

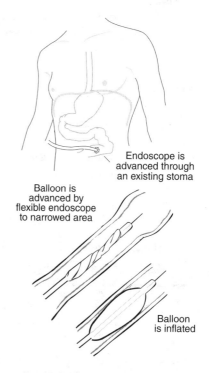

Endoscope is advanced through an existing stoma

Balloon is advanced by flexible endoscope to narrowed area

Balloon is inflated

Explanation

An ileostomy is an artificial opening (called a stoma) created in the abdomen. The physician performs endoscopy through ileostomy and dilates strictures by balloon catheter. The physician places the endoscope into the ileostomy and advances the endoscope into the small intestine. The lumen of the ileum, the last part of the small intestine, is visualized. Areas of stenosis are identified and a balloon catheter is passed to the point of constriction and a little beyond. The balloon is inflated to the appropriate diameter and gradually withdrawn through the stenosed area, stretching the walls of the bowel at the strictured area. The endoscope is withdrawn at the completion of the procedure.

Coding Tips

Report the appropriate endoscopy for each anatomic site examined. Surgical endoscopy includes diagnostic endoscopy; however, diagnostic endoscopy can be identified separately when performed at the same surgical session as an open procedure. For multiple strictures treated with transendoscopic balloon dilations during the same session, report 44381 with modifier 59 or an X{EPSU} modifier for each additional stricture. For diagnostic endoscopic evaluation of the small intestinal pouch, with or without brushing or washing, see 44385; with biopsy, single or multiple, see 44386. For colonoscopy through stoma, with or without brushing or washing, see 44388; with biopsy, single or multiple, see 44389. For Ileoscopy, through stoma, with placement of an endoscopic stent, see 44384. Bleeding that occurs as the result of an endoscopic procedure, and controlled during the same operative session, is not reported separately. Do not report 44381 with 44380 or 44384. If fluoroscopic guidance is used, see 74360.

ICD-10-CM Diagnostic Codes

C17.2	Malignant neoplasm of ileum
C78.4	Secondary malignant neoplasm of small intestine
C7A.012	Malignant carcinoid tumor of the ileum
D3A.012	Benign carcinoid tumor of the ileum

K50.012	Crohn's disease of small intestine with intestinal obstruction
K50.812	Crohn's disease of both small and large intestine with intestinal obstruction
K56.49	Other impaction of intestine
K56.51	Intestinal adhesions [bands], with partial obstruction
K56.52	Intestinal adhesions [bands] with complete obstruction
K56.690	Other partial intestinal obstruction
K56.691	Other complete intestinal obstruction
K91.31	Postprocedural partial intestinal obstruction
K91.32	Postprocedural complete intestinal obstruction
K91.89	Other postprocedural complications and disorders of digestive system
Q41.2	Congenital absence, atresia and stenosis of ileum
Q41.8	Congenital absence, atresia and stenosis of other specified parts of small intestine

AMA: 44381 2018,Jan,8; 2017,Jan,8; 2016,Jan,13; 2015,Jan,16

Relative Value Units/Medicare Edits

Non-Facility RVU	Work	PE	MP	Total
44381	1.38	29.46	0.17	31.01
Facility RVU	**Work**	**PE**	**MP**	**Total**
44381	1.38	0.88	0.17	2.43

	FUD	Status	MUE	Modifiers				IOM Reference
44381	0	A	1(3)	51	N/A	N/A	N/A	None

* with documentation

Terms To Know

dilation. Artificial increase in the diameter of an opening or lumen made by medication or by instrumentation.

guidewire. Flexible metal instrument designed to lead another instrument in its proper course.

ileostomy. Artificial surgical opening that brings the end of the ileum out through the abdominal wall to the skin surface for the diversion of feces through a stoma.

lumen. Space inside an intestine, artery, vein, duct, or tube.

stenosis. Narrowing or constriction of a passage.

stent. Tube to provide support in a body cavity or lumen.

stricture. Narrowing of an anatomical structure.

44384

44384   Ileoscopy, through stoma; with placement of endoscopic stent (includes pre- and post-dilation and guide wire passage, when performed)

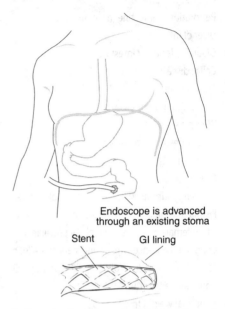

Endoscope is advanced through an existing stoma

Stent   GI lining

An ileoscopy is performed with transendoscopic stent placement, including predilation

Explanation

The physician uses an endoscope through an ileostomy to view the ileum and places an endoscopic stent. The physician places the endoscope into the ileostomy and advances the endoscope into the small intestine. The lumen of the ileum is visualized. The endoscope is placed at the site of an obstruction or stricture and the necessary stent length is determined. The stent (endoprosthesis) is introduced into the site of the obstruction. Using a commercial delivery system, a plastic covering over the stent is removed and the stent self-deploys, shoring-up the walls at a specific site in the ileum. When necessary, a balloon catheter is placed into the stent and gently inflated to more fully deploy the stent. The delivery system and endoscope are removed. This code includes dilation before and after stent placement, as well as guidewire passage when performed.

Coding Tips

Bleeding that occurs as the result of an endoscopic procedure, and controlled during the same operative session, is not reported separately. If fluoroscopic guidance is used, see 74360. For placement of a transendoscopic stent via small intestinal endoscopy, see 44379. Do not report 44384 with 44380 or 44381.

ICD-10-CM Diagnostic Codes

C17.2	Malignant neoplasm of ileum
C78.4	Secondary malignant neoplasm of small intestine
C7A.012	Malignant carcinoid tumor of the ileum
D13.39	Benign neoplasm of other parts of small intestine
D3A.012	Benign carcinoid tumor of the ileum
K50.012	Crohn's disease of small intestine with intestinal obstruction
K50.812	Crohn's disease of both small and large intestine with intestinal obstruction
K56.49	Other impaction of intestine

K56.51	Intestinal adhesions [bands], with partial obstruction
K56.52	Intestinal adhesions [bands] with complete obstruction
K56.690	Other partial intestinal obstruction
K56.691	Other complete intestinal obstruction
K91.31	Postprocedural partial intestinal obstruction
K91.32	Postprocedural complete intestinal obstruction
K91.81	Other intraoperative complications of digestive system
K91.89	Other postprocedural complications and disorders of digestive system
Q41.2	Congenital absence, atresia and stenosis of ileum
Q41.8	Congenital absence, atresia and stenosis of other specified parts of small intestine

AMA: 44384 2018,Jan,8; 2017,Jan,8; 2016,Jan,13; 2015,Jan,16

Relative Value Units/Medicare Edits

Non-Facility RVU	Work	PE	MP	Total
44384	2.85	1.3	0.34	4.49
Facility RVU	**Work**	**PE**	**MP**	**Total**
44384	2.85	1.3	0.34	4.49

	FUD	Status	MUE	Modifiers				IOM Reference
44384	0	A	1(3)	51	N/A	N/A	N/A	None

* with documentation

Terms To Know

dilation. Artificial increase in the diameter of an opening or lumen made by medication or by instrumentation.

guidewire. Flexible metal instrument designed to lead another instrument in its proper course.

ileostomy. Artificial surgical opening that brings the end of the ileum out through the abdominal wall to the skin surface for the diversion of feces through a stoma.

ileum. Lower portion of the small intestine, from the jejunum to the cecum.

lumen. Space inside an intestine, artery, vein, duct, or tube.

obstruction. Blockage that prevents normal function of the valve or structure.

stent. Tube to provide support in a body cavity or lumen.

stricture. Narrowing of an anatomical structure.

44385-44386

| 44385 | Endoscopic evaluation of small intestinal pouch (eg, Kock pouch, ileal reservoir [S or J]); diagnostic, including collection of specimen(s) by brushing or washing, when performed (separate procedure) |
| 44386 | with biopsy, single or multiple |

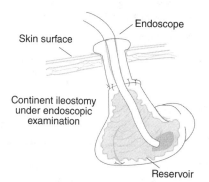

Specimens may be collected by brushing, washing, or biopsy

Explanation

The physician performs endoscopic evaluation of an intestinal pouch and may obtain brushings or washings (44385) or biopsies (44386). The physician places the endoscope into the pouch, through the anus or abdominal wall stoma. The lumen of the pouch is visualized and brushings or washings or biopsies may be obtained. The endoscope is withdrawn at the completion of the procedure.

Coding Tips

Note that 44385, a separate procedure by definition, is usually a component of a more complex service and is not identified separately. When performed alone or with other unrelated procedures/services it may be reported. If performed alone, list the code; if performed with other procedures/services, list the code and append modifier 59 or an X{EPSU} modifier. Report the appropriate endoscopy for each anatomic site examined. Surgical endoscopy includes diagnostic endoscopy; however, diagnostic endoscopy can be identified separately when performed at the same surgical session as an open procedure. For ileoscopy through stoma, with or without brushing or washing, see 44380; with biopsy, single or multiple, see 44382; with transendoscopic balloon dilation, see 44381; with placement of endoscopic stent, see 44384. For colonoscopy through stoma, with or without brushing or washing, see 44388; with biopsy, single or multiple, see 44389. Bleeding that occurs as the result of an endoscopic procedure, and controlled during the same operative session, is not reported separately. Do not report 44385 and 44386 together.

ICD-10-CM Diagnostic Codes

K56.51	Intestinal adhesions [bands], with partial obstruction
K56.52	Intestinal adhesions [bands] with complete obstruction
K56.690	Other partial intestinal obstruction
K56.691	Other complete intestinal obstruction
K58.9	Irritable bowel syndrome without diarrhea
K63.0	Abscess of intestine
K63.1	Perforation of intestine (nontraumatic)
K63.2	Fistula of intestine
K63.3	Ulcer of intestine
K63.81	Dieulafoy lesion of intestine
K91.31	Postprocedural partial intestinal obstruction

K91.32	Postprocedural complete intestinal obstruction
K91.850	Pouchitis
K91.858	Other complications of intestinal pouch
K91.89	Other postprocedural complications and disorders of digestive system
K94.11	Enterostomy hemorrhage
K94.12	Enterostomy infection
K94.13	Enterostomy malfunction
K94.19	Other complications of enterostomy

AMA: 44385 2018,Jan,8; 2017,Jan,8; 2016,Jan,13; 2015,Jan,16 **44386** 2018,Jan,8; 2017,Jan,8; 2016,Jan,13; 2015,Jan,16

Relative Value Units/Medicare Edits

Non-Facility RVU	Work	PE	MP	Total
44385	1.2	5.09	0.15	6.44
44386	1.5	7.87	0.17	9.54
Facility RVU	Work	PE	MP	Total
44385	1.2	0.74	0.15	2.09
44386	1.5	0.91	0.17	2.58

	FUD	Status	MUE	Modifiers				IOM Reference
44385	0	A	1(3)	51	N/A	N/A	N/A	None
44386	0	A	1(2)	51	N/A	N/A	N/A	

* with documentation

Terms To Know

biopsy. Tissue or fluid removed for diagnostic purposes through analysis of the cells in the biopsy material.

brush. Tool used to gather cell samples or clean a body part.

Kock procedure. Surgical procedure in which the physician forms a reservoir of distal ileum (Kock pouch) and brings it through the abdominal wall onto the skin as a continent ileostomy.

lumen. Space inside an intestine, artery, vein, duct, or tube.

reservoir. Space or body cavity for storage of liquid.

specimen. Tissue cells or sample of fluid taken for analysis, pathologic examination, and diagnosis.

stoma. Opening created in the abdominal wall from an internal organ or structure for diversion of waste elimination, drainage, and access.

44388-44389

44388	Colonoscopy through stoma; diagnostic, including collection of specimen(s) by brushing or washing, when performed (separate procedure)
44389	with biopsy, single or multiple

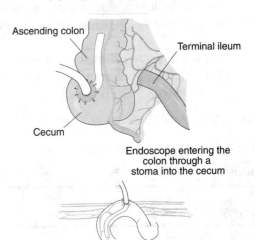

Ascending colon

Terminal ileum

Cecum

Endoscope entering the colon through a stoma into the cecum

Specimens may be collected by brushing, washing, or biopsy

Explanation

The physician performs colonoscopy through an abdominal wall colostomy. The physician places the endoscope into the colostomy and advances the endoscope into the colon. The lumen of the colon is visualized and brushings or washings (44388) or biopsies (44389) may be obtained. The endoscope is withdrawn at the completion of the procedure.

Coding Tips

Note that 44388, a separate procedure by definition, is usually a component of a more complex service and is not identified separately. When performed alone or with other unrelated procedures it may be reported. If performed alone, list the code; if performed with other procedures, list the code and append modifier 59 or an X{EPSU} modifier. Report the appropriate endoscopy for each anatomic site examined. Surgical endoscopy includes diagnostic endoscopy; however, diagnostic endoscopy can be identified separately when performed at the same surgical session as an open procedure. Do not report 44388–44389 together. Do not report 44388 in addition to 44390–44408 or 44389 with 44403 for the same lesion.

ICD-10-CM Diagnostic Codes

C18.2	Malignant neoplasm of ascending colon
C18.3	Malignant neoplasm of hepatic flexure
C18.4	Malignant neoplasm of transverse colon
C18.5	Malignant neoplasm of splenic flexure
C18.6	Malignant neoplasm of descending colon
C18.7	Malignant neoplasm of sigmoid colon
C49.A4	Gastrointestinal stromal tumor of large intestine
C78.5	Secondary malignant neoplasm of large intestine and rectum
C7A.022	Malignant carcinoid tumor of the ascending colon
C7A.023	Malignant carcinoid tumor of the transverse colon
C7A.024	Malignant carcinoid tumor of the descending colon
C7A.025	Malignant carcinoid tumor of the sigmoid colon
D01.0	Carcinoma in situ of colon

D01.49	Carcinoma in situ of other parts of intestine
D12.2	Benign neoplasm of ascending colon
D12.3	Benign neoplasm of transverse colon
D12.4	Benign neoplasm of descending colon
D12.5	Benign neoplasm of sigmoid colon
D37.4	Neoplasm of uncertain behavior of colon
D3A.022	Benign carcinoid tumor of the ascending colon
D3A.023	Benign carcinoid tumor of the transverse colon
D3A.024	Benign carcinoid tumor of the descending colon
D3A.025	Benign carcinoid tumor of the sigmoid colon
D50.0	Iron deficiency anemia secondary to blood loss (chronic)
K50.111	Crohn's disease of large intestine with rectal bleeding
K50.112	Crohn's disease of large intestine with intestinal obstruction
K50.114	Crohn's disease of large intestine with abscess
K50.811	Crohn's disease of both small and large intestine with rectal bleeding
K50.814	Crohn's disease of both small and large intestine with abscess
K51.012	Ulcerative (chronic) pancolitis with intestinal obstruction
K51.013	Ulcerative (chronic) pancolitis with fistula
K51.311	Ulcerative (chronic) rectosigmoiditis with rectal bleeding
K51.312	Ulcerative (chronic) rectosigmoiditis with intestinal obstruction
K51.313	Ulcerative (chronic) rectosigmoiditis with fistula
K51.314	Ulcerative (chronic) rectosigmoiditis with abscess
K51.411	Inflammatory polyps of colon with rectal bleeding
K51.412	Inflammatory polyps of colon with intestinal obstruction
K51.413	Inflammatory polyps of colon with fistula
K51.414	Inflammatory polyps of colon with abscess
K51.418	Inflammatory polyps of colon with other complication
K51.511	Left sided colitis with rectal bleeding
K51.513	Left sided colitis with fistula
K51.514	Left sided colitis with abscess
K51.813	Other ulcerative colitis with fistula
K51.814	Other ulcerative colitis with abscess
K52.0	Gastroenteritis and colitis due to radiation
K52.1	Toxic gastroenteritis and colitis
K52.82	Eosinophilic colitis
K55.041	Focal (segmental) acute infarction of large intestine
K55.042	Diffuse acute infarction of large intestine
K55.21	Angiodysplasia of colon with hemorrhage
K56.51	Intestinal adhesions [bands], with partial obstruction
K56.52	Intestinal adhesions [bands] with complete obstruction
K57.21	Diverticulitis of large intestine with perforation and abscess with bleeding
K57.31	Diverticulosis of large intestine without perforation or abscess with bleeding
K57.33	Diverticulitis of large intestine without perforation or abscess with bleeding
K57.40	Diverticulitis of both small and large intestine with perforation and abscess without bleeding
K58.0	Irritable bowel syndrome with diarrhea
K58.9	Irritable bowel syndrome without diarrhea
K59.01	Slow transit constipation
K59.02	Outlet dysfunction constipation

K59.31	Toxic megacolon
K63.0	Abscess of intestine
K63.1	Perforation of intestine (nontraumatic)
K63.2	Fistula of intestine
K63.3	Ulcer of intestine
K63.5	Polyp of colon
K63.81	Dieulafoy lesion of intestine
M35.08	Sjögren syndrome with gastrointestinal involvement
Q43.1	Hirschsprung's disease
R62.7	Adult failure to thrive ⒜
R63.4	Abnormal weight loss
R63.6	Underweight
Z12.11	Encounter for screening for malignant neoplasm of colon

AMA: **44388** 2018,Jan,8; 2017,Jan,8; 2016,Jan,13; 2015,Jan,16 **44389** 2018,Jan,8; 2017,Jan,8; 2016,Jan,13; 2015,Jan,16

Relative Value Units/Medicare Edits

Non-Facility RVU	Work	PE	MP	Total
44388	2.72	6.39	0.39	9.5
44389	3.02	9.13	0.38	12.53
Facility RVU	Work	PE	MP	Total
44388	2.72	1.45	0.39	4.56
44389	3.02	1.61	0.38	5.01

	FUD	Status	MUE	Modifiers				IOM Reference
44388	0	A	1(3)	51	N/A	N/A	N/A	None
44389	0	A	1(2)	51	N/A	N/A	N/A	

* with documentation

44390

44390   Colonoscopy through stoma; with removal of foreign body(s)

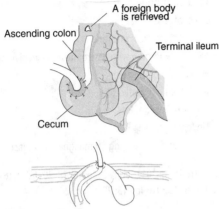

An endoscope is advanced through an existing colostomy in order to remove a foreign body

Explanation

The physician performs colonoscopy through an abdominal wall colostomy and removes a foreign body(s). The physician places the endoscope into the colostomy and advances the endoscope into the colon. The lumen of the colon is visualized. The foreign body(s) is isolated and grasped with a snare or forceps (placed through the endoscope) and removed. The endoscope is withdrawn at the completion of the procedure.

Coding Tips

Report the appropriate endoscopy for each anatomic site examined. Surgical endoscopy includes a diagnostic endoscopy; however, diagnostic endoscopy can be identified separately when performed at the same surgical session as an open procedure. Report fluoroscopic guidance with 76000, when performed. For a small intestinal endoscopy, enteroscopy beyond the second portion of the duodenum, not including the ileum, with removal of a foreign body, see 44363. For colonoscopy flexible, with removal of a foreign body, see 45379. Do not report 44390 with 44388.

ICD-10-CM Diagnostic Codes

T18.4XXA	Foreign body in colon, initial encounter
T18.8XXA	Foreign body in other parts of alimentary tract, initial encounter
Z43.3	Encounter for attention to colostomy

AMA: 44390 2018,Jan,8; 2017,Jan,8; 2016,Jan,13; 2015,Jan,16

Relative Value Units/Medicare Edits

Non-Facility RVU	Work	PE	MP	Total
44390	3.74	8.05	0.41	12.2
Facility RVU	Work	PE	MP	Total
44390	3.74	1.97	0.41	6.12

	FUD	Status	MUE	Modifiers				IOM Reference
44390	0	A	1(3)	51	N/A	N/A	N/A	None

* with documentation

44391

44391   Colonoscopy through stoma; with control of bleeding, any method

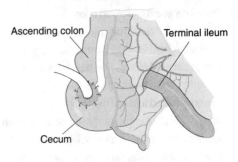

Endoscope entering the colon through a stoma to the cecum

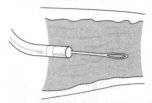

Bleeding may be controlled by any method

Explanation

The physician performs colonoscopy through an abdominal wall colostomy and controls an area of bleeding. The physician places the endoscope into the colostomy and advances the endoscope into the colon. The lumen of the colon is visualized and the area of bleeding is identified and controlled. The endoscope is withdrawn at the completion of the procedure.

Coding Tips

Surgical endoscopy includes diagnostic endoscopy; however, diagnostic endoscopy can be identified separately when performed at the same surgical session as an open procedure. For a small intestinal endoscopy, without ileum, with control of bleeding, any method, see 44366; including ileum, see 44378. For flexible colonoscopy with control of bleeding, see 45382. Do not report 44391 in addition to 44388 or with 44404 for the same lesion.

ICD-10-CM Diagnostic Codes

C17.2	Malignant neoplasm of ileum
C17.3	Meckel's diverticulum, malignant
C18.0	Malignant neoplasm of cecum
C18.1	Malignant neoplasm of appendix
C18.2	Malignant neoplasm of ascending colon
C18.3	Malignant neoplasm of hepatic flexure
C18.4	Malignant neoplasm of transverse colon
C18.5	Malignant neoplasm of splenic flexure
C18.6	Malignant neoplasm of descending colon
C18.7	Malignant neoplasm of sigmoid colon
C19	Malignant neoplasm of rectosigmoid junction
C20	Malignant neoplasm of rectum
C78.5	Secondary malignant neoplasm of large intestine and rectum
C7A.012	Malignant carcinoid tumor of the ileum
C7A.020	Malignant carcinoid tumor of the appendix
C7A.021	Malignant carcinoid tumor of the cecum
C7A.022	Malignant carcinoid tumor of the ascending colon

C7A.023	Malignant carcinoid tumor of the transverse colon
C7A.024	Malignant carcinoid tumor of the descending colon
C7A.025	Malignant carcinoid tumor of the sigmoid colon
D01.0	Carcinoma in situ of colon
D12.0	Benign neoplasm of cecum
D12.1	Benign neoplasm of appendix
D12.2	Benign neoplasm of ascending colon
D12.3	Benign neoplasm of transverse colon
D12.4	Benign neoplasm of descending colon
D12.5	Benign neoplasm of sigmoid colon
D37.4	Neoplasm of uncertain behavior of colon
D3A.012	Benign carcinoid tumor of the ileum
D3A.020	Benign carcinoid tumor of the appendix
D3A.021	Benign carcinoid tumor of the cecum
D3A.022	Benign carcinoid tumor of the ascending colon
D3A.023	Benign carcinoid tumor of the transverse colon
D3A.024	Benign carcinoid tumor of the descending colon
D3A.025	Benign carcinoid tumor of the sigmoid colon
K50.011	Crohn's disease of small intestine with rectal bleeding
K50.111	Crohn's disease of large intestine with rectal bleeding
K50.811	Crohn's disease of both small and large intestine with rectal bleeding
K51.011	Ulcerative (chronic) pancolitis with rectal bleeding
K51.211	Ulcerative (chronic) proctitis with rectal bleeding
K51.311	Ulcerative (chronic) rectosigmoiditis with rectal bleeding
K51.411	Inflammatory polyps of colon with rectal bleeding
K51.511	Left sided colitis with rectal bleeding
K52.0	Gastroenteritis and colitis due to radiation
K55.041	Focal (segmental) acute infarction of large intestine
K55.042	Diffuse acute infarction of large intestine
K55.1	Chronic vascular disorders of intestine
K55.21	Angiodysplasia of colon with hemorrhage
K57.21	Diverticulitis of large intestine with perforation and abscess with bleeding
K57.31	Diverticulosis of large intestine without perforation or abscess with bleeding
K57.33	Diverticulitis of large intestine without perforation or abscess with bleeding
K57.41	Diverticulitis of both small and large intestine with perforation and abscess with bleeding
K57.51	Diverticulosis of both small and large intestine without perforation or abscess with bleeding
K57.53	Diverticulitis of both small and large intestine without perforation or abscess with bleeding
K63.1	Perforation of intestine (nontraumatic)
K63.81	Dieulafoy lesion of intestine
K92.1	Melena
Q43.0	Meckel's diverticulum (displaced) (hypertrophic)

AMA: **44391** 2018,Jan,8; 2017,Jan,8; 2016,Jan,13; 2015,Jan,16

Relative Value Units/Medicare Edits

Non-Facility RVU	Work	PE	MP	Total
44391	4.12	15.88	0.46	20.46
Facility RVU	**Work**	**PE**	**MP**	**Total**
44391	4.12	2.12	0.46	6.7

	FUD	Status	MUE	Modifiers				IOM Reference
44391	0	A	1(3)	51	N/A	N/A	N/A	None

* with documentation

Terms To Know

colonoscopy. Visual inspection of the colon using a fiberoptic scope.

colostomy. Artificial surgical opening anywhere along the length of the colon to the skin surface for the diversion of feces.

Dieulafoy lesion. Abnormally large submucosal artery protruding through a defect in the stomach mucosa or intestines that can cause massive and life-threatening hemorrhaging.

lumen. Space inside an intestine, artery, vein, duct, or tube.

malignant neoplasm. Any cancerous tumor or lesion exhibiting uncontrolled tissue growth that can progressively invade other parts of the body with its disease-generating cells.

Meckel's diverticulum. Congenital, abnormal remnant of embryonic digestive system development that leaves a sacculation or outpouching from the wall of the small intestine near the terminal part of the ileum made of acid-secreting tissue as in the stomach.

stoma. Opening created in the abdominal wall from an internal organ or structure for diversion of waste elimination, drainage, and access.

Intestines

44392-44394 [44401]

44392 Colonoscopy through stoma; with removal of tumor(s), polyp(s), or other lesion(s) by hot biopsy forceps

44401 Colonoscopy through stoma; with ablation of tumor(s), polyp(s), or other lesion(s) (includes pre-and post-dilation and guide wire passage, when performed)

44394 with removal of tumor(s), polyp(s), or other lesion(s) by snare technique

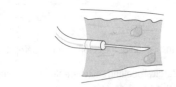

Tumors, polyps, or other lesions are removed by ablation

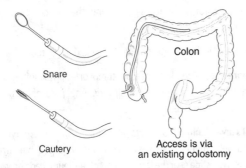

Snare

Cautery

Colon

Access is via an existing colostomy

Explanation

The physician performs colonoscopy through an abdominal wall colostomy and removes a tumor, polyp, or other lesion with hot biopsy forceps. The physician places the endoscope into the colostomy and advances the endoscope into the colon. The lumen of the colon is visualized and the tumor, polyp, or lesion is identified and removed with hot biopsy forceps. The endoscope is withdrawn at the completion of the procedure. Report 44401 for ablation by other method, including dilation before and after the procedure, as well as guidewire passage when performed. Report 44394 for removal of a lesion by snare technique.

Coding Tips

For colonoscopy through stoma with removal of tumors, polyps, or lesions by hot biopsy forceps, see 44392; snare technique, see 44394; ablation by any other method, see 44401; with endoscopic mucosal resection, see 44403. Do not report 44392, 44394, or 44401 when reporting 44388. Do not report 44401 in addition to 44405 or 44394 with 44403 for the same lesion.

ICD-10-CM Diagnostic Codes

C17.2	Malignant neoplasm of ileum
C18.0	Malignant neoplasm of cecum
C18.1	Malignant neoplasm of appendix
C18.2	Malignant neoplasm of ascending colon
C18.3	Malignant neoplasm of hepatic flexure
C18.4	Malignant neoplasm of transverse colon
C18.5	Malignant neoplasm of splenic flexure
C18.6	Malignant neoplasm of descending colon
C18.7	Malignant neoplasm of sigmoid colon
C18.8	Malignant neoplasm of overlapping sites of colon
C19	Malignant neoplasm of rectosigmoid junction
C20	Malignant neoplasm of rectum
C49.A4	Gastrointestinal stromal tumor of large intestine
C78.4	Secondary malignant neoplasm of small intestine
C78.5	Secondary malignant neoplasm of large intestine and rectum
C7A.012	Malignant carcinoid tumor of the ileum
C7A.020	Malignant carcinoid tumor of the appendix
C7A.021	Malignant carcinoid tumor of the cecum
C7A.022	Malignant carcinoid tumor of the ascending colon
C7A.023	Malignant carcinoid tumor of the transverse colon
C7A.024	Malignant carcinoid tumor of the descending colon
C7A.025	Malignant carcinoid tumor of the sigmoid colon
C7A.026	Malignant carcinoid tumor of the rectum
D01.0	Carcinoma in situ of colon
D01.1	Carcinoma in situ of rectosigmoid junction
D01.2	Carcinoma in situ of rectum
D01.3	Carcinoma in situ of anus and anal canal
D01.49	Carcinoma in situ of other parts of intestine
D01.7	Carcinoma in situ of other specified digestive organs
D12.0	Benign neoplasm of cecum
D12.1	Benign neoplasm of appendix
D12.2	Benign neoplasm of ascending colon
D12.3	Benign neoplasm of transverse colon
D12.4	Benign neoplasm of descending colon
D12.5	Benign neoplasm of sigmoid colon
D13.39	Benign neoplasm of other parts of small intestine
D37.3	Neoplasm of uncertain behavior of appendix
D37.4	Neoplasm of uncertain behavior of colon
D37.5	Neoplasm of uncertain behavior of rectum
D3A.012	Benign carcinoid tumor of the ileum
D3A.020	Benign carcinoid tumor of the appendix
D3A.021	Benign carcinoid tumor of the cecum
D3A.022	Benign carcinoid tumor of the ascending colon
D3A.023	Benign carcinoid tumor of the transverse colon
D3A.024	Benign carcinoid tumor of the descending colon
D3A.025	Benign carcinoid tumor of the sigmoid colon
D3A.026	Benign carcinoid tumor of the rectum
D49.0	Neoplasm of unspecified behavior of digestive system
K51.40	Inflammatory polyps of colon without complications
K51.411	Inflammatory polyps of colon with rectal bleeding
K51.412	Inflammatory polyps of colon with intestinal obstruction
K51.413	Inflammatory polyps of colon with fistula
K51.414	Inflammatory polyps of colon with abscess
K51.418	Inflammatory polyps of colon with other complication
K55.20	Angiodysplasia of colon without hemorrhage
K55.21	Angiodysplasia of colon with hemorrhage
K56.51	Intestinal adhesions [bands], with partial obstruction
K56.52	Intestinal adhesions [bands] with complete obstruction
K63.5	Polyp of colon
K63.81	Dieulafoy lesion of intestine
K63.89	Other specified diseases of intestine
K92.1	Melena
Q43.2	Other congenital functional disorders of colon

| Q43.8 | Other specified congenital malformations of intestine |
| R93.3 | Abnormal findings on diagnostic imaging of other parts of digestive tract |

AMA: 44392 2018,Jan,8; 2017,Jan,8; 2016,Jan,13; 2015,Jan,16 **44394** 2018,Jan,8; 2017,Jan,8; 2016,Jan,13; 2015,Jan,16 **44401** 2018,Jan,8; 2017,Jan,8; 2016,Jan,13; 2015,Jan,16

Relative Value Units/Medicare Edits

Non-Facility RVU	Work	PE	MP	Total
44392	3.53	7.58	0.49	11.6
44401	4.34	77.43	0.46	82.23
44394	4.03	8.72	0.49	13.24
Facility RVU	Work	PE	MP	Total
44392	3.53	1.76	0.49	5.78
44401	4.34	2.24	0.46	7.04
44394	4.03	2.03	0.49	6.55

	FUD	Status	MUE	Modifiers				IOM Reference
44392	0	A	1(2)	51	N/A	N/A	N/A	None
44401	0	A	1(2)	51	N/A	N/A	N/A	
44394	0	A	1(2)	51	N/A	N/A	N/A	

* with documentation

Terms To Know

ablation. Removal or destruction of tissue by cutting, electrical energy, chemical substances, or excessive heat application.

dilation. Artificial increase in the diameter of an opening or lumen made by medication or by instrumentation.

forceps. Tool used for grasping or compressing tissue.

guidewire. Flexible metal instrument designed to lead another instrument in its proper course.

hot biopsy. Using forceps technique, simultaneously excises and fulgurates polyps; avoids the bleeding associated with cold-forceps biopsy; and preserves the specimen for histologic examination (in contrast, a simple fulguration of the polyp destroys it).

polyp. Small growth on a stalk-like attachment projecting from a mucous membrane.

snare. Wire used as a loop to excise a polyp or lesion.

stoma. Opening created in the abdominal wall from an internal organ or structure for diversion of waste elimination, drainage, and access.

tumor. Pathological swelling or enlargement; a neoplastic growth of uncontrolled, abnormal multiplication of cells.

44402

| 44402 | Colonoscopy through stoma; with endoscopic stent placement (including pre- and post-dilation and guide wire passage, when performed) |

A colonoscopy is performed with delivery through an existing surgically created stoma

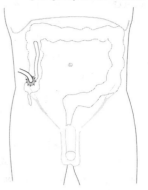

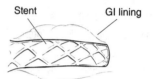

Stent   GI lining

Explanation

The physician uses a colonoscope to examine the colon through an abdominal wall colostomy and places an endoscopic stent. The physician places the endoscope into the colostomy and advances the endoscope into the colon. The lumen of the colon is visualized. The endoscope is placed at the site of an obstruction or stricture and the necessary stent length is determined. The stent (endoprosthesis) is introduced into the site of the obstruction. Using a commercial delivery system, a plastic covering over the stent is removed and the stent self-deploys, shoring-up the walls at a specific site in the large intestine. When necessary, a balloon catheter is placed into the stent and gently inflated to more fully deploy the stent. The delivery system and colonoscope are removed. This code includes dilation before and after stent placement, as well as guidewire passage when performed.

Coding Tips

Report fluoroscopic guidance with 74360, if performed. For colonoscopy with endoscopic stent placement, see 45389. Do not report 44402 with 44388 or 44405.

ICD-10-CM Diagnostic Codes

C17.2	Malignant neoplasm of ileum
C18.0	Malignant neoplasm of cecum
C18.1	Malignant neoplasm of appendix
C18.2	Malignant neoplasm of ascending colon
C18.3	Malignant neoplasm of hepatic flexure
C18.4	Malignant neoplasm of transverse colon
C18.5	Malignant neoplasm of splenic flexure
C18.6	Malignant neoplasm of descending colon
C18.7	Malignant neoplasm of sigmoid colon
C18.8	Malignant neoplasm of overlapping sites of colon
C19	Malignant neoplasm of rectosigmoid junction

C49.A4	Gastrointestinal stromal tumor of large intestine
C78.4	Secondary malignant neoplasm of small intestine
C78.5	Secondary malignant neoplasm of large intestine and rectum
C7A.012	Malignant carcinoid tumor of the ileum
C7A.020	Malignant carcinoid tumor of the appendix
C7A.021	Malignant carcinoid tumor of the cecum
C7A.022	Malignant carcinoid tumor of the ascending colon
C7A.023	Malignant carcinoid tumor of the transverse colon
C7A.024	Malignant carcinoid tumor of the descending colon
C7A.025	Malignant carcinoid tumor of the sigmoid colon
D49.0	Neoplasm of unspecified behavior of digestive system
K50.012	Crohn's disease of small intestine with intestinal obstruction
K50.112	Crohn's disease of large intestine with intestinal obstruction
K50.812	Crohn's disease of both small and large intestine with intestinal obstruction
K51.012	Ulcerative (chronic) pancolitis with intestinal obstruction
K51.212	Ulcerative (chronic) proctitis with intestinal obstruction
K51.312	Ulcerative (chronic) rectosigmoiditis with intestinal obstruction
K51.412	Inflammatory polyps of colon with intestinal obstruction
K51.512	Left sided colitis with intestinal obstruction
K51.812	Other ulcerative colitis with intestinal obstruction
K56.49	Other impaction of intestine
K56.51	Intestinal adhesions [bands], with partial obstruction
K56.52	Intestinal adhesions [bands] with complete obstruction
K56.690	Other partial intestinal obstruction
K56.691	Other complete intestinal obstruction
K91.31	Postprocedural partial intestinal obstruction
K91.32	Postprocedural complete intestinal obstruction
K91.89	Other postprocedural complications and disorders of digestive system
Q41.8	Congenital absence, atresia and stenosis of other specified parts of small intestine
Q42.0	Congenital absence, atresia and stenosis of rectum with fistula
Q42.1	Congenital absence, atresia and stenosis of rectum without fistula
Q42.8	Congenital absence, atresia and stenosis of other parts of large intestine
R93.3	Abnormal findings on diagnostic imaging of other parts of digestive tract

AMA: **44402** 2018,Jan,8; 2017,Jan,8; 2016,Jan,13; 2015,Jan,16

Relative Value Units/Medicare Edits

Non-Facility RVU	Work	PE	MP	Total
44402	4.7	2.4	0.49	7.59
Facility RVU	Work	PE	MP	Total
44402	4.7	2.4	0.49	7.59

	FUD	Status	MUE	Modifiers			IOM Reference
44402	0	A	1(3)	51	N/A	N/A	N/A	None

* with documentation

44403-44404

44403	Colonoscopy through stoma; with endoscopic mucosal resection
44404	with directed submucosal injection(s), any substance

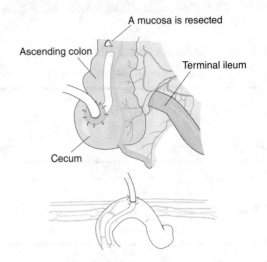

An endoscope is advanced through an existing colostomy in order to perform a mucosal resection or submucosal injections

Explanation

The physician uses a colonoscope to examine the colon through an abdominal wall colostomy. The physician places the endoscope into the colostomy and advances into the colon. The lumen of the colon is visualized with an instrument containing a camera and light. The scope is directed to the affected area. In 44403, a special needle is used to administer fluid under the polyp to elevate the polyp allowing for the removal from the bowel lining. Removal may be done by snare, cutting out, or suction and typically includes cautery of the attached blood vessels. The tissue is sent to pathology for analysis and the scope is withdrawn at the completion of the procedure. In 44404, the physician injects a substance into the submucosa, directed at specific areas through the scope, while viewing the colon. Submucosal saline injections, for instance, may be done before polypectomy using snare and electrocautery to greatly enhance the effectiveness of resection for large sessile colorectal polyps. The scope is withdrawn at the completion of the procedure.

Coding Tips

Do not report 44403 with 44388 or in addition to 44389, 44394, or 44404 for the same lesion. Do not report 44404 with 44388 or in addition to 44391 or 44403 for the same lesion.

ICD-10-CM Diagnostic Codes

C17.2	Malignant neoplasm of ileum
C18.0	Malignant neoplasm of cecum
C18.1	Malignant neoplasm of appendix
C18.2	Malignant neoplasm of ascending colon
C18.3	Malignant neoplasm of hepatic flexure
C18.4	Malignant neoplasm of transverse colon
C18.5	Malignant neoplasm of splenic flexure
C18.6	Malignant neoplasm of descending colon
C18.7	Malignant neoplasm of sigmoid colon
C18.8	Malignant neoplasm of overlapping sites of colon
C49.A4	Gastrointestinal stromal tumor of large intestine
C78.4	Secondary malignant neoplasm of small intestine

C78.5	Secondary malignant neoplasm of large intestine and rectum
C7A.012	Malignant carcinoid tumor of the ileum
C7A.020	Malignant carcinoid tumor of the appendix
C7A.021	Malignant carcinoid tumor of the cecum
C7A.022	Malignant carcinoid tumor of the ascending colon
C7A.023	Malignant carcinoid tumor of the transverse colon
C7A.024	Malignant carcinoid tumor of the descending colon
C7A.025	Malignant carcinoid tumor of the sigmoid colon
D01.0	Carcinoma in situ of colon
D01.49	Carcinoma in situ of other parts of intestine
D12.0	Benign neoplasm of cecum
D12.1	Benign neoplasm of appendix
D12.2	Benign neoplasm of ascending colon
D12.3	Benign neoplasm of transverse colon
D12.4	Benign neoplasm of descending colon
D12.5	Benign neoplasm of sigmoid colon
D13.39	Benign neoplasm of other parts of small intestine
D37.1	Neoplasm of uncertain behavior of stomach
D37.2	Neoplasm of uncertain behavior of small intestine
D37.3	Neoplasm of uncertain behavior of appendix
D37.4	Neoplasm of uncertain behavior of colon
D37.5	Neoplasm of uncertain behavior of rectum
D3A.012	Benign carcinoid tumor of the ileum
D3A.020	Benign carcinoid tumor of the appendix
D3A.021	Benign carcinoid tumor of the cecum
D3A.022	Benign carcinoid tumor of the ascending colon
D3A.023	Benign carcinoid tumor of the transverse colon
D3A.024	Benign carcinoid tumor of the descending colon
D3A.025	Benign carcinoid tumor of the sigmoid colon
D49.0	Neoplasm of unspecified behavior of digestive system
K51.40	Inflammatory polyps of colon without complications
K51.411	Inflammatory polyps of colon with rectal bleeding
K51.412	Inflammatory polyps of colon with intestinal obstruction
K51.413	Inflammatory polyps of colon with fistula
K51.414	Inflammatory polyps of colon with abscess
K51.418	Inflammatory polyps of colon with other complication
K62.1	Rectal polyp
K63.5	Polyp of colon
K63.81	Dieulafoy lesion of intestine
R93.3	Abnormal findings on diagnostic imaging of other parts of digestive tract

AMA: 44403 2019,Dec,14; 2018,Jan,8; 2017,Jan,8; 2016,Jan,13; 2015,Jan,16
44404 2018,Jan,8; 2017,Jan,8; 2016,Jan,13; 2015,Jan,16

Relative Value Units/Medicare Edits

Non-Facility RVU	Work	PE	MP	Total
44403	5.5	2.75	0.59	8.84
44404	3.02	9.22	0.37	12.61
Facility RVU	Work	PE	MP	Total
44403	5.5	2.75	0.59	8.84
44404	3.02	1.61	0.37	5.0

	FUD	Status	MUE	Modifiers				IOM Reference
44403	0	A	1(3)	51	N/A	N/A	N/A	None
44404	0	A	1(3)	51	N/A	N/A	N/A	

* with documentation

Terms To Know

carcinoid tumor. Specific type of slow-growing neuroendocrine tumors. Carcinoid tumors occur most commonly in the hormone producing cells of the gastrointestinal tracts and can also occur in the pancreas, testes, ovaries, or lungs.

colostomy. Artificial surgical opening anywhere along the length of the colon to the skin surface for the diversion of feces.

electrocautery. Division or cutting of tissue using high-frequency electrical current to produce heat, which destroys cells.

polyp. Small growth on a stalk-like attachment projecting from a mucous membrane.

snare. Wire used as a loop to excise a polyp or lesion.

stoma. Opening created in the abdominal wall from an internal organ or structure for diversion of waste elimination, drainage, and access.

44405

44405 Colonoscopy through stoma; with transendoscopic balloon dilation

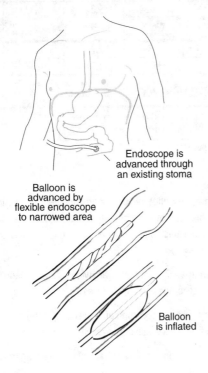

Endoscope is advanced through an existing stoma

Balloon is advanced by flexible endoscope to narrowed area

Balloon is inflated

Explanation

The physician uses a colonoscope to examine the colon through an abdominal wall colostomy and dilates strictures by balloon catheter. The physician places the endoscope into the colostomy and advances into the colon. The lumen of the colon is visualized. Areas of stenosis are identified and a balloon catheter is passed to the point of constriction and a little beyond. The balloon is inflated to the appropriate diameter and gradually withdrawn through the stenosed area, stretching the walls of the strictured area. The scope is withdrawn at the completion of the procedure.

Coding Tips

Surgical endoscopy includes diagnostic endoscopy; however, diagnostic endoscopy can be identified separately when performed at the same surgical session as an open procedure. When fluoroscopic guidance is performed, report 74360. For multiple strictures treated with transendoscopic balloon dilations during the same session, report 44405 with modifier 59 or an X{EPSU} modifier for each additional stricture. Do not report 44405 with 44388, 44401, or 44402.

ICD-10-CM Diagnostic Codes

K50.012	Crohn's disease of small intestine with intestinal obstruction
K50.112	Crohn's disease of large intestine with intestinal obstruction
K50.812	Crohn's disease of both small and large intestine with intestinal obstruction
K51.012	Ulcerative (chronic) pancolitis with intestinal obstruction
K51.212	Ulcerative (chronic) proctitis with intestinal obstruction
K51.312	Ulcerative (chronic) rectosigmoiditis with intestinal obstruction
K51.412	Inflammatory polyps of colon with intestinal obstruction
K51.512	Left sided colitis with intestinal obstruction
K51.812	Other ulcerative colitis with intestinal obstruction
K56.1	Intussusception

K56.2	Volvulus
K56.49	Other impaction of intestine
K56.51	Intestinal adhesions [bands], with partial obstruction
K56.52	Intestinal adhesions [bands] with complete obstruction
K56.690	Other partial intestinal obstruction
K56.691	Other complete intestinal obstruction
K91.31	Postprocedural partial intestinal obstruction
K91.32	Postprocedural complete intestinal obstruction
K91.89	Other postprocedural complications and disorders of digestive system
Q42.0	Congenital absence, atresia and stenosis of rectum with fistula
Q42.1	Congenital absence, atresia and stenosis of rectum without fistula
Q42.8	Congenital absence, atresia and stenosis of other parts of large intestine

AMA: **44405** 2018,Jan,8; 2017,Jan,8; 2016,Jan,13; 2015,Jan,16

Relative Value Units/Medicare Edits

Non-Facility RVU	Work	PE	MP	Total
44405	3.23	13.75	0.34	17.32
Facility RVU	**Work**	**PE**	**MP**	**Total**
44405	3.23	1.75	0.34	5.32

	FUD	Status	MUE	Modifiers				IOM Reference
44405	0	A	1(3)	51	N/A	N/A	N/A	None

* with documentation

Terms To Know

colostomy. Artificial surgical opening anywhere along the length of the colon to the skin surface for the diversion of feces.

endoscopy. Visual inspection of the body using a fiberoptic scope.

lumen. Space inside an intestine, artery, vein, duct, or tube.

obstruction. Blockage that prevents normal function of the valve or structure.

stenosis. Narrowing or constriction of a passage.

stricture. Narrowing of an anatomical structure.

44406-44407

44406 Colonoscopy through stoma; with endoscopic ultrasound examination, limited to the sigmoid, descending, transverse, or ascending colon and cecum and adjacent structures

44407 with transendoscopic ultrasound guided intramural or transmural fine needle aspiration/biopsy(s), includes endoscopic ultrasound examination limited to the sigmoid, descending, transverse, or ascending colon and cecum and adjacent structures

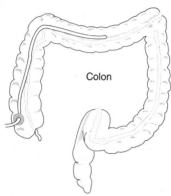

Colon

An endoscope with ultrasound transducer delivered through an existing stoma into the colon

Explanation

In 44406, the physician uses a flexible colonoscope to examine the colon and perform an endoscopic ultrasound (EUS) examination. Ultrasound and endoscopic imaging techniques are combined in this diagnostic modality. An endoscope equipped with an ultrasound transducer at the tip is inserted into the colon through an abdominal wall colostomy. The lumen of the colon is visualized and the probe tip is guided next to the area of concern. Sound waves are sent out from the transducer and reflect back to a receiving unit at varying speeds as they pass through different densities of tissue. The waves are converted to electrical pulses displayed as a picture on screen. Using ultrasound from within the endoscope instead of transcutaneously shortens the distance between the source and the target lesion and produces greater clarity from high frequency, high-resolution sound waves that have a short penetration distance. EUS is currently the most accurate method of staging cancer within the gastrointestinal tract. In 44407, the physician uses a colonoscope to examine the colon and perform a transendoscopic ultrasound guided intramural or transmural fine needle aspiration (FNA)/biopsy(s). An endoscope equipped with an ultrasound transducer at the tip is inserted into the colon through an abdominal wall colostomy. The lumen of the colon is visualized and the probe tip is guided next to the area of concern. Sound waves are sent out from the transducer and reflect back to a receiving unit at varying speeds as they pass through different densities of tissue. The waves are converted to electrical pulses displayed as a picture on screen. An FNA needle is passed through the scope to the site of the lesion, lymph node, or tumor and a fine needle aspiration/biopsy(s) is taken of the abnormal tissue or fluid within the colon wall or through the intestinal wall. These codes are used for examination of the colon, cecum, and surrounding structures only.

Coding Tips

Surgical endoscopy includes diagnostic endoscopy; however, diagnostic endoscopy can be identified separately when performed at the same surgical session as an open procedure. Colonoscopy involves examination of the entire colon, from the rectum to the cecum, and may also include the terminal ileum. Report the appropriate endoscopy for each anatomic site examined. Do not report 44406–44407 with 44388, 76975, or each other. Do not report 44407 with 76942. These codes may only be reported once per session.

ICD-10-CM Diagnostic Codes

C18.0	Malignant neoplasm of cecum
C18.1	Malignant neoplasm of appendix
C18.2	Malignant neoplasm of ascending colon
C18.3	Malignant neoplasm of hepatic flexure
C18.4	Malignant neoplasm of transverse colon
C18.5	Malignant neoplasm of splenic flexure
C18.6	Malignant neoplasm of descending colon
C18.7	Malignant neoplasm of sigmoid colon
C18.8	Malignant neoplasm of overlapping sites of colon
C19	Malignant neoplasm of rectosigmoid junction
C49.A4	Gastrointestinal stromal tumor of large intestine
C78.5	Secondary malignant neoplasm of large intestine and rectum
C7A.020	Malignant carcinoid tumor of the appendix
C7A.021	Malignant carcinoid tumor of the cecum
C7A.022	Malignant carcinoid tumor of the ascending colon
C7A.023	Malignant carcinoid tumor of the transverse colon
C7A.024	Malignant carcinoid tumor of the descending colon
C7A.025	Malignant carcinoid tumor of the sigmoid colon
D01.0	Carcinoma in situ of colon
D01.1	Carcinoma in situ of rectosigmoid junction
D12.0	Benign neoplasm of cecum
D12.1	Benign neoplasm of appendix
D12.2	Benign neoplasm of ascending colon
D12.3	Benign neoplasm of transverse colon
D12.4	Benign neoplasm of descending colon
D12.5	Benign neoplasm of sigmoid colon
D12.7	Benign neoplasm of rectosigmoid junction
D37.4	Neoplasm of uncertain behavior of colon
D3A.020	Benign carcinoid tumor of the appendix
D3A.021	Benign carcinoid tumor of the cecum
D3A.022	Benign carcinoid tumor of the ascending colon
D3A.023	Benign carcinoid tumor of the transverse colon
D3A.024	Benign carcinoid tumor of the descending colon
D3A.025	Benign carcinoid tumor of the sigmoid colon
K50.111	Crohn's disease of large intestine with rectal bleeding
K50.112	Crohn's disease of large intestine with intestinal obstruction
K50.113	Crohn's disease of large intestine with fistula
K50.114	Crohn's disease of large intestine with abscess
K50.811	Crohn's disease of both small and large intestine with rectal bleeding
K50.812	Crohn's disease of both small and large intestine with intestinal obstruction
K50.813	Crohn's disease of both small and large intestine with fistula
K50.814	Crohn's disease of both small and large intestine with abscess
K51.411	Inflammatory polyps of colon with rectal bleeding
K51.412	Inflammatory polyps of colon with intestinal obstruction
K51.413	Inflammatory polyps of colon with fistula
K51.414	Inflammatory polyps of colon with abscess
K51.418	Inflammatory polyps of colon with other complication

K51.811	Other ulcerative colitis with rectal bleeding
K51.812	Other ulcerative colitis with intestinal obstruction
K51.813	Other ulcerative colitis with fistula
K51.814	Other ulcerative colitis with abscess
K55.041	Focal (segmental) acute infarction of large intestine
K55.042	Diffuse acute infarction of large intestine
K55.1	Chronic vascular disorders of intestine
K55.20	Angiodysplasia of colon without hemorrhage
K55.21	Angiodysplasia of colon with hemorrhage
K58.0	Irritable bowel syndrome with diarrhea
K58.9	Irritable bowel syndrome without diarrhea
K59.01	Slow transit constipation
K59.02	Outlet dysfunction constipation
K59.31	Toxic megacolon
K63.0	Abscess of intestine
K63.1	Perforation of intestine (nontraumatic)
K63.2	Fistula of intestine
K63.3	Ulcer of intestine
K63.4	Enteroptosis
K63.5	Polyp of colon
K63.81	Dieulafoy lesion of intestine
K92.1	Melena
M35.08	Sjögren syndrome with gastrointestinal involvement
Q43.1	Hirschsprung's disease
R62.7	Adult failure to thrive Ⓐ
R63.4	Abnormal weight loss
R63.6	Underweight

AMA: 44406 2018,Jan,8; 2017,Jan,8; 2016,Jan,13; 2015,Jan,16 **44407** 2018,Jan,8; 2017,Jan,8; 2016,Jan,13; 2015,Jan,16

Relative Value Units/Medicare Edits

Non-Facility RVU	Work	PE	MP	Total
44406	4.1	2.13	0.44	6.67
44407	4.96	2.51	0.53	8.0
Facility RVU	Work	PE	MP	Total
44406	4.1	2.13	0.44	6.67
44407	4.96	2.51	0.53	8.0

	FUD	Status	MUE	Modifiers				IOM Reference
44406	0	A	1(3)	51	N/A	N/A	N/A	None
44407	0	A	1(2)	51	N/A	N/A	N/A	

* with documentation

44408

44408 Colonoscopy through stoma; with decompression (for pathologic distention) (eg, volvulus, megacolon), including placement of decompression tube, when performed

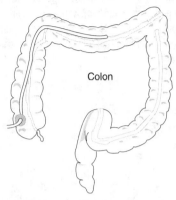

Colon

An endoscope is delivered through an existing stoma into the colon

Explanation

The physician uses a colonoscope to examine the colon through an abdominal wall colostomy to decompress a pathologic distention, such as a volvulus or megacolon. The physician places the endoscope into the colostomy and advances into the colon. The lumen of the colon is visualized. The scope is advanced into the area of distention decompressing it as the scope passes through the lumen. The scope is withdrawn at the completion of the procedure. This procedure includes placement of a decompression tube when utilized.

Coding Tips

Report the appropriate endoscopy for each anatomic site examined. Surgical endoscopy includes diagnostic endoscopy; however, diagnostic endoscopy can be identified separately when performed at the same surgical session as an open procedure. Note that endoscopic reduction of volvulus is performed more frequently using a rigid proctoscope. Do not report 44408 with 44388. Report once per session only.

ICD-10-CM Diagnostic Codes

K56.2	Volvulus
K59.31	Toxic megacolon
K59.39	Other megacolon

AMA: 44408 2018,Jan,8; 2017,Jan,8; 2016,Jan,13; 2015,Jan,16

Relative Value Units/Medicare Edits

Non-Facility RVU	Work	PE	MP	Total
44408	4.14	2.15	0.45	6.74
Facility RVU	Work	PE	MP	Total
44408	4.14	2.15	0.45	6.74

	FUD	Status	MUE	Modifiers				IOM Reference
44408	0	A	1(3)	51	N/A	N/A	N/A	None

* with documentation

44500

44500 Introduction of long gastrointestinal tube (eg, Miller-Abbott) (separate procedure)

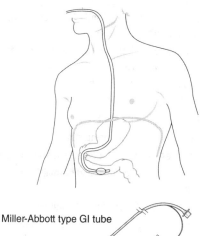

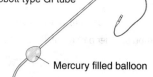

Miller-Abbott type GI tube

Mercury filled balloon

A long Miller-Abbott style gastrointestinal tube is introduced into the GI tract. It is a double lumen tube; one line is open for decompression and the other delivers a liquid filled balloon

Explanation

A long, Miller-Abbott style gastrointestinal tube with a mercury-filled balloon at the bottom is introduced, usually nasally, and used to clear gastrointestinal strictures. The patient is seated lower than the person performing the procedure and the dilator is placed in the posterior pharynx. The patient swallows and the tube and balloon are carried into the small intestine. The balloon is inflated and withdrawn until resistance is encountered. The balloon is partially deflated, withdrawn a little more, and re-inflated. This process is repeated several times to achieve dilation of the stricture. This procedure may be done without fluoroscopy or with fluoroscopy by instilling a diluted contrast into the balloon.

Coding Tips

This separate procedure, by definition, is usually a component of a more complex service and is not identified separately. When performed alone or with other unrelated procedures/services it may be reported. If performed alone, list the code; if performed with other procedures/services, list the code and append modifier 59 or an X{EPSU} modifier. As exempt from modifier 51, this code is not subject to multiple procedure rules. No reimbursement reduction or modifier 51 is applied. Radiological supervision and interpretation is reported with 74340, when performed. For naso- or oro-gastric tube placement, see 43752.

ICD-10-CM Diagnostic Codes

K22.2	Esophageal obstruction
K31.1	Adult hypertrophic pyloric stenosis △
K31.2	Hourglass stricture and stenosis of stomach
K31.3	Pylorospasm, not elsewhere classified
K31.5	Obstruction of duodenum
K31.89	Other diseases of stomach and duodenum
K56.0	Paralytic ileus
K56.1	Intussusception
K56.2	Volvulus
K56.49	Other impaction of intestine
K56.51	Intestinal adhesions [bands], with partial obstruction
K56.52	Intestinal adhesions [bands] with complete obstruction
K56.690	Other partial intestinal obstruction
K56.691	Other complete intestinal obstruction
K91.31	Postprocedural partial intestinal obstruction
K91.32	Postprocedural complete intestinal obstruction
Q40.0	Congenital hypertrophic pyloric stenosis
Q40.2	Other specified congenital malformations of stomach
Q41.0	Congenital absence, atresia and stenosis of duodenum
Q41.1	Congenital absence, atresia and stenosis of jejunum
Q41.2	Congenital absence, atresia and stenosis of ileum
Q41.8	Congenital absence, atresia and stenosis of other specified parts of small intestine
Q43.3	Congenital malformations of intestinal fixation
Q43.8	Other specified congenital malformations of intestine

AMA: **44500** 2020,Aug,9; 2018,Jan,8; 2017,Jan,8; 2016,Sep,9; 2016,Jan,13; 2015,Jan,16

Relative Value Units/Medicare Edits

Non-Facility RVU	Work	PE	MP	Total
44500	0.39	0.14	0.04	0.57
Facility RVU	**Work**	**PE**	**MP**	**Total**
44500	0.39	0.14	0.04	0.57

	FUD	Status	MUE	Modifiers				IOM Reference
44500	0	A	1(3)	N/A	N/A	N/A	80*	None

* with documentation

44602-44603

44602 Suture of small intestine (enterorrhaphy) for perforated ulcer, diverticulum, wound, injury or rupture; single perforation
44603   multiple perforations

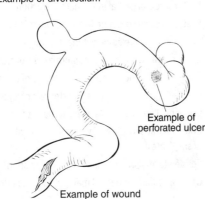

Depiction of small intestine segment showing various conditions requiring suture repair

Example of diverticulum

Example of perforated ulcer

Example of wound

Explanation

The physician performs suture closure of a single small bowel perforation. The physician makes an abdominal incision. Next, the abdomen is explored and the small bowel perforation is identified and repaired with sutures. The incision is closed. Report 44603 for multiple perforations.

Coding Tips

For suture of large intestine, single or multiple perforations, without colostomy, see 44604; with colostomy, see 44605.

ICD-10-CM Diagnostic Codes

K26.0	Acute duodenal ulcer with hemorrhage
K26.1	Acute duodenal ulcer with perforation
K26.2	Acute duodenal ulcer with both hemorrhage and perforation
K26.4	Chronic or unspecified duodenal ulcer with hemorrhage
K26.5	Chronic or unspecified duodenal ulcer with perforation
K26.6	Chronic or unspecified duodenal ulcer with both hemorrhage and perforation
K28.0	Acute gastrojejunal ulcer with hemorrhage
K28.1	Acute gastrojejunal ulcer with perforation
K28.2	Acute gastrojejunal ulcer with both hemorrhage and perforation
K28.4	Chronic or unspecified gastrojejunal ulcer with hemorrhage
K28.5	Chronic or unspecified gastrojejunal ulcer with perforation
K28.6	Chronic or unspecified gastrojejunal ulcer with both hemorrhage and perforation
K31.89	Other diseases of stomach and duodenum
K50.011	Crohn's disease of small intestine with rectal bleeding
K50.012	Crohn's disease of small intestine with intestinal obstruction
K50.018	Crohn's disease of small intestine with other complication
K50.811	Crohn's disease of both small and large intestine with rectal bleeding
K50.812	Crohn's disease of both small and large intestine with intestinal obstruction
K50.818	Crohn's disease of both small and large intestine with other complication
K57.00	Diverticulitis of small intestine with perforation and abscess without bleeding
K57.01	Diverticulitis of small intestine with perforation and abscess with bleeding
K57.40	Diverticulitis of both small and large intestine with perforation and abscess without bleeding
K57.41	Diverticulitis of both small and large intestine with perforation and abscess with bleeding
K63.1	Perforation of intestine (nontraumatic)
K63.3	Ulcer of intestine
K63.81	Dieulafoy lesion of intestine
K63.89	Other specified diseases of intestine
S36.410A	Primary blast injury of duodenum, initial encounter
S36.418A	Primary blast injury of other part of small intestine, initial encounter
S36.420A	Contusion of duodenum, initial encounter
S36.428A	Contusion of other part of small intestine, initial encounter
S36.430A	Laceration of duodenum, initial encounter
S36.438A	Laceration of other part of small intestine, initial encounter

AMA: 44602 2020,Feb,13

Relative Value Units/Medicare Edits

Non-Facility RVU	Work	PE	MP	Total
44602	24.72	11.17	5.63	41.52
44603	28.16	13.31	6.19	47.66
Facility RVU	**Work**	**PE**	**MP**	**Total**
44602	24.72	11.17	5.63	41.52
44603	28.16	13.31	6.19	47.66

	FUD	Status	MUE	Modifiers				IOM Reference
44602	90	A	1(2)	51	N/A	62*	80	None
44603	90	A	1(2)	51	N/A	62*	80	

* with documentation

Terms To Know

diverticulum. Pouch or sac in the walls of an organ or canal.

perforation. Hole in an object, organ, or tissue, or the act of punching or boring holes through a part.

ulcer. Open sore or excavating lesion of skin or the tissue on the surface of an organ from the sloughing of chronically inflamed and necrosing tissue.

Intestines

44604-44605

44604 Suture of large intestine (colorrhaphy) for perforated ulcer, diverticulum, wound, injury or rupture (single or multiple perforations); without colostomy
44605 with colostomy

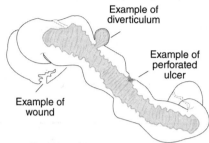

Example of diverticulum

Example of perforated ulcer

Example of wound

Depiction of large intestine segment showing various conditions requiring suture repair

Explanation

The physician performs suture closure of a colon perforation. The physician makes an abdominal incision. Next, the abdomen is explored and the colon perforation is identified and repaired with sutures. In 44605, a loop or end of colon proximal to the repair is brought out through a separate incision on the abdominal wall onto the skin as a colostomy. The initial incision is closed.

Coding Tips

If significant additional time and effort are documented, append modifier 22 and submit a cover letter and operative report. Intraoperative colonic lavage is reported with 44701, when performed. For suture of the small intestine, single perforation, see 44602; multiple perforations, see 44603. For gastrorrhaphy, suture of perforated duodenal or gastric ulcer, wound, or injury, see 43840. For excision of Meckel's diverticulum (diverticulectomy) or omphalomesenteric duct, see 44800.

ICD-10-CM Diagnostic Codes

K50.111	Crohn's disease of large intestine with rectal bleeding
K50.112	Crohn's disease of large intestine with intestinal obstruction
K50.118	Crohn's disease of large intestine with other complication
K50.811	Crohn's disease of both small and large intestine with rectal bleeding
K50.812	Crohn's disease of both small and large intestine with intestinal obstruction
K50.818	Crohn's disease of both small and large intestine with other complication
K51.011	Ulcerative (chronic) pancolitis with rectal bleeding
K51.012	Ulcerative (chronic) pancolitis with intestinal obstruction
K51.013	Ulcerative (chronic) pancolitis with fistula
K51.014	Ulcerative (chronic) pancolitis with abscess
K51.018	Ulcerative (chronic) pancolitis with other complication
K51.311	Ulcerative (chronic) rectosigmoiditis with rectal bleeding
K51.312	Ulcerative (chronic) rectosigmoiditis with intestinal obstruction
K51.313	Ulcerative (chronic) rectosigmoiditis with fistula
K51.314	Ulcerative (chronic) rectosigmoiditis with abscess
K56.2	Volvulus
K57.20	Diverticulitis of large intestine with perforation and abscess without bleeding
K57.21	Diverticulitis of large intestine with perforation and abscess with bleeding
K57.40	Diverticulitis of both small and large intestine with perforation and abscess without bleeding
K57.41	Diverticulitis of both small and large intestine with perforation and abscess with bleeding
K63.1	Perforation of intestine (nontraumatic)
K63.2	Fistula of intestine
K63.3	Ulcer of intestine
K63.81	Dieulafoy lesion of intestine
K63.89	Other specified diseases of intestine
K92.89	Other specified diseases of the digestive system
P78.0	Perinatal intestinal perforation 🔲
S36.510A	Primary blast injury of ascending [right] colon, initial encounter
S36.511A	Primary blast injury of transverse colon, initial encounter
S36.512A	Primary blast injury of descending [left] colon, initial encounter
S36.513A	Primary blast injury of sigmoid colon, initial encounter
S36.518A	Primary blast injury of other part of colon, initial encounter
S36.530A	Laceration of ascending [right] colon, initial encounter
S36.531A	Laceration of transverse colon, initial encounter
S36.532A	Laceration of descending [left] colon, initial encounter
S36.533A	Laceration of sigmoid colon, initial encounter
S36.538A	Laceration of other part of colon, initial encounter
Z05.5	Observation and evaluation of newborn for suspected gastrointestinal condition ruled out 🔲

AMA: **44604** 2014,Jan,11 **44605** 2014,Jan,11

Relative Value Units/Medicare Edits

Non-Facility RVU	Work	PE	MP	Total
44604	18.16	8.97	4.02	31.15
44605	22.08	11.34	4.81	38.23
Facility RVU	**Work**	**PE**	**MP**	**Total**
44604	18.16	8.97	4.02	31.15
44605	22.08	11.34	4.81	38.23

	FUD	Status	MUE	Modifiers				IOM Reference
44604	90	A	1(2)	51	N/A	62*	80	None
44605	90	A	1(2)	51	N/A	62*	80	

* with documentation

44615

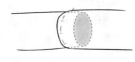

44615 Intestinal stricturoplasty (enterotomy and enterorrhaphy) with or without dilation, for intestinal obstruction

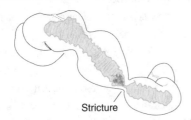

Bowel above
obstruction may
become distended

Schematic of
circular enterorrhaphy

Stricture

Depicted is large intestine segment
showing stricture and impacted waste

Explanation

The physician performs an abdominal incision to gain access to the site of an intestinal narrowing (stricture). Once identified, the intestinal stricture is incised (enterotomy) in a longitudinal manner. The physician may find it necessary or prudent to dilate the stenotic intestine to complete proper repair. The intestine is repaired or sutured. The two divided portions of the incised intestine may be reapproximated after one segment is drawn into the other (invagination) end to end (enterorrhaphy). The abdominal incision is sutured or stapled closed.

Coding Tips

For suture of the small intestine (enterorrhaphy) for perforated ulcer, diverticulum, wound, injury, or rupture, see 44602–44603.

ICD-10-CM Diagnostic Codes

K50.012	Crohn's disease of small intestine with intestinal obstruction
K50.112	Crohn's disease of large intestine with intestinal obstruction
K50.812	Crohn's disease of both small and large intestine with intestinal obstruction
K51.012	Ulcerative (chronic) pancolitis with intestinal obstruction
K51.212	Ulcerative (chronic) proctitis with intestinal obstruction
K51.312	Ulcerative (chronic) rectosigmoiditis with intestinal obstruction
K51.412	Inflammatory polyps of colon with intestinal obstruction
K51.512	Left sided colitis with intestinal obstruction
K51.812	Other ulcerative colitis with intestinal obstruction
K56.51	Intestinal adhesions [bands], with partial obstruction
K56.52	Intestinal adhesions [bands] with complete obstruction
K56.690	Other partial intestinal obstruction
K56.691	Other complete intestinal obstruction
K91.2	Postsurgical malabsorption, not elsewhere classified
K91.31	Postprocedural partial intestinal obstruction
K91.32	Postprocedural complete intestinal obstruction
Q41.0	Congenital absence, atresia and stenosis of duodenum
Q41.1	Congenital absence, atresia and stenosis of jejunum
Q41.2	Congenital absence, atresia and stenosis of ileum
Q41.8	Congenital absence, atresia and stenosis of other specified parts of small intestine
Q42.0	Congenital absence, atresia and stenosis of rectum with fistula
Q42.1	Congenital absence, atresia and stenosis of rectum without fistula
Q42.2	Congenital absence, atresia and stenosis of anus with fistula
Q42.3	Congenital absence, atresia and stenosis of anus without fistula
Q42.8	Congenital absence, atresia and stenosis of other parts of large intestine
Q43.2	Other congenital functional disorders of colon

AMA: **44615** 2014,Jan,11

Relative Value Units/Medicare Edits

Non-Facility RVU	Work	PE	MP	Total
44615	18.16	9.42	3.99	31.57
Facility RVU	**Work**	**PE**	**MP**	**Total**
44615	18.16	9.42	3.99	31.57

	FUD	Status	MUE	Modifiers				IOM Reference
44615	90	A	3(3)	51	N/A	62*	80	None

* with documentation

Terms To Know

anastomosis. Surgically created connection between ducts, blood vessels, or bowel segments to allow flow from one to the other.

dilation. Artificial increase in the diameter of an opening or lumen made by medication or by instrumentation.

incision. Act of cutting into tissue or an organ.

intestinal or peritoneal adhesions with obstruction. Abnormal fibrous band growths joining separate tissues in the peritoneum or intestine, causing blockage.

stenosis. Narrowing or constriction of a passage.

stricture. Narrowing of an anatomical structure.

suture. Numerous stitching techniques employed in wound closure.

buried suture. Continuous or interrupted suture placed under the skin for a layered closure.

continuous suture. Running stitch with tension evenly distributed across a single strand to provide a leakproof closure line.

interrupted suture. Series of single stitches with tension isolated at each stitch, in which all stitches are not affected if one becomes loose, and the isolated sutures cannot act as a wick to transport an infection.

purse-string suture. Continuous suture placed around a tubular structure and tightened, to reduce or close the lumen.

retention suture. Secondary stitching that bridges the primary suture, providing support for the primary repair; a plastic or rubber bolster may be placed over the primary repair and under the retention sutures.

44620-44626

44620 Closure of enterostomy, large or small intestine;
44625   with resection and anastomosis other than colorectal
44626   with resection and colorectal anastomosis (eg, closure of Hartmann type procedure)

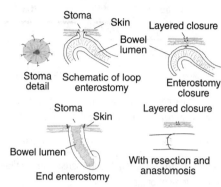

An enterostomy is closed, requiring resection of a segment of bowel and anastomosis to restore continuity

Explanation

The physician takes down and closes an enterostomy (stoma) of the small intestine or colon. The physician makes an incision around the stoma or a separate abdominal incision may be made. Next, the stoma is mobilized and taken down from the abdominal wall and the stoma is closed. The abdominal incisions are closed. In 44625, the stoma is resected and anastomosis, other than colorectal, is completed. Report 44626 for both resection of the intestine and a colorectal anastomosis, or a reconnection of the colon and rectum.

Coding Tips

For enterectomy, resection of small intestine, single resection and anastomosis, see 44120; each additional resection and anastomosis, see 44121; with enterostomy, see 44125. For laparoscopic closure of enterostomy, large or small intestine with resection and anastomosis, see 44227. For placement of an enterostomy or cecostomy tube (e.g., for decompression or feeding), see 44300.

ICD-10-CM Diagnostic Codes

K56.51	Intestinal adhesions [bands], with partial obstruction
K56.52	Intestinal adhesions [bands] with complete obstruction
K94.01	Colostomy hemorrhage
K94.02	Colostomy infection
K94.03	Colostomy malfunction
K94.09	Other complications of colostomy
K94.11	Enterostomy hemorrhage
K94.12	Enterostomy infection
K94.13	Enterostomy malfunction
K94.19	Other complications of enterostomy
Z43.2	Encounter for attention to ileostomy
Z43.3	Encounter for attention to colostomy
Z43.4	Encounter for attention to other artificial openings of digestive tract

AMA: **44620** 2014,Jan,11 **44625** 2014,Jan,11 **44626** 2014,Jan,11

Relative Value Units/Medicare Edits

Non-Facility RVU	Work	PE	MP	Total
44620	14.43	8.04	2.98	25.45
44625	17.28	9.06	3.35	29.69
44626	27.9	13.02	6.04	46.96
Facility RVU	Work	PE	MP	Total
44620	14.43	8.04	2.98	25.45
44625	17.28	9.06	3.35	29.69
44626	27.9	13.02	6.04	46.96

	FUD	Status	MUE	Modifiers				IOM Reference
44620	90	A	2(3)	51	N/A	62*	80	None
44625	90	A	1(3)	51	N/A	62*	80	
44626	90	A	1(3)	51	N/A	62*	80	

* with documentation

Terms To Know

anastomosis. Surgically created connection between ducts, blood vessels, or bowel segments to allow flow from one to the other.

colostomy. Artificial surgical opening anywhere along the length of the colon to the skin surface for the diversion of feces.

enterostomy. Surgically created opening into the intestine through the abdominal wall.

Hartmann procedure. The lower part of the sigmoid colon and/or the upper part of the rectum is excised. The descending colon is manipulated and sutured to the skin to create a colostomy. The proximal end of the descending colon is oversewn and a pouch is formed.

ileostomy. Artificial surgical opening that brings the end of the ileum out through the abdominal wall to the skin surface for the diversion of feces through a stoma.

resection. Surgical removal of a part or all of an organ or body part.

stoma. Opening created in the abdominal wall from an internal organ or structure for diversion of waste elimination, drainage, and access.

Intestines

44640

44640 Closure of intestinal cutaneous fistula

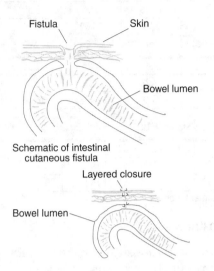

Fistula   Skin

Bowel lumen

Schematic of intestinal cutaneous fistula

Layered closure

Bowel lumen

Explanation

The physician takes down and closes an intestinal cutaneous fistula. The physician makes an abdominal incision. Next, the bowel is mobilized and the fistula is identified and taken down from the abdominal wall and skin. The segment of bowel containing the fistula is resected and the bowel ends reapproximated with staples or sutures. The abdominal wall incisions are closed.

Coding Tips

For closure of an enteroenteric or an enterocolic fistula, see 44650; enterovesical, without intestinal or bladder resection, see 44660; renocolic, see 50525–50526; gastrocolic, see 43880; rectovesical fistula, see 45800–45805.

ICD-10-CM Diagnostic Codes

K31.6	Fistula of stomach and duodenum
K50.013	Crohn's disease of small intestine with fistula
K50.113	Crohn's disease of large intestine with fistula
K50.813	Crohn's disease of both small and large intestine with fistula
K51.013	Ulcerative (chronic) pancolitis with fistula
K51.213	Ulcerative (chronic) proctitis with fistula
K51.313	Ulcerative (chronic) rectosigmoiditis with fistula
K51.413	Inflammatory polyps of colon with fistula
K51.513	Left sided colitis with fistula
K51.813	Other ulcerative colitis with fistula
K63.2	Fistula of intestine
Q43.8	Other specified congenital malformations of intestine
Q79.59	Other congenital malformations of abdominal wall
T81.83XA	Persistent postprocedural fistula, initial encounter

AMA: 44640 2014,Jan,11

Relative Value Units/Medicare Edits

Non-Facility RVU	Work	PE	MP	Total
44640	24.2	11.7	5.2	41.1
Facility RVU	**Work**	**PE**	**MP**	**Total**
44640	24.2	11.7	5.2	41.1

	FUD	Status	MUE	Modifiers				IOM Reference
44640	90	A	2(3)	51	N/A	62*	80	None

* with documentation

Terms To Know

anastomosis. Surgically created connection between ducts, blood vessels, or bowel segments to allow flow from one to the other.

anomaly. Irregularity in the structure or position of an organ or tissue.

congenital. Present at birth, occurring through heredity or an influence during gestation up to the moment of birth.

cutaneous. Relating to the skin.

duodenum. First portion of the small intestine connected to the stomach at the pylorus and extending to the jejunum.

fistula. Abnormal tube-like passage between two body cavities or organs or from an organ to the outside surface.

lumen. Space inside an intestine, artery, vein, duct, or tube.

resect. Cutting out or removing a portion or all of a bone, organ, or other structure.

skin. Outer protective covering of the body composed of the epidermis and dermis, situated above the subcutaneous tissues.

suture. Numerous stitching techniques employed in wound closure.

buried suture. Continuous or interrupted suture placed under the skin for a layered closure.

continuous suture. Running stitch with tension evenly distributed across a single strand to provide a leakproof closure line.

interrupted suture. Series of single stitches with tension isolated at each stitch, in which all stitches are not affected if one becomes loose, and the isolated sutures cannot act as a wick to transport an infection.

purse-string suture. Continuous suture placed around a tubular structure and tightened, to reduce or close the lumen.

retention suture. Secondary stitching that bridges the primary suture, providing support for the primary repair; a plastic or rubber bolster may be placed over the primary repair and under the retention sutures.

Intestines

44650

44650 Closure of enteroenteric or enterocolic fistula

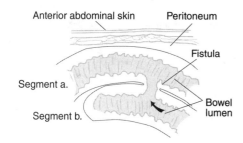

Anterior abdominal skin — Peritoneum
Fistula
Segment a.
Segment b.
Bowel lumen

Explanation

The physician closes a connection (fistula) between loops of small bowel or between the small bowel and colon. The physician makes an abdominal incision. Next, the enteroenteric or enterocolic fistula is identified and divided. The ends of the fistula may be closed with sutures or the segments of bowel involved with the fistula may be resected and the bowel ends reapproximated in order to completely remove the involved areas. The incision is closed.

Coding Tips

For closure of an intestinal cutaneous fistula, see 44640; enterovesical, without intestinal or bladder resection, see 44660; renocolic, abdominal approach, see 50525; thoracic, see 50526; gastrocolic, see 43880; rectovesical, see 45800–45805.

ICD-10-CM Diagnostic Codes

K31.6	Fistula of stomach and duodenum
K31.89	Other diseases of stomach and duodenum
K50.013	Crohn's disease of small intestine with fistula
K50.113	Crohn's disease of large intestine with fistula
K50.813	Crohn's disease of both small and large intestine with fistula
K51.013	Ulcerative (chronic) pancolitis with fistula
K51.213	Ulcerative (chronic) proctitis with fistula
K51.313	Ulcerative (chronic) rectosigmoiditis with fistula
K51.413	Inflammatory polyps of colon with fistula
K51.513	Left sided colitis with fistula
K51.813	Other ulcerative colitis with fistula
K63.2	Fistula of intestine
Q43.8	Other specified congenital malformations of intestine
Q79.59	Other congenital malformations of abdominal wall
T81.83XA	Persistent postprocedural fistula, initial encounter

AMA: **44650** 2014,Jan,11

Relative Value Units/Medicare Edits

Non-Facility RVU	Work	PE	MP	Total
44650	25.12	11.94	5.29	42.35
Facility RVU	**Work**	**PE**	**MP**	**Total**
44650	25.12	11.94	5.29	42.35

	FUD	Status	MUE	Modifiers				IOM Reference
44650	90	A	2(3)	51	N/A	62*	80	None

* with documentation

44660-44661

44660 Closure of enterovesical fistula; without intestinal or bladder resection
44661 with intestine and/or bladder resection

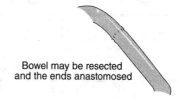

Bowel may be resected
and the ends anastomosed

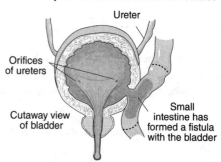

Bladder may be resected and closed with sutures

Ureter
Orifices of ureters
Cutaway view of bladder
Small intestine has formed a fistula with the bladder

An enterovesical fistula (communication between bowel and bladder) is repaired

Explanation

The physician closes a connection between the small bowel and bladder (enterovesical fistula). The physician makes an abdominal incision. Next, the enterovesical fistula is identified and divided. The ends of the fistula are closed with sutures. In 44661, the connection of the fistula to the bladder is resected and the bladder is closed with sutures; the segment of intestine containing the fistula is resected and the ends are reapproximated. The incision is closed.

Coding Tips

For closure of an intestinal cutaneous fistula, see 44640; enteroenteric or an enterocolic, see 44650; renocolic, abdominal approach, see 50525; thoracic approach, see 50526; gastrocolic, see 43880; rectovesical, see 45800–45805.

ICD-10-CM Diagnostic Codes

K38.3	Fistula of appendix
N32.1	Vesicointestinal fistula
N32.2	Vesical fistula, not elsewhere classified
N49.8	Inflammatory disorders of other specified male genital organs ♂
Q64.73	Congenital urethrorectal fistula
Q64.79	Other congenital malformations of bladder and urethra
Q64.8	Other specified congenital malformations of urinary system
T81.83XA	Persistent postprocedural fistula, initial encounter

AMA: **44660** 2014,Jan,11 **44661** 2014,Jan,11

Relative Value Units/Medicare Edits

Non-Facility RVU	Work	PE	MP	Total
44660	23.91	11.07	4.2	39.18
44661	27.35	12.61	5.51	45.47
Facility RVU	Work	PE	MP	Total
44660	23.91	11.07	4.2	39.18
44661	27.35	12.61	5.51	45.47

	FUD	Status	MUE	Modifiers				IOM Reference
44660	90	A	1(3)	51	N/A	62*	80	None
44661	90	A	1(3)	51	N/A	62*	80	

* with documentation

Terms To Know

congenital anomaly. Abnormality that is present at birth that may be the result of genetic factors, teratogens, or other conditions that affect the fetus in utero. The abnormalities may be readily apparent at birth or may remain undiscovered until some point after birth.

enterovesical fistula. Abnormal communication between the small intestine and the bladder.

fistula. Abnormal tube-like passage between two body cavities or organs or from an organ to the outside surface.

regional enteritis. Chronic inflammation of unknown origin affecting the ileum and/or colon.

resection. Surgical removal of a part or all of an organ or body part.

vesico-. Relating to the bladder.

44680

44680   Intestinal plication (separate procedure)

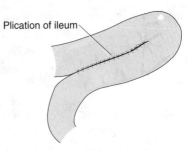

Plication of ileum

A segment of intestine is plicated or folded upon itself and held with sutures

Explanation

The physician folds the intestine upon itself and attaches the edges with sutures for anchoring purposes. The physician makes an abdominal incision. Next, the bowel is folded upon itself and the edges are plicated with sutures without making an anastomosis to anchor the bowel in place. The incision is closed.

Coding Tips

This separate procedure by definition is usually a component of a more complex service and is not identified separately. When performed alone or with other unrelated procedures/services it may be reported. If performed alone, list the code; if performed with other procedures/services, list the code and append modifier 59 or an X{EPSU} modifier.

ICD-10-CM Diagnostic Codes

K56.1	Intussusception
K56.2	Volvulus
K56.49	Other impaction of intestine
K56.51	Intestinal adhesions [bands], with partial obstruction
K56.52	Intestinal adhesions [bands] with complete obstruction
K56.690	Other partial intestinal obstruction
K56.691	Other complete intestinal obstruction
K91.2	Postsurgical malabsorption, not elsewhere classified
K91.31	Postprocedural partial intestinal obstruction
K91.32	Postprocedural complete intestinal obstruction
Q41.0	Congenital absence, atresia and stenosis of duodenum
Q41.1	Congenital absence, atresia and stenosis of jejunum
Q41.2	Congenital absence, atresia and stenosis of ileum
Q41.8	Congenital absence, atresia and stenosis of other specified parts of small intestine
Q42.0	Congenital absence, atresia and stenosis of rectum with fistula
Q42.1	Congenital absence, atresia and stenosis of rectum without fistula
Q42.2	Congenital absence, atresia and stenosis of anus with fistula
Q42.3	Congenital absence, atresia and stenosis of anus without fistula
Q42.8	Congenital absence, atresia and stenosis of other parts of large intestine
Q43.8	Other specified congenital malformations of intestine
Q45.8	Other specified congenital malformations of digestive system

AMA: 44680 2014,Jan,11

Relative Value Units/Medicare Edits

Non-Facility RVU	Work	PE	MP	Total
44680	17.96	9.54	4.39	31.89
Facility RVU	Work	PE	MP	Total
44680	17.96	9.54	4.39	31.89

	FUD	Status	MUE	Modifiers				IOM Reference
44680	90	A	1(3)	51	N/A	62*	80	None

* with documentation

Terms To Know

anastomosis. Surgically created connection between ducts, blood vessels, or bowel segments to allow flow from one to the other.

closure. Repairing an incision or wound by suture or other means.

complication. Condition arising after the beginning of observation and treatment that modifies the course of the patient's illness or the medical care required, or an undesired result or misadventure in medical care.

congenital. Present at birth, occurring through heredity or an influence during gestation up to the moment of birth.

ileum. Lower portion of the small intestine, from the jejunum to the cecum.

incision. Act of cutting into tissue or an organ.

intestinal or peritoneal adhesions with obstruction. Abnormal fibrous band growths joining separate tissues in the peritoneum or intestine, causing blockage.

intussusception. Prolapse of one section of intestine into the lumen of an adjacent section of the bowel. This condition, which occurs mainly in children, causes pain, vomiting, and mucous passed from the rectum and requires surgical intervention.

obstruction. Blockage that prevents normal function of the valve or structure.

plication. Surgical technique involving folding, tucking, or pleating to reduce the size of a hollow structure or organ.

stenosis. Narrowing or constriction of a passage.

volvulus. Twisting, knotting, or entanglement of the bowel on itself that may quickly compromise oxygen supply to the intestinal tissues. A volvulus usually occurs at the sigmoid and ileocecal areas of the intestines.

44700

44700   Exclusion of small intestine from pelvis by mesh or other prosthesis, or native tissue (eg, bladder or omentum)

The small bowel is surgically excluded from the pelvis

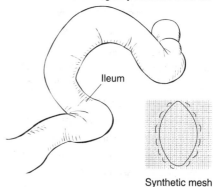

Ileum

Synthetic mesh

Explanation

Prior to implementing radiation therapy, the physician uses mesh, other prosthesis, or native tissue (bladder or omentum) to lift and fix the small intestine away from the site of radiation therapy. An abdominal incision is made. If mesh or other prosthetic material is used, it is sutured into place. If native tissue is used, a sling is fashioned and sutured into place. The incision is sutured closed.

Coding Tips

This procedure is performed on patients with malignant neoplasms of pelvic organs and is used to move healthy bowel from the radiation site so that it will not be damaged by radiation therapy. For therapeutic radiation clinical treatment, see the Radiation Oncology section of the CPT book.

ICD-10-CM Diagnostic Codes

C16.0	Malignant neoplasm of cardia
C16.1	Malignant neoplasm of fundus of stomach
C16.2	Malignant neoplasm of body of stomach
C16.3	Malignant neoplasm of pyloric antrum
C16.4	Malignant neoplasm of pylorus
C17.3	Meckel's diverticulum, malignant
C18.0	Malignant neoplasm of cecum
C18.1	Malignant neoplasm of appendix
C18.2	Malignant neoplasm of ascending colon
C18.3	Malignant neoplasm of hepatic flexure
C18.4	Malignant neoplasm of transverse colon
C18.5	Malignant neoplasm of splenic flexure
C18.6	Malignant neoplasm of descending colon
C18.7	Malignant neoplasm of sigmoid colon
C20	Malignant neoplasm of rectum
C21.1	Malignant neoplasm of anal canal
C21.2	Malignant neoplasm of cloacogenic zone
C48.1	Malignant neoplasm of specified parts of peritoneum
C51.0	Malignant neoplasm of labium majus ♀
C51.1	Malignant neoplasm of labium minus ♀
C51.2	Malignant neoplasm of clitoris ♀
C52	Malignant neoplasm of vagina ♀

C53.0	Malignant neoplasm of endocervix ♀	
C53.1	Malignant neoplasm of exocervix ♀	
C54.0	Malignant neoplasm of isthmus uteri ♀	
C54.1	Malignant neoplasm of endometrium ♀	
C54.2	Malignant neoplasm of myometrium ♀	
C54.3	Malignant neoplasm of fundus uteri ♀	
C56.1	Malignant neoplasm of right ovary ♀ ☑	
C56.2	Malignant neoplasm of left ovary ♀ ☑	
C56.3	Malignant neoplasm of bilateral ovaries ♀ ☑	
C57.01	Malignant neoplasm of right fallopian tube ♀ ☑	
C57.02	Malignant neoplasm of left fallopian tube ♀ ☑	
C57.11	Malignant neoplasm of right broad ligament ♀ ☑	
C57.12	Malignant neoplasm of left broad ligament ♀ ☑	
C57.21	Malignant neoplasm of right round ligament ♀ ☑	
C57.22	Malignant neoplasm of left round ligament ♀ ☑	
C57.3	Malignant neoplasm of parametrium ♀	
C57.7	Malignant neoplasm of other specified female genital organs ♀	
C57.8	Malignant neoplasm of overlapping sites of female genital organs ♀	
C61	Malignant neoplasm of prostate ♂	
C64.1	Malignant neoplasm of right kidney, except renal pelvis ☑	
C64.2	Malignant neoplasm of left kidney, except renal pelvis ☑	
C65.1	Malignant neoplasm of right renal pelvis ☑	
C65.2	Malignant neoplasm of left renal pelvis ☑	
C66.1	Malignant neoplasm of right ureter ☑	
C66.2	Malignant neoplasm of left ureter ☑	
C67.0	Malignant neoplasm of trigone of bladder	
C67.1	Malignant neoplasm of dome of bladder	
C67.2	Malignant neoplasm of lateral wall of bladder	
C67.3	Malignant neoplasm of anterior wall of bladder	
C67.4	Malignant neoplasm of posterior wall of bladder	
C67.5	Malignant neoplasm of bladder neck	
C67.6	Malignant neoplasm of ureteric orifice	
C67.7	Malignant neoplasm of urachus	
C68.0	Malignant neoplasm of urethra	
C68.1	Malignant neoplasm of paraurethral glands	
C78.5	Secondary malignant neoplasm of large intestine and rectum	
C78.6	Secondary malignant neoplasm of retroperitoneum and peritoneum	
C79.01	Secondary malignant neoplasm of right kidney and renal pelvis ☑	
C79.02	Secondary malignant neoplasm of left kidney and renal pelvis ☑	
C79.11	Secondary malignant neoplasm of bladder	
C79.61	Secondary malignant neoplasm of right ovary ♀ ☑	
C79.62	Secondary malignant neoplasm of left ovary ♀ ☑	
C79.63	Secondary malignant neoplasm of bilateral ovaries ♀ ☑	
C7A.020	Malignant carcinoid tumor of the appendix	
C7A.021	Malignant carcinoid tumor of the cecum	
C7A.022	Malignant carcinoid tumor of the ascending colon	
C7A.023	Malignant carcinoid tumor of the transverse colon	
C7A.024	Malignant carcinoid tumor of the descending colon	
C7A.025	Malignant carcinoid tumor of the sigmoid colon	
C7A.026	Malignant carcinoid tumor of the rectum	

C7A.092	Malignant carcinoid tumor of the stomach
C7B.04	Secondary carcinoid tumors of peritoneum
C81.06	Nodular lymphocyte predominant Hodgkin lymphoma, intrapelvic lymph nodes
C81.46	Lymphocyte-rich Hodgkin lymphoma, intrapelvic lymph nodes
C82.56	Diffuse follicle center lymphoma, intrapelvic lymph nodes
C84.Z6	Other mature T/NK-cell lymphomas, intrapelvic lymph nodes
C85.26	Mediastinal (thymic) large B-cell lymphoma, intrapelvic lymph nodes
C85.86	Other specified types of non-Hodgkin lymphoma, intrapelvic lymph nodes

AMA: 44700 2014,Jan,11

Relative Value Units/Medicare Edits

Non-Facility RVU	Work	PE	MP	Total
44700	17.48	8.91	2.86	29.25
Facility RVU	**Work**	**PE**	**MP**	**Total**
44700	17.48	8.91	2.86	29.25

	FUD	Status	MUE	Modifiers				IOM Reference
44700	90	A	1(2)	51	N/A	62*	80	None

* with documentation

Terms To Know

carcinoid tumor. Specific type of slow-growing neuroendocrine tumors. Carcinoid tumors occur most commonly in the hormone producing cells of the gastrointestinal tracts and can also occur in the pancreas, testes, ovaries, or lungs.

cautery. Destruction or burning of tissue by means of a hot instrument, an electric current, or a caustic chemical, such as silver nitrate.

lesion. Area of damaged tissue that has lost continuity or function, due to disease or trauma. Lesions may be located on internal structures such as the brain, nerves, or kidneys, or visible on the skin.

malignant neoplasm. Any cancerous tumor or lesion exhibiting uncontrolled tissue growth that can progressively invade other parts of the body with its disease-generating cells.

mesh. Synthetic fabric used as a prosthetic patch in hernia repair.

omentum. Fold of peritoneal tissue suspended between the stomach and neighboring visceral organs of the abdominal cavity.

prosthesis. Device that replaces all or part of an internal body organ or replaces all or part of the function of a permanently inoperative or malfunctioning internal body organ.

44701

| + | **44701** | Intraoperative colonic lavage (List separately in addition to code for primary procedure) |

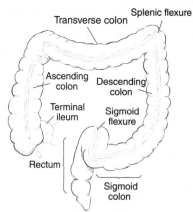

In the course of an operative session the colon is lavaged or irrigated

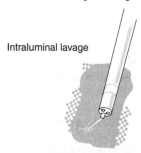

Intraluminal lavage

Explanation

The patient's colon is flushed during a surgical procedure. A Foley catheter is inserted into the cecum through which the irrigation is performed. A noncrushing bowel clamp is placed across the terminal ilium to prevent the lavage fluid from flowing into the small intestine. An intravenous infusion set is connected to the catheter and a clear, corrugated scavenger tube is inserted in the distal bowel and secured in place. A closed irrigation system is created by securing a large bag to the free end of the tube, draped over the patient to the side. The colon is lavaged with warm, isotonic saline solution for 15 to 30 minutes until the flow through the tube is seen to be clear.

Coding Tips

Report 44701 in addition to 44140, 44145, 44150, or 44604. Do not report 44701 when reporting 44300 or 44950–44960.

ICD-10-CM Diagnostic Codes

This/these CPT code(s) are add-on code(s). See the primary procedure code that this code is performed with for your ICD-10-CM code selections.

AMA: **44701** 2014,Jan,11

Relative Value Units/Medicare Edits

Non-Facility RVU	Work	PE	MP	Total
44701	3.1	1.15	0.74	4.99
Facility RVU	**Work**	**PE**	**MP**	**Total**
44701	3.1	1.15	0.74	4.99

	FUD	Status	MUE	Modifiers				IOM Reference
44701	N/A	A	1(2)	N/A	N/A	62*	80	None

* with documentation

Terms To Know

clamp. Tool used to grip, compress, join, or fasten body parts.

distal. Located farther away from a specified reference point or the trunk.

Foley catheter. Temporary indwelling urethral catheter held in place in the bladder by an inflated balloon containing fluid or air.

ileum. Lower portion of the small intestine, from the jejunum to the cecum.

infusion. Introduction of a therapeutic fluid, other than blood, into the bloodstream.

intra. Within.

intravenous. Within a vein or veins.

irrigation. To wash out or cleanse a body cavity, wound, or tissue with water or other fluid.

lavage. Washing.

lumen. Space inside an intestine, artery, vein, duct, or tube.

small intestine. First portion of intestine connecting to the pylorus at the proximal end and consisting of the duodenum, jejunum, and ileum.

tube. Long, hollow cylindrical instrument or body structure.

44705

44705 Preparation of fecal microbiota for instillation, including assessment of donor specimen

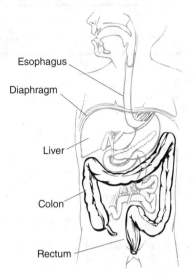

Esophagus

Diaphragm

Liver

Colon

Rectum

Microbiota is instilled in the digestive tract

Intestines

Explanation

Fecal microbiota transplantation (FMT) is the process of instilling fecal matter from a donor to a patient to treat a Clostridium difficile (C. diff) infection, most commonly. The donor stool is thinned using a normal saline solution and filtered for use in a nasogastric tube or an enema application. This code includes the screening protocol of the donor specimen for C. diff and other enteric bacterial pathogens and any ova or parasites.

Coding Tips

Do not report 44705 with 74283. For fecal instillation via enema or oro- or nasogastric tube, see 44799. Medicare and some other payers may require G0455 be reported for this service.

ICD-10-CM Diagnostic Codes

A04.71	Enterocolitis due to Clostridium difficile, recurrent
A04.72	Enterocolitis due to Clostridium difficile, not specified as recurrent
K50.011	Crohn's disease of small intestine with rectal bleeding
K50.012	Crohn's disease of small intestine with intestinal obstruction
K50.013	Crohn's disease of small intestine with fistula
K50.014	Crohn's disease of small intestine with abscess
K50.018	Crohn's disease of small intestine with other complication
K50.111	Crohn's disease of large intestine with rectal bleeding
K50.112	Crohn's disease of large intestine with intestinal obstruction
K50.113	Crohn's disease of large intestine with fistula
K50.114	Crohn's disease of large intestine with abscess
K50.118	Crohn's disease of large intestine with other complication
K51.00	Ulcerative (chronic) pancolitis without complications
K51.011	Ulcerative (chronic) pancolitis with rectal bleeding
K51.012	Ulcerative (chronic) pancolitis with intestinal obstruction
K51.013	Ulcerative (chronic) pancolitis with fistula
K51.014	Ulcerative (chronic) pancolitis with abscess
K51.018	Ulcerative (chronic) pancolitis with other complication
K51.80	Other ulcerative colitis without complications
K51.811	Other ulcerative colitis with rectal bleeding
K51.812	Other ulcerative colitis with intestinal obstruction
K51.813	Other ulcerative colitis with fistula
K51.814	Other ulcerative colitis with abscess
K51.818	Other ulcerative colitis with other complication
K55.021	Focal (segmental) acute infarction of small intestine
K55.022	Diffuse acute infarction of small intestine
K55.031	Focal (segmental) acute (reversible) ischemia of large intestine
K55.032	Diffuse acute (reversible) ischemia of large intestine
K55.041	Focal (segmental) acute infarction of large intestine
K55.042	Diffuse acute infarction of large intestine
K58.0	Irritable bowel syndrome with diarrhea
K58.1	Irritable bowel syndrome with constipation
K58.2	Mixed irritable bowel syndrome
K58.8	Other irritable bowel syndrome
K59.01	Slow transit constipation
K59.02	Outlet dysfunction constipation
K59.03	Drug induced constipation
K59.04	Chronic idiopathic constipation
K59.09	Other constipation

Associated HCPCS Codes

G0455	Preparation with instillation of fecal microbiota by any method, including assessment of donor specimen

AMA: **44705** 2018,Jan,8; 2017,Jan,8; 2016,Jan,13; 2015,Jan,16

Relative Value Units/Medicare Edits

Non-Facility RVU	Work	PE	MP	Total
44705	1.42	1.72	0.13	3.27
Facility RVU	**Work**	**PE**	**MP**	**Total**
44705	1.42	0.55	0.13	2.1

	FUD	Status	MUE	Modifiers				IOM Reference
44705	N/A	I	1(3)	N/A	N/A	N/A	N/A	None

* with documentation

Terms To Know

colitis. Inflammation of the colon, caused by an infection or external influences such as laxatives, radiation, or antibiotics.

instillation. Administering a liquid slowly over time, drop by drop.

nasogastric tube. Long, hollow, cylindrical catheter made of soft rubber or plastic that is inserted through the nose down into the stomach, and is used for feeding, instilling medication, or withdrawing gastric contents.

44715

44715 Backbench standard preparation of cadaver or living donor intestine allograft prior to transplantation, including mobilization and fashioning of the superior mesenteric artery and vein

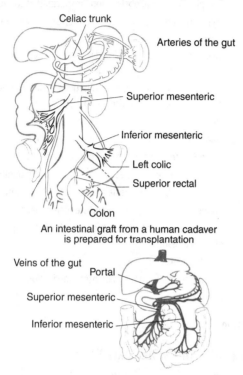

An intestinal graft from a human cadaver is prepared for transplantation

Explanation

The physician performs a standard backbench preparation of an intestine allograft requiring mobilizing and fashioning of the superior mesenteric artery and vein. Backbench or back table preparation refers to procedures performed on the intestine allograft to prepare the allograft for transplant. Removal of the small intestine graft requires careful dissection of the superior mesenteric artery (SMA) and superior mesenteric vein (SMV). Backbench or back table preparation of the SMA or SMV is required when the pedicles are too short. When a cadaver donor is used, the SMA and/or SMV are lengthened using free vascular grafts from the iliac or carotid arteries and veins that were procured from the cadaver. The physician performs the grafting procedure prior to transplantation of the intestine allograft.

Coding Tips

For backbench reconstruction of a cadaver or living donor intestine allograft prior to transplantation, venous anastomosis, see 44720; arterial anastomosis, see 44721.

ICD-10-CM Diagnostic Codes

C17.0	Malignant neoplasm of duodenum
C17.1	Malignant neoplasm of jejunum
C17.2	Malignant neoplasm of ileum
C17.3	Meckel's diverticulum, malignant
C17.8	Malignant neoplasm of overlapping sites of small intestine
C7A.010	Malignant carcinoid tumor of the duodenum
C7A.011	Malignant carcinoid tumor of the jejunum
C7A.012	Malignant carcinoid tumor of the ileum
K31.5	Obstruction of duodenum
K31.6	Fistula of stomach and duodenum
K50.012	Crohn's disease of small intestine with intestinal obstruction
K50.013	Crohn's disease of small intestine with fistula
K50.014	Crohn's disease of small intestine with abscess
K50.112	Crohn's disease of large intestine with intestinal obstruction
K50.812	Crohn's disease of both small and large intestine with intestinal obstruction
K50.813	Crohn's disease of both small and large intestine with fistula
K50.814	Crohn's disease of both small and large intestine with abscess
K51.012	Ulcerative (chronic) pancolitis with intestinal obstruction
K51.212	Ulcerative (chronic) proctitis with intestinal obstruction
K51.312	Ulcerative (chronic) rectosigmoiditis with intestinal obstruction
K55.061	Focal (segmental) acute infarction of intestine, part unspecified
K55.062	Diffuse acute infarction of intestine, part unspecified
K55.1	Chronic vascular disorders of intestine
K56.2	Volvulus
K56.601	Complete intestinal obstruction, unspecified as to cause
K57.01	Diverticulitis of small intestine with perforation and abscess with bleeding
K57.40	Diverticulitis of both small and large intestine with perforation and abscess without bleeding
K57.51	Diverticulosis of both small and large intestine without perforation or abscess with bleeding
P77.1	Stage 1 necrotizing enterocolitis in newborn **N**
P77.2	Stage 2 necrotizing enterocolitis in newborn **N**
P77.3	Stage 3 necrotizing enterocolitis in newborn **N**
Q41.0	Congenital absence, atresia and stenosis of duodenum
Q41.1	Congenital absence, atresia and stenosis of jejunum
Q41.2	Congenital absence, atresia and stenosis of ileum
Q41.8	Congenital absence, atresia and stenosis of other specified parts of small intestine
Q43.1	Hirschsprung's disease
Q43.3	Congenital malformations of intestinal fixation
Q79.3	Gastroschisis

AMA: 44715 2014,Jan,11

Relative Value Units/Medicare Edits

Non-Facility RVU	Work	PE	MP	Total
44715	0.0	0.0	0.0	0.0
Facility RVU	**Work**	**PE**	**MP**	**Total**
44715	0.0	0.0	0.0	0.0

	FUD	Status	MUE	Modifiers				IOM Reference
44715	N/A	C	1(2)	51	N/A	62*	80	None

* with documentation

Intestines

44720

44720 Backbench reconstruction of cadaver or living donor intestine allograft prior to transplantation; venous anastomosis, each

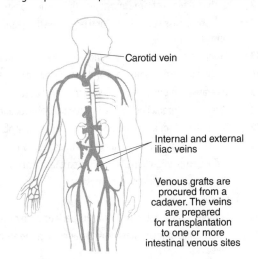

Carotid vein

Internal and external iliac veins

Venous grafts are procured from a cadaver. The veins are prepared for transplantation to one or more intestinal venous sites

Explanation

The physician performs a backbench preparation of an intestine allograft requiring venous anastomosis. Backbench or back table preparation refers to procedures performed on the intestine allograft to prepare the allograft for transplant. The physician procures venous grafts from the iliac or carotid veins of the cadaver. The physician applies the venous grafts to one or more venous sites on the intestine. Report 44720 for each venous anastomosis.

Coding Tips

For backbench standard preparation of a cadaver or living donor intestine allograft prior to transplantation, superior mesenteric artery and vein, see 44715. For backbench reconstruction of a cadaver or living donor intestine allograft prior to transplantation, arterial anastomosis, see 44721.

ICD-10-CM Diagnostic Codes

C17.0	Malignant neoplasm of duodenum
C17.1	Malignant neoplasm of jejunum
C17.2	Malignant neoplasm of ileum
C17.3	Meckel's diverticulum, malignant
C17.8	Malignant neoplasm of overlapping sites of small intestine
C7A.010	Malignant carcinoid tumor of the duodenum
C7A.011	Malignant carcinoid tumor of the jejunum
C7A.012	Malignant carcinoid tumor of the ileum
K31.5	Obstruction of duodenum
K31.6	Fistula of stomach and duodenum
K50.012	Crohn's disease of small intestine with intestinal obstruction
K50.013	Crohn's disease of small intestine with fistula
K50.014	Crohn's disease of small intestine with abscess
K50.112	Crohn's disease of large intestine with intestinal obstruction
K50.812	Crohn's disease of both small and large intestine with intestinal obstruction
K50.813	Crohn's disease of both small and large intestine with fistula
K50.814	Crohn's disease of both small and large intestine with abscess
K51.012	Ulcerative (chronic) pancolitis with intestinal obstruction
K51.212	Ulcerative (chronic) proctitis with intestinal obstruction
K51.312	Ulcerative (chronic) rectosigmoiditis with intestinal obstruction
K55.061	Focal (segmental) acute infarction of intestine, part unspecified
K55.062	Diffuse acute infarction of intestine, part unspecified
K55.1	Chronic vascular disorders of intestine
K56.2	Volvulus
K56.601	Complete intestinal obstruction, unspecified as to cause
K57.01	Diverticulitis of small intestine with perforation and abscess with bleeding
K57.40	Diverticulitis of both small and large intestine with perforation and abscess without bleeding
K57.51	Diverticulosis of both small and large intestine without perforation or abscess with bleeding
P77.1	Stage 1 necrotizing enterocolitis in newborn N
P77.2	Stage 2 necrotizing enterocolitis in newborn N
P77.3	Stage 3 necrotizing enterocolitis in newborn N
Q41.0	Congenital absence, atresia and stenosis of duodenum
Q41.1	Congenital absence, atresia and stenosis of jejunum
Q41.2	Congenital absence, atresia and stenosis of ileum
Q41.8	Congenital absence, atresia and stenosis of other specified parts of small intestine
Q43.1	Hirschsprung's disease
Q43.3	Congenital malformations of intestinal fixation
Q79.3	Gastroschisis

AMA: 44720 2014,Jan,11

Relative Value Units/Medicare Edits

Non-Facility RVU	Work	PE	MP	Total
44720	5.0	1.85	1.24	8.09
Facility RVU	**Work**	**PE**	**MP**	**Total**
44720	5.0	1.85	1.24	8.09

	FUD	Status	MUE	Modifiers				IOM Reference
44720	N/A	A	2(3)	51	N/A	62*	80	None

* with documentation

44721

44721 Backbench reconstruction of cadaver or living donor intestine allograft prior to transplantation; arterial anastomosis, each

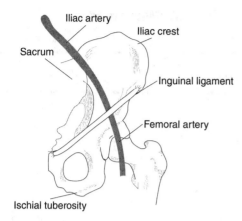

Iliac artery
Iliac crest
Sacrum
Inguinal ligament
Femoral artery
Ischial tuberosity

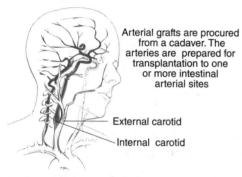

Arterial grafts are procured from a cadaver. The arteries are prepared for transplantation to one or more intestinal arterial sites

External carotid
Internal carotid

Explanation

The physician performs a backbench preparation of an intestine allograft requiring arterial anastomosis. Backbench or back table preparation refers to procedures performed on the intestine allograft to prepare the allograft for transplant. The physician procures arterial grafts from the iliac or carotid arteries of the cadaver. The physician applies the arterial grafts to one or more arterial sites on the intestine. Report 44721 for each arterial anastomosis.

Coding Tips

For backbench standard preparation of a cadaver or living donor intestine allograft prior to transplantation, superior mesenteric artery and vein, see 44715. For backbench reconstruction of a cadaver or living donor intestine allograft prior to transplantation, venous anastomosis, see 44720.

ICD-10-CM Diagnostic Codes

C17.0	Malignant neoplasm of duodenum
C17.1	Malignant neoplasm of jejunum
C17.2	Malignant neoplasm of ileum
C17.3	Meckel's diverticulum, malignant
C17.8	Malignant neoplasm of overlapping sites of small intestine
C7A.010	Malignant carcinoid tumor of the duodenum
C7A.011	Malignant carcinoid tumor of the jejunum
C7A.012	Malignant carcinoid tumor of the ileum
K31.5	Obstruction of duodenum
K31.6	Fistula of stomach and duodenum
K50.012	Crohn's disease of small intestine with intestinal obstruction
K50.013	Crohn's disease of small intestine with fistula
K50.014	Crohn's disease of small intestine with abscess
K50.112	Crohn's disease of large intestine with intestinal obstruction
K50.812	Crohn's disease of both small and large intestine with intestinal obstruction
K50.813	Crohn's disease of both small and large intestine with fistula
K50.814	Crohn's disease of both small and large intestine with abscess
K51.012	Ulcerative (chronic) pancolitis with intestinal obstruction
K51.212	Ulcerative (chronic) proctitis with intestinal obstruction
K51.312	Ulcerative (chronic) rectosigmoiditis with intestinal obstruction
K55.061	Focal (segmental) acute infarction of intestine, part unspecified
K55.062	Diffuse acute infarction of intestine, part unspecified
K55.1	Chronic vascular disorders of intestine
K56.2	Volvulus
K56.601	Complete intestinal obstruction, unspecified as to cause
K57.01	Diverticulitis of small intestine with perforation and abscess with bleeding
K57.40	Diverticulitis of both small and large intestine with perforation and abscess without bleeding
K57.51	Diverticulosis of both small and large intestine without perforation or abscess with bleeding
P77.1	Stage 1 necrotizing enterocolitis in newborn **N**
P77.2	Stage 2 necrotizing enterocolitis in newborn **N**
P77.3	Stage 3 necrotizing enterocolitis in newborn **N**
Q41.0	Congenital absence, atresia and stenosis of duodenum
Q41.1	Congenital absence, atresia and stenosis of jejunum
Q41.2	Congenital absence, atresia and stenosis of ileum
Q41.8	Congenital absence, atresia and stenosis of other specified parts of small intestine
Q43.1	Hirschsprung's disease
Q43.3	Congenital malformations of intestinal fixation
Q79.3	Gastroschisis

AMA: **44721** 2018,Jan,8; 2017,Jan,8; 2016,Jan,13; 2015,Jan,16

Relative Value Units/Medicare Edits

Non-Facility RVU	Work	PE	MP	Total
44721	7.0	2.59	1.72	11.31
Facility RVU	**Work**	**PE**	**MP**	**Total**
44721	7.0	2.59	1.72	11.31

	FUD	Status	MUE	Modifiers				IOM Reference
44721	N/A	A	2(3)	51	N/A	62*	80	None

* with documentation

Terms To Know

allograft. Graft from one individual to another of the same species.

anastomosis. Surgically created connection between ducts, blood vessels, or bowel segments to allow flow from one to the other.

cadaver. Dead body.

donor. Person from whom tissues or organs are removed for transplantation.

44800

44800 Excision of Meckel's diverticulum (diverticulectomy) or omphalomesenteric duct

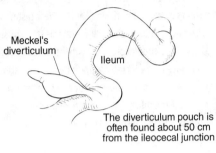

Meckel's diverticulum

Ileum

The diverticulum pouch is often found about 50 cm from the ileocecal junction

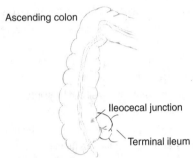

Ascending colon

Ileocecal junction

Terminal ileum

Meckel's diverticulum is a common condition, occurring in about 3 percent of people

Explanation

The physician excises a Meckel's diverticulum or an omphalomesenteric duct. The physician makes an abdominal incision. Next, the Meckel's diverticulum in the terminal ileum or the omphalomesenteric duct connecting the terminal ileum to the umbilicus is identified. The Meckel's diverticulum or omphalomesenteric duct is excised and the defect in the ileum is closed with sutures or staples or the segment of ileum may be excised and reapproximated. The incision is closed.

Coding Tips

For excision of a lesion of the mesentery, see 44820. For suture of the mesentery, see 44850. For suture of a small intestine (enterorrhaphy) for perforated ulcer, diverticulum, wound, injury, or rupture, single perforation, see 44602; for multiple perforations, see 44603. For suture of the large intestine (colorrhaphy) for perforated ulcer, diverticulum, wound, injury, or rupture, single or multiple perforations, without colostomy, see 44604; with colostomy, see 44605. For enterectomy, resection of the small intestine, single resection and anastomosis, see 44120; for each additional resection and anastomosis, see 44121; with enterostomy, see 44125.

ICD-10-CM Diagnostic Codes

C17.3	Meckel's diverticulum, malignant
C78.4	Secondary malignant neoplasm of small intestine
D01.49	Carcinoma in situ of other parts of intestine
D13.39	Benign neoplasm of other parts of small intestine
D37.2	Neoplasm of uncertain behavior of small intestine
K56.51	Intestinal adhesions [bands], with partial obstruction
K56.52	Intestinal adhesions [bands] with complete obstruction
K56.690	Other partial intestinal obstruction
K56.691	Other complete intestinal obstruction
K91.31	Postprocedural partial intestinal obstruction
K91.32	Postprocedural complete intestinal obstruction
Q43.0	Meckel's diverticulum (displaced) (hypertrophic)
Q43.8	Other specified congenital malformations of intestine

AMA: **44800** 2014,Jan,11

Relative Value Units/Medicare Edits

Non-Facility RVU	Work	PE	MP	Total
44800	12.05	8.05	2.69	22.79
Facility RVU	**Work**	**PE**	**MP**	**Total**
44800	12.05	8.05	2.69	22.79

	FUD	Status	MUE	Modifiers				IOM Reference
44800	90	A	1(3)	51	N/A	62*	80	None

* with documentation

Terms To Know

closure. Repairing an incision or wound by suture or other means.

defect. Imperfection, flaw, or absence.

excision. Surgical removal of an organ or tissue.

ileum. Lower portion of the small intestine, from the jejunum to the cecum.

incision. Act of cutting into tissue or an organ.

malignant. Any condition tending to progress toward death, specifically an invasive tumor with a loss of cellular differentiation that has the ability to spread or metastasize to other body areas.

Meckel's diverticulum. Congenital, abnormal remnant of embryonic digestive system development that leaves a sacculation or outpouching from the wall of the small intestine near the terminal part of the ileum made of acid-secreting tissue as in the stomach.

neoplasm. New abnormal growth, tumor.

secondary. Second in order of occurrence or importance, or appearing during the course of another disease or condition.

44820

44820 Excision of lesion of mesentery (separate procedure)

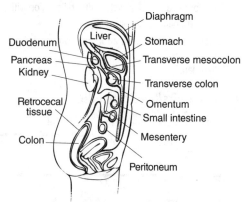

The mesentery is a double layer of peritoneal tissue enclosing most of the internal organs and anchoring them to the abdominal wall

Explanation

The physician excises a lesion in the mesentery. The physician makes an abdominal incision. Next, the lesion in the mesentery is identified. The lesion is removed by shelling it out of the mesentery, resecting a portion of the mesentery with the lesion, or resecting a segment of bowel and mesentery to include the lesion with reapproximation of the bowel. The incision is closed.

Coding Tips

This separate procedure, by definition, is usually a component of a more complex service and is not identified separately. When performed alone or with other unrelated procedures/services it may be reported. If performed alone, list the code; if performed with other procedures/ services, list the code and append modifier 59 or an X{EPSU} modifier. For excision of Meckel's diverticulum (diverticulectomy) or omphalomesenteric duct, see 44800. For suture of the small intestine (enterorrhaphy) for perforated ulcer, diverticulum, wound, injury, or rupture, single perforation, see 44602; for multiple perforations, see 44603. For suture of the large intestine (colorrhaphy) for perforated ulcer, diverticulum, wound, injury, or rupture, single or multiple perforations, without colostomy, see 44604; with colostomy, see 44605. For enterectomy, resection of the small intestine, single resection and anastomosis, see 44120; for each additional resection and anastomosis, see 44121; with enterostomy, see 44125.

ICD-10-CM Diagnostic Codes

A18.31	Tuberculous peritonitis
C48.1	Malignant neoplasm of specified parts of peritoneum
C48.8	Malignant neoplasm of overlapping sites of retroperitoneum and peritoneum
C78.6	Secondary malignant neoplasm of retroperitoneum and peritoneum
C7B.04	Secondary carcinoid tumors of peritoneum
D19.1	Benign neoplasm of mesothelial tissue of peritoneum
D20.0	Benign neoplasm of soft tissue of retroperitoneum
D20.1	Benign neoplasm of soft tissue of peritoneum
I88.0	Nonspecific mesenteric lymphadenitis
K55.021	Focal (segmental) acute infarction of small intestine
K55.022	Diffuse acute infarction of small intestine
K55.041	Focal (segmental) acute infarction of large intestine
K55.042	Diffuse acute infarction of large intestine
K55.1	Chronic vascular disorders of intestine
K65.0	Generalized (acute) peritonitis
K65.1	Peritoneal abscess
K65.2	Spontaneous bacterial peritonitis
K65.3	Choleperitonitis
K65.4	Sclerosing mesenteritis
K65.8	Other peritonitis
K66.8	Other specified disorders of peritoneum
Q43.3	Congenital malformations of intestinal fixation

AMA: 44820 2014,Jan,11

Relative Value Units/Medicare Edits

Non-Facility RVU	Work	PE	MP	Total
44820	13.73	7.97	3.14	24.84
Facility RVU	**Work**	**PE**	**MP**	**Total**
44820	13.73	7.97	3.14	24.84

	FUD	Status	MUE	Modifiers				IOM Reference
44820	90	A	1(3)	51	N/A	62*	80	None

* with documentation

Terms To Know

adhesion. Abnormal fibrous connection between two structures, soft tissue or bony structures, that may occur as the result of surgery, infection, or trauma.

effusion. Escape of fluid from within a body cavity.

lesion. Area of damaged tissue that has lost continuity or function, due to disease or trauma.

mesentery. Two layers of peritoneum that fold to surround the organs and attach to the abdominal wall.

44850

44850 Suture of mesentery (separate procedure)

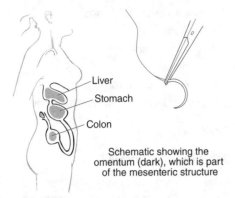

Schematic showing the omentum (dark), which is part of the mesenteric structure

Explanation

The physician repairs a defect in the mesentery with sutures. The physician makes an abdominal incision. Next, the mesenteric defect is identified and closed with sutures. The incision is closed.

Coding Tips

This separate procedure by definition is usually a component of a more complex service and is not identified separately. When performed alone or with other unrelated procedures/services it may be reported. If performed alone, list the code; if performed with other procedures/services, list the code and append modifier 59 or an X{EPSU} modifier. For suture of the small intestine (enterorrhaphy) for perforated ulcer, diverticulum, wound, injury, or rupture, single perforation, see 44602; for multiple perforations, see 44603. For suture of the large intestine (colorrhaphy) for perforated ulcer, diverticulum, wound, injury, or rupture, single or multiple perforations, without colostomy, see 44604; with colostomy, see 44605. For reduction or repair of an internal hernia, see 44050.

ICD-10-CM Diagnostic Codes

S31.620A   Laceration with foreign body of abdominal wall, right upper quadrant with penetration into peritoneal cavity, initial encounter ☑

S31.621A   Laceration with foreign body of abdominal wall, left upper quadrant with penetration into peritoneal cavity, initial encounter ☑

S31.622A   Laceration with foreign body of abdominal wall, epigastric region with penetration into peritoneal cavity, initial encounter

S31.623A   Laceration with foreign body of abdominal wall, right lower quadrant with penetration into peritoneal cavity, initial encounter ☑

S31.624A   Laceration with foreign body of abdominal wall, left lower quadrant with penetration into peritoneal cavity, initial encounter ☑

S31.625A   Laceration with foreign body of abdominal wall, periumbilic region with penetration into peritoneal cavity, initial encounter

S31.650A   Open bite of abdominal wall, right upper quadrant with penetration into peritoneal cavity, initial encounter ☑

S31.651A   Open bite of abdominal wall, left upper quadrant with penetration into peritoneal cavity, initial encounter ☑

S31.652A   Open bite of abdominal wall, epigastric region with penetration into peritoneal cavity, initial encounter

S31.653A   Open bite of abdominal wall, right lower quadrant with penetration into peritoneal cavity, initial encounter ☑

S31.654A   Open bite of abdominal wall, left lower quadrant with penetration into peritoneal cavity, initial encounter ☑

S31.655A   Open bite of abdominal wall, periumbilic region with penetration into peritoneal cavity, initial encounter

S36.893A   Laceration of other intra-abdominal organs, initial encounter

AMA: 44850 2014,Jan,11

Relative Value Units/Medicare Edits

Non-Facility RVU	Work	PE	MP	Total
44850	12.11	7.22	2.74	22.07
Facility RVU	**Work**	**PE**	**MP**	**Total**
44850	12.11	7.22	2.74	22.07

	FUD	Status	MUE	Modifiers				IOM Reference
44850	90	A	1(3)	51	N/A	62*	80	None

* with documentation

Terms To Know

defect. Imperfection, flaw, or absence.

mesentery. Two layers of peritoneum that fold to surround the organs and attach to the abdominal wall.

open wound. Opening or break of the skin.

suture. Numerous stitching techniques employed in wound closure.

buried suture. Continuous or interrupted suture placed under the skin for a layered closure.

continuous suture. Running stitch with tension evenly distributed across a single strand to provide a leakproof closure line.

interrupted suture. Series of single stitches with tension isolated at each stitch, in which all stitches are not affected if one becomes loose, and the isolated sutures cannot act as a wick to transport an infection.

purse-string suture. Continuous suture placed around a tubular structure and tightened, to reduce or close the lumen.

retention suture. Secondary stitching that bridges the primary suture, providing support for the primary repair; a plastic or rubber bolster may be placed over the primary repair and under the retention sutures.

44900

44900   Incision and drainage of appendiceal abscess, open

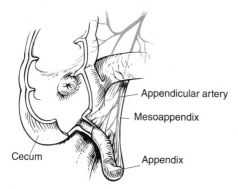

Surgical access to an abscessed appendix and the
open incision and drainage of the infection

Explanation

The physician drains an appendiceal abscess. The physician makes an
abdominal incision. Next, the abscess near the appendix is identified and
incised and drained. A drain may be left in the abscess cavity. The abdominal
wall incision is closed and the skin incision may be left open to heal secondarily.

Coding Tips

For appendectomy, open, see 44950; laparoscopic approach, see 44970; open
approach, performed for an indicated purpose at the time of another major
procedure (not as a separate procedure), see 44955; for ruptured appendix
with abscess or generalized peritonitis, see 44960. For percutaneous,
image-guided drainage of an appendiceal abscess, via catheter, see 49406.

ICD-10-CM Diagnostic Codes

K35.21	Acute appendicitis with generalized peritonitis, with abscess
K35.33	Acute appendicitis with perforation and localized peritonitis, with abscess
K36	Other appendicitis

AMA: **44900** 2014,Jan,11

Relative Value Units/Medicare Edits

Non-Facility RVU	Work	PE	MP	Total
44900	12.57	7.6	3.08	23.25
Facility RVU	Work	PE	MP	Total
44900	12.57	7.6	3.08	23.25

	FUD	Status	MUE	Modifiers				IOM Reference
44900	90	A	1(2)	51	N/A	62*	80	None

* with documentation

44950-44955

44950   Appendectomy;
+   44955   when done for indicated purpose at time of other major
procedure (not as separate procedure) (List separately in
addition to code for primary procedure)

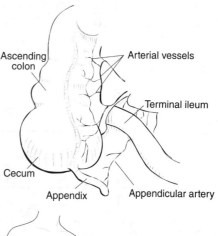

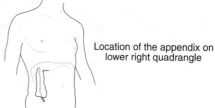

Location of the appendix on
lower right quadrangle

Explanation

The physician removes the appendix through an abdominal incision. The
appendix is identified and mobilized, its blood supply is divided and the
appendix is transected and removed. The incision is closed. Report 44955
when the procedure is performed at the same time as another major procedure.

Coding Tips

An incidental appendectomy performed at the time of another intra-abdominal
surgery is not reported separately. For those rare instances where it is necessary
to report incidental appendectomy, append modifier 52 to 44950. For
appendectomy for ruptured appendix with abscess or generalized peritonitis,
see 44960. For laparoscopic appendectomy, see 44970.

ICD-10-CM Diagnostic Codes

C18.1	Malignant neoplasm of appendix
C7A.020	Malignant carcinoid tumor of the appendix
D12.1	Benign neoplasm of appendix
D37.3	Neoplasm of uncertain behavior of appendix
K35.20	Acute appendicitis with generalized peritonitis, without abscess
K35.21	Acute appendicitis with generalized peritonitis, with abscess
K35.30	Acute appendicitis with localized peritonitis, without perforation or gangrene
K35.31	Acute appendicitis with localized peritonitis and gangrene, without perforation
K35.32	Acute appendicitis with perforation and localized peritonitis, without abscess
K35.33	Acute appendicitis with perforation and localized peritonitis, with abscess
K35.890	Other acute appendicitis without perforation or gangrene
K35.891	Other acute appendicitis without perforation, with gangrene

Appendix

K36	Other appendicitis
K38.0	Hyperplasia of appendix
K38.1	Appendicular concretions
K38.2	Diverticulum of appendix
K38.3	Fistula of appendix
K38.8	Other specified diseases of appendix
R10.823	Right lower quadrant rebound abdominal tenderness
R19.03	Right lower quadrant abdominal swelling, mass and lump

AMA: 44950 2018,Jan,8; 2017,Jan,8; 2016,Jan,13; 2015,Jan,16 **44955** 2018,Jan,8; 2017,Jan,8; 2016,Jan,13; 2015,Jan,16

Relative Value Units/Medicare Edits

Non-Facility RVU	Work	PE	MP	Total
44950	10.6	5.92	2.5	19.02
44955	1.53	0.6	0.32	2.45
Facility RVU	**Work**	**PE**	**MP**	**Total**
44950	10.6	5.92	2.5	19.02
44955	1.53	0.6	0.32	2.45

	FUD	Status	MUE	Modifiers				IOM Reference
44950	90	A	1(2)	51	N/A	62*	80	None
44955	N/A	A	1(2)	N/A	N/A	62*	80	

* with documentation

Terms To Know

abscess. Circumscribed collection of pus resulting from bacteria, frequently associated with swelling and other signs of inflammation.

appendicitis. Inflammation and infection of the appendix. In the acute stage of the disease, common symptoms include severe pain in the right lower quadrant of the abdomen, nausea, and vomiting.

gangrene. Death of tissue, usually resulting from a loss of vascular supply, followed by a bacterial attack or onset of disease.

hyperplasia of appendix. Increase in the size and number of cells in the appendix.

laparoscopy. Direct visualization of the peritoneal cavity, outer fallopian tubes, uterus, and ovaries utilizing a laparoscope, a thin, flexible fiberoptic tube.

perforation. Hole in an object, organ, or tissue, or the act of punching or boring holes through a part.

peritonitis. Inflammation and infection within the peritoneal cavity, the space between the membrane lining the abdominopelvic walls and covering the internal organs.

transection. Transverse dissection; to cut across a long axis; cross section.

44960

44960   Appendectomy; for ruptured appendix with abscess or generalized peritonitis

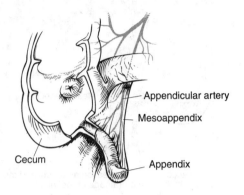

- Appendicular artery
- Mesoappendix
- Cecum
- Appendix

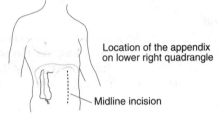

Location of the appendix on lower right quadrangle

Midline incision

Explanation

The physician removes a perforated appendix. The physician makes an abdominal incision. The appendix is identified and mobilized, its blood supply is divided, and the appendix is transected and removed. The abscess cavity is debrided and irrigated. The incision is closed.

Coding Tips

When 44960 is performed with another separately identifiable procedure, the highest dollar value code is listed as the primary procedure and subsequent procedures are appended with modifier 51. Appendectomy, see 44950; when performed for an indicated purpose at the time of another major procedure (not as a separate procedure), see 44955. For laparoscopic approach, see 44970.

ICD-10-CM Diagnostic Codes

| K35.20 | Acute appendicitis with generalized peritonitis, without abscess |
| K35.21 | Acute appendicitis with generalized peritonitis, with abscess |

AMA: 44960 2019,Dec,12; 2018,Jan,8; 2017,Jan,8; 2016,Jan,13; 2015,Jan,16

Relative Value Units/Medicare Edits

Non-Facility RVU	Work	PE	MP	Total
44960	14.5	7.99	3.46	25.95
Facility RVU	**Work**	**PE**	**MP**	**Total**
44960	14.5	7.99	3.46	25.95

	FUD	Status	MUE	Modifiers				IOM Reference
44960	90	A	1(2)	51	N/A	62*	80	None

* with documentation

44970

44970 Laparoscopy, surgical, appendectomy

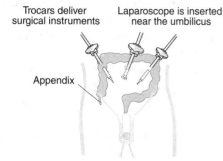

Trocars deliver surgical instruments
Laparoscope is inserted near the umbilicus
Appendix

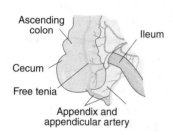

Ascending colon
Ileum
Cecum
Free tenia
Appendix and appendicular artery

Explanation

The physician performs a laparoscopic appendectomy. The physician places a trocar at the umbilicus and insufflates the abdomen. The laparoscope is placed through the umbilical port and additional trocars are placed into the abdominal cavity. The appendix is identified, dissected from surrounding structures, and its blood supply divided. The appendix is transected with staples or suture and removed. The trocars are removed and the incisions are closed.

Coding Tips

Surgical laparoscopy always includes diagnostic laparoscopy. To report a diagnostic laparoscopy (peritoneoscopy) (separate procedure) only, see 49320. For open appendectomy, see 44950; when performed for an indicated purpose at the time of another major procedure (not as a separate procedure), see 44955; for a ruptured appendix with abscess or generalized peritonitis, see 44960.

ICD-10-CM Diagnostic Codes

C18.1	Malignant neoplasm of appendix
C78.5	Secondary malignant neoplasm of large intestine and rectum
C7A.020	Malignant carcinoid tumor of the appendix
D12.1	Benign neoplasm of appendix
D37.3	Neoplasm of uncertain behavior of appendix
K35.20	Acute appendicitis with generalized peritonitis, without abscess
K35.21	Acute appendicitis with generalized peritonitis, with abscess
K35.30	Acute appendicitis with localized peritonitis, without perforation or gangrene
K35.31	Acute appendicitis with localized peritonitis and gangrene, without perforation
K35.32	Acute appendicitis with perforation and localized peritonitis, without abscess
K35.33	Acute appendicitis with perforation and localized peritonitis, with abscess
K35.890	Other acute appendicitis without perforation or gangrene
K35.891	Other acute appendicitis without perforation, with gangrene
K36	Other appendicitis
K38.0	Hyperplasia of appendix
K38.1	Appendicular concretions
K38.2	Diverticulum of appendix
K38.3	Fistula of appendix
K38.8	Other specified diseases of appendix
R10.813	Right lower quadrant abdominal tenderness
R10.823	Right lower quadrant rebound abdominal tenderness

AMA: 44970 2019,Dec,12; 2018,Jan,8; 2017,Jan,8; 2016,Jan,13; 2015,Mar,3; 2015,Jan,16

Relative Value Units/Medicare Edits

Non-Facility RVU	Work	PE	MP	Total
44970	9.45	6.13	2.24	17.82
Facility RVU	**Work**	**PE**	**MP**	**Total**
44970	9.45	6.13	2.24	17.82

	FUD	Status	MUE	Modifiers				IOM Reference
44970	90	A	1(2)	51	N/A	62	80	None

* with documentation

Terms To Know

abscess. Circumscribed collection of pus resulting from bacteria, frequently associated with swelling and other signs of inflammation. Abscesses may be punctured or aspirated or the physician may perform an incision and drainage.

acute. Sudden, severe. Documentation and reporting of an acute condition is important to establishing medical necessity.

appendicitis. Inflammation and infection of the appendix. In the acute stage of the disease, common symptoms include severe pain in the right lower quadrant of the abdomen, nausea, and vomiting.

dissect. Cut apart or separate tissue for surgical purposes or for visual or microscopic study.

gangrene. Death of tissue, usually resulting from a loss of vascular supply, followed by a bacterial attack or onset of disease.

hyperplasia of appendix. Increase in the size and number of cells in the appendix.

insufflation. Blowing air or gas into a body cavity.

laparoscopy. Direct visualization of the peritoneal cavity, outer fallopian tubes, uterus, and ovaries utilizing a laparoscope, a thin, flexible fiberoptic tube.

neoplasm. New abnormal growth, tumor.

transection. Transverse dissection; to cut across a long axis; cross section.

Appendix

45000

45000   Transrectal drainage of pelvic abscess

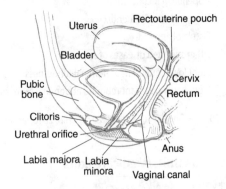

Uterus
Rectouterine pouch
Bladder
Cervix
Pubic bone
Rectum
Clitoris
Urethral orifice
Anus
Labia majora
Labia minora
Vaginal canal

Lateral schematic showing
the female rectoperineal area

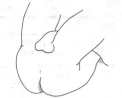

Incision is made in the rectum to
access an abscess of the pelvis

Explanation

The physician drains a pelvic abscess through the rectum. The physician identifies the area of abscess through the rectum by palpation or preoperative localizing studies. Next, a transanal incision is made through the rectum into the abscess cavity and the abscess is irrigated and drained. The incision is left open to drain.

Coding Tips

For incision and drainage of a submucosal abscess, rectum, see 45005; deep supralevator, pelvirectal, or retrorectal abscess, see 45020. For image-guided drainage of a pelvic abscess, via catheter, transrectally, see 49407.

ICD-10-CM Diagnostic Codes

A54.09	Other gonococcal infection of lower genitourinary tract
A54.1	Gonococcal infection of lower genitourinary tract with periurethral and accessory gland abscess
A54.24	Gonococcal female pelvic inflammatory disease ♀
A54.29	Other gonococcal genitourinary infections
A56.01	Chlamydial cystitis and urethritis
A56.09	Other chlamydial infection of lower genitourinary tract
A56.11	Chlamydial female pelvic inflammatory disease ♀
A56.19	Other chlamydial genitourinary infection
A56.3	Chlamydial infection of anus and rectum
A60.1	Herpesviral infection of perianal skin and rectum
K50.114	Crohn's disease of large intestine with abscess
K50.118	Crohn's disease of large intestine with other complication
K50.814	Crohn's disease of both small and large intestine with abscess
K51.014	Ulcerative (chronic) pancolitis with abscess
K51.214	Ulcerative (chronic) proctitis with abscess
K51.314	Ulcerative (chronic) rectosigmoiditis with abscess
K51.414	Inflammatory polyps of colon with abscess
K51.514	Left sided colitis with abscess
K51.814	Other ulcerative colitis with abscess
K57.00	Diverticulitis of small intestine with perforation and abscess without bleeding
K57.01	Diverticulitis of small intestine with perforation and abscess with bleeding
K57.20	Diverticulitis of large intestine with perforation and abscess without bleeding
K57.21	Diverticulitis of large intestine with perforation and abscess with bleeding
K57.32	Diverticulitis of large intestine without perforation or abscess without bleeding
K57.40	Diverticulitis of both small and large intestine with perforation and abscess without bleeding
K57.41	Diverticulitis of both small and large intestine with perforation and abscess with bleeding
K57.52	Diverticulitis of both small and large intestine without perforation or abscess without bleeding
K61.5	Supralevator abscess
K63.0	Abscess of intestine
K65.0	Generalized (acute) peritonitis
K65.1	Peritoneal abscess
K65.2	Spontaneous bacterial peritonitis
K65.3	Choleperitonitis
K65.4	Sclerosing mesenteritis
K65.8	Other peritonitis
K67	Disorders of peritoneum in infectious diseases classified elsewhere
K68.19	Other retroperitoneal abscess
N70.01	Acute salpingitis ♀
N70.02	Acute oophoritis ♀
N70.03	Acute salpingitis and oophoritis ♀
N70.11	Chronic salpingitis ♀
N70.12	Chronic oophoritis ♀
N70.13	Chronic salpingitis and oophoritis ♀
N71.0	Acute inflammatory disease of uterus ♀
N71.1	Chronic inflammatory disease of uterus ♀
N72	Inflammatory disease of cervix uteri ♀
N73.0	Acute parametritis and pelvic cellulitis ♀
N73.1	Chronic parametritis and pelvic cellulitis ♀
N73.3	Female acute pelvic peritonitis ♀
N73.4	Female chronic pelvic peritonitis ♀
N73.6	Female pelvic peritoneal adhesions (postinfective) ♀
N73.8	Other specified female pelvic inflammatory diseases ♀
N74	Female pelvic inflammatory disorders in diseases classified elsewhere ♀
N76.0	Acute vaginitis ♀
N76.1	Subacute and chronic vaginitis ♀
N76.5	Ulceration of vagina ♀
N76.81	Mucositis (ulcerative) of vagina and vulva ♀
N76.89	Other specified inflammation of vagina and vulva ♀
N77.1	Vaginitis, vulvitis and vulvovaginitis in diseases classified elsewhere ♀
O03.0	Genital tract and pelvic infection following incomplete spontaneous abortion Ⓜ ♀

Rectum

O04.5	Genital tract and pelvic infection following (induced) termination of pregnancy Ⓜ ♀	
O07.0	Genital tract and pelvic infection following failed attempted termination of pregnancy Ⓜ ♀	
O08.0	Genital tract and pelvic infection following ectopic and molar pregnancy Ⓜ ♀	
O08.82	Sepsis following ectopic and molar pregnancy Ⓜ ♀	

AMA: 45000 2014,Jan,11

Relative Value Units/Medicare Edits

Non-Facility RVU	Work	PE	MP	Total
45000	6.3	5.13	1.1	12.53
Facility RVU	**Work**	**PE**	**MP**	**Total**
45000	6.3	5.13	1.1	12.53

	FUD	Status	MUE	Modifiers				IOM Reference
45000	90	A	1(3)	51	N/A	N/A	N/A	None

* with documentation

Terms To Know

abscess. Circumscribed collection of pus resulting from bacteria, frequently associated with swelling and other signs of inflammation.

colitis. Inflammation of mucous membranes of the colon.

peritonitis. Inflammation and infection within the peritoneal cavity, the space between the membrane lining the abdominopelvic walls and covering the internal organs.

salpingitis. Inflammation of the fallopian tubes, usually caused by a bacterial infection and occurring in conjunction with inflammation of the ovaries (oophoritis).

45005

45005   Incision and drainage of submucosal abscess, rectum

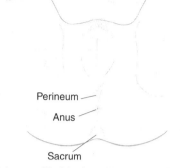

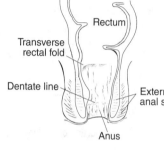

A transanal incision is made into the rectum to access a submucosal abscess of the rectum

Explanation

The physician drains a submucosal rectal abscess. The physician identifies the area of abscess in the rectum. Next, a transanal incision is made through the rectal lining into the abscess cavity and the abscess is drained. The incision is left open to drain.

Coding Tips

For incision and drainage of deep supralevator, pelvirectal, or retrorectal abscess, report 45020. Transrectal drainage of a pelvic abscess is reported with code 45000. For image-guided drainage of a pelvic abscess, via catheter, transrectally, see 49407.

ICD-10-CM Diagnostic Codes

A54.6	Gonococcal infection of anus and rectum
A56.3	Chlamydial infection of anus and rectum
A60.1	Herpesviral infection of perianal skin and rectum
K51.214	Ulcerative (chronic) proctitis with abscess
K61.0	Anal abscess
K61.1	Rectal abscess
K61.2	Anorectal abscess
K61.31	Horseshoe abscess
K61.39	Other ischiorectal abscess
K61.4	Intrasphincteric abscess

AMA: 45005 2014,Jan,11

Rectum

Relative Value Units/Medicare Edits

Non-Facility RVU	Work	PE	MP	Total
45005	2.02	6.81	0.43	9.26
Facility RVU	Work	PE	MP	Total
45005	2.02	2.38	0.43	4.83

	FUD	Status	MUE	Modifiers				IOM Reference
45005	10	A	1(3)	51	N/A	N/A	N/A	None

* with documentation

Terms To Know

abscess. Circumscribed collection of pus resulting from bacteria, frequently associated with swelling and other signs of inflammation.

drain. Device that creates a channel to allow fluid from a cavity, wound, or infected area to exit the body.

incision and drainage. Cutting open body tissue for the removal of tissue fluids or infected discharge from a wound or cavity.

infection. Presence of microorganisms in body tissues that may result in cellular damage.

mucosa. Moist tissue lining the mouth (buccal mucosa), stomach (gastric mucosa), intestines, and respiratory tract.

rectal. Pertaining to the rectum, the end portion of the large intestine.

sub. Below.

transverse. Crosswise at right angles to the long axis of a structure or part.

45020

45020   Incision and drainage of deep supralevator, pelvirectal, or retrorectal abscess

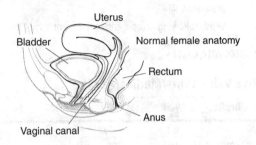

Deep abscesses can form around the rectum as it exits the peritoneum

Explanation

The physician drains an abscess above the pelvic floor or behind the rectum through the rectum. The physician identifies the area of abscess by palpation or preoperative localizing studies. Next, a transanal incision is made through the rectum into the abscess cavity and the abscess is drained. The incision is left open to drain.

Coding Tips

For transrectal drainage of a pelvic abscess, see 45000. For incision and drainage of a submucosal rectal abscess, see 45005. For incision and drainage of perianal abscess, superficial, see 46050. For incision and drainage of ischiorectal or intramural abscess, with fistulectomy or fistulotomy, submuscular, with or without placement of seton, see 46060. For image-guided drainage of a pelvic abscess, via catheter, transrectally, see 49407.

ICD-10-CM Diagnostic Codes

A54.09	Other gonococcal infection of lower genitourinary tract
A54.1	Gonococcal infection of lower genitourinary tract with periurethral and accessory gland abscess
A54.24	Gonococcal female pelvic inflammatory disease ♀
A54.29	Other gonococcal genitourinary infections
A56.01	Chlamydial cystitis and urethritis
A56.09	Other chlamydial infection of lower genitourinary tract
A56.11	Chlamydial female pelvic inflammatory disease ♀
A56.19	Other chlamydial genitourinary infection
A56.3	Chlamydial infection of anus and rectum
A60.1	Herpesviral infection of perianal skin and rectum
K50.114	Crohn's disease of large intestine with abscess
K50.814	Crohn's disease of both small and large intestine with abscess
K51.014	Ulcerative (chronic) pancolitis with abscess
K51.214	Ulcerative (chronic) proctitis with abscess
K51.314	Ulcerative (chronic) rectosigmoiditis with abscess
K51.414	Inflammatory polyps of colon with abscess
K51.514	Left sided colitis with abscess
K51.814	Other ulcerative colitis with abscess
K57.00	Diverticulitis of small intestine with perforation and abscess without bleeding
K57.01	Diverticulitis of small intestine with perforation and abscess with bleeding

Rectum

K57.20	Diverticulitis of large intestine with perforation and abscess without bleeding
K57.21	Diverticulitis of large intestine with perforation and abscess with bleeding
K57.40	Diverticulitis of both small and large intestine with perforation and abscess without bleeding
K57.41	Diverticulitis of both small and large intestine with perforation and abscess with bleeding
K61.0	Anal abscess
K61.1	Rectal abscess
K61.2	Anorectal abscess
K61.31	Horseshoe abscess
K61.39	Other ischiorectal abscess
K61.4	Intrasphincteric abscess
K61.5	Supralevator abscess
K63.0	Abscess of intestine
K65.0	Generalized (acute) peritonitis
K65.1	Peritoneal abscess
K65.2	Spontaneous bacterial peritonitis
K65.3	Choleperitonitis
K65.4	Sclerosing mesenteritis
K65.8	Other peritonitis
K68.11	Postprocedural retroperitoneal abscess
K68.19	Other retroperitoneal abscess
N70.01	Acute salpingitis ♀
N70.02	Acute oophoritis ♀
N70.03	Acute salpingitis and oophoritis ♀
N70.11	Chronic salpingitis ♀
N70.12	Chronic oophoritis ♀
N70.13	Chronic salpingitis and oophoritis ♀
N71.0	Acute inflammatory disease of uterus ♀
N71.1	Chronic inflammatory disease of uterus ♀
N72	Inflammatory disease of cervix uteri ♀
N73.0	Acute parametritis and pelvic cellulitis ♀
N73.1	Chronic parametritis and pelvic cellulitis ♀
N73.3	Female acute pelvic peritonitis ♀
N73.4	Female chronic pelvic peritonitis ♀
N73.6	Female pelvic peritoneal adhesions (postinfective) ♀
N73.8	Other specified female pelvic inflammatory diseases ♀
N74	Female pelvic inflammatory disorders in diseases classified elsewhere ♀
N75.0	Cyst of Bartholin's gland ♀
N76.0	Acute vaginitis ♀
N76.1	Subacute and chronic vaginitis ♀
N77.1	Vaginitis, vulvitis and vulvovaginitis in diseases classified elsewhere ♀
O03.0	Genital tract and pelvic infection following incomplete spontaneous abortion Ⓜ ♀
O04.5	Genital tract and pelvic infection following (induced) termination of pregnancy Ⓜ ♀
O07.0	Genital tract and pelvic infection following failed attempted termination of pregnancy Ⓜ ♀
O08.0	Genital tract and pelvic infection following ectopic and molar pregnancy Ⓜ ♀

AMA: 45020 2014,Jan,11

Relative Value Units/Medicare Edits

Non-Facility RVU	Work	PE	MP	Total
45020	8.56	6.63	1.76	16.95
Facility RVU	**Work**	**PE**	**MP**	**Total**
45020	8.56	6.63	1.76	16.95

	FUD	Status	MUE	Modifiers				IOM Reference
45020	90	A	1(3)	51	N/A	N/A	N/A	None

* with documentation

Terms To Know

abscess. Circumscribed collection of pus resulting from bacteria, frequently associated with swelling and other signs of inflammation.

cellulitis. Infection of the skin and subcutaneous tissues, most often caused by Staphylococcus or Streptococcus bacteria secondary to a cutaneous lesion. Progression of the inflammation may lead to abscess and tissue death, or even systemic infection-like bacteremia.

chronic. Persistent, continuing, or recurring.

incision and drainage. Cutting open body tissue for the removal of tissue fluids or infected discharge from a wound or cavity.

infection. Presence of microorganisms in body tissues that may result in cellular damage.

localization. Limitation to one area.

Rectum

45100

45100 Biopsy of anorectal wall, anal approach (eg, congenital megacolon)

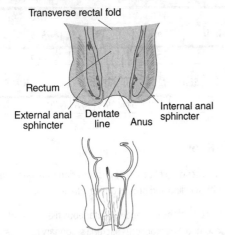

A biopsy sample is collected from the rectal wall using an anal approach

Explanation

The physician performs a biopsy of the rectal wall using a transanal approach. The physician performs an incisional biopsy or a suction biopsy of the low rectal wall. The biopsy may be closed with sutures.

Coding Tips

An excisional biopsy is not reported separately when a therapeutic excision is performed during the same surgical session. If a specimen is transported to an outside laboratory, report 99000 for handling or conveyance. Endoscopic biopsy is reported with 45305.

ICD-10-CM Diagnostic Codes

A54.6	Gonococcal infection of anus and rectum
A56.3	Chlamydial infection of anus and rectum
A60.1	Herpesviral infection of perianal skin and rectum
C19	Malignant neoplasm of rectosigmoid junction
C20	Malignant neoplasm of rectum
C21.1	Malignant neoplasm of anal canal
C21.2	Malignant neoplasm of cloacogenic zone
C21.8	Malignant neoplasm of overlapping sites of rectum, anus and anal canal
C78.5	Secondary malignant neoplasm of large intestine and rectum
C7A.026	Malignant carcinoid tumor of the rectum
D01.1	Carcinoma in situ of rectosigmoid junction
D01.2	Carcinoma in situ of rectum
D01.3	Carcinoma in situ of anus and anal canal
D12.7	Benign neoplasm of rectosigmoid junction
D12.8	Benign neoplasm of rectum
D12.9	Benign neoplasm of anus and anal canal
D3A.026	Benign carcinoid tumor of the rectum
D49.0	Neoplasm of unspecified behavior of digestive system
E85.81	Light chain (AL) amyloidosis
E85.82	Wild-type transthyretin-related (ATTR) amyloidosis
E85.89	Other amyloidosis
K50.10	Crohn's disease of large intestine without complications
K50.111	Crohn's disease of large intestine with rectal bleeding
K50.112	Crohn's disease of large intestine with intestinal obstruction
K50.113	Crohn's disease of large intestine with fistula
K50.114	Crohn's disease of large intestine with abscess
K50.118	Crohn's disease of large intestine with other complication
K50.80	Crohn's disease of both small and large intestine without complications
K50.811	Crohn's disease of both small and large intestine with rectal bleeding
K50.812	Crohn's disease of both small and large intestine with intestinal obstruction
K50.813	Crohn's disease of both small and large intestine with fistula
K50.814	Crohn's disease of both small and large intestine with abscess
K50.818	Crohn's disease of both small and large intestine with other complication
K51.00	Ulcerative (chronic) pancolitis without complications
K51.011	Ulcerative (chronic) pancolitis with rectal bleeding
K51.012	Ulcerative (chronic) pancolitis with intestinal obstruction
K51.013	Ulcerative (chronic) pancolitis with fistula
K51.014	Ulcerative (chronic) pancolitis with abscess
K51.018	Ulcerative (chronic) pancolitis with other complication
K51.20	Ulcerative (chronic) proctitis without complications
K51.211	Ulcerative (chronic) proctitis with rectal bleeding
K51.212	Ulcerative (chronic) proctitis with intestinal obstruction
K51.213	Ulcerative (chronic) proctitis with fistula
K51.214	Ulcerative (chronic) proctitis with abscess
K51.218	Ulcerative (chronic) proctitis with other complication
K51.30	Ulcerative (chronic) rectosigmoiditis without complications
K51.311	Ulcerative (chronic) rectosigmoiditis with rectal bleeding
K51.312	Ulcerative (chronic) rectosigmoiditis with intestinal obstruction
K51.313	Ulcerative (chronic) rectosigmoiditis with fistula
K51.314	Ulcerative (chronic) rectosigmoiditis with abscess
K51.318	Ulcerative (chronic) rectosigmoiditis with other complication
K51.50	Left sided colitis without complications
K51.511	Left sided colitis with rectal bleeding
K51.512	Left sided colitis with intestinal obstruction
K51.513	Left sided colitis with fistula
K51.514	Left sided colitis with abscess
K51.518	Left sided colitis with other complication
K51.80	Other ulcerative colitis without complications
K51.811	Other ulcerative colitis with rectal bleeding
K51.812	Other ulcerative colitis with intestinal obstruction
K51.813	Other ulcerative colitis with fistula
K51.814	Other ulcerative colitis with abscess
K51.818	Other ulcerative colitis with other complication
K55.011	Focal (segmental) acute (reversible) ischemia of small intestine
K55.012	Diffuse acute (reversible) ischemia of small intestine
K55.021	Focal (segmental) acute infarction of small intestine
K55.022	Diffuse acute infarction of small intestine
K55.031	Focal (segmental) acute (reversible) ischemia of large intestine
K55.032	Diffuse acute (reversible) ischemia of large intestine
K55.041	Focal (segmental) acute infarction of large intestine
K55.042	Diffuse acute infarction of large intestine

Rectum

K55.051	Focal (segmental) acute (reversible) ischemia of intestine, part unspecified
K55.052	Diffuse acute (reversible) ischemia of intestine, part unspecified
K55.1	Chronic vascular disorders of intestine
K55.20	Angiodysplasia of colon without hemorrhage
K55.8	Other vascular disorders of intestine
K57.20	Diverticulitis of large intestine with perforation and abscess without bleeding
K57.21	Diverticulitis of large intestine with perforation and abscess with bleeding
K57.30	Diverticulosis of large intestine without perforation or abscess without bleeding
K57.31	Diverticulosis of large intestine without perforation or abscess with bleeding
K57.32	Diverticulitis of large intestine without perforation or abscess without bleeding
K57.33	Diverticulitis of large intestine without perforation or abscess with bleeding
K57.40	Diverticulitis of both small and large intestine with perforation and abscess without bleeding
K57.41	Diverticulitis of both small and large intestine with perforation and abscess with bleeding
K57.50	Diverticulosis of both small and large intestine without perforation or abscess without bleeding
K57.51	Diverticulosis of both small and large intestine without perforation or abscess with bleeding
K57.52	Diverticulitis of both small and large intestine without perforation or abscess without bleeding
K57.53	Diverticulitis of both small and large intestine without perforation or abscess with bleeding
K58.0	Irritable bowel syndrome with diarrhea
K58.1	Irritable bowel syndrome with constipation
K58.2	Mixed irritable bowel syndrome
K58.8	Other irritable bowel syndrome
K58.9	Irritable bowel syndrome without diarrhea
K61.0	Anal abscess
K61.1	Rectal abscess
K61.2	Anorectal abscess
K61.31	Horseshoe abscess
K61.39	Other ischiorectal abscess
K61.4	Intrasphincteric abscess
K62.3	Rectal prolapse
K62.4	Stenosis of anus and rectum
K62.5	Hemorrhage of anus and rectum
K62.6	Ulcer of anus and rectum
K62.7	Radiation proctitis
K62.82	Dysplasia of anus
K62.89	Other specified diseases of anus and rectum
K92.1	Melena
Q43.1	Hirschsprung's disease
Q43.2	Other congenital functional disorders of colon

AMA: 45100 2014,Jan,11

Relative Value Units/Medicare Edits

Non-Facility RVU	Work	PE	MP	Total
45100	4.04	4.08	0.74	8.86
Facility RVU	**Work**	**PE**	**MP**	**Total**
45100	4.04	4.08	0.74	8.86

	FUD	Status	MUE	Modifiers				IOM Reference
45100	90	A	2(3)	51	N/A	N/A	N/A	None

* with documentation

Terms To Know

approach. Method or anatomical location used to gain access to a body organ or specific area for procedures.

biopsy. Tissue or fluid removed for diagnostic purposes through analysis of the cells in the biopsy material.

Crohn's disease. Chronic inflammation of the gastrointestinal tract characterized by chronic granulomatous disease, most commonly affecting the intestines and the terminal ileum.

megacolon. Enlargement or dilation of the large intestines or the colon.

neoplasm. New abnormal growth, tumor.

pancolitis. Severe form of ulcerative colitis, where inflammation affects the entire colon. May be caused by infection or external influences such as laxatives, radiation, or antibiotics.

45108

45108 Anorectal myomectomy

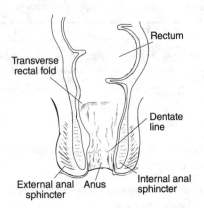

The muscular lining of the anorectal area is surgically accessed via the anus. A tumor or area of muscle is excised and the access incision is closed

Explanation

The physician removes a muscle tumor or a section of muscle from the anorectum. The physician identifies the anorectal muscle tumor or area of interest. A transanal incision is made through the rectal wall and the tumor or identified area of muscle is excised. The incision is closed by approximating the muscle edges and closing the incision in the rectal lining.

Coding Tips

For excision of a rectal tumor by proctotomy, transsacral or transcoccygeal approach, see 45160. For excision of a rectal tumor via transanal approach, not including muscularis propria (e.g., full thickness), see 45171; including muscularis propria, see 45172. Destruction of a rectal tumor, any method, transanal approach, is reported with 45190.

ICD-10-CM Diagnostic Codes

C19	Malignant neoplasm of rectosigmoid junction
C20	Malignant neoplasm of rectum
C21.1	Malignant neoplasm of anal canal
C21.2	Malignant neoplasm of cloacogenic zone
C21.8	Malignant neoplasm of overlapping sites of rectum, anus and anal canal
C49.A5	Gastrointestinal stromal tumor of rectum
C78.5	Secondary malignant neoplasm of large intestine and rectum
C7A.026	Malignant carcinoid tumor of the rectum
D01.1	Carcinoma in situ of rectosigmoid junction
D01.2	Carcinoma in situ of rectum
D01.3	Carcinoma in situ of anus and anal canal
D12.7	Benign neoplasm of rectosigmoid junction
D12.8	Benign neoplasm of rectum
D12.9	Benign neoplasm of anus and anal canal
D3A.026	Benign carcinoid tumor of the rectum
K59.01	Slow transit constipation
K59.02	Outlet dysfunction constipation
K59.03	Drug induced constipation
K59.04	Chronic idiopathic constipation
K59.09	Other constipation

K62.4	Stenosis of anus and rectum
K62.7	Radiation proctitis
K62.82	Dysplasia of anus
K62.89	Other specified diseases of anus and rectum
Q42.0	Congenital absence, atresia and stenosis of rectum with fistula
Q42.1	Congenital absence, atresia and stenosis of rectum without fistula
Q42.2	Congenital absence, atresia and stenosis of anus with fistula
Q42.3	Congenital absence, atresia and stenosis of anus without fistula
Q43.1	Hirschsprung's disease
R15.0	Incomplete defecation
R15.1	Fecal smearing
R15.2	Fecal urgency
R15.9	Full incontinence of feces

AMA: 45108 2014,Jan,11

Relative Value Units/Medicare Edits

Non-Facility RVU	Work	PE	MP	Total
45108	5.12	4.68	1.25	11.05
Facility RVU	**Work**	**PE**	**MP**	**Total**
45108	5.12	4.68	1.25	11.05

	FUD	Status	MUE	Modifiers				IOM Reference
45108	90	A	1(2)	51	N/A	62*	N/A	None

* with documentation

Terms To Know

benign. Mild or nonmalignant in nature.

closure. Repairing an incision or wound by suture or other means.

excision. Surgical removal of an organ or tissue.

incision. Act of cutting into tissue or an organ.

malignant. Any condition tending to progress toward death, specifically an invasive tumor with a loss of cellular differentiation that has the ability to spread or metastasize to other body areas.

myomectomy. Excision of a benign lesion of the muscle.

neoplasm. New abnormal growth, tumor.

tumor. Pathological swelling or enlargement; a neoplastic growth of uncontrolled, abnormal multiplication of cells.

Rectum

45110

45110 Proctectomy; complete, combined abdominoperineal, with colostomy

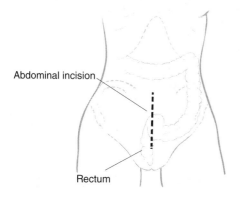

The anus and rectum are removed through the perineum. The approach is combined abdominoperineal

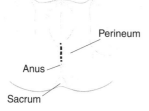

Explanation

The physician removes the entire rectum and anus and forms a colostomy. The physician makes an abdominal incision. The proximal rectum is mobilized within the abdomen to the level of the sphincter muscles and the colon is divided above the pelvic brim. An incision is made around the anus from a perineal approach and the anus and distal rectum are dissected free of surrounding structures and the anus and rectum are removed. The proximal end of colon is brought out through a separate incision on the abdominal wall as a colostomy. The abdominal and perineal incisions are closed.

Coding Tips

For laparoscopic approach, see 45395. For proctectomy, combined abdominoperineal pull-through procedure (e.g., colo-anal anastomosis), see 45112. For partial proctectomy with rectal mucosectomy, ileoanal anastomosis, creation of ileal reservoir (S or J), with or without loop ileostomy, see 45113; for partial proctectomy with anastomosis, abdominal and transsacral approach, see 45114; for transsacral approach only, see 45116.

ICD-10-CM Diagnostic Codes

C18.2	Malignant neoplasm of ascending colon
C18.3	Malignant neoplasm of hepatic flexure
C18.4	Malignant neoplasm of transverse colon
C18.5	Malignant neoplasm of splenic flexure
C18.6	Malignant neoplasm of descending colon
C18.7	Malignant neoplasm of sigmoid colon
C18.8	Malignant neoplasm of overlapping sites of colon
C19	Malignant neoplasm of rectosigmoid junction
C20	Malignant neoplasm of rectum
C21.1	Malignant neoplasm of anal canal
C21.2	Malignant neoplasm of cloacogenic zone
C21.8	Malignant neoplasm of overlapping sites of rectum, anus and anal canal
C49.A5	Gastrointestinal stromal tumor of rectum
C78.5	Secondary malignant neoplasm of large intestine and rectum
C7A.022	Malignant carcinoid tumor of the ascending colon
C7A.023	Malignant carcinoid tumor of the transverse colon
C7A.024	Malignant carcinoid tumor of the descending colon
C7A.025	Malignant carcinoid tumor of the sigmoid colon
C7A.026	Malignant carcinoid tumor of the rectum
D01.0	Carcinoma in situ of colon
D01.1	Carcinoma in situ of rectosigmoid junction
D01.2	Carcinoma in situ of rectum
D12.2	Benign neoplasm of ascending colon
D12.3	Benign neoplasm of transverse colon
D12.4	Benign neoplasm of descending colon
D12.5	Benign neoplasm of sigmoid colon
D37.4	Neoplasm of uncertain behavior of colon
D37.5	Neoplasm of uncertain behavior of rectum
D3A.022	Benign carcinoid tumor of the ascending colon
D3A.023	Benign carcinoid tumor of the transverse colon
D3A.024	Benign carcinoid tumor of the descending colon
D3A.025	Benign carcinoid tumor of the sigmoid colon
D3A.026	Benign carcinoid tumor of the rectum
K50.111	Crohn's disease of large intestine with rectal bleeding
K50.112	Crohn's disease of large intestine with intestinal obstruction
K50.113	Crohn's disease of large intestine with fistula
K50.114	Crohn's disease of large intestine with abscess
K50.118	Crohn's disease of large intestine with other complication
K51.011	Ulcerative (chronic) pancolitis with rectal bleeding
K51.012	Ulcerative (chronic) pancolitis with intestinal obstruction
K51.013	Ulcerative (chronic) pancolitis with fistula
K51.014	Ulcerative (chronic) pancolitis with abscess
K51.018	Ulcerative (chronic) pancolitis with other complication
K51.211	Ulcerative (chronic) proctitis with rectal bleeding
K51.212	Ulcerative (chronic) proctitis with intestinal obstruction
K51.213	Ulcerative (chronic) proctitis with fistula
K51.214	Ulcerative (chronic) proctitis with abscess
K51.218	Ulcerative (chronic) proctitis with other complication
K51.311	Ulcerative (chronic) rectosigmoiditis with rectal bleeding
K51.312	Ulcerative (chronic) rectosigmoiditis with intestinal obstruction
K51.313	Ulcerative (chronic) rectosigmoiditis with fistula
K51.314	Ulcerative (chronic) rectosigmoiditis with abscess
K51.318	Ulcerative (chronic) rectosigmoiditis with other complication
K51.411	Inflammatory polyps of colon with rectal bleeding
K51.412	Inflammatory polyps of colon with intestinal obstruction
K51.413	Inflammatory polyps of colon with fistula
K51.414	Inflammatory polyps of colon with abscess
K51.418	Inflammatory polyps of colon with other complication
K51.511	Left sided colitis with rectal bleeding
K51.512	Left sided colitis with intestinal obstruction
K51.513	Left sided colitis with fistula
K51.514	Left sided colitis with abscess
K51.518	Left sided colitis with other complication

Rectum

K51.811	Other ulcerative colitis with rectal bleeding	
K51.812	Other ulcerative colitis with intestinal obstruction	
K51.813	Other ulcerative colitis with fistula	
K51.814	Other ulcerative colitis with abscess	
K51.818	Other ulcerative colitis with other complication	
K55.011	Focal (segmental) acute (reversible) ischemia of small intestine	
K55.012	Diffuse acute (reversible) ischemia of small intestine	
K55.021	Focal (segmental) acute infarction of small intestine	
K55.022	Diffuse acute infarction of small intestine	
K55.031	Focal (segmental) acute (reversible) ischemia of large intestine	
K55.032	Diffuse acute (reversible) ischemia of large intestine	
K55.041	Focal (segmental) acute infarction of large intestine	
K55.042	Diffuse acute infarction of large intestine	
K55.051	Focal (segmental) acute (reversible) ischemia of intestine, part unspecified	
K55.052	Diffuse acute (reversible) ischemia of intestine, part unspecified	
K55.1	Chronic vascular disorders of intestine	
K55.8	Other vascular disorders of intestine	
K62.2	Anal prolapse	
K62.3	Rectal prolapse	
K62.82	Dysplasia of anus	
K63.5	Polyp of colon	
Q43.1	Hirschsprung's disease	
Q43.2	Other congenital functional disorders of colon	

AMA: 45110 2014,Jan,11

Relative Value Units/Medicare Edits

Non-Facility RVU	Work	PE	MP	Total
45110	30.76	17.33	5.58	53.67
Facility RVU	Work	PE	MP	Total
45110	30.76	17.33	5.58	53.67

	FUD	Status	MUE	Modifiers				IOM Reference
45110	90	A	1(2)	51	N/A	62*	80	None

* with documentation

Terms To Know

colostomy. Artificial surgical opening anywhere along the length of the colon to the skin surface for the diversion of feces.

45111

45111   Proctectomy; partial resection of rectum, transabdominal approach

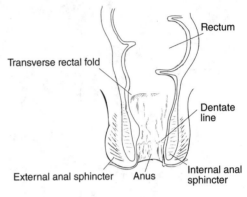

The rectum is partially removed. Access is abdominal

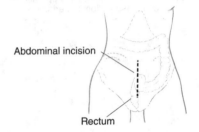

Explanation

The physician removes the proximal rectum using an open transabdominal approach. The physician makes an abdominal incision. The distal colon and rectum are mobilized and divided proximal and distal to the segment of interest and that portion of the rectum is removed. The distal end of the colon is approximated to the remaining rectum or may be closed with sutures or staples. The abdominal incision is closed.

Coding Tips

For partial proctectomy with anastomosis, abdominal and transsacral approach, see 45114; for transsacral approach only, see 45116.

ICD-10-CM Diagnostic Codes

C18.2	Malignant neoplasm of ascending colon
C18.3	Malignant neoplasm of hepatic flexure
C18.4	Malignant neoplasm of transverse colon
C18.5	Malignant neoplasm of splenic flexure
C18.6	Malignant neoplasm of descending colon
C18.7	Malignant neoplasm of sigmoid colon
C18.8	Malignant neoplasm of overlapping sites of colon
C19	Malignant neoplasm of rectosigmoid junction
C20	Malignant neoplasm of rectum
C21.1	Malignant neoplasm of anal canal
C21.2	Malignant neoplasm of cloacogenic zone
C21.8	Malignant neoplasm of overlapping sites of rectum, anus and anal canal
C49.A5	Gastrointestinal stromal tumor of rectum
C78.5	Secondary malignant neoplasm of large intestine and rectum
C7A.022	Malignant carcinoid tumor of the ascending colon
C7A.023	Malignant carcinoid tumor of the transverse colon

Rectum

C7A.024	Malignant carcinoid tumor of the descending colon
C7A.025	Malignant carcinoid tumor of the sigmoid colon
C7A.026	Malignant carcinoid tumor of the rectum
D01.0	Carcinoma in situ of colon
D01.1	Carcinoma in situ of rectosigmoid junction
D01.2	Carcinoma in situ of rectum
D12.2	Benign neoplasm of ascending colon
D12.3	Benign neoplasm of transverse colon
D12.4	Benign neoplasm of descending colon
D12.5	Benign neoplasm of sigmoid colon
D37.4	Neoplasm of uncertain behavior of colon
D37.5	Neoplasm of uncertain behavior of rectum
D3A.022	Benign carcinoid tumor of the ascending colon
D3A.023	Benign carcinoid tumor of the transverse colon
D3A.024	Benign carcinoid tumor of the descending colon
D3A.025	Benign carcinoid tumor of the sigmoid colon
D3A.026	Benign carcinoid tumor of the rectum
K50.111	Crohn's disease of large intestine with rectal bleeding
K50.112	Crohn's disease of large intestine with intestinal obstruction
K50.113	Crohn's disease of large intestine with fistula
K50.114	Crohn's disease of large intestine with abscess
K50.118	Crohn's disease of large intestine with other complication
K51.011	Ulcerative (chronic) pancolitis with rectal bleeding
K51.012	Ulcerative (chronic) pancolitis with intestinal obstruction
K51.013	Ulcerative (chronic) pancolitis with fistula
K51.014	Ulcerative (chronic) pancolitis with abscess
K51.018	Ulcerative (chronic) pancolitis with other complication
K51.211	Ulcerative (chronic) proctitis with rectal bleeding
K51.212	Ulcerative (chronic) proctitis with intestinal obstruction
K51.213	Ulcerative (chronic) proctitis with fistula
K51.214	Ulcerative (chronic) proctitis with abscess
K51.218	Ulcerative (chronic) proctitis with other complication
K51.311	Ulcerative (chronic) rectosigmoiditis with rectal bleeding
K51.312	Ulcerative (chronic) rectosigmoiditis with intestinal obstruction
K51.313	Ulcerative (chronic) rectosigmoiditis with fistula
K51.314	Ulcerative (chronic) rectosigmoiditis with abscess
K51.318	Ulcerative (chronic) rectosigmoiditis with other complication
K51.411	Inflammatory polyps of colon with rectal bleeding
K51.412	Inflammatory polyps of colon with intestinal obstruction
K51.413	Inflammatory polyps of colon with fistula
K51.414	Inflammatory polyps of colon with abscess
K51.418	Inflammatory polyps of colon with other complication
K51.511	Left sided colitis with rectal bleeding
K51.512	Left sided colitis with intestinal obstruction
K51.513	Left sided colitis with fistula
K51.514	Left sided colitis with abscess
K51.518	Left sided colitis with other complication
K51.811	Other ulcerative colitis with rectal bleeding
K51.812	Other ulcerative colitis with intestinal obstruction
K51.813	Other ulcerative colitis with fistula
K51.814	Other ulcerative colitis with abscess
K51.818	Other ulcerative colitis with other complication
K55.011	Focal (segmental) acute (reversible) ischemia of small intestine
K55.012	Diffuse acute (reversible) ischemia of small intestine
K55.021	Focal (segmental) acute infarction of small intestine
K55.022	Diffuse acute infarction of small intestine
K55.031	Focal (segmental) acute (reversible) ischemia of large intestine
K55.032	Diffuse acute (reversible) ischemia of large intestine
K55.041	Focal (segmental) acute infarction of large intestine
K55.042	Diffuse acute infarction of large intestine
K55.051	Focal (segmental) acute (reversible) ischemia of intestine, part unspecified
K55.052	Diffuse acute (reversible) ischemia of intestine, part unspecified
K55.1	Chronic vascular disorders of intestine
K55.8	Other vascular disorders of intestine
K62.2	Anal prolapse
K62.3	Rectal prolapse
K62.82	Dysplasia of anus
K63.5	Polyp of colon
Q43.1	Hirschsprung's disease
Q43.2	Other congenital functional disorders of colon

AMA: **45111** 2014,Jan,11

Relative Value Units/Medicare Edits

Non-Facility RVU	Work	PE	MP	Total
45111	18.01	10.37	3.57	31.95
Facility RVU	Work	PE	MP	Total
45111	18.01	10.37	3.57	31.95

	FUD	Status	MUE	Modifiers				IOM Reference
45111	90	A	1(2)	51	N/A	62*	80	None

* with documentation

Terms To Know

closure. Repairing an incision or wound by suture or other means.

distal. Located farther away from a specified reference point or the trunk.

proximal. Located closest to a specified reference point, usually the midline or trunk.

resection. Surgical removal of a part or all of an organ or body part.

45112

45112 Proctectomy, combined abdominoperineal, pull-through procedure (eg, colo-anal anastomosis)

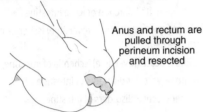

Colon is mobilized via abdominal incision

Anus and rectum are pulled through perineum incision and resected

The entire rectum and anus are removed via combined abdominal and perineal incisions

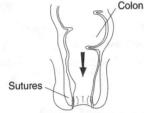

The mobilized colon is pulled through the perineal incision and fashioned into a neorectum and anus

Explanation

The physician removes the rectum and performs an anastomosis between the colon and the anus. The physician makes an abdominal incision. The distal colon and rectum are mobilized within the abdomen to the level of the sphincter muscles. The colon is divided above the pelvic brim and the rectum at the level of the sphincter muscles and removed. The mucosa may be stripped from the remaining distal rectum from a perineal approach. The distal colon is pulled through the sphincter complex and approximated to the anus with sutures. The incision is closed.

Coding Tips

For proctectomy, complete, combined abdominoperineal, with colostomy, see 45110; for partial resection of rectum, transabdominal approach, see 45111. For proctectomy, partial, with rectal mucosectomy, ileoanal anastomosis, creation of ileal reservoir (S or J), with or without loop ileostomy, see 45113. For proctectomy, partial, with anastomosis, abdominal and transsacral approach, see 45114; for transsacral approach only (Kraske type), see 45116. For colo-anal anastomosis with colonic reservoir or pouch, see, 45119. For proctectomy, complete (for congenital megacolon), abdominal and perineal approach, with pull-through procedure and anastomosis (e.g., Swenson, Duhamel, or Soave type operation), see 45120; with subtotal or total colectomy, with multiple biopsies, see 45121. For proctectomy, partial, without anastomosis, perineal approach, see 45123.

ICD-10-CM Diagnostic Codes

C19	Malignant neoplasm of rectosigmoid junction
C20	Malignant neoplasm of rectum
C21.1	Malignant neoplasm of anal canal
C21.2	Malignant neoplasm of cloacogenic zone
C21.8	Malignant neoplasm of overlapping sites of rectum, anus and anal canal
C49.A5	Gastrointestinal stromal tumor of rectum
C78.5	Secondary malignant neoplasm of large intestine and rectum
C7A.026	Malignant carcinoid tumor of the rectum
D01.1	Carcinoma in situ of rectosigmoid junction
D01.2	Carcinoma in situ of rectum
D37.5	Neoplasm of uncertain behavior of rectum
D3A.026	Benign carcinoid tumor of the rectum
K50.111	Crohn's disease of large intestine with rectal bleeding
K50.112	Crohn's disease of large intestine with intestinal obstruction
K50.113	Crohn's disease of large intestine with fistula
K50.114	Crohn's disease of large intestine with abscess
K50.118	Crohn's disease of large intestine with other complication
K51.211	Ulcerative (chronic) proctitis with rectal bleeding
K51.212	Ulcerative (chronic) proctitis with intestinal obstruction
K51.213	Ulcerative (chronic) proctitis with fistula
K51.214	Ulcerative (chronic) proctitis with abscess
K51.218	Ulcerative (chronic) proctitis with other complication
K51.311	Ulcerative (chronic) rectosigmoiditis with rectal bleeding
K51.312	Ulcerative (chronic) rectosigmoiditis with intestinal obstruction
K51.313	Ulcerative (chronic) rectosigmoiditis with fistula
K51.314	Ulcerative (chronic) rectosigmoiditis with abscess
K51.318	Ulcerative (chronic) rectosigmoiditis with other complication
K55.041	Focal (segmental) acute infarction of large intestine
K55.042	Diffuse acute infarction of large intestine
K55.1	Chronic vascular disorders of intestine
K55.8	Other vascular disorders of intestine
K62.2	Anal prolapse
K62.3	Rectal prolapse
K62.82	Dysplasia of anus
Q43.1	Hirschsprung's disease
Q43.2	Other congenital functional disorders of colon

AMA: **45112** 2014,Jan,11

Relative Value Units/Medicare Edits

Non-Facility RVU	Work	PE	MP	Total
45112	33.18	15.7	5.58	54.46
Facility RVU	**Work**	**PE**	**MP**	**Total**
45112	33.18	15.7	5.58	54.46

	FUD	Status	MUE	Modifiers				IOM Reference
45112	90	A	1(2)	51	N/A	62*	80	None

* with documentation

Terms To Know

Hirschsprung's disease. Congenital enlargement or dilation of the colon, with the absence of nerve cells in a segment of colon distally that causes the inability to defecate.

prolapse. Falling, sliding, or sinking of an organ from its normal location in the body.

regional enteritis. Chronic inflammation of unknown origin affecting the ileum and/or colon.

Rectum

45113

45113 Proctectomy, partial, with rectal mucosectomy, ileoanal anastomosis, creation of ileal reservoir (S or J), with or without loop ileostomy

The mucosal lining of the distal rectum and anus is surgically stripped prior to pulling through and suturing the newly formed ileal pouch

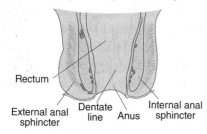

Example of J-shaped pouch

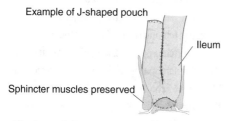

The reservoir is anastomosed to the anus, often at the dentate line, creating a neorectum. A loop colostomy may also be created well above this site to eliminate waste during the healing period

Explanation

The physician removes the proximal rectum, strips the mucosa from the distal rectum and performs an anastomosis between an ileal pouch and the anus. The physician makes an abdominal incision. The distal colon and rectum are mobilized within the abdomen to the level of the sphincter muscles. The colon is divided above the pelvic brim and the rectum is divided above the sphincter muscles and removed. The mucosa of the distal rectum is stripped from a perineal approach. The distal ileum is folded upon itself and approximated in order to form a reservoir. The ileal pouch is pulled through the remaining muscular cuff of distal rectum and sutured to the anus. A loop ileostomy may be formed proximal to the anastomosis. The incision is closed.

Coding Tips

For proctectomy, complete, combined abdominoperineal, with colostomy, see 45110; for partial resection of rectum, transabdominal approach, see 45111. For proctectomy, combined abdominoperineal, pull-through procedure (e.g., colo-anal anastomosis), see 45112. For proctectomy, partial, with anastomosis, abdominal and transsacral approach, see 45114; for transsacral approach only (Kraske type), see 45116. For proctectomy, complete (for congenital megacolon), abdominal and perineal approach, with pull-through procedure and anastomosis (e.g., Swenson, Duhamel, or Soave type operation), see 45120; with subtotal or total colectomy, with multiple biopsies, see 45121. For proctectomy, partial, without anastomosis, perineal approach, see 45123.

ICD-10-CM Diagnostic Codes

C19	Malignant neoplasm of rectosigmoid junction
C20	Malignant neoplasm of rectum
C21.1	Malignant neoplasm of anal canal
C21.2	Malignant neoplasm of cloacogenic zone
C21.8	Malignant neoplasm of overlapping sites of rectum, anus and anal canal
C49.A5	Gastrointestinal stromal tumor of rectum
C78.5	Secondary malignant neoplasm of large intestine and rectum
C7A.026	Malignant carcinoid tumor of the rectum
D01.1	Carcinoma in situ of rectosigmoid junction
D01.2	Carcinoma in situ of rectum
D37.5	Neoplasm of uncertain behavior of rectum
D3A.026	Benign carcinoid tumor of the rectum
K50.111	Crohn's disease of large intestine with rectal bleeding
K50.112	Crohn's disease of large intestine with intestinal obstruction
K50.113	Crohn's disease of large intestine with fistula
K50.114	Crohn's disease of large intestine with abscess
K50.118	Crohn's disease of large intestine with other complication
K51.211	Ulcerative (chronic) proctitis with rectal bleeding
K51.212	Ulcerative (chronic) proctitis with intestinal obstruction
K51.213	Ulcerative (chronic) proctitis with fistula
K51.214	Ulcerative (chronic) proctitis with abscess
K51.218	Ulcerative (chronic) proctitis with other complication
K51.311	Ulcerative (chronic) rectosigmoiditis with rectal bleeding
K51.312	Ulcerative (chronic) rectosigmoiditis with intestinal obstruction
K51.313	Ulcerative (chronic) rectosigmoiditis with fistula
K51.314	Ulcerative (chronic) rectosigmoiditis with abscess
K51.318	Ulcerative (chronic) rectosigmoiditis with other complication
K55.041	Focal (segmental) acute infarction of large intestine
K55.042	Diffuse acute infarction of large intestine
K55.1	Chronic vascular disorders of intestine
K55.8	Other vascular disorders of intestine
K62.2	Anal prolapse
K62.3	Rectal prolapse
K62.82	Dysplasia of anus
Q43.1	Hirschsprung's disease
Q43.2	Other congenital functional disorders of colon

AMA: 45113 2014,Jan,11

Relative Value Units/Medicare Edits

Non-Facility RVU	Work	PE	MP	Total
45113	33.22	17.08	4.25	54.55
Facility RVU	**Work**	**PE**	**MP**	**Total**
45113	33.22	17.08	4.25	54.55

	FUD	Status	MUE	Modifiers				IOM Reference
45113	90	A	1(2)	51	N/A	62*	80	None

* with documentation

Terms To Know

anastomosis. Surgically created connection between ducts, blood vessels, or bowel segments to allow flow from one to the other.

ileostomy. Artificial surgical opening that brings the end of the ileum out through the abdominal wall to the skin surface for the diversion of feces through a stoma.

proctectomy. Surgical resection of the rectum.

45114-45116

45114 Proctectomy, partial, with anastomosis; abdominal and transsacral approach
45116 transsacral approach only (Kraske type)

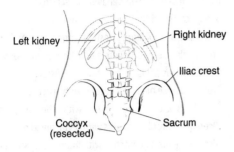

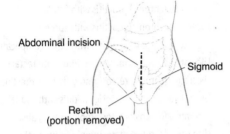

A portion of the rectum is resected and the remaining ends brought together and anastomosed

Explanation

The physician removes a portion of the rectum through a combined abdominal and transsacral approach (45114). The physician makes an abdominal incision. The proximal rectum and distal colon are mobilized and the colon is divided above the pelvic brim. An incision is made posteriorly at the junction of the sacrum and coccyx. The coccyx is excised. Dissection is continued posteriorly to further mobilize the rectum. The rectum is divided distally and the excised segment is removed. The distal end of colon is approximated to the remaining rectal stump with sutures or staples. The incisions are closed. Report 45116 when performed via the transsacral approach only.

Coding Tips

For proctectomy, complete, combined abdominoperineal, with colostomy, see 45110; for partial resection of the rectum, transabdominal approach, see 45111. For proctectomy, combined abdominoperineal, pull-through procedure (e.g., coloanal anastomosis), see 45112. For proctectomy, partial, with rectal mucosectomy, ileoanal anastomosis, creation of ileal reservoir (S or J), with or without loop ileostomy, see 45113. For proctectomy, complete (for congenital megacolon), abdominal and perineal approach, with pull-through procedure and anastomosis (e.g., Swenson, Duhamel, or Soave type operation), see 45120; with subtotal or total colectomy, with multiple biopsies, see 45121. For proctectomy, partial, without anastomosis, perineal approach, see 45123.

ICD-10-CM Diagnostic Codes

C19	Malignant neoplasm of rectosigmoid junction
C20	Malignant neoplasm of rectum
C21.1	Malignant neoplasm of anal canal
C21.2	Malignant neoplasm of cloacogenic zone
C21.8	Malignant neoplasm of overlapping sites of rectum, anus and anal canal
C49.A5	Gastrointestinal stromal tumor of rectum
C78.5	Secondary malignant neoplasm of large intestine and rectum
C7A.026	Malignant carcinoid tumor of the rectum
D01.1	Carcinoma in situ of rectosigmoid junction
D01.2	Carcinoma in situ of rectum
D37.5	Neoplasm of uncertain behavior of rectum
D3A.026	Benign carcinoid tumor of the rectum
K50.10	Crohn's disease of large intestine without complications
K50.111	Crohn's disease of large intestine with rectal bleeding
K50.112	Crohn's disease of large intestine with intestinal obstruction
K50.113	Crohn's disease of large intestine with fistula
K50.114	Crohn's disease of large intestine with abscess
K50.118	Crohn's disease of large intestine with other complication
K51.20	Ulcerative (chronic) proctitis without complications
K51.211	Ulcerative (chronic) proctitis with rectal bleeding
K51.212	Ulcerative (chronic) proctitis with intestinal obstruction
K51.213	Ulcerative (chronic) proctitis with fistula
K51.214	Ulcerative (chronic) proctitis with abscess
K51.218	Ulcerative (chronic) proctitis with other complication
K51.30	Ulcerative (chronic) rectosigmoiditis without complications
K51.311	Ulcerative (chronic) rectosigmoiditis with rectal bleeding
K51.312	Ulcerative (chronic) rectosigmoiditis with intestinal obstruction
K51.313	Ulcerative (chronic) rectosigmoiditis with fistula
K51.314	Ulcerative (chronic) rectosigmoiditis with abscess
K51.318	Ulcerative (chronic) rectosigmoiditis with other complication
K51.80	Other ulcerative colitis without complications
K55.041	Focal (segmental) acute infarction of large intestine
K55.042	Diffuse acute infarction of large intestine
K55.1	Chronic vascular disorders of intestine
K55.8	Other vascular disorders of intestine
K62.2	Anal prolapse
K62.3	Rectal prolapse
K62.82	Dysplasia of anus
Q43.1	Hirschsprung's disease
Q43.2	Other congenital functional disorders of colon

AMA: **45114** 2014,Jan,11 **45116** 2014,Jan,11

Relative Value Units/Medicare Edits

Non-Facility RVU	Work	PE	MP	Total
45114	30.79	15.42	7.55	53.76
45116	27.72	13.72	3.54	44.98
Facility RVU	**Work**	**PE**	**MP**	**Total**
45114	30.79	15.42	7.55	53.76
45116	27.72	13.72	3.54	44.98

	FUD	Status	MUE	Modifiers				IOM Reference
45114	90	A	1(2)	51	N/A	62*	80	None
45116	90	A	1(2)	51	N/A	62*	80	

* with documentation

45119

45119 Proctectomy, combined abdominoperineal pull-through procedure (eg, colo-anal anastomosis), with creation of colonic reservoir (eg, J-pouch), with diverting enterostomy when performed

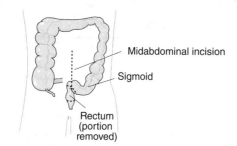

Midabdominal incision
Sigmoid
Rectum (portion removed)

Combined transperineal and abdominal approach

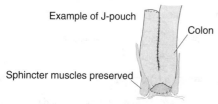

Example of J-pouch
Colon
Sphincter muscles preserved

A reservoir is fashioned and a portion pulled through the anus, often at the dentate line, creating a neorectum. A loop colostomy may also be created well above this site to eliminate waste during the healing period

Explanation

The physician surgically removes the rectum. The physician makes an abdominal incision, and the distal part of the diseased colon and rectum are mobilized down to the level of the anal sphincter muscles. The rectum is incised at the level of the sphincter muscles while the colon is incised above the pelvic brim where it is disease free. The diseased colon and rectum are removed. The free end of the distal colon is brought through the sphincter complex and approximated with the anus to form a colo-anal anastomosis. The distal colon is folded and sutured in such a way as to create a colonic reservoir pouch. The physician may elect to bring a loop or end of the colon through a separate abdominal incision to create a stoma (enterostomy). The incisions are sutured closed.

Coding Tips

For a pull-through procedure without creation of a colonic reservoir, see 45112. For a complete proctectomy for congenital megacolon, see 44120–44121. For laparoscopic approach, see 45397.

ICD-10-CM Diagnostic Codes

C19	Malignant neoplasm of rectosigmoid junction
C20	Malignant neoplasm of rectum
C21.1	Malignant neoplasm of anal canal
C21.2	Malignant neoplasm of cloacogenic zone
C21.8	Malignant neoplasm of overlapping sites of rectum, anus and anal canal
C49.A5	Gastrointestinal stromal tumor of rectum
C78.5	Secondary malignant neoplasm of large intestine and rectum
C7A.026	Malignant carcinoid tumor of the rectum
D01.1	Carcinoma in situ of rectosigmoid junction
D01.2	Carcinoma in situ of rectum
D37.5	Neoplasm of uncertain behavior of rectum

D3A.026	Benign carcinoid tumor of the rectum
K50.111	Crohn's disease of large intestine with rectal bleeding
K50.112	Crohn's disease of large intestine with intestinal obstruction
K50.113	Crohn's disease of large intestine with fistula
K50.114	Crohn's disease of large intestine with abscess
K50.118	Crohn's disease of large intestine with other complication
K51.20	Ulcerative (chronic) proctitis without complications
K51.211	Ulcerative (chronic) proctitis with rectal bleeding
K51.212	Ulcerative (chronic) proctitis with intestinal obstruction
K51.213	Ulcerative (chronic) proctitis with fistula
K51.214	Ulcerative (chronic) proctitis with abscess
K51.218	Ulcerative (chronic) proctitis with other complication
K51.311	Ulcerative (chronic) rectosigmoiditis with rectal bleeding
K51.312	Ulcerative (chronic) rectosigmoiditis with intestinal obstruction
K51.313	Ulcerative (chronic) rectosigmoiditis with fistula
K51.314	Ulcerative (chronic) rectosigmoiditis with abscess
K51.318	Ulcerative (chronic) rectosigmoiditis with other complication
K55.041	Focal (segmental) acute infarction of large intestine
K55.042	Diffuse acute infarction of large intestine
K55.1	Chronic vascular disorders of intestine
K55.8	Other vascular disorders of intestine
K62.2	Anal prolapse
K62.3	Rectal prolapse
K62.82	Dysplasia of anus
Q43.1	Hirschsprung's disease
Q43.2	Other congenital functional disorders of colon

AMA: **45119** 2018,Jan,8; 2017,Jan,8; 2016,Jan,13; 2015,Jan,16

Relative Value Units/Medicare Edits

Non-Facility RVU	Work	PE	MP	Total
45119	33.48	17.18	4.27	54.93
Facility RVU	**Work**	**PE**	**MP**	**Total**
45119	33.48	17.18	4.27	54.93

	FUD	Status	MUE	Modifiers				IOM Reference
45119	90	A	1(2)	51	N/A	62*	80	None

* with documentation

Terms To Know

anastomosis. Surgically created connection between ducts, blood vessels, or bowel segments to allow flow from one to the other.

neoplasm. New abnormal growth, tumor.

45120

45120 Proctectomy, complete (for congenital megacolon), abdominal and perineal approach; with pull-through procedure and anastomosis (eg, Swenson, Duhamel, or Soave type operation)

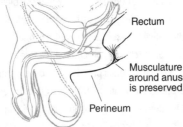

Abdominal and perineal incisions are used

Rectum

Musculature around anus is preserved

Perineum

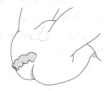

Soave type procedure involves stripping anal mucosa before the colon is pulled through

Explanation

The physician removes or bypasses the diseased rectal segment and performs an anastomosis of the colon and anus. The physician makes an abdominal incision. The rectum and distal colon are mobilized and the colon is divided just proximal to the diseased rectal segment. The rectal segment may be removed and the distal colon pulled through the sphincter complex and approximated to the anus with sutures from a perineal approach. Alternatively, the distal colon may be pulled down and approximated to the anus with sutures, bypassing the diseased rectal segment with a combined longitudinal anastomosis between the colon and the diseased rectal segment. The incision is closed.

Coding Tips

For proctectomy, complete, combined abdominoperineal, with colostomy, see 45110; for partial resection of rectum, transabdominal approach, see 45111. For proctectomy, combined abdominoperineal, pull-through procedure (e.g., colo-anal anastomosis), see 45112. For proctectomy, partial, with rectal mucosectomy, ileoanal anastomosis, creation of ileal reservoir (S or J), with or without loop ileostomy, see 45113. For proctectomy, complete (for congenital megacolon), abdominal and perineal approach, with subtotal or total colectomy, with multiple biopsies, see 45121. For proctectomy, partial, without anastomosis, perineal approach, see 45123.

ICD-10-CM Diagnostic Codes

Q43.1   Hirschsprung's disease

AMA: 45120 2014,Jan,11

Relative Value Units/Medicare Edits

Non-Facility RVU	Work	PE	MP	Total
45120	26.4	14.47	6.46	47.33
Facility RVU	**Work**	**PE**	**MP**	**Total**
45120	26.4	14.47	6.46	47.33

	FUD	Status	MUE	Modifiers				IOM Reference
45120	90	A	1(2)	51	N/A	62*	80	None

* with documentation

Terms To Know

anastomosis. Surgically created connection between ducts, blood vessels, or bowel segments to allow flow from one to the other.

bypass. Auxiliary or diverted route to maintain continuous flow.

closure. Repairing an incision or wound by suture or other means.

congenital. Present at birth, occurring through heredity or an influence during gestation up to the moment of birth.

distal. Located farther away from a specified reference point or the trunk.

Hirschsprung's disease. Congenital enlargement or dilation of the colon, with the absence of nerve cells in a segment of colon distally that causes the inability to defecate.

incision. Act of cutting into tissue or an organ.

mucous membranes. Thin sheets of tissue that secrete mucous and absorb water, salt, and other solutes. Mucous membranes cover or line cavities or canals of the body that open to the outside, such as linings of the mouth, respiratory and genitourinary passages, and the digestive tube.

perineal. Pertaining to the pelvic floor area between the thighs; the diamond-shaped area bordered by the pubic symphysis in front, the ischial tuberosities on the sides, and the coccyx in back.

proximal. Located closest to a specified reference point, usually the midline or trunk.

resect. Cutting out or removing a portion or all of a bone, organ, or other structure.

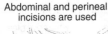

Rectum

45121

45121   Proctectomy, complete (for congenital megacolon), abdominal and perineal approach; with subtotal or total colectomy, with multiple biopsies

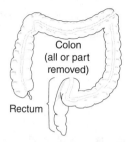

Colon
(all or part
removed)

Rectum

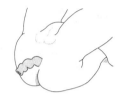

The remaining healthy bowel segment, colon or ileum, is "pulled through" the perineal incision

Explanation

The physician removes the rectum and part or all of the colon, and performs an anastomosis of the remaining colon or ileum and anus. The physician makes an abdominal incision. Multiple biopsies are taken of the colon wall to determine the level of disease. The involved rectum and colon are mobilized and removed. The remaining segment of colon or ileum is pulled through the sphincter complex and approximated to the anus with sutures from a perineal approach. Alternatively, the colon or ileum may be pulled down and approximated to the anus with sutures, bypassing a small remaining rectal segment with a combined longitudinal anastomosis to the rectal segment. The incision is closed.

Coding Tips

For proctectomy, complete, combined abdominoperineal, with colostomy, see 45110; for partial resection of rectum, transabdominal approach, see 45111. For proctectomy, combined abdominoperineal, pull-through procedure (e.g., colo-anal anastomosis), see 45112. For proctectomy, partial, with rectal mucosectomy, ileoanal anastomosis, creation of ileal reservoir (S or J), with or without loop ileostomy, see 45113. For proctectomy, complete (for congenital megacolon), abdominal and perineal approach, with pull-through procedure and anastomosis (e.g., Swenson, Duhamel, or Soave type operation), see 45120. For proctectomy, partial, without anastomosis, perineal approach, see 45123.

ICD-10-CM Diagnostic Codes

Q43.1   Hirschsprung's disease

AMA: 45121 2014,Jan,11

Relative Value Units/Medicare Edits

Non-Facility RVU	Work	PE	MP	Total
45121	29.08	15.47	7.11	51.66
Facility RVU	Work	PE	MP	Total
45121	29.08	15.47	7.11	51.66

	FUD	Status	MUE	Modifiers				IOM Reference
45121	90	A	1(2)	51	N/A	62*	80	None

* with documentation

Terms To Know

anastomosis. Surgically created connection between ducts, blood vessels, or bowel segments to allow flow from one to the other.

biopsy. Tissue or fluid removed for diagnostic purposes through analysis of the cells in the biopsy material.

closure. Repairing an incision or wound by suture or other means.

congenital. Present at birth, occurring through heredity or an influence during gestation up to the moment of birth.

Hirschsprung's disease. Congenital enlargement or dilation of the colon, with the absence of nerve cells in a segment of colon distally that causes the inability to defecate.

ileum. Lower portion of the small intestine, from the jejunum to the cecum.

incision. Act of cutting into tissue or an organ.

perineal. Pertaining to the pelvic floor area between the thighs; the diamond-shaped area bordered by the pubic symphysis in front, the ischial tuberosities on the sides, and the coccyx in back.

resection. Surgical removal of a part or all of an organ or body part.

Rectum

45123

45123 Proctectomy, partial, without anastomosis, perineal approach

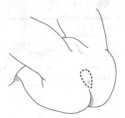

A perineal approach is used to resect a portion of the rectum

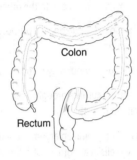

Colon

Rectum

Explanation

The physician removes a portion of the rectum through a perineal approach. The physician makes an incision around the anus. Dissection is continued around the anus to mobilize the anus and distal rectum. The anus and distal rectum are removed. A proximal colostomy may be formed. The incision is closed.

Coding Tips

For a partial proctectomy with rectal mucosectomy, ileoanal anastomosis, creation of ileal reservoir (S or J), with or without loop ileostomy, see 45113. For a partial proctectomy with anastomosis, abdominal and transsacral approach, see 45114; transsacral approach only (Kraske type), see 45116.

ICD-10-CM Diagnostic Codes

C19	Malignant neoplasm of rectosigmoid junction
C20	Malignant neoplasm of rectum
C21.1	Malignant neoplasm of anal canal
C21.2	Malignant neoplasm of cloacogenic zone
C21.8	Malignant neoplasm of overlapping sites of rectum, anus and anal canal
C49.A5	Gastrointestinal stromal tumor of rectum
C78.5	Secondary malignant neoplasm of large intestine and rectum
C7A.026	Malignant carcinoid tumor of the rectum
D01.1	Carcinoma in situ of rectosigmoid junction
D01.2	Carcinoma in situ of rectum
D37.5	Neoplasm of uncertain behavior of rectum
D3A.026	Benign carcinoid tumor of the rectum
K50.111	Crohn's disease of large intestine with rectal bleeding
K50.112	Crohn's disease of large intestine with intestinal obstruction
K50.113	Crohn's disease of large intestine with fistula
K50.114	Crohn's disease of large intestine with abscess
K50.118	Crohn's disease of large intestine with other complication

K51.211	Ulcerative (chronic) proctitis with rectal bleeding
K51.212	Ulcerative (chronic) proctitis with intestinal obstruction
K51.213	Ulcerative (chronic) proctitis with fistula
K51.214	Ulcerative (chronic) proctitis with abscess
K51.218	Ulcerative (chronic) proctitis with other complication
K51.311	Ulcerative (chronic) rectosigmoiditis with rectal bleeding
K51.312	Ulcerative (chronic) rectosigmoiditis with intestinal obstruction
K51.313	Ulcerative (chronic) rectosigmoiditis with fistula
K51.314	Ulcerative (chronic) rectosigmoiditis with abscess
K51.318	Ulcerative (chronic) rectosigmoiditis with other complication
K55.041	Focal (segmental) acute infarction of large intestine
K55.042	Diffuse acute infarction of large intestine
K55.1	Chronic vascular disorders of intestine
K55.8	Other vascular disorders of intestine
K62.2	Anal prolapse
K62.3	Rectal prolapse
K62.82	Dysplasia of anus
Q43.1	Hirschsprung's disease
Q43.2	Other congenital functional disorders of colon

AMA: 45123 2014,Jan,11

Relative Value Units/Medicare Edits

Non-Facility RVU	Work	PE	MP	Total
45123	18.86	10.64	3.14	32.64
Facility RVU	**Work**	**PE**	**MP**	**Total**
45123	18.86	10.64	3.14	32.64

	FUD	Status	MUE	Modifiers				IOM Reference
45123	90	A	1(2)	51	N/A	62*	80	None

* with documentation

Terms To Know

approach. Method or anatomical location used to gain access to a body organ or specific area for procedures.

colostomy. Artificial surgical opening anywhere along the length of the colon to the skin surface for the diversion of feces.

dissection. Separating by cutting tissue or body structures apart.

neoplasm. New abnormal growth, tumor.

perineal. Pertaining to the pelvic floor area between the thighs; the diamond-shaped area bordered by the pubic symphysis in front, the ischial tuberosities on the sides, and the coccyx in back.

prolapse. Falling, sliding, or sinking of an organ from its normal location in the body.

proximal. Located closest to a specified reference point, usually the midline or trunk.

resect. Cutting out or removing a portion or all of a bone, organ, or other structure.

Rectum

45126

45126 Pelvic exenteration for colorectal malignancy, with proctectomy (with or without colostomy), with removal of bladder and ureteral transplantations, and/or hysterectomy, or cervicectomy, with or without removal of tube(s), with or without removal of ovary(s), or any combination thereof

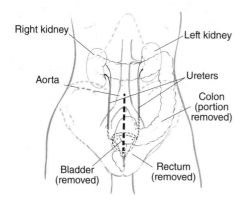

Right kidney / Left kidney / Aorta / Ureters / Colon (portion removed) / Bladder (removed) / Rectum (removed)

Explanation

The physician removes pelvic organs, with or without a colostomy, due to cancer of the colon and rectum. The physician makes an abdominal incision. The distal colon and rectum are mobilized and divided proximal and distal to the segment of interest. The pelvic organs are dissected free of surrounding structures and removed. The colon and rectum may be reapproximated or the proximal end of the colon may be brought out through a separate incision on the abdominal wall as a colostomy and the remaining rectum closed with staples or sutures. The initial incision is closed. In males the procedure may include removal of the prostate and bladder. In a female the procedure may include removal of the bladder and also the uterus, cervix, fallopian tubes, and/or ovaries depending upon the extent of the disease.

Coding Tips

Pelvic exenteration performed for a gynecologic malignancy should be reported with 58240; for lower urinary tract or male genital malignancy, see, 51597.

ICD-10-CM Diagnostic Codes

C18.0	Malignant neoplasm of cecum
C18.1	Malignant neoplasm of appendix
C18.2	Malignant neoplasm of ascending colon
C18.3	Malignant neoplasm of hepatic flexure
C18.4	Malignant neoplasm of transverse colon
C18.5	Malignant neoplasm of splenic flexure
C18.6	Malignant neoplasm of descending colon
C18.7	Malignant neoplasm of sigmoid colon
C18.8	Malignant neoplasm of overlapping sites of colon
C19	Malignant neoplasm of rectosigmoid junction
C20	Malignant neoplasm of rectum
C21.1	Malignant neoplasm of anal canal
C21.2	Malignant neoplasm of cloacogenic zone
C21.8	Malignant neoplasm of overlapping sites of rectum, anus and anal canal
C49.A4	Gastrointestinal stromal tumor of large intestine
C49.A5	Gastrointestinal stromal tumor of rectum

C78.5	Secondary malignant neoplasm of large intestine and rectum
C7A.020	Malignant carcinoid tumor of the appendix
C7A.021	Malignant carcinoid tumor of the cecum
C7A.022	Malignant carcinoid tumor of the ascending colon
C7A.023	Malignant carcinoid tumor of the transverse colon
C7A.024	Malignant carcinoid tumor of the descending colon
C7A.025	Malignant carcinoid tumor of the sigmoid colon
C7A.026	Malignant carcinoid tumor of the rectum
K62.7	Radiation proctitis
K62.89	Other specified diseases of anus and rectum
K63.0	Abscess of intestine
K65.0	Generalized (acute) peritonitis
K68.19	Other retroperitoneal abscess
K68.9	Other disorders of retroperitoneum

AMA: 45126 2014,Jan,11

Relative Value Units/Medicare Edits

Non-Facility RVU	Work	PE	MP	Total
45126	49.1	23.65	7.55	80.3
Facility RVU	**Work**	**PE**	**MP**	**Total**
45126	49.1	23.65	7.55	80.3

	FUD	Status	MUE	Modifiers				IOM Reference
45126	90	A	1(2)	51	N/A	62*	80	None

* with documentation

Terms To Know

colostomy. Artificial surgical opening anywhere along the length of the colon to the skin surface for the diversion of feces.

dissect. Cut apart or separate tissue for surgical purposes or for visual or microscopic study.

distal. Located farther away from a specified reference point or the trunk.

division. Separating into two or more parts.

exenteration. Surgical removal of the entire contents of a body cavity, such as the pelvis or orbit.

malignant. Any condition tending to progress toward death, specifically an invasive tumor with a loss of cellular differentiation that has the ability to spread or metastasize to other body areas.

proximal. Located closest to a specified reference point, usually the midline or trunk.

Rectum

45130-45135

45130 Excision of rectal procidentia, with anastomosis; perineal approach
45135 abdominal and perineal approach

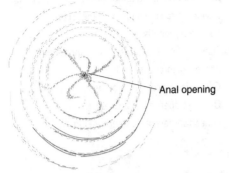

Prolapsed rectum (procidentia) forms concentric folds of tissue outside the perineum

Anal opening

The descended rectum is resected and redundant tissue eliminated. The remaining rectum may require fixation to surrounding structures to prevent future prolapse

Explanation

The physician removes a rectal prolapse through a combined abdominal and perineal approach. The physician makes an abdominal incision. The proximal colon and rectum are mobilized. The rectum and colon are prolapsed through the anus. A circular incision is made through the distal rectum at the anorectal junction from a perineal approach. The mesentery and blood supply to the prolapsed rectum is divided and the segment is telescoped out through the anus. The proximal rectum or colon is divided and the prolapsed segment is removed. The proximal end of rectum or colon is approximated the anus with sutures or staples. The incision is closed. Report 45130 when only a perineal approach is used.

Coding Tips

For perirectal injection of sclerosing solution for prolapse, see 45520. For reduction of procidentia under anesthesia, see 45900. For proctopexy for prolapse, abdominal approach, see 45540; perineal, see 45541; with sigmoid resection, abdominal approach, see 45550.

ICD-10-CM Diagnostic Codes

K62.3   Rectal prolapse

AMA: 45130 2014,Jan,11 **45135** 2014,Jan,11

Relative Value Units/Medicare Edits

Non-Facility RVU	Work	PE	MP	Total
45130	18.5	10.19	2.98	31.67
45135	22.36	12.5	2.85	37.71
Facility RVU	**Work**	**PE**	**MP**	**Total**
45130	18.5	10.19	2.98	31.67
45135	22.36	12.5	2.85	37.71

	FUD	Status	MUE	Modifiers				IOM Reference
45130	90	A	1(2)	51	N/A	62*	80	None
45135	90	A	1(2)	51	N/A	62*	80	

* with documentation

45136

45136 Excision of ileoanal reservoir with ileostomy

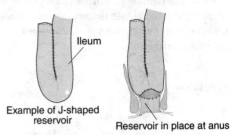

Ileum

Example of J-shaped reservoir

Reservoir in place at anus

The terminal ileum had been formed into an S-shaped or J-shaped reservoir. The reservoir is removed in this procedure

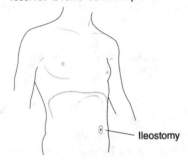

Ileostomy

Explanation

The physician excises an ileoanal reservoir and creates an ileostomy. The physician makes an abdominal incision. Dissection is carried down to the site of the ileoanal reservoir. The reservoir is excised at the level where the ileum was previously anastomosed to the anus. The anus is closed. The loose end of the ileum may be trimmed. A disk of skin is excised from the abdominal wall and the terminal ileum is brought out through the split rectus muscle and the opening in the abdomen to form a stoma on the abdominal wall. An anastomosis is performed via the transanal approach and the full thickness of the ileum is sutured to the anal canal. Interrupted sutures complete the ileostomy construction.

Coding Tips

Do not report 45136 with 44005 or 44310. For proctectomy, partial, with rectal mucosectomy, ileoanal anastomosis, creation of ileal reservoir (S or J), with or without loop ileostomy, see 45113.

ICD-10-CM Diagnostic Codes

C18.0	Malignant neoplasm of cecum
C18.1	Malignant neoplasm of appendix
C18.2	Malignant neoplasm of ascending colon
C18.3	Malignant neoplasm of hepatic flexure
C18.4	Malignant neoplasm of transverse colon
C18.5	Malignant neoplasm of splenic flexure
C18.6	Malignant neoplasm of descending colon
C18.7	Malignant neoplasm of sigmoid colon
C18.8	Malignant neoplasm of overlapping sites of colon
C19	Malignant neoplasm of rectosigmoid junction
C78.5	Secondary malignant neoplasm of large intestine and rectum
C7A.020	Malignant carcinoid tumor of the appendix
C7A.021	Malignant carcinoid tumor of the cecum

C7A.022	Malignant carcinoid tumor of the ascending colon	
C7A.023	Malignant carcinoid tumor of the transverse colon	
C7A.024	Malignant carcinoid tumor of the descending colon	
C7A.025	Malignant carcinoid tumor of the sigmoid colon	
D01.0	Carcinoma in situ of colon	
D01.1	Carcinoma in situ of rectosigmoid junction	
D01.2	Carcinoma in situ of rectum	
D01.49	Carcinoma in situ of other parts of intestine	
D12.0	Benign neoplasm of cecum	
D12.1	Benign neoplasm of appendix	
D12.2	Benign neoplasm of ascending colon	
D12.3	Benign neoplasm of transverse colon	
D12.4	Benign neoplasm of descending colon	
D12.5	Benign neoplasm of sigmoid colon	
D12.7	Benign neoplasm of rectosigmoid junction	
D12.8	Benign neoplasm of rectum	
D37.3	Neoplasm of uncertain behavior of appendix	
D37.4	Neoplasm of uncertain behavior of colon	
D37.5	Neoplasm of uncertain behavior of rectum	
D3A.020	Benign carcinoid tumor of the appendix	
D3A.021	Benign carcinoid tumor of the cecum	
D3A.022	Benign carcinoid tumor of the ascending colon	
D3A.023	Benign carcinoid tumor of the transverse colon	
D3A.024	Benign carcinoid tumor of the descending colon	
D3A.025	Benign carcinoid tumor of the sigmoid colon	
D3A.026	Benign carcinoid tumor of the rectum	
D49.0	Neoplasm of unspecified behavior of digestive system	
K50.111	Crohn's disease of large intestine with rectal bleeding	
K50.112	Crohn's disease of large intestine with intestinal obstruction	
K50.113	Crohn's disease of large intestine with fistula	
K50.114	Crohn's disease of large intestine with abscess	
K50.118	Crohn's disease of large intestine with other complication	
K50.812	Crohn's disease of both small and large intestine with intestinal obstruction	
K50.813	Crohn's disease of both small and large intestine with fistula	
K50.814	Crohn's disease of both small and large intestine with abscess	
K51.00	Ulcerative (chronic) pancolitis without complications	
K51.011	Ulcerative (chronic) pancolitis with rectal bleeding	
K51.012	Ulcerative (chronic) pancolitis with intestinal obstruction	
K51.013	Ulcerative (chronic) pancolitis with fistula	
K51.014	Ulcerative (chronic) pancolitis with abscess	
K51.018	Ulcerative (chronic) pancolitis with other complication	
K51.211	Ulcerative (chronic) proctitis with rectal bleeding	
K51.212	Ulcerative (chronic) proctitis with intestinal obstruction	
K51.213	Ulcerative (chronic) proctitis with fistula	
K51.214	Ulcerative (chronic) proctitis with abscess	
K51.218	Ulcerative (chronic) proctitis with other complication	
K51.311	Ulcerative (chronic) rectosigmoiditis with rectal bleeding	
K51.312	Ulcerative (chronic) rectosigmoiditis with intestinal obstruction	
K51.313	Ulcerative (chronic) rectosigmoiditis with fistula	
K51.314	Ulcerative (chronic) rectosigmoiditis with abscess	
K51.318	Ulcerative (chronic) rectosigmoiditis with other complication	
K51.511	Left sided colitis with rectal bleeding	

K51.512	Left sided colitis with intestinal obstruction
K51.513	Left sided colitis with fistula
K51.514	Left sided colitis with abscess
K51.518	Left sided colitis with other complication
K51.811	Other ulcerative colitis with rectal bleeding
K51.812	Other ulcerative colitis with intestinal obstruction
K51.813	Other ulcerative colitis with fistula
K51.814	Other ulcerative colitis with abscess
K51.818	Other ulcerative colitis with other complication
K55.041	Focal (segmental) acute infarction of large intestine
K55.042	Diffuse acute infarction of large intestine
K55.1	Chronic vascular disorders of intestine
K59.81	Ogilvie syndrome
K63.1	Perforation of intestine (nontraumatic)
K63.5	Polyp of colon
K63.89	Other specified diseases of intestine
P77.1	Stage 1 necrotizing enterocolitis in newborn **N**
P77.2	Stage 2 necrotizing enterocolitis in newborn **N**
P77.3	Stage 3 necrotizing enterocolitis in newborn **N**

AMA: 45136 2014,Jan,11

Relative Value Units/Medicare Edits

Non-Facility RVU	Work	PE	MP	Total
45136	30.82	17.47	3.95	52.24
Facility RVU	**Work**	**PE**	**MP**	**Total**
45136	30.82	17.47	3.95	52.24

	FUD	Status	MUE	Modifiers				IOM Reference
45136	90	A	1(2)	51	N/A	62*	80	None

* with documentation

Terms To Know

anastomosis. Surgically created connection between ducts, blood vessels, or bowel segments to allow flow from one to the other.

approach. Method or anatomical location used to gain access to a body organ or specific area for procedures.

dissection. (dis. apart; -section, act of cutting) Separating by cutting tissue or body structures apart.

excision. Surgical removal of an organ or tissue.

ileostomy. Artificial surgical opening that brings the end of the ileum out through the abdominal wall to the skin surface for the diversion of feces through a stoma.

ileum. Lower portion of the small intestine, from the jejunum to the cecum.

reservoir. Space or body cavity for storage of liquid.

stoma. Opening created in the abdominal wall from an internal organ or structure for diversion of waste elimination, drainage, and access.

Rectum

45150

45150   Division of stricture of rectum

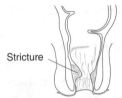

An anal stricture is divided. The approach is usually from the anus and incisions are placed horizontally around the circumference of the restricted area

Explanation

The physician performs division of a rectal stricture. The physician makes longitudinal incisions in the scar tissue in one or more places circumferentially around the strictured area of the rectal mucosa. A dilatation of the strictured area may be performed. In addition, the internal anal sphincter may be incised as part of the procedure.

Coding Tips

For perirectal injection of sclerosing solution for prolapse, see 45520. For reduction of procidentia under anesthesia, see 45900. For proctopexy for prolapse, abdominal approach, see 45540; for perineal approach, see 45541. For proctopexy combined with sigmoid resection, abdominal approach, see 45550.

ICD-10-CM Diagnostic Codes

K62.4   Stenosis of anus and rectum

AMA: 45150 2014,Jan,11

Relative Value Units/Medicare Edits

Non-Facility RVU	Work	PE	MP	Total
45150	5.85	5.22	1.44	12.51
Facility RVU	**Work**	**PE**	**MP**	**Total**
45150	5.85	5.22	1.44	12.51

	FUD	Status	MUE	Modifiers				IOM Reference
45150	90	A	1(2)	51	N/A	N/A	80*	None

* with documentation

45160

45160   Excision of rectal tumor by proctotomy, transsacral or transcoccygeal approach

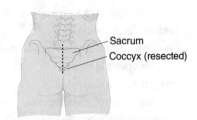

A rectal tumor is excised through removal of a portion of the rectum (proctotomy)

Explanation

The physician removes a rectal tumor through a transsacral or transcoccygeal approach. The physician makes an incision at the junction of the sacrum and coccyx. The coccyx is excised and dissection is continued posteriorly to mobilize the rectum. The tumor is identified, an incision is made in the rectum (proctotomy), and the tumor is excised. The rectum is closed with sutures or staples. The initial incision is closed.

Coding Tips

Excision of a rectal tumor by transanal approach is reported with 45171–45172; destruction by transanal approach, see 45190. For proctosigmoidoscopy, rigid, with removal of a single tumor, polyp, or other lesion by hot biopsy forceps or bipolar cautery, see 45308; with removal of a single tumor, polyp, or other lesion by snare technique, see 45309; with removal of multiple tumors, polyps, or other lesions by hot biopsy forceps, bipolar cautery, or snare technique, see 45315; ablation of tumors, polyps, or other lesions, see 45320.

ICD-10-CM Diagnostic Codes

C19	Malignant neoplasm of rectosigmoid junction
C20	Malignant neoplasm of rectum
C21.2	Malignant neoplasm of cloacogenic zone
C21.8	Malignant neoplasm of overlapping sites of rectum, anus and anal canal
C49.A5	Gastrointestinal stromal tumor of rectum
C78.5	Secondary malignant neoplasm of large intestine and rectum
C7A.026	Malignant carcinoid tumor of the rectum
D01.1	Carcinoma in situ of rectosigmoid junction
D01.2	Carcinoma in situ of rectum
D01.7	Carcinoma in situ of other specified digestive organs
D12.7	Benign neoplasm of rectosigmoid junction
D12.8	Benign neoplasm of rectum
D37.5	Neoplasm of uncertain behavior of rectum
D3A.026	Benign carcinoid tumor of the rectum
D49.0	Neoplasm of unspecified behavior of digestive system

AMA: 45160 2014,Jan,11

Coding Companion for General Surgery/Gastroenterology

Rectum

Relative Value Units/Medicare Edits

Non-Facility RVU	Work	PE	MP	Total
45160	16.33	10.04	4.01	30.38
Facility RVU	Work	PE	MP	Total
45160	16.33	10.04	4.01	30.38

	FUD	Status	MUE	Modifiers				IOM Reference
45160	90	A	1(3)	51	N/A	62*	80	None

* with documentation

Terms To Know

approach. Method or anatomical location used to gain access to a body organ or specific area for procedures. The approach is not coded separately although it may be a specified component of the procedure, such as laparoscopic versus incisional, or spinal procedures in which the amount of dissection required to expose the spine significantly alters with the site of approach.

coccyx. Lowest extremity of the vertebral column, formed by the fusion of three to five rudimentary vertebral segments under the sacrum.

excision. Surgical removal of an organ or tissue.

sacrum. Lower portion of the spine composed of five fused vertebrae designated as S1-S5.

tumor. Pathological swelling or enlargement; a neoplastic growth of uncontrolled, abnormal multiplication of cells.

45171-45172

45171 Excision of rectal tumor, transanal approach; not including muscularis propria (ie, partial thickness)
45172 including muscularis propria (ie, full thickness)

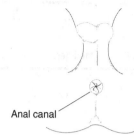

Anal canal

A rectal tumor is excised through removal of a portion of the rectum (proctotomy)

Explanation

The physician removes a rectal tumor through a transanal approach. The physician explores the anal canal and exposes the tumor. Report 45171 for a partial thickness excision (one that excludes the muscularis propria) and 45172 for a full thickness excision (including the muscularis propria). The defect in the rectum is closed with sutures.

Coding Tips

For destruction of a rectal tumor by transanal approach, see 45190. For excision of a rectal tumor by proctotomy, transsacral or transcoccygeal approach, report 45160. To report a transanal endoscopic microsurgical (e.g., TEMS) excision of a rectal tumor, including muscularis propria (e.g., full thickness), see 0184T.

ICD-10-CM Diagnostic Codes

C19	Malignant neoplasm of rectosigmoid junction
C20	Malignant neoplasm of rectum
C21.2	Malignant neoplasm of cloacogenic zone
C21.8	Malignant neoplasm of overlapping sites of rectum, anus and anal canal
C49.A5	Gastrointestinal stromal tumor of rectum
C78.5	Secondary malignant neoplasm of large intestine and rectum
C7A.026	Malignant carcinoid tumor of the rectum
D01.1	Carcinoma in situ of rectosigmoid junction
D01.2	Carcinoma in situ of rectum
D01.7	Carcinoma in situ of other specified digestive organs
D12.7	Benign neoplasm of rectosigmoid junction
D12.8	Benign neoplasm of rectum
D37.5	Neoplasm of uncertain behavior of rectum
D3A.026	Benign carcinoid tumor of the rectum
D49.0	Neoplasm of unspecified behavior of digestive system

AMA: 45171 2018,Jan,8; 2017,Jan,8; 2016,Jan,13; 2015,Jan,16 **45172** 2018,Jan,8; 2018,Feb,11; 2017,Jan,8; 2016,Jan,13; 2015,Jan,16

Rectum

Relative Value Units/Medicare Edits

Non-Facility RVU	Work	PE	MP	Total
45171	8.13	8.72	1.49	18.34
45172	12.13	10.18	2.05	24.36
Facility RVU	Work	PE	MP	Total
45171	8.13	8.72	1.49	18.34
45172	12.13	10.18	2.05	24.36

	FUD	Status	MUE	Modifiers				IOM Reference
45171	90	A	2(3)	51	N/A	62*	80	None
45172	90	A	2(3)	51	N/A	62*	80	

* with documentation

Terms To Know

defect. Imperfection, flaw, or absence.

excision. Surgical removal of an organ or tissue.

full thickness. Consisting of skin and subcutaneous tissue.

malignant neoplasm. Any cancerous tumor or lesion exhibiting uncontrolled tissue growth that can progressively invade other parts of the body with its disease-generating cells.

tumor. Pathological swelling or enlargement; a neoplastic growth of uncontrolled, abnormal multiplication of cells.

45190

45190 Destruction of rectal tumor (eg, electrodesiccation, electrosurgery, laser ablation, laser resection, cryosurgery) transanal approach

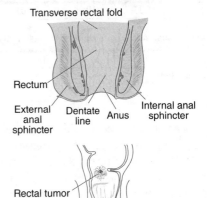

A rectal tumor is approached from the anus and destroyed

Explanation

The physician performs destruction of a rectal tumor from a transanal approach. The physician explores the anal canal and exposes the tumor. The tumor is ablated by electrosurgery, laser, freezing (cryosurgery), or some other method.

Coding Tips

For excision of a rectal tumor by proctotomy, transsacral or transcoccygeal approach, see 45160. For excision of a rectal tumor, transanal approach, not including muscularis propria (e.g., full thickness), see 45171; including muscularis propria, see 45172.

ICD-10-CM Diagnostic Codes

C19	Malignant neoplasm of rectosigmoid junction
C20	Malignant neoplasm of rectum
C21.2	Malignant neoplasm of cloacogenic zone
C21.8	Malignant neoplasm of overlapping sites of rectum, anus and anal canal
C49.A5	Gastrointestinal stromal tumor of rectum
C78.5	Secondary malignant neoplasm of large intestine and rectum
C7A.026	Malignant carcinoid tumor of the rectum
D01.1	Carcinoma in situ of rectosigmoid junction
D01.2	Carcinoma in situ of rectum
D12.7	Benign neoplasm of rectosigmoid junction
D12.8	Benign neoplasm of rectum
D37.5	Neoplasm of uncertain behavior of rectum
D3A.026	Benign carcinoid tumor of the rectum

AMA: **45190** 2018,Jan,8; 2017,Jan,8; 2016,Jan,13; 2015,Jan,16

Rectum

Relative Value Units/Medicare Edits

Non-Facility RVU	Work	PE	MP	Total
45190	10.42	8.79	1.62	20.83
Facility RVU	Work	PE	MP	Total
45190	10.42	8.79	1.62	20.83

	FUD	Status	MUE	Modifiers				IOM Reference
45190	90	A	1(3)	51	N/A	62*	N/A	None

* with documentation

Terms To Know

ablation. Removal or destruction of a body part or tissue or its function. Ablation may be performed by surgical means, hormones, drugs, radiofrequency, heat, chemical application, or other methods.

anomaly. Irregularity in the structure or position of an organ or tissue.

carcinoma in situ. Malignancy that arises from the cells of the vessel, gland, or organ of origin that remains confined to that site or has not invaded neighboring tissue.

cryosurgery. Application of intense cold, usually produced using liquid nitrogen, to locally freeze diseased or unwanted tissue and induce tissue necrosis without causing harm to adjacent tissue.

destruction. Ablation or eradication of a structure or tissue.

electrocautery. Division or cutting of tissue using high-frequency electrical current to produce heat, which destroys cells.

laser surgery. Use of concentrated, sharply defined light beams to cut, cauterize, coagulate, seal, or vaporize tissue.

45300-45305

45300	Proctosigmoidoscopy, rigid; diagnostic, with or without collection of specimen(s) by brushing or washing (separate procedure)
45303	with dilation (eg, balloon, guide wire, bougie)
45305	with biopsy, single or multiple

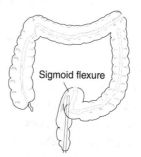

Sigmoid flexure

A rigid proctosigmoid examination is performed. Usually access beyond the sigmoid flexure is limited due to the rigidity of the scope

Explanation

The physician performs rigid proctosigmoidoscopy in addition to other procedures. The physician inserts the rigid proctosigmoidoscope into the anus and advances the scope. The sigmoid colon and rectal lumen are visualized. Brushings or washings may be obtained (45300), a stricture may be identified and dilated with a balloon or device (45303) or biopsies may be obtained of suspicious areas (45305). The proctosigmoidoscope is removed at the completion of the procedure.

Coding Tips

Note that 45300 is a separate procedure by definition and is usually a component of a more complex service and is not identified separately. When performed alone or with other unrelated procedures/services it may be reported. Surgical endoscopy includes diagnostic endoscopy; however, diagnostic endoscopy can be identified separately when performed at the same surgical session as an open procedure. Proctosigmoidoscopy codes are reported only when a rigid proctoscope (stiff hollow tube-like instrument) is used. If a flexible instrument is used, flexible sigmoidoscopy codes should be reported. For radiological supervision and interpretation related to dilation of a stricture, see 74360.

ICD-10-CM Diagnostic Codes

C18.7	Malignant neoplasm of sigmoid colon
C19	Malignant neoplasm of rectosigmoid junction
C20	Malignant neoplasm of rectum
C21.1	Malignant neoplasm of anal canal
C21.2	Malignant neoplasm of cloacogenic zone
C49.A4	Gastrointestinal stromal tumor of large intestine
C49.A5	Gastrointestinal stromal tumor of rectum
C7A.025	Malignant carcinoid tumor of the sigmoid colon
C7A.026	Malignant carcinoid tumor of the rectum
D01.0	Carcinoma in situ of colon
D01.1	Carcinoma in situ of rectosigmoid junction
D01.2	Carcinoma in situ of rectum
D01.3	Carcinoma in situ of anus and anal canal
D12.5	Benign neoplasm of sigmoid colon
D12.7	Benign neoplasm of rectosigmoid junction

Rectum

D12.8	Benign neoplasm of rectum
D12.9	Benign neoplasm of anus and anal canal
D37.4	Neoplasm of uncertain behavior of colon
D37.5	Neoplasm of uncertain behavior of rectum
D3A.025	Benign carcinoid tumor of the sigmoid colon
D3A.026	Benign carcinoid tumor of the rectum
K50.111	Crohn's disease of large intestine with rectal bleeding
K50.112	Crohn's disease of large intestine with intestinal obstruction
K50.812	Crohn's disease of both small and large intestine with intestinal obstruction
K50.813	Crohn's disease of both small and large intestine with fistula
K50.814	Crohn's disease of both small and large intestine with abscess
K51.011	Ulcerative (chronic) pancolitis with rectal bleeding
K51.012	Ulcerative (chronic) pancolitis with intestinal obstruction
K51.014	Ulcerative (chronic) pancolitis with abscess
K51.212	Ulcerative (chronic) proctitis with intestinal obstruction
K51.213	Ulcerative (chronic) proctitis with fistula
K51.214	Ulcerative (chronic) proctitis with abscess
K51.312	Ulcerative (chronic) rectosigmoiditis with intestinal obstruction
K51.314	Ulcerative (chronic) rectosigmoiditis with abscess
K51.411	Inflammatory polyps of colon with rectal bleeding
K51.412	Inflammatory polyps of colon with intestinal obstruction
K51.413	Inflammatory polyps of colon with fistula
K51.414	Inflammatory polyps of colon with abscess
K51.512	Left sided colitis with intestinal obstruction
K51.513	Left sided colitis with fistula
K51.514	Left sided colitis with abscess
K52.0	Gastroenteritis and colitis due to radiation
K52.1	Toxic gastroenteritis and colitis
K52.21	Food protein-induced enterocolitis syndrome
K52.22	Food protein-induced enteropathy
K52.82	Eosinophilic colitis
K55.041	Focal (segmental) acute infarction of large intestine
K55.042	Diffuse acute infarction of large intestine
K55.1	Chronic vascular disorders of intestine
K55.20	Angiodysplasia of colon without hemorrhage
K55.21	Angiodysplasia of colon with hemorrhage
K56.1	Intussusception
K56.2	Volvulus
K56.51	Intestinal adhesions [bands], with partial obstruction
K56.52	Intestinal adhesions [bands] with complete obstruction
K57.21	Diverticulitis of large intestine with perforation and abscess with bleeding
K57.31	Diverticulosis of large intestine without perforation or abscess with bleeding
K57.32	Diverticulitis of large intestine without perforation or abscess without bleeding
K57.40	Diverticulitis of both small and large intestine with perforation and abscess without bleeding
K57.41	Diverticulitis of both small and large intestine with perforation and abscess with bleeding
K58.0	Irritable bowel syndrome with diarrhea
K58.9	Irritable bowel syndrome without diarrhea
K59.01	Slow transit constipation

K59.02	Outlet dysfunction constipation
K59.1	Functional diarrhea
K60.3	Anal fistula
K60.4	Rectal fistula
K60.5	Anorectal fistula
K61.0	Anal abscess
K61.1	Rectal abscess
K61.2	Anorectal abscess
K61.31	Horseshoe abscess
K61.39	Other ischiorectal abscess
K61.4	Intrasphincteric abscess
K62.0	Anal polyp
K62.1	Rectal polyp
K62.2	Anal prolapse
K62.3	Rectal prolapse
K62.5	Hemorrhage of anus and rectum
K62.6	Ulcer of anus and rectum
K62.7	Radiation proctitis
K63.5	Polyp of colon
K64.0	First degree hemorrhoids
K64.1	Second degree hemorrhoids
K64.2	Third degree hemorrhoids
K64.3	Fourth degree hemorrhoids
M35.08	Sjögren syndrome with gastrointestinal involvement
Q42.0	Congenital absence, atresia and stenosis of rectum with fistula
Q42.1	Congenital absence, atresia and stenosis of rectum without fistula
Q42.2	Congenital absence, atresia and stenosis of anus with fistula
Q42.3	Congenital absence, atresia and stenosis of anus without fistula
Q43.1	Hirschsprung's disease

AMA: **45300** 2018,Jan,8; 2017,Jan,8; 2016,Jan,13; 2015,Jan,16 **45303** 2018,Jan,8; 2017,Jan,8; 2016,Jan,13; 2015,Jan,16 **45305** 2018,Jan,8; 2017,Jan,8; 2016,Jan,13; 2015,Jan,16

Relative Value Units/Medicare Edits

Non-Facility RVU	Work	PE	MP	Total
45300	0.8	2.99	0.13	3.92
45303	1.4	28.46	0.21	30.07
45305	1.15	4.06	0.2	5.41
Facility RVU	Work	PE	MP	Total
45300	0.8	0.48	0.13	1.41
45303	1.4	0.85	0.21	2.46
45305	1.15	0.78	0.2	2.13

	FUD	Status	MUE	Modifiers				IOM Reference
45300	0	A	1(3)	51	N/A	N/A	N/A	None
45303	0	A	1(3)	51	N/A	N/A	N/A	
45305	0	A	1(2)	51	N/A	N/A	N/A	

* with documentation

45307

45307 Proctosigmoidoscopy, rigid; with removal of foreign body

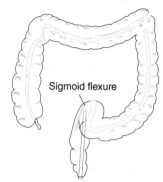

A rigid proctosigmoid examination is performed. Usually access beyond the sigmoid flexure is limited due to the rigidity of the scope

Sigmoid flexure

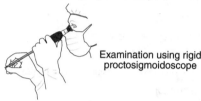

Examination using rigid proctosigmoidoscope

Explanation

The physician performs rigid proctosigmoidoscopy and removes a foreign body. The physician inserts the rigid proctosigmoidoscope into the anus and advances the scope. The sigmoid colon and rectal lumen are visualized and the foreign body is identified. The foreign body is removed by a snare or forceps inserted through the scope. The proctosigmoidoscope is removed at the completion of the procedure.

Coding Tips

Report the appropriate endoscopy for each anatomic site examined. Surgical endoscopy includes diagnostic endoscopy; however, diagnostic endoscopy can be identified separately when performed at the same surgical session as an open procedure. Proctosigmoidoscopy codes are reported only when a rigid proctoscope (stiff hollow tube-like instrument) is used. If a flexible instrument is used, flexible sigmoidoscopy codes should be reported. For sigmoidoscopy, flexible, with removal of a foreign body, see 45332. For colonoscopy, flexible, with removal of a foreign body, see 45379. For anoscopy, with removal of a foreign body, see 46608.

ICD-10-CM Diagnostic Codes

K62.5	Hemorrhage of anus and rectum
K62.89	Other specified diseases of anus and rectum
K92.1	Melena
T18.4XXA	Foreign body in colon, initial encounter
T18.5XXA	Foreign body in anus and rectum, initial encounter

AMA: **45307** 2018,Jan,8; 2017,Jan,8; 2016,Jan,13; 2015,Jan,16

Relative Value Units/Medicare Edits

Non-Facility RVU	Work	PE	MP	Total
45307	1.6	4.26	0.21	6.07
Facility RVU	**Work**	**PE**	**MP**	**Total**
45307	1.6	0.98	0.21	2.79

	FUD	Status	MUE	Modifiers				IOM Reference
45307	0	A	1(3)	51	N/A	N/A	80*	None

* with documentation

Terms To Know

endoscopy. Visual inspection of the body using a fiberoptic scope.

forceps. Tool used for grasping or compressing tissue.

foreign body. Any object or substance found in an organ and tissue that does not belong under normal circumstances.

hemorrhage. Internal or external bleeding with loss of significant amounts of blood.

lumen. Space inside an intestine, artery, vein, duct, or tube.

proctosigmoidoscope. Instrument used for examination of the sigmoid colon and rectum.

sigmoidoscopy. Endoscopic examination of the entire rectum and sigmoid colon, often including a portion of the descending colon and usually performed with a flexible fiberoptic scope in conjunction with a surgical procedure.

snare. Wire used as a loop to excise a polyp or lesion.

45308-45315

45308 Proctosigmoidoscopy, rigid; with removal of single tumor, polyp, or other lesion by hot biopsy forceps or bipolar cautery

45309 with removal of single tumor, polyp, or other lesion by snare technique

45315 with removal of multiple tumors, polyps, or other lesions by hot biopsy forceps, bipolar cautery or snare technique

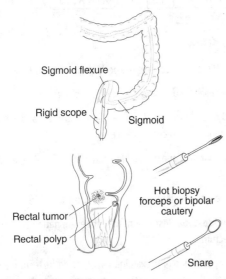

Sigmoid flexure

Rigid scope

Sigmoid

Rectal tumor

Rectal polyp

Hot biopsy forceps or bipolar cautery

Snare

Single or multiple tumors, polyps, or other lesions are removed by hot biopsy, bipolar cautery, or snare technique

Explanation

The physician performs rigid proctosigmoidoscopy and removes a tumor, polyp, or other lesion. The physician inserts the rigid proctosigmoidoscope into the anus and advances the scope. The sigmoid colon and rectal lumen are visualized and the tumor(s), polyp(s) or other lesion(s) is identified and removed by hot biopsy forceps or cautery (45308), snare technique (45309), or a combination of both techniques (45315). The proctosigmoidoscope is removed at the completion of the procedure.

Coding Tips

Surgical endoscopy includes diagnostic endoscopy; however, diagnostic endoscopy can be identified separately when performed at the same surgical session as an open procedure. Proctosigmoidoscopy codes are reported only when a rigid proctoscope (stiff hollow tube-like instrument) is used. If a flexible instrument is used, flexible sigmoidoscopy codes should be reported. For sigmoidoscopy, flexible, with removal of tumors, polyps, or other lesions by hot biopsy forceps, see 45333; by snare technique, see 45338. For anoscopy, with removal of a tumor, polyp, or other lesion, see 46610–46612.

ICD-10-CM Diagnostic Codes

C18.7	Malignant neoplasm of sigmoid colon
C18.8	Malignant neoplasm of overlapping sites of colon
C19	Malignant neoplasm of rectosigmoid junction
C20	Malignant neoplasm of rectum
C21.1	Malignant neoplasm of anal canal
C21.2	Malignant neoplasm of cloacogenic zone
C21.8	Malignant neoplasm of overlapping sites of rectum, anus and anal canal
C49.A4	Gastrointestinal stromal tumor of large intestine
C49.A5	Gastrointestinal stromal tumor of rectum
C78.5	Secondary malignant neoplasm of large intestine and rectum
C7A.025	Malignant carcinoid tumor of the sigmoid colon
C7A.026	Malignant carcinoid tumor of the rectum
D01.0	Carcinoma in situ of colon
D01.1	Carcinoma in situ of rectosigmoid junction
D01.2	Carcinoma in situ of rectum
D01.3	Carcinoma in situ of anus and anal canal
D12.5	Benign neoplasm of sigmoid colon
D12.7	Benign neoplasm of rectosigmoid junction
D12.8	Benign neoplasm of rectum
D12.9	Benign neoplasm of anus and anal canal
D37.4	Neoplasm of uncertain behavior of colon
D37.5	Neoplasm of uncertain behavior of rectum
D3A.025	Benign carcinoid tumor of the sigmoid colon
D3A.026	Benign carcinoid tumor of the rectum
K62.0	Anal polyp
K62.1	Rectal polyp
K62.5	Hemorrhage of anus and rectum
K62.82	Dysplasia of anus
K62.89	Other specified diseases of anus and rectum
K63.5	Polyp of colon

AMA: 45308 2018,Jan,8; 2017,Jan,8; 2016,Jan,13; 2015,Jan,16 **45309** 2018,Jan,8; 2017,Jan,8; 2016,Jan,13; 2015,Jan,16 **45315** 2018,Jan,8; 2017,Jan,8; 2016,Jan,13; 2015,Jan,16

Relative Value Units/Medicare Edits

Non-Facility RVU	Work	PE	MP	Total
45308	1.3	4.54	0.32	6.16
45309	1.4	4.61	0.34	6.35
45315	1.7	4.75	0.43	6.88
Facility RVU	**Work**	**PE**	**MP**	**Total**
45308	1.3	0.85	0.32	2.47
45309	1.4	0.89	0.34	2.63
45315	1.7	1.0	0.43	3.13

	FUD	Status	MUE	Modifiers				IOM Reference
45308	0	A	1(2)	51	N/A	N/A	N/A	None
45309	0	A	1(2)	51	N/A	N/A	N/A	
45315	0	A	1(2)	51	N/A	N/A	N/A	

* with documentation

Rectum

45317

45317 Proctosigmoidoscopy, rigid; with control of bleeding (eg, injection, bipolar cautery, unipolar cautery, laser, heater probe, stapler, plasma coagulator)

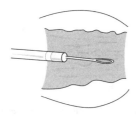

Bleeding in the sigmoid and/or rectum is controlled using any of a variety of techniques

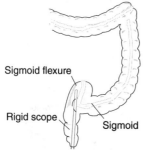

Sigmoid flexure

Rigid scope

Sigmoid

A rigid endoscopic procedure of the rectum and sigmoid is performed

Explanation

The physician performs rigid proctosigmoidoscopy and controls an area of bleeding. The physician inserts the rigid proctosigmoidoscope into the anus and advances the scope. The sigmoid colon and rectal lumen are visualized and the area of bleeding is identified and controlled. A variety of methods can be used to control bleeding, including injection, bipolar cautery, unipolar cautery, laser, heater probe, stapler, or plasma coagulator. The proctosigmoidoscope is removed at the completion of the procedure.

Coding Tips

Report the appropriate endoscopy for each anatomic site examined. Surgical endoscopy includes diagnostic endoscopy; however, diagnostic endoscopy can be identified separately when performed at the same surgical session as an open procedure. Proctosigmoidoscopy codes are reported only when a rigid proctoscope (stiff hollow tube-like instrument) is used. If a flexible instrument is used, flexible sigmoidoscopy codes should be reported. For sigmoidoscopy flexible, with control of bleeding, see 45334. For colonoscopy, flexible, with control of bleeding, see 45382. For anoscopy, with control of bleeding, see 46614.

ICD-10-CM Diagnostic Codes

C18.7	Malignant neoplasm of sigmoid colon
C19	Malignant neoplasm of rectosigmoid junction
C20	Malignant neoplasm of rectum
C21.1	Malignant neoplasm of anal canal
C21.2	Malignant neoplasm of cloacogenic zone
C21.8	Malignant neoplasm of overlapping sites of rectum, anus and anal canal
C49.A4	Gastrointestinal stromal tumor of large intestine
C49.A5	Gastrointestinal stromal tumor of rectum
C78.5	Secondary malignant neoplasm of large intestine and rectum
C7A.025	Malignant carcinoid tumor of the sigmoid colon
C7A.026	Malignant carcinoid tumor of the rectum
D01.0	Carcinoma in situ of colon
D01.1	Carcinoma in situ of rectosigmoid junction
D01.2	Carcinoma in situ of rectum
D01.3	Carcinoma in situ of anus and anal canal
D12.5	Benign neoplasm of sigmoid colon
D12.7	Benign neoplasm of rectosigmoid junction
D12.8	Benign neoplasm of rectum
D12.9	Benign neoplasm of anus and anal canal
D37.4	Neoplasm of uncertain behavior of colon
D37.5	Neoplasm of uncertain behavior of rectum
D3A.025	Benign carcinoid tumor of the sigmoid colon
D3A.026	Benign carcinoid tumor of the rectum
K50.111	Crohn's disease of large intestine with rectal bleeding
K50.811	Crohn's disease of both small and large intestine with rectal bleeding
K51.011	Ulcerative (chronic) pancolitis with rectal bleeding
K51.211	Ulcerative (chronic) proctitis with rectal bleeding
K51.311	Ulcerative (chronic) rectosigmoiditis with rectal bleeding
K51.411	Inflammatory polyps of colon with rectal bleeding
K51.511	Left sided colitis with rectal bleeding
K51.811	Other ulcerative colitis with rectal bleeding
K55.011	Focal (segmental) acute (reversible) ischemia of small intestine
K55.012	Diffuse acute (reversible) ischemia of small intestine
K55.021	Focal (segmental) acute infarction of small intestine
K55.022	Diffuse acute infarction of small intestine
K55.031	Focal (segmental) acute (reversible) ischemia of large intestine
K55.032	Diffuse acute (reversible) ischemia of large intestine
K55.041	Focal (segmental) acute infarction of large intestine
K55.042	Diffuse acute infarction of large intestine
K55.051	Focal (segmental) acute (reversible) ischemia of intestine, part unspecified
K55.052	Diffuse acute (reversible) ischemia of intestine, part unspecified
K55.1	Chronic vascular disorders of intestine
K55.21	Angiodysplasia of colon with hemorrhage
K57.21	Diverticulitis of large intestine with perforation and abscess with bleeding
K57.31	Diverticulosis of large intestine without perforation or abscess with bleeding
K57.32	Diverticulitis of large intestine without perforation or abscess without bleeding
K57.33	Diverticulitis of large intestine without perforation or abscess with bleeding
K62.5	Hemorrhage of anus and rectum
K62.7	Radiation proctitis
K62.82	Dysplasia of anus
K62.89	Other specified diseases of anus and rectum
K92.1	Melena
S36.63XA	Laceration of rectum, initial encounter

AMA: 45317 2018,Jan,8; 2017,Jan,8; 2016,Jan,13; 2015,Jan,16

Relative Value Units/Medicare Edits

Non-Facility RVU	Work	PE	MP	Total
45317	1.9	4.39	0.26	6.55
Facility RVU	Work	PE	MP	Total
45317	1.9	1.05	0.26	3.21

	FUD	Status	MUE	Modifiers				IOM Reference
45317	0	A	1(3)	51	N/A	N/A	N/A	None

* with documentation

Terms To Know

angiodysplasia. Vascular abnormalities, with or without bleeding.

cautery. Destruction or burning of tissue by means of a hot instrument, an electric current, or a caustic chemical, such as silver nitrate.

coagulation. Clot formation.

diverticulosis. Saclike pouches of the mucous membrane lining the intestine, herniating through the muscular wall of the colon, and occurring without inflammation.

fistula. Abnormal tube-like passage between two body cavities or organs or from an organ to the outside surface.

malignant. Any condition tending to progress toward death, specifically an invasive tumor with a loss of cellular differentiation that has the ability to spread or metastasize to other body areas.

ulcerative colitis. Chronic recurrent inflammation of the large intestine (colon) causing mucosal and submucosal ulceration of unknown cause, and leading to symptoms of abdominal pain, diarrhea with passage of non-fecal discharges, and rectal bleeding.

45320

45320 Proctosigmoidoscopy, rigid; with ablation of tumor(s), polyp(s), or other lesion(s) not amenable to removal by hot biopsy forceps, bipolar cautery or snare technique (eg, laser)

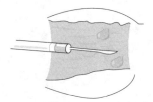

Tumors, polyps, or other lesions are ablated from the rectum/sigmoid region of the colon

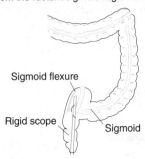

Sigmoid flexure

Rigid scope   Sigmoid

Explanation

The physician performs rigid proctosigmoidoscopy and ablation of a tumor polyp or other lesion. The physician inserts the proctosigmoidoscope into the anus and advances the scope. The lumen of the sigmoid colon and rectum that visualized and the tumor, polyp, or other lesion is identified and ablation performed. The proctosigmoidoscope is removed at the completion of the procedure.

Coding Tips

Report the appropriate endoscopy for each anatomic site examined. Surgical endoscopy includes diagnostic endoscopy; however, diagnostic endoscopy can be identified separately when performed at the same surgical session as an open procedure. Proctosigmoidoscopy codes are reported only when a rigid proctoscope (stiff hollow tube-like instrument) is used. If a flexible instrument is used, flexible sigmoidoscopy codes should be reported. For flexible sigmoidoscopy with ablation of tumors, polyps, or other lesions, see 45346. For colonoscopy, flexible, with ablation of tumors, polyps, or other lesions, see 45388. For anoscopy, with ablation of tumors, polyps, or other lesions, see 46615.

ICD-10-CM Diagnostic Codes

C18.7	Malignant neoplasm of sigmoid colon
C18.8	Malignant neoplasm of overlapping sites of colon
C19	Malignant neoplasm of rectosigmoid junction
C20	Malignant neoplasm of rectum
C21.1	Malignant neoplasm of anal canal
C21.2	Malignant neoplasm of cloacogenic zone
C21.8	Malignant neoplasm of overlapping sites of rectum, anus and anal canal
C49.A4	Gastrointestinal stromal tumor of large intestine
C49.A5	Gastrointestinal stromal tumor of rectum
C78.5	Secondary malignant neoplasm of large intestine and rectum
C7A.025	Malignant carcinoid tumor of the sigmoid colon

C7A.026	Malignant carcinoid tumor of the rectum
D01.0	Carcinoma in situ of colon
D01.1	Carcinoma in situ of rectosigmoid junction
D01.2	Carcinoma in situ of rectum
D01.3	Carcinoma in situ of anus and anal canal
D12.5	Benign neoplasm of sigmoid colon
D12.7	Benign neoplasm of rectosigmoid junction
D12.8	Benign neoplasm of rectum
D12.9	Benign neoplasm of anus and anal canal
D37.4	Neoplasm of uncertain behavior of colon
D37.5	Neoplasm of uncertain behavior of rectum
D3A.025	Benign carcinoid tumor of the sigmoid colon
D3A.026	Benign carcinoid tumor of the rectum
D49.0	Neoplasm of unspecified behavior of digestive system
K62.0	Anal polyp
K62.1	Rectal polyp
K62.5	Hemorrhage of anus and rectum
K62.82	Dysplasia of anus
K63.5	Polyp of colon

AMA: 45320 2018,Jan,8; 2017,Jan,8; 2016,Jan,13; 2015,Jan,16

Relative Value Units/Medicare Edits

Non-Facility RVU	Work	PE	MP	Total
45320	1.68	4.66	0.42	6.76
Facility RVU	Work	PE	MP	Total
45320	1.68	0.99	0.42	3.09

	FUD	Status	MUE	Modifiers				IOM Reference
45320	0	A	1(2)	51	N/A	N/A	N/A	None

* with documentation

Terms To Know

ablation. Removal or destruction of tissue by cutting, electrical energy, chemical substances, or excessive heat application.

benign. Mild or nonmalignant in nature.

lesion. Area of damaged tissue that has lost continuity or function, due to disease or trauma.

lumen. Space inside an intestine, artery, vein, duct, or tube.

malignant. Any condition tending to progress toward death, specifically an invasive tumor with a loss of cellular differentiation that has the ability to spread or metastasize to other body areas.

polyp. Small growth on a stalk-like attachment projecting from a mucous membrane.

tumor. Pathological swelling or enlargement; a neoplastic growth of uncontrolled, abnormal multiplication of cells.

45321

45321   Proctosigmoidoscopy, rigid; with decompression of volvulus

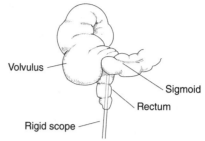

A rigid proctosigmoidoscope is inserted into the anus and a volvulus of the rectum or sigmoid is decompressed

Explanation

The physician performs rigid proctosigmoidoscopy and decompresses a sigmoid volvulus. The physician inserts the proctosigmoidoscope into the anus and advances the scope. The lumen of the sigmoid colon and rectum is visualized. The proctosigmoidoscope is advanced into the volvulus, decompressing the volvulus as it passes through the bowel lumen. The proctosigmoidoscope is removed at the completion of the procedure.

Coding Tips

Report the appropriate endoscopy for each anatomic site examined. Surgical endoscopy includes diagnostic endoscopy; however, diagnostic endoscopy can be identified separately when performed at the same surgical session as an open procedure. Proctosigmoidoscopy codes are reported only when a rigid proctoscope (stiff hollow tube-like instrument) is used. If a flexible instrument is used, flexible sigmoidoscopy codes should be reported. For sigmoidoscopy, flexible, with decompression of volvulus, any method, see 45337.

ICD-10-CM Diagnostic Codes

K56.2   Volvulus

AMA: 45321 2018,Jan,8; 2017,Jan,8; 2016,Jan,13; 2015,Jan,16

Relative Value Units/Medicare Edits

Non-Facility RVU	Work	PE	MP	Total
45321	1.65	0.98	0.42	3.05
Facility RVU	Work	PE	MP	Total
45321	1.65	0.98	0.42	3.05

	FUD	Status	MUE	Modifiers				IOM Reference
45321	0	A	1(2)	51	N/A	N/A	N/A	None

* with documentation

Rectum

45327

45327 Proctosigmoidoscopy, rigid; with transendoscopic stent placement (includes predilation)

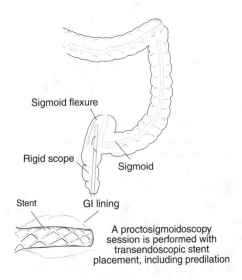

A proctosigmoidoscopy session is performed with transendoscopic stent placement, including predilation

Explanation

The physician uses a rigid proctosigmoidoscopy to examine the rectum and sigmoid colon and places a transendoscopic stent. The physician inserts the rigid proctosigmoidoscope into the anus and advances the scope. The sigmoid colon and rectal lumen are visualized. The endoscope is placed at the site of an obstruction or stricture and the necessary stent length is determined. The stent (endoprosthesis) is introduced into the site of the obstruction. Using a commercial delivery system, a plastic covering over the stent is removed and the stent self-deploys, shoring up the walls at a specific site in the sigmoid colon. When necessary, a balloon catheter is placed into the stent and gently inflated to more fully deploy the stent. The delivery system and endoscope are removed.

Coding Tips

Report the appropriate endoscopy for each anatomic site examined. Surgical endoscopy includes diagnostic endoscopy; however, diagnostic endoscopy can be identified separately when performed at the same surgical session as an open procedure. Proctosigmoidoscopy codes are reported only when a rigid proctoscope (stiff hollow tube-like instrument) is used. If a flexible instrument is used, flexible sigmoidoscopy codes should be reported. For endoscopic stent placement through sigmoidoscopy, see 45347.

ICD-10-CM Diagnostic Codes

K50.112	Crohn's disease of large intestine with intestinal obstruction
K50.812	Crohn's disease of both small and large intestine with intestinal obstruction
K51.012	Ulcerative (chronic) pancolitis with intestinal obstruction
K51.212	Ulcerative (chronic) proctitis with intestinal obstruction
K51.312	Ulcerative (chronic) rectosigmoiditis with intestinal obstruction
K51.412	Inflammatory polyps of colon with intestinal obstruction
K51.512	Left sided colitis with intestinal obstruction
K51.812	Other ulcerative colitis with intestinal obstruction
K56.51	Intestinal adhesions [bands], with partial obstruction
K56.52	Intestinal adhesions [bands] with complete obstruction
K56.690	Other partial intestinal obstruction

K56.691	Other complete intestinal obstruction
K91.31	Postprocedural partial intestinal obstruction
K91.32	Postprocedural complete intestinal obstruction
K91.89	Other postprocedural complications and disorders of digestive system
Q42.0	Congenital absence, atresia and stenosis of rectum with fistula
Q42.1	Congenital absence, atresia and stenosis of rectum without fistula
Q42.2	Congenital absence, atresia and stenosis of anus with fistula
Q42.3	Congenital absence, atresia and stenosis of anus without fistula
Q42.8	Congenital absence, atresia and stenosis of other parts of large intestine

AMA: **45327** 2018,Jan,8; 2017,Jan,8; 2016,Jan,13; 2015,Jan,16

Relative Value Units/Medicare Edits

Non-Facility RVU	Work	PE	MP	Total
45327	1.9	1.07	0.46	3.43
Facility RVU	**Work**	**PE**	**MP**	**Total**
45327	1.9	1.07	0.46	3.43

	FUD	Status	MUE	Modifiers				IOM Reference
45327	0	A	1(2)	51	N/A	N/A	N/A	None

* with documentation

Terms To Know

atresia. Congenital closure or absence of a tubular organ or an opening to the body surface.

intestinal or peritoneal adhesions with obstruction. Abnormal fibrous band growths joining separate tissues in the peritoneum or intestine, causing blockage.

lumen. Space inside an intestine, artery, vein, duct, or tube.

malignant. Any condition tending to progress toward death, specifically an invasive tumor with a loss of cellular differentiation that has the ability to spread or metastasize to other body areas.

obstruction. Blockage that prevents normal function of the valve or structure.

stenosis. Narrowing or constriction of a passage.

Rectum

45330-45331

45330 Sigmoidoscopy, flexible; diagnostic, including collection of specimen(s) by brushing or washing, when performed (separate procedure)

45331 with biopsy, single or multiple

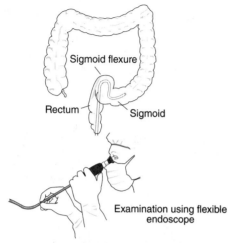

Sigmoid flexure

Rectum

Sigmoid

Examination using flexible endoscope

Specimen(s) may be collected by brushing, washing, or biopsy

Explanation

The physician performs flexible sigmoidoscopy and may obtain brushings, washings, or biopsies. The physician inserts the sigmoidoscope into the anus and advances the scope through the rectum and into the sigmoid colon. The lumen of the sigmoid colon and rectum are visualized. In 45330, brushings and washings may be obtained. In 45331, biopsies are obtained with forceps placed through the scope. The sigmoidoscope is withdrawn at the completion of the procedure.

Coding Tips

Note that 45330, a separate procedure by definition, is usually a component of a more complex service and is not identified separately. When performed alone or with other unrelated procedures/services it may be reported. If performed alone, list the code; if performed with other procedures/services, list the code and append modifier 59 or an X{EPSU} modifier. Report the appropriate endoscopy for each anatomic site examined. Surgical endoscopy includes diagnostic endoscopy; however, diagnostic endoscopy can be identified separately when performed at the same surgical session as an open procedure. Flexible sigmoidoscopy includes an examination of the entire rectum, sigmoid colon, and may include a portion of the descending colon. When examination of the rectum and sigmoid colon is performed using a rigid proctoscope (stiff hollow tube-like instrument), see 45300 or 45305. Bleeding that occurs as the result of an endoscopic procedure, and controlled during the same operative session, is not reported separately. Do not report 45330 with 45331–45342, 45346–45347, or 45349–45350. Do not report 45331 in addition to 45349 for the same lesion.

ICD-10-CM Diagnostic Codes

C18.6	Malignant neoplasm of descending colon
C18.7	Malignant neoplasm of sigmoid colon
C19	Malignant neoplasm of rectosigmoid junction
C20	Malignant neoplasm of rectum
C21.1	Malignant neoplasm of anal canal
C21.2	Malignant neoplasm of cloacogenic zone
C49.A4	Gastrointestinal stromal tumor of large intestine
C78.5	Secondary malignant neoplasm of large intestine and rectum
C7A.025	Malignant carcinoid tumor of the sigmoid colon
C7A.026	Malignant carcinoid tumor of the rectum
D01.0	Carcinoma in situ of colon
D01.1	Carcinoma in situ of rectosigmoid junction
D01.2	Carcinoma in situ of rectum
D12.5	Benign neoplasm of sigmoid colon
D12.7	Benign neoplasm of rectosigmoid junction
D12.8	Benign neoplasm of rectum
D37.4	Neoplasm of uncertain behavior of colon
D37.5	Neoplasm of uncertain behavior of rectum
D3A.025	Benign carcinoid tumor of the sigmoid colon
D3A.026	Benign carcinoid tumor of the rectum
K50.111	Crohn's disease of large intestine with rectal bleeding
K50.112	Crohn's disease of large intestine with intestinal obstruction
K50.113	Crohn's disease of large intestine with fistula
K50.114	Crohn's disease of large intestine with abscess
K50.811	Crohn's disease of both small and large intestine with rectal bleeding
K50.812	Crohn's disease of both small and large intestine with intestinal obstruction
K50.813	Crohn's disease of both small and large intestine with fistula
K50.814	Crohn's disease of both small and large intestine with abscess
K51.311	Ulcerative (chronic) rectosigmoiditis with rectal bleeding
K51.312	Ulcerative (chronic) rectosigmoiditis with intestinal obstruction
K51.313	Ulcerative (chronic) rectosigmoiditis with fistula
K51.314	Ulcerative (chronic) rectosigmoiditis with abscess
K51.411	Inflammatory polyps of colon with rectal bleeding
K51.412	Inflammatory polyps of colon with intestinal obstruction
K51.413	Inflammatory polyps of colon with fistula
K51.414	Inflammatory polyps of colon with abscess
K51.511	Left sided colitis with rectal bleeding
K51.512	Left sided colitis with intestinal obstruction
K51.513	Left sided colitis with fistula
K51.514	Left sided colitis with abscess
K51.811	Other ulcerative colitis with rectal bleeding
K51.812	Other ulcerative colitis with intestinal obstruction
K51.813	Other ulcerative colitis with fistula
K51.814	Other ulcerative colitis with abscess
K52.82	Eosinophilic colitis
K55.031	Focal (segmental) acute (reversible) ischemia of large intestine
K55.032	Diffuse acute (reversible) ischemia of large intestine
K55.041	Focal (segmental) acute infarction of large intestine
K55.042	Diffuse acute infarction of large intestine
K55.1	Chronic vascular disorders of intestine
K55.20	Angiodysplasia of colon without hemorrhage
K55.21	Angiodysplasia of colon with hemorrhage
K56.2	Volvulus
K57.21	Diverticulitis of large intestine with perforation and abscess with bleeding

Rectum

K57.31	Diverticulosis of large intestine without perforation or abscess with bleeding	
K57.33	Diverticulitis of large intestine without perforation or abscess with bleeding	
K57.40	Diverticulitis of both small and large intestine with perforation and abscess without bleeding	
K57.50	Diverticulosis of both small and large intestine without perforation or abscess without bleeding	
K57.53	Diverticulitis of both small and large intestine without perforation or abscess with bleeding	
K58.0	Irritable bowel syndrome with diarrhea	
K59.01	Slow transit constipation	
K59.02	Outlet dysfunction constipation	
K59.1	Functional diarrhea	
K60.4	Rectal fistula	
K60.5	Anorectal fistula	
K61.1	Rectal abscess	
K61.2	Anorectal abscess	
K61.31	Horseshoe abscess	
K61.39	Other ischiorectal abscess	
K61.4	Intrasphincteric abscess	
K61.5	Supralevator abscess	
K62.1	Rectal polyp	
K62.3	Rectal prolapse	
K62.5	Hemorrhage of anus and rectum	
K62.7	Radiation proctitis	
K62.82	Dysplasia of anus	
K63.5	Polyp of colon	
K64.0	First degree hemorrhoids	
K64.1	Second degree hemorrhoids	
K64.2	Third degree hemorrhoids	
K64.3	Fourth degree hemorrhoids	
M35.08	Sjögren syndrome with gastrointestinal involvement	
Q43.1	Hirschsprung's disease	

AMA: 45330 2018,Jan,8; 2017,Jan,8; 2016,Jan,13; 2016,Feb,13; 2015,Sep,12; 2015,Jan,16 **45331** 2018,Jan,8; 2017,Jan,8; 2016,Jan,13; 2016,Feb,13; 2015,Jan,16

Relative Value Units/Medicare Edits

Non-Facility RVU	Work	PE	MP	Total
45330	0.84	4.65	0.11	5.6
45331	1.14	7.5	0.14	8.78
Facility RVU	Work	PE	MP	Total
45330	0.84	0.67	0.11	1.62
45331	1.14	0.81	0.14	2.09

	FUD	Status	MUE	Modifiers				IOM Reference
45330	0	A	1(3)	51	N/A	N/A	N/A	None
45331	0	A	1(2)	51	N/A	N/A	N/A	

* with documentation

45332

45332   Sigmoidoscopy, flexible; with removal of foreign body(s)

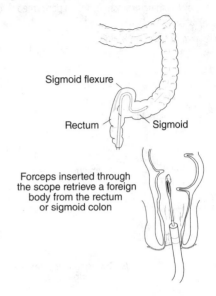

Sigmoid flexure

Rectum   Sigmoid

Forceps inserted through the scope retrieve a foreign body from the rectum or sigmoid colon

Explanation

The physician performs flexible sigmoidoscopy and removes a foreign body(s). The physician inserts the sigmoidoscope into the anus and advances the scope through the rectum and into the sigmoid colon. The lumen of the sigmoid colon and rectum are visualized. The foreign body(s) is identified and removed with a snare or forceps placed through the sigmoidoscope. The sigmoidoscope is withdrawn at the completion of the procedure.

Coding Tips

Report the appropriate endoscopy for each anatomic site examined. Surgical endoscopy includes diagnostic endoscopy; however, diagnostic endoscopy can be identified separately when performed at the same surgical session as an open procedure. If fluoroscopic guidance is used, see 76000. Flexible sigmoidoscopy includes an examination of the entire rectum, sigmoid colon, and may include a portion of the descending colon. When examination of the rectum and sigmoid colon with removal of a foreign body is performed using a rigid proctoscope (stiff hollow tube-like instrument), see 45307. For colonoscopy, flexible, proximal to splenic flexure, with removal of a foreign body, see 45379. For anoscopy, with removal of a foreign body, see 46608. Bleeding that occurs as the result of an endoscopic procedure, and is controlled during the same operative session, is not reported separately. Do not report 45332 in conjunction with 45330.

ICD-10-CM Diagnostic Codes

T18.4XXA	Foreign body in colon, initial encounter
T18.5XXA	Foreign body in anus and rectum, initial encounter

AMA: 45332 2018,Jan,8; 2017,Jan,8; 2016,Jan,13; 2016,Feb,13; 2015,Jan,16

Relative Value Units/Medicare Edits

Non-Facility RVU	Work	PE	MP	Total
45332	1.76	6.4	0.22	8.38
Facility RVU	Work	PE	MP	Total
45332	1.76	1.07	0.22	3.05

	FUD	Status	MUE	Modifiers				IOM Reference
45332	0	A	1(3)	51	N/A	N/A	N/A	None

* with documentation

Terms To Know

endoscopy. Visual inspection of the body using a fiberoptic scope.

forceps. Tool used for grasping or compressing tissue.

foreign body. Any object or substance found in an organ and tissue that does not belong under normal circumstances.

lumen. Space inside an intestine, artery, vein, duct, or tube.

sigmoidoscopy. Endoscopic examination of the entire rectum and sigmoid colon, often including a portion of the descending colon and usually performed with a flexible fiberoptic scope in conjunction with a surgical procedure.

snare. Wire used as a loop to excise a polyp or lesion.

45333

45333   Sigmoidoscopy, flexible; with removal of tumor(s), polyp(s), or other lesion(s) by hot biopsy forceps

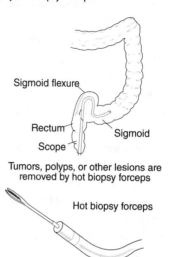

Tumors, polyps, or other lesions are removed by hot biopsy forceps

Hot biopsy forceps

Explanation

The physician performs flexible sigmoidoscopy and removes a tumor, polyp, or other lesion. The physician inserts the sigmoidoscope into the anus and advances the scope through the rectum and into the sigmoid colon. The lumen of the sigmoid colon and rectum are visualized and the tumor, polyp, or other lesion is identified and removed with hot biopsy forceps. The sigmoidoscope is withdrawn at the completion of the procedure.

Coding Tips

Report the appropriate endoscopy for each anatomic site examined. Surgical endoscopy includes diagnostic endoscopy; however, diagnostic endoscopy can be identified separately when performed at the same surgical session as an open procedure. Note that 45333 is reported only once regardless of the number of lesions removed. Flexible sigmoidoscopy includes an examination of the entire rectum, sigmoid colon, and may include a portion of the descending colon. When examination of the rectum and sigmoid colon with removal of a lesion is performed using a rigid proctoscope (stiff hollow tube-like instrument), use 45308 for removal of a single tumor, polyp, or other lesion by hot biopsy forceps or bipolar cautery; 45315 for removal of multiple lesions by these techniques. If submucosal injection (any substance) is performed prior to lesion removal, report 45335 for the submucosal injection in addition to 45333. For colonoscopy, flexible, with removal of tumors, polyps, or other lesions, by hot biopsy forceps, see 45384. Bleeding that occurs as the result of an endoscopic procedure, and controlled during the same operative session, is not reported separately. Do not report 45333 with 45330.

ICD-10-CM Diagnostic Codes

C18.7	Malignant neoplasm of sigmoid colon
C18.8	Malignant neoplasm of overlapping sites of colon
C19	Malignant neoplasm of rectosigmoid junction
C20	Malignant neoplasm of rectum
C21.2	Malignant neoplasm of cloacogenic zone
C21.8	Malignant neoplasm of overlapping sites of rectum, anus and anal canal
C49.A4	Gastrointestinal stromal tumor of large intestine
C78.5	Secondary malignant neoplasm of large intestine and rectum
C7A.025	Malignant carcinoid tumor of the sigmoid colon

Rectum

C7A.026	Malignant carcinoid tumor of the rectum	
D01.0	Carcinoma in situ of colon	
D01.1	Carcinoma in situ of rectosigmoid junction	
D01.2	Carcinoma in situ of rectum	
D01.49	Carcinoma in situ of other parts of intestine	
D12.5	Benign neoplasm of sigmoid colon	
D12.7	Benign neoplasm of rectosigmoid junction	
D12.8	Benign neoplasm of rectum	
D37.4	Neoplasm of uncertain behavior of colon	
D37.5	Neoplasm of uncertain behavior of rectum	
D3A.025	Benign carcinoid tumor of the sigmoid colon	
D3A.026	Benign carcinoid tumor of the rectum	
D49.0	Neoplasm of unspecified behavior of digestive system	
K51.40	Inflammatory polyps of colon without complications	
K51.411	Inflammatory polyps of colon with rectal bleeding	
K51.412	Inflammatory polyps of colon with intestinal obstruction	
K51.413	Inflammatory polyps of colon with fistula	
K51.414	Inflammatory polyps of colon with abscess	
K51.418	Inflammatory polyps of colon with other complication	
K55.20	Angiodysplasia of colon without hemorrhage	
K55.21	Angiodysplasia of colon with hemorrhage	
K62.1	Rectal polyp	
K62.6	Ulcer of anus and rectum	
K62.89	Other specified diseases of anus and rectum	
K63.5	Polyp of colon	

AMA: **45333** 2018,Jan,8; 2017,Jan,8; 2016,Jan,13; 2016,Feb,13; 2015,Jan,16

Relative Value Units/Medicare Edits

Non-Facility RVU	Work	PE	MP	Total
45333	1.55	8.32	0.21	10.08
Facility RVU	Work	PE	MP	Total
45333	1.55	0.97	0.21	2.73

	FUD	Status	MUE	Modifiers				IOM Reference
45333	0	A	1(2)	51	N/A	N/A	N/A	None

* with documentation

45334

45334 Sigmoidoscopy, flexible; with control of bleeding, any method

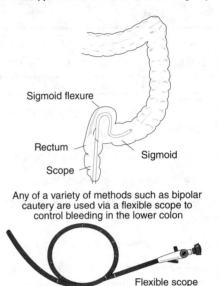

Sigmoid flexure

Rectum

Scope

Sigmoid

Any of a variety of methods such as bipolar cautery are used via a flexible scope to control bleeding in the lower colon

Flexible scope

Explanation

The physician performs flexible sigmoidoscopy and controls an area of bleeding. The physician inserts the sigmoidoscope into the anus and advances the scope through the rectum and into the sigmoid colon. The lumen of the sigmoid colon and rectum are visualized and the area of bleeding is controlled. A variety of methods can be used to control bleeding, including medication application and cauterization. The sigmoidoscope is withdrawn at the completion of the procedure.

Coding Tips

Report the appropriate endoscopy for each anatomic site examined. Surgical endoscopy includes diagnostic endoscopy; however, diagnostic endoscopy can be identified separately when performed at the same surgical session as an open procedure. Flexible sigmoidoscopy includes an examination of the entire rectum, sigmoid colon, and may include a portion of the descending colon. When examination of the rectum and sigmoid colon with control of bleeding is performed using a rigid proctoscope (stiff hollow tube-like instrument), see 45317. For colonoscopy, flexible, with control of bleeding, see 45382. For anoscopy, with control of bleeding, see 46614. Bleeding that occurs as the result of an endoscopic procedure, and controlled during the same operative session, is not reported separately. Do not report 45334 with 45330 or in addition to 45335 or 45350 for the same lesion.

ICD-10-CM Diagnostic Codes

C18.7	Malignant neoplasm of sigmoid colon
C18.8	Malignant neoplasm of overlapping sites of colon
C19	Malignant neoplasm of rectosigmoid junction
C20	Malignant neoplasm of rectum
C21.1	Malignant neoplasm of anal canal
C21.2	Malignant neoplasm of cloacogenic zone
C21.8	Malignant neoplasm of overlapping sites of rectum, anus and anal canal
C49.A4	Gastrointestinal stromal tumor of large intestine
C78.5	Secondary malignant neoplasm of large intestine and rectum
C7A.025	Malignant carcinoid tumor of the sigmoid colon

C7A.026	Malignant carcinoid tumor of the rectum
D01.0	Carcinoma in situ of colon
D01.1	Carcinoma in situ of rectosigmoid junction
D01.2	Carcinoma in situ of rectum
D01.3	Carcinoma in situ of anus and anal canal
D01.49	Carcinoma in situ of other parts of intestine
D12.5	Benign neoplasm of sigmoid colon
D12.7	Benign neoplasm of rectosigmoid junction
D12.8	Benign neoplasm of rectum
D12.9	Benign neoplasm of anus and anal canal
D37.4	Neoplasm of uncertain behavior of colon
D37.5	Neoplasm of uncertain behavior of rectum
D3A.025	Benign carcinoid tumor of the sigmoid colon
D3A.026	Benign carcinoid tumor of the rectum
K50.111	Crohn's disease of large intestine with rectal bleeding
K50.811	Crohn's disease of both small and large intestine with rectal bleeding
K51.011	Ulcerative (chronic) pancolitis with rectal bleeding
K51.211	Ulcerative (chronic) proctitis with rectal bleeding
K51.311	Ulcerative (chronic) rectosigmoiditis with rectal bleeding
K51.411	Inflammatory polyps of colon with rectal bleeding
K51.511	Left sided colitis with rectal bleeding
K51.811	Other ulcerative colitis with rectal bleeding
K55.011	Focal (segmental) acute (reversible) ischemia of small intestine
K55.012	Diffuse acute (reversible) ischemia of small intestine
K55.021	Focal (segmental) acute infarction of small intestine
K55.022	Diffuse acute infarction of small intestine
K55.031	Focal (segmental) acute (reversible) ischemia of large intestine
K55.032	Diffuse acute (reversible) ischemia of large intestine
K55.041	Focal (segmental) acute infarction of large intestine
K55.042	Diffuse acute infarction of large intestine
K55.051	Focal (segmental) acute (reversible) ischemia of intestine, part unspecified
K55.052	Diffuse acute (reversible) ischemia of intestine, part unspecified
K55.1	Chronic vascular disorders of intestine
K55.21	Angiodysplasia of colon with hemorrhage
K55.8	Other vascular disorders of intestine
K57.21	Diverticulitis of large intestine with perforation and abscess with bleeding
K57.31	Diverticulosis of large intestine without perforation or abscess with bleeding
K57.33	Diverticulitis of large intestine without perforation or abscess with bleeding
K57.41	Diverticulitis of both small and large intestine with perforation and abscess with bleeding
K57.51	Diverticulosis of both small and large intestine without perforation or abscess with bleeding
K57.53	Diverticulitis of both small and large intestine without perforation or abscess with bleeding
K62.5	Hemorrhage of anus and rectum
K62.7	Radiation proctitis
K62.89	Other specified diseases of anus and rectum
K64.0	First degree hemorrhoids
K64.1	Second degree hemorrhoids

K64.2	Third degree hemorrhoids
K64.3	Fourth degree hemorrhoids
K64.8	Other hemorrhoids
K92.1	Melena

AMA: 45334 2018,Jan,8; 2017,Jan,8; 2016,Jan,13; 2016,Feb,13; 2015,Jan,16

Relative Value Units/Medicare Edits

Non-Facility RVU	Work	PE	MP	Total
45334	2.0	13.83	0.22	16.05
Facility RVU	**Work**	**PE**	**MP**	**Total**
45334	2.0	1.19	0.22	3.41

	FUD	Status	MUE	Modifiers				IOM Reference
45334	0	A	1(3)	51	N/A	N/A	N/A	None

* with documentation

Terms To Know

hemorrhage. Internal or external bleeding with loss of significant amounts of blood.

malignant. Any condition tending to progress toward death, specifically an invasive tumor with a loss of cellular differentiation that has the ability to spread or metastasize to other body areas.

neoplasm. New abnormal growth, tumor.

thrombosed hemorrhoid. Dilated, varicose vein in the anal region that has clotted blood within it.

Rectum

45335

45335 Sigmoidoscopy, flexible; with directed submucosal injection(s), any substance

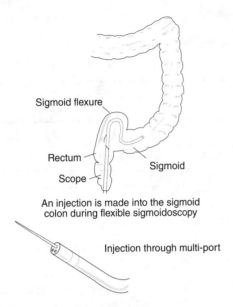

Sigmoid flexure

Rectum

Scope

Sigmoid

An injection is made into the sigmoid colon during flexible sigmoidoscopy

Injection through multi-port

Explanation

The physician performs flexible sigmoidoscopy and injects a substance into the submucosa, directed at specific areas through the scope while viewing the colon. The physician inserts the sigmoidoscope into the anus and advances the scope into the sigmoid colon. The lumen of the sigmoid colon and rectum are visualized. Submucosal saline injections, for instance, may be done before polypectomy using snare and electrocautery to greatly enhance the effectiveness of resection for large sessile colorectal polyps.

Coding Tips

Report the appropriate endoscopy for each anatomic site examined. Surgical endoscopy includes diagnostic endoscopy; however, diagnostic endoscopy can be identified separately when performed at the same surgical session as an open procedure. When submucosal injection is performed at the time of lesion removal, the submucosal injection is reported separately. Report 45335 only once regardless of the number of injections performed. For colonoscopy, flexible, with a directed submucosal injection, see 45381. Bleeding that occurs as the result of an endoscopic procedure, and controlled during the same operative session, is not reported separately. Do not report 45335 with 45330 or in addition to 45334 or 45349 for the same lesion.

ICD-10-CM Diagnostic Codes

C18.6	Malignant neoplasm of descending colon
C18.7	Malignant neoplasm of sigmoid colon
C18.8	Malignant neoplasm of overlapping sites of colon
C19	Malignant neoplasm of rectosigmoid junction
C20	Malignant neoplasm of rectum
C21.1	Malignant neoplasm of anal canal
C21.2	Malignant neoplasm of cloacogenic zone
C21.8	Malignant neoplasm of overlapping sites of rectum, anus and anal canal
C49.A4	Gastrointestinal stromal tumor of large intestine
D01.0	Carcinoma in situ of colon
D01.1	Carcinoma in situ of rectosigmoid junction
D01.2	Carcinoma in situ of rectum
D01.3	Carcinoma in situ of anus and anal canal
D12.4	Benign neoplasm of descending colon
D12.5	Benign neoplasm of sigmoid colon
D12.7	Benign neoplasm of rectosigmoid junction
D12.8	Benign neoplasm of rectum
D12.9	Benign neoplasm of anus and anal canal
D37.4	Neoplasm of uncertain behavior of colon
D37.5	Neoplasm of uncertain behavior of rectum
D37.8	Neoplasm of uncertain behavior of other specified digestive organs
D3A.025	Benign carcinoid tumor of the sigmoid colon
D3A.026	Benign carcinoid tumor of the rectum
K51.40	Inflammatory polyps of colon without complications
K51.411	Inflammatory polyps of colon with rectal bleeding
K51.412	Inflammatory polyps of colon with intestinal obstruction
K51.413	Inflammatory polyps of colon with fistula
K51.414	Inflammatory polyps of colon with abscess
K51.418	Inflammatory polyps of colon with other complication
K62.0	Anal polyp
K62.1	Rectal polyp
K62.89	Other specified diseases of anus and rectum
K63.5	Polyp of colon
K63.89	Other specified diseases of intestine

AMA: **45335** 2018,Jan,8; 2017,Jan,8; 2016,Jan,13; 2016,Feb,13; 2015,Jan,16

Relative Value Units/Medicare Edits

Non-Facility RVU	Work	PE	MP	Total
45335	1.04	7.61	0.14	8.79
Facility RVU	**Work**	**PE**	**MP**	**Total**
45335	1.04	0.76	0.14	1.94

	FUD	Status	MUE	Modifiers				IOM Reference
45335	0	A	1(2)	51	N/A	N/A	N/A	None

* with documentation

Rectum

45337

45337 Sigmoidoscopy, flexible; with decompression (for pathologic distention) (eg, volvulus, megacolon), including placement of decompression tube, when performed

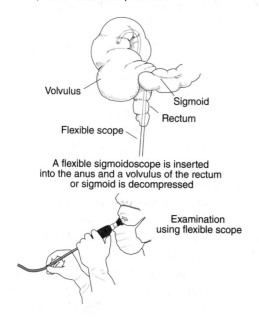

Volvulus
Sigmoid
Rectum
Flexible scope

A flexible sigmoidoscope is inserted into the anus and a volvulus of the rectum or sigmoid is decompressed

Examination using flexible scope

Explanation

The physician performs flexible sigmoidoscopy with decompression of a pathological distention, such as a volvulus or megacolon. The physician inserts the sigmoidoscope into the anus and advances the scope through the rectum and into the sigmoid colon. The lumen of the sigmoid colon and rectum are visualized. The sigmoidoscope is advanced into the area of distention decompressing it as the scope passes through the bowel lumen. The sigmoidoscope is withdrawn at the completion of the procedure. This procedure includes placement of a decompression tube when utilized.

Coding Tips

Report the appropriate endoscopy for each anatomic site examined. Surgical endoscopy includes diagnostic endoscopy; however, diagnostic endoscopy can be identified separately when performed at the same surgical session as an open procedure. Flexible sigmoidoscopy includes an examination of the entire rectum, sigmoid colon, and may include a portion of the descending colon. When examination of the rectum and sigmoid colon with decompression of volvulus is performed using a rigid proctoscope (stiff hollow tube-like instrument), see 45321. Note that endoscopic reduction of a pathologic distention (e.g., volvulus) is performed more frequently using a rigid proctoscope. Only when the area of distention cannot be reached by rigid proctoscope is flexible sigmoidoscopic decompression attempted. Bleeding that occurs as the result of an endoscopic procedure, and controlled during the same operative session, is not reported separately. Do not report 45337 with 45330. This service should only be reported once per session.

ICD-10-CM Diagnostic Codes

K56.2	Volvulus
K59.31	Toxic megacolon
K59.39	Other megacolon

AMA: 45337 2018,Jan,8; 2017,Jan,8; 2016,Jan,13; 2016,Feb,13; 2015,Jan,16

Relative Value Units/Medicare Edits

Non-Facility RVU	Work	PE	MP	Total
45337	2.1	0.99	0.26	3.35
Facility RVU	**Work**	**PE**	**MP**	**Total**
45337	2.1	0.99	0.26	3.35

	FUD	Status	MUE	Modifiers			IOM Reference
45337	0	A	1(2)	51	N/A	N/A	N/A	None

* with documentation

Terms To Know

decompression. Release of pressure.

dilation. Artificial increase in the diameter of an opening or lumen made by medication or by instrumentation.

distention. Enlarged or expanded due to pressure from inside.

lumen. Space inside an intestine, artery, vein, duct, or tube.

megacolon. Enlargement or dilation of the large intestines or the colon.

obstruction. Blockage that prevents normal function of the valve or structure.

pathological. Pertaining to, or relating to, disease.

sigmoidoscopy. Endoscopic examination of the entire rectum and sigmoid colon, often including a portion of the descending colon and usually performed with a flexible fiberoptic scope in conjunction with a surgical procedure.

volvulus. Twisting, knotting, or entanglement of the bowel on itself that may quickly compromise oxygen supply to the intestinal tissues. A volvulus usually occurs at the sigmoid and ileocecal areas of the intestines.

Rectum

● New   ▲ Revised   + Add On   ★ Telemedicine   AMA: CPT Assist   [Resequenced]   ☑ Laterality   © 2021 Optum360, LLC

Coding Companion for General Surgery/Gastroenterology

591

45338 [45346]

45338 Sigmoidoscopy, flexible; with removal of tumor(s), polyp(s), or other lesion(s) by snare technique

45346 Sigmoidoscopy, flexible; with ablation of tumor(s), polyp(s), or other lesion(s) (includes pre- and post-dilation and guide wire passage, when performed)

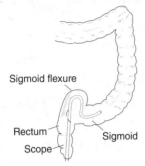

Sigmoid flexure

Rectum

Sigmoid

Scope

A flexible sigmoidoscopy is performed to remove or ablate tumors or other lesions

Explanation

The physician performs flexible sigmoidoscopy and removes tumors, polyps, or other lesions. The physician inserts the sigmoidoscope into the anus and advances the scope through the rectum and into the sigmoid colon. The lumen of the sigmoid colon and rectum are visualized. The tumor, polyp, or other lesions are identified and removed by snare technique in 45338 or by ablation in 45346. The sigmoidoscope is withdrawn at the completion of the procedure. Code 45346 includes dilation before and after with utilization of a guidewire, if employed.

Coding Tips

Report the appropriate endoscopy for each anatomic site examined. Surgical endoscopy includes diagnostic endoscopy; however, diagnostic endoscopy can be identified separately when performed at the same surgical session as an open procedure. Flexible sigmoidoscopy includes an examination of the entire rectum, sigmoid colon, and may include a portion of the descending colon. When examination of the rectum and sigmoid colon with removal of a lesion is performed using a rigid proctoscope (stiff hollow tube-like instrument), for snare technique, see 45309; ablation, see 45320; with endoscopic mucosal resection, see 45349. If submucosal injection (any substance) is performed prior to lesion removal, report 45335 for the submucosal injection in addition to these codes. For colonoscopy, flexible, with ablation of tumors, polyps, or other lesions, see 45388. For anoscopy, with ablation of tumors, polyps, or other lesions not amenable to removal by hot biopsy forceps, bipolar cautery, or snare technique, see 46615. Bleeding that occurs as the result of an endoscopic procedure, and controlled during the same operative session, is not reported separately. Do not report 45338 or 45346 with 45330. Do not report 45338 in addition to 45349 or 45346 in addition to 45340 for the same lesion.

ICD-10-CM Diagnostic Codes

C18.6	Malignant neoplasm of descending colon
C18.7	Malignant neoplasm of sigmoid colon
C18.8	Malignant neoplasm of overlapping sites of colon
C19	Malignant neoplasm of rectosigmoid junction
C20	Malignant neoplasm of rectum
C21.1	Malignant neoplasm of anal canal
C21.2	Malignant neoplasm of cloacogenic zone
C21.8	Malignant neoplasm of overlapping sites of rectum, anus and anal canal
C49.A4	Gastrointestinal stromal tumor of large intestine
C78.5	Secondary malignant neoplasm of large intestine and rectum
C7A.025	Malignant carcinoid tumor of the sigmoid colon
C7A.026	Malignant carcinoid tumor of the rectum
D01.0	Carcinoma in situ of colon
D01.1	Carcinoma in situ of rectosigmoid junction
D01.2	Carcinoma in situ of rectum
D01.3	Carcinoma in situ of anus and anal canal
D01.49	Carcinoma in situ of other parts of intestine
D12.4	Benign neoplasm of descending colon
D12.5	Benign neoplasm of sigmoid colon
D12.7	Benign neoplasm of rectosigmoid junction
D12.8	Benign neoplasm of rectum
D12.9	Benign neoplasm of anus and anal canal
D37.4	Neoplasm of uncertain behavior of colon
D37.5	Neoplasm of uncertain behavior of rectum
D3A.025	Benign carcinoid tumor of the sigmoid colon
D3A.026	Benign carcinoid tumor of the rectum
D49.0	Neoplasm of unspecified behavior of digestive system
K51.40	Inflammatory polyps of colon without complications
K51.411	Inflammatory polyps of colon with rectal bleeding
K51.412	Inflammatory polyps of colon with intestinal obstruction
K51.413	Inflammatory polyps of colon with fistula
K51.414	Inflammatory polyps of colon with abscess
K51.418	Inflammatory polyps of colon with other complication
K55.20	Angiodysplasia of colon without hemorrhage
K55.21	Angiodysplasia of colon with hemorrhage
K62.0	Anal polyp
K62.1	Rectal polyp
K62.5	Hemorrhage of anus and rectum
K62.6	Ulcer of anus and rectum
K62.82	Dysplasia of anus
K62.89	Other specified diseases of anus and rectum
K63.5	Polyp of colon
K63.89	Other specified diseases of intestine

AMA: **45338** 2018,Jan,8; 2017,Jan,8; 2016,Jan,13; 2016,Feb,13; 2015,Jan,16
45346 2018,Jan,8; 2017,Jan,8; 2016,Jan,13; 2016,Feb,13; 2015,Jan,16

Relative Value Units/Medicare Edits

Non-Facility RVU	Work	PE	MP	Total
45338	2.05	6.77	0.25	9.07
45346	2.81	76.84	0.32	79.97
Facility RVU	**Work**	**PE**	**MP**	**Total**
45338	2.05	1.2	0.25	3.5
45346	2.81	1.54	0.32	4.67

	FUD	Status	MUE	Modifiers				IOM Reference
45338	0	A	1(2)	51	N/A	N/A	N/A	None
45346	0	A	1(2)	51	N/A	N/A	N/A	

* with documentation

Rectum

45340

45340 Sigmoidoscopy, flexible; with transendoscopic balloon dilation

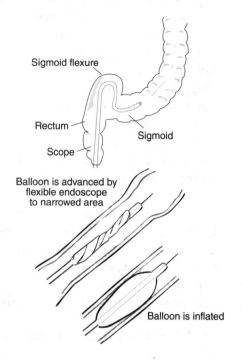

Sigmoid flexure

Rectum

Scope

Sigmoid

Balloon is advanced by flexible endoscope to narrowed area

Balloon is inflated

Explanation

The physician performs flexible sigmoidoscopy and dilates strictures by balloon catheter. The physician inserts the sigmoidoscope into the anus and advances the scope through the rectum and into the sigmoid colon. The lumen of the sigmoid colon and rectum are visualized. Areas of stenosis are identified and a balloon catheter is passed to the point of constriction and a little beyond. The balloon is inflated to the appropriate diameter and gradually withdrawn through the stenosed area, stretching the walls of the bowel at the strictured area. The scope is withdrawn at the completion of the procedure.

Coding Tips

Report the appropriate endoscopy for each anatomic site examined. Surgical endoscopy includes diagnostic endoscopy; however, diagnostic endoscopy can be identified separately when performed at the same surgical session as an open procedure. If fluoroscopic guidance is used, see 74360. For multiple strictures treated with transendoscopic balloon dilations during the same session, report 45340 with modifier 59 or an X{EPSU} modifier for each additional stricture. For colonoscopy, flexible, with transendoscopic balloon dilation, one or more strictures, see 45386. Bleeding that occurs as the result of an endoscopic procedure, and is controlled during the same operative session, is not reported separately. Do not report 45340 with 45330, 45346, or 45347.

ICD-10-CM Diagnostic Codes

K50.112	Crohn's disease of large intestine with intestinal obstruction
K50.812	Crohn's disease of both small and large intestine with intestinal obstruction
K51.012	Ulcerative (chronic) pancolitis with intestinal obstruction
K51.212	Ulcerative (chronic) proctitis with intestinal obstruction
K51.312	Ulcerative (chronic) rectosigmoiditis with intestinal obstruction
K51.412	Inflammatory polyps of colon with intestinal obstruction
K51.512	Left sided colitis with intestinal obstruction
K51.812	Other ulcerative colitis with intestinal obstruction
K56.1	Intussusception
K56.2	Volvulus
K56.51	Intestinal adhesions [bands], with partial obstruction
K56.52	Intestinal adhesions [bands] with complete obstruction
K56.690	Other partial intestinal obstruction
K56.691	Other complete intestinal obstruction
K91.31	Postprocedural partial intestinal obstruction
K91.32	Postprocedural complete intestinal obstruction
Q42.0	Congenital absence, atresia and stenosis of rectum with fistula
Q42.1	Congenital absence, atresia and stenosis of rectum without fistula
Q42.2	Congenital absence, atresia and stenosis of anus with fistula
Q42.3	Congenital absence, atresia and stenosis of anus without fistula
Q42.8	Congenital absence, atresia and stenosis of other parts of large intestine

AMA: 45340 2018,Jan,8; 2017,Jan,8; 2016,Jan,13; 2016,Feb,13; 2015,Jan,16

Relative Value Units/Medicare Edits

Non-Facility RVU	Work	PE	MP	Total
45340	1.25	12.98	0.16	14.39
Facility RVU	**Work**	**PE**	**MP**	**Total**
45340	1.25	0.85	0.16	2.26

	FUD	Status	MUE	Modifiers				IOM Reference
45340	0	A	1(2)	51	N/A	N/A	N/A	None

* with documentation

Terms To Know

atresia. Congenital closure or absence of a tubular organ or an opening to the body surface.

balloon catheter. Any catheter equipped with an inflatable balloon at the end to hold it in place in a body cavity or to be used for dilation of a vessel lumen.

congenital. Present at birth, occurring through heredity or an influence during gestation up to the moment of birth.

dilation. Artificial increase in the diameter of an opening or lumen made by medication or by instrumentation.

intestinal or peritoneal adhesions with obstruction. Abnormal fibrous band growths joining separate tissues in the peritoneum or intestine, causing blockage.

lumen. Space inside an intestine, artery, vein, duct, or tube.

obstruction. Blockage that prevents normal function of the valve or structure.

stenosis. Narrowing or constriction of a passage.

stricture. Narrowing of an anatomical structure.

45341

45341   Sigmoidoscopy, flexible; with endoscopic ultrasound examination

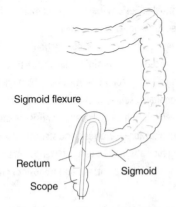

Sigmoid flexure

Rectum

Scope

Sigmoid

A flexible sigmoidoscopy is performed
with an endoscopic ultrasound

Explanation

The physician uses a flexible sigmoidoscopy to examine the rectum and
sigmoid colon and performs an endoscopic ultrasound examination. The
physician inserts the sigmoidoscopy into the anus and advances the scope
into the sigmoid colon. The lumen of the sigmoid colon and rectum are
visualized. The sigmoidoscope is removed and replaced with an
echoendoscope or an ultrasound probe is passed through the already placed
sigmoidoscope. The echoendoscope or ultrasound probe is fitted with a
water-filled balloon near the tip; the tip contains a transducer that picks-up
the ultrasound frequency and relays it to a processor, outside of the body. The
water-filled tip is positioned in the sigmoid colon, against the colon wall next
to the area of interest. The area is scanned and an ultrasound image is projected
through the processor to a monitor in real-time. When the ultrasound
examination is complete the echoendoscope, or esophagoscope and
ultrasound probes are removed.

Coding Tips

Report the appropriate endoscopy for each anatomic site examined. Surgical
endoscopy includes diagnostic endoscopy; however, diagnostic endoscopy
can be identified separately when performed at the same surgical session as
an open procedure. This service should only be reported once per session.
Bleeding that occurs as the result of an endoscopic procedure, and controlled
during the same operative session, is not reported separately. For
esophagoscopy with endoscopic ultrasound examination, see 43231. Do not
report 45341 with 45330, 45342, 76872, or 76975.

ICD-10-CM Diagnostic Codes

C18.6	Malignant neoplasm of descending colon
C18.7	Malignant neoplasm of sigmoid colon
C19	Malignant neoplasm of rectosigmoid junction
C20	Malignant neoplasm of rectum
C21.1	Malignant neoplasm of anal canal
C49.A4	Gastrointestinal stromal tumor of large intestine
C49.A5	Gastrointestinal stromal tumor of rectum
C78.5	Secondary malignant neoplasm of large intestine and rectum
C7A.024	Malignant carcinoid tumor of the descending colon
C7A.025	Malignant carcinoid tumor of the sigmoid colon
C7A.026	Malignant carcinoid tumor of the rectum

D01.0	Carcinoma in situ of colon
D01.1	Carcinoma in situ of rectosigmoid junction
D01.2	Carcinoma in situ of rectum
D01.3	Carcinoma in situ of anus and anal canal
D01.49	Carcinoma in situ of other parts of intestine
D12.4	Benign neoplasm of descending colon
D12.5	Benign neoplasm of sigmoid colon
D12.7	Benign neoplasm of rectosigmoid junction
D12.8	Benign neoplasm of rectum
D12.9	Benign neoplasm of anus and anal canal
D37.4	Neoplasm of uncertain behavior of colon
D37.5	Neoplasm of uncertain behavior of rectum
D3A.024	Benign carcinoid tumor of the descending colon
D3A.025	Benign carcinoid tumor of the sigmoid colon
D3A.026	Benign carcinoid tumor of the rectum
K50.10	Crohn's disease of large intestine without complications
K50.111	Crohn's disease of large intestine with rectal bleeding
K50.112	Crohn's disease of large intestine with intestinal obstruction
K50.113	Crohn's disease of large intestine with fistula
K50.114	Crohn's disease of large intestine with abscess
K50.811	Crohn's disease of both small and large intestine with rectal bleeding
K50.812	Crohn's disease of both small and large intestine with intestinal obstruction
K50.813	Crohn's disease of both small and large intestine with fistula
K50.814	Crohn's disease of both small and large intestine with abscess
K51.011	Ulcerative (chronic) pancolitis with rectal bleeding
K51.012	Ulcerative (chronic) pancolitis with intestinal obstruction
K51.013	Ulcerative (chronic) pancolitis with fistula
K51.014	Ulcerative (chronic) pancolitis with abscess
K51.20	Ulcerative (chronic) proctitis without complications
K51.211	Ulcerative (chronic) proctitis with rectal bleeding
K51.212	Ulcerative (chronic) proctitis with intestinal obstruction
K51.213	Ulcerative (chronic) proctitis with fistula
K51.214	Ulcerative (chronic) proctitis with abscess
K51.30	Ulcerative (chronic) rectosigmoiditis without complications
K51.311	Ulcerative (chronic) rectosigmoiditis with rectal bleeding
K51.312	Ulcerative (chronic) rectosigmoiditis with intestinal obstruction
K51.313	Ulcerative (chronic) rectosigmoiditis with fistula
K51.314	Ulcerative (chronic) rectosigmoiditis with abscess
K51.40	Inflammatory polyps of colon without complications
K51.411	Inflammatory polyps of colon with rectal bleeding
K51.412	Inflammatory polyps of colon with intestinal obstruction
K51.413	Inflammatory polyps of colon with fistula
K51.414	Inflammatory polyps of colon with abscess
K51.511	Left sided colitis with rectal bleeding
K51.512	Left sided colitis with intestinal obstruction
K51.513	Left sided colitis with fistula
K51.514	Left sided colitis with abscess
K51.80	Other ulcerative colitis without complications
K51.811	Other ulcerative colitis with rectal bleeding
K51.812	Other ulcerative colitis with intestinal obstruction
K51.813	Other ulcerative colitis with fistula

Rectum

K51.814	Other ulcerative colitis with abscess
K52.82	Eosinophilic colitis
K52.89	Other specified noninfective gastroenteritis and colitis
K55.031	Focal (segmental) acute (reversible) ischemia of large intestine
K55.032	Diffuse acute (reversible) ischemia of large intestine
K55.041	Focal (segmental) acute infarction of large intestine
K55.042	Diffuse acute infarction of large intestine
K55.1	Chronic vascular disorders of intestine
K55.20	Angiodysplasia of colon without hemorrhage
K55.21	Angiodysplasia of colon with hemorrhage
K56.2	Volvulus
K56.51	Intestinal adhesions [bands], with partial obstruction
K56.52	Intestinal adhesions [bands] with complete obstruction
K56.690	Other partial intestinal obstruction
K56.691	Other complete intestinal obstruction
K57.20	Diverticulitis of large intestine with perforation and abscess without bleeding
K57.21	Diverticulitis of large intestine with perforation and abscess with bleeding
K57.30	Diverticulosis of large intestine without perforation or abscess without bleeding
K57.31	Diverticulosis of large intestine without perforation or abscess with bleeding
K57.32	Diverticulitis of large intestine without perforation or abscess without bleeding
K57.33	Diverticulitis of large intestine without perforation or abscess with bleeding
K57.40	Diverticulitis of both small and large intestine with perforation and abscess without bleeding
K57.41	Diverticulitis of both small and large intestine with perforation and abscess with bleeding
K57.50	Diverticulosis of both small and large intestine without perforation or abscess without bleeding
K57.51	Diverticulosis of both small and large intestine without perforation or abscess with bleeding
K57.52	Diverticulitis of both small and large intestine without perforation or abscess without bleeding
K57.53	Diverticulitis of both small and large intestine without perforation or abscess with bleeding
K58.0	Irritable bowel syndrome with diarrhea
K58.9	Irritable bowel syndrome without diarrhea
K59.1	Functional diarrhea
K60.3	Anal fistula
K60.4	Rectal fistula
K60.5	Anorectal fistula
K61.0	Anal abscess
K61.1	Rectal abscess
K61.2	Anorectal abscess
K61.31	Horseshoe abscess
K61.39	Other ischiorectal abscess
K61.5	Supralevator abscess
K62.1	Rectal polyp
K62.2	Anal prolapse
K62.3	Rectal prolapse

K62.4	Stenosis of anus and rectum
K62.5	Hemorrhage of anus and rectum
K62.6	Ulcer of anus and rectum
K62.7	Radiation proctitis
K62.82	Dysplasia of anus
K62.89	Other specified diseases of anus and rectum
K63.0	Abscess of intestine
K63.5	Polyp of colon
K64.0	First degree hemorrhoids
K64.1	Second degree hemorrhoids
K64.2	Third degree hemorrhoids
K64.3	Fourth degree hemorrhoids
K91.31	Postprocedural partial intestinal obstruction
K91.32	Postprocedural complete intestinal obstruction
K92.1	Melena
M35.08	Sjögren syndrome with gastrointestinal involvement
Q42.0	Congenital absence, atresia and stenosis of rectum with fistula
Q42.1	Congenital absence, atresia and stenosis of rectum without fistula
Q42.2	Congenital absence, atresia and stenosis of anus with fistula
Q42.3	Congenital absence, atresia and stenosis of anus without fistula
Q42.8	Congenital absence, atresia and stenosis of other parts of large intestine
Q43.1	Hirschsprung's disease
Q43.2	Other congenital functional disorders of colon
Q43.3	Congenital malformations of intestinal fixation
Q43.4	Duplication of intestine
Q43.6	Congenital fistula of rectum and anus

AMA: **45341** 2018,Jan,8; 2017,Jan,8; 2016,Jan,13; 2016,Feb,13; 2015,Jan,16

Relative Value Units/Medicare Edits

Non-Facility RVU	Work	PE	MP	Total
45341	2.12	1.25	0.23	3.6
Facility RVU	**Work**	**PE**	**MP**	**Total**
45341	2.12	1.25	0.23	3.6

	FUD	Status	MUE	Modifiers				IOM Reference
45341	0	A	1(2)	51	N/A	N/A	N/A	None

* with documentation

45342

45342 Sigmoidoscopy, flexible; with transendoscopic ultrasound guided intramural or transmural fine needle aspiration/biopsy(s)

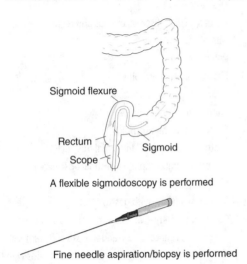

Sigmoid flexure

Rectum

Scope

Sigmoid

A flexible sigmoidoscopy is performed

Fine needle aspiration/biopsy is performed

Explanation

The physician uses a flexible sigmoidoscopy to examine the rectum and sigmoid colon and performs a transendoscopic ultrasound guided intramural or transmural fine needle aspiration/biopsy. The physician inserts the sigmoidoscopy into the anus and advances the scope into the sigmoid colon. The lumen of the sigmoid colon and rectum are visualized. The sigmoidoscope may be removed. A radial scanning echoendoscope is inserted and ultrasound scanning is performed, or an ultrasound probe is passed through the already placed endoscope. The site for a fine needle aspiration biopsy is determined. If a radial scanning echoendoscope is used it is removed and is replaced with a curvilinear array echoendoscope. The echoendoscope or ultrasound probe is fitted with a water-filled balloon near the tip; the tip contains a transducer that picks up the ultrasound frequency and relays it to a processor, outside of the body. The water-filled tip is positioned in the sigmoid colon against the colon wall next to the predetermined fine needle aspiration (FNA) biopsy site. The area is scanned and an ultrasound image is projected through the processor to a monitor in real-time. An FNA needle is passed through the scope to the biopsy site and a biopsy is taken of the tissue or the needle is inserted through the wall of the tissue into the lesion, or other structure, such as a lymph node. The area is biopsied. When the FNA is complete the echoendoscope or sigmoidoscope and ultrasound probes are removed.

Coding Tips

Surgical endoscopy includes diagnostic endoscopy; however, diagnostic endoscopy can be identified separately when performed at the same surgical session as an open procedure. Report this service only once per session. Bleeding that occurs as the result of an endoscopic procedure, and controlled during the same operative session, is not reported separately. For transrectal ultrasound utilizing rigid probe device, see 76872. For interpretation of specimen, see 88172–88173. Do not report 45342 with 45330, 45341, 76872, 76942, or 76975.

ICD-10-CM Diagnostic Codes

C18.6	Malignant neoplasm of descending colon
C18.7	Malignant neoplasm of sigmoid colon
C19	Malignant neoplasm of rectosigmoid junction
C20	Malignant neoplasm of rectum
C21.1	Malignant neoplasm of anal canal
C21.2	Malignant neoplasm of cloacogenic zone
C49.A4	Gastrointestinal stromal tumor of large intestine
C49.A5	Gastrointestinal stromal tumor of rectum
C78.5	Secondary malignant neoplasm of large intestine and rectum
C7A.024	Malignant carcinoid tumor of the descending colon
C7A.025	Malignant carcinoid tumor of the sigmoid colon
C7A.026	Malignant carcinoid tumor of the rectum
D01.0	Carcinoma in situ of colon
D01.1	Carcinoma in situ of rectosigmoid junction
D01.2	Carcinoma in situ of rectum
D01.3	Carcinoma in situ of anus and anal canal
D12.4	Benign neoplasm of descending colon
D12.5	Benign neoplasm of sigmoid colon
D12.7	Benign neoplasm of rectosigmoid junction
D12.8	Benign neoplasm of rectum
D12.9	Benign neoplasm of anus and anal canal
D37.4	Neoplasm of uncertain behavior of colon
D37.5	Neoplasm of uncertain behavior of rectum
D37.8	Neoplasm of uncertain behavior of other specified digestive organs
D3A.024	Benign carcinoid tumor of the descending colon
D3A.025	Benign carcinoid tumor of the sigmoid colon
D3A.026	Benign carcinoid tumor of the rectum
K50.10	Crohn's disease of large intestine without complications
K50.111	Crohn's disease of large intestine with rectal bleeding
K50.112	Crohn's disease of large intestine with intestinal obstruction
K50.113	Crohn's disease of large intestine with fistula
K50.114	Crohn's disease of large intestine with abscess
K50.118	Crohn's disease of large intestine with other complication
K50.811	Crohn's disease of both small and large intestine with rectal bleeding
K50.812	Crohn's disease of both small and large intestine with intestinal obstruction
K50.813	Crohn's disease of both small and large intestine with fistula
K50.814	Crohn's disease of both small and large intestine with abscess
K51.20	Ulcerative (chronic) proctitis without complications
K51.211	Ulcerative (chronic) proctitis with rectal bleeding
K51.212	Ulcerative (chronic) proctitis with intestinal obstruction
K51.213	Ulcerative (chronic) proctitis with fistula
K51.214	Ulcerative (chronic) proctitis with abscess
K51.218	Ulcerative (chronic) proctitis with other complication
K51.311	Ulcerative (chronic) rectosigmoiditis with rectal bleeding
K51.312	Ulcerative (chronic) rectosigmoiditis with intestinal obstruction
K51.313	Ulcerative (chronic) rectosigmoiditis with fistula
K51.314	Ulcerative (chronic) rectosigmoiditis with abscess
K51.318	Ulcerative (chronic) rectosigmoiditis with other complication
K51.411	Inflammatory polyps of colon with rectal bleeding
K51.412	Inflammatory polyps of colon with intestinal obstruction
K51.413	Inflammatory polyps of colon with fistula
K51.414	Inflammatory polyps of colon with abscess
K51.511	Left sided colitis with rectal bleeding
K51.512	Left sided colitis with intestinal obstruction

N Newborn: 0   **P** Pediatric: 0-17   **M** Maternity: 9-64   **A** Adult: 15-124   ♂ Male Only   ♀ Female Only

Coding Companion for General Surgery/Gastroenterology

Rectum

K51.513	Left sided colitis with fistula
K51.514	Left sided colitis with abscess
K51.518	Left sided colitis with other complication
K51.80	Other ulcerative colitis without complications
K51.811	Other ulcerative colitis with rectal bleeding
K51.812	Other ulcerative colitis with intestinal obstruction
K51.813	Other ulcerative colitis with fistula
K51.814	Other ulcerative colitis with abscess
K52.0	Gastroenteritis and colitis due to radiation
K52.1	Toxic gastroenteritis and colitis
K52.82	Eosinophilic colitis
K52.89	Other specified noninfective gastroenteritis and colitis
K55.031	Focal (segmental) acute (reversible) ischemia of large intestine
K55.032	Diffuse acute (reversible) ischemia of large intestine
K55.041	Focal (segmental) acute infarction of large intestine
K55.042	Diffuse acute infarction of large intestine
K55.1	Chronic vascular disorders of intestine
K55.20	Angiodysplasia of colon without hemorrhage
K55.21	Angiodysplasia of colon with hemorrhage
K55.8	Other vascular disorders of intestine
K57.20	Diverticulitis of large intestine with perforation and abscess without bleeding
K57.21	Diverticulitis of large intestine with perforation and abscess with bleeding
K57.30	Diverticulosis of large intestine without perforation or abscess without bleeding
K57.31	Diverticulosis of large intestine without perforation or abscess with bleeding
K57.32	Diverticulitis of large intestine without perforation or abscess without bleeding
K57.33	Diverticulitis of large intestine without perforation or abscess with bleeding
K57.40	Diverticulitis of both small and large intestine with perforation and abscess without bleeding
K57.41	Diverticulitis of both small and large intestine with perforation and abscess with bleeding
K57.50	Diverticulosis of both small and large intestine without perforation or abscess without bleeding
K57.51	Diverticulosis of both small and large intestine without perforation or abscess with bleeding
K57.52	Diverticulitis of both small and large intestine without perforation or abscess without bleeding
K57.53	Diverticulitis of both small and large intestine without perforation or abscess with bleeding
K62.0	Anal polyp
K62.1	Rectal polyp
K62.6	Ulcer of anus and rectum
K62.7	Radiation proctitis
K62.82	Dysplasia of anus
K62.89	Other specified diseases of anus and rectum
K63.5	Polyp of colon
K63.89	Other specified diseases of intestine
K92.1	Melena
K92.89	Other specified diseases of the digestive system

| M35.08 | Sjögren syndrome with gastrointestinal involvement |

AMA: 45342 2018,Jan,8; 2017,Jan,8; 2016,Jan,13; 2016,Feb,13; 2015,Jan,16

Relative Value Units/Medicare Edits

Non-Facility RVU	Work	PE	MP	Total
45342	2.98	1.64	0.32	4.94
Facility RVU	**Work**	**PE**	**MP**	**Total**
45342	2.98	1.64	0.32	4.94

	FUD	Status	MUE	Modifiers				IOM Reference
45342	0	A	1(2)	51	N/A	N/A	N/A	None

* with documentation

Terms To Know

fine needle aspiration. 22- or 25-gauge needle attached to a syringe is inserted into a lesion/tissue and a few cells are aspirated for biopsy and diagnostic study. Aspiration is also used to remove fluid from a benign cyst.

intramural. Within the wall of an organ.

lumen. Space inside an intestine, artery, vein, duct, or tube.

sigmoidoscopy. Endoscopic examination of the entire rectum and sigmoid colon, often including a portion of the descending colon and usually performed with a flexible fiberoptic scope in conjunction with a surgical procedure.

transducer. Apparatus that transfers or translates one type of energy into another, such as converting pressure to an electrical signal.

ultrasound. Imaging using ultra-high sound frequency bounced off body structures.

45347

45347 Sigmoidoscopy, flexible; with placement of endoscopic stent (includes pre- and post-dilation and guide wire passage, when performed)

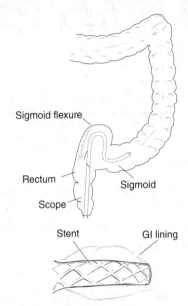

A sigmoidoscopy session is performed with endoscopic stent placement, including pre- and postdilation

Explanation

The physician performs flexible sigmoidoscopy to examine the rectum and sigmoid colon and places an endoscopic stent. The physician inserts the sigmoidoscope into the anus and advances the scope through the rectum and into the sigmoid colon. The lumen of the sigmoid colon and rectum are visualized. The endoscope is placed at the site of an obstruction or stricture and the necessary stent length is determined. The stent (endoprosthesis) is introduced into the site of the obstruction. Using a commercial delivery system, a plastic covering over the stent is removed and the stent self-deploys, shoring-up the walls at a specific site in the sigmoid colon. When necessary, a balloon catheter is placed into the stent and gently inflated to more fully deploy the stent. The delivery system and endoscope are removed. This code includes dilation before and after the procedure and utilization of a guidewire, if employed.

Coding Tips

Surgical endoscopy includes diagnostic endoscopy; however, diagnostic endoscopy can be identified separately when performed at the same surgical session as an open procedure. Flexible sigmoidoscopy includes an examination of the entire rectum, sigmoid colon, and may include a portion of the descending colon. When examination of the rectum and sigmoid colon with transendoscopic stent placement is performed using a rigid proctoscope (stiff hollow tube-like instrument), see 45327. Bleeding that occurs as the result of an endoscopic procedure, and controlled during the same operative session, is not reported separately. Do not report 45347 with 45330 or 45340. If fluoroscopic guidance is used, see 74360.

ICD-10-CM Diagnostic Codes

C18.7	Malignant neoplasm of sigmoid colon
C18.8	Malignant neoplasm of overlapping sites of colon
C19	Malignant neoplasm of rectosigmoid junction
C20	Malignant neoplasm of rectum
C21.2	Malignant neoplasm of cloacogenic zone
C21.8	Malignant neoplasm of overlapping sites of rectum, anus and anal canal
C78.5	Secondary malignant neoplasm of large intestine and rectum
K50.112	Crohn's disease of large intestine with intestinal obstruction
K50.812	Crohn's disease of both small and large intestine with intestinal obstruction
K51.012	Ulcerative (chronic) pancolitis with intestinal obstruction
K51.212	Ulcerative (chronic) proctitis with intestinal obstruction
K51.312	Ulcerative (chronic) rectosigmoiditis with intestinal obstruction
K51.412	Inflammatory polyps of colon with intestinal obstruction
K51.512	Left sided colitis with intestinal obstruction
K51.812	Other ulcerative colitis with intestinal obstruction
K56.1	Intussusception
K56.2	Volvulus
K56.51	Intestinal adhesions [bands], with partial obstruction
K56.52	Intestinal adhesions [bands] with complete obstruction
K56.690	Other partial intestinal obstruction
K56.691	Other complete intestinal obstruction
K62.4	Stenosis of anus and rectum
K91.31	Postprocedural partial intestinal obstruction
K91.32	Postprocedural complete intestinal obstruction
Q42.0	Congenital absence, atresia and stenosis of rectum with fistula
Q42.1	Congenital absence, atresia and stenosis of rectum without fistula
Q42.8	Congenital absence, atresia and stenosis of other parts of large intestine

AMA: 45347 2018,Jan,8; 2017,Jan,8; 2016,Jan,13; 2016,Feb,13; 2015,Jan,16

Relative Value Units/Medicare Edits

Non-Facility RVU	Work	PE	MP	Total
45347	2.72	1.47	0.3	4.49
Facility RVU	**Work**	**PE**	**MP**	**Total**
45347	2.72	1.47	0.3	4.49

	FUD	Status	MUE	Modifiers				IOM Reference
45347	0	A	1(3)	51	N/A	N/A	N/A	None

* with documentation

Terms To Know

dilation. Artificial increase in the diameter of an opening or lumen made by medication or by instrumentation.

sigmoidoscopy. Endoscopic examination of the entire rectum and sigmoid colon, often including a portion of the descending colon and usually performed with a flexible fiberoptic scope in conjunction with a surgical procedure.

stent. Tube to provide support in a body cavity or lumen.

stricture. Narrowing of an anatomical structure.

Rectum

45349

45349 Sigmoidoscopy, flexible; with endoscopic mucosal resection

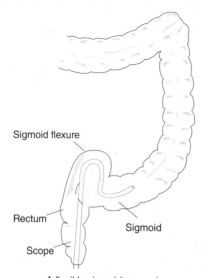

Sigmoid flexure

Rectum

Scope

Sigmoid

A flexible sigmoidoscopy is
performed and the mucosa is resected

Explanation

The physician inserts the sigmoidoscope into the anus and advances the scope through the rectum and into the sigmoid colon. The lumen of the sigmoid colon and rectum are visualized. The scope is directed to the affected area. A special needle is used to administer fluid under the polyp, elevating the polyp and allowing its removal from the bowel lining. Removal may be done by snare, cutting out, or suction and typically includes cautery of the attached blood vessels. The tissue is sent to pathology for analysis and the scope is withdrawn at the completion of the procedure.

Coding Tips

Surgical endoscopy includes diagnostic endoscopy; however, diagnostic endoscopy can be identified separately when performed at the same surgical session as an open procedure. Bleeding that occurs as the result of an endoscopic procedure, and controlled during the same operative session, is not reported separately. Do not report 45349 with 45330 or in addition to 45331, 45335, 45338, or 45350 for the same lesion.

ICD-10-CM Diagnostic Codes

C18.7	Malignant neoplasm of sigmoid colon
C18.8	Malignant neoplasm of overlapping sites of colon
C19	Malignant neoplasm of rectosigmoid junction
C20	Malignant neoplasm of rectum
C21.2	Malignant neoplasm of cloacogenic zone
C21.8	Malignant neoplasm of overlapping sites of rectum, anus and anal canal
C78.5	Secondary malignant neoplasm of large intestine and rectum
C7A.025	Malignant carcinoid tumor of the sigmoid colon
C7A.026	Malignant carcinoid tumor of the rectum
D01.0	Carcinoma in situ of colon
D01.1	Carcinoma in situ of rectosigmoid junction
D01.2	Carcinoma in situ of rectum
D01.49	Carcinoma in situ of other parts of intestine
D12.5	Benign neoplasm of sigmoid colon
D12.7	Benign neoplasm of rectosigmoid junction
D12.8	Benign neoplasm of rectum
D37.4	Neoplasm of uncertain behavior of colon
D37.5	Neoplasm of uncertain behavior of rectum
D3A.025	Benign carcinoid tumor of the sigmoid colon
D3A.026	Benign carcinoid tumor of the rectum
D49.0	Neoplasm of unspecified behavior of digestive system
K51.40	Inflammatory polyps of colon without complications
K51.411	Inflammatory polyps of colon with rectal bleeding
K51.412	Inflammatory polyps of colon with intestinal obstruction
K51.413	Inflammatory polyps of colon with fistula
K51.414	Inflammatory polyps of colon with abscess
K51.418	Inflammatory polyps of colon with other complication
K62.1	Rectal polyp
K62.89	Other specified diseases of anus and rectum
K63.5	Polyp of colon

AMA: **45349** 2020,May,13; 2019,Dec,14; 2018,Jan,8; 2017,Jan,8; 2016,Jan,13; 2015,Jan,16

Relative Value Units/Medicare Edits

Non-Facility RVU	Work	PE	MP	Total
45349	3.52	1.86	0.39	5.77
Facility RVU	**Work**	**PE**	**MP**	**Total**
45349	3.52	1.86	0.39	5.77

	FUD	Status	MUE	Modifiers				IOM Reference
45349	0	A	1(3)	51	N/A	N/A	N/A	None

* with documentation

Terms To Know

lumen. Space inside an intestine, artery, vein, duct, or tube.

sigmoidoscopy. Endoscopic examination of the entire rectum and sigmoid colon, often including a portion of the descending colon and usually performed with a flexible fiberoptic scope in conjunction with a surgical procedure.

stent. Tube to provide support in a body cavity or lumen.

suction. Vacuum evacuation of fluid or tissue.

Rectum

45350

45350   Sigmoidoscopy, flexible; with band ligation(s) (eg, hemorrhoids)

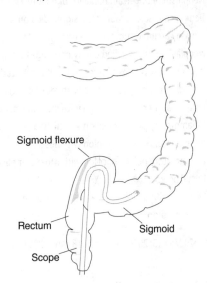

Sigmoid flexure

Rectum

Sigmoid

Scope

Explanation

The physician uses a flexible sigmoidoscope to examine the rectum and sigmoid colon and perform band ligation for hemorrhoids. The physician inserts the sigmoidoscope into the anus and advances the scope through the rectum and into the sigmoid colon. The lumen of the sigmoid colon and rectum are visualized. The scope is directed to the affected area. The physician identifies the hemorrhoid. The hemorrhoid is ligated at its base with a rubber band. The hemorrhoid tissue is allowed to slough over time.

Coding Tips

Surgical endoscopy includes diagnostic endoscopy; however, diagnostic endoscopy can be identified separately when performed at the same surgical session as an open procedure. This service should only be reported once per session. For control of active bleeding with band ligation, see 45334. Bleeding that occurs as the result of an endoscopic procedure, and controlled during the same operative session, is not reported separately. Do not report 45350 with 45330, 45349, or 46221 or in addition to 45334 for the same lesion.

ICD-10-CM Diagnostic Codes

K64.0	First degree hemorrhoids
K64.1	Second degree hemorrhoids
K64.2	Third degree hemorrhoids
K64.3	Fourth degree hemorrhoids
K64.8	Other hemorrhoids

AMA: 45350 2020,Feb,11; 2018,Jan,8; 2017,Jan,8; 2016,Jan,13; 2015,Jan,16

Relative Value Units/Medicare Edits

Non-Facility RVU	Work	PE	MP	Total
45350	1.68	18.66	0.21	20.55
Facility RVU	**Work**	**PE**	**MP**	**Total**
45350	1.68	1.04	0.21	2.93

	FUD	Status	MUE	Modifiers				IOM Reference
45350	0	A	1(2)	51	N/A	N/A	N/A	None

* with documentation

45378

45378   Colonoscopy, flexible; diagnostic, including collection of specimen(s) by brushing or washing, when performed (separate procedure)

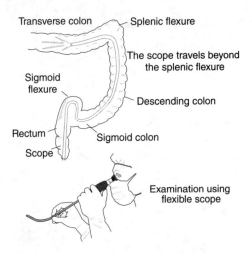

Transverse colon — Splenic flexure

The scope travels beyond the splenic flexure

Sigmoid flexure

Descending colon

Rectum

Sigmoid colon

Scope

Examination using flexible scope

Explanation

The physician performs flexible colonoscopy and may obtain brushings or washings. The physician inserts the colonoscope into the anus and advances the scope through the colon to the cecum. The lumen of the colon and rectum are visualized. Brushings or washings may be obtained. The colonoscope is withdrawn at the completion of the procedure.

Coding Tips

This separate procedure, by definition, is usually a component of a more complex service and is not identified separately. When performed alone or with other unrelated procedures/services it may be reported. If performed with other procedures/services, list the code with modifier 59 or an X{EPSU} modifier. Surgical endoscopy always includes diagnostic endoscopy. However, diagnostic endoscopy can be identified separately when performed at the same surgical session as an open procedure. Bleeding that occurs as the result of an endoscopic procedure, and controlled during the same operative session, is not reported separately. Report a colonoscopy with decompression of a pathologic distention with 45393. Do not report 45378 with 45379–45393 or 45398.

ICD-10-CM Diagnostic Codes

C18.0	Malignant neoplasm of cecum
C18.2	Malignant neoplasm of ascending colon
C18.3	Malignant neoplasm of hepatic flexure
C18.4	Malignant neoplasm of transverse colon
C18.5	Malignant neoplasm of splenic flexure
C18.6	Malignant neoplasm of descending colon
C18.7	Malignant neoplasm of sigmoid colon
C49.A4	Gastrointestinal stromal tumor of large intestine
C78.5	Secondary malignant neoplasm of large intestine and rectum
C7A.022	Malignant carcinoid tumor of the ascending colon
C7A.023	Malignant carcinoid tumor of the transverse colon
C7A.024	Malignant carcinoid tumor of the descending colon
C7A.025	Malignant carcinoid tumor of the sigmoid colon
D01.0	Carcinoma in situ of colon
D12.2	Benign neoplasm of ascending colon

D12.3	Benign neoplasm of transverse colon
D12.4	Benign neoplasm of descending colon
D12.5	Benign neoplasm of sigmoid colon
D37.4	Neoplasm of uncertain behavior of colon
D3A.022	Benign carcinoid tumor of the ascending colon
D3A.023	Benign carcinoid tumor of the transverse colon
D3A.024	Benign carcinoid tumor of the descending colon
D3A.025	Benign carcinoid tumor of the sigmoid colon
D49.0	Neoplasm of unspecified behavior of digestive system
K50.10	Crohn's disease of large intestine without complications
K50.111	Crohn's disease of large intestine with rectal bleeding
K50.112	Crohn's disease of large intestine with intestinal obstruction
K50.113	Crohn's disease of large intestine with fistula
K50.114	Crohn's disease of large intestine with abscess
K50.811	Crohn's disease of both small and large intestine with rectal bleeding
K50.812	Crohn's disease of both small and large intestine with intestinal obstruction
K50.813	Crohn's disease of both small and large intestine with fistula
K50.814	Crohn's disease of both small and large intestine with abscess
K51.011	Ulcerative (chronic) pancolitis with rectal bleeding
K51.012	Ulcerative (chronic) pancolitis with intestinal obstruction
K51.013	Ulcerative (chronic) pancolitis with fistula
K51.014	Ulcerative (chronic) pancolitis with abscess
K51.311	Ulcerative (chronic) rectosigmoiditis with rectal bleeding
K51.312	Ulcerative (chronic) rectosigmoiditis with intestinal obstruction
K51.313	Ulcerative (chronic) rectosigmoiditis with fistula
K51.314	Ulcerative (chronic) rectosigmoiditis with abscess
K51.411	Inflammatory polyps of colon with rectal bleeding
K51.412	Inflammatory polyps of colon with intestinal obstruction
K51.413	Inflammatory polyps of colon with fistula
K51.414	Inflammatory polyps of colon with abscess
K51.50	Left sided colitis without complications
K51.511	Left sided colitis with rectal bleeding
K51.512	Left sided colitis with intestinal obstruction
K51.513	Left sided colitis with fistula
K51.514	Left sided colitis with abscess
K52.0	Gastroenteritis and colitis due to radiation
K52.1	Toxic gastroenteritis and colitis
K55.041	Focal (segmental) acute infarction of large intestine
K55.042	Diffuse acute infarction of large intestine
K55.21	Angiodysplasia of colon with hemorrhage
K56.41	Fecal impaction
K56.51	Intestinal adhesions [bands], with partial obstruction
K56.52	Intestinal adhesions [bands] with complete obstruction
K57.20	Diverticulitis of large intestine with perforation and abscess without bleeding
K57.21	Diverticulitis of large intestine with perforation and abscess with bleeding
K57.30	Diverticulosis of large intestine without perforation or abscess without bleeding
K57.33	Diverticulitis of large intestine without perforation or abscess with bleeding

K57.41	Diverticulitis of both small and large intestine with perforation and abscess with bleeding
K57.50	Diverticulosis of both small and large intestine without perforation or abscess without bleeding
K59.01	Slow transit constipation
K63.0	Abscess of intestine
K63.1	Perforation of intestine (nontraumatic)
K63.2	Fistula of intestine
K63.3	Ulcer of intestine
K63.5	Polyp of colon
K63.81	Dieulafoy lesion of intestine
K92.1	Melena
M35.08	Sjögren syndrome with gastrointestinal involvement
Q43.1	Hirschsprung's disease
R62.7	Adult failure to thrive ▲
R63.4	Abnormal weight loss
Z03.821	Encounter for observation for suspected ingested foreign body ruled out
Z03.823	Encounter for observation for suspected inserted (injected) foreign body ruled out
Z12.11	Encounter for screening for malignant neoplasm of colon

Associated HCPCS Codes

| G0105 | Colorectal cancer screening; colonoscopy on individual at high risk |
| G0121 | Colorectal cancer screening; colonoscopy on individual not meeting criteria for high risk |

AMA: **45378** 2018,Jan,7; 2018,Jan,8; 2017,Sep,14; 2017,Jan,8; 2016,Jan,13; 2015,Sep,12; 2015,Jan,16

Relative Value Units/Medicare Edits

Non-Facility RVU	Work	PE	MP	Total
45378	3.26	6.56	0.41	10.23
Facility RVU	**Work**	**PE**	**MP**	**Total**
45378	3.26	1.73	0.41	5.4

	FUD	Status	MUE	Modifiers				IOM Reference
45378	0	A	1(3)	51	N/A	N/A	N/A	None

* with documentation

45379

45379 Colonoscopy, flexible; with removal of foreign body(s)

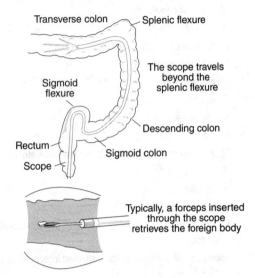

A flexible scope is inserted for foreign body removal

Explanation

The physician performs flexible colonoscopy and removes a foreign body(s). The physician inserts the colonoscope into the anus and advances the scope through the colon to the cecum. The lumen of the colon and rectum are visualized. The foreign body(s) is identified and removed by forceps or snare placed through the colonoscope. The colonoscope is withdrawn at the completion of the procedure.

Coding Tips

Report the appropriate endoscopy for each anatomic site examined. Surgical endoscopy includes diagnostic endoscopy; however, diagnostic endoscopy can be identified separately when performed at the same surgical session as an open procedure. Colonoscopy involves examination of the entire colon, from the rectum to the cecum, and may also include the terminal ileum. An incomplete colonoscopy with full colonoscopy preparation is reported with the colonoscopy code and modifier 52. For colonoscopy through stoma, with removal of a foreign body, see 44390. For proctosigmoidoscopy, rigid, with removal of a foreign body, see 45307. For sigmoidoscopy, flexible, with removal of a foreign body, see 45332. If fluoroscopic guidance is performed, see 76000. Bleeding that occurs as the result of an endoscopic procedure, and controlled during the same operative session, is not reported separately. Do not report 45379 with 45378.

ICD-10-CM Diagnostic Codes

T18.4XXA   Foreign body in colon, initial encounter
T18.8XXA   Foreign body in other parts of alimentary tract, initial encounter

AMA: 45379 2018,Jan,8; 2017,Jan,8; 2016,Jan,13; 2015,Jan,16

Relative Value Units/Medicare Edits

Non-Facility RVU	Work	PE	MP	Total
45379	4.28	8.32	0.49	13.09
Facility RVU	**Work**	**PE**	**MP**	**Total**
45379	4.28	2.17	0.49	6.94

	FUD	Status	MUE	Modifiers			IOM Reference
45379	0	A	1(3)	51	N/A	N/A	N/A	None

* with documentation

Terms To Know

endoscopy. Visual inspection of the body using a fiberoptic scope.

forceps. Tool used for grasping or compressing tissue.

foreign body. Any object or substance found in an organ and tissue that does not belong under normal circumstances.

lumen. Space inside an intestine, artery, vein, duct, or tube.

snare. Wire used as a loop to excise a polyp or lesion.

stoma. Opening created in the abdominal wall from an internal organ or structure for diversion of waste elimination, drainage, and access.

45380

45380 Colonoscopy, flexible; with biopsy, single or multiple

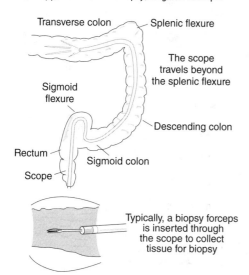

Transverse colon — Splenic flexure

The scope travels beyond the splenic flexure

Sigmoid flexure

Descending colon

Rectum

Sigmoid colon

Scope

Typically, a biopsy forceps is inserted through the scope to collect tissue for biopsy

A flexible scope is inserted for biopsy

Explanation

The physician performs flexible colonoscopy and obtains tissue samples. The physician inserts the colonoscope into the anus and advances the scope through the colon to the cecum. The lumen of the colon and rectum are visualized and biopsies are obtained. The colonoscope is withdrawn at the completion of the procedure.

Coding Tips

Report the appropriate endoscopy for each anatomical site examined. Surgical endoscopy always includes diagnostic endoscopy; however, diagnostic endoscopy can be identified separately when performed at the same surgical session as an open procedure. Colonoscopy involves examination of the entire colon, from the rectum to the cecum, and may also include the terminal ileum. An incomplete colonoscopy with full colonoscopy preparation is reported with the colonoscopy code and modifier 52. Bleeding that occurs as the result of an endoscopic procedure, and controlled during the same operative session, is not reported separately. Do not report 45380 with 45378 or in addition to 45390 for the same lesion.

ICD-10-CM Diagnostic Codes

C18.0	Malignant neoplasm of cecum
C18.1	Malignant neoplasm of appendix
C18.2	Malignant neoplasm of ascending colon
C18.3	Malignant neoplasm of hepatic flexure
C18.4	Malignant neoplasm of transverse colon
C18.5	Malignant neoplasm of splenic flexure
C18.6	Malignant neoplasm of descending colon
C18.7	Malignant neoplasm of sigmoid colon
C19	Malignant neoplasm of rectosigmoid junction
C20	Malignant neoplasm of rectum
C49.A4	Gastrointestinal stromal tumor of large intestine
C49.A5	Gastrointestinal stromal tumor of rectum
C78.5	Secondary malignant neoplasm of large intestine and rectum
C7A.020	Malignant carcinoid tumor of the appendix
C7A.021	Malignant carcinoid tumor of the cecum
C7A.022	Malignant carcinoid tumor of the ascending colon
C7A.023	Malignant carcinoid tumor of the transverse colon
C7A.024	Malignant carcinoid tumor of the descending colon
C7A.025	Malignant carcinoid tumor of the sigmoid colon
C7A.026	Malignant carcinoid tumor of the rectum
D01.0	Carcinoma in situ of colon
D01.1	Carcinoma in situ of rectosigmoid junction
D01.49	Carcinoma in situ of other parts of intestine
D12.0	Benign neoplasm of cecum
D12.1	Benign neoplasm of appendix
D12.2	Benign neoplasm of ascending colon
D12.3	Benign neoplasm of transverse colon
D12.4	Benign neoplasm of descending colon
D12.5	Benign neoplasm of sigmoid colon
D12.7	Benign neoplasm of rectosigmoid junction
D37.3	Neoplasm of uncertain behavior of appendix
D37.4	Neoplasm of uncertain behavior of colon
D37.5	Neoplasm of uncertain behavior of rectum
D3A.020	Benign carcinoid tumor of the appendix
D3A.021	Benign carcinoid tumor of the cecum
D3A.022	Benign carcinoid tumor of the ascending colon
D3A.023	Benign carcinoid tumor of the transverse colon
D3A.024	Benign carcinoid tumor of the descending colon
D3A.025	Benign carcinoid tumor of the sigmoid colon
D3A.026	Benign carcinoid tumor of the rectum
D49.0	Neoplasm of unspecified behavior of digestive system
K50.10	Crohn's disease of large intestine without complications
K50.111	Crohn's disease of large intestine with rectal bleeding
K50.112	Crohn's disease of large intestine with intestinal obstruction
K50.113	Crohn's disease of large intestine with fistula
K50.114	Crohn's disease of large intestine with abscess
K50.811	Crohn's disease of both small and large intestine with rectal bleeding
K50.812	Crohn's disease of both small and large intestine with intestinal obstruction
K50.813	Crohn's disease of both small and large intestine with fistula
K50.814	Crohn's disease of both small and large intestine with abscess
K51.011	Ulcerative (chronic) pancolitis with rectal bleeding
K51.012	Ulcerative (chronic) pancolitis with intestinal obstruction
K51.013	Ulcerative (chronic) pancolitis with fistula
K51.014	Ulcerative (chronic) pancolitis with abscess
K51.311	Ulcerative (chronic) rectosigmoiditis with rectal bleeding
K51.312	Ulcerative (chronic) rectosigmoiditis with intestinal obstruction
K51.313	Ulcerative (chronic) rectosigmoiditis with fistula
K51.314	Ulcerative (chronic) rectosigmoiditis with abscess
K51.411	Inflammatory polyps of colon with rectal bleeding
K51.412	Inflammatory polyps of colon with intestinal obstruction
K51.413	Inflammatory polyps of colon with fistula
K51.414	Inflammatory polyps of colon with abscess
K51.50	Left sided colitis without complications
K51.511	Left sided colitis with rectal bleeding
K51.512	Left sided colitis with intestinal obstruction
K51.513	Left sided colitis with fistula

Rectum

K51.514	Left sided colitis with abscess
K52.0	Gastroenteritis and colitis due to radiation
K52.1	Toxic gastroenteritis and colitis
K52.21	Food protein-induced enterocolitis syndrome
K52.22	Food protein-induced enteropathy
K55.031	Focal (segmental) acute (reversible) ischemia of large intestine
K55.032	Diffuse acute (reversible) ischemia of large intestine
K55.041	Focal (segmental) acute infarction of large intestine
K55.042	Diffuse acute infarction of large intestine
K55.21	Angiodysplasia of colon with hemorrhage
K56.41	Fecal impaction
K56.51	Intestinal adhesions [bands], with partial obstruction
K56.52	Intestinal adhesions [bands] with complete obstruction
K56.690	Other partial intestinal obstruction
K56.691	Other complete intestinal obstruction
K59.01	Slow transit constipation
K62.1	Rectal polyp
K62.5	Hemorrhage of anus and rectum
K63.5	Polyp of colon
K63.81	Dieulafoy lesion of intestine
K91.31	Postprocedural partial intestinal obstruction
K91.32	Postprocedural complete intestinal obstruction
K92.1	Melena
M35.08	Sjögren syndrome with gastrointestinal involvement
R19.4	Change in bowel habit
R62.7	Adult failure to thrive A
R63.4	Abnormal weight loss
Z12.11	Encounter for screening for malignant neoplasm of colon

AMA: 45380 2018,Jan,8; 2017,Jan,8; 2016,Jan,13; 2015,Jan,16

Relative Value Units/Medicare Edits

Non-Facility RVU	Work	PE	MP	Total
45380	3.56	9.25	0.42	13.23
Facility RVU	Work	PE	MP	Total
45380	3.56	1.87	0.42	5.85

	FUD	Status	MUE	Modifiers				IOM Reference
45380	0	A	1(2)	51	N/A	N/A	N/A	None

* with documentation

45381

45381   Colonoscopy, flexible; with directed submucosal injection(s), any substance

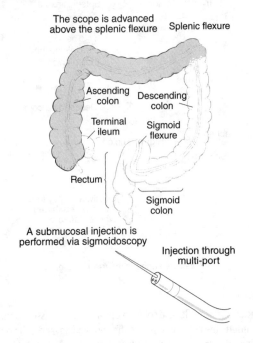

The scope is advanced above the splenic flexure — Splenic flexure
Ascending colon — Descending colon
Terminal ileum — Sigmoid flexure
Rectum
Sigmoid colon
A submucosal injection is performed via sigmoidoscopy
Injection through multi-port

Explanation

The physician performs flexible colonoscopy and injects a substance into the submucosa, directed at specific areas through the scope, while viewing the colon. The physician inserts the colonoscope into the anus and advances the scope through the colon to the cecum. The lumen of the colon is visualized. Submucosal saline injections, for instance, may be done before polypectomy using snare and electrocautery to greatly enhance the effectiveness of resection for large sessile colorectal polyps.

Coding Tips

Surgical endoscopy includes diagnostic endoscopy; however, diagnostic endoscopy can be identified separately when performed at the same surgical session as an open procedure. Report 45381 once regardless of the number of injections performed. For flexible sigmoidoscopy with directed submucosal injection(s), any substance, see 45335. Bleeding that occurs as the result of an endoscopic procedure, and controlled during the same operative session, is not reported separately. Do not report 45381 with 45378 or in addition to 45382 or 45390 for the same lesion.

ICD-10-CM Diagnostic Codes

C17.2	Malignant neoplasm of ileum
C18.0	Malignant neoplasm of cecum
C18.1	Malignant neoplasm of appendix
C18.2	Malignant neoplasm of ascending colon
C18.3	Malignant neoplasm of hepatic flexure
C18.4	Malignant neoplasm of transverse colon
C18.5	Malignant neoplasm of splenic flexure
C18.6	Malignant neoplasm of descending colon
C18.7	Malignant neoplasm of sigmoid colon
C18.8	Malignant neoplasm of overlapping sites of colon
C19	Malignant neoplasm of rectosigmoid junction
C20	Malignant neoplasm of rectum

C21.2	Malignant neoplasm of cloacogenic zone
C21.8	Malignant neoplasm of overlapping sites of rectum, anus and anal canal
C49.A4	Gastrointestinal stromal tumor of large intestine
C49.A5	Gastrointestinal stromal tumor of rectum
C78.4	Secondary malignant neoplasm of small intestine
C78.5	Secondary malignant neoplasm of large intestine and rectum
C7A.012	Malignant carcinoid tumor of the ileum
C7A.020	Malignant carcinoid tumor of the appendix
C7A.021	Malignant carcinoid tumor of the cecum
C7A.022	Malignant carcinoid tumor of the ascending colon
C7A.023	Malignant carcinoid tumor of the transverse colon
C7A.024	Malignant carcinoid tumor of the descending colon
C7A.025	Malignant carcinoid tumor of the sigmoid colon
C7A.026	Malignant carcinoid tumor of the rectum
D01.0	Carcinoma in situ of colon
D01.1	Carcinoma in situ of rectosigmoid junction
D01.2	Carcinoma in situ of rectum
D01.49	Carcinoma in situ of other parts of intestine
D12.0	Benign neoplasm of cecum
D12.1	Benign neoplasm of appendix
D12.2	Benign neoplasm of ascending colon
D12.3	Benign neoplasm of transverse colon
D12.4	Benign neoplasm of descending colon
D12.5	Benign neoplasm of sigmoid colon
D12.7	Benign neoplasm of rectosigmoid junction
D12.8	Benign neoplasm of rectum
D37.3	Neoplasm of uncertain behavior of appendix
D37.4	Neoplasm of uncertain behavior of colon
D37.5	Neoplasm of uncertain behavior of rectum
D3A.020	Benign carcinoid tumor of the appendix
D3A.021	Benign carcinoid tumor of the cecum
D3A.022	Benign carcinoid tumor of the ascending colon
D3A.023	Benign carcinoid tumor of the transverse colon
D3A.024	Benign carcinoid tumor of the descending colon
D3A.025	Benign carcinoid tumor of the sigmoid colon
D3A.026	Benign carcinoid tumor of the rectum
D49.0	Neoplasm of unspecified behavior of digestive system
K51.40	Inflammatory polyps of colon without complications
K51.411	Inflammatory polyps of colon with rectal bleeding
K51.412	Inflammatory polyps of colon with intestinal obstruction
K51.413	Inflammatory polyps of colon with fistula
K51.414	Inflammatory polyps of colon with abscess
K51.418	Inflammatory polyps of colon with other complication
K62.1	Rectal polyp
K63.5	Polyp of colon

AMA: **45381** 2018,Jan,8; 2017,Jan,8; 2017,Jan,6; 2016,Jan,13; 2015,Jan,16

Relative Value Units/Medicare Edits

Non-Facility RVU	Work	PE	MP	Total
45381	3.56	9.36	0.42	13.34
Facility RVU	**Work**	**PE**	**MP**	**Total**
45381	3.56	1.87	0.42	5.85

	FUD	Status	MUE	Modifiers				IOM Reference
45381	0	A	1(2)	51	N/A	N/A	N/A	None

* with documentation

Terms To Know

benign lesion. Neoplasm or change in tissue that is not cancerous (nonmalignant).

carcinoid tumor. Specific type of slow-growing neuroendocrine tumors. Carcinoid tumors occur most commonly in the hormone producing cells of the gastrointestinal tracts and can also occur in the pancreas, testes, ovaries, or lungs.

injection. Forcing a liquid substance into a body part such as a joint or muscle.

lumen. Space inside an intestine, artery, vein, duct, or tube.

malignant neoplasm. Any cancerous tumor or lesion exhibiting uncontrolled tissue growth that can progressively invade other parts of the body with its disease-generating cells.

polyp. Small growth on a stalk-like attachment projecting from a mucous membrane.

resection. Surgical removal of a part or all of an organ or body part.

45382

45382 Colonoscopy, flexible; with control of bleeding, any method

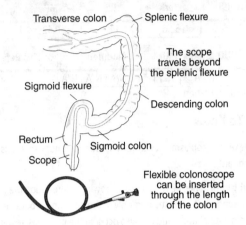

Transverse colon — Splenic flexure

The scope travels beyond the splenic flexure

Sigmoid flexure

Descending colon

Rectum

Sigmoid colon

Scope

Flexible colonoscope can be inserted through the length of the colon

Explanation

The physician performs flexible colonoscopy and controls an area of bleeding. The physician inserts the colonoscope into the anus and advances the scope through the colon to the cecum. The lumen of the colon and rectum are visualized and the area of bleeding is identified and controlled. A variety of methods can be used to control the bleeding, including medication application, laser, heat, or electric probe. The colonoscope is withdrawn at the completion of the procedure.

Coding Tips

Surgical endoscopy includes diagnostic endoscopy; however, diagnostic endoscopy can be identified separately when performed at the same surgical session as an open procedure. Colonoscopy involves examination of the entire colon, from the rectum to the cecum, and may also include the terminal ileum. An incomplete colonoscopy with full colonoscopy preparation is reported with the colonoscopy code and modifier 52. For colonoscopy through stoma, with control of bleeding, see 44391. For proctosigmoidoscopy, rigid, with control of bleeding, see 45317. For sigmoidoscopy, flexible, with control of bleeding, see 45334. Bleeding that occurs as the result of an endoscopic procedure, and controlled during the same operative session, is not reported separately. Do not report 45382 with 45378 or in addition to 45381 or 45398 for the same lesion.

ICD-10-CM Diagnostic Codes

C17.2	Malignant neoplasm of ileum
C17.3	Meckel's diverticulum, malignant
C18.0	Malignant neoplasm of cecum
C18.1	Malignant neoplasm of appendix
C18.2	Malignant neoplasm of ascending colon
C18.3	Malignant neoplasm of hepatic flexure
C18.4	Malignant neoplasm of transverse colon
C18.5	Malignant neoplasm of splenic flexure
C18.6	Malignant neoplasm of descending colon
C18.7	Malignant neoplasm of sigmoid colon
C18.8	Malignant neoplasm of overlapping sites of colon
C19	Malignant neoplasm of rectosigmoid junction
C20	Malignant neoplasm of rectum
C21.8	Malignant neoplasm of overlapping sites of rectum, anus and anal canal

C78.4	Secondary malignant neoplasm of small intestine
C78.5	Secondary malignant neoplasm of large intestine and rectum
C7A.012	Malignant carcinoid tumor of the ileum
C7A.020	Malignant carcinoid tumor of the appendix
C7A.021	Malignant carcinoid tumor of the cecum
C7A.022	Malignant carcinoid tumor of the ascending colon
C7A.023	Malignant carcinoid tumor of the transverse colon
C7A.024	Malignant carcinoid tumor of the descending colon
C7A.025	Malignant carcinoid tumor of the sigmoid colon
C7A.026	Malignant carcinoid tumor of the rectum
D01.0	Carcinoma in situ of colon
D01.1	Carcinoma in situ of rectosigmoid junction
D01.2	Carcinoma in situ of rectum
D01.49	Carcinoma in situ of other parts of intestine
D12.0	Benign neoplasm of cecum
D12.1	Benign neoplasm of appendix
D12.2	Benign neoplasm of ascending colon
D12.3	Benign neoplasm of transverse colon
D12.4	Benign neoplasm of descending colon
D12.5	Benign neoplasm of sigmoid colon
D12.7	Benign neoplasm of rectosigmoid junction
D12.8	Benign neoplasm of rectum
D37.4	Neoplasm of uncertain behavior of colon
D37.5	Neoplasm of uncertain behavior of rectum
D3A.012	Benign carcinoid tumor of the ileum
D3A.020	Benign carcinoid tumor of the appendix
D3A.021	Benign carcinoid tumor of the cecum
D3A.022	Benign carcinoid tumor of the ascending colon
D3A.023	Benign carcinoid tumor of the transverse colon
D3A.024	Benign carcinoid tumor of the descending colon
D3A.025	Benign carcinoid tumor of the sigmoid colon
D3A.026	Benign carcinoid tumor of the rectum
K50.011	Crohn's disease of small intestine with rectal bleeding
K50.111	Crohn's disease of large intestine with rectal bleeding
K50.811	Crohn's disease of both small and large intestine with rectal bleeding
K51.011	Ulcerative (chronic) pancolitis with rectal bleeding
K51.211	Ulcerative (chronic) proctitis with rectal bleeding
K51.311	Ulcerative (chronic) rectosigmoiditis with rectal bleeding
K51.411	Inflammatory polyps of colon with rectal bleeding
K51.511	Left sided colitis with rectal bleeding
K51.811	Other ulcerative colitis with rectal bleeding
K52.0	Gastroenteritis and colitis due to radiation
K52.1	Toxic gastroenteritis and colitis
K52.21	Food protein-induced enterocolitis syndrome
K52.22	Food protein-induced enteropathy
K52.81	Eosinophilic gastritis or gastroenteritis
K52.82	Eosinophilic colitis
K52.89	Other specified noninfective gastroenteritis and colitis
K55.031	Focal (segmental) acute (reversible) ischemia of large intestine
K55.032	Diffuse acute (reversible) ischemia of large intestine
K55.041	Focal (segmental) acute infarction of large intestine
K55.042	Diffuse acute infarction of large intestine

N Newborn: 0   **P** Pediatric: 0-17   **M** Maternity: 9-64   **A** Adult: 15-124   ♂ Male Only   ♀ Female Only

Rectum

K55.1	Chronic vascular disorders of intestine	
K55.21	Angiodysplasia of colon with hemorrhage	
K55.8	Other vascular disorders of intestine	
K57.21	Diverticulitis of large intestine with perforation and abscess with bleeding	
K57.31	Diverticulosis of large intestine without perforation or abscess with bleeding	
K57.33	Diverticulitis of large intestine without perforation or abscess with bleeding	
K57.41	Diverticulitis of both small and large intestine with perforation and abscess with bleeding	
K57.51	Diverticulosis of both small and large intestine without perforation or abscess with bleeding	
K57.53	Diverticulitis of both small and large intestine without perforation or abscess with bleeding	
K62.5	Hemorrhage of anus and rectum	
K62.7	Radiation proctitis	
K62.89	Other specified diseases of anus and rectum	
K63.1	Perforation of intestine (nontraumatic)	
K63.3	Ulcer of intestine	
K63.5	Polyp of colon	
K63.81	Dieulafoy lesion of intestine	
K63.89	Other specified diseases of intestine	
K92.1	Melena	
Q27.33	Arteriovenous malformation of digestive system vessel	
Q43.0	Meckel's diverticulum (displaced) (hypertrophic)	

AMA: **45382** 2018,Jan,8; 2017,Jan,8; 2016,Jan,13; 2015,Jan,16

Relative Value Units/Medicare Edits

Non-Facility RVU	Work	PE	MP	Total
45382	4.66	16.07	0.51	21.24
Facility RVU	**Work**	**PE**	**MP**	**Total**
45382	4.66	2.36	0.51	7.53

	FUD	Status	MUE	Modifiers				IOM Reference
45382	0	A	1(3)	51	N/A	N/A	N/A	None

* with documentation

45384-45385 [45388]

45388	Colonoscopy, flexible; with ablation of tumor(s), polyp(s), or other lesion(s) (includes pre- and post-dilation and guide wire passage, when performed)
45384	with removal of tumor(s), polyp(s), or other lesion(s) by hot biopsy forceps
45385	with removal of tumor(s), polyp(s), or other lesion(s) by snare technique

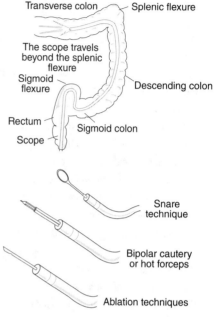

Tumors, polyps, or other lesions are removed by any of a variety of techniques

Explanation

In 45384, the physician performs flexible colonoscopy and removes a tumor, polyp, or other lesion. The physician inserts the colonoscope into the anus and advances the scope through the colon to the cecum. The lumen of the colon and rectum are visualized. The tumor, polyp, or other lesions are identified and removed by hot biopsy forceps. The colonoscope is withdrawn at the completion of the procedure. Report 45385 for removal by snare technique and 45388 for ablation by laser or other method.

Coding Tips

Report the appropriate endoscopy for each anatomic site examined. Surgical endoscopy includes a diagnostic endoscopy; however, diagnostic endoscopy can be identified separately when performed at the same surgical session as an open procedure. For proctosigmoidoscopy, rigid, with removal of multiple tumors, polyps, or lesions by hot biopsy forceps, bipolar cautery, or snare technique, see 45315; for ablation by any other method, see 45320. For sigmoidoscopy, flexible, with removal of tumors, polyps, or lesions by hot biopsy forceps, see 45333; by snare technique, see 45338; for ablation by any other method, see 45346. Colonoscopy with endoscopic mucosal resection is reported with 45390. Bleeding that occurs as the result of an endoscopic procedure, and controlled during the same operative session, is not reported separately. Do not report 45385 with 45390. Do not report 45388 in addition to 45386 when performed on the same lesion. Do not report 45384–45385 and 45388 with 45378.

ICD-10-CM Diagnostic Codes

C17.2	Malignant neoplasm of ileum

Rectum

C18.0	Malignant neoplasm of cecum	K51.412	Inflammatory polyps of colon with intestinal obstruction
C18.1	Malignant neoplasm of appendix	K51.413	Inflammatory polyps of colon with fistula
C18.2	Malignant neoplasm of ascending colon	K51.414	Inflammatory polyps of colon with abscess
C18.3	Malignant neoplasm of hepatic flexure	K51.418	Inflammatory polyps of colon with other complication
C18.4	Malignant neoplasm of transverse colon	K55.20	Angiodysplasia of colon without hemorrhage

C18.0 Malignant neoplasm of cecum
C18.1 Malignant neoplasm of appendix
C18.2 Malignant neoplasm of ascending colon
C18.3 Malignant neoplasm of hepatic flexure
C18.4 Malignant neoplasm of transverse colon
C18.5 Malignant neoplasm of splenic flexure
C18.6 Malignant neoplasm of descending colon
C18.7 Malignant neoplasm of sigmoid colon
C18.8 Malignant neoplasm of overlapping sites of colon
C19 Malignant neoplasm of rectosigmoid junction
C20 Malignant neoplasm of rectum
C21.8 Malignant neoplasm of overlapping sites of rectum, anus and anal canal
C49.A4 Gastrointestinal stromal tumor of large intestine
C49.A5 Gastrointestinal stromal tumor of rectum
C78.4 Secondary malignant neoplasm of small intestine
C78.5 Secondary malignant neoplasm of large intestine and rectum
C7A.012 Malignant carcinoid tumor of the ileum
C7A.020 Malignant carcinoid tumor of the appendix
C7A.021 Malignant carcinoid tumor of the cecum
C7A.022 Malignant carcinoid tumor of the ascending colon
C7A.023 Malignant carcinoid tumor of the transverse colon
C7A.024 Malignant carcinoid tumor of the descending colon
C7A.025 Malignant carcinoid tumor of the sigmoid colon
C7A.026 Malignant carcinoid tumor of the rectum
D01.0 Carcinoma in situ of colon
D01.1 Carcinoma in situ of rectosigmoid junction
D01.2 Carcinoma in situ of rectum
D12.0 Benign neoplasm of cecum
D12.1 Benign neoplasm of appendix
D12.2 Benign neoplasm of ascending colon
D12.3 Benign neoplasm of transverse colon
D12.4 Benign neoplasm of descending colon
D12.5 Benign neoplasm of sigmoid colon
D12.7 Benign neoplasm of rectosigmoid junction
D12.8 Benign neoplasm of rectum
D13.39 Benign neoplasm of other parts of small intestine
D37.3 Neoplasm of uncertain behavior of appendix
D37.4 Neoplasm of uncertain behavior of colon
D37.5 Neoplasm of uncertain behavior of rectum
D37.8 Neoplasm of uncertain behavior of other specified digestive organs
D3A.012 Benign carcinoid tumor of the ileum
D3A.020 Benign carcinoid tumor of the appendix
D3A.021 Benign carcinoid tumor of the cecum
D3A.022 Benign carcinoid tumor of the ascending colon
D3A.023 Benign carcinoid tumor of the transverse colon
D3A.024 Benign carcinoid tumor of the descending colon
D3A.025 Benign carcinoid tumor of the sigmoid colon
D3A.026 Benign carcinoid tumor of the rectum
D49.0 Neoplasm of unspecified behavior of digestive system
K51.40 Inflammatory polyps of colon without complications
K51.411 Inflammatory polyps of colon with rectal bleeding

K51.412 Inflammatory polyps of colon with intestinal obstruction
K51.413 Inflammatory polyps of colon with fistula
K51.414 Inflammatory polyps of colon with abscess
K51.418 Inflammatory polyps of colon with other complication
K55.20 Angiodysplasia of colon without hemorrhage
K62.1 Rectal polyp
K62.89 Other specified diseases of anus and rectum
K63.5 Polyp of colon
K92.1 Melena
R93.3 Abnormal findings on diagnostic imaging of other parts of digestive tract
Z12.11 Encounter for screening for malignant neoplasm of colon

AMA: **45384** 2018,Jan,8; 2017,Jan,8; 2016,Jan,13; 2015,Jun,10; 2015,Jan,16 **45385** 2018,Jan,8; 2017,Jan,6; 2017,Jan,8; 2016,Jan,13; 2015,Jan,16 **45388** 2018,Jan,8; 2017,Jan,8; 2016,Jan,13; 2015,Jan,16

Relative Value Units/Medicare Edits

Non-Facility RVU	Work	PE	MP	Total
45388	4.88	79.44	0.59	84.91
45384	4.07	10.23	0.56	14.86
45385	4.57	8.62	0.51	13.7
Facility RVU	**Work**	**PE**	**MP**	**Total**
45388	4.88	2.41	0.59	7.88
45384	4.07	2.01	0.56	6.64
45385	4.57	2.31	0.51	7.39

	FUD	Status	MUE	Modifiers				IOM Reference
45388	0	A	1(2)	51	N/A	N/A	N/A	None
45384	0	A	1(2)	51	N/A	N/A	N/A	
45385	0	A	1(2)	51	N/A	N/A	N/A	

* with documentation

Terms To Know

dilation. Artificial increase in the diameter of an opening or lumen made by medication or by instrumentation.

polyp. Small growth on a stalk-like attachment projecting from a mucous membrane.

tumor. Pathological swelling or enlargement; a neoplastic growth of uncontrolled, abnormal multiplication of cells.

45386

45386 Colonoscopy, flexible; with transendoscopic balloon dilation

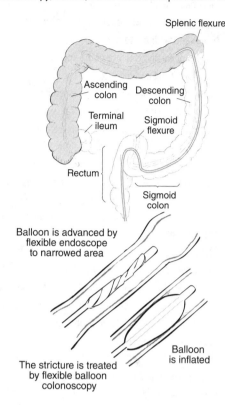

Splenic flexure

Ascending colon
Descending colon
Terminal ileum
Sigmoid flexure
Rectum
Sigmoid colon

Balloon is advanced by flexible endoscope to narrowed area

Balloon is inflated

The stricture is treated by flexible balloon colonoscopy

Explanation

The physician performs flexible colonoscopy and dilates strictures by balloon catheter. The physician inserts the colonoscope into the anus and advances the scope through the colon to the cecum. The lumen of the colon is visualized. Areas of stenosis are identified and a balloon catheter is passed to the point of constriction and a little beyond. The balloon is inflated to the appropriate diameter and gradually withdrawn through the stenosed area, stretching the walls of the bowel at the strictured area. The scope is withdrawn at the completion of the procedure.

Coding Tips

Report the appropriate endoscopy for each anatomic site examined. Surgical endoscopy includes diagnostic endoscopy; however, diagnostic endoscopy can be identified separately when performed at the same surgical session as an open procedure. Colonoscopy involves examination of the entire colon, from the rectum to the cecum, and may also include the terminal ileum. An incomplete colonoscopy with full colonoscopy preparation is reported with the colonoscopy code and modifier 52. For flexible sigmoidoscopy with transendoscopic balloon dilation, see 45340. For multiple strictures treated with transendoscopic balloon dilations during the same session, report 45386 with modifier 59 or an X{EPSU} modifier for each additional stricture dilated. If fluoroscopic guidance is used, see 74360. For endoscopic stent placement, see 45389. Bleeding that occurs as the result of an endoscopic procedure, and controlled during the same operative session, is not reported separately. Do not report 45386 with 45378, 45388, or 45389.

ICD-10-CM Diagnostic Codes

K50.112	Crohn's disease of large intestine with intestinal obstruction
K50.812	Crohn's disease of both small and large intestine with intestinal obstruction
K51.012	Ulcerative (chronic) pancolitis with intestinal obstruction
K51.212	Ulcerative (chronic) proctitis with intestinal obstruction
K51.312	Ulcerative (chronic) rectosigmoiditis with intestinal obstruction
K51.412	Inflammatory polyps of colon with intestinal obstruction
K51.512	Left sided colitis with intestinal obstruction
K51.812	Other ulcerative colitis with intestinal obstruction
K56.1	Intussusception
K56.2	Volvulus
K56.49	Other impaction of intestine
K56.51	Intestinal adhesions [bands], with partial obstruction
K56.52	Intestinal adhesions [bands] with complete obstruction
K56.690	Other partial intestinal obstruction
K56.691	Other complete intestinal obstruction
K91.31	Postprocedural partial intestinal obstruction
K91.32	Postprocedural complete intestinal obstruction
K91.89	Other postprocedural complications and disorders of digestive system
Q42.0	Congenital absence, atresia and stenosis of rectum with fistula
Q42.1	Congenital absence, atresia and stenosis of rectum without fistula
Q42.8	Congenital absence, atresia and stenosis of other parts of large intestine

AMA: **45386** 2018,Jan,8; 2017,Jan,8; 2016,Jan,13; 2015,Jan,16

Relative Value Units/Medicare Edits

Non-Facility RVU	Work	PE	MP	Total
45386	3.77	14.77	0.45	18.99
Facility RVU	**Work**	**PE**	**MP**	**Total**
45386	3.77	1.94	0.45	6.16

	FUD	Status	MUE	Modifiers				IOM Reference
45386	0	A	1(2)	51	N/A	N/A	N/A	None

* with documentation

Terms To Know

atresia. Congenital closure or absence of a tubular organ or an opening to the body surface.

congenital. Present at birth, occurring through heredity or an influence during gestation up to the moment of birth.

constriction. Narrowed or squeezed portion of a tubular or luminal structure, such as a duct, vessel, or tube (e.g., esophagus). The narrowing can be a defect that is occurring naturally, or one that is surgically induced for therapeutic reasons.

Rectum

45389

45389 Colonoscopy, flexible; with endoscopic stent placement (includes pre- and post-dilation and guide wire passage, when performed)

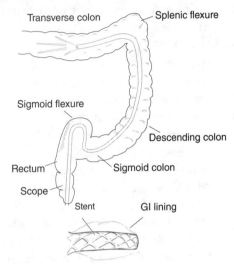

A colonoscopy session is performed with endoscopic stent placement, including pre- and postdilation

Explanation

The physician uses a colonoscope to examine the colon and place an endoscopic stent. The physician inserts the flexible endoscope into the anus and advances the scope through the colon to the cecum. The lumen of the colon is visualized. The endoscope is placed at the site of an obstruction or stricture and the necessary stent length is determined. If the area is partially occluded or obstructed, a balloon-tipped catheter is inserted through the scope and the balloon is inflated to dilate the area before stent placement. The stent (endoprosthesis) is introduced to the site of the lesion by a stent-carrying catheter inserted through the scope. The plastic covering over the stent is removed and the stent self-deploys, shoring-up the walls at the target site in the colon. When necessary, a balloon catheter is placed into the stent and gently inflated to more fully deploy the stent. The delivery system and endoscope are removed at the completion of the procedure. This code reports dilation before and after the procedure and utilization of a guidewire, if employed.

Coding Tips

Surgical endoscopy includes diagnostic endoscopy; however, diagnostic endoscopy can be identified separately when performed at the same surgical session as an open procedure. If fluoroscopic guidance is used, see 74360. Bleeding that occurs as the result of an endoscopic procedure, and controlled during the same operative session, is not reported separately. Do not report 45389 with 45378 or 45386.

ICD-10-CM Diagnostic Codes

C17.2	Malignant neoplasm of ileum
C18.0	Malignant neoplasm of cecum
C18.1	Malignant neoplasm of appendix
C18.2	Malignant neoplasm of ascending colon
C18.3	Malignant neoplasm of hepatic flexure
C18.4	Malignant neoplasm of transverse colon
C18.5	Malignant neoplasm of splenic flexure
C18.6	Malignant neoplasm of descending colon
C18.7	Malignant neoplasm of sigmoid colon
C18.8	Malignant neoplasm of overlapping sites of colon
C19	Malignant neoplasm of rectosigmoid junction
C20	Malignant neoplasm of rectum
C78.4	Secondary malignant neoplasm of small intestine
C7A.012	Malignant carcinoid tumor of the ileum
C7A.020	Malignant carcinoid tumor of the appendix
C7A.021	Malignant carcinoid tumor of the cecum
C7A.022	Malignant carcinoid tumor of the ascending colon
C7A.023	Malignant carcinoid tumor of the transverse colon
C7A.024	Malignant carcinoid tumor of the descending colon
C7A.025	Malignant carcinoid tumor of the sigmoid colon
D49.0	Neoplasm of unspecified behavior of digestive system
K50.012	Crohn's disease of small intestine with intestinal obstruction
K50.112	Crohn's disease of large intestine with intestinal obstruction
K50.812	Crohn's disease of both small and large intestine with intestinal obstruction
K51.012	Ulcerative (chronic) pancolitis with intestinal obstruction
K51.212	Ulcerative (chronic) proctitis with intestinal obstruction
K51.312	Ulcerative (chronic) rectosigmoiditis with intestinal obstruction
K51.412	Inflammatory polyps of colon with intestinal obstruction
K51.512	Left sided colitis with intestinal obstruction
K56.51	Intestinal adhesions [bands], with partial obstruction
K56.52	Intestinal adhesions [bands] with complete obstruction
K56.690	Other partial intestinal obstruction
K56.691	Other complete intestinal obstruction
K91.31	Postprocedural partial intestinal obstruction
K91.32	Postprocedural complete intestinal obstruction
Q42.0	Congenital absence, atresia and stenosis of rectum with fistula
Q42.1	Congenital absence, atresia and stenosis of rectum without fistula

AMA: **45389** 2018,Jan,8; 2017,Jan,8; 2016,Jan,13; 2015,Jan,16

Relative Value Units/Medicare Edits

Non-Facility RVU	Work	PE	MP	Total
45389	5.24	2.6	0.59	8.43
Facility RVU	**Work**	**PE**	**MP**	**Total**
45389	5.24	2.6	0.59	8.43

	FUD	Status	MUE	Modifiers				IOM Reference
45389	0	A	1(3)	51	N/A	N/A	N/A	None

* with documentation

Rectum

45391

45391 Colonoscopy, flexible; with endoscopic ultrasound examination limited to the rectum, sigmoid, descending, transverse, or ascending colon and cecum, and adjacent structures

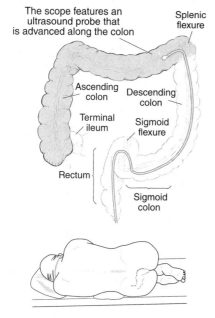

The scope features an ultrasound probe that is advanced along the colon

Splenic flexure

Ascending colon

Descending colon

Terminal ileum

Sigmoid flexure

Rectum

Sigmoid colon

Position of patient for colonoscopy

Explanation

The physician uses a flexible colonoscope to examine the colon and perform an endoscopic ultrasound (EUS) examination. Ultrasound and endoscopic imaging techniques are combined in this diagnostic modality. A flexible fiberoptic endoscope equipped with an ultrasound transducer at the tip is inserted into the anus and the scope is advanced through the colon to the cecum. The lumen of the colon is visualized and the probe tip is guided next to the area of concern. Sound waves are sent out from the transducer and reflect back to a receiving unit at varying speeds as they pass through different densities of tissue. The waves are converted to electrical pulses displayed as a picture on screen. Using ultrasound from within the endoscope instead of transcutaneously shortens the distance between the source and the target lesion and produces greater clarity from high frequency, high-resolution sound waves that have a short penetration distance. EUS is currently the most accurate method of staging cancer within the gastrointestinal tract.

Coding Tips

Report the appropriate endoscopy for each anatomic site examined. Surgical endoscopy includes diagnostic endoscopy; however, diagnostic endoscopy can be identified separately when performed at the same surgical session as an open procedure. Colonoscopy involves examination of the entire colon, from the rectum to the cecum, and may also include the terminal ileum. An incomplete colonoscopy with full colonoscopy preparation is reported with the colonoscopy code and modifier 52. Bleeding that occurs as the result of an endoscopic procedure, and controlled during the same operative session, is not reported separately. Report 45391 only once per session. Do not report 45391 with 45378, 45392, 76872, or 76975.

ICD-10-CM Diagnostic Codes

C18.0	Malignant neoplasm of cecum
C18.2	Malignant neoplasm of ascending colon
C18.3	Malignant neoplasm of hepatic flexure
C18.4	Malignant neoplasm of transverse colon
C18.5	Malignant neoplasm of splenic flexure
C18.6	Malignant neoplasm of descending colon
C18.7	Malignant neoplasm of sigmoid colon
C19	Malignant neoplasm of rectosigmoid junction
C20	Malignant neoplasm of rectum
C21.8	Malignant neoplasm of overlapping sites of rectum, anus and anal canal
C49.A4	Gastrointestinal stromal tumor of large intestine
C49.A5	Gastrointestinal stromal tumor of rectum
C78.5	Secondary malignant neoplasm of large intestine and rectum
C7A.021	Malignant carcinoid tumor of the cecum
C7A.022	Malignant carcinoid tumor of the ascending colon
C7A.023	Malignant carcinoid tumor of the transverse colon
C7A.024	Malignant carcinoid tumor of the descending colon
C7A.025	Malignant carcinoid tumor of the sigmoid colon
C7A.026	Malignant carcinoid tumor of the rectum
D01.0	Carcinoma in situ of colon
D01.1	Carcinoma in situ of rectosigmoid junction
D01.2	Carcinoma in situ of rectum
D01.49	Carcinoma in situ of other parts of intestine
D12.0	Benign neoplasm of cecum
D12.2	Benign neoplasm of ascending colon
D12.3	Benign neoplasm of transverse colon
D12.4	Benign neoplasm of descending colon
D12.5	Benign neoplasm of sigmoid colon
D12.7	Benign neoplasm of rectosigmoid junction
D12.8	Benign neoplasm of rectum
D37.4	Neoplasm of uncertain behavior of colon
D37.5	Neoplasm of uncertain behavior of rectum
D3A.020	Benign carcinoid tumor of the appendix
D3A.021	Benign carcinoid tumor of the cecum
D3A.022	Benign carcinoid tumor of the ascending colon
D3A.023	Benign carcinoid tumor of the transverse colon
D3A.024	Benign carcinoid tumor of the descending colon
D3A.025	Benign carcinoid tumor of the sigmoid colon
D3A.026	Benign carcinoid tumor of the rectum
K50.10	Crohn's disease of large intestine without complications
K50.111	Crohn's disease of large intestine with rectal bleeding
K50.112	Crohn's disease of large intestine with intestinal obstruction
K50.113	Crohn's disease of large intestine with fistula
K50.114	Crohn's disease of large intestine with abscess
K50.811	Crohn's disease of both small and large intestine with rectal bleeding
K50.812	Crohn's disease of both small and large intestine with intestinal obstruction
K50.813	Crohn's disease of both small and large intestine with fistula
K50.814	Crohn's disease of both small and large intestine with abscess
K51.40	Inflammatory polyps of colon without complications
K51.411	Inflammatory polyps of colon with rectal bleeding
K51.412	Inflammatory polyps of colon with intestinal obstruction
K51.413	Inflammatory polyps of colon with fistula

K51.414	Inflammatory polyps of colon with abscess
K51.511	Left sided colitis with rectal bleeding
K51.512	Left sided colitis with intestinal obstruction
K51.513	Left sided colitis with fistula
K51.514	Left sided colitis with abscess
K51.811	Other ulcerative colitis with rectal bleeding
K51.812	Other ulcerative colitis with intestinal obstruction
K51.813	Other ulcerative colitis with fistula
K51.814	Other ulcerative colitis with abscess
K55.031	Focal (segmental) acute (reversible) ischemia of large intestine
K55.032	Diffuse acute (reversible) ischemia of large intestine
K55.041	Focal (segmental) acute infarction of large intestine
K55.042	Diffuse acute infarction of large intestine
K55.1	Chronic vascular disorders of intestine
K55.20	Angiodysplasia of colon without hemorrhage
K55.21	Angiodysplasia of colon with hemorrhage
K55.8	Other vascular disorders of intestine
K58.0	Irritable bowel syndrome with diarrhea
K58.9	Irritable bowel syndrome without diarrhea
K59.01	Slow transit constipation
K59.02	Outlet dysfunction constipation
K59.09	Other constipation
K59.31	Toxic megacolon
K62.1	Rectal polyp
K62.89	Other specified diseases of anus and rectum
K63.0	Abscess of intestine
K63.1	Perforation of intestine (nontraumatic)
K63.2	Fistula of intestine
K63.3	Ulcer of intestine
K63.4	Enteroptosis
K63.5	Polyp of colon
K63.81	Dieulafoy lesion of intestine
K92.1	Melena
M35.08	Sjögren syndrome with gastrointestinal involvement
Q43.1	Hirschsprung's disease
Q43.2	Other congenital functional disorders of colon
R63.4	Abnormal weight loss

AMA: 45391 2018,Jan,8; 2017,Jan,8; 2016,Jan,13; 2015,Jan,16

Relative Value Units/Medicare Edits

Non-Facility RVU	Work	PE	MP	Total
45391	4.64	2.36	0.48	7.48
Facility RVU	Work	PE	MP	Total
45391	4.64	2.36	0.48	7.48

	FUD	Status	MUE	Modifiers				IOM Reference
45391	0	A	1(2)	51	N/A	N/A	N/A	None

* with documentation

45392

45392 Colonoscopy, flexible; with transendoscopic ultrasound guided intramural or transmural fine needle aspiration/biopsy(s), includes endoscopic ultrasound examination limited to the rectum, sigmoid, descending, transverse, or ascending colon and cecum, and adjacent structures

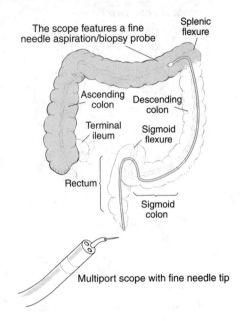

The scope features a fine needle aspiration/biopsy probe

Multiport scope with fine needle tip

Explanation

The physician uses a flexible colonoscope to examine the colon and perform a transendoscopic, ultrasound-guided intramural or transmural fine needle aspiration (FNA)/biopsy(s). A flexible fiberoptic endoscope equipped with an ultrasound transducer at the tip is inserted into the anus and the scope is advanced through the colon to the cecum. The lumen of the colon is visualized and the probe tip is guided to the area of concern. Sound waves are sent out from the transducer and reflect back to a receiving unit at varying speeds as they pass through different densities of tissue. The waves are converted to electrical pulses displayed as a picture on screen. An FNA needle is passed through the scope to the site of the lesion, lymph node, or tumor and a fine needle aspiration/biopsy(s) is taken of the abnormal tissue or fluid within the colon wall or through the intestinal wall. The instruments are removed.

Coding Tips

Report the appropriate endoscopy for each anatomic site examined. Surgical endoscopy includes diagnostic endoscopy; however, diagnostic endoscopy can be identified separately when performed at the same surgical session as an open procedure. Colonoscopy involves examination of the entire colon, from the rectum to the cecum, and may also include the terminal ileum. To report an incomplete colonoscopy with full colonoscopy preparation, use the colonoscopy code with modifier 52. Report 45392 only once per session. Bleeding that occurs as the result of an endoscopic procedure, and controlled during the same operative session, is not reported separately. Do not report 45392 with 45378, 45391, 76872, 76942, or 76975.

ICD-10-CM Diagnostic Codes

C18.0	Malignant neoplasm of cecum
C18.2	Malignant neoplasm of ascending colon
C18.3	Malignant neoplasm of hepatic flexure
C18.4	Malignant neoplasm of transverse colon

C18.5	Malignant neoplasm of splenic flexure
C18.6	Malignant neoplasm of descending colon
C18.7	Malignant neoplasm of sigmoid colon
C19	Malignant neoplasm of rectosigmoid junction
C20	Malignant neoplasm of rectum
C21.8	Malignant neoplasm of overlapping sites of rectum, anus and anal canal
C49.A4	Gastrointestinal stromal tumor of large intestine
C49.A5	Gastrointestinal stromal tumor of rectum
C78.5	Secondary malignant neoplasm of large intestine and rectum
C7A.021	Malignant carcinoid tumor of the cecum
C7A.022	Malignant carcinoid tumor of the ascending colon
C7A.023	Malignant carcinoid tumor of the transverse colon
C7A.024	Malignant carcinoid tumor of the descending colon
C7A.025	Malignant carcinoid tumor of the sigmoid colon
C7A.026	Malignant carcinoid tumor of the rectum
D01.0	Carcinoma in situ of colon
D01.1	Carcinoma in situ of rectosigmoid junction
D01.2	Carcinoma in situ of rectum
D01.49	Carcinoma in situ of other parts of intestine
D12.0	Benign neoplasm of cecum
D12.2	Benign neoplasm of ascending colon
D12.3	Benign neoplasm of transverse colon
D12.4	Benign neoplasm of descending colon
D12.5	Benign neoplasm of sigmoid colon
D12.7	Benign neoplasm of rectosigmoid junction
D12.8	Benign neoplasm of rectum
D37.4	Neoplasm of uncertain behavior of colon
D37.5	Neoplasm of uncertain behavior of rectum
D3A.020	Benign carcinoid tumor of the appendix
D3A.021	Benign carcinoid tumor of the cecum
D3A.022	Benign carcinoid tumor of the ascending colon
D3A.023	Benign carcinoid tumor of the transverse colon
D3A.024	Benign carcinoid tumor of the descending colon
D3A.025	Benign carcinoid tumor of the sigmoid colon
D3A.026	Benign carcinoid tumor of the rectum
K50.10	Crohn's disease of large intestine without complications
K50.111	Crohn's disease of large intestine with rectal bleeding
K50.112	Crohn's disease of large intestine with intestinal obstruction
K50.113	Crohn's disease of large intestine with fistula
K50.114	Crohn's disease of large intestine with abscess
K50.811	Crohn's disease of both small and large intestine with rectal bleeding
K50.812	Crohn's disease of both small and large intestine with intestinal obstruction
K50.813	Crohn's disease of both small and large intestine with fistula
K50.814	Crohn's disease of both small and large intestine with abscess
K51.40	Inflammatory polyps of colon without complications
K51.411	Inflammatory polyps of colon with rectal bleeding
K51.412	Inflammatory polyps of colon with intestinal obstruction
K51.413	Inflammatory polyps of colon with fistula
K51.414	Inflammatory polyps of colon with abscess
K51.511	Left sided colitis with rectal bleeding
K51.512	Left sided colitis with intestinal obstruction
K51.513	Left sided colitis with fistula
K51.514	Left sided colitis with abscess
K51.811	Other ulcerative colitis with rectal bleeding
K51.812	Other ulcerative colitis with intestinal obstruction
K51.813	Other ulcerative colitis with fistula
K51.814	Other ulcerative colitis with abscess
K55.031	Focal (segmental) acute (reversible) ischemia of large intestine
K55.032	Diffuse acute (reversible) ischemia of large intestine
K55.041	Focal (segmental) acute infarction of large intestine
K55.042	Diffuse acute infarction of large intestine
K55.1	Chronic vascular disorders of intestine
K55.20	Angiodysplasia of colon without hemorrhage
K55.21	Angiodysplasia of colon with hemorrhage
K55.8	Other vascular disorders of intestine
K58.0	Irritable bowel syndrome with diarrhea
K58.9	Irritable bowel syndrome without diarrhea
K59.01	Slow transit constipation
K59.02	Outlet dysfunction constipation
K59.09	Other constipation
K59.31	Toxic megacolon
K62.1	Rectal polyp
K62.89	Other specified diseases of anus and rectum
K63.0	Abscess of intestine
K63.1	Perforation of intestine (nontraumatic)
K63.2	Fistula of intestine
K63.3	Ulcer of intestine
K63.4	Enteroptosis
K63.5	Polyp of colon
K63.81	Dieulafoy lesion of intestine
K92.1	Melena
M35.08	Sjögren syndrome with gastrointestinal involvement
Q43.1	Hirschsprung's disease
Q43.2	Other congenital functional disorders of colon
R63.4	Abnormal weight loss

AMA: 45392 2018,Jan,8; 2017,Jan,8; 2016,Jan,13; 2015,Jan,16

Relative Value Units/Medicare Edits

Non-Facility RVU	Work	PE	MP	Total
45392	5.5	2.74	0.63	8.87
Facility RVU	Work	PE	MP	Total
45392	5.5	2.74	0.63	8.87

	FUD	Status	MUE	Modifiers				IOM Reference
45392	0	A	1(2)	51	N/A	N/A	N/A	None

* with documentation

Rectum

[45390]

45390 Colonoscopy, flexible; with endoscopic mucosal resection

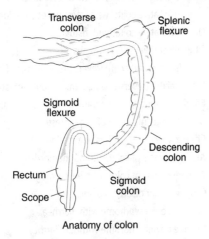

Anatomy of colon

Explanation

The physician uses a flexible colonoscope to examine the colon. The physician inserts the colonoscope into the anus and advances the scope through the colon to the cecum. The lumen of the colon and rectum are visualized with an instrument containing a camera and light. The scope is directed to the affected area. A special needle is used to administer fluid under the polyp to elevate the polyp allowing for the removal from the bowel lining. Removal may be done by snare, cutting out, or suction and typically includes cautery of the attached blood vessels. The tissue is sent to pathology for analysis and the scope is withdrawn at the completion of the procedure.

Coding Tips

Surgical endoscopy includes diagnostic endoscopy; however, diagnostic endoscopy can be identified separately when performed at the same surgical session as an open procedure. Bleeding that occurs as the result of an endoscopic procedure, and controlled during the same operative session, is not reported separately. Do not report 45390 with 45378 or in addition to 45380, 45381, 45385, or 45398 for the same lesion.

ICD-10-CM Diagnostic Codes

C17.2	Malignant neoplasm of ileum
C18.0	Malignant neoplasm of cecum
C18.2	Malignant neoplasm of ascending colon
C18.3	Malignant neoplasm of hepatic flexure
C18.4	Malignant neoplasm of transverse colon
C18.5	Malignant neoplasm of splenic flexure
C18.6	Malignant neoplasm of descending colon
C18.7	Malignant neoplasm of sigmoid colon
C18.8	Malignant neoplasm of overlapping sites of colon
C19	Malignant neoplasm of rectosigmoid junction
C20	Malignant neoplasm of rectum
C78.5	Secondary malignant neoplasm of large intestine and rectum
C7A.012	Malignant carcinoid tumor of the ileum
C7A.021	Malignant carcinoid tumor of the cecum
C7A.022	Malignant carcinoid tumor of the ascending colon
C7A.023	Malignant carcinoid tumor of the transverse colon
C7A.024	Malignant carcinoid tumor of the descending colon
C7A.025	Malignant carcinoid tumor of the sigmoid colon
C7A.026	Malignant carcinoid tumor of the rectum
D01.0	Carcinoma in situ of colon
D01.49	Carcinoma in situ of other parts of intestine
D12.0	Benign neoplasm of cecum
D12.2	Benign neoplasm of ascending colon
D12.3	Benign neoplasm of transverse colon
D12.4	Benign neoplasm of descending colon
D12.5	Benign neoplasm of sigmoid colon
D12.7	Benign neoplasm of rectosigmoid junction
D12.8	Benign neoplasm of rectum
D13.39	Benign neoplasm of other parts of small intestine
D37.4	Neoplasm of uncertain behavior of colon
D37.5	Neoplasm of uncertain behavior of rectum
D3A.012	Benign carcinoid tumor of the ileum
D3A.021	Benign carcinoid tumor of the cecum
D3A.022	Benign carcinoid tumor of the ascending colon
D3A.023	Benign carcinoid tumor of the transverse colon
D3A.024	Benign carcinoid tumor of the descending colon
D3A.025	Benign carcinoid tumor of the sigmoid colon
D3A.026	Benign carcinoid tumor of the rectum
D49.0	Neoplasm of unspecified behavior of digestive system
K51.40	Inflammatory polyps of colon without complications
K51.411	Inflammatory polyps of colon with rectal bleeding
K51.412	Inflammatory polyps of colon with intestinal obstruction
K51.413	Inflammatory polyps of colon with fistula
K51.414	Inflammatory polyps of colon with abscess
K51.418	Inflammatory polyps of colon with other complication
K63.3	Ulcer of intestine
K63.5	Polyp of colon
K63.81	Dieulafoy lesion of intestine
R93.3	Abnormal findings on diagnostic imaging of other parts of digestive tract

AMA: 45390 2020,May,13; 2019,Dec,14; 2018,Jan,8; 2017,Jan,6; 2017,Jan,8; 2016,Jan,13; 2015,Jan,16

Relative Value Units/Medicare Edits

Non-Facility RVU	Work	PE	MP	Total
45390	6.04	2.98	0.64	9.66
Facility RVU	**Work**	**PE**	**MP**	**Total**
45390	6.04	2.98	0.64	9.66

	FUD	Status	MUE	Modifiers				IOM Reference
45390	0	A	1(3)	51	N/A	N/A	N/A	None

* with documentation

Terms To Know

colonoscopy. Visual inspection of the colon using a fiberoptic scope.

neoplasm. New abnormal growth, tumor.

resection. Surgical removal of a part or all of an organ or body part.

Coding Companion for General Surgery/Gastroenterology

Rectum

45393

45393 Colonoscopy, flexible; with decompression (for pathologic distention) (eg, volvulus, megacolon), including placement of decompression tube, when performed

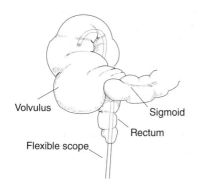

Explanation

The physician uses a flexible colonoscope to examine the colon and decompress a pathologic distention such as a volvulus or megacolon. The physician inserts the scope into the anus and advances the scope into the colon. The lumen of the colon and rectum are visualized. The scope is advanced into the area of distention decompressing it as the scope passes through the lumen. The scope is withdrawn at the completion of the procedure. This procedure includes placement of a decompression tube when utilized.

Coding Tips

Report the appropriate endoscopy for each anatomic site examined. Surgical endoscopy includes diagnostic endoscopy; however, diagnostic endoscopy can be identified separately when performed at the same surgical session as an open procedure. Colonoscopy involves examination of the entire colon, from the rectum to the cecum, and may also include the terminal ileum. When examination of the rectum and sigmoid colon with decompression of volvulus is performed using a rigid proctoscope (stiff hollow tube-like instrument), see 45321. Note that endoscopic reduction of the volvulus is performed more frequently using a rigid proctoscope. Only when the volvulus cannot be reached by rigid proctoscope is flexible colonoscopy decompression attempted. Bleeding that occurs as the result of an endoscopic procedure, and controlled during the same operative session, is not reported separately. Report 45393 only once per session. Do not report 45393 with 45378.

ICD-10-CM Diagnostic Codes

K56.2	Volvulus
K59.31	Toxic megacolon
K59.39	Other megacolon

AMA: 45393 2018,Jan,8; 2017,Jan,8; 2016,Jan,13; 2015,Jan,16

Relative Value Units/Medicare Edits

Non-Facility RVU	Work	PE	MP	Total
45393	4.68	2.1	0.59	7.37
Facility RVU	**Work**	**PE**	**MP**	**Total**
45393	4.68	2.1	0.59	7.37

	FUD	Status	MUE	Modifiers				IOM Reference
45393	0	A	1(3)	51	N/A	N/A	N/A	None

* with documentation

[45398]

45398 Colonoscopy, flexible; with band ligation(s) (eg, hemorrhoids)

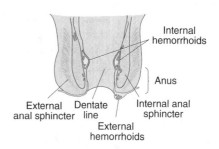

Explanation

The physician uses a flexible colonoscope to examine the rectum and colon and perform band ligation for hemorrhoids. The physician inserts the scope into the anus and advances the scope into the colon. The lumen of the colon and rectum are visualized. The scope is directed to the affected area. The physician identifies the hemorrhoid. The hemorrhoid is ligated at its base with a rubber band. The hemorrhoid tissue is allowed to slough over time.

Coding Tips

Surgical endoscopy includes diagnostic endoscopy; however, diagnostic endoscopy can be identified separately when performed at the same surgical session as an open procedure. For control of active bleeding with band ligation, see 45382. Bleeding that occurs as the result of an endoscopic procedure, and controlled during the same operative session, is not reported separately. Report 45398 only once per session. Do not report 45398 with 45378, 45390, or 46221 or in addition to 45382 for the same lesion.

ICD-10-CM Diagnostic Codes

K64.0	First degree hemorrhoids
K64.1	Second degree hemorrhoids
K64.2	Third degree hemorrhoids
K64.3	Fourth degree hemorrhoids
K64.8	Other hemorrhoids

AMA: 45398 2020,Feb,11; 2018,Jan,8; 2018,Jan,7; 2017,Sep,14; 2017,Jan,8; 2016,Jan,13; 2015,Jan,16

Relative Value Units/Medicare Edits

Non-Facility RVU	Work	PE	MP	Total
45398	4.2	20.44	0.59	25.23
Facility RVU	**Work**	**PE**	**MP**	**Total**
45398	4.2	2.06	0.59	6.85

	FUD	Status	MUE	Modifiers				IOM Reference
45398	0	A	1(2)	51	N/A	N/A	N/A	None

* with documentation

Terms To Know

hemorrhoid. Dilated, varicose vein in the anal region caused by continually increased venous pressure. Reversed blood flow and clotted blood within a vein that extends beyond the anus.

45395-45397

45395 Laparoscopy, surgical; proctectomy, complete, combined abdominoperineal, with colostomy

45397 proctectomy, combined abdominoperineal pull-through procedure (eg, colo-anal anastomosis), with creation of colonic reservoir (eg, J-pouch), with diverting enterostomy, when performed

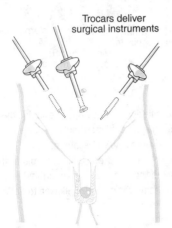

Trocars deliver surgical instruments

A complete, combined abdominoperineal proctectomy is performed laparoscopically with colostomy. The creation of colonic reservoir with diverting enterostomy

Explanation

With the patient under general anesthesia, the physician places a trocar at the umbilicus into the abdomen and insufflates the abdominal cavity. The physician places a laparoscope through the umbilical incision and additional trocars are placed, through which the surgical instruments are inserted. The physician mobilizes the sigmoid colon, tractions it upward, and incises the right pelvic peritoneum. Dissection and ligation are carried out on the inferior mesenteric artery and inferior mesenteric vein. The dissection is carried into the retrorectal space by using cautery scissors. The peritoneum is incised on both sides of the rectum and also anteriorly at the pouch of Douglas, and the mesorectum is mobilized off the sacrum. The physician frees the rectum from the posterior vaginal wall or the prostate and seminal vesicles. After the rectum is totally mobilized, a loop of sigmoid colon is brought through the small incision in a lower quadrant port, where it may be transected outside the body. The distal part is sutured shut and returned to the cavity and the stoma is matured. The specimen is removed en bloc during the perineal phase of the resection performed in a conventional fashion. The laparoscopic instruments are removed and the incisions are sutured. In 45397, the free end of the distal colon is brought through the sphincter complex and approximated with the anus to form a colo-anal anastomosis. The distal colon is folded and sutured in such a way as to create a colonic reservoir pouch. The physician may elect to bring a loop or end of the colon through a separate abdominal incision to create a stoma (diverting enterostomy).

Coding Tips

Surgical laparoscopy always includes diagnostic laparoscopy; the diagnostic laparoscopy should not be reported separately. For diagnostic laparoscopy only, see 49320. For open proctectomy, complete, with colostomy, see 45110; combined abdominoperineal pull-through procedure (e.g., colo-anal anastomosis), with creation of a colonic reservoir (e.g., J-pouch), with diverting enterostomy, see 45119.

ICD-10-CM Diagnostic Codes

C18.0	Malignant neoplasm of cecum
C18.1	Malignant neoplasm of appendix
C18.2	Malignant neoplasm of ascending colon
C18.3	Malignant neoplasm of hepatic flexure
C18.4	Malignant neoplasm of transverse colon
C18.5	Malignant neoplasm of splenic flexure
C18.6	Malignant neoplasm of descending colon
C18.7	Malignant neoplasm of sigmoid colon
C18.8	Malignant neoplasm of overlapping sites of colon
C19	Malignant neoplasm of rectosigmoid junction
C20	Malignant neoplasm of rectum
C21.1	Malignant neoplasm of anal canal
C21.2	Malignant neoplasm of cloacogenic zone
C21.8	Malignant neoplasm of overlapping sites of rectum, anus and anal canal
C78.5	Secondary malignant neoplasm of large intestine and rectum
C7A.022	Malignant carcinoid tumor of the ascending colon
C7A.023	Malignant carcinoid tumor of the transverse colon
C7A.024	Malignant carcinoid tumor of the descending colon
C7A.025	Malignant carcinoid tumor of the sigmoid colon
C7A.026	Malignant carcinoid tumor of the rectum
D01.0	Carcinoma in situ of colon
D01.1	Carcinoma in situ of rectosigmoid junction
D01.2	Carcinoma in situ of rectum
D12.2	Benign neoplasm of ascending colon
D12.3	Benign neoplasm of transverse colon
D12.4	Benign neoplasm of descending colon
D12.5	Benign neoplasm of sigmoid colon
D37.4	Neoplasm of uncertain behavior of colon
D37.5	Neoplasm of uncertain behavior of rectum
D3A.022	Benign carcinoid tumor of the ascending colon
D3A.023	Benign carcinoid tumor of the transverse colon
D3A.024	Benign carcinoid tumor of the descending colon
D3A.025	Benign carcinoid tumor of the sigmoid colon
D3A.026	Benign carcinoid tumor of the rectum
K50.111	Crohn's disease of large intestine with rectal bleeding
K50.112	Crohn's disease of large intestine with intestinal obstruction
K50.113	Crohn's disease of large intestine with fistula
K50.114	Crohn's disease of large intestine with abscess
K50.118	Crohn's disease of large intestine with other complication
K51.011	Ulcerative (chronic) pancolitis with rectal bleeding
K51.012	Ulcerative (chronic) pancolitis with intestinal obstruction
K51.013	Ulcerative (chronic) pancolitis with fistula
K51.014	Ulcerative (chronic) pancolitis with abscess
K51.018	Ulcerative (chronic) pancolitis with other complication
K51.211	Ulcerative (chronic) proctitis with rectal bleeding
K51.212	Ulcerative (chronic) proctitis with intestinal obstruction
K51.213	Ulcerative (chronic) proctitis with fistula
K51.214	Ulcerative (chronic) proctitis with abscess
K51.218	Ulcerative (chronic) proctitis with other complication
K51.311	Ulcerative (chronic) rectosigmoiditis with rectal bleeding
K51.312	Ulcerative (chronic) rectosigmoiditis with intestinal obstruction

Rectum

K51.313	Ulcerative (chronic) rectosigmoiditis with fistula
K51.314	Ulcerative (chronic) rectosigmoiditis with abscess
K51.318	Ulcerative (chronic) rectosigmoiditis with other complication
K51.411	Inflammatory polyps of colon with rectal bleeding
K51.412	Inflammatory polyps of colon with intestinal obstruction
K51.413	Inflammatory polyps of colon with fistula
K51.414	Inflammatory polyps of colon with abscess
K51.418	Inflammatory polyps of colon with other complication
K51.511	Left sided colitis with rectal bleeding
K51.512	Left sided colitis with intestinal obstruction
K51.513	Left sided colitis with fistula
K51.514	Left sided colitis with abscess
K51.518	Left sided colitis with other complication
K51.811	Other ulcerative colitis with rectal bleeding
K51.812	Other ulcerative colitis with intestinal obstruction
K51.813	Other ulcerative colitis with fistula
K51.814	Other ulcerative colitis with abscess
K51.818	Other ulcerative colitis with other complication
K55.031	Focal (segmental) acute (reversible) ischemia of large intestine
K55.032	Diffuse acute (reversible) ischemia of large intestine
K55.041	Focal (segmental) acute infarction of large intestine
K55.042	Diffuse acute infarction of large intestine
K55.1	Chronic vascular disorders of intestine
K62.2	Anal prolapse
K62.3	Rectal prolapse
K62.82	Dysplasia of anus
Q43.1	Hirschsprung's disease

AMA: **45395** 2018,Jan,8; 2017,Jan,8; 2016,Jan,13; 2015,Jan,16 **45397** 2018,Jan,8; 2017,Jan,8; 2016,Jan,13; 2015,Jan,16

Relative Value Units/Medicare Edits

Non-Facility RVU	Work	PE	MP	Total
45395	33.0	18.83	5.67	57.5
45397	36.5	19.94	5.81	62.25
Facility RVU	Work	PE	MP	Total
45395	33.0	18.83	5.67	57.5
45397	36.5	19.94	5.81	62.25

	FUD	Status	MUE	Modifiers				IOM Reference
45395	90	A	1(2)	51	N/A	62*	80	None
45397	90	A	1(2)	51	N/A	62*	80	

* with documentation

45400-45402

45400	Laparoscopy, surgical; proctopexy (for prolapse)
45402	proctopexy (for prolapse), with sigmoid resection

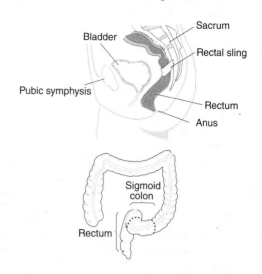

Explanation

The physician performs a laparoscopic proctopexy (or rectopexy) for correction of rectal prolapse. With the patient under general anesthesia, the physician places trocars into the abdomen and insufflates the abdominal cavity. Using a laparoscope, the physician completely mobilizes the rectum down to the pelvic floor and attaches the rectum to the sacrum using polypropylene mesh. The mesh is initially stapled to the sacral hollow and sutured on both sides of the rectum. The trocars are removed and the incisions are closed with sutures. In 45402, a laparoscopic sigmoid resection is performed in conjunction with the proctopexy. Using a laparoscope, the physician mobilizes the sigmoid colon and rectum. The redundant segment of sigmoid colon and rectum are excised and an anastomosis is created between the remaining bowel ends with sutures or staples. Following laparoscopic proctopexy as described above, the trocars are removed and the incision closed with sutures.

Coding Tips

Surgical laparoscopy always includes diagnostic laparoscopy; the diagnostic laparoscopy should not be reported separately. For proctopexy, abdominal approach, see 45540; perineal approach, see 45541. Proctopexy with sigmoid resection, via abdominal approach, is reported with 45550.

ICD-10-CM Diagnostic Codes

K57.20	Diverticulitis of large intestine with perforation and abscess without bleeding
K57.21	Diverticulitis of large intestine with perforation and abscess with bleeding
K57.30	Diverticulosis of large intestine without perforation or abscess without bleeding
K57.31	Diverticulosis of large intestine without perforation or abscess with bleeding
K57.32	Diverticulitis of large intestine without perforation or abscess without bleeding
K57.33	Diverticulitis of large intestine without perforation or abscess with bleeding
K57.40	Diverticulitis of both small and large intestine with perforation and abscess without bleeding

Rectum

K57.41	Diverticulitis of both small and large intestine with perforation and abscess with bleeding		
K57.50	Diverticulosis of both small and large intestine without perforation or abscess without bleeding		
K57.52	Diverticulitis of both small and large intestine without perforation or abscess without bleeding		
K59.31	Toxic megacolon		
K59.39	Other megacolon		
K62.3	Rectal prolapse		
Q43.8	Other specified congenital malformations of intestine		

AMA: 45400 2018,Jan,8; 2017,Jan,8; 2016,Jan,13; 2015,Jan,16 **45402** 2018,Jan,8; 2017,Jan,8; 2016,Jan,13; 2015,Jan,16

Relative Value Units/Medicare Edits

Non-Facility RVU	Work	PE	MP	Total
45400	19.44	10.56	3.11	33.11
45402	26.51	13.2	4.52	44.23
Facility RVU	**Work**	**PE**	**MP**	**Total**
45400	19.44	10.56	3.11	33.11
45402	26.51	13.2	4.52	44.23

	FUD	Status	MUE	Modifiers				IOM Reference
45400	90	A	1(2)	51	N/A	62*	80	None
45402	90	A	1(2)	51	N/A	62*	80	

* with documentation

Terms To Know

anastomosis. Surgically created connection between ducts, blood vessels, or bowel segments to allow flow from one to the other.

laparoscopy. Direct visualization of the peritoneal cavity, outer fallopian tubes, uterus, and ovaries utilizing a laparoscope, a thin, flexible fiberoptic tube.

prolapse. Falling, sliding, or sinking of an organ from its normal location in the body.

resection. Surgical removal of a part or all of an organ or body part.

stenosis. Narrowing or constriction of a passage.

Rectum

45500

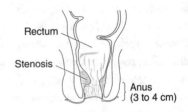

45500 Proctoplasty; for stenosis

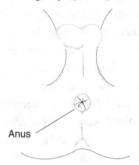

A stenotic stricture of the anal-rectal area is surgically repaired (proctoplasty)

Explanation

The physician performs proctoplasty for an area of stenosis. The physician makes a longitudinal incision through the scar tissue at the anorectal junction or may completely excise the scar tissue to an area of normal mucosa. The surrounding perianal skin is undermined and mobilized in one of several possible fashions as a flap. The flap is approximated to the normal mucosa at the edges of the incised or excised scar, thus closing the wound.

Coding Tips

Proctoplasty for prolapse of mucous membrane is reported with 45505. Report proctosigmoidoscopy, rigid, with dilation, with 45303. For anoscopy with dilation, any method, see 46604. For anoplasty, plastic operation for stricture, adult, see 46700; infant, see 46705.

ICD-10-CM Diagnostic Codes

K62.4	Stenosis of anus and rectum
Q42.0	Congenital absence, atresia and stenosis of rectum with fistula
Q42.1	Congenital absence, atresia and stenosis of rectum without fistula

AMA: 45500 2014,Jan,11

Relative Value Units/Medicare Edits

Non-Facility RVU	Work	PE	MP	Total
45500	7.73	7.29	1.89	16.91
Facility RVU	**Work**	**PE**	**MP**	**Total**
45500	7.73	7.29	1.89	16.91

	FUD	Status	MUE	Modifiers				IOM Reference
45500	90	A	1(2)	51	N/A	N/A	80*	None

* with documentation

45505

45505 Proctoplasty; for prolapse of mucous membrane

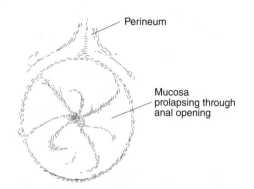

Perineum

Mucosa prolapsing through anal opening

Explanation

The physician performs proctoplasty for an area of prolapse of rectal mucosa (ectropion). The physician makes a circular incision just proximal to the prolapsing mucosa and mobilizes the redundant mucosa. An incision is made out onto the perianal skin to form a flap of skin on the right and left sides of the anus adjacent to the mobilized mucosa. The mucosa is excised and the flaps of skin are advanced into the anal canal. The mucosal edges are reapproximated in their normal anatomic position with sutures. The skin incisions are closed completing the procedure.

Coding Tips

There are several procedures for treating rectal prolapse. In this procedure, only the rectal mucosa is involved. Treatment involves surgical excision and plastic repair of the mucosa only. For perirectal injection of sclerosing solution, see 45520. Proctopexy, abdominal approach, see 45540; perineal approach, see 45541. For proctopexy with sigmoid resection, abdominal approach, report 45550.

ICD-10-CM Diagnostic Codes

K62.2	Anal prolapse
K62.3	Rectal prolapse

AMA: 45505 2018,Jan,8; 2017,Jan,8; 2016,Jan,13; 2015,Mar,9; 2015,Jan,16

Relative Value Units/Medicare Edits

Non-Facility RVU	Work	PE	MP	Total
45505	8.36	7.92	1.46	17.74
Facility RVU	**Work**	**PE**	**MP**	**Total**
45505	8.36	7.92	1.46	17.74

	FUD	Status	MUE	Modifiers				IOM Reference
45505	90	A	1(2)	51	N/A	N/A	N/A	None

* with documentation

45520

45520 Perirectal injection of sclerosing solution for prolapse

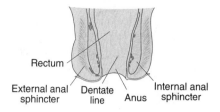

Rectum

External anal sphincter   Dentate line   Anus   Internal anal sphincter

The internal sphincter is an involuntary muscle and relaxes only upon stimulation from parasympathetic nerves. The external sphincter is voluntary. Together with the puborectalis muscle they form the anal ring

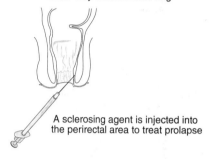

A sclerosing agent is injected into the perirectal area to treat prolapse

Explanation

The physician performs sclerotherapy for rectal prolapse. The physician identifies the anorectal ring. Sclerosing solution is injected into the submucosa of the rectum circumferentially just above the anorectal ring.

Coding Tips

Code 45520 should be reported only once per surgical session regardless of the number of injections administered. There are several methods for treating a rectal prolapse. For proctoplasty of mucous membrane, see 45505. Proctopexy, abdominal approach, see 45540; perineal approach, see 45541. Proctopexy, with sigmoid resection, abdominal approach is reported with 45550. Check with the specific payer to determine coverage.

ICD-10-CM Diagnostic Codes

K62.3	Rectal prolapse

AMA: 45520 2018,Jan,8; 2017,Jan,8; 2016,Jan,13; 2015,Jan,16

Relative Value Units/Medicare Edits

Non-Facility RVU	Work	PE	MP	Total
45520	0.55	4.37	0.06	4.98
Facility RVU	**Work**	**PE**	**MP**	**Total**
45520	0.55	0.54	0.06	1.15

	FUD	Status	MUE	Modifiers				IOM Reference
45520	0	A	1(2)	51	N/A	N/A	N/A	None

* with documentation

45540-45541

45540   Proctopexy (eg, for prolapse); abdominal approach
45541   perineal approach

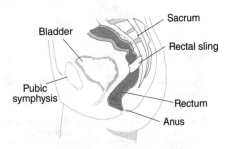

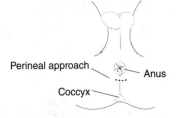

To repair rectal prolapse, the rectum is surgically accessed and mobilized. Its muscular posterior wall is sutured to the sacrum

Explanation

The physician approximates the rectum to the sacrum (proctopexy) for rectal prolapse via two different approaches; an abdominal incision in 45540 or a transverse incision between the anus and coccyx in 45541. The rectum is completely mobilized from the sacrum and placed in upward tension to remove any redundancy. The rectum is reapproximated to the sacrum with sutures or a mesh may be wrapped around the rectum and attached to the sacrum. The incisions are closed.

Coding Tips

Proctopexy codes should be selected based on approach and extent of the procedure. The procedures above involve fixation of the rectum to the sacrum, differentiated by the approach. For laparoscopic proctopexy, see 45400. Proctopexy combined with sigmoid resection, abdominal approach, is reported with 45550.

ICD-10-CM Diagnostic Codes

K62.3   Rectal prolapse

AMA: 45540 2014,Jan,11 **45541** 2014,Jan,11

Relative Value Units/Medicare Edits

Non-Facility RVU	Work	PE	MP	Total
45540	18.12	9.79	3.02	30.93
45541	14.85	10.17	2.84	27.86
Facility RVU	Work	PE	MP	Total
45540	18.12	9.79	3.02	30.93
45541	14.85	10.17	2.84	27.86

	FUD	Status	MUE	Modifiers				IOM Reference
45540	90	A	1(2)	51	N/A	62*	80	None
45541	90	A	1(2)	51	N/A	62*	80	

* with documentation

45550

45550   Proctopexy (eg, for prolapse); with sigmoid resection, abdominal approach

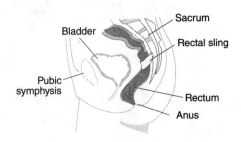

A proctopexy is performed in combination with resection of all or a portion of the sigmoid colon

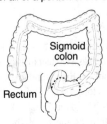

Explanation

The physician approximates the rectum to the sacrum and performs a sigmoid colon resection. The physician makes an abdominal incision. The sigmoid colon and rectum are mobilized. The redundant segment of sigmoid colon and rectum is excised and an anastomosis is created between the remaining bowel ends with sutures or staples. The rectum is approximated to the sacrum with sutures. The incision is closed.

Coding Tips

Proctopexy codes should be selected based on approach and extent of the procedure. For proctopexy, abdominal approach, see 45540; perineal approach, see 45541. Laparoscopic proctopexy is reported with 45400; with sigmoid resection, see 45402.

ICD-10-CM Diagnostic Codes

K57.20	Diverticulitis of large intestine with perforation and abscess without bleeding
K57.21	Diverticulitis of large intestine with perforation and abscess with bleeding
K57.30	Diverticulosis of large intestine without perforation or abscess without bleeding
K57.31	Diverticulosis of large intestine without perforation or abscess with bleeding
K57.32	Diverticulitis of large intestine without perforation or abscess without bleeding
K57.33	Diverticulitis of large intestine without perforation or abscess with bleeding
K57.40	Diverticulitis of both small and large intestine with perforation and abscess without bleeding
K57.41	Diverticulitis of both small and large intestine with perforation and abscess with bleeding
K57.50	Diverticulosis of both small and large intestine without perforation or abscess without bleeding

Coding Companion for General Surgery/Gastroenterology

K57.52	Diverticulitis of both small and large intestine without perforation or abscess without bleeding
K59.31	Toxic megacolon
K59.39	Other megacolon
K62.3	Rectal prolapse
Q43.8	Other specified congenital malformations of intestine

AMA: 45550 2014,Jan,11

Relative Value Units/Medicare Edits

Non-Facility RVU	Work	PE	MP	Total
45550	24.8	13.73	4.42	42.95
Facility RVU	**Work**	**PE**	**MP**	**Total**
45550	24.8	13.73	4.42	42.95

	FUD	Status	MUE	Modifiers				IOM Reference
45550	90	A	1(2)	51	N/A	62*	80	None

* with documentation

Terms To Know

anastomosis. Surgically created connection between ducts, blood vessels, or bowel segments to allow flow from one to the other.

approach. Method or anatomical location used to gain access to a body organ or specific area for procedures. The approach is not coded separately although it may be a specified component of the procedure, such as laparoscopic versus incisional, or spinal procedures in which the amount of dissection required to expose the spine significantly alters with the site of approach.

closure. Repairing an incision or wound by suture or other means.

incision. Act of cutting into tissue or an organ.

prolapse. Falling, sliding, or sinking of an organ from its normal location in the body.

resection. Surgical removal of a part or all of an organ or body part.

sacrum. Lower portion of the spine composed of five fused vertebrae designated as S1-S5.

45560

| 45560 | Repair of rectocele (separate procedure) |

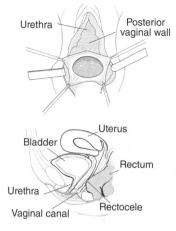

Rectum descends and protrudes through posterior wall of vagina

Explanation

The physician repairs a rectocele, a herniation of the rectum against the vaginal wall. The physician makes an incision in the mucosa of the posterior vaginal wall over the rectocele. The rectocele is dissected free of surrounding structures and the levator muscles are identified. The rectum is plicated to surrounding fascia with multiple sutures and the levator muscles are reapproximated. The vaginal mucosa is excised and the incision is closed.

Coding Tips

This separate procedure by definition is usually a component of a more complex service and is not identified separately. When performed alone or with other unrelated procedures it may be reported. If performed alone, list the code; if performed with other procedures/services, list the code and append modifier 59 or an X{EPSU} modifier. Posterior colporrhaphy, repair of a rectocele, with or without perineorrhaphy, is reported with 57250. For combined anteroposterior colporrhaphy, see 57260; with enterocele repair, see 57265.

ICD-10-CM Diagnostic Codes

| K62.3 | Rectal prolapse |
| N81.6 | Rectocele ♀ |

AMA: 45560 2014,Jan,11

Relative Value Units/Medicare Edits

Non-Facility RVU	Work	PE	MP	Total
45560	11.5	7.12	1.73	20.35
Facility RVU	**Work**	**PE**	**MP**	**Total**
45560	11.5	7.12	1.73	20.35

	FUD	Status	MUE	Modifiers				IOM Reference
45560	90	A	1(2)	51	N/A	62*	80	None

* with documentation

45562-45563

45562 Exploration, repair, and presacral drainage for rectal injury;
45563   with colostomy

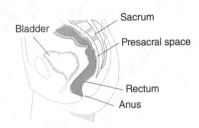

The rectum is repaired as necessary and drainage is provided from the presacral space (between the posterior rectum and the sacrum)

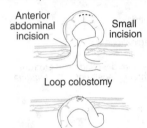

Loop colostomy

A temporary colostomy may also be performed

Explanation

The physician explores, repairs, and drains a rectal injury. The physician makes an abdominal incision. The rectal injury is explored and repaired with sutures if possible. An incision is made between the coccyx and anus in 45562. In 45563, a loop or end of sigmoid colon is brought through a separate incision on the abdominal wall as a colostomy and an incision is made between the coccyx and anus. Drains are placed in the presacral space in both procedures. The abdominal incisions are closed.

Coding Tips

The procedure described above may vary depending on the nature and extent of the rectal injury. If significant additional time and effort is documented, append modifier 22 and submit a cover letter and operative report. For transrectal drainage of an abscess, see 45000. Incision and drainage, submucosal abscess, rectum, see 45005; deep supralevator, pelvirectal or retrorectal, see 45020.

ICD-10-CM Diagnostic Codes

S36.61XA   Primary blast injury of rectum, initial encounter
S36.62XA   Contusion of rectum, initial encounter
S36.63XA   Laceration of rectum, initial encounter
S36.69XA   Other injury of rectum, initial encounter

AMA: 45562 2014,Jan,11 **45563** 2014,Jan,11

Relative Value Units/Medicare Edits

Non-Facility RVU	Work	PE	MP	Total
45562	17.98	11.72	3.62	33.32
45563	26.38	16.43	6.44	49.25
Facility RVU	Work	PE	MP	Total
45562	17.98	11.72	3.62	33.32
45563	26.38	16.43	6.44	49.25

	FUD	Status	MUE	Modifiers				IOM Reference
45562	90	A	1(2)	51	N/A	62*	80	None
45563	90	A	1(2)	51	N/A	62*	80	

* with documentation

Terms To Know

absorbable sutures. Strands used for suture or repair of tissue prepared from collagen or a synthetic polymer and capable of being absorbed by tissue over time.

drain. Device that creates a channel to allow fluid from a cavity, wound, or infected area to exit the body.

exploration. Examination for diagnostic purposes.

nonabsorbable sutures. Strands of natural or synthetic material that resist absorption into living tissue and are removed once healing is under way. Nonabsorbable sutures are commonly used to close skin wounds and repair tendons or collagenous tissue.

repair. Surgical closure of a wound. The wound may be a result of injury/trauma or it may be a surgically created defect. Repairs are divided into three categories: simple, intermediate, and complex.

sacrum. Lower portion of the spine composed of five fused vertebrae designated as S1-S5.

suture. Numerous stitching techniques employed in wound closure.

buried suture. Continuous or interrupted suture placed under the skin for a layered closure.

continuous suture. Running stitch with tension evenly distributed across a single strand to provide a leakproof closure line.

interrupted suture. Series of single stitches with tension isolated at each stitch, in which all stitches are not affected if one becomes loose, and the isolated sutures cannot act as a wick to transport an infection.

purse-string suture. Continuous suture placed around a tubular structure and tightened, to reduce or close the lumen.

retention suture. Secondary stitching that bridges the primary suture, providing support for the primary repair; a plastic or rubber bolster may be placed over the primary repair and under the retention sutures.

Rectum

45800-45805

45800 Closure of rectovesical fistula;
45805   with colostomy

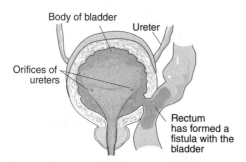

Closure of rectovesical fistula, a communication between rectum and bladder. A colostomy may also be performed during the same surgical session

Explanation

The physician closes a connection between the rectum and the bladder (rectovesical fistula). The physician makes an abdominal incision. The sigmoid colon and rectum are mobilized and the connection between the rectum and bladder is identified and divided. The fistulous openings in the rectum and bladder are debrided and closed with sutures. In 45805, a proximal colostomy is also created. The involved segment of colon or rectum may be excised. A loop or end of sigmoid colon proximal to the involved area is brought out through a separate incision on the abdominal wall as a colostomy. Abdominal incisions are closed.

Coding Tips

In order to select the correct procedure code, it is necessary to identify which structures the fistula connects. In this case, the fistula connects the rectum and the bladder. For closure of a rectourethral fistula, see 45820; with colostomy, see 45825.

ICD-10-CM Diagnostic Codes

N32.1   Vesicointestinal fistula

AMA: **45800** 2014,Jan,11 **45805** 2014,Jan,11

Relative Value Units/Medicare Edits

Non-Facility RVU	Work	PE	MP	Total
45800	20.31	12.42	4.96	37.69
45805	23.32	14.65	5.7	43.67
Facility RVU	**Work**	**PE**	**MP**	**Total**
45800	20.31	12.42	4.96	37.69
45805	23.32	14.65	5.7	43.67

	FUD	Status	MUE	Modifiers				IOM Reference
45800	90	A	1(3)	51	N/A	62*	80	None
45805	90	A	1(3)	51	N/A	62*	80	

* with documentation

45820-45825

45820 Closure of rectourethral fistula;
45825   with colostomy

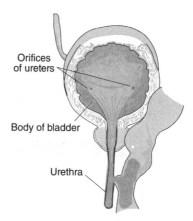

Rectum has formed a fistula with the urethra

Explanation

The physician closes a rectourethral fistula. The physician makes an abdominal incision. The rectum is dissected from the prostate and the fistula is identified and divided. The fistulous opening in the rectum is closed with sutures and the opening in the urethra may be closed or left open. A pedicle of omentum is usually mobilized and placed between the areas of repair. In 45825, loop or end of proximal colon is brought through a separate incision on the abdominal wall as a colostomy. The incision is closed. As an alternate method to 45820, an incision may be made between the anus and urethra from a perineal approach and dissection continued between the rectum and urethra. The fistula is identified and divided and the openings in the rectum and urethra are closed.

Coding Tips

In order to select the correct procedure code, it is necessary to identify which structures the fistula connects. In this case, the fistula connects the rectum and the urethra. For closure of a rectovesical fistula, see 45800; with colostomy, see 45805.

ICD-10-CM Diagnostic Codes

N36.0   Urethral fistula
Q64.73   Congenital urethrorectal fistula

AMA: **45820** 2014,Jan,11 **45825** 2014,Jan,11

Relative Value Units/Medicare Edits

Non-Facility RVU	Work	PE	MP	Total
45820	20.37	12.44	4.97	37.78
45825	24.17	15.62	5.92	45.71
Facility RVU	**Work**	**PE**	**MP**	**Total**
45820	20.37	12.44	4.97	37.78
45825	24.17	15.62	5.92	45.71

	FUD	Status	MUE	Modifiers				IOM Reference
45820	90	A	1(3)	51	N/A	62*	80	None
45825	90	A	1(3)	51	N/A	62*	80	

* with documentation

45900

45900 Reduction of procidentia (separate procedure) under anesthesia

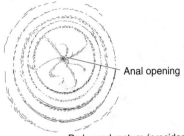

Anal opening

Prolapsed rectum (procidentia)
forms concentric folds
of tissue outside the perineum

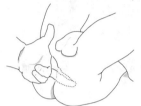

Explanation

The physician reduces a rectal prolapse (procidentia) to a patient under general anesthesia. The physician performs a manual reduction of an incarcerated rectal prolapse by pushing the prolapsed segment into the anus under the relaxation of anesthesia.

Coding Tips

This separate procedure by definition is usually a component of a more complex service and is not identified separately. When performed alone or with other unrelated procedures it may be reported. If performed alone, list the code; if performed with other procedures/services, list the code and append modifier 59 or an X{EPSU} modifier.

ICD-10-CM Diagnostic Codes

K62.2	Anal prolapse
K62.3	Rectal prolapse

AMA: **45900** 2014,Jan,11

Relative Value Units/Medicare Edits

Non-Facility RVU	Work	PE	MP	Total
45900	2.99	2.57	0.74	6.3
Facility RVU	**Work**	**PE**	**MP**	**Total**
45900	2.99	2.57	0.74	6.3

	FUD	Status	MUE	Modifiers				IOM Reference
45900	10	A	1(2)	51	N/A	N/A	80*	None

* with documentation

45905

45905 Dilation of anal sphincter (separate procedure) under anesthesia other than local

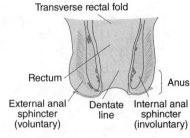

Transverse rectal fold

Rectum

Anus

External anal
sphincter
(voluntary)

Dentate
line

Internal anal
sphincter
(involuntary)

Digital dilation of anal sphincter
under anesthesia other than local

Explanation

The physician dilates the anal sphincter under anesthesia. The physician performs dilation of the anal sphincter digitally or with a dilating instrument under the relaxation of anesthesia.

Coding Tips

This separate procedure by definition is usually a component of a more complex service and is not identified separately. When performed alone or with other unrelated procedures it may be reported. If performed alone, list the code; if performed with other procedures/services, list the code and append modifier 59 or an X{EPSU} modifier.

ICD-10-CM Diagnostic Codes

C21.1	Malignant neoplasm of anal canal
C21.2	Malignant neoplasm of cloacogenic zone
C21.8	Malignant neoplasm of overlapping sites of rectum, anus and anal canal
D12.9	Benign neoplasm of anus and anal canal
K59.01	Slow transit constipation
K59.02	Outlet dysfunction constipation
K59.03	Drug induced constipation
K59.04	Chronic idiopathic constipation
K59.09	Other constipation
K59.4	Anal spasm
K60.0	Acute anal fissure
K60.1	Chronic anal fissure
K61.0	Anal abscess
K61.2	Anorectal abscess
K62.4	Stenosis of anus and rectum
K62.89	Other specified diseases of anus and rectum
K64.0	First degree hemorrhoids
K64.1	Second degree hemorrhoids
K64.2	Third degree hemorrhoids
K64.3	Fourth degree hemorrhoids
K64.8	Other hemorrhoids
Q42.2	Congenital absence, atresia and stenosis of anus with fistula
Q42.3	Congenital absence, atresia and stenosis of anus without fistula

AMA: **45905** 2014,Jan,11

N Newborn: 0   **P** Pediatric: 0-17   **M** Maternity: 9-64   **A** Adult: 15-124   ♂ Male Only   ♀ Female Only   CPT © 2021 American Medical Association. All Rights Reserved.

Coding Companion for General Surgery/Gastroenterology

Rectum

Relative Value Units/Medicare Edits

Non-Facility RVU	Work	PE	MP	Total
45905	2.35	2.21	0.42	4.98
Facility RVU	Work	PE	MP	Total
45905	2.35	2.21	0.42	4.98

	FUD	Status	MUE	Modifiers				IOM Reference
45905	10	A	1(2)	51	N/A	N/A	N/A	None

* with documentation

Terms To Know

abscess. Circumscribed collection of pus resulting from bacteria, frequently associated with swelling and other signs of inflammation.

anal fissure. Slit, crack, or tear of the anal mucosa that can cause pain, bleeding, and infection.

atresia. Congenital closure or absence of a tubular organ or an opening to the body surface.

benign. Mild or nonmalignant in nature.

congenital. Present at birth, occurring through heredity or an influence during gestation up to the moment of birth.

dilation. Artificial increase in the diameter of an opening or lumen made by medication or by instrumentation.

fistula. Abnormal tube-like passage between two body cavities or organs or from an organ to the outside surface.

general anesthesia. State of unconsciousness produced by an anesthetic agent or agents, inducing amnesia by blocking the awareness center in the brain, and rendering the patient unable to control protective reflexes, such as breathing.

hemorrhoid. Dilated, varicose vein in the anal region caused by continually increased venous pressure. Reversed blood flow and clotted blood within a vein that extends beyond the anus.

malignant. Any condition tending to progress toward death, specifically an invasive tumor with a loss of cellular differentiation that has the ability to spread or metastasize to other body areas.

neoplasm. New abnormal growth, tumor.

spasm. Involuntary muscle contraction.

stenosis. Narrowing or constriction of a passage.

45910

45910   Dilation of rectal stricture (separate procedure) under anesthesia other than local

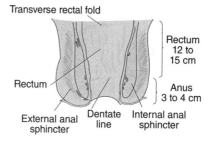

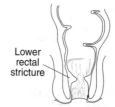

A rectal stricture is dilated while the patient is under general anesthesia

Explanation

The physician dilates a rectal stricture under anesthesia. The physician performs dilation of a rectal stricture digitally or with a dilating instrument under the relaxation of anesthesia.

Coding Tips

This separate procedure by definition is usually a component of a more complex service and is not identified separately. When performed alone or with other unrelated procedures it may be reported. If performed alone, list the code; if performed with other procedures/services, list the code and append modifier 59 or an X{EPSU} modifier.

ICD-10-CM Diagnostic Codes

K62.4	Stenosis of anus and rectum
Q42.0	Congenital absence, atresia and stenosis of rectum with fistula
Q42.1	Congenital absence, atresia and stenosis of rectum without fistula

AMA: 45910 2014,Jan,11

Relative Value Units/Medicare Edits

Non-Facility RVU	Work	PE	MP	Total
45910	2.85	2.33	0.46	5.64
Facility RVU	Work	PE	MP	Total
45910	2.85	2.33	0.46	5.64

	FUD	Status	MUE	Modifiers				IOM Reference
45910	10	A	1(2)	51	N/A	N/A	N/A	None

* with documentation

Rectum

45915

45915   Removal of fecal impaction or foreign body (separate procedure) under anesthesia

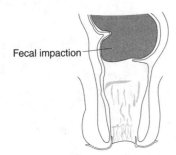

A fecal impaction or foreign body of the rectum is removed while the patient is under a general anesthesia

Explanation

The physician removes a foreign body or fecal impaction under anesthesia. The physician performs removal of a foreign body or fecal impaction manually or with an instrument under the relaxation of anesthesia.

Coding Tips

This separate procedure by definition is usually a component of a more complex service and is not identified separately. When performed alone or with other unrelated procedures it may be reported. If performed alone, list the code; if performed with other procedures/services, list the code and append modifier 59 or an X{EPSU} modifier.

ICD-10-CM Diagnostic Codes

K56.41	Fecal impaction
K56.49	Other impaction of intestine
K56.690	Other partial intestinal obstruction
K56.691	Other complete intestinal obstruction
T18.5XXA	Foreign body in anus and rectum, initial encounter

AMA: **45915** 2018,Jan,8; 2017,Jan,8; 2016,Jan,13; 2015,Jan,16

Relative Value Units/Medicare Edits

Non-Facility RVU	Work	PE	MP	Total
45915	3.19	6.89	0.56	10.64
Facility RVU	**Work**	**PE**	**MP**	**Total**
45915	3.19	3.08	0.56	6.83

	FUD	Status	MUE	Modifiers				IOM Reference
45915	10	A	1(2)	51	N/A	N/A	N/A	None

* with documentation

45990

45990   Anorectal exam, surgical, requiring anesthesia (general, spinal, or epidural), diagnostic

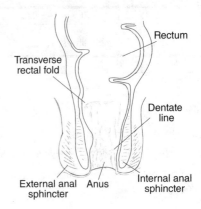

Explanation

The physician performs a diagnostic anorectal exam. The patient is placed under general, spinal or epidural anesthesia. The physician examines the external perineal area. A pelvic examination is performed when appropriate. A digital rectal exam is performed. An anoscope is inserted into the rectum. The anal canal and distal rectum are visualized. The anoscope is removed and a rigid proctosigmoidoscope is inserted into the anus and advanced. The sigmoid colon and rectal lumen are visualized. The proctosigmoidoscope is removed.

Coding Tips

This procedure includes an external perineal exam, digital rectal exam, pelvic exam (when appropriate), diagnostic anoscopy, and diagnostic rigid proctoscopy. If at any time during the diagnostic exam a surgical procedure is undertaken, report the procedure code only. Do not report 45990 with 45300-45327, 46600, 57410, or 99170.

ICD-10-CM Diagnostic Codes

C19	Malignant neoplasm of rectosigmoid junction
C20	Malignant neoplasm of rectum
C21.1	Malignant neoplasm of anal canal
C21.2	Malignant neoplasm of cloacogenic zone
C21.8	Malignant neoplasm of overlapping sites of rectum, anus and anal canal
C78.5	Secondary malignant neoplasm of large intestine and rectum
C7A.026	Malignant carcinoid tumor of the rectum
D01.1	Carcinoma in situ of rectosigmoid junction
D01.2	Carcinoma in situ of rectum
D01.3	Carcinoma in situ of anus and anal canal
D12.7	Benign neoplasm of rectosigmoid junction
D12.8	Benign neoplasm of rectum
D12.9	Benign neoplasm of anus and anal canal
D37.5	Neoplasm of uncertain behavior of rectum
D3A.026	Benign carcinoid tumor of the rectum
K56.41	Fecal impaction
K56.51	Intestinal adhesions [bands], with partial obstruction
K56.52	Intestinal adhesions [bands] with complete obstruction
K59.01	Slow transit constipation

K59.02	Outlet dysfunction constipation
K59.03	Drug induced constipation
K59.04	Chronic idiopathic constipation
K60.3	Anal fistula
K60.4	Rectal fistula
K60.5	Anorectal fistula
K61.0	Anal abscess
K61.1	Rectal abscess
K61.2	Anorectal abscess
K61.31	Horseshoe abscess
K61.39	Other ischiorectal abscess
K61.4	Intrasphincteric abscess
K61.5	Supralevator abscess
K62.0	Anal polyp
K62.1	Rectal polyp
K62.2	Anal prolapse
K62.3	Rectal prolapse
K62.5	Hemorrhage of anus and rectum
K62.6	Ulcer of anus and rectum
K62.82	Dysplasia of anus
K64.0	First degree hemorrhoids
K64.1	Second degree hemorrhoids
K64.2	Third degree hemorrhoids
K64.3	Fourth degree hemorrhoids
K64.4	Residual hemorrhoidal skin tags
K64.5	Perianal venous thrombosis
K64.8	Other hemorrhoids
K92.1	Melena
R15.0	Incomplete defecation
R15.1	Fecal smearing
R15.2	Fecal urgency
R15.9	Full incontinence of feces
R19.5	Other fecal abnormalities

AMA: 45990 2018,Jan,8; 2017,Jan,8; 2016,Jan,13; 2015,Jan,16

Relative Value Units/Medicare Edits

Non-Facility RVU	Work	PE	MP	Total
45990	1.8	0.98	0.3	3.08
Facility RVU	**Work**	**PE**	**MP**	**Total**
45990	1.8	0.98	0.3	3.08

	FUD	Status	MUE	Modifiers				IOM Reference
45990	0	A	1(2)	51	N/A	62*	80*	None

* with documentation

46020

46020   Placement of seton

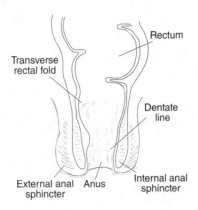

A seton is placed in the rectum

Explanation

The physician makes an incision in the anal opening. A suture is passed and the seton is securely tied using a rubber band, or similar technique. A nylon suture is threaded around the sphincter and tied loosely. An elastic band is secured to the suture and a safety pin is attached. The pin is taped to the patient's thigh and the patient is instructed to adjust the amount of pull to produce minimal discomfort until the seton cuts through.

Coding Tips

Do not report 46020 with 46060, 46280, or 46600. For removal of an anal seton, other marker, see 46030. Surgical trays, A4550, are not separately reimbursed by Medicare; however, other third-party payers may cover them. Check with the specific payer to determine coverage.

ICD-10-CM Diagnostic Codes

K51.213	Ulcerative (chronic) proctitis with fistula
K51.313	Ulcerative (chronic) rectosigmoiditis with fistula
K60.3	Anal fistula
K60.4	Rectal fistula
K60.5	Anorectal fistula
K61.4	Intrasphincteric abscess
T81.83XA	Persistent postprocedural fistula, initial encounter

AMA: 46020 2014,Jan,11

Relative Value Units/Medicare Edits

Non-Facility RVU	Work	PE	MP	Total
46020	3.0	4.92	0.53	8.45
Facility RVU	**Work**	**PE**	**MP**	**Total**
46020	3.0	3.5	0.53	7.03

	FUD	Status	MUE	Modifiers			IOM Reference
46020	10	A	2(3)	51	N/A	N/A	N/A	None

* with documentation

46030

46030   Removal of anal seton, other marker

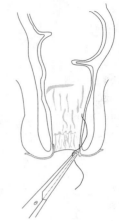

Seton under removal from anus

Explanation

The physician removes an anal seton or other marker. The physician identifies the seton stitch or other marker at the anal verge. The seton is divided and removed. The external anal sphincter at the level of the seton may be divided.

Coding Tips

Placement of a seton is reported with 46020. For transrectal drainage of abscess pelvic, see 45000; submucosal, rectum, see 45005; deep, supralevator, pelvirectal, or retrorectal, see 45020. For incision and drainage of abscess, intramural, intramuscular, or submucosal, transanal, under anesthesia, see 46045; superficial, perianal, see 46050; submuscular, ischiorectal or intramural, with fistulectomy or fistulotomy, with or without placement of seton, see 46060.

ICD-10-CM Diagnostic Codes

K51.213	Ulcerative (chronic) proctitis with fistula
K51.313	Ulcerative (chronic) rectosigmoiditis with fistula
K60.3	Anal fistula
K60.4	Rectal fistula
K60.5	Anorectal fistula
K61.4	Intrasphincteric abscess
T81.83XA	Persistent postprocedural fistula, initial encounter

AMA: 46030 2014,Jan,11

Relative Value Units/Medicare Edits

Non-Facility RVU	Work	PE	MP	Total
46030	1.26	3.09	0.21	4.56
Facility RVU	**Work**	**PE**	**MP**	**Total**
46030	1.26	1.17	0.21	2.64

	FUD	Status	MUE	Modifiers			IOM Reference
46030	10	A	1(3)	51	N/A	N/A	80*	None

* with documentation

Anus

46040

46040　Incision and drainage of ischiorectal and/or perirectal abscess (separate procedure)

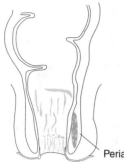
Perianal abscess

Explanation

The physician drains a perirectal or ischiorectal abscess. The physician identifies the location of the abscess. The perianal skin over the abscess is incised and the abscess cavity is opened and drained. The incision is packed open for continued drainage.

Coding Tips

This separate procedure by definition is usually a component of a more complex service and is not identified separately. When performed alone or with other unrelated procedures/services it may be reported. If performed alone, list the code; if performed with other procedures, list the code and append modifier 59 or an X{EPSU} modifier. Drainage of abscess codes are selected by site and surgical approach. For transrectal drainage of abscess pelvic, see 45000; submucosal, rectum, see 45005; deep, supralevator, pelvirectal, or retrorectal, see 45020. For incision and drainage of abscess, intramural, intramuscular, or submucosal, transanal, under anesthesia, see 46045; superficial, perianal, see 46050; submuscular, ischiorectal or intramural, with fistulectomy or fistulotomy, with or without placement of seton, see 46060.

ICD-10-CM Diagnostic Codes

K61.0	Anal abscess
K61.1	Rectal abscess
K61.2	Anorectal abscess
K61.31	Horseshoe abscess
K61.39	Other ischiorectal abscess
K61.4	Intrasphincteric abscess

AMA: 46040 2014,Jan,11

Relative Value Units/Medicare Edits

Non-Facility RVU	Work	PE	MP	Total
46040	5.37	10.18	1.12	16.67
Facility RVU	**Work**	**PE**	**MP**	**Total**
46040	5.37	6.06	1.12	12.55

	FUD	Status	MUE	Modifiers				IOM Reference
46040	90	A	2(3)	51	N/A	N/A	N/A	None

* with documentation

46045

46045　Incision and drainage of intramural, intramuscular, or submucosal abscess, transanal, under anesthesia

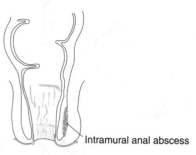
Intramural anal abscess

Incision and drainage is performed

Explanation

The physician drains a perirectal abscess in the intramural, intramuscular, or submucosal position. The physician identifies the location of the abscess in relation to the sphincter muscles. The perianal skin or rectal mucosa over the abscess is incised. Dissection is carried through muscle if necessary and the abscess cavity is opened and drained. The incision is packed open for continued drainage.

Coding Tips

Drainage of abscess codes are selected by abscess site and surgical approach. For transrectal drainage of abscess pelvic, see 45000; submucosal, rectum, see 45005; deep, supralevator, pelvirectal, or retrorectal, see 45020. For incision and drainage of abscess, ischiorectal and or perirectal, see 46040; perianal, see 46050; submuscular, ischiorectal or intramural, with fistulectomy or fistulotomy, with or without placement of seton, see 46060.

ICD-10-CM Diagnostic Codes

K51.214	Ulcerative (chronic) proctitis with abscess
K51.314	Ulcerative (chronic) rectosigmoiditis with abscess
K61.0	Anal abscess
K61.1	Rectal abscess
K61.2	Anorectal abscess
K61.31	Horseshoe abscess
K61.39	Other ischiorectal abscess
K61.4	Intrasphincteric abscess

AMA: 46045 2014,Jan,11

Relative Value Units/Medicare Edits

Non-Facility RVU	Work	PE	MP	Total
46045	5.87	6.03	1.15	13.05
Facility RVU	**Work**	**PE**	**MP**	**Total**
46045	5.87	6.03	1.15	13.05

	FUD	Status	MUE	Modifiers				IOM Reference
46045	90	A	2(3)	51	N/A	N/A	N/A	None

* with documentation

Anus

46050

46050   Incision and drainage, perianal abscess, superficial

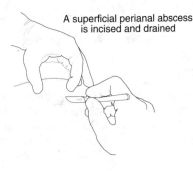

Rectum

External anal sphincter

Dentate line

Superficial anal abscess

A superficial perianal abscess is incised and drained

Explanation

The physician drains a superficial perianal abscess. The physician identifies the location of the abscess. The perianal skin over the abscess is incised and the abscess cavity is opened and drained. The incision is packed open for continued drainage.

Coding Tips

Drainage of abscess codes are selected by abscess site and surgical approach. For transrectal drainage of abscess pelvic, see 45000; submucosal, rectum, see 45005; deep, supralevator, pelvirectal, or retrorectal, see 45020. For incision and drainage of abscess, ischiorectal and or perirectal, see 46040; intramural, intramuscular, or submucosal, transanal, under anesthesia, see 46045; submuscular, ischiorectal or intramural, with fistulectomy or fistulotomy, with or without placement of seton, see 46060.

ICD-10-CM Diagnostic Codes

K61.0   Anal abscess
K61.2   Anorectal abscess
K61.4   Intrasphincteric abscess

AMA: 46050 2014,Jan,11

Relative Value Units/Medicare Edits

Non-Facility RVU	Work	PE	MP	Total
46050	1.24	5.55	0.25	7.04
Facility RVU	**Work**	**PE**	**MP**	**Total**
46050	1.24	1.46	0.25	2.95

	FUD	Status	MUE	Modifiers				IOM Reference
46050	10	A	2(3)	51	N/A	N/A	N/A	None

* with documentation

46060

46060   Incision and drainage of ischiorectal or intramural abscess, with fistulectomy or fistulotomy, submuscular, with or without placement of seton

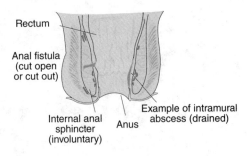

Rectum

Anal fistula (cut open or cut out)

Internal anal sphincter (involuntary)

Anus

Example of intramural abscess (drained)

Explanation

The physician drains an ischiorectal or intramural perirectal abscess with fistulectomy or fistulotomy and may place a seton. The physician identifies the location of the abscess and the internal and external openings of the anal fistula in relation to the sphincter muscles. An incision is made in the perianal skin over the abscess and the abscess cavity is opened and drained. The mucosa, skin, and internal sphincter muscle overlying the fistula is incised and the fistula is completely unroofed or may be excised. If the fistula goes beneath the external sphincter muscle, a stitch (seton) may be placed through the fistula tract to allow drainage and preserve continence. The incision is left open to drain and the abscess cavity is packed open for continued drainage.

Coding Tips

Do not report this code with 46020. Drainage of abscess codes are selected by abscess site and surgical approach. For transrectal drainage of abscess pelvic, see 45000; submucosal, rectum, see 45005; deep, supralevator, pelvirectal, or retrorectal, see 45020. For incision and drainage of abscess, ischiorectal and or perirectal, see 46040; intramural, intramuscular, or submucosal, transanal, under anesthesia, see 46045; superficial, perianal, see 46050.

ICD-10-CM Diagnostic Codes

K51.213   Ulcerative (chronic) proctitis with fistula
K51.313   Ulcerative (chronic) rectosigmoiditis with fistula
K60.4   Rectal fistula
K60.5   Anorectal fistula
K61.1   Rectal abscess
K61.2   Anorectal abscess
K61.31   Horseshoe abscess
K61.39   Other ischiorectal abscess
K61.4   Intrasphincteric abscess
Q43.6   Congenital fistula of rectum and anus
T81.83XA   Persistent postprocedural fistula, initial encounter

AMA: 46060 2014,Jan,11

Anus

Relative Value Units/Medicare Edits

Non-Facility RVU	Work	PE	MP	Total
46060	6.37	6.82	1.15	14.34
Facility RVU	Work	PE	MP	Total
46060	6.37	6.82	1.15	14.34

	FUD	Status	MUE	Modifiers				IOM Reference
46060	90	A	2(3)	51	N/A	N/A	N/A	None

* with documentation

Terms To Know

abscess. Circumscribed collection of pus resulting from bacteria, frequently associated with swelling and other signs of inflammation.

fistula. Abnormal tube-like passage between two body cavities or organs or from an organ to the outside surface.

intramural. Within the wall of an organ.

packing. Material placed into a cavity or wound, such as gels, gauze, pads, and sponges.

seton. Finely spun thread or other fine material for leading the passage of wider instruments through a fistula, canal, or sinus tract.

sphincter. Ring-like band of muscle that surrounds a bodily opening, constricting and relaxing as required for normal physiological functioning.

unroof. To remove the top, roof, or covering.

46080

46080   Sphincterotomy, anal, division of sphincter (separate procedure)

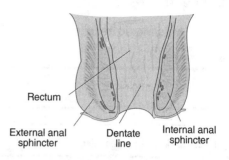

Rectum

External anal sphincter

Dentate line

Internal anal sphincter

Explanation

The physician divides the anal sphincter. The patient is placed in jackknife or lithotomy position. The physician performs digital and instrumental dilation of the anus with exposure of the patient's anal canal. A small incision is made between the muscle layers of the anus and internal muscle is divided without opening the lining of the anus.

Coding Tips

This separate procedure by definition is usually a component of a more complex service and is not identified separately. When performed alone or with other unrelated procedures it may be reported. If performed alone, list the code; if performed with other procedures/services, list the code and append modifier 59 or an X{EPSU} modifier. For fissurectomy including sphincterotomy, when performed, see 46200.

ICD-10-CM Diagnostic Codes

K59.01	Slow transit constipation
K59.02	Outlet dysfunction constipation
K59.4	Anal spasm
K60.0	Acute anal fissure
K60.1	Chronic anal fissure
K62.0	Anal polyp
K62.4	Stenosis of anus and rectum
K64.0	First degree hemorrhoids
K64.1	Second degree hemorrhoids
K64.2	Third degree hemorrhoids
K64.3	Fourth degree hemorrhoids
K64.4	Residual hemorrhoidal skin tags
K64.8	Other hemorrhoids
Q42.2	Congenital absence, atresia and stenosis of anus with fistula
Q42.3	Congenital absence, atresia and stenosis of anus without fistula
Q43.5	Ectopic anus
Q43.6	Congenital fistula of rectum and anus
S30.3XXA	Contusion of anus, initial encounter
S30.817A	Abrasion of anus, initial encounter
S30.827A	Blister (nonthermal) of anus, initial encounter
S30.857A	Superficial foreign body of anus, initial encounter
S30.877A	Other superficial bite of anus, initial encounter
S31.831A	Laceration without foreign body of anus, initial encounter
S31.832A	Laceration with foreign body of anus, initial encounter
S31.833A	Puncture wound without foreign body of anus, initial encounter

Anus

S31.834A   Puncture wound with foreign body of anus, initial encounter
S31.835A   Open bite of anus, initial encounter
T18.5XXA   Foreign body in anus and rectum, initial encounter

AMA: **46080** 2014,Jan,11

Relative Value Units/Medicare Edits

Non-Facility RVU	Work	PE	MP	Total
46080	2.52	5.51	0.48	8.51
Facility RVU	**Work**	**PE**	**MP**	**Total**
46080	2.52	1.65	0.48	4.65

	FUD	Status	MUE	Modifiers				IOM Reference
46080	10	A	1(2)	51	N/A	N/A	N/A	None

* with documentation

Terms To Know

congenital. Present at birth, occurring through heredity or an influence during gestation up to the moment of birth.

fissure. Deep furrow, groove, or cleft in tissue structures.

fistula. Abnormal tube-like passage between two body cavities or organs or from an organ to the outside surface.

stenosis. Narrowing or constriction of a passage.

46083

46083   Incision of thrombosed hemorrhoid, external

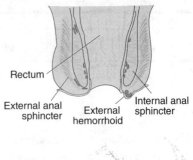

Rectum

External anal sphincter   External hemorrhoid   Internal anal sphincter

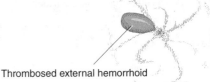

Thrombosed external hemorrhoid

Explanation

The physician performs incision of a thrombosed external hemorrhoid. The physician identifies the thrombosed external hemorrhoid. An incision is made in the skin over the hemorrhoid and the thrombus is removed. The incision is left open for continued drainage.

Coding Tips

Code 46083 may be reported for each external thrombosed hemorrhoid that is excised. Selection of codes for hemorrhoid treatment depends on the site of the hemorrhoid (internal or external) and the nature of the surgical procedure (injection, destruction, incision, ligation, or excision). For excision of external anal papilla or tag, single, see 46220; multiple, see 46230. For hemorrhoidectomy, external, two or more columns/groups, see 46250; internal by rubber band(s) ligation, see 46221. For excision of an external thrombosed hemorrhoid, see 46320. Injection of a hemorrhoidal sclerosing agent is reported with 46500.

ICD-10-CM Diagnostic Codes

K64.1   Second degree hemorrhoids
K64.2   Third degree hemorrhoids
K64.3   Fourth degree hemorrhoids
K64.4   Residual hemorrhoidal skin tags
K64.5   Perianal venous thrombosis
K64.8   Other hemorrhoids

AMA: **46083** 2018,Jan,8; 2017,Jan,8; 2016,Jan,13; 2015,Jan,16

Relative Value Units/Medicare Edits

Non-Facility RVU	Work	PE	MP	Total
46083	1.45	4.51	0.26	6.22
Facility RVU	**Work**	**PE**	**MP**	**Total**
46083	1.45	1.51	0.26	3.22

	FUD	Status	MUE	Modifiers				IOM Reference
46083	10	A	2(3)	51	N/A	N/A	N/A	None

* with documentation

Anus

46200

46200   Fissurectomy, including sphincterotomy, when performed

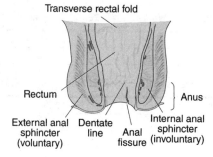

Transverse rectal fold

Rectum

Anus

External anal sphincter (voluntary)   Dentate line   Anal fissure   Internal anal sphincter (involuntary)

An anal fissure is a skin tear in the most distal part of the anus, from the dentate line to the anal verge

Explanation

The physician excises a fissure (fissurectomy) and may perform a sphincterotomy. The physician identifies the anal fissure and the internal sphincter muscle by palpation. An incision is made around the fissure, dissecting it free of underlying sphincter muscle, and the fissure is excised. The internal sphincter muscle may be incised, usually in a lateral position away from the fissure. The incision is usually left open to allow drainage.

Coding Tips

Fissurectomy is frequently performed in conjunction with other procedures. For hemorrhoidectomy with fissurectomy, see 46257 and 46261; and fistulectomy, see 46258 and 46262.

ICD-10-CM Diagnostic Codes

K60.0	Acute anal fissure
K60.1	Chronic anal fissure
K62.4	Stenosis of anus and rectum
K62.5	Hemorrhage of anus and rectum
Q43.6	Congenital fistula of rectum and anus

AMA: **46200** 2014,Jan,11

Relative Value Units/Medicare Edits

Non-Facility RVU	Work	PE	MP	Total
46200	3.59	10.05	0.62	14.26
Facility RVU	Work	PE	MP	Total
46200	3.59	5.72	0.62	9.93

	FUD	Status	MUE	Modifiers				IOM Reference
46200	90	A	1(3)	51	N/A	N/A	N/A	None

* with documentation

46221

46221   Hemorrhoidectomy, internal, by rubber band ligation(s)

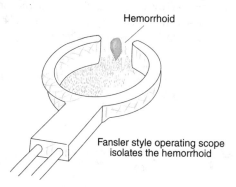

Hemorrhoid

Fansler style operating scope isolates the hemorrhoid

The hemorrhoid is ligated

Explanation

The physician performs hemorrhoidectomy by tying off (ligating) an internal hemorrhoid. The physician identifies the internal hemorrhoid. The hemorrhoid is ligated at its base with a rubber band. The hemorrhoid tissue is allowed to slough over time.

Coding Tips

Selection of codes for hemorrhoid treatment depends on the site of the hemorrhoid (internal or external) and the nature of the surgical procedure (injection, destruction, incision, ligation, or excision). For incision of an external thrombosed hemorrhoid, see 46083; for excision, see 46320. For excision of an external anal papilla or tag, single, see 46220; multiple, see 46230. For external hemorrhoidectomy, two or more columns/groups, see 46250. For injection of a hemorrhoidal sclerosing agent, see 46500. For ligation of internal hemorrhoids by other than rubber band, without imaging guidance, single hemorrhoid column/group, see 46945; two or more hemorrhoid columns/groups, see 46946. Do not report 46221 with 45350, 45398, or 46948.

ICD-10-CM Diagnostic Codes

K64.0	First degree hemorrhoids
K64.1	Second degree hemorrhoids
K64.2	Third degree hemorrhoids
K64.3	Fourth degree hemorrhoids
K64.5	Perianal venous thrombosis
K64.8	Other hemorrhoids

AMA: **46221** 2020,Feb,11; 2018,Jan,8; 2018,Jan,7; 2017,Sep,14; 2017,Jan,8; 2016,Jan,13; 2015,Jan,16; 2015,Apr,10

Relative Value Units/Medicare Edits

Non-Facility RVU	Work	PE	MP	Total
46221	2.36	5.91	0.33	8.6
Facility RVU	Work	PE	MP	Total
46221	2.36	3.03	0.33	5.72

	FUD	Status	MUE	Modifiers				IOM Reference
46221	10	A	1(2)	51	N/A	N/A	N/A	None

* with documentation

Anus

[46945, 46946]

46945   Hemorrhoidectomy, internal, by ligation other than rubber band; single hemorrhoid column/group, without imaging guidance
46946   Hemorrhoidectomy, internal, by ligation other than rubber band; 2 or more hemorrhoid columns/groups, without imaging guidance

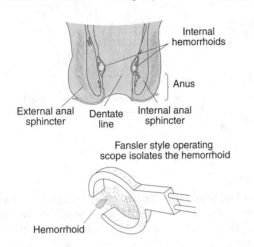

Explanation

The physician performs ligation (tying off) of internal hemorrhoids using methods other than rubber bands. The physician explores the anal canal and identifies the hemorrhoid column(s). Report 46945 for ligation of a single hemorrhoid column or group and 46946 for ligation of two or more columns or groups.

Coding Tips

Selection of codes for hemorrhoid treatment depends on the site of the hemorrhoid (internal or external) and the nature of the surgical procedure (injection, destruction, incision, ligation, or excision). For incision of an external thrombosed hemorrhoid, see 46083; for excision, see 46320. For hemorrhoidectomy by rubber band ligature, see 46221. For excision of an external anal papilla or tag, single, see 46220; for multiple, see 46230. For external hemorrhoidectomy, two or more columns/groups, see 46250. For injection of a hemorrhoidal sclerosing agent, see 46500. Do not report 46945-46946 with 46948, 76872, 76942, or 76998.

ICD-10-CM Diagnostic Codes

K64.0	First degree hemorrhoids
K64.1	Second degree hemorrhoids
K64.2	Third degree hemorrhoids
K64.3	Fourth degree hemorrhoids
K64.5	Perianal venous thrombosis
K64.8	Other hemorrhoids

AMA: **46945** 2020,Feb,11; 2018,Jan,8; 2017,Jan,8; 2016,Jan,13; 2015,Apr,10
46946 2020,Feb,11; 2018,Jan,8; 2017,Jan,8; 2016,Jan,13; 2015,Apr,10

Relative Value Units/Medicare Edits

Non-Facility RVU	Work	PE	MP	Total
46945	3.69	5.77	0.61	10.07
46946	4.5	6.12	0.71	11.33
Facility RVU	**Work**	**PE**	**MP**	**Total**
46945	3.69	5.77	0.61	10.07
46946	4.5	6.12	0.71	11.33

	FUD	Status	MUE	Modifiers				IOM Reference
46945	90	A	1(2)	51	N/A	N/A	N/A	None
46946	90	A	1(2)	51	N/A	N/A	N/A	

* with documentation

Terms To Know

anal papilla. Skin tag protruding up from the area between the skin and the inside lining of the anus. Anal papillae frequently occur with anal fissures and are often detected during a digital examination of the anus or with a scope.

exploration. Examination for diagnostic purposes.

hemorrhoid. Dilated, varicose vein in the anal region caused by continually increased venous pressure. Reversed blood flow and clotted blood within a vein that extends beyond the anus.

ligation. Tying off a blood vessel or duct with a suture or a soft, thin wire.

thrombosed hemorrhoid. Dilated, varicose vein in the anal region that has clotted blood within it.

Coding Companion for General Surgery/Gastroenterology

Anus

[46948]

46948   Hemorrhoidectomy, internal, by transanal hemorrhoidal dearterialization, 2 or more hemorrhoid columns/groups, including ultrasound guidance, with mucopexy, when performed

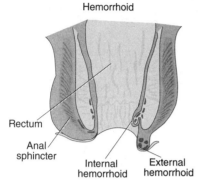

Internal transanal hemorrhoids are dearterialized

Explanation

The physician performs transanal dearterialization of two or more hemorrhoid groups or columns as an alternative to excisional hemorrhoidectomy or stapled hemorrhoidopexy. With the patient under general anesthesia or IV sedation with infiltration of a local anesthetic, the physician identifies the arteries supplying blood to the hemorrhoids utilizing a proctoscope coupled with a Doppler transducer. In order to interrupt the blood supply to the hemorrhoid, each selected artery is tied off (ligated) using a 2-0 absorbable suture. Mucopexy, or lifting and suturing of prolapsed mucosal membranes, may also be performed in cases of redundant prolapse.

Coding Tips

For ligation of internal hemorrhoids by other than rubber band, without imaging guidance, single hemorrhoid column or group, see 46945; for two or more hemorrhoid columns or groups, see 46946. For transanal dearterialization of a single hemorrhoid column or group, see 46999. Do not report 46948 with 76872, 76942, or 76998.

ICD-10-CM Diagnostic Codes

K64.0	First degree hemorrhoids
K64.1	Second degree hemorrhoids
K64.2	Third degree hemorrhoids
K64.3	Fourth degree hemorrhoids
K64.8	Other hemorrhoids

AMA: 46948 2020,Feb,11

Relative Value Units/Medicare Edits

Non-Facility RVU	Work	PE	MP	Total
46948	5.57	6.58	1.1	13.25
Facility RVU	Work	PE	MP	Total
46948	5.57	6.58	1.1	13.25

	FUD	Status	MUE	Modifiers				IOM Reference
46948	90	A	1(2)	51	N/A	N/A	N/A	None

* with documentation

[46220]

46220   Excision of single external papilla or tag, anus

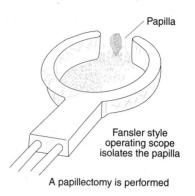

A papillectomy is performed

Explanation

The physician performs excision of a single external anal papilla or skin tag. The physician identifies the anal skin tag or papilla, which is usually associated with the external edge of a fissure or fistula. An incision is made around the skin tag or papilla and the lesion is dissected from the underlying sphincter muscle and removed. The incision is closed with sutures or may be left partially open to drain.

Coding Tips

For excision of multiple external anal papillae or tags, see 46230. Hemorrhoidectomy, external, 2 or more columns/groups is reported with 46250. For internal hemorrhoidectomy by rubber band(s) ligation, see 46221. For incision of external thrombosed hemorrhoid, see 46083; excision, see 46320. Report injection of a hemorrhoidal sclerosing agent with 46500. Surgical trays, A4550, are not separately reimbursed by Medicare; however, other third-party payers may cover them. Check with the specific payer to determine coverage.

ICD-10-CM Diagnostic Codes

K62.0	Anal polyp
K62.82	Dysplasia of anus
K64.4	Residual hemorrhoidal skin tags

AMA: 46220 2014,Jan,11

Relative Value Units/Medicare Edits

Non-Facility RVU	Work	PE	MP	Total
46220	1.61	5.49	0.28	7.38
Facility RVU	Work	PE	MP	Total
46220	1.61	1.65	0.28	3.54

	FUD	Status	MUE	Modifiers				IOM Reference
46220	10	A	1(2)	51	N/A	N/A	N/A	None

* with documentation

Terms To Know

anal papilla. Skin tag protruding up from the area between the skin and the inside lining of the anus. Anal papillae frequently occur with anal fissures and are often detected during a digital examination of the anus or with a scope.

benign. Mild or nonmalignant in nature.

46230

46230　Excision of multiple external papillae or tags, anus

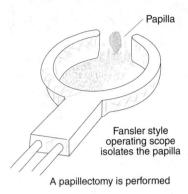

Papilla

Fansler style
operating scope
isolates the papilla

A papillectomy is performed

Explanation
The physician performs an excision of multiple external anal papillae or tags. Papillae are often associated with the external edge of an anal fissure or fistula. Once the physician has identified the external tags or papillae, incisions are made around the lesions. The lesions are dissected from the underlying sphincter muscle and removed. The incisions are closed with sutures or may be left partially open to drain.

Coding Tips
For excision of a single external anal papilla or tag, see 46220. For external hemorrhoidectomy, 2 or more columns/groups, see 46250. To report incision of an external thrombosed hemorrhoid, see 46083; excision, see 46320. Internal hemorrhoidectomy by rubber band(s) ligation is reported with code 46221. For injection of a hemorrhoidal sclerosing agent, see 46500.

ICD-10-CM Diagnostic Codes
K62.0	Anal polyp
K62.82	Dysplasia of anus
K64.4	Residual hemorrhoidal skin tags

AMA: 46230 2014,Jan,11

Relative Value Units/Medicare Edits
Non-Facility RVU	Work	PE	MP	Total
46230	2.62	6.16	0.44	9.22
Facility RVU	Work	PE	MP	Total
46230	2.62	2.02	0.44	5.08

	FUD	Status	MUE	Modifiers				IOM Reference
46230	10	A	1(2)	51	N/A	N/A	N/A	None

* with documentation

[46320]

46320　Excision of thrombosed hemorrhoid, external

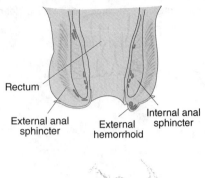

Rectum

External anal
sphincter

External
hemorrhoid

Internal anal
sphincter

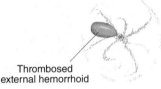

Thrombosed
external hemorrhoid

Explanation
The physician performs an excision of an external hemorrhoid that has become clotted with blood (thrombosed). Following appropriate anesthesia, the physician exposes the thrombosed external hemorrhoid. The hemorrhoid is completely excised with a scalpel. The site of the excision may be closed or left open to allow continued drainage.

Coding Tips
Selection of codes depends on the site of the hemorrhoid (internal or external) and the nature of the surgical procedure (injection, destruction, incision, ligation, excision, excision with other procedures). For excision of external anal papilla or tag, single, see 46220; multiple, see 46230. For an internal hemorrhoidectomy by rubber band ligation(s), see 46221. For external hemorrhoidectomy, 2 or more columns/groups, see 46250. To report an internal and external hemorrhoidectomy, single column or group, see 46255.

ICD-10-CM Diagnostic Codes
K62.5	Hemorrhage of anus and rectum
K62.89	Other specified diseases of anus and rectum
K64.1	Second degree hemorrhoids
K64.2	Third degree hemorrhoids
K64.3	Fourth degree hemorrhoids
K64.5	Perianal venous thrombosis
K64.8	Other hemorrhoids

AMA: 46320 2014,Jan,11

Relative Value Units/Medicare Edits
Non-Facility RVU	Work	PE	MP	Total
46320	1.64	4.39	0.28	6.31
Facility RVU	Work	PE	MP	Total
46320	1.64	1.4	0.28	3.32

	FUD	Status	MUE	Modifiers				IOM Reference
46320	10	A	2(3)	51	N/A	N/A	N/A	None

* with documentation

Anus

46250

46250   Hemorrhoidectomy, external, 2 or more columns/groups

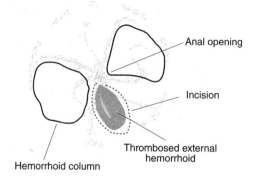

- Anal opening
- Incision
- Thrombosed external hemorrhoid
- Hemorrhoid column

Explanation

The physician performs an excision of external hemorrhoids. The physician identifies the external hemorrhoids. Incisions are made around the hemorrhoids and the lesions are dissected from the underlying sphincter muscle and removed. The incisions are closed with sutures.

Coding Tips

Selection of codes for hemorrhoid treatment depends on the site of the hemorrhoid (internal or external) and the nature of the surgical procedure (injection, destruction, incision, ligation, or excision). For hemorrhoidectomy, external, single column/group, see 46999. For incision of an external thrombosed hemorrhoid, see 46083; for excision, see 46320. For excision of an external anal papilla or tag, single, see 46220; multiple, see 46230. For internal hemorrhoidectomy by rubber band(s) ligation, see 46221. For injection of a hemorrhoidal sclerosing agent, see 46500. Do not report 46250 with 46948.

ICD-10-CM Diagnostic Codes

K64.0	First degree hemorrhoids
K64.1	Second degree hemorrhoids
K64.2	Third degree hemorrhoids
K64.3	Fourth degree hemorrhoids
K64.4	Residual hemorrhoidal skin tags
K64.5	Perianal venous thrombosis
K64.8	Other hemorrhoids

AMA: **46250** 2014,Jan,11

Relative Value Units/Medicare Edits

Non-Facility RVU	Work	PE	MP	Total
46250	4.25	9.48	0.75	14.48
Facility RVU	**Work**	**PE**	**MP**	**Total**
46250	4.25	4.45	0.75	9.45

	FUD	Status	MUE	Modifiers				IOM Reference
46250	90	A	1(2)	51	N/A	N/A	N/A	None

* with documentation

46255-46258

46255   Hemorrhoidectomy, internal and external, single column/group;
46257   with fissurectomy
46258   with fistulectomy, including fissurectomy, when performed

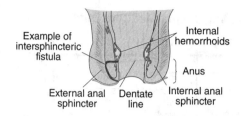

- Example of intersphincteric fistula
- Internal hemorrhoids
- Anus
- External anal sphincter
- Dentate line
- Internal anal sphincter

Removal of hemorrhoids. A fissurectomy or fistulectomy may also be performed

Explanation

The physician performs excision of a single column or group of internal and external hemorrhoids. The physician explores the anal canal and identifies the hemorrhoid column. An incision is made in the rectal mucosa around the hemorrhoids and the lesions are dissected from the underlying sphincter muscles and removed. The incisions are closed with sutures. In 46257, hemorrhoidectomy with an associated fissure is performed. An incision is made around the fissure and the fissure is dissected from the underlying sphincter muscles and excised. In 46258, hemorrhoidectomy with associated fistulectomy and a possible fissurectomy is performed. If the fistula is in the same plane as the hemorrhoid, a single incision is made in the mucosa around the lesions and the lesions are dissected from the underlying sphincter muscles and removed. If the lesions are in different planes, separate incisions are used to excise the lesions. If a fissure is present it may be excised in a similar manner. The incisions are closed with sutures.

Coding Tips

Selection of codes for hemorrhoid treatment depends on the site of the hemorrhoid (internal or external) and the nature of the surgical procedure (injection, destruction, incision, ligation, or excision). For hemorrhoidectomy, internal/external, two or more columns/groups, see 46260; with fissurectomy, see 46261; with fistulectomy, including fissurectomy, when performed, see 46262. For excision of a single external anal papilla or tag, see 46220; multiple, see 46230. For incision of an external thrombosed hemorrhoid, see 46083; excision, see 46320. For internal hemorrhoidectomy by rubber band(s) ligation, see 46221. For injection of a hemorrhoidal sclerosing agent, see 46500. Do not report 46255–46258 with 46948.

ICD-10-CM Diagnostic Codes

K60.0	Acute anal fissure
K60.1	Chronic anal fissure
K60.3	Anal fistula
K60.4	Rectal fistula
K60.5	Anorectal fistula
K62.5	Hemorrhage of anus and rectum
K62.82	Dysplasia of anus
K62.89	Other specified diseases of anus and rectum
K64.0	First degree hemorrhoids
K64.1	Second degree hemorrhoids
K64.2	Third degree hemorrhoids
K64.3	Fourth degree hemorrhoids

Anus

K64.4	Residual hemorrhoidal skin tags
K64.5	Perianal venous thrombosis
K64.8	Other hemorrhoids
Q43.6	Congenital fistula of rectum and anus

AMA: 46255 2018,Jan,8; 2017,Jan,8; 2016,Jan,13; 2015,Jan,16

Relative Value Units/Medicare Edits

Non-Facility RVU	Work	PE	MP	Total
46255	4.96	9.88	0.91	15.75
46257	5.76	5.87	1.03	12.66
46258	6.41	6.21	1.57	14.19
Facility RVU	Work	PE	MP	Total
46255	4.96	4.7	0.91	10.57
46257	5.76	5.87	1.03	12.66
46258	6.41	6.21	1.57	14.19

	FUD	Status	MUE	Modifiers				IOM Reference
46255	90	A	1(2)	51	N/A	N/A	N/A	None
46257	90	A	1(2)	51	N/A	N/A	N/A	
46258	90	A	1(2)	51	N/A	N/A	80*	

* with documentation

Terms To Know

external thrombosed hemorrhoid. Reversed blood flow and clotted blood within a vein that extends beyond the anus.

fissure. Deep furrow, groove, or cleft in tissue structures.

fistula. Abnormal tube-like passage between two body cavities or organs or from an organ to the outside surface.

hemorrhoid. Dilated, varicose vein in the anal region caused by continually increased venous pressure. Reversed blood flow and clotted blood within a vein that extends beyond the anus.

46260-46262

46260	Hemorrhoidectomy, internal and external, 2 or more columns/groups;
46261	with fissurectomy
46262	with fistulectomy, including fissurectomy, when performed

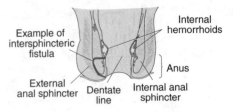

Removal is complex or extensive. A fissurectomy or fistulectomy may also be performed

Explanation

The physician performs excision of two or more columns or groups of internal and external hemorrhoids. The physician explores the anal canal and identifies the hemorrhoid columns. Incisions are made in the rectal mucosa around the hemorrhoid columns. The lesions are dissected from the underlying sphincter muscles and removed. The incisions are closed with sutures. In 46261, hemorrhoidectomy is performed as described above and an associated fissure is excised. In 46262, an associated fistulectomy and a possible fissurectomy are performed in addition to the hemorrhoidectomy.

Coding Tips

Selection of codes for hemorrhoid treatment depends on the site of the hemorrhoid (internal or external) and the nature of the surgical procedure (injection, destruction, incision, ligation, or excision). For hemorrhoidectomy, internal/external, single column/group, see 46255; with fissurectomy, see 46257; with fistulectomy, including fissurectomy, when performed, see 46258. Hemorrhoidectomy, external, two or more columns/groups, is reported with 46250. For excision of an external anal papilla or tag, single, see 46220; multiple, see 46230. For incision of an external thrombosed hemorrhoid, see 46083; excision, see 46320. For an internal hemorrhoidectomy by rubber band(s) ligation, see 46221. For injection of a hemorrhoidal sclerosing agent, see 46500. Do not report 46260–46262 with 46948.

ICD-10-CM Diagnostic Codes

K60.0	Acute anal fissure
K60.1	Chronic anal fissure
K60.3	Anal fistula
K60.4	Rectal fistula
K60.5	Anorectal fistula
K62.5	Hemorrhage of anus and rectum
K62.82	Dysplasia of anus
K62.89	Other specified diseases of anus and rectum
K64.0	First degree hemorrhoids
K64.1	Second degree hemorrhoids
K64.2	Third degree hemorrhoids
K64.3	Fourth degree hemorrhoids
K64.4	Residual hemorrhoidal skin tags
K64.5	Perianal venous thrombosis
K64.8	Other hemorrhoids
Q43.6	Congenital fistula of rectum and anus

AMA: 46262 2018,Jan,8; 2017,Jan,8; 2016,Jan,13; 2015,Jan,16

Anus

Relative Value Units/Medicare Edits

Non-Facility RVU	Work	PE	MP	Total
46260	6.73	6.25	1.28	14.26
46261	7.76	6.43	1.31	15.5
46262	7.91	7.29	1.36	16.56

Facility RVU	Work	PE	MP	Total
46260	6.73	6.25	1.28	14.26
46261	7.76	6.43	1.31	15.5
46262	7.91	7.29	1.36	16.56

	FUD	Status	MUE	Modifiers				IOM Reference
46260	90	A	1(2)	51	N/A	N/A	N/A	None
46261	90	A	1(2)	51	N/A	N/A	N/A	
46262	90	A	1(2)	51	N/A	N/A	N/A	

* with documentation

Terms To Know

dissect. Cut apart or separate tissue for surgical purposes or for visual or microscopic study.

dysplasia. Abnormality or alteration in the size, shape, and organization of cells from their normal pattern of development.

excise. Remove or cut out.

external thrombosed hemorrhoid. Reversed blood flow and clotted blood within a vein that extends beyond the anus.

fissure. Deep furrow, groove, or cleft in tissue structures.

fistula. Abnormal tube-like passage between two body cavities or organs or from an organ to the outside surface.

hemorrhoid. Dilated, varicose vein in the anal region caused by continually increased venous pressure. Reversed blood flow and clotted blood within a vein that extends beyond the anus.

46270-46285

46270	Surgical treatment of anal fistula (fistulectomy/fistulotomy); subcutaneous
46275	intersphincteric
46280	transsphincteric, suprasphincteric, extrasphincteric or multiple, including placement of seton, when performed
46285	second stage

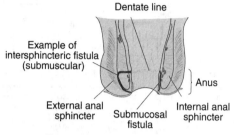

Dentate line

Example of intersphincteric fistula (submuscular)

Anus

External anal sphincter

Submucosal fistula

Internal anal sphincter

Removal is complex or multiple

An anal fistula is treated by incision (fistulotomy) or by excision (fistulectomy)

Explanation

In 46270, the physician excises or incises a subcutaneous anal fistula. The physician explores the anal canal and identifies the location of the fistula in relation to the sphincter muscles. The skin and subcutaneous tissue overlying the fistula is excised or incised to open the fistula tract. The incision is usually left open to allow continued drainage. Report 46275 for excision or incision of an intersphincteric anal fistula. Surgical treatment, via excision or incision, of a transsphincteric, suprasphincteric, extrasphincteric, or multiple anal fistula is reported with 46280 and includes seton placement, when performed. Report 46285 for a second stage excision or incision of an anal fistula.

Coding Tips

Do not report 46280 with 46020. For a fistulectomy performed with a hemorrhoidectomy, see 46258 and 46262. For closure of an anal fistula with a rectal advancement flap, see 46288.

ICD-10-CM Diagnostic Codes

K60.3	Anal fistula
K60.4	Rectal fistula
K60.5	Anorectal fistula
Q43.6	Congenital fistula of rectum and anus
T81.83XA	Persistent postprocedural fistula, initial encounter

AMA: **46270** 2014,Jan,11 **46275** 2014,Jan,11 **46280** 2014,Jan,11 **46285** 2014,Jan,11

Anus

Relative Value Units/Medicare Edits

Non-Facility RVU	Work	PE	MP	Total
46270	4.92	10.19	0.94	16.05
46275	5.42	10.52	0.93	16.87
46280	6.39	6.66	1.09	14.14
46285	5.42	10.46	0.92	16.8
Facility RVU	**Work**	**PE**	**MP**	**Total**
46270	4.92	5.95	0.94	11.81
46275	5.42	6.07	0.93	12.42
46280	6.39	6.66	1.09	14.14
46285	5.42	6.08	0.92	12.42

	FUD	Status	MUE	Modifiers				IOM Reference
46270	90	A	1(3)	51	N/A	N/A	N/A	None
46275	90	A	1(3)	51	N/A	N/A	N/A	
46280	90	A	1(2)	51	N/A	N/A	N/A	
46285	90	A	1(3)	51	N/A	N/A	N/A	

* with documentation

Terms To Know

congenital. Present at birth, occurring through heredity or an influence during gestation up to the moment of birth.

drain. Device that creates a channel to allow fluid from a cavity, wound, or infected area to exit the body.

excision. Surgical removal of an organ or tissue.

fistula. Abnormal tube-like passage between two body cavities or organs or from an organ to the outside surface.

mucous membranes. Thin sheets of tissue that secrete mucous and absorb water, salt, and other solutes. Mucous membranes cover or line cavities or canals of the body that open to the outside, such as linings of the mouth, respiratory and genitourinary passages, and the digestive tube.

seton. Finely spun thread or other fine material for leading the passage of wider instruments through a fistula, canal, or sinus tract.

subcutaneous tissue. Sheet or wide band of adipose (fat) and areolar connective tissue in two layers attached to the dermis.

46288

46288   Closure of anal fistula with rectal advancement flap

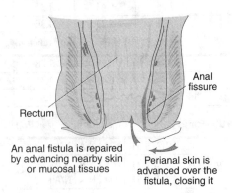

An anal fistula is repaired by advancing nearby skin or mucosal tissues

Perianal skin is advanced over the fistula, closing it

Rectum

Anal fissure

Explanation

The physician excises an anal fistula and closes the defect with a rectal advancement flap. The physician explores the anal canal and identifies the location of the fistula in relation to the sphincter muscles. The fistula tract is excised. An incision is made onto the perianal skin and a wedge of skin and subcutaneous tissue are mobilized and advanced into the defect created by the excision of the fistula. The incisions are closed with sutures.

Coding Tips

For surgical closure of an anal fistula, subcutaneous, see 46270; intersphincteric, see 46275, trans-, supra-, or extrasphincteric, or multiple, with placement of seton, when performed, see 46280; second stage, see 46285. Fistulectomy performed with hemorrhoidectomy is reported with see 46258 or 46262.

ICD-10-CM Diagnostic Codes

K60.3	Anal fistula
K60.4	Rectal fistula
K60.5	Anorectal fistula
Q43.6	Congenital fistula of rectum and anus
T81.83XA	Persistent postprocedural fistula, initial encounter

AMA: 46288 2014,Jan,11

Relative Value Units/Medicare Edits

Non-Facility RVU	Work	PE	MP	Total
46288	7.81	7.3	1.3	16.41
Facility RVU	**Work**	**PE**	**MP**	**Total**
46288	7.81	7.3	1.3	16.41

	FUD	Status	MUE	Modifiers				IOM Reference
46288	90	A	1(3)	51	N/A	N/A	N/A	None

* with documentation

Anus

46500

46500 Injection of sclerosing solution, hemorrhoids

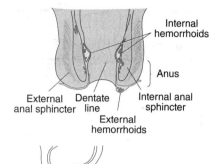

Internal hemorrhoids

Anus

External anal sphincter
Dentate line
Internal anal sphincter
External hemorrhoids

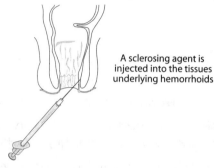

A sclerosing agent is injected into the tissues underlying hemorrhoids

Explanation

The physician performs sclerotherapy of internal hemorrhoids. The physician explores the anal canal and identifies the hemorrhoid columns. Sclerosing solution is injected into the submucosa of the rectal wall under the hemorrhoid columns.

Coding Tips

For hemorrhoidectomy, external, two or more columns/groups, see 46250; single column/group, see 46999; internal/external, single column/group, see 46255; with fissurectomy, see 46257; with fistulectomy, including fissurectomy, when performed, see 46258. Incision of a thrombosed external hemorrhoid is reported with 46083; excision, see 46320. For excision of an external anal papilla or tag, single, see 46220; multiple, see 46230. Internal hemorrhoidectomy by rubber band(s) ligation is reported with 46221. For destruction of internal hemorrhoids by thermal energy, see 46930. Hemorrhoidopexy by stapling is reported with 46947. Surgical trays, A4550, are not separately reimbursed by Medicare; however, other third-party payers may cover them. Check with the specific payer to determine coverage.

ICD-10-CM Diagnostic Codes

K64.0	First degree hemorrhoids
K64.1	Second degree hemorrhoids
K64.2	Third degree hemorrhoids
K64.3	Fourth degree hemorrhoids
K64.8	Other hemorrhoids

AMA: 46500 2018,Jan,8; 2017,Jan,8; 2016,Jan,13; 2015,Jan,16

Relative Value Units/Medicare Edits

Non-Facility RVU	Work	PE	MP	Total
46500	1.74	7.52	0.26	9.52
Facility RVU	Work	PE	MP	Total
46500	1.74	3.53	0.26	5.53

	FUD	Status	MUE	Modifiers				IOM Reference
46500	10	A	1(2)	51	N/A	N/A	N/A	None

* with documentation

Terms To Know

hemorrhoid. Dilated, varicose vein in the anal region caused by continually increased venous pressure. Reversed blood flow and clotted blood within a vein that extends beyond the anus.

injection. Forcing a liquid substance into a body part such as a joint or muscle.

rectal. Pertaining to the rectum, the end portion of the large intestine.

sclerotherapy. Injection of a chemical agent that will irritate, inflame, and cause fibrosis in a vein, eventually obliterating hemorrhoids or varicose veins.

thrombosed hemorrhoid. Dilated, varicose vein in the anal region that has clotted blood within it.

Anus

46505

46505   Chemodenervation of internal anal sphincter

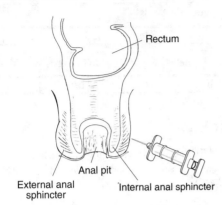

Botulinum toxin is injected into anal tissue to reduce
pain or spasm or to promote healing

Explanation

The physician utilizes chemodenervation (the use of chemical agents, including neurotoxins) to provide selective weakening of certain muscles or muscle groups by causing a neuromuscular blockade. Chemodenervation works by introducing a substance used to block the transfer of chemicals at the presynaptic membrane. Botulinum toxin type A (BTX-A, Botox®) is the most common substance used. To treat chronic anal fissures, the physician injects BTX-A into the internal anal sphincter. This permits chemical denervation of the anal sphincter and promotes healing of the fissure.

Coding Tips

For chemodenervation of other muscles, see 64612, 64616, 64617, or 64642–64647. Report destruction of nerve by neurolytic agent with code 64630. This code reports the injection service only. Supplies used when providing this procedure may be reported with the appropriate HCPCS level II "J" code. Check with the specific payer to determine coverage.

ICD-10-CM Diagnostic Codes

K59.01	Slow transit constipation
K59.02	Outlet dysfunction constipation
K59.03	Drug induced constipation
K59.04	Chronic idiopathic constipation
K59.09	Other constipation
K60.0	Acute anal fissure
K60.1	Chronic anal fissure
K62.5	Hemorrhage of anus and rectum
K62.6	Ulcer of anus and rectum
K62.89	Other specified diseases of anus and rectum
K64.0	First degree hemorrhoids
K64.1	Second degree hemorrhoids
K64.2	Third degree hemorrhoids
K64.3	Fourth degree hemorrhoids
K64.8	Other hemorrhoids

AMA: 46505 2019,Apr,9; 2018,Jan,8; 2017,Jan,8; 2016,Jan,13; 2015,Jan,16

Relative Value Units/Medicare Edits

Non-Facility RVU	Work	PE	MP	Total
46505	3.18	5.62	0.52	9.32
Facility RVU	Work	PE	MP	Total
46505	3.18	3.69	0.52	7.39

	FUD	Status	MUE	Modifiers				IOM Reference
46505	10	A	1(2)	51	50	N/A	N/A	None

* with documentation

Terms To Know

anal fissure. Slit, crack, or tear of the anal mucosa that can cause pain, bleeding, and infection.

BTX. Botulinum toxin.

dysplasia. Abnormality or alteration in the size, shape, and organization of cells from their normal pattern of development.

injection. Forcing a liquid substance into a body part such as a joint or muscle.

sphincter. Ring-like band of muscle that surrounds a bodily opening, constricting and relaxing as required for normal physiological functioning.

ulcer. Open sore or excavating lesion of skin or the tissue on the surface of an organ from the sloughing of chronically inflamed and necrosing tissue.

Anus

46600-46601

46600 Anoscopy; diagnostic, including collection of specimen(s) by brushing or washing, when performed (separate procedure)

46601 diagnostic, with high-resolution magnification (HRA) (eg, colposcope, operating microscope) and chemical agent enhancement, including collection of specimen(s) by brushing or washing, when performed

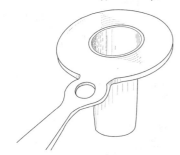

Hirschman type anoscope

Any of several types of scopes may be inserted into the anal-rectal column. The anus and distal rectum are visualized

Explanation

In 46600, the physician performs anoscopy and may obtain brushings or washings. The physician inserts the anoscope into the anus and advances the scope. The anal canal and distal rectal mucosa are visualized and brushings or washings may be obtained. In 46601, the physician performs a diagnostic examination of the anal canal using high resolution anoscopy (HRA), frequently indicated for patients with abnormal anal cytology. The physician examines the anal canal using a thin round tube (anoscope) and a high resolution magnifying instrument (colposcope). A mild acidic liquid may be applied to the anal canal to facilitate evaluation of any abnormal or dysplastic tissue as it causes abnormal tissue to turn white. Code 46601 includes specimens obtained by brushing or washing, when performed. The anoscope is withdrawn at the completion of the procedure.

Coding Tips

Note that 46600, a separate procedure by definition, is usually a component of a more complex service and is not identified separately. When performed alone or with other unrelated procedures/services it may be reported; if performed with other procedures/services, list the code and append modifier 59 or an X{EPSU} modifier. Report the appropriate endoscopy for each anatomical site examined. Surgical endoscopy always includes diagnostic endoscopy. However, diagnostic endoscopy can be identified separately when performed at the same surgical session as an open procedure. Diagnostic high resolution anoscopy (HRA) is reported with 46601. Do not report 46600 with 46020–46947 or in addition to 0184T when performed in the same operative session. Do not report 46601 with 69990.

ICD-10-CM Diagnostic Codes

C20	Malignant neoplasm of rectum
C21.1	Malignant neoplasm of anal canal
C21.2	Malignant neoplasm of cloacogenic zone
C21.8	Malignant neoplasm of overlapping sites of rectum, anus and anal canal
C49.A5	Gastrointestinal stromal tumor of rectum
C7A.026	Malignant carcinoid tumor of the rectum
D01.2	Carcinoma in situ of rectum
D01.3	Carcinoma in situ of anus and anal canal
D12.8	Benign neoplasm of rectum
D12.9	Benign neoplasm of anus and anal canal
D37.8	Neoplasm of uncertain behavior of other specified digestive organs
D3A.026	Benign carcinoid tumor of the rectum
D49.0	Neoplasm of unspecified behavior of digestive system
K51.20	Ulcerative (chronic) proctitis without complications
K51.211	Ulcerative (chronic) proctitis with rectal bleeding
K51.212	Ulcerative (chronic) proctitis with intestinal obstruction
K51.214	Ulcerative (chronic) proctitis with abscess
K51.218	Ulcerative (chronic) proctitis with other complication
K59.01	Slow transit constipation
K59.02	Outlet dysfunction constipation
K59.03	Drug induced constipation
K59.04	Chronic idiopathic constipation
K59.09	Other constipation
K59.4	Anal spasm
K60.0	Acute anal fissure
K60.1	Chronic anal fissure
K60.3	Anal fistula
K60.4	Rectal fistula
K60.5	Anorectal fistula
K61.0	Anal abscess
K61.1	Rectal abscess
K61.2	Anorectal abscess
K61.31	Horseshoe abscess
K61.39	Other ischiorectal abscess
K61.4	Intrasphincteric abscess
K61.5	Supralevator abscess
K62.0	Anal polyp
K62.1	Rectal polyp
K62.2	Anal prolapse
K62.3	Rectal prolapse
K62.4	Stenosis of anus and rectum
K62.5	Hemorrhage of anus and rectum
K62.6	Ulcer of anus and rectum
K62.7	Radiation proctitis
K62.82	Dysplasia of anus
K62.89	Other specified diseases of anus and rectum
K64.0	First degree hemorrhoids
K64.1	Second degree hemorrhoids
K64.2	Third degree hemorrhoids
K64.3	Fourth degree hemorrhoids
K64.4	Residual hemorrhoidal skin tags
K64.5	Perianal venous thrombosis
K64.8	Other hemorrhoids
K92.1	Melena
K92.89	Other specified diseases of the digestive system
L29.0	Pruritus ani
M35.08	Sjögren syndrome with gastrointestinal involvement
Q42.2	Congenital absence, atresia and stenosis of anus with fistula
Q42.3	Congenital absence, atresia and stenosis of anus without fistula

Anus

R15.0	Incomplete defecation
R15.1	Fecal smearing
R15.2	Fecal urgency
R15.9	Full incontinence of feces
Z12.12	Encounter for screening for malignant neoplasm of rectum

AMA: 46600 2018,Jan,8; 2018,Jan,7; 2017,Jan,8; 2016,Jan,13; 2015,Jan,16
46601 2018,Oct,11; 2016,Feb,12

Relative Value Units/Medicare Edits

Non-Facility RVU	Work	PE	MP	Total
46600	0.55	2.93	0.09	3.57
46601	1.6	2.66	0.22	4.48
Facility RVU	**Work**	**PE**	**MP**	**Total**
46600	0.55	0.54	0.09	1.18
46601	1.6	0.96	0.22	2.78

	FUD	Status	MUE	Modifiers				IOM Reference
46600	0	A	1(3)	51	N/A	N/A	N/A	None
46601	0	A	1(3)	51	N/A	N/A	N/A	

* with documentation

Terms To Know

anoscopy. Endoscopic diagnostic procedure in which an anoscope is inserted through the anus and advanced. The anal canal and distal rectal mucosa are visualized and brushings or washings may be obtained.

distal. Located farther away from a specified reference point or the trunk.

dysplasia. Abnormality or alteration in the size, shape, and organization of cells from their normal pattern of development.

mucosa. Moist tissue lining the mouth (buccal mucosa), stomach (gastric mucosa), intestines, and respiratory tract.

46604

46604 Anoscopy; with dilation (eg, balloon, guide wire, bougie)

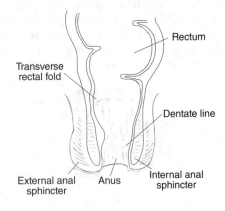

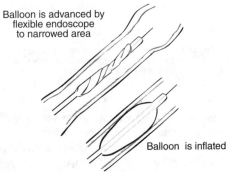

Balloon is advanced by flexible endoscope to narrowed area

Balloon is inflated

Explanation

The physician performs anoscopy and performs anal dilation. The physician inserts the anoscope into the anus and advances the scope. The anal canal and distal rectal mucosa are visualized. Dilation of the anal sphincter or a distal stricture is performed with the anoscope, digitally, or by some other instrument. The anoscope is withdrawn at the completion of the procedure.

Coding Tips

Report the appropriate endoscopy for each anatomic site examined. Surgical endoscopy always includes a diagnostic endoscopy. However, diagnostic endoscopy can be identified separately when performed at the same surgical session as an open procedure. A biopsy is not separately reportable when performed with excision of a lesion. For high-resolution anoscopy (HRA), diagnostic, see 46601; with biopsy, see 46607. When medically necessary, report moderate (conscious) sedation provided by the performing provider with 99151–99153. When provided by another provider, report 99155–99157.

ICD-10-CM Diagnostic Codes

C20	Malignant neoplasm of rectum
C21.1	Malignant neoplasm of anal canal
C21.2	Malignant neoplasm of cloacogenic zone
C21.8	Malignant neoplasm of overlapping sites of rectum, anus and anal canal
C49.A5	Gastrointestinal stromal tumor of rectum
C7A.026	Malignant carcinoid tumor of the rectum
D01.1	Carcinoma in situ of rectosigmoid junction
D01.2	Carcinoma in situ of rectum
D01.3	Carcinoma in situ of anus and anal canal
D12.8	Benign neoplasm of rectum

Anus

D12.9	Benign neoplasm of anus and anal canal	
D37.8	Neoplasm of uncertain behavior of other specified digestive organs	
D3A.026	Benign carcinoid tumor of the rectum	
D49.0	Neoplasm of unspecified behavior of digestive system	
K51.20	Ulcerative (chronic) proctitis without complications	
K51.211	Ulcerative (chronic) proctitis with rectal bleeding	
K51.212	Ulcerative (chronic) proctitis with intestinal obstruction	
K51.214	Ulcerative (chronic) proctitis with abscess	
K51.218	Ulcerative (chronic) proctitis with other complication	
K51.30	Ulcerative (chronic) rectosigmoiditis without complications	
K51.311	Ulcerative (chronic) rectosigmoiditis with rectal bleeding	
K51.312	Ulcerative (chronic) rectosigmoiditis with intestinal obstruction	
K51.314	Ulcerative (chronic) rectosigmoiditis with abscess	
K51.318	Ulcerative (chronic) rectosigmoiditis with other complication	
K59.01	Slow transit constipation	
K59.02	Outlet dysfunction constipation	
K59.03	Drug induced constipation	
K59.04	Chronic idiopathic constipation	
K59.09	Other constipation	
K59.4	Anal spasm	
K60.0	Acute anal fissure	
K60.1	Chronic anal fissure	
K60.3	Anal fistula	
K60.4	Rectal fistula	
K60.5	Anorectal fistula	
K61.4	Intrasphincteric abscess	
K62.0	Anal polyp	
K62.1	Rectal polyp	
K62.2	Anal prolapse	
K62.3	Rectal prolapse	
K62.4	Stenosis of anus and rectum	
K62.5	Hemorrhage of anus and rectum	
K62.6	Ulcer of anus and rectum	
K62.7	Radiation proctitis	
K62.82	Dysplasia of anus	
K62.89	Other specified diseases of anus and rectum	
K64.5	Perianal venous thrombosis	
K92.1	Melena	
K92.89	Other specified diseases of the digestive system	
L29.0	Pruritus ani	
Q42.2	Congenital absence, atresia and stenosis of anus with fistula	
Q42.3	Congenital absence, atresia and stenosis of anus without fistula	
R15.0	Incomplete defecation	
R15.1	Fecal smearing	
R15.2	Fecal urgency	
R15.9	Full incontinence of feces	
Z12.12	Encounter for screening for malignant neoplasm of rectum	

AMA: 46604 2018,Jan,8; 2017,Jan,8; 2016,Jan,13; 2015,Jan,16

Relative Value Units/Medicare Edits

Non-Facility RVU	Work	PE	MP	Total
46604	1.03	19.96	0.16	21.15
Facility RVU	Work	PE	MP	Total
46604	1.03	0.72	0.16	1.91

	FUD	Status	MUE	Modifiers				IOM Reference
46604	0	A	1(2)	51	N/A	N/A	N/A	None

* with documentation

Terms To Know

balloon catheter. Any catheter equipped with an inflatable balloon at the end to hold it in place in a body cavity or to be used for dilation of a vessel lumen.

bougie. Probe used to dilate or calibrate a body part.

fissure. Deep furrow, groove, or cleft in tissue structures.

fistula. Abnormal tube-like passage between two body cavities or organs or from an organ to the outside surface.

melena. Passage of blood in the stool. The stool is black and tarry in appearance due to the presence of blood within the intestine. Melena is often a symptom of a more serious condition.

mucosa. Moist tissue lining the mouth (buccal mucosa), stomach (gastric mucosa), intestines, and respiratory tract.

stricture. Narrowing of an anatomical structure.

Anus

Coding Companion for General Surgery/Gastroenterology

645

46606-46607

46606 Anoscopy; with biopsy, single or multiple
46607   with high-resolution magnification (HRA) (eg, colposcope, operating microscope) and chemical agent enhancement, with biopsy, single or multiple

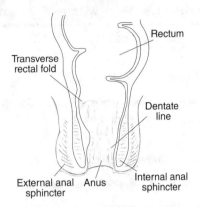

Rectum
Transverse rectal fold
Dentate line
External anal sphincter
Anus
Internal anal sphincter

Explanation

In 46606, the physician performs anoscopy and obtains tissue samples by biopsy. The physician inserts the anoscope into the anus and advances the scope. The anal canal and distal rectal mucosa are visualized and tissue samples are obtained. The anoscope is withdrawn at the completion of the procedure. In 46607, the examination is performed using high resolution anoscopy (HRA), frequently indicated for patients with abnormal anal cytology. The physician examines the anal canal using a thin round tube (anoscope) and a high resolution magnifying instrument (colposcope). A mild acidic liquid may be applied to the anal canal to facilitate evaluation of any abnormal or dysplastic tissue as it causes abnormal tissue to turn white. The anoscope is withdrawn at the completion of the procedure. Both codes include biopsy.

Coding Tips

Report the appropriate endoscopy for each anatomical site examined. Surgical endoscopy always includes diagnostic endoscopy. However, diagnostic endoscopy can be identified separately when performed at the same surgical session as an open procedure. A biopsy is not reported separately when performed with excision of a lesion. For high-resolution anoscopy (HRA), diagnostic, see 46601. Do not report 46607 with 69990.

ICD-10-CM Diagnostic Codes

C20	Malignant neoplasm of rectum
C21.1	Malignant neoplasm of anal canal
C21.2	Malignant neoplasm of cloacogenic zone
C21.8	Malignant neoplasm of overlapping sites of rectum, anus and anal canal
C49.A5	Gastrointestinal stromal tumor of rectum
C7A.026	Malignant carcinoid tumor of the rectum
D01.1	Carcinoma in situ of rectosigmoid junction
D01.2	Carcinoma in situ of rectum
D01.3	Carcinoma in situ of anus and anal canal
D12.8	Benign neoplasm of rectum
D12.9	Benign neoplasm of anus and anal canal
D37.8	Neoplasm of uncertain behavior of other specified digestive organs
D3A.026	Benign carcinoid tumor of the rectum
K51.20	Ulcerative (chronic) proctitis without complications
K51.211	Ulcerative (chronic) proctitis with rectal bleeding
K51.212	Ulcerative (chronic) proctitis with intestinal obstruction
K51.214	Ulcerative (chronic) proctitis with abscess
K51.218	Ulcerative (chronic) proctitis with other complication
K51.30	Ulcerative (chronic) rectosigmoiditis without complications
K51.311	Ulcerative (chronic) rectosigmoiditis with rectal bleeding
K51.312	Ulcerative (chronic) rectosigmoiditis with intestinal obstruction
K51.314	Ulcerative (chronic) rectosigmoiditis with abscess
K51.318	Ulcerative (chronic) rectosigmoiditis with other complication
K59.01	Slow transit constipation
K59.02	Outlet dysfunction constipation
K59.03	Drug induced constipation
K59.04	Chronic idiopathic constipation
K59.09	Other constipation
K59.4	Anal spasm
K60.0	Acute anal fissure
K60.1	Chronic anal fissure
K60.3	Anal fistula
K60.4	Rectal fistula
K60.5	Anorectal fistula
K61.0	Anal abscess
K61.1	Rectal abscess
K61.2	Anorectal abscess
K61.31	Horseshoe abscess
K61.39	Other ischiorectal abscess
K61.4	Intrasphincteric abscess
K61.5	Supralevator abscess
K62.0	Anal polyp
K62.1	Rectal polyp
K62.2	Anal prolapse
K62.3	Rectal prolapse
K62.4	Stenosis of anus and rectum
K62.5	Hemorrhage of anus and rectum
K62.6	Ulcer of anus and rectum
K62.7	Radiation proctitis
K62.82	Dysplasia of anus
K62.89	Other specified diseases of anus and rectum
K64.5	Perianal venous thrombosis
K92.1	Melena
K92.89	Other specified diseases of the digestive system
L29.0	Pruritus ani
M35.08	Sjögren syndrome with gastrointestinal involvement
Q42.2	Congenital absence, atresia and stenosis of anus with fistula
Q42.3	Congenital absence, atresia and stenosis of anus without fistula
R15.0	Incomplete defecation
R15.1	Fecal smearing
R15.2	Fecal urgency
R15.9	Full incontinence of feces
Z12.12	Encounter for screening for malignant neoplasm of rectum

AMA: 46606 2019,Sep,10; 2018,Jan,8; 2017,Jan,8; 2016,Jan,13; 2015,Jan,16
46607 2019,Dec,12; 2018,Oct,11; 2016,Feb,12

Anus

Relative Value Units/Medicare Edits

Non-Facility RVU	Work	PE	MP	Total
46606	1.2	7.15	0.21	8.56
46607	2.2	3.74	0.32	6.26
Facility RVU	Work	PE	MP	Total
46606	1.2	0.8	0.21	2.21
46607	2.2	1.22	0.32	3.74

	FUD	Status	MUE	Modifiers				IOM Reference
46606	0	A	1(2)	51	N/A	N/A	N/A	None
46607	0	A	1(2)	51	N/A	N/A	N/A	

* with documentation

Terms To Know

anoscopy. Endoscopic diagnostic procedure in which an anoscope is inserted through the anus and advanced. The anal canal and distal rectal mucosa are visualized and brushings or washings may be obtained.

biopsy. Tissue or fluid removed for diagnostic purposes through analysis of the cells in the biopsy material.

distal. Located farther away from a specified reference point or the trunk.

dysplasia. Abnormality or alteration in the size, shape, and organization of cells from their normal pattern of development.

mucosa. Moist tissue lining the mouth (buccal mucosa), stomach (gastric mucosa), intestines, and respiratory tract.

operating microscope. Compound microscope with two or more lens systems or several grouped lenses in one unit that provides magnifying power to the surgeon up to 40X.

specimen. Tissue cells or sample of fluid taken for analysis, pathologic examination, and diagnosis.

tissue. Group of similar cells with a similar function that form definite structures and organs. Tissue types include epithelial tissue, muscle tissue, connective tissue, and nervous tissue.

46608

46608   Anoscopy; with removal of foreign body

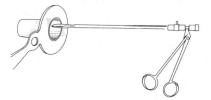

A grasping forceps is manipulated through the anoscope and a foreign body is removed from the anal canal

Explanation

The physician performs anoscopy and removes a foreign body. The physician inserts the anoscope through the anus and advances the scope. The anal canal and distal rectal mucosa are visualized. The foreign body is identified and removed with a snare or forceps placed through the anoscope. The anoscope is withdrawn at the completion of the procedure.

Coding Tips

Report the appropriate endoscopy for each anatomic site examined. Surgical endoscopy includes diagnostic endoscopy; however, diagnostic endoscopy can be identified separately when performed at the same surgical session as an open procedure. For removal of fecal impaction or foreign body, under anesthesia, see 45915. Supplies used when providing this procedure may be reported with the appropriate HCPCS level II code. Check with the specific payer to determine coverage.

ICD-10-CM Diagnostic Codes

K59.4	Anal spasm
K62.5	Hemorrhage of anus and rectum
K62.89	Other specified diseases of anus and rectum
S30.857A	Superficial foreign body of anus, initial encounter
S31.832A	Laceration with foreign body of anus, initial encounter
S31.834A	Puncture wound with foreign body of anus, initial encounter
T18.5XXA	Foreign body in anus and rectum, initial encounter

AMA: **46608** 2018,Jan,8; 2017,Jan,8; 2016,Jan,13; 2015,Jan,16

Relative Value Units/Medicare Edits

Non-Facility RVU	Work	PE	MP	Total
46608	1.3	7.38	0.32	9.0
Facility RVU	Work	PE	MP	Total
46608	1.3	0.85	0.32	2.47

	FUD	Status	MUE	Modifiers				IOM Reference
46608	0	A	1(3)	51	N/A	N/A	N/A	None

* with documentation

Anus

46610-46612

46610 Anoscopy; with removal of single tumor, polyp, or other lesion by hot biopsy forceps or bipolar cautery

46611 with removal of single tumor, polyp, or other lesion by snare technique

46612 with removal of multiple tumors, polyps, or other lesions by hot biopsy forceps, bipolar cautery or snare technique

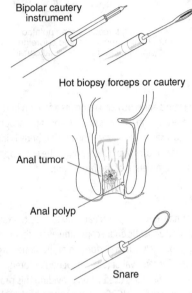

Bipolar cautery instrument

Hot biopsy forceps or cautery

Anal tumor

Anal polyp

Snare

Explanation

The physician performs anoscopy and removes a tumor, polyp, or other lesion. The physician inserts the anoscope into the anus and advances the scope. The anal canal and distal rectal mucosa are visualized. The tumor, polyp, or other lesion is identified and removed by hot biopsy forceps or cautery in 46610; multiple lesions by the same methods in 46612 or snare technique in 46611. The anoscope is withdrawn at the completion of the procedure.

Coding Tips

Report the appropriate endoscopy for each anatomic site examined. Surgical endoscopy includes diagnostic endoscopy; however, diagnostic endoscopy can be identified separately when performed at the same surgical session as an open procedure. Biopsy is not reported separately when performed with excision of a lesion. For anoscopy with ablation of single or multiple tumors, polyps, or other lesions, not amenable to removal by hot biopsy forceps, bipolar cautery, or snare technique, see 46615.

ICD-10-CM Diagnostic Codes

C20	Malignant neoplasm of rectum
C21.1	Malignant neoplasm of anal canal
C21.2	Malignant neoplasm of cloacogenic zone
C21.8	Malignant neoplasm of overlapping sites of rectum, anus and anal canal
C49.A5	Gastrointestinal stromal tumor of rectum
C7A.026	Malignant carcinoid tumor of the rectum
D01.2	Carcinoma in situ of rectum
D01.3	Carcinoma in situ of anus and anal canal
D01.49	Carcinoma in situ of other parts of intestine
D01.7	Carcinoma in situ of other specified digestive organs
D12.8	Benign neoplasm of rectum
D12.9	Benign neoplasm of anus and anal canal
D37.8	Neoplasm of uncertain behavior of other specified digestive organs
D3A.026	Benign carcinoid tumor of the rectum
D49.0	Neoplasm of unspecified behavior of digestive system
K62.0	Anal polyp
K62.1	Rectal polyp
K62.5	Hemorrhage of anus and rectum
K62.6	Ulcer of anus and rectum
K62.82	Dysplasia of anus
K62.89	Other specified diseases of anus and rectum

AMA: **46610** 2018,Jan,8; 2017,Jan,8; 2016,Jan,13; 2015,Jan,16 **46611** 2018,Jan,8; 2017,Jan,8; 2016,Jan,13; 2015,Jan,16 **46612** 2018,Jan,8; 2017,Jan,8; 2016,Jan,13; 2015,Jan,16

Relative Value Units/Medicare Edits

Non-Facility RVU	Work	PE	MP	Total
46610	1.28	6.97	0.23	8.48
46611	1.3	5.29	0.19	6.78
46612	1.5	8.47	0.37	10.34
Facility RVU	Work	PE	MP	Total
46610	1.28	0.83	0.23	2.34
46611	1.3	0.85	0.19	2.34
46612	1.5	0.93	0.37	2.8

	FUD	Status	MUE	Modifiers				IOM Reference
46610	0	A	1(2)	51	N/A	N/A	N/A	None
46611	0	A	1(2)	51	N/A	N/A	N/A	
46612	0	A	1(2)	51	N/A	N/A	N/A	

* with documentation

Terms To Know

anoscopy. Endoscopic diagnostic procedure in which an anoscope is inserted through the anus and advanced. The anal canal and distal rectal mucosa are visualized and brushings or washings may be obtained.

cautery. Destruction or burning of tissue by means of a hot instrument, an electric current, or a caustic chemical, such as silver nitrate.

hot biopsy. Using forceps technique, simultaneously excises and fulgurates polyps; avoids the bleeding associated with cold-forceps biopsy; and preserves the specimen for histologic examination (in contrast, a simple fulguration of the polyp destroys it).

mucosa. Moist tissue lining the mouth (buccal mucosa), stomach (gastric mucosa), intestines, and respiratory tract.

snare. Wire used as a loop to excise a polyp or lesion.

Anus

46614

46614 Anoscopy; with control of bleeding (eg, injection, bipolar cautery, unipolar cautery, laser, heater probe, stapler, plasma coagulator)

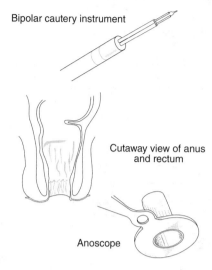

Bipolar cautery instrument

Cutaway view of anus and rectum

Anoscope

Explanation

The physician performs anoscopy and controls an area of bleeding. The physician inserts the anoscope into the anus and advances the scope. The anal canal and distal rectal mucosa are visualized. The area of bleeding is identified and controlled. The anoscope is withdrawn at the completion of the procedure.

Coding Tips

Report the appropriate endoscopy for each anatomic site examined. Surgical endoscopy includes diagnostic endoscopy. Endoscopy procedures with control of bleeding: proctosigmoidoscopy, rigid, see 45317; sigmoidoscopy, flexible, see 45334; colonoscopy, flexible, see 45382.

ICD-10-CM Diagnostic Codes

C20	Malignant neoplasm of rectum
C21.1	Malignant neoplasm of anal canal
C21.2	Malignant neoplasm of cloacogenic zone
C21.8	Malignant neoplasm of overlapping sites of rectum, anus and anal canal
C78.5	Secondary malignant neoplasm of large intestine and rectum
C7A.026	Malignant carcinoid tumor of the rectum
D01.2	Carcinoma in situ of rectum
D01.3	Carcinoma in situ of anus and anal canal
D01.49	Carcinoma in situ of other parts of intestine
D12.8	Benign neoplasm of rectum
D12.9	Benign neoplasm of anus and anal canal
D37.5	Neoplasm of uncertain behavior of rectum
D3A.026	Benign carcinoid tumor of the rectum
K50.111	Crohn's disease of large intestine with rectal bleeding
K50.811	Crohn's disease of both small and large intestine with rectal bleeding
K51.011	Ulcerative (chronic) pancolitis with rectal bleeding
K51.211	Ulcerative (chronic) proctitis with rectal bleeding
K51.311	Ulcerative (chronic) rectosigmoiditis with rectal bleeding
K51.411	Inflammatory polyps of colon with rectal bleeding
K51.511	Left sided colitis with rectal bleeding
K51.811	Other ulcerative colitis with rectal bleeding
K55.031	Focal (segmental) acute (reversible) ischemia of large intestine
K55.032	Diffuse acute (reversible) ischemia of large intestine
K55.041	Focal (segmental) acute infarction of large intestine
K55.042	Diffuse acute infarction of large intestine
K55.1	Chronic vascular disorders of intestine
K55.8	Other vascular disorders of intestine
K62.5	Hemorrhage of anus and rectum
K62.6	Ulcer of anus and rectum
K62.82	Dysplasia of anus
K62.89	Other specified diseases of anus and rectum
K64.0	First degree hemorrhoids
K64.1	Second degree hemorrhoids
K64.2	Third degree hemorrhoids
K64.3	Fourth degree hemorrhoids
K64.4	Residual hemorrhoidal skin tags
K64.5	Perianal venous thrombosis
K64.8	Other hemorrhoids
K92.1	Melena
S31.831A	Laceration without foreign body of anus, initial encounter
S31.832A	Laceration with foreign body of anus, initial encounter
S31.833A	Puncture wound without foreign body of anus, initial encounter
S31.834A	Puncture wound with foreign body of anus, initial encounter
S31.835A	Open bite of anus, initial encounter
S36.61XA	Primary blast injury of rectum, initial encounter
S36.69XA	Other injury of rectum, initial encounter

AMA: **46614** 2018,Jan,8; 2017,Jan,8; 2016,Jan,13; 2015,Jan,16

Relative Value Units/Medicare Edits

Non-Facility RVU	Work	PE	MP	Total
46614	1.0	3.86	0.15	5.01
Facility RVU	**Work**	**PE**	**MP**	**Total**
46614	1.0	0.71	0.15	1.86

	FUD	Status	MUE	Modifiers				IOM Reference
46614	0	A	1(3)	51	N/A	N/A	N/A	None

* with documentation

46615

46615 Anoscopy; with ablation of tumor(s), polyp(s), or other lesion(s) not amenable to removal by hot biopsy forceps, bipolar cautery or snare technique

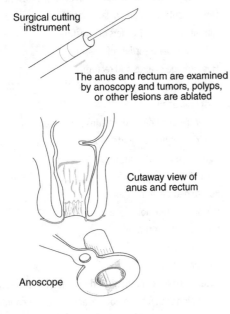

Surgical cutting instrument

The anus and rectum are examined by anoscopy and tumors, polyps, or other lesions are ablated

Cutaway view of anus and rectum

Anoscope

Explanation

The physician performs anoscopy and performs ablation of a tumor, polyp, or other lesion. The physician inserts the anoscope through the anus and advances the scope. The anal canal and distal rectal mucosa are visualized. The tumor, polyp, or other lesion is identified and ablation of the lesion is performed. The anoscope is withdrawn at the completion of the procedure.

Coding Tips

Surgical endoscopy always includes diagnostic endoscopy. For anoscopy with removal of a single tumor, polyp, or other lesion by hot biopsy forceps or bipolar cautery, see 46610; multiple lesions by same techniques, see 46612; single lesion by snare technique, see 46611; with control of bleeding, see 46614.

ICD-10-CM Diagnostic Codes

C20	Malignant neoplasm of rectum
C21.1	Malignant neoplasm of anal canal
C21.2	Malignant neoplasm of cloacogenic zone
C21.8	Malignant neoplasm of overlapping sites of rectum, anus and anal canal
C49.A5	Gastrointestinal stromal tumor of rectum
C7A.026	Malignant carcinoid tumor of the rectum
D01.2	Carcinoma in situ of rectum
D01.3	Carcinoma in situ of anus and anal canal
D01.49	Carcinoma in situ of other parts of intestine
D01.7	Carcinoma in situ of other specified digestive organs
D12.8	Benign neoplasm of rectum
D12.9	Benign neoplasm of anus and anal canal
D37.8	Neoplasm of uncertain behavior of other specified digestive organs
D3A.026	Benign carcinoid tumor of the rectum

D49.0	Neoplasm of unspecified behavior of digestive system
K62.0	Anal polyp
K62.1	Rectal polyp
K62.5	Hemorrhage of anus and rectum
K62.6	Ulcer of anus and rectum
K62.82	Dysplasia of anus
K62.89	Other specified diseases of anus and rectum

AMA: 46615 2018,Jan,8; 2017,Jan,8; 2016,Jan,13; 2015,Jan,16

Relative Value Units/Medicare Edits

Non-Facility RVU	Work	PE	MP	Total
46615	1.5	3.67	0.19	5.36
Facility RVU	**Work**	**PE**	**MP**	**Total**
46615	1.5	0.97	0.19	2.66

	FUD	Status	MUE	Modifiers				IOM Reference
46615	0	A	1(2)	51	N/A	N/A	N/A	None

* with documentation

Terms To Know

ablation. Removal or destruction of a body part or tissue or its function. Ablation may be performed by surgical means, hormones, drugs, radiofrequency, heat, chemical application, or other methods.

carcinoma in situ. Malignancy that arises from the cells of the vessel, gland, or organ of origin that remains confined to that site or has not invaded neighboring tissue.

cautery. Destruction or burning of tissue by means of a hot instrument, an electric current, or a caustic chemical, such as silver nitrate.

forceps. Tool used for grasping or compressing tissue.

neoplasm. New abnormal growth, tumor.

polyp. Small growth on a stalk-like attachment projecting from a mucous membrane.

snare. Wire used as a loop to excise a polyp or lesion.

ulcer. Open sore or excavating lesion of skin or the tissue on the surface of an organ from the sloughing of chronically inflamed and necrosing tissue.

46700-46705

46700   Anoplasty, plastic operation for stricture; adult
46705   infant

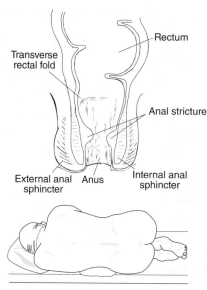

An anal stricture is repaired on an adult

Explanation

The physician performs anoplasty for an anal stricture in an adult. The physician explores the anal canal and identifies the stricture. An incision is made in the scar of the stricture and a portion of the stricture is excised. Incisions are extended onto the perianal skin and subcutaneous tissue and skin flaps are mobilized and advanced into the defects created by the scar excision. The flaps are sutured to the surrounding skin and anoderm thus closing the defect. Report 47605 when the patient is an infant.

Coding Tips

For simple incision of an anal septum, infant, see 46070. Do not append modifier 63 to 46705 as the description or nature of the procedure includes infants up to 4 kg.

ICD-10-CM Diagnostic Codes

K59.01	Slow transit constipation
K59.02	Outlet dysfunction constipation
K59.03	Drug induced constipation
K59.04	Chronic idiopathic constipation
K59.09	Other constipation
K62.4	Stenosis of anus and rectum
K62.89	Other specified diseases of anus and rectum
Q42.2	Congenital absence, atresia and stenosis of anus with fistula
Q42.3	Congenital absence, atresia and stenosis of anus without fistula
Q42.8	Congenital absence, atresia and stenosis of other parts of large intestine

AMA: **46700** 2014,Jan,11 **46705** 2014,Jan,11

Relative Value Units/Medicare Edits

Non-Facility RVU	Work	PE	MP	Total
46700	9.81	8.03	1.53	19.37
46705	7.43	7.71	1.82	16.96
Facility RVU	Work	PE	MP	Total
46700	9.81	8.03	1.53	19.37
46705	7.43	7.71	1.82	16.96

	FUD	Status	MUE	Modifiers			IOM Reference
46700	90	A	1(2)	51	N/A	N/A	N/A	None
46705	90	A	1(2)	51	N/A	62*	80	

* with documentation

Terms To Know

atresia. Congenital closure or absence of a tubular organ or an opening to the body surface.

congenital. Present at birth, occurring through heredity or an influence during gestation up to the moment of birth.

defect. Imperfection, flaw, or absence.

excision. Surgical removal of an organ or tissue.

exploration. Examination for diagnostic purposes.

incision. Act of cutting into tissue or an organ.

rectal. Pertaining to the rectum, the end portion of the large intestine.

scar tissue. Fibrous connective tissue that forms around a wounded area or injury, composed mainly of fibroblasts or collagenous fibers.

stenosis. Narrowing or constriction of a passage.

stricture. Narrowing of an anatomical structure.

subcutaneous tissue. Sheet or wide band of adipose (fat) and areolar connective tissue in two layers attached to the dermis.

Anus

46706-46707

46706　Repair of anal fistula with fibrin glue
46707　Repair of anorectal fistula with plug (eg, porcine small intestine submucosa [SIS])

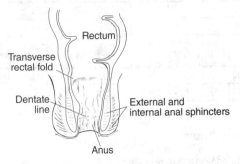

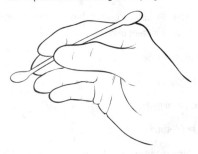

Fissures that form in the anus
are repaired with fibrin glue or plug

Explanation

The physician repairs an anal fistula using fibrin glue (46706). Fibrin glue is made with human fibrinogen pooled from the plasma of long-term donors under control methods that avoid passing infection to the recipient. The glue is composed of two components, usually applied through double lumen catheters to guide the component injections separately to the tissue and must be applied at a temperature of 37° C. The fistula is localized and cannulated and then prepped for the glue. The margins and canal of the fistula are de-epithelialized with electrocoagulation and/or roughening the fistulous canal with a brush. Some bleeding actually improves the adhesion of the fibrin clot. The gluing is done so as to completely fill the defect and around the borders of the fistula, sealing it with a clot. Fibrin glue only works on tissue capable of local regeneration for wound healing since the glue does not actually function as a seal or a plug, but provides the substrate for fibroblasts to move in. After about four weeks, the glued surface is replaced by scar tissue and the fibrin glue totally decomposes. Mechanical stress must be avoided while this stage is developing. In 46707, the physician treats an anorectal fistula or artificial communication from the anus or rectum to the skin with a porcine small intestine submucosa (SIS) plug. The patient is in a prone position. Using a sterile probe, the physician identifies the primary fistula opening by advancing the probe through the secondary fistula opening. The fistula is irrigated. The fistula plug is introduced through the internal (primary) fistula opening and threaded into the fistula until the internal opening is occluded. The plug is trimmed flush with the mucosal wall of the anus or colon and also trimmed flush at the secondary site. Each end of the plug is secured with resorbable sutures.

Coding Tips

Fistulectomy performed with hemorrhoidectomy is reported with codes 46258 and 46262. For surgical treatment of an anal fistula (fistulectomy/fistulotomy), see 46270–46285. For closure of anal fistula with a rectal advancement flap, see 46288.

ICD-10-CM Diagnostic Codes

K60.3　Anal fistula
K60.5　Anorectal fistula
T81.83XA　Persistent postprocedural fistula, initial encounter

AMA: 46707 2018,Jan,8; 2017,Jan,8; 2016,Jan,13; 2015,Jan,16

Relative Value Units/Medicare Edits

Non-Facility RVU	Work	PE	MP	Total
46706	2.44	2.23	0.61	5.28
46707	6.39	7.0	1.57	14.96
Facility RVU	**Work**	**PE**	**MP**	**Total**
46706	2.44	2.23	0.61	5.28
46707	6.39	7.0	1.57	14.96

	FUD	Status	MUE	Modifiers				IOM Reference
46706	10	A	1(3)	51	N/A	N/A	N/A	None
46707	90	A	1(3)	51	N/A	N/A	80*	

* with documentation

Terms To Know

anal fistula. Abnormal opening on the skin surface near the anus, which may connect with the rectum.

cannulation. Insertion of a flexible length of hollow tubing into a blood vessel, duct, or body cavity, usually for extracorporeal circulation or chemotherapy infusion to a particular region of the body.

closure. Repairing an incision or wound by suture or other means.

coagulation. Clot formation.

defect. Imperfection, flaw, or absence.

irrigate. Washing out, lavage.

lumen. Space inside an intestine, artery, vein, duct, or tube.

prone. Lying face downward.

regeneration. Process of reproducing or regrowing tissue.

repair. Surgical closure of a wound. The wound may be a result of injury/trauma or it may be a surgically created defect. Repairs are divided into three categories: simple, intermediate, and complex.

scar tissue. Fibrous connective tissue that forms around a wounded area or injury, composed mainly of fibroblasts or collagenous fibers.

Anus

46710-46712

46710 Repair of ileoanal pouch fistula/sinus (eg, perineal or vaginal), pouch advancement; transperineal approach
46712 Repair of ileoanal pouch fistula/sinus (eg, perineal or vaginal), pouch advancement; combined transperineal and transabdominal approach

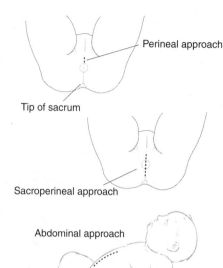

Perineal approach

Tip of sacrum

Sacroperineal approach

Abdominal approach

Explanation

The physician repairs an ileoanal pouch fistula or sinus by pouch advancement using a transperineal or combined transperineal and transabdominal approach. An ileoanal pouch is created as a place for the storage of stool in patients that have had their large intestines removed due to disease. The pouch is connected to the anus, allowing the patient to have a bowel movement into the anus rather than needing a colostomy bag. If a drainage tract (fistula or sinus) erodes from an ileoanal pouch to the perineal area or into the vagina, it can be repaired by dissecting the tract from its external origin, the skin of the perineum or the lining of the vagina, to its source at the ileoanal pouch, and closing the tissues. In 46710, the tract is dissected (removed) and closed starting in the perineal area. In 46712, the tract is dissected (removed) using an approach that combines dissection starting in the perineal area moving toward the pouch along with an incision in the lower abdominal wall that allows access to the ileoanal pouch internally. In both cases, any damage done to the pouch is repaired (pouch advancement).

Coding Tips

For repair of low imperforate anus, with anoperineal fistula, see 46715; with transposition of anoperineal or anovestibular fistula, see 46716. These procedures may be performed during multiple surgical sessions as a staged procedure. To indicate that this is a staged or related procedure performed during the postoperative period by the same physician, append modifier 58.

ICD-10-CM Diagnostic Codes

K63.2	Fistula of intestine
K91.850	Pouchitis
K91.858	Other complications of intestinal pouch
K91.89	Other postprocedural complications and disorders of digestive system
N82.4	Other female intestinal-genital tract fistulae ♀
N82.8	Other female genital tract fistulae ♀
T81.83XA	Persistent postprocedural fistula, initial encounter

AMA: **46710** 2018,Jan,8; 2017,Jan,8; 2016,Jan,13; 2015,Jan,16 **46712** 2018,Jan,8; 2017,Jan,8; 2016,Jan,13; 2015,Jan,16

Relative Value Units/Medicare Edits

Non-Facility RVU	Work	PE	MP	Total
46710	17.14	11.69	4.2	33.03
46712	36.45	20.65	8.92	66.02
Facility RVU	**Work**	**PE**	**MP**	**Total**
46710	17.14	11.69	4.2	33.03
46712	36.45	20.65	8.92	66.02

	FUD	Status	MUE	Modifiers				IOM Reference
46710	90	A	1(3)	51	N/A	62*	80	None
46712	90	A	1(3)	51	N/A	62*	80	

* with documentation

Terms To Know

approach. Method or anatomical location used to gain access to a body organ or specific area for procedures.

dissect. Cut apart or separate tissue for surgical purposes or for visual or microscopic study.

fistula. Abnormal tube-like passage between two body cavities or organs or from an organ to the outside surface.

perineal. Pertaining to the pelvic floor area between the thighs; the diamond-shaped area bordered by the pubic symphysis in front, the ischial tuberosities on the sides, and the coccyx in back.

repair. Surgical closure of a wound. The wound may be a result of injury/trauma or it may be a surgically created defect. Repairs are divided into three categories: simple, intermediate, and complex.

sinus. Open space, cavity, or channel within the body or abnormal cavity, fistula, or channel created by a localized infection to allow the escape of pus.

Anus

46715-46716

46715 Repair of low imperforate anus; with anoperineal fistula (cut-back procedure)
46716 with transposition of anoperineal or anovestibular fistula

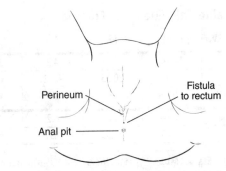

Perineum

Fistula to rectum

Anal pit

An imperforate anus and fistula are repaired

Explanation

The physician performs an incision to open a low imperforate anus ("cutback" procedure). The physician exposes the perineum and identifies the fistulous opening to the imperforate anus. An incision is made through the fistula into the anus onto the skin thus opening the anus. The anus is usually dilated with Hegar dilators. The incision is usually left open to heal. In 46716, the physician transposes an ectopic anal orifice. The imperforate anus has usually been previously incised and opened. The physician makes an incision around the anus. Dissection is continued circumferentially around the distal rectum. Next, a cruciate incision is made over the usual site of the anus and an opening is created through the subcutaneous tissue and what remains of the external sphincter. The rectum is tunneled down through the new orifice and sutured to the new location. The incision at the previous anal site is closed.

Coding Tips

Code selection depends on the site of the closure (low, high), the type of repair, the surgical approach, and the presence/absence and site of the fistula. For repair of a high imperforate anus without fistula, perineal or sacroperineal approach, see 46730; combined transabdominal and sacroperineal approaches, see 46735; with rectourethral or rectovaginal fistula, perineal or sacroperineal approach, see 46740; combined transabdominal and sacroperineal approaches, see 46742. Do not append modifier 63 to these codes as the description or nature of the procedure includes infants up to 4 kg.

ICD-10-CM Diagnostic Codes

Q42.0	Congenital absence, atresia and stenosis of rectum with fistula
Q42.2	Congenital absence, atresia and stenosis of anus with fistula
Q42.3	Congenital absence, atresia and stenosis of anus without fistula
Q43.6	Congenital fistula of rectum and anus

AMA: 46715 2014,Jan,11 **46716** 2014,Jan,11

Relative Value Units/Medicare Edits

Non-Facility RVU	Work	PE	MP	Total
46715	7.62	7.03	1.88	16.53
46716	17.54	14.61	4.31	36.46
Facility RVU	**Work**	**PE**	**MP**	**Total**
46715	7.62	7.03	1.88	16.53
46716	17.54	14.61	4.31	36.46

	FUD	Status	MUE	Modifiers				IOM Reference
46715	90	A	1(2)	51	N/A	N/A	80	None
46716	90	A	1(2)	51	N/A	62*	80	

* with documentation

Terms To Know

anomaly. Irregularity in the structure or position of an organ or tissue.

atresia. Congenital closure or absence of a tubular organ or an opening to the body surface.

circumferential. Pertaining to the perimeter of an object or body.

closure. Repairing an incision or wound by suture or other means.

congenital. Present at birth, occurring through heredity or an influence during gestation up to the moment of birth.

dilation. Artificial increase in the diameter of an opening or lumen made by medication or by instrumentation.

dissect. Cut apart or separate tissue for surgical purposes or for visual or microscopic study.

fistula. Abnormal tube-like passage between two body cavities or organs or from an organ to the outside surface.

incision. Act of cutting into tissue or an organ.

perineal. Pertaining to the pelvic floor area between the thighs; the diamond-shaped area bordered by the pubic symphysis in front, the ischial tuberosities on the sides, and the coccyx in back.

skin. Outer protective covering of the body composed of the epidermis and dermis, situated above the subcutaneous tissues.

stenosis. Narrowing or constriction of a passage.

subcutaneous tissue. Sheet or wide band of adipose (fat) and areolar connective tissue in two layers attached to the dermis.

Anus (side tab)

46730-46735

46730   Repair of high imperforate anus without fistula; perineal or sacroperineal approach

46735   combined transabdominal and sacroperineal approaches

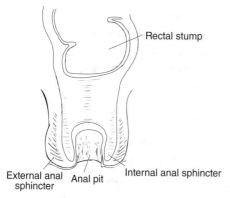

Rectal stump

External anal sphincter   Anal pit   Internal anal sphincter

A high imperforate anus is repaired

Explanation

In 46730, the physician repairs a high imperforate anus through a perineal or sacroperineal approach. The physician makes an incision at the usual site of the anus. Dissection is continued through the external sphincter. The puborectalis muscle is identified and dissection is carried through the muscle to identify and mobilize the rectal stump. The rectal stump is pulled through the sphincter complex, opened, and sutured to the sphincter and skin creating an anal opening. Alternately, a posterior midline sacral incision may be made initially. Dissection is carried superiorly, the puborectalis muscle is identified and a tract is formed through the puborectalis sling to the new anal opening. A perineal incision is made and the rectal stump mobilized and pulled through the sphincter complex onto the skin as described above. In 46735, the physician repairs an imperforate anus by combined transabdominal and sacroperineal approaches. The physician makes a posterior midline incision on the sacrum and removes the coccyx. The puborectalis muscle is identified and a tract is made through the puborectalis sling to the future anal site. Next, the physician makes an abdominal incision and mobilizes the distal colon and rectum. The rectum is divided and the mucosa is stripped from the distal rectum. An incision is made in the bottom of the rectal muscle pouch and the proximal rectum or colon is pulled through the muscular floor and puborectalis sling to the new anal site. A skin incision is made at the new anal site and the end of the colon is sutured to the sphincter muscles and skin creating a new anus. The incisions are closed.

Coding Tips

Code selection depends on the site of the closure (low, high), the type of repair, the surgical approach, and the presence/absence and site of the fistula. For repair of low imperforate anus, with anoperineal fistula, see 46715; with transposition of anoperineal or anovestibular fistula, see 46716. For repair of a high imperforate anus with rectourethral or rectovaginal fistula, perineal or sacroperineal approach, see 46740; combined transabdominal and sacroperineal approaches, see 46742. Do not append modifier 63 to these codes as the description or nature of the procedure includes infants up to 4 kg.

ICD-10-CM Diagnostic Codes

Q42.3   Congenital absence, atresia and stenosis of anus without fistula

AMA: **46730** 2014,Jan,11 **46735** 2014,Jan,11

Relative Value Units/Medicare Edits

Non-Facility RVU	Work	PE	MP	Total
46730	30.65	20.57	7.5	58.72
46735	36.14	22.61	8.84	67.59
Facility RVU	Work	PE	MP	Total
46730	30.65	20.57	7.5	58.72
46735	36.14	22.61	8.84	67.59

	FUD	Status	MUE	Modifiers				IOM Reference
46730	90	A	1(2)	51	N/A	62*	80	None
46735	90	A	1(2)	51	N/A	62*	80	

* with documentation

Terms To Know

anomaly. Irregularity in the structure or position of an organ or tissue.

approach. Method or anatomical location used to gain access to a body organ or specific area for procedures.

atresia. Congenital closure or absence of a tubular organ or an opening to the body surface.

closure. Repairing an incision or wound by suture or other means.

congenital. Present at birth, occurring through heredity or an influence during gestation up to the moment of birth.

dissect. Cut apart or separate tissue for surgical purposes or for visual or microscopic study.

fistula. Abnormal tube-like passage between two body cavities or organs or from an organ to the outside surface.

incision. Act of cutting into tissue or an organ.

mucous membranes. Thin sheets of tissue that secrete mucous and absorb water, salt, and other solutes. Mucous membranes cover or line cavities or canals of the body that open to the outside, such as linings of the mouth, respiratory and genitourinary passages, and the digestive tube.

perineal. Pertaining to the pelvic floor area between the thighs; the diamond-shaped area bordered by the pubic symphysis in front, the ischial tuberosities on the sides, and the coccyx in back.

stenosis. Narrowing or constriction of a passage.

Anus

46740-46742

46740 Repair of high imperforate anus with rectourethral or rectovaginal fistula; perineal or sacroperineal approach

46742 combined transabdominal and sacroperineal approaches

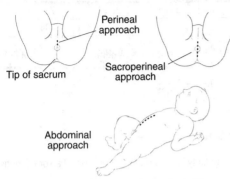

Perineal approach

Tip of sacrum

Sacroperineal approach

Abdominal approach

A high imperforate anus is repaired with a rectovaginal (shown) or rectourethral fistula

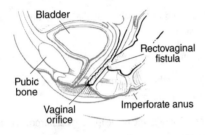

Bladder

Rectovaginal fistula

Pubic bone

Vaginal orifice

Imperforate anus

Explanation

In 46740, the physician repairs a high imperforate anus with a urethral or vaginal fistula through a perineal or sacroperineal approach. The physician makes an incision at the usual site of the anus. Dissection is continued through the external sphincter. The puborectalis muscle is identified and dissection is carried through the muscle to identify and mobilize the rectal stump. The urethral or vaginal fistula is identified, divided, and closed with sutures. The rectal stump is pulled through the sphincter complex, opened and sutured to the sphincter muscles and skin creating a new anal orifice. A posterior midline sacral incision may be made initially. Dissection is carried superiorly, the puborectalis muscle is identified and a tract is formed through the puborectalis sling to the new anal opening. A perineal incision is made at the site of the new anal opening. The rectal stump is mobilized, the fistula identified and divided, and the rectum pulled through the sphincter complex onto the skin as described above. In 46742, a combined transabdominal and sacroperineal approach is used. The physician makes a posterior midline incision on the sacrum and removes the coccyx. The puborectalis muscle is identified and a tract is developed through the puborectalis sling to the future anal site. Next, the physician makes an abdominal incision and mobilizes the distal colon and rectum. The rectum is divided, the mucosa is stripped from the distal rectum, and the urethral or vaginal fistula is identified and closed with sutures. An incision is made in the bottom of the rectal muscle pouch and the proximal rectum or colon is pulled through the muscular floor and puborectalis sling to the new anal site. A skin incision is made at the new anal site and the end of the colon is sutured to the sphincter muscles and skin creating a new anus. The incisions are closed.

Coding Tips

Code selection depends on the site of the closure (low, high), the type of repair, the surgical approach, and the presence/absence and site of the fistula. For repair of a high imperforate anus without fistula, perineal or sacroperineal

approach, see 46730; combined transabdominal and sacroperineal approaches, see 46735. Repair of low imperforate anus, with anoperineal fistula, is reported with 46715; with transposition of anoperineal or anovestibular fistula, see 46716. Do not append modifier 63 to these codes as the description or nature of the procedure includes infants up to 4 kg.

ICD-10-CM Diagnostic Codes

N36.0	Urethral fistula
N82.3	Fistula of vagina to large intestine ♀
Q42.2	Congenital absence, atresia and stenosis of anus with fistula
Q52.2	Congenital rectovaginal fistula ♀
Q64.73	Congenital urethrorectal fistula

AMA: 46740 2014,Jan,11 **46742** 2014,Jan,11

Relative Value Units/Medicare Edits

Non-Facility RVU	Work	PE	MP	Total
46740	33.9	21.88	8.28	64.06
46742	40.14	24.09	9.81	74.04
Facility RVU	**Work**	**PE**	**MP**	**Total**
46740	33.9	21.88	8.28	64.06
46742	40.14	24.09	9.81	74.04

	FUD	Status	MUE	Modifiers				IOM Reference
46740	90	A	1(2)	51	N/A	62*	80	None
46742	90	A	1(2)	51	N/A	62*	80	

* with documentation

Terms To Know

atresia. Congenital closure or absence of a tubular organ or an opening to the body surface.

closure. Repairing an incision or wound by suture or other means.

congenital. Present at birth, occurring through heredity or an influence during gestation up to the moment of birth.

dissect. Cut apart or separate tissue for surgical purposes or for visual or microscopic study.

fistula. Abnormal tube-like passage between two body cavities or organs or from an organ to the outside surface.

incision. Act of cutting into tissue or an organ.

mucous membranes. Thin sheets of tissue that secrete mucous and absorb water, salt, and other solutes. Mucous membranes cover or line cavities or canals of the body that open to the outside, such as linings of the mouth, respiratory and genitourinary passages, and the digestive tube.

perineal. Pertaining to the pelvic floor area between the thighs; the diamond-shaped area bordered by the pubic symphysis in front, the ischial tuberosities on the sides, and the coccyx in back.

stenosis. Narrowing or constriction of a passage.

N Newborn: 0　**P** Pediatric: 0-17　**M** Maternity: 9-64　**A** Adult: 15-124　♂ Male Only　♀ Female Only　CPT © 2021 American Medical Association. All Rights Reserved.

Anus

46744-46748

46744 Repair of cloacal anomaly by anorectovaginoplasty and urethroplasty, sacroperineal approach
46746 Repair of cloacal anomaly by anorectovaginoplasty and urethroplasty, combined abdominal and sacroperineal approach;
46748 with vaginal lengthening by intestinal graft or pedicle flaps

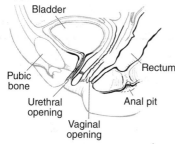

Persistent cloaca: common urinary, fecal, and reproductive passage

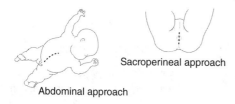

Abdominal approach | Sacroperineal approach

Explanation

The physician repairs a cloacal anomaly. The patient is placed in a lithotomy position. The physician either makes a small incision in the perineum (46744) or uses a combined abdominal and sacroperineal approach (46746). The bladder, urethra, and vagina are dissected free of each other. A new rectum is formed by interposing muscle posterior to the rectum. The surgeon may also create separate openings, dividing membranes for the urethra, vagina, and rectum by using intestinal grafts, pedicle flaps, and free skin grafts to lengthen the vagina as an additional procedure (46748). The incision is closed with sutures.

Coding Tips

Coding surgical repair of cloacal anomaly is dependent on the approach (sacroperineal or combined abdominal/sacroperineal) and the need for intestinal grafting or pedicle flaps. Do not append modifier 63 to 46744 as the description or nature of the procedure includes infants up to 4 kg.

ICD-10-CM Diagnostic Codes

Q43.7   Persistent cloaca

AMA: **46744** 2014,Jan,11 **46746** 2014,Jan,11 **46748** 2014,Jan,11

Relative Value Units/Medicare Edits

Non-Facility RVU	Work	PE	MP	Total
46744	58.94	31.17	14.4	104.51
46746	65.44	33.71	16.01	115.16
46748	71.42	35.93	17.47	124.82
Facility RVU	**Work**	**PE**	**MP**	**Total**
46744	58.94	31.17	14.4	104.51
46746	65.44	33.71	16.01	115.16
46748	71.42	35.93	17.47	124.82

	FUD	Status	MUE	Modifiers				IOM Reference
46744	90	A	1(2)	51	N/A	62*	80	None
46746	90	A	1(2)	51	N/A	62*	80	
46748	90	A	1(2)	51	N/A	62*	80	

* with documentation

Terms To Know

anomaly. Irregularity in the structure or position of an organ or tissue.

approach. Method or anatomical location used to gain access to a body organ or specific area for procedures.

cloacal anomaly. Congenital anomaly resulting from the failure of one common urinary, anal, and reproductive vaginal passage of the early embryonic stage to develop into the properly divided rectal and urogenital sections.

congenital. Present at birth, occurring through heredity or an influence during gestation up to the moment of birth.

dissect. Cut apart or separate tissue for surgical purposes or for visual or microscopic study.

fistula. Abnormal tube-like passage between two body cavities or organs or from an organ to the outside surface.

free graft. Unattached piece of skin and tissue moved to another part of the body and sutured into place to repair a defect.

graft. Tissue implant from another part of the body or another person.

lithotomy position. Common position patients may be placed in for some surgical procedures and examinations involving the pelvis and/or lower abdomen. The patient is placed supine (on their back), hips and knees flexed, thighs apart, with feet supported in raised stirrups.

pedicle flap. Full-thickness skin and subcutaneous tissue for grafting that remains partially attached to the donor site by a pedicle or stem in which the blood vessels supplying the flap remain intact.

perineal. Pertaining to the pelvic floor area between the thighs; the diamond-shaped area bordered by the pubic symphysis in front, the ischial tuberosities on the sides, and the coccyx in back.

posterior. Located in the back part or caudal end of the body.

urethra. Small tube lined with mucous membrane that leads from the bladder to the exterior of the body.

Anus

46750-46751

46750 Sphincteroplasty, anal, for incontinence or prolapse; adult
46751 child

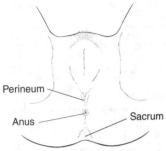

Perineum

Anus

Sacrum

The anal sphincters are surgically corrected for incontinence or prolapse

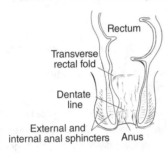

Rectum

Transverse rectal fold

Dentate line

External and internal anal sphincters

Anus

Explanation

The physician performs anal sphincteroplasty for prolapse or incontinence in an adult. The physician makes a transverse incision anterior to the anus. Dissection is carried through subcutaneous tissues to expose the anal canal. The external anal sphincter muscle is dissected from the internal sphincter in the anterior plane and divided in the midline. The ends of the external sphincter are wrapped around the anal canal in an overlapping fashion and approximated with sutures. The incision is closed. Report 46751 when the procedure is performed on a child.

Coding Tips

For sphincteroplasty, anal, for incontinence, adult, muscle transplant, see 46760; levator muscle imbrication (Park posterior anal repair), see 46761. Proctoplasty for prolapse of a mucous membrane, see 45505. For proctopexy, abdominal approach, see 45540; perineal approach, see 45541. Graft (Thiersch operation) for rectal incontinence and/or prolapse is reported with 46753; removal of Thiersch wire or suture, anal canal, see 46754.

ICD-10-CM Diagnostic Codes

K62.3	Rectal prolapse
K62.81	Anal sphincter tear (healed) (nontraumatic) (old)
R15.0	Incomplete defecation
R15.1	Fecal smearing
R15.2	Fecal urgency
R15.9	Full incontinence of feces

AMA: 46750 2014,Jan,11 **46751** 2014,Jan,11

Relative Value Units/Medicare Edits

Non-Facility RVU	Work	PE	MP	Total
46750	12.15	8.14	1.88	22.17
46751	9.3	8.3	2.27	19.87
Facility RVU	**Work**	**PE**	**MP**	**Total**
46750	12.15	8.14	1.88	22.17
46751	9.3	8.3	2.27	19.87

	FUD	Status	MUE	Modifiers				IOM Reference
46750	90	A	1(2)	51	N/A	62*	80	100-03,230.10
46751	90	A	1(2)	51	N/A	62*	80	

* with documentation

Terms To Know

closure. Repairing an incision or wound by suture or other means.

dissect. Cut apart or separate tissue for surgical purposes or for visual or microscopic study.

incision. Act of cutting into tissue or an organ.

incontinence. Inability to control urination or defecation.

perineal. Pertaining to the pelvic floor area between the thighs; the diamond-shaped area bordered by the pubic symphysis in front, the ischial tuberosities on the sides, and the coccyx in back.

prolapse. Falling, sliding, or sinking of an organ from its normal location in the body.

rectal. Pertaining to the rectum, the end portion of the large intestine.

sacrum. Lower portion of the spine composed of five fused vertebrae designated as S1-S5.

sphincteroplasty. Surgical repair done to correct, augment, or improve the muscular function of a sphincter, such as the anus or intestines.

subcutaneous tissue. Sheet or wide band of adipose (fat) and areolar connective tissue in two layers attached to the dermis.

suture. Numerous stitching techniques employed in wound closure.

buried suture. Continuous or interrupted suture placed under the skin for a layered closure.

continuous suture. Running stitch with tension evenly distributed across a single strand to provide a leakproof closure line.

interrupted suture. Series of single stitches with tension isolated at each stitch, in which all stitches are not affected if one becomes loose, and the isolated sutures cannot act as a wick to transport an infection.

purse-string suture. Continuous suture placed around a tubular structure and tightened, to reduce or close the lumen.

retention suture. Secondary stitching that bridges the primary suture, providing support for the primary repair; a plastic or rubber bolster may be placed over the primary repair and under the retention sutures.

transverse. Crosswise at right angles to the long axis of a structure or part.

Anus

46753

46753   Graft (Thiersch operation) for rectal incontinence and/or prolapse

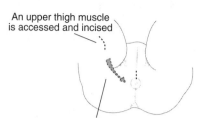

An upper thigh muscle is accessed and incised

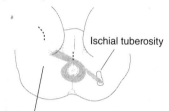

The muscle is pulled subcutaneously through to the perianal area

Ischial tuberosity

The muscle is wrapped around the anal canal and its fibrous end attached to an ischial tuberosity

Explanation

The physician places a wire, suture, or muscular graft around the anus for rectal prolapse or incontinence (Thiersch procedure). The physician makes incisions on opposite sides of the anus in the lateral perianal subcutaneous tissue. A wire, suture, or muscular graft mobilized from the thigh is wrapped around the anus in the subcutaneous space and secured in place. The incisions are closed.

Coding Tips

Proctoplasty for prolapse of mucous membrane, see 45505. For proctopexy, abdominal approach, see 45540; perineal approach, see 45541. Removal of Thiersch wire or suture, anal canal is reported with 46754.

ICD-10-CM Diagnostic Codes

K62.3	Rectal prolapse
R15.0	Incomplete defecation
R15.1	Fecal smearing
R15.2	Fecal urgency
R15.9	Full incontinence of feces

AMA: **46753** 2014,Jan,11

Relative Value Units/Medicare Edits

Non-Facility RVU	Work	PE	MP	Total
46753	8.89	7.38	2.17	18.44
Facility RVU	**Work**	**PE**	**MP**	**Total**
46753	8.89	7.38	2.17	18.44

	FUD	Status	MUE	Modifiers				IOM Reference
46753	90	A	1(2)	51	N/A	N/A	N/A	100-03,230.10

* with documentation

46754

46754   Removal of Thiersch wire or suture, anal canal

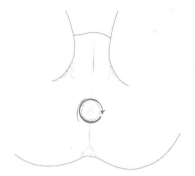

Wire or suture material encircles the anal canal

Explanation

The physician removes a wire or suture that has been placed around the anal canal for rectal prolapse or incontinence. The physician makes incisions in the lateral perianal subcutaneous tissue. The wire or suture that is encircling the anus is identified, divided, and removed. The incisions are closed.

Coding Tips

For removal of an anal seton or other marker, see 46030. Graft (Thiersch operation) for rectal incontinence and/or prolapse is reported with 46753.

ICD-10-CM Diagnostic Codes

Z48.02	Encounter for removal of sutures
Z48.815	Encounter for surgical aftercare following surgery on the digestive system
Z48.89	Encounter for other specified surgical aftercare

AMA: **46754** 2014,Jan,11

Relative Value Units/Medicare Edits

Non-Facility RVU	Work	PE	MP	Total
46754	3.01	6.69	0.39	10.09
Facility RVU	**Work**	**PE**	**MP**	**Total**
46754	3.01	3.56	0.39	6.96

	FUD	Status	MUE	Modifiers				IOM Reference
46754	10	A	1(3)	51	N/A	N/A	80*	None

* with documentation

Anus

46760

46760 Sphincteroplasty, anal, for incontinence, adult; muscle transplant

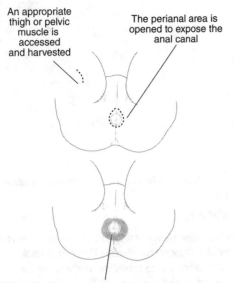

An appropriate thigh or pelvic muscle is accessed and harvested

The perianal area is opened to expose the anal canal

The muscle is grafted as necessary to sphincter muscle or other muscle to restore continence

Explanation

The physician performs an anal sphincteroplasty with a muscular graft for incontinence in an adult. The physician makes a transverse incision anterior to the anus. Dissection is carried through subcutaneous tissue to expose the anal canal and the remaining external sphincter muscle is dissected from the internal sphincter. A muscle from the thigh is mobilized and tunneled to the perineum. The muscle is wrapped around the anal canal and approximated with sutures. The incisions are closed.

Coding Tips

Sphincteroplasty, anal, for incontinence or prolapse, adult, see 46750; child, see 46751; with levator muscle imbrication (Park posterior and repair), see 46761.

ICD-10-CM Diagnostic Codes

K62.81	Anal sphincter tear (healed) (nontraumatic) (old)
R15.0	Incomplete defecation
R15.1	Fecal smearing
R15.2	Fecal urgency
R15.9	Full incontinence of feces

AMA: 46760 2014,Jan,11

Relative Value Units/Medicare Edits

Non-Facility RVU	Work	PE	MP	Total
46760	17.45	12.47	2.22	32.14
Facility RVU	Work	PE	MP	Total
46760	17.45	12.47	2.22	32.14

	FUD	Status	MUE	Modifiers				IOM Reference
46760	90	A	1(2)	51	N/A	62*	80	100-03,230.10

* with documentation

46761

46761 Sphincteroplasty, anal, for incontinence, adult; levator muscle imbrication (Park posterior anal repair)

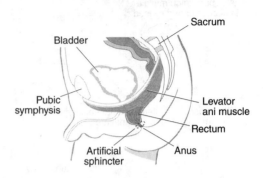

Sacrum
Bladder
Pubic symphysis
Levator ani muscle
Rectum
Artificial sphincter
Anus

Explanation

The physician performs sphincteroplasty with levator muscle imbrication for incontinence in an adult (Park repair). The physician makes a transverse incision anterior to the anus. Dissection is carried through the subcutaneous tissue to expose the anal canal. The external sphincter muscle is dissected from the internal sphincter and dissection is continued between the sphincters to expose the puborectalis muscle (levator). The edges of the puborectalis muscle are imbricated around the anal canal with sutures. The external sphincter muscle is imbricated around the anal canal with sutures. The incision is closed.

Coding Tips

For sphincteroplasty, anal, for incontinence or prolapse, adult, see 46750; child, see 46751. For sphincteroplasty, anal, for incontinence, adult, with muscle transplant, see 46760.

ICD-10-CM Diagnostic Codes

K62.81	Anal sphincter tear (healed) (nontraumatic) (old)
R15.0	Incomplete defecation
R15.1	Fecal smearing
R15.2	Fecal urgency
R15.9	Full incontinence of feces

AMA: 46761 2014,Jan,11

Relative Value Units/Medicare Edits

Non-Facility RVU	Work	PE	MP	Total
46761	15.29	9.33	2.44	27.06
Facility RVU	Work	PE	MP	Total
46761	15.29	9.33	2.44	27.06

	FUD	Status	MUE	Modifiers				IOM Reference
46761	90	A	1(2)	51	N/A	62*	80	None

* with documentation

Terms To Know

sphincteroplasty. Surgical repair done to correct, augment, or improve the muscular function of a sphincter, such as the anus or intestines.

Anus

[46947]

46947 Hemorrhoidopexy (eg, for prolapsing internal hemorrhoids) by stapling

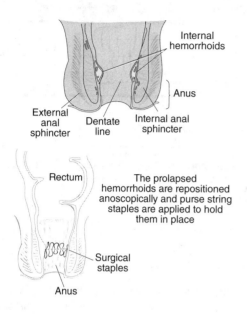

Internal hemorrhoids

Anus

External anal sphincter

Dentate line

Internal anal sphincter

Rectum

The prolapsed hemorrhoids are repositioned anoscopically and purse string staples are applied to hold them in place

Surgical staples

Anus

Explanation

The physician performs a stapled hemorrhoidopexy for prolapsing internal hemorrhoids. After having fleet enemas or oral preparation for cleansing the colon, the patient is sedated and given local or spinal anesthesia. A circular anal dilator is inserted that reduces the prolapsed anal tissue. The center obturator piece is removed and the prolapsed mucosa falls into the dilator lumen. An anoscope is inserted through the dilator that pushes the mucosa back against the rectal wall for 270 degrees of rotation. The other tissue protrudes through a window in the scope through which a purse string suture is made, containing only mucous membrane. The anoscope is rotated until a purse-string suture is completed around the anal circumference. A circular stapler is positioned proximal to the suture. The ends are tied externally. With traction on the purse string suture, the prolapsed mucosa is brought into the casing of the circular stapler, which is fired to release two staggered rows of staples while a circular knife removes a column of redundant mucosa from the upper anal canal. The staple line is examined and instruments are removed.

Coding Tips

Internal hemorrhoidectomy by rubber band(s) ligation is reported with 46221; by ligation other than rubber band, single hemorrhoid column or group, see 46945; two or more hemorrhoid columns/groups, see 46946. For injection of a hemorrhoidal sclerosing agent, see 46500. Destruction of internal hemorrhoids by thermal energy is reported with 46930.

ICD-10-CM Diagnostic Codes

K64.0	First degree hemorrhoids
K64.1	Second degree hemorrhoids
K64.2	Third degree hemorrhoids
K64.3	Fourth degree hemorrhoids
K64.8	Other hemorrhoids

AMA: **46947** 2018,Jan,8; 2017,Jan,8; 2016,Jan,13; 2015,Jan,16

Relative Value Units/Medicare Edits

Non-Facility RVU	Work	PE	MP	Total
46947	5.57	4.69	1.16	11.42
Facility RVU	**Work**	**PE**	**MP**	**Total**
46947	5.57	4.69	1.16	11.42

	FUD	Status	MUE	Modifiers				IOM Reference
46947	90	A	1(2)	51	N/A	N/A	N/A	None

* with documentation

Terms To Know

anoscope. Short speculum for examining the anal canal and lower rectum.

hemorrhoid. Dilated, varicose vein in the anal region caused by continually increased venous pressure. Reversed blood flow and clotted blood within a vein that extends beyond the anus.

mucosa. Moist tissue lining the mouth (buccal mucosa), stomach (gastric mucosa), intestines, and respiratory tract.

prolapse. Falling, sliding, or sinking of an organ from its normal location in the body.

proximal. Located closest to a specified reference point, usually the midline or trunk.

purse-string suture. Continuous suture placed around a tubular structure and tightened, to reduce or close the lumen.

traction. Drawing out or holding tension on an area by applying a direct therapeutic pulling force.

46900-46916

46900 Destruction of lesion(s), anus (eg, condyloma, papilloma, molluscum contagiosum, herpetic vesicle), simple; chemical
46910 electrodesiccation
46916 cryosurgery

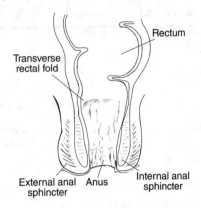

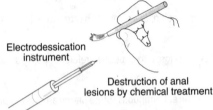

Electrodessication instrument

Destruction of anal lesions by chemical treatment

Minor lesions of the anal canal are destroyed using any of a variety of methods

Explanation

The physician performs destruction of anal lesions with chemicals in 46900. The physician exposes the perianal skin and identifies the lesions. The lesions are painted with destructive chemicals. In 46910, the physician performs destruction of anal lesions with electrodesiccation. The physician exposes the perianal skin and identifies the lesions. The lesions are destroyed with cautery. In 46916, the physician performs destruction of anal lesions with cryosurgery. The physician exposes the perianal skin and identifies the lesions. The lesions are frozen and destroyed, usually with liquid nitrogen.

Coding Tips

For simple destruction by laser, see 46917; surgical excision, see 46922; extensive, by any method, see 46924. Destruction of internal hemorrhoids by thermal energy is reported with 46930.

ICD-10-CM Diagnostic Codes

A54.6	Gonococcal infection of anus and rectum
A56.3	Chlamydial infection of anus and rectum
A60.1	Herpesviral infection of perianal skin and rectum
A63.0	Anogenital (venereal) warts
A63.8	Other specified predominantly sexually transmitted diseases
A66.1	Multiple papillomata and wet crab yaws
B00.89	Other herpesviral infection
B07.8	Other viral warts
B08.1	Molluscum contagiosum
B08.8	Other specified viral infections characterized by skin and mucous membrane lesions
D12.9	Benign neoplasm of anus and anal canal

K62.82	Dysplasia of anus
K62.89	Other specified diseases of anus and rectum

AMA: **46910** 2019,Dec,12

Relative Value Units/Medicare Edits

Non-Facility RVU	Work	PE	MP	Total
46900	1.91	4.99	0.25	7.15
46910	1.91	5.78	0.3	7.99
46916	1.91	5.53	0.19	7.63
Facility RVU	**Work**	**PE**	**MP**	**Total**
46900	1.91	1.81	0.25	3.97
46910	1.91	1.74	0.3	3.95
46916	1.91	2.01	0.19	4.11

	FUD	Status	MUE	Modifiers				IOM Reference
46900	10	A	1(2)	51	N/A	N/A	N/A	None
46910	10	A	1(2)	51	N/A	N/A	N/A	
46916	10	A	1(2)	51	N/A	N/A	N/A	

* with documentation

Terms To Know

chemosurgery. Application of chemical agents to destroy tissue, originally referring to the in situ chemical fixation of premalignant or malignant lesions to facilitate surgical excision.

condyloma. Infectious tumor-like growth caused by the human papilloma virus, with a branching connective tissue core and epithelial covering that occurs on the skin and mucous membranes of the perianal region and external genitalia.

cryosurgery. Application of intense cold, usually produced using liquid nitrogen, to locally freeze diseased or unwanted tissue and induce tissue necrosis without causing harm to adjacent tissue.

destruction. Ablation or eradication of a structure or tissue.

electrosurgery. Use of electric currents to generate heat in performing surgery.

lesion. Area of damaged tissue that has lost continuity or function, due to disease or trauma.

molluscum contagiosum. Common, benign, viral skin infection, usually self-limiting, that appears as a gray or flesh-colored umbilicated lesion by itself or in groups, and later becomes white with an expulsable core containing the replication bodies. It is often transmitted sexually in adults, by autoinoculation, or close contact in children.

tissue. Group of similar cells with a similar function that form definite structures and organs. Tissue types include epithelial tissue, muscle tissue, connective tissue, and nervous tissue.

Anus

46917-46924

46917 Destruction of lesion(s), anus (eg, condyloma, papilloma, molluscum contagiosum, herpetic vesicle), simple; laser surgery
46922   surgical excision
46924 Destruction of lesion(s), anus (eg, condyloma, papilloma, molluscum contagiosum, herpetic vesicle), extensive (eg, laser surgery, electrosurgery, cryosurgery, chemosurgery)

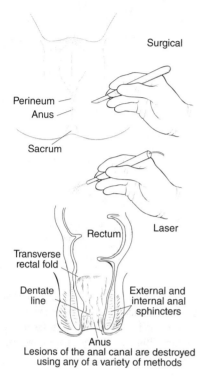

Lesions of the anal canal are destroyed using any of a variety of methods

Explanation

The physician performs destruction of anal lesions with laser therapy in 46917. The physician exposes the perianal skin and identifies the lesions. The lesions are destroyed by laser ablation or laser excision. In 46922, the physician performs destruction of anal lesions by excision. The physician exposes the perianal skin and identifies the lesions. The lesions are surgically excised. The incisions are closed. In 46924, destruction of extensive anal lesions is performed by various methods, such as laser surgery, electrosurgery, cryosurgery, or chemosurgery.

Coding Tips

For simple destruction by chemical, see 46900; electrodesiccation, see 46910; cryosurgery, see 46916. Destruction of internal hemorrhoids by thermal energy is reported with 46930.

ICD-10-CM Diagnostic Codes

A54.6	Gonococcal infection of anus and rectum
A56.3	Chlamydial infection of anus and rectum
A60.1	Herpesviral infection of perianal skin and rectum
A63.0	Anogenital (venereal) warts
A63.8	Other specified predominantly sexually transmitted diseases
A66.1	Multiple papillomata and wet crab yaws
B00.89	Other herpesviral infection
B07.8	Other viral warts
B08.1	Molluscum contagiosum
B08.8	Other specified viral infections characterized by skin and mucous membrane lesions
D12.9	Benign neoplasm of anus and anal canal
K62.5	Hemorrhage of anus and rectum
K62.82	Dysplasia of anus
K62.89	Other specified diseases of anus and rectum

AMA: **46917** 2014,Jan,11 **46922** 2014,Jan,11 **46924** 2014,Jan,11

Relative Value Units/Medicare Edits

Non-Facility RVU	Work	PE	MP	Total
46917	1.91	10.87	0.3	13.08
46922	1.91	7.1	0.34	9.35
46924	2.81	13.47	0.43	16.71
Facility RVU	**Work**	**PE**	**MP**	**Total**
46917	1.91	1.53	0.3	3.74
46922	1.91	1.76	0.34	4.01
46924	2.81	2.04	0.43	5.28

	FUD	Status	MUE		Modifiers			IOM Reference
46917	10	A	1(2)	51	N/A	N/A	N/A	100-03,140.5
46922	10	A	1(2)	51	N/A	N/A	N/A	
46924	10	A	1(2)	51	N/A	N/A	N/A	

* with documentation

Terms To Know

chemosurgery. Application of chemical agents to destroy tissue, originally referring to the in situ chemical fixation of premalignant or malignant lesions to facilitate surgical excision.

condyloma. Infectious tumor-like growth caused by the human papilloma virus, with a branching connective tissue core and epithelial covering that occurs on the skin and mucous membranes of the perianal region and external genitalia.

cryosurgery. Application of intense cold, usually produced using liquid nitrogen, to locally freeze diseased or unwanted tissue and induce tissue necrosis without causing harm to adjacent tissue.

destruction. Ablation or eradication of a structure or tissue.

electrosurgery. Use of electric currents to generate heat in performing surgery.

laser surgery. Use of concentrated, sharply defined light beams to cut, cauterize, coagulate, seal, or vaporize tissue.

molluscum contagiosum. Common, benign, viral skin infection, usually self-limiting, that appears as a gray or flesh-colored umbilicated lesion by itself or in groups, and later becomes white with an expulsable core containing the replication bodies. It is often transmitted sexually in adults, by autoinoculation, or close contact in children.

papilloma. Benign skin neoplasm with small branchings from the epithelial surface.

Anus

46930

46930 Destruction of internal hemorrhoid(s) by thermal energy (eg, infrared coagulation, cautery, radiofrequency)

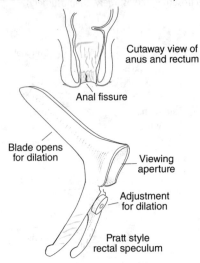

Internal hemorrhoids are destroyed using thermal energy

Explanation

The physician destroys internal hemorrhoids using various forms of thermal energy. The physician explores the anal canal and identifies the hemorrhoid columns. The hemorrhoids may be destroyed by clamping and cauterization, by employing high-frequency radio waves (radiofrequency), or by infrared or laser coagulation, which causes the hemorrhoidal tissue to harden, deteriorate, and form scar tissue as the area heals. The hemorrhoidal remnants may be removed.

Coding Tips

Internal hemorrhoidectomy by rubber band(s) ligation is reported with 46221; by ligation other than rubber band, single hemorrhoid column or group, see 46945; two or more hemorrhoid columns/groups, see 46946. For injection of a hemorrhoidal sclerosing agent, see 46500. For hemorrhoidopexy by stapling for internal prolapsed hemorrhoids, see 46947.

ICD-10-CM Diagnostic Codes

K64.0	First degree hemorrhoids
K64.1	Second degree hemorrhoids
K64.2	Third degree hemorrhoids
K64.3	Fourth degree hemorrhoids
K64.8	Other hemorrhoids

AMA: 46930 2018,Jan,8; 2017,Jan,8; 2016,Jul,8; 2016,Jan,13; 2015,Apr,10

Relative Value Units/Medicare Edits

Non-Facility RVU	Work	PE	MP	Total
46930	1.61	4.74	0.21	6.56
Facility RVU	Work	PE	MP	Total
46930	1.61	2.69	0.21	4.51

	FUD	Status	MUE	Modifiers				IOM Reference
46930	90	A	1(2)	51	N/A	N/A	80*	None

* with documentation

46940-46942

46940 Curettage or cautery of anal fissure, including dilation of anal sphincter (separate procedure); initial
46942 subsequent

An anal fissure is treated by curettage or cauterization, including dilation of the anal sphincter

Cutaway view of anus and rectum

Anal fissure

Blade opens for dilation

Viewing aperture

Adjustment for dilation

Pratt style rectal speculum

Explanation

The physician performs an initial (46940) or subsequent (46942) curettage or cautery of an anal fissure with dilation of the anal sphincter. The physician exposes the perianal area and identifies the fissure. The fissure is debrided with curettage or cautery. The anal sphincter is manually dilated.

Coding Tips

These separate procedures by definition are usually a component of a more complex service and are not identified separately. When performed alone or with other unrelated procedures/services they may be reported. If performed alone, list the code; if performed with other procedures/services, list the code and append modifier 59 or an X{EPSU} modifier.

ICD-10-CM Diagnostic Codes

K59.01	Slow transit constipation
K59.02	Outlet dysfunction constipation
K59.03	Drug induced constipation
K59.04	Chronic idiopathic constipation
K59.09	Other constipation
K60.0	Acute anal fissure
K60.1	Chronic anal fissure
K62.5	Hemorrhage of anus and rectum
K62.89	Other specified diseases of anus and rectum

AMA: 46940 2014,Jan,11 **46942** 2014,Jan,11

Anus

Relative Value Units/Medicare Edits

Non-Facility RVU	Work	PE	MP	Total
46940	2.35	5.14	0.34	7.83
46942	2.07	5.1	0.28	7.45
Facility RVU	**Work**	**PE**	**MP**	**Total**
46940	2.35	1.56	0.34	4.25
46942	2.07	1.45	0.28	3.8

	FUD	Status	MUE	Modifiers				IOM Reference
46940	10	A	1(2)	51	N/A	N/A	N/A	None
46942	10	A	1(3)	51	N/A	N/A	80*	

* with documentation

Terms To Know

anal fissure. Slit, crack, or tear of the anal mucosa that can cause pain, bleeding, and infection.

cautery. Destruction or burning of tissue by means of a hot instrument, an electric current, or a caustic chemical, such as silver nitrate.

constipation. Infrequent or incomplete and difficult bowel movements.

curettage. Removal of tissue by scraping.

debride. To remove all foreign objects and devitalized or infected tissue from a burn or wound to prevent infection and promote healing.

destruction. Ablation or eradication of a structure or tissue.

dilation. Artificial increase in the diameter of an opening or lumen made by medication or by instrumentation.

excision. Surgical removal of an organ or tissue.

lesion. Area of damaged tissue that has lost continuity or function, due to disease or trauma. Lesions may be located on internal structures such as the brain, nerves, or kidneys, or visible on the skin.

speculum. Tool used to enlarge the opening of any canal or cavity.

sphincter. Ring-like band of muscle that surrounds a bodily opening, constricting and relaxing as required for normal physiological functioning.

Anus

47000-47001

47000 Biopsy of liver, needle; percutaneous
+ 47001 when done for indicated purpose at time of other major procedure (List separately in addition to code for primary procedure)

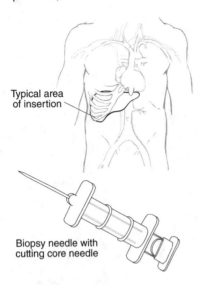

Typical area of insertion

Biopsy needle with cutting core needle

A biopsy specimen from the liver is collected percutaneously by needle

Explanation

The physician takes tissue from the liver for examination. In 47000, the physician uses separately reportable ultrasound guidance to place a hollow bore needle between the ribs on the patient's right side. The liver biopsy is sent for pathology for separately reportable activity. Report 47001 when a liver biopsy is performed incidental to another major procedure.

Coding Tips

Report 47001 in addition to 47000 when performed for an indicated purpose at the same time as another major procedure. For fine needle aspiration performed with these procedures, see 10004–10012 and 10021. Imaging guidance is reported with 76942, 77002, 77012, or 77021, when performed. Evaluation of fine needle aspirate, when performed, is reported with 88172–88173.

ICD-10-CM Diagnostic Codes

B00.81	Herpesviral hepatitis
B15.0	Hepatitis A with hepatic coma
B15.9	Hepatitis A without hepatic coma
B16.0	Acute hepatitis B with delta-agent with hepatic coma
B16.1	Acute hepatitis B with delta-agent without hepatic coma
B16.2	Acute hepatitis B without delta-agent with hepatic coma
B16.9	Acute hepatitis B without delta-agent and without hepatic coma
B17.0	Acute delta-(super) infection of hepatitis B carrier
B17.10	Acute hepatitis C without hepatic coma
B17.11	Acute hepatitis C with hepatic coma
B17.2	Acute hepatitis E
B18.0	Chronic viral hepatitis B with delta-agent
B18.1	Chronic viral hepatitis B without delta-agent
B18.2	Chronic viral hepatitis C
B25.1	Cytomegaloviral hepatitis

B94.2	Sequelae of viral hepatitis
C22.0	Liver cell carcinoma
C22.1	Intrahepatic bile duct carcinoma
C22.2	Hepatoblastoma
C22.3	Angiosarcoma of liver
C22.4	Other sarcomas of liver
C22.7	Other specified carcinomas of liver
C78.7	Secondary malignant neoplasm of liver and intrahepatic bile duct
C7B.02	Secondary carcinoid tumors of liver
C80.2	Malignant neoplasm associated with transplanted organ
D01.5	Carcinoma in situ of liver, gallbladder and bile ducts
D13.4	Benign neoplasm of liver
D13.5	Benign neoplasm of extrahepatic bile ducts
D37.6	Neoplasm of uncertain behavior of liver, gallbladder and bile ducts
D47.Z1	Post-transplant lymphoproliferative disorder (PTLD)
D47.Z2	Castleman disease
E80.4	Gilbert syndrome
E80.5	Crigler-Najjar syndrome
E80.6	Other disorders of bilirubin metabolism
E83.01	Wilson's disease
E83.110	Hereditary hemochromatosis
E83.111	Hemochromatosis due to repeated red blood cell transfusions
E88.01	Alpha-1-antitrypsin deficiency
K70.0	Alcoholic fatty liver △
K70.10	Alcoholic hepatitis without ascites △
K70.11	Alcoholic hepatitis with ascites △
K70.2	Alcoholic fibrosis and sclerosis of liver △
K70.30	Alcoholic cirrhosis of liver without ascites △
K70.31	Alcoholic cirrhosis of liver with ascites △
K70.40	Alcoholic hepatic failure without coma △
K70.41	Alcoholic hepatic failure with coma △
K71.0	Toxic liver disease with cholestasis
K71.10	Toxic liver disease with hepatic necrosis, without coma
K71.11	Toxic liver disease with hepatic necrosis, with coma
K71.2	Toxic liver disease with acute hepatitis
K71.3	Toxic liver disease with chronic persistent hepatitis
K71.4	Toxic liver disease with chronic lobular hepatitis
K71.50	Toxic liver disease with chronic active hepatitis without ascites
K71.51	Toxic liver disease with chronic active hepatitis with ascites
K71.7	Toxic liver disease with fibrosis and cirrhosis of liver
K71.8	Toxic liver disease with other disorders of liver
K72.00	Acute and subacute hepatic failure without coma
K72.01	Acute and subacute hepatic failure with coma
K72.10	Chronic hepatic failure without coma
K72.11	Chronic hepatic failure with coma
K74.01	Hepatic fibrosis, early fibrosis
K74.02	Hepatic fibrosis, advanced fibrosis
K74.1	Hepatic sclerosis
K74.2	Hepatic fibrosis with hepatic sclerosis
K74.3	Primary biliary cirrhosis
K74.4	Secondary biliary cirrhosis
K74.69	Other cirrhosis of liver

K75.0	Abscess of liver
K75.1	Phlebitis of portal vein
K75.2	Nonspecific reactive hepatitis
K75.4	Autoimmune hepatitis
K75.81	Nonalcoholic steatohepatitis (NASH)
K76.0	Fatty (change of) liver, not elsewhere classified
K76.1	Chronic passive congestion of liver
K76.2	Central hemorrhagic necrosis of liver
K76.3	Infarction of liver
K76.4	Peliosis hepatis
K76.5	Hepatic veno-occlusive disease
K76.6	Portal hypertension
K76.7	Hepatorenal syndrome
K76.81	Hepatopulmonary syndrome
K91.82	Postprocedural hepatic failure
K91.83	Postprocedural hepatorenal syndrome
P78.81	Congenital cirrhosis (of liver) Ⓝ
Q44.6	Cystic disease of liver
Q44.7	Other congenital malformations of liver
R16.0	Hepatomegaly, not elsewhere classified
R16.2	Hepatomegaly with splenomegaly, not elsewhere classified
T86.41	Liver transplant rejection
T86.42	Liver transplant failure
T86.43	Liver transplant infection
T86.49	Other complications of liver transplant
Z48.23	Encounter for aftercare following liver transplant

AMA: 47000 2019,Apr,4; 2018,Jan,8; 2017,Jan,8; 2016,Jan,13; 2015,Jan,16
47001 2018,Jan,8; 2017,Jan,8; 2016,Jan,13; 2015,Jan,16

Relative Value Units/Medicare Edits

Non-Facility RVU	Work	PE	MP	Total
47000	1.65	7.51	0.15	9.31
47001	1.9	0.7	0.45	3.05
Facility RVU	**Work**	**PE**	**MP**	**Total**
47000	1.65	0.76	0.15	2.56
47001	1.9	0.7	0.45	3.05

	FUD	Status	MUE	Modifiers				IOM Reference
47000	0	A	3(3)	51	N/A	N/A	N/A	None
47001	N/A	A	3(3)	N/A	N/A	62*	N/A	
* with documentation								

47010

47010 Hepatotomy, for open drainage of abscess or cyst, 1 or 2 stages

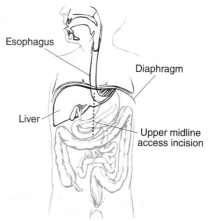

The liver is surgically accessed and incised for open drainage of an abscess or cyst

Explanation

The physician incises the liver to drain an abscess or a cyst, sometimes taking one or two stages. The physician exposes the liver via an upper midline incision. The cyst is incised and suctioned with care to not contaminate the abdomen with purulent matter. Cultures and pathology are sent in a separately reported activity. The incision is closed.

Coding Tips

For laparotomy with aspiration and/or injection of hepatic parasitic cysts or abscesses, see 47015. For wedge biopsy of the liver, see 47100. For marsupialization of a cyst or an abscess, see 47300. For percutaneous image-guided drainage of a hepatic abscess or cyst, via catheter, see 49405.

ICD-10-CM Diagnostic Codes

A06.4	Amebic liver abscess
B67.0	Echinococcus granulosus infection of liver
B67.5	Echinococcus multilocularis infection of liver
K75.0	Abscess of liver
K75.89	Other specified inflammatory liver diseases
K76.89	Other specified diseases of liver
K77	Liver disorders in diseases classified elsewhere
Q44.6	Cystic disease of liver

AMA: 47010 2014,Jan,11

Relative Value Units/Medicare Edits

Non-Facility RVU	Work	PE	MP	Total
47010	19.4	11.94	4.58	35.92
Facility RVU	**Work**	**PE**	**MP**	**Total**
47010	19.4	11.94	4.58	35.92

	FUD	Status	MUE	Modifiers				IOM Reference
47010	90	A	1(3)	51	N/A	62*	80	None
* with documentation								

Liver

47015

47015   Laparotomy, with aspiration and/or injection of hepatic parasitic (eg, amoebic or echinococcal) cyst(s) or abscess(es)

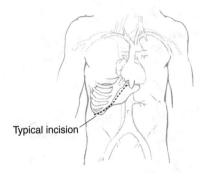

An abdominal incision is made (laparotomy) and the liver accessed. Parasitic cysts or abscesses are aspirated

Explanation

The physician performs aspiration or injection of liver parasitic cysts or abscesses. The physician makes an abdominal incision. The liver is mobilized and the parasitic cysts or abscesses are identified. The remaining abdominal contents are packed off with sponges for protection. The cysts are aspirated with a needle and syringe or unroofed and aspirated and may be injected with a hypertonic solution. The abdominal incision is closed.

Coding Tips

For open drainage of an abscess or a cyst, see 47010. For marsupialization of a cyst or an abscess, see 47300. For percutaneous, image-guided drainage of a hepatic abscess or cyst, via catheter, see 49405.

ICD-10-CM Diagnostic Codes

A06.4	Amebic liver abscess
B67.0	Echinococcus granulosus infection of liver
B67.5	Echinococcus multilocularis infection of liver

AMA: 47015 2014,Jan,11

Relative Value Units/Medicare Edits

Non-Facility RVU	Work	PE	MP	Total
47015	18.5	11.58	4.53	34.61
Facility RVU	Work	PE	MP	Total
47015	18.5	11.58	4.53	34.61

	FUD	Status	MUE	Modifiers				IOM Reference
47015	90	A	1(2)	51	N/A	62*	80	None

* with documentation

Terms To Know

abscess. Circumscribed collection of pus resulting from bacteria, frequently associated with swelling and other signs of inflammation.

echinococcosis. Infection caused by larval forms of tapeworms of the genus *Echinococcus*.

47100

47100   Biopsy of liver, wedge

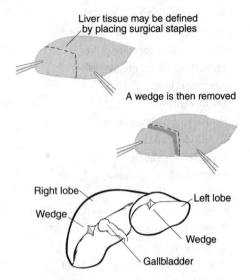

Liver tissue may be defined by placing surgical staples

A wedge is then removed

Right lobe — Left lobe — Wedge — Wedge — Gallbladder

Explanation

The physician takes a wedge-shaped section of liver tissue for biopsy. The physician exposes the abdomen via an upper abdominal incision through skin, fascia, and muscle. Interrupted mattress sutures are placed on the edge of the liver lobe. A pie-shaped wedge of the liver is resected and sent for pathology in a separately reportable activity. Electrocautery is used to obtain hemostasis of the liver edge. The abdominal incision is closed with layered sutures.

Coding Tips

For percutaneous needle biopsy, liver, see 47000; performed at time of other major procedure, see 47001.

ICD-10-CM Diagnostic Codes

B00.81	Herpesviral hepatitis
B15.0	Hepatitis A with hepatic coma
B15.9	Hepatitis A without hepatic coma
B16.0	Acute hepatitis B with delta-agent with hepatic coma
B16.1	Acute hepatitis B with delta-agent without hepatic coma
B16.2	Acute hepatitis B without delta-agent with hepatic coma
B16.9	Acute hepatitis B without delta-agent and without hepatic coma
B17.0	Acute delta-(super) infection of hepatitis B carrier
B17.10	Acute hepatitis C without hepatic coma
B17.11	Acute hepatitis C with hepatic coma
B17.2	Acute hepatitis E
B18.0	Chronic viral hepatitis B with delta-agent
B18.1	Chronic viral hepatitis B without delta-agent
B18.2	Chronic viral hepatitis C
B18.8	Other chronic viral hepatitis
B25.1	Cytomegaloviral hepatitis
B94.2	Sequelae of viral hepatitis
C22.0	Liver cell carcinoma
C22.1	Intrahepatic bile duct carcinoma
C22.2	Hepatoblastoma

Liver

C22.3	Angiosarcoma of liver
C78.7	Secondary malignant neoplasm of liver and intrahepatic bile duct
C7B.02	Secondary carcinoid tumors of liver
C80.2	Malignant neoplasm associated with transplanted organ
D01.5	Carcinoma in situ of liver, gallbladder and bile ducts
D13.4	Benign neoplasm of liver
D37.6	Neoplasm of uncertain behavior of liver, gallbladder and bile ducts
D47.Z1	Post-transplant lymphoproliferative disorder (PTLD)
D47.Z2	Castleman disease
E80.4	Gilbert syndrome
E80.5	Crigler-Najjar syndrome
E83.01	Wilson's disease
E83.110	Hereditary hemochromatosis
E83.111	Hemochromatosis due to repeated red blood cell transfusions
E88.01	Alpha-1-antitrypsin deficiency
K70.0	Alcoholic fatty liver △
K70.10	Alcoholic hepatitis without ascites △
K70.11	Alcoholic hepatitis with ascites △
K70.2	Alcoholic fibrosis and sclerosis of liver △
K70.30	Alcoholic cirrhosis of liver without ascites △
K70.31	Alcoholic cirrhosis of liver with ascites △
K70.40	Alcoholic hepatic failure without coma △
K70.41	Alcoholic hepatic failure with coma △
K71.0	Toxic liver disease with cholestasis
K71.10	Toxic liver disease with hepatic necrosis, without coma
K71.11	Toxic liver disease with hepatic necrosis, with coma
K71.2	Toxic liver disease with acute hepatitis
K71.3	Toxic liver disease with chronic persistent hepatitis
K71.4	Toxic liver disease with chronic lobular hepatitis
K71.50	Toxic liver disease with chronic active hepatitis without ascites
K71.51	Toxic liver disease with chronic active hepatitis with ascites
K71.6	Toxic liver disease with hepatitis, not elsewhere classified
K71.7	Toxic liver disease with fibrosis and cirrhosis of liver
K72.00	Acute and subacute hepatic failure without coma
K72.01	Acute and subacute hepatic failure with coma
K72.10	Chronic hepatic failure without coma
K72.11	Chronic hepatic failure with coma
K74.01	Hepatic fibrosis, early fibrosis
K74.02	Hepatic fibrosis, advanced fibrosis
K74.1	Hepatic sclerosis
K74.2	Hepatic fibrosis with hepatic sclerosis
K74.3	Primary biliary cirrhosis
K74.4	Secondary biliary cirrhosis
K75.0	Abscess of liver
K75.1	Phlebitis of portal vein
K75.3	Granulomatous hepatitis, not elsewhere classified
K75.4	Autoimmune hepatitis
K75.81	Nonalcoholic steatohepatitis (NASH)
K76.1	Chronic passive congestion of liver
K76.2	Central hemorrhagic necrosis of liver
K76.3	Infarction of liver

K76.4	Peliosis hepatis
K76.5	Hepatic veno-occlusive disease
K76.6	Portal hypertension
K76.7	Hepatorenal syndrome
K76.81	Hepatopulmonary syndrome
K91.82	Postprocedural hepatic failure
K91.83	Postprocedural hepatorenal syndrome
P78.81	Congenital cirrhosis (of liver) ◼
Q44.6	Cystic disease of liver
Q44.7	Other congenital malformations of liver
R63.4	Abnormal weight loss
R94.5	Abnormal results of liver function studies
T86.41	Liver transplant rejection
T86.42	Liver transplant failure
T86.43	Liver transplant infection
T86.49	Other complications of liver transplant

AMA: 47100 2014,Jan,11

Relative Value Units/Medicare Edits

Non-Facility RVU	Work	PE	MP	Total
47100	12.91	9.21	3.05	25.17
Facility RVU	Work	PE	MP	Total
47100	12.91	9.21	3.05	25.17

	FUD	Status	MUE	Modifiers				IOM Reference
47100	90	A	3(3)	51	N/A	62*	80	None

* with documentation

Liver

47120-47130

47120 Hepatectomy, resection of liver; partial lobectomy
47122   trisegmentectomy
47125   total left lobectomy
47130   total right lobectomy

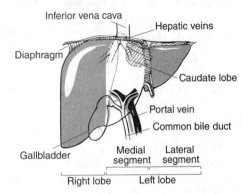

Explanation

The physician removes a section of liver, or lobectomy. The physician exposes the liver via an upper midline incision through skin, fascia, and muscle. The fibrous connections of the liver to the diaphragm are divided and the portal structures are controlled. The portal and hepatic vessels associated with the affected lobe are divided. The portal structures are clamped. The liver parenchyma is divided by pressure or coagulation hemostasis. The portal clamp is removed and hemostasis is assured before the abdomen is closed with sutures. Report 47120 if a partial lobectomy is performed; report 47122 if a trisegmentectomy is performed; report 47125 if a total left lobectomy is performed; and report 47130 if a total right lobectomy is performed.

Coding Tips

For donor hepatectomy, see 47133 and 47140–47142. For liver allotransplantation, see 47135.

ICD-10-CM Diagnostic Codes

C22.0	Liver cell carcinoma
C22.1	Intrahepatic bile duct carcinoma
C22.2	Hepatoblastoma
C22.3	Angiosarcoma of liver
C78.7	Secondary malignant neoplasm of liver and intrahepatic bile duct
C7B.02	Secondary carcinoid tumors of liver
C80.2	Malignant neoplasm associated with transplanted organ
D01.5	Carcinoma in situ of liver, gallbladder and bile ducts
D13.4	Benign neoplasm of liver
D13.5	Benign neoplasm of extrahepatic bile ducts
D37.6	Neoplasm of uncertain behavior of liver, gallbladder and bile ducts
D3A.098	Benign carcinoid tumors of other sites
D47.Z2	Castleman disease
E80.5	Crigler-Najjar syndrome
E85.81	Light chain (AL) amyloidosis
E85.82	Wild-type transthyretin-related (ATTR) amyloidosis
E85.89	Other amyloidosis
K70.0	Alcoholic fatty liver 🅰
K70.10	Alcoholic hepatitis without ascites 🅰
K70.11	Alcoholic hepatitis with ascites 🅰
K70.2	Alcoholic fibrosis and sclerosis of liver 🅰
K70.30	Alcoholic cirrhosis of liver without ascites 🅰
K70.31	Alcoholic cirrhosis of liver with ascites 🅰
K70.40	Alcoholic hepatic failure without coma 🅰
K70.41	Alcoholic hepatic failure with coma 🅰
K71.0	Toxic liver disease with cholestasis
K71.10	Toxic liver disease with hepatic necrosis, without coma
K71.11	Toxic liver disease with hepatic necrosis, with coma
K71.2	Toxic liver disease with acute hepatitis
K71.3	Toxic liver disease with chronic persistent hepatitis
K71.4	Toxic liver disease with chronic lobular hepatitis
K71.50	Toxic liver disease with chronic active hepatitis without ascites
K71.51	Toxic liver disease with chronic active hepatitis with ascites
K71.6	Toxic liver disease with hepatitis, not elsewhere classified
K71.7	Toxic liver disease with fibrosis and cirrhosis of liver
K72.00	Acute and subacute hepatic failure without coma
K72.01	Acute and subacute hepatic failure with coma
K72.10	Chronic hepatic failure without coma
K72.11	Chronic hepatic failure with coma
K73.0	Chronic persistent hepatitis, not elsewhere classified
K73.1	Chronic lobular hepatitis, not elsewhere classified
K73.2	Chronic active hepatitis, not elsewhere classified
K74.1	Hepatic sclerosis
K74.2	Hepatic fibrosis with hepatic sclerosis
K74.3	Primary biliary cirrhosis
K74.4	Secondary biliary cirrhosis
K76.1	Chronic passive congestion of liver
K76.2	Central hemorrhagic necrosis of liver
K76.3	Infarction of liver
K76.4	Peliosis hepatis
K76.5	Hepatic veno-occlusive disease
K76.6	Portal hypertension
K83.5	Biliary cyst
P78.81	Congenital cirrhosis (of liver) 🅽
P78.84	Gestational alloimmune liver disease
Q44.6	Cystic disease of liver
R16.0	Hepatomegaly, not elsewhere classified
R16.2	Hepatomegaly with splenomegaly, not elsewhere classified
S36.112A	Contusion of liver, initial encounter
S36.114A	Minor laceration of liver, initial encounter
S36.115A	Moderate laceration of liver, initial encounter
S36.116A	Major laceration of liver, initial encounter

AMA: **47120** 2018,Jan,8; 2017,Jan,8; 2016,Oct,11; 2016,Jan,13; 2015,Jan,16

Relative Value Units/Medicare Edits

Non-Facility RVU	Work	PE	MP	Total
47120	39.01	20.77	9.22	69.0
47122	59.48	27.49	13.99	100.96
47125	53.04	25.11	12.61	90.76
47130	57.19	26.77	13.62	97.58
Facility RVU	**Work**	**PE**	**MP**	**Total**
47120	39.01	20.77	9.22	69.0
47122	59.48	27.49	13.99	100.96
47125	53.04	25.11	12.61	90.76
47130	57.19	26.77	13.62	97.58

	FUD	Status	MUE	Modifiers				IOM Reference
47120	90	A	2(3)	51	N/A	62*	80	None
47122	90	A	1(2)	51	N/A	62*	80	
47125	90	A	1(2)	51	N/A	62*	80	
47130	90	A	1(2)	51	N/A	62*	80	

* with documentation

Terms To Know

cirrhosis of liver. Chronic disease of the liver that characteristically produces intertwining bands of fibrotic tissue that change the normal structure of the lobes of the liver and destroys normal cells, which then regenerate into nodules and cause the liver to stop functioning over time. This form of cirrhosis is not alcohol related.

fascia. Fibrous sheet or band of tissue that envelops organs, muscles, and groupings of muscles.

hemostasis. Interruption of blood flow or the cessation or arrest of bleeding.

jaundice. Increased bilirubin and deposits of bile pigment in the skin and sclera, causing a yellow tint.

lobectomy. Excision of a lobe of an organ such as the liver, thyroid, lung, or brain.

malignant neoplasm. Any cancerous tumor or lesion exhibiting uncontrolled tissue growth that can progressively invade other parts of the body with its disease-generating cells.

resection. Surgical removal of a part or all of an organ or body part.

47140

47140   Donor hepatectomy (including cold preservation), from living donor; left lateral segment only (segments II and III)

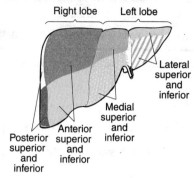

The left lateral portion of liver is removed from a living donor

Explanation

Surgeons remove the left lateral portion only (segments II and III) of the liver from a living donor, who is oftentimes a parent of compatible blood type donating to an infant or young child. Bilateral subcostal incisions are made to the xiphoid and the peritoneum is entered. The liver is exposed and mobilized. The left hepatic vein is exposed, adhesions are removed, and the porta hepatis is encircled with a drain. The left hepatic artery is dissected free and looped. The gastrohepatic ligament is transected and any aberrant left hepatic arteries within it are dissected to the left gastric artery. The left lateral segment of the liver is now reflected forward and ligaments are dissected away. The left portal vein is dissected and encircled. The left bile duct is identified and the left hepatic duct is transected, along with any multiple bile ducts within the liver, while preserving blood supply to the main bile duct. Ultrasound is used to locate the left and middle hepatic veins and the left hepatic vein is dissected and encircled. The liver's resection lines are marked with cautery. Vessels and bile ducts within this area are sutured and divided. The liver is resected and hemostasis maintained with a laser coagulator. Clamps are applied to the left hepatic artery, hepatic vein, and portal vein. The left lateral segment is removed and perfused with preservative solution for transplant. The clamped vessels and the left bile duct are sutured. The liver is checked for complete hemostasis and any bile leaks before closing. The tissue is preserved for transplantation into the recipient. The organ remains under refrigeration, packed in a sealable container with some preserving solution and kept on ice in a suitable carrier.

Coding Tips

Liver transplantation involves three distinct components: donor hepatectomy, backbench work, and recipient liver allotransplantation. Code 47140 reports a living donor hepatectomy, left lateral segment (II and III) only. For a total left lobectomy (segments II, III, and IV), see 47141; total right lobectomy (segments V, VI, VII, and VIII), see 47142. Living donor hepatectomy includes harvesting and cold preservation of the graft (perfusing with cold preservation solution and cold maintenance) and preoperative, intraoperative, and postoperative care of the donor. For donor hepatectomy from a cadaver donor, see 47133. For liver allotransplantation, orthotopic, partial or whole, living donor or cadaver, any age, see 47135. For backbench preparation, see 47143–47147.

ICD-10-CM Diagnostic Codes

Z52.6   Liver donor

AMA: 47140 2018,Jan,8; 2017,Jan,8; 2016,Jan,13; 2015,Jan,16

Liver

Relative Value Units/Medicare Edits

Non-Facility RVU	Work	PE	MP	Total
47140	59.4	31.29	14.52	105.21
Facility RVU	**Work**	**PE**	**MP**	**Total**
47140	59.4	31.29	14.52	105.21

	FUD	Status	MUE	Modifiers				IOM Reference
47140	90	A	1(2)	51	N/A	62*	80	None

* with documentation

Terms To Know

allograft. Graft from one individual to another of the same species.

atresia. Congenital closure or absence of a tubular organ or an opening to the body surface.

cirrhosis. Disease of the liver that has the characteristics of intertwining band of fibrous tissue that divides the parenchyma into micro- and macronodular areas, which cause the liver to stop functioning over time.

dissect. Cut apart or separate tissue for surgical purposes or for visual or microscopic study.

donor. Person from whom tissues or organs are removed for transplantation.

lateral. On/to the side.

malignant. Any condition tending to progress toward death, specifically an invasive tumor with a loss of cellular differentiation that has the ability to spread or metastasize to other body areas.

neoplasm. New abnormal growth, tumor.

orthotopic transplant. Movement or replacement of an organ or tissue in which the patient's nonfunctioning organ is removed.

47141

47141   Donor hepatectomy (including cold preservation), from living donor; total left lobectomy (segments II, III and IV)

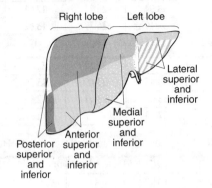

The total left lobe of liver
is removed from a living donor

Explanation

Surgeons remove the whole left lobe (segments II, III, and IV) of the liver from a living donor, who is oftentimes a parent of compatible blood type donating to an infant or young child. Bilateral subcostal incisions are made to the xiphoid and the peritoneum is entered. The liver is exposed and mobilized. The left hepatic vein is exposed, adhesions are removed, and the porta hepatis is encircled with a drain. The left hepatic artery is dissected free and looped. The gastrohepatic ligament is transected and any aberrant left hepatic arteries within it are dissected to the left gastric artery. The left lateral segment of the liver is now reflected forward and ligaments are dissected away. The left portal vein is dissected and encircled. The left bile duct is identified. A cholecystectomy and cholangiogram are performed with catheter insertion into the cystic duct. The left hepatic duct is transected, along with any multiple bile ducts within the liver, while preserving blood supply to the main bile duct. Ultrasound is used to locate the left and middle hepatic veins, which are dissected and encircled. The liver's resection lines are marked with cautery. Vessels and bile ducts within this area are sutured and divided. The liver is resected and hemostasis is maintained with a laser coagulator. Clamps are applied to the left hepatic artery, hepatic vein, and portal vein. The total left lobe of the liver is removed and perfused with preservative solution for transplant. The clamped vessels and the left bile duct are sutured. The liver is checked for complete hemostasis and any bile leaks before closing. A final cholangiogram is performed, the catheter is removed, and the cystic duct is sutured. The tissue is preserved for transplantation into the recipient. The organ remains under refrigeration, packed in a sealable container with some preserving solution and kept on ice in a suitable carrier.

Coding Tips

Liver transplantation involves three distinct components: donor hepatectomy, backbench work, and recipient liver allotransplantation. Code 47140 reports a living donor hepatectomy, left lateral segment (II and III) only. For a total left lobectomy (segments II, III, and IV), see 47141; total right lobectomy (segments V, VI, VII, and VIII), see 47142. Living donor hepatectomy includes harvesting and cold preservation of the graft (perfusing with cold preservation solution and cold maintenance) and preoperative, intraoperative, and postoperative care of the donor. For donor hepatectomy from a cadaver donor, see 47133. For liver allotransplantation, orthotopic, partial or whole, living donor or cadaver, any age, see 47135. For backbench preparation, see 47143–47147.

Coding Companion for General Surgery/Gastroenterology

Liver

ICD-10-CM Diagnostic Codes

Z52.6   Liver donor

AMA: **47141** 2014,Jan,11

Relative Value Units/Medicare Edits

Non-Facility RVU	Work	PE	MP	Total
47141	71.5	36.82	17.47	125.79
Facility RVU	**Work**	**PE**	**MP**	**Total**
47141	71.5	36.82	17.47	125.79

	FUD	Status	MUE	Modifiers				IOM Reference
47141	90	A	1(2)	51	N/A	62*	80	None

* with documentation

Terms To Know

allograft. Graft from one individual to another of the same species.

artery. Vessel through which oxygenated blood passes away from the heart to any part of the body.

dissect. Cut apart or separate tissue for surgical purposes or for visual or microscopic study.

hemostasis. Interruption of blood flow or the cessation or arrest of bleeding.

orthotopic transplant. Movement or replacement of an organ or tissue in which the patient's nonfunctioning organ is removed.

resection. Surgical removal of a part or all of an organ or body part.

transection. Transverse dissection; to cut across a long axis; cross section.

47142

47142   Donor hepatectomy (including cold preservation), from living donor; total right lobectomy (segments V, VI, VII and VIII)

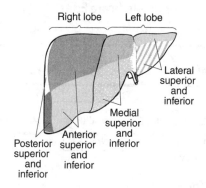

The total right lobe of liver is removed from a living donor

Explanation

Surgeons remove the whole right lobe (segments V, VI, VII, and VIII) of the liver from a living donor, who is oftentimes a parent of compatible blood type donating to an infant or young child. Bilateral subcostal incisions are made to the xiphoid and the peritoneum is entered. The liver is exposed and mobilized. Ligaments on the right are divided and dissection is continued to the inferior vena cava. Adhesions are removed and the porta hepatis is encircled with a drain. The right hepatic artery is dissected free and looped. A cholecystectomy and cholangiogram are performed with catheter insertion into the cystic duct. The right portal vein is dissected and encircled. The right bile ducts are identified. The right hepatic duct is transected within the liver parenchyma, along with any multiple bile ducts, while preserving blood supply to the main bile duct. The caudate lobe must be mobilized from the inferior vena cava. All accessory hepatic veins are ligated and ultrasound is used to locate the right and middle hepatic veins. The right hepatic vein is dissected and encircled. The liver's resection lines are marked with cautery. Vessels and bile ducts within this area are sutured and divided, maintaining the veins from segments V and VIII, and the liver is resected. Hemostasis is maintained with a laser coagulator. Clamps are applied to the right hepatic artery, hepatic vein, and portal vein. The right lobe of the liver is removed and perfused with preservative solution for transplant. The clamped vessels and the right bile duct are sutured. The liver is checked for complete hemostasis and any bile leaks before closing. A final cholangiogram is performed, the catheter is removed, and the cystic duct is sutured. The tissue is preserved for transplantation into the recipient. The organ remains under refrigeration, packed in a sealable container with some preserving solution and kept on ice in a suitable carrier.

Coding Tips

Liver transplantation involves three distinct components: donor hepatectomy, backbench work, and recipient liver allotransplantation. Code 47140 reports a living donor hepatectomy, left lateral segment (II and III) only. For a total left lobectomy (segments II, III, and IV), see 47141; total right lobectomy (segments V, VI, VII, and VIII), see 47142. A living donor hepatectomy includes harvesting and cold preservation of the graft (perfusing with cold preservation solution and cold maintenance) and preoperative, intraoperative, and postoperative care of the donor. For a donor hepatectomy from a cadaver donor, see 47133. For liver allotransplantation, orthotopic, partial or whole, living donor or cadaver, any age, see 47135. For backbench preparation, see 47143–47147.

Liver

ICD-10-CM Diagnostic Codes

Z52.6   Liver donor

AMA: **47142** 2014,Jan,11

Relative Value Units/Medicare Edits

Non-Facility RVU	Work	PE	MP	Total
47142	79.44	39.76	19.43	138.63
Facility RVU	**Work**	**PE**	**MP**	**Total**
47142	79.44	39.76	19.43	138.63

	FUD	Status	MUE	Modifiers				IOM Reference
47142	90	A	1(2)	51	N/A	62*	80	None

* with documentation

Terms To Know

adhesion. Abnormal fibrous connection between two structures, soft tissue or bony structures, that may occur as the result of surgery, infection, or trauma.

artery. Vessel through which oxygenated blood passes away from the heart to any part of the body.

cadaver. Dead body.

donor. Person from whom tissues or organs are removed for transplantation.

hemostasis. Interruption of blood flow or the cessation or arrest of bleeding.

mobilization. Therapy that consists of small passive movements, usually applied as a series of gentle stretches in a smooth, rhythmic fashion to the individual vertebrae. The movements are applied at various locations on each of the affected vertebrae, and at various angles, directed at relieving restriction in movement at any particular level of the spine. Mobilization stretches stiff joints to restore range. It also relieves pain. For example, it is especially effective with arthritic joints.

vena cava. Main venous trunk that empties into the right atrium from both the lower and upper regions, beginning at the junction of the common iliac veins inferiorly and the two brachiocephalic veins superiorly.

47143

47143   Backbench standard preparation of cadaver donor whole liver graft prior to allotransplantation, including cholecystectomy, if necessary, and dissection and removal of surrounding soft tissues to prepare the vena cava, portal vein, hepatic artery, and common bile duct for implantation; without trisegment or lobe split

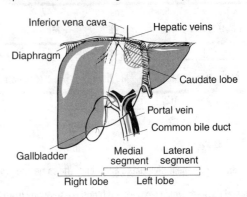

Explanation

The physician performs a standard backbench preparation of cadaver donor whole liver graft without trisegment or lobe split prior to allotransplantation. Backbench or back table preparation refers to procedures performed on the donor organ following procurement to prepare the donor organ for transplant. After removal from the body, the liver is flushed with a preserving solution and packed. The superfluous tissues that accompany the liver when it is removed en bloc are removed. If the gallbladder has been removed with the liver, it is dissected free. Next, any necessary vascular reconstruction procedures are performed with the arteries being the most common sites of reconstruction. The goal of the physician is to provide a single common inflow vessel of sufficient length so that only one anastomosis is required in the recipient. Arterial grafting is performed using previously procured iliac artery grafts as required to accomplish this goal. Other vessels, including the vena cava and portal vein, are prepared and grafting performed as needed. All vessels and grafts are tested for patency and integrity by flushing with preservation solution. Next, the common bile duct is inspected and residual tissue removed. Following liver preparation, the internal iliac arteries and veins are prepared for use as arterial and venous grafts in the recipient. When all residual tissue has been removed, vascular grafting performed as needed, and the common bile duct prepared, the liver is ready for transplant.

Coding Tips

Liver transplantation involves three distinct components: donor hepatectomy, backbench work, and recipient liver allotransplantation. Do not report 47143 with 47120–47125, 47600, or 47610. Code 47140 reports a living donor hepatectomy, left lateral segment (II and III) only. For a total left lobectomy (segments II, III, and IV), see 47141; total right lobectomy (segments V, VI, VII, and VIII), see 47142. A living donor hepatectomy includes harvesting and cold preservation of the graft (perfusing with cold preservation solution and cold maintenance) and preoperative, intraoperative, and postoperative care of the donor. For donor hepatectomy from a cadaver donor, see 47133. For liver allotransplantation, orthotopic, partial or whole, living donor or cadaver, any age, see 47135. For backbench preparation, see 47143–47147.

ICD-10-CM Diagnostic Codes

The application of this code is too broad to adequately present ICD-10-CM diagnostic code links here. Refer to your ICD-10-CM book.

AMA: **47143** 2018,Jan,8; 2017,Jan,8; 2016,Jan,13; 2015,Jan,16

Relative Value Units/Medicare Edits

Non-Facility RVU	Work	PE	MP	Total
47143	0.0	0.0	0.0	0.0
Facility RVU	Work	PE	MP	Total
47143	0.0	0.0	0.0	0.0

	FUD	Status	MUE	Modifiers				IOM Reference
47143	N/A	C	1(2)	51	N/A	62*	80	None

* with documentation

Terms To Know

anastomosis. Surgically created connection between ducts, blood vessels, or bowel segments to allow flow from one to the other.

backbench preparation. Procedures performed on a donor organ following procurement to prepare the organ for transplant into the recipient. Excess fat and other tissue may be removed, the organ may be perfused, and vital arteries may be sized, repaired, or modified to fit the patient. These procedures are done on a back table in the operating room before transplantation can begin.

cadaver. Dead body.

donor. Person from whom tissues or organs are removed for transplantation.

patency. State of a tube-like structure or conduit being open and unobstructed.

reconstruction. Recreating, restoring, or rebuilding a body part or organ.

47144

47144   Backbench standard preparation of cadaver donor whole liver graft prior to allotransplantation, including cholecystectomy, if necessary, and dissection and removal of surrounding soft tissues to prepare the vena cava, portal vein, hepatic artery, and common bile duct for implantation; with trisegment split of whole liver graft into 2 partial liver grafts (ie, left lateral segment [segments II and III] and right trisegment [segments I and IV through VIII])

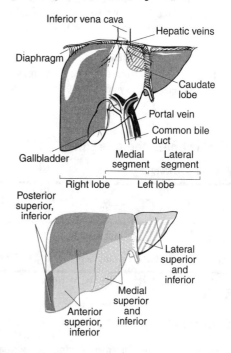

Explanation

The physician performs a standard backbench preparation of cadaver donor whole liver graft with trisegment split of whole liver graft into two partial liver grafts prior to allotransplantation. Backbench or back table preparation refers to procedures performed on the donor organ following procurement to prepare the donor organ for transplant. After removal from the body, the liver is flushed with a preserving solution and packed. The superfluous tissues that accompany the liver when it is removed en bloc are removed. If the gallbladder has been removed with the liver, it is dissected free. In split liver transplants, the liver can be split prior to procurement (in situ) or during the back table preparation (ex situ). If an ex situ split is required, it is performed at this time. A trisegment split involves dividing the liver through the falciform ligament to create a small left lateral segment graft for a child and a large extended right lobe graft for an adult. Next, any necessary vascular reconstruction procedures are performed, with the arteries being the most common sites of reconstruction. The goal of the physician is to construct a single common inflow vessel of sufficient length in the donor liver segments so that only one anastomosis is required in the recipient. Arterial grafting is performed using previously procured iliac artery grafts as required to accomplish this goal. Other vessels, including the vena cava and portal vein, are prepared and venous grafting performed as needed. All vessels and grafts are tested for patency and integrity by flushing with preservation solution. Next, the common bile duct is inspected and residual tissue removed. Following liver preparation, the internal iliac arteries and veins are prepared for use as arterial and venous grafts in the recipient. When all residual tissue has been removed, vascular grafting performed as needed, and the common bile duct prepared, the liver segments are ready for transplant.

Liver

Coding Tips

Liver transplantation involves three distinct components: donor hepatectomy, backbench work, and recipient liver allotransplantation. Do not report 47144 with 47120–47125, 47600, or 47610. Code 47140 reports a living donor hepatectomy, left lateral segment (II and III) only. For a total left lobectomy (segments II, III, and IV), see 47141; total right lobectomy (segments V, VI, VII, and VIII), see 47142. A living donor hepatectomy includes harvesting and cold preservation of the graft (perfusing with cold preservation solution and cold maintenance) and preoperative, intraoperative, and postoperative care of the donor. For a donor hepatectomy from a cadaver donor, see 47133. For a liver allotransplantation, orthotopic, partial or whole, living donor or cadaver, any age, see 47135. For backbench preparation, see 47143–47147.

ICD-10-CM Diagnostic Codes

The application of this code is too broad to adequately present ICD-10-CM diagnostic code links here. Refer to your ICD-10-CM book.

AMA: **47144** 2014,Jan,11

Relative Value Units/Medicare Edits

Non-Facility RVU	Work	PE	MP	Total
47144	0.0	0.0	0.0	0.0
Facility RVU	**Work**	**PE**	**MP**	**Total**
47144	0.0	0.0	0.0	0.0

	FUD	Status	MUE	Modifiers				IOM Reference
47144	90	C	1(2)	51	N/A	62*	80	None

* with documentation

Terms To Know

backbench preparation. Procedures performed on a donor organ following procurement to prepare the organ for transplant into the recipient. Excess fat and other tissue may be removed, the organ may be perfused, and vital arteries may be sized, repaired, or modified to fit the patient. These procedures are done on a back table in the operating room before transplantation can begin.

dissection. (dis. apart; -section, act of cutting) Separating by cutting tissue or body structures apart.

graft. Tissue implant from another part of the body or another person.

patency. State of a tube-like structure or conduit being open and unobstructed.

reconstruction. Recreating, restoring, or rebuilding a body part or organ.

transplant. Insertion of an organ or tissue from one person or site into another.

47145

47145 Backbench standard preparation of cadaver donor whole liver graft prior to allotransplantation, including cholecystectomy, if necessary, and dissection and removal of surrounding soft tissues to prepare the vena cava, portal vein, hepatic artery, and common bile duct for implantation; with lobe split of whole liver graft into 2 partial liver grafts (ie, left lobe [segments II, III, and IV] and right lobe [segments I and V through VIII])

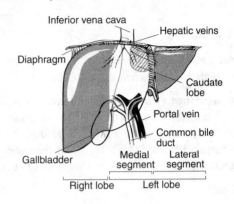

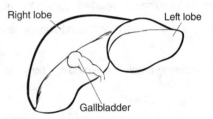

Explanation

The physician performs a standard backbench preparation of cadaver donor whole liver graft with lobe split of whole liver graft into two partial liver grafts prior to allotransplantation. Backbench or back table preparation refers to procedures performed on the donor organ following procurement to prepare the donor organ for transplant. After removal from the body, the liver is flushed with a preserving solution and packed. The superfluous tissues that accompany the liver when it is removed en bloc are removed. If the gallbladder has been removed with the liver, it is dissected free. In split liver transplants, the liver can be split prior to procurement (in situ) or during the back table preparation (ex situ). If an ex situ split is required, it is performed at this time. A lobe split involves dividing the liver through the main portal fissure and gallbladder bed to create right and left lobe grafts. Next, any necessary vascular reconstruction procedures are performed, with the arteries being the most common sites of reconstruction. The goal of the physician is to construct a single common inflow vessel of sufficient length in the two donor liver lobes so that only one anastomosis is required in the recipient. Arterial grafting is performed using previously procured iliac artery grafts as required to accomplish this goal. Other vessels, including the vena cava and portal vein, are prepared and venous grafting performed as needed. All vessels and grafts are tested for patency and integrity by flushing with preservation solution. Next, the common bile duct is inspected and residual tissue removed. Following liver preparation, the internal iliac arteries and veins are prepared for use as arterial and venous grafts in the recipient. When all residual tissue has been removed, vascular grafting performed as needed, and the common bile duct prepared, the two liver lobes are ready for transplant.

Liver

Coding Tips

Liver transplantation involves three distinct components: donor hepatectomy, backbench work, and recipient liver allotransplantation. Do not report 47145 with 47120–47125, 47600, or 47610. Code 47140 reports a living donor hepatectomy, left lateral segment (II and III) only. For a total left lobectomy (segments II, III, and IV), see 47141; total right lobectomy (segments V, VI, VII, and VIII), see 47142. A living donor hepatectomy includes harvesting and cold preservation of the graft (perfusing with cold preservation solution and cold maintenance) and preoperative, intraoperative, and postoperative care of the donor. For donor hepatectomy from a cadaver donor, see 47133. For liver allotransplantation, orthotopic, partial or whole, living donor or cadaver, any age, see 47135. For backbench preparation, see 47143–47147.

ICD-10-CM Diagnostic Codes

The application of this code is too broad to adequately present ICD-10-CM diagnostic code links here. Refer to your ICD-10-CM book.

AMA: **47145** 2014,Jan,11

Relative Value Units/Medicare Edits

Non-Facility RVU	Work	PE	MP	Total
47145	0.0	0.0	0.0	0.0
Facility RVU	Work	PE	MP	Total
47145	0.0	0.0	0.0	0.0

	FUD	Status	MUE	Modifiers				IOM Reference
47145	N/A	C	1(2)	51	N/A	62*	80	None

* with documentation

Terms To Know

backbench preparation. Procedures performed on a donor organ following procurement to prepare the organ for transplant into the recipient. Excess fat and other tissue may be removed, the organ may be perfused, and vital arteries may be sized, repaired, or modified to fit the patient. These procedures are done on a back table in the operating room before transplantation can begin.

donor. Person from whom tissues or organs are removed for transplantation.

en bloc. In total.

graft. Tissue implant from another part of the body or another person.

reconstruction. Recreating, restoring, or rebuilding a body part or organ.

transplant. Insertion of an organ or tissue from one person or site into another.

47146

47146   Backbench reconstruction of cadaver or living donor liver graft prior to allotransplantation; venous anastomosis, each

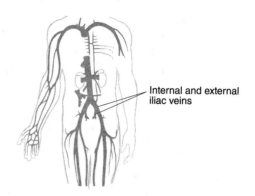

Internal and external iliac veins

Explanation

The physician performs venous anastomosis during a backbench reconstruction of cadaver or living donor liver graft prior to allotransplantation. Previously procured iliac vein grafts from the liver donor are anastomosed to the veins of the donor liver as required. Multiple grafts may be required depending on anatomical variations found in the liver donor. Code 47146 is reported for each venous graft performed.

Coding Tips

Liver transplantation involves three distinct components: donor hepatectomy, backbench work, and recipient liver allotransplantation. Do not report 47146 with 47120–47125, 47600, or 47610. Code 47140 reports a living donor hepatectomy, left lateral segment (II and III) only. For a total left lobectomy (segments II, III, and IV), see 47141; total right lobectomy (segments V, VI, VII, and VIII), see 47142. A living donor hepatectomy includes harvesting and cold preservation of the graft (perfusing with cold preservation solution and cold maintenance) and preoperative, intraoperative, and postoperative care of the donor. For a donor hepatectomy from a cadaver donor, see 47133. For liver allotransplantation, orthotopic, partial or whole, living donor or cadaver, any age, see 47135. For backbench preparation, see 47143–47147.

ICD-10-CM Diagnostic Codes

The application of this code is too broad to adequately present ICD-10-CM diagnostic code links here. Refer to your ICD-10-CM book.

AMA: **47146** 2014,Jan,11

Relative Value Units/Medicare Edits

Non-Facility RVU	Work	PE	MP	Total
47146	6.0	2.22	1.44	9.66
Facility RVU	Work	PE	MP	Total
47146	6.0	2.22	1.44	9.66

	FUD	Status	MUE	Modifiers				IOM Reference
47146	N/A	A	2(3)	51	N/A	62*	80	None

* with documentation

Liver

47147

47147   Backbench reconstruction of cadaver or living donor liver graft prior
         to allotransplantation; arterial anastomosis, each

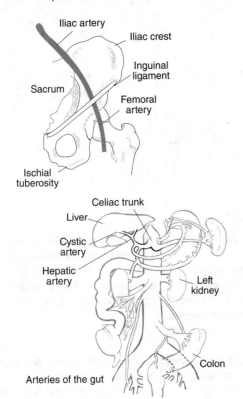

Explanation

The physician performs arterial anastomosis during a backbench reconstruction
of cadaver or living donor liver graft prior to allotransplantation. Previously
procured iliac artery grafts from the liver donor are anastomosed to the arteries
of the donor liver as required. Multiple grafts may be required depending on
anatomical variations found in the liver donor. Code 47147 is reported for
each artery graft performed.

Coding Tips

Liver transplantation involves three distinct components: donor hepatectomy,
backbench work, and recipient liver allotransplantation. Do not report 47147
with 47120–47125, 47600, or 47610. Code 47140 reports a living donor
hepatectomy, left lateral segment (II and III) only. For a total left lobectomy
(segments II, III, and IV), see 47141; total right lobectomy (segments V, VI, VII,
and VIII), see 47142. A living donor hepatectomy includes harvesting and cold
preservation of the graft (perfusing with cold preservation solution and cold
maintenance) and preoperative, intraoperative, and postoperative care of the
donor. For donor hepatectomy from a cadaver donor, see 47133. For liver
allotransplantation, orthotopic, partial or whole, living donor or cadaver, any
age, see 47135. For backbench preparation, see 47143–47147.

ICD-10-CM Diagnostic Codes

The application of this code is too broad to adequately present ICD-10-CM
diagnostic code links here. Refer to your ICD-10-CM book.

AMA: 47147 2014,Jan,11

Relative Value Units/Medicare Edits

Non-Facility RVU	Work	PE	MP	Total
47147	7.0	2.57	1.66	11.23
Facility RVU	Work	PE	MP	Total
47147	7.0	2.57	1.66	11.23

	FUD	Status	MUE	Modifiers				IOM Reference
47147	N/A	A	1(3)	51	N/A	62*	80	None

* with documentation

Terms To Know

anastomosis. Surgically created connection between ducts, blood vessels,
or bowel segments to allow flow from one to the other.

artery. Vessel through which oxygenated blood passes away from the heart
to any part of the body.

backbench preparation. Procedures performed on a donor organ following
procurement to prepare the organ for transplant into the recipient. Excess fat
and other tissue may be removed, the organ may be perfused, and vital arteries
may be sized, repaired, or modified to fit the patient. These procedures are
done on a back table in the operating room before transplantation can begin.

cadaver. Dead body.

donor. Person from whom tissues or organs are removed for transplantation.

graft. Tissue implant from another part of the body or another person.

lobectomy. Excision of a lobe of an organ such as the liver, thyroid, lung, or
brain.

reconstruction. Recreating, restoring, or rebuilding a body part or organ.

transplant. Insertion of an organ or tissue from one person or site into another.

Liver

47300

47300   Marsupialization of cyst or abscess of liver

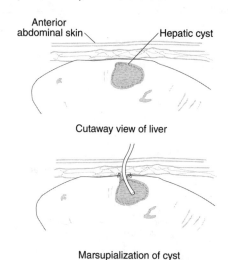

Cutaway view of liver

Marsupialization of cyst

Explanation

The physician creates a pouch with the lining of a cyst on the liver. The physician exposes the liver via an upper midline abdominal incision through skin, fascia, and muscles. The cyst is incised and suctioned with care not to contaminate the abdomen. Electrocautery is used to resect the cyst wall to allow open drainage into the abdomen. The abdominal incision is closed with sutures.

Coding Tips

For open drainage of an abscess or cyst, see 47010. For percutaneous, image-guided drainage of a hepatic abscess or cyst, via catheter, see 49405. For laparotomy with aspiration and/or injection of hepatic parasitic cysts or abscesses, see 47015.

ICD-10-CM Diagnostic Codes

A06.4   Amebic liver abscess
B67.0   Echinococcus granulosus infection of liver
B67.5   Echinococcus multilocularis infection of liver
K75.0   Abscess of liver
K75.89   Other specified inflammatory liver diseases
K76.89   Other specified diseases of liver
K77   Liver disorders in diseases classified elsewhere
Q44.6   Cystic disease of liver

AMA: **47300** 2014,Jan,11

Relative Value Units/Medicare Edits

Non-Facility RVU	Work	PE	MP	Total
47300	18.14	11.17	4.33	33.64
Facility RVU	Work	PE	MP	Total
47300	18.14	11.17	4.33	33.64

	FUD	Status	MUE	Modifiers				IOM Reference
47300	90	A	2(3)	51	N/A	62*	80	None

* with documentation

47350-47362

47350   Management of liver hemorrhage; simple suture of liver wound or injury
47360   complex suture of liver wound or injury, with or without hepatic artery ligation
47361   exploration of hepatic wound, extensive debridement, coagulation and/or suture, with or without packing of liver
47362   re-exploration of hepatic wound for removal of packing

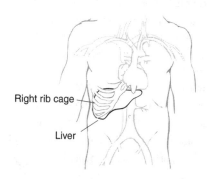

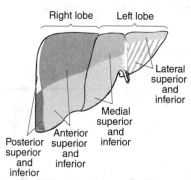

Explanation

The physician sutures a liver wound to control the bleeding or repair damage. In 47350, the physician exposes the liver via an upper midline abdominal incision. The abdomen is packed to control bleeding. The patient is stabilized hemodynamically. The liver is systematically exposed with pressure on bleeding points. The liver tissue is divided to expose the points of bleeding and the bleeding is controlled by ligation of bleeding vessels. The abdominal incision is closed. Report 47360 if the procedure requires a complex suture of liver wound or injury, with or without hepatic artery ligation; report 47361 if the procedure requires an exploration of a hepatic wound, extensive debridement, coagulation, and/or suture, with or without packing of the liver; and report 47362 if the procedure is a re-exploration of hepatic wound for removal of packing.

Coding Tips

Coding management of a liver hemorrhage and related repair is dependent on the extent of the injury (simple, complex, complex requiring extensive debridement, coagulation, and/or suturing).

ICD-10-CM Diagnostic Codes

K91.61   Intraoperative hemorrhage and hematoma of a digestive system organ or structure complicating a digestive system procedure
K91.62   Intraoperative hemorrhage and hematoma of a digestive system organ or structure complicating other procedure
K91.71   Accidental puncture and laceration of a digestive system organ or structure during a digestive system procedure

Liver

K91.72	Accidental puncture and laceration of a digestive system organ or structure during other procedure
K91.840	Postprocedural hemorrhage of a digestive system organ or structure following a digestive system procedure
K91.841	Postprocedural hemorrhage of a digestive system organ or structure following other procedure
K91.870	Postprocedural hematoma of a digestive system organ or structure following a digestive system procedure
K91.871	Postprocedural hematoma of a digestive system organ or structure following other procedure
K91.872	Postprocedural seroma of a digestive system organ or structure following a digestive system procedure
K91.873	Postprocedural seroma of a digestive system organ or structure following other procedure
S36.112A	Contusion of liver, initial encounter
S36.114A	Minor laceration of liver, initial encounter
S36.115A	Moderate laceration of liver, initial encounter
S36.116A	Major laceration of liver, initial encounter
S36.118A	Other injury of liver, initial encounter

AMA: 47350 2020,Oct,14 **47360** 2020,Oct,14 **47361** 2020,Oct,14 **47362** 2020,Jan,6

Relative Value Units/Medicare Edits

Non-Facility RVU	Work	PE	MP	Total
47350	22.49	12.75	5.27	40.51
47360	31.31	16.66	7.65	55.62
47361	52.6	24.48	12.11	89.19
47362	23.54	13.58	5.13	42.25
Facility RVU	Work	PE	MP	Total
47350	22.49	12.75	5.27	40.51
47360	31.31	16.66	7.65	55.62
47361	52.6	24.48	12.11	89.19
47362	23.54	13.58	5.13	42.25

	FUD	Status	MUE	Modifiers				IOM Reference
47350	90	A	1(3)	51	N/A	62*	80	None
47360	90	A	1(3)	51	N/A	62*	80	
47361	90	A	1(3)	51	N/A	62*	80	
47362	90	A	1(3)	51	N/A	62*	80	

* with documentation

Terms To Know

coagulation. Clot formation.

debridement. Removal of dead or contaminated tissue and foreign matter from a wound.

hemorrhage. Internal or external bleeding with loss of significant amounts of blood.

ligation. Tying off a blood vessel or duct with a suture or a soft, thin wire.

packing. Material placed into a cavity or wound, such as gels, gauze, pads, and sponges.

47370-47371

47370	Laparoscopy, surgical, ablation of 1 or more liver tumor(s); radiofrequency
47371	cryosurgical

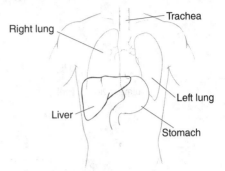

Liver tumors are ablated laparoscopically by radiofrequency or cryosurgery

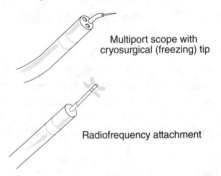

Multiport scope with cryosurgical (freezing) tip

Radiofrequency attachment

Explanation

The physician places a laparoscope via a small periumbilical port or through a small incision in the right upper quadrant, and an additional port is placed in the right upper quadrant under direct vision. Adhesions are lysed and ligamentous attachments divided to mobilize the liver. The physician examines all the parietal and visceral peritoneal surfaces, the lesser sac, the omentum, and the viscera. The gastrohepatic omentum is opened for inspection of the caudate lobe, followed by sequential laparoscopic ultrasonographic examination of all eight liver segments using an ultrasonic probe. Radiofrequency ablation is performed using a 15-gauge needle with a retractable curved electrode placed percutaneously into the abdomen at the place overlying the area of interest under direct vision. The needle is directed into the center of the lesion under real-time ultrasound guidance, tines are deployed, and alternating current is delivered to ablate the tumor. Upon completion of ablation, the probe tract is cauterized and the needle withdrawn. In microwave ablation, which is also part of the radiofrequency spectrum, microwaves are delivered from the needle to create a small region of heat that destroys the targeted cells. Report 47371 if ablation is accomplished using a cool-tipped multiple probe electrode.

Coding Tips

Do not report these codes more than once during a surgical session unless a different method of ablation (e.g., cryosurgical and radiofrequency) is performed. Imaging guidance is reported with 76940, when performed. For open ablation of one or more liver tumors, radiofrequency, see 47380; cryosurgery, see 47381; percutaneous, see 47382.

ICD-10-CM Diagnostic Codes

C22.0	Liver cell carcinoma

C22.1	Intrahepatic bile duct carcinoma
C22.2	Hepatoblastoma
C22.3	Angiosarcoma of liver
C22.4	Other sarcomas of liver
C22.7	Other specified carcinomas of liver
C78.7	Secondary malignant neoplasm of liver and intrahepatic bile duct
C7B.02	Secondary carcinoid tumors of liver
C7B.8	Other secondary neuroendocrine tumors
D01.5	Carcinoma in situ of liver, gallbladder and bile ducts
D13.4	Benign neoplasm of liver
D13.5	Benign neoplasm of extrahepatic bile ducts
D37.6	Neoplasm of uncertain behavior of liver, gallbladder and bile ducts
K76.89	Other specified diseases of liver

AMA: **47370** 2018,Jan,8; 2017,Jan,8; 2016,Jan,13; 2015,Jan,16

Relative Value Units/Medicare Edits

Non-Facility RVU	Work	PE	MP	Total
47370	20.8	11.22	4.95	36.97
47371	20.8	11.37	5.08	37.25
Facility RVU	**Work**	**PE**	**MP**	**Total**
47370	20.8	11.22	4.95	36.97
47371	20.8	11.37	5.08	37.25

	FUD	Status	MUE	Modifiers				IOM Reference
47370	90	A	1(2)	51	N/A	62*	80	None
47371	90	A	1(2)	51	N/A	62*	80	

* with documentation

Terms To Know

ablation. Removal or destruction of a body part or tissue or its function. Ablation may be performed by surgical means, hormones, drugs, radiofrequency, heat, chemical application, or other methods.

adhesion. Abnormal fibrous connection between two structures, soft tissue or bony structures, that may occur as the result of surgery, infection, or trauma.

carcinoid tumor. Specific type of slow-growing neuroendocrine tumors. Carcinoid tumors occur most commonly in the hormone producing cells of the gastrointestinal tracts and can also occur in the pancreas, testes, ovaries, or lungs.

carcinoma. Malignant growth of epithelial cells in the coverings and linings of organs and tissues. The cells tend to spread to other locations via the bloodstream or lymphatic channels.

cryosurgery. Application of intense cold, usually produced using liquid nitrogen, to locally freeze diseased or unwanted tissue and induce tissue necrosis without causing harm to adjacent tissue.

lesion. Area of damaged tissue that has lost continuity or function, due to disease or trauma. Lesions may be located on internal structures such as the brain, nerves, or kidneys, or visible on the skin.

47380-47381

47380 Ablation, open, of 1 or more liver tumor(s); radiofrequency
47381 cryosurgical

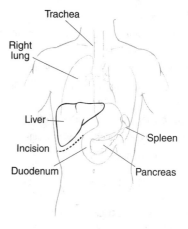

Explanation

The physician performs radiofrequency ablation of a liver tumor via an open laparotomy. Grounding pads are placed on the patient's legs. The physician performs a midline laparotomy. Dissection is carried down to the liver. Under direct visualization, a needle-electrode, with an insulated shaft and an uninsulated distal tip, is inserted into the tumor. Each treatment session has about 10 to 15 minutes of active ablation. The energy at the needle tip causes ionic agitation and frictional heat in the surrounding tissue, which, when hot enough, leads to cell death and coagulative necrosis. This results in a 3 to 5.5 cm sphere of dead tissue per treatment session. In large tumors, the physician may create more than one sphere next to each other to try to turn the tumor edges in three dimensions. A small margin of normal tissue next to the tumor is also burned, as a precaution to destroy all tumor cells. The tumor cells are not removed, but are gradually replaced by fibrosis and scar tissue. One method uses a needle-within-a-needle electrode system with an inner needle that expands once placed into the tumor. In 47381, the physician performs cryosurgical ablation of a liver tumor. The physician performs a laparotomy. Dissection is carrier down to the liver. Cryosurgical probes are inserted into the liver tumor. The cryosurgical probes rapidly freeze (liquid nitrogen at -196°C or nitrous oxide at -89.5°C) the area being treated, the liver tissue is slowly thawed, and repeated cycles of freezing and thawing are immediately performed. Cryogen may also be applied directly into or on to the tumor by probe, direct application, spraying, or by pouring. The incision is closed with layered sutures.

Coding Tips

Imaging guidance is reported with 76940, when performed. Report percutaneous ablation of one or more liver tumors via radiofrequency with 47382; via cryoablation, see 47383. For laparoscopic ablation of one or more liver tumors, radiofrequency, see 47370; cryosurgery, see 47371.

ICD-10-CM Diagnostic Codes

C22.0	Liver cell carcinoma
C22.1	Intrahepatic bile duct carcinoma
C22.2	Hepatoblastoma
C22.3	Angiosarcoma of liver
C22.4	Other sarcomas of liver
C22.7	Other specified carcinomas of liver

Liver

C78.7	Secondary malignant neoplasm of liver and intrahepatic bile duct
C7A.1	Malignant poorly differentiated neuroendocrine tumors
C7A.8	Other malignant neuroendocrine tumors
C7B.02	Secondary carcinoid tumors of liver
C7B.8	Other secondary neuroendocrine tumors
D01.5	Carcinoma in situ of liver, gallbladder and bile ducts
D13.4	Benign neoplasm of liver
D13.5	Benign neoplasm of extrahepatic bile ducts
D37.6	Neoplasm of uncertain behavior of liver, gallbladder and bile ducts
D3A.098	Benign carcinoid tumors of other sites
D49.0	Neoplasm of unspecified behavior of digestive system
K76.89	Other specified diseases of liver

AMA: **47380** 2018,Jan,8; 2017,Jan,8; 2016,Jan,13; 2015,Jan,16

Relative Value Units/Medicare Edits

Non-Facility RVU	Work	PE	MP	Total
47380	24.56	12.52	5.57	42.65
47381	24.88	12.88	6.09	43.85
Facility RVU	**Work**	**PE**	**MP**	**Total**
47380	24.56	12.52	5.57	42.65
47381	24.88	12.88	6.09	43.85

	FUD	Status	MUE	Modifiers				IOM Reference
47380	90	A	1(2)	51	N/A	62*	80	None
47381	90	A	1(2)	51	N/A	62*	80	

* with documentation

Terms To Know

ablation. Removal or destruction of tissue by cutting, electrical energy, chemical substances, or excessive heat application.

cryosurgery. Application of intense cold, usually produced using liquid nitrogen, to locally freeze diseased or unwanted tissue and induce tissue necrosis without causing harm to adjacent tissue.

fibrosis. Formation of fibrous tissue as part of the restorative process.

radiofrequency ablation. To destroy by electromagnetic wave frequencies.

sarcoma. Malignant tumor arising in connective tissue, bone, cartilage, or striated muscle that spreads to neighboring tissue through the bloodstream.

47382-47383

47382   Ablation, 1 or more liver tumor(s), percutaneous, radiofrequency
47383   Ablation, 1 or more liver tumor(s), percutaneous, cryoablation

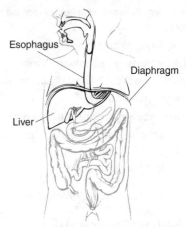

Liver tumors are ablated percutaneously

Explanation

Intravenous sedation is administered and grounding pads are placed on the patient's legs. A needle-electrode, with an insulated shaft and an uninsulated distal tip, is inserted through the skin and directly into the tumor. Ultrasound, CT scan, or MRI guide the needles to the correct spot and monitor treatment. Each treatment session has about 10 to 15 minutes of active ablation. Report 47382 when the energy at the needle tip causes ionic agitation and frictional heat in the surrounding tissue, which, when hot enough, leads to cell death and coagulative necrosis. This results in a 3 to 5.5 cm sphere of dead tissue per treatment session. In large tumors, the physician may create more than one sphere next to each other to try to turn the tumor edges in three dimensions. A small margin of normal tissue next to the tumor is also burned, as a precaution to destroy all tumor cells. The tumor cells are not removed, but are gradually replaced by fibrosis and scar tissue. One method uses a needle-within-a-needle electrode system with an inner needle that expands once placed into the tumor. Report 47383 when the physician performs cryosurgical ablation of a liver tumor. Cryosurgical probes are inserted into the liver tumor. The cryosurgical probes rapidly freeze the area being treated (liquid nitrogen at -196°C or nitrous oxide at -89.5°C), the liver tissue is slowly thawed, and repeated cycles of freezing and thawing are immediately performed. Cryogen may also be applied directly into or onto the tumor by probe, direct application, spraying, or pouring.

Coding Tips

Imaging guidance and monitoring, when performed, is reported with 76940, 77013, or 77022. For laparoscopic ablation of one or more liver tumors, radiofrequency, see 47370; cryosurgery, see 47371. Report open ablation of one or more liver tumors via radiofrequency with 47380; via cryosurgical, see 47381.

ICD-10-CM Diagnostic Codes

C22.0	Liver cell carcinoma
C22.1	Intrahepatic bile duct carcinoma
C22.2	Hepatoblastoma
C22.3	Angiosarcoma of liver
C22.4	Other sarcomas of liver
C22.7	Other specified carcinomas of liver

Liver

C78.7	Secondary malignant neoplasm of liver and intrahepatic bile duct
C7A.1	Malignant poorly differentiated neuroendocrine tumors
C7A.8	Other malignant neuroendocrine tumors
C7B.02	Secondary carcinoid tumors of liver
C7B.8	Other secondary neuroendocrine tumors
D01.5	Carcinoma in situ of liver, gallbladder and bile ducts
D13.4	Benign neoplasm of liver
D13.5	Benign neoplasm of extrahepatic bile ducts
D37.6	Neoplasm of uncertain behavior of liver, gallbladder and bile ducts
D3A.098	Benign carcinoid tumors of other sites
D49.0	Neoplasm of unspecified behavior of digestive system
K76.89	Other specified diseases of liver

AMA: **47382** 2018,Jan,8; 2017,Jan,8; 2016,Jan,13; 2015,Jan,16 **47383** 2018,Jan,8; 2017,Jan,8; 2016,Jan,13; 2015,Jan,16

Relative Value Units/Medicare Edits

Non-Facility RVU	Work	PE	MP	Total
47382	14.97	108.3	1.34	124.61
47383	8.88	187.57	0.77	197.22
Facility RVU	**Work**	**PE**	**MP**	**Total**
47382	14.97	5.04	1.34	21.35
47383	8.88	3.26	0.77	12.91

	FUD	Status	MUE	Modifiers				IOM Reference
47382	10	A	1(2)	51	N/A	N/A	N/A	None
47383	10	A	1(2)	51	N/A	N/A	N/A	

* with documentation

Terms To Know

cryosurgery. Application of intense cold, usually produced using liquid nitrogen, to locally freeze diseased or unwanted tissue and induce tissue necrosis without causing harm to adjacent tissue.

radiofrequency ablation. To destroy by electromagnetic wave frequencies.

Liver

47400

47400 Hepaticotomy or hepaticostomy with exploration, drainage, or removal of calculus

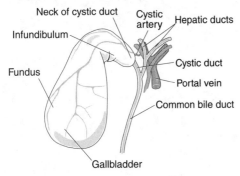

Neck of cystic duct

Cystic artery

Hepatic ducts

Infundibulum

Cystic duct

Fundus

Portal vein

Common bile duct

Gallbladder

A calculus may be removed through an incision into the common bile duct

Explanation

The physician makes a midline abdominal incision. The physician makes an incision into the hepatic duct and surgically creates an artificial opening. The physician performs exploration, drainage, or removal of calculus from the hepatic duct. The hepatic duct is closed primarily or around a tube for continued drainage. If a drainage tube is placed, a separate incision is made in the abdominal wall through which the drainage tube is positioned. The abdominal incisions are closed.

Coding Tips

Do not confuse hepaticotomy or hepaticostomy with hepatotomy, which is used to describe an incision into the liver itself. For hepatotomy, see 47010. For percutaneous, image-guided drainage of a hepatic abscess or cyst, via catheter, see 49405.

ICD-10-CM Diagnostic Codes

K80.32	Calculus of bile duct with acute cholangitis without obstruction
K80.33	Calculus of bile duct with acute cholangitis with obstruction
K80.34	Calculus of bile duct with chronic cholangitis without obstruction
K80.35	Calculus of bile duct with chronic cholangitis with obstruction
K80.36	Calculus of bile duct with acute and chronic cholangitis without obstruction
K80.37	Calculus of bile duct with acute and chronic cholangitis with obstruction
K80.42	Calculus of bile duct with acute cholecystitis without obstruction
K80.43	Calculus of bile duct with acute cholecystitis with obstruction
K80.44	Calculus of bile duct with chronic cholecystitis without obstruction
K80.45	Calculus of bile duct with chronic cholecystitis with obstruction
K80.46	Calculus of bile duct with acute and chronic cholecystitis without obstruction
K80.47	Calculus of bile duct with acute and chronic cholecystitis with obstruction
K80.50	Calculus of bile duct without cholangitis or cholecystitis without obstruction
K80.51	Calculus of bile duct without cholangitis or cholecystitis with obstruction
K80.62	Calculus of gallbladder and bile duct with acute cholecystitis without obstruction
K80.63	Calculus of gallbladder and bile duct with acute cholecystitis with obstruction
K80.64	Calculus of gallbladder and bile duct with chronic cholecystitis without obstruction
K80.65	Calculus of gallbladder and bile duct with chronic cholecystitis with obstruction
K80.66	Calculus of gallbladder and bile duct with acute and chronic cholecystitis without obstruction
K80.67	Calculus of gallbladder and bile duct with acute and chronic cholecystitis with obstruction
K80.70	Calculus of gallbladder and bile duct without cholecystitis without obstruction
K80.71	Calculus of gallbladder and bile duct without cholecystitis with obstruction
K80.80	Other cholelithiasis without obstruction
K80.81	Other cholelithiasis with obstruction
K83.1	Obstruction of bile duct

AMA: 47400 2014,Jan,11

Relative Value Units/Medicare Edits

Non-Facility RVU	Work	PE	MP	Total
47400	36.36	18.54	8.89	63.79
Facility RVU	**Work**	**PE**	**MP**	**Total**
47400	36.36	18.54	8.89	63.79

	FUD	Status	MUE	Modifiers				IOM Reference
47400	90	A	1(3)	51	N/A	62*	80	None

* with documentation

Terms To Know

calculus. Abnormal, stone-like concretion of calcium, cholesterol, mineral salts, or other substances that forms in any part of the body.

cholecystitis. Inflammation of the gallbladder. Acute cholecystitis is most often the result of an obstruction at the outlet of the gallbladder, with consequent edema and congestion that can progress to serious cases of gangrene and perforation. Chronic cholecystitis is a mild symptomatic inflammation of the gallbladder that continues over a long period. Acute and chronic forms may also occur together.

drain. Device that creates a channel to allow fluid from a cavity, wound, or infected area to exit the body.

exploration. Examination for diagnostic purposes.

obstruction. Blockage that prevents normal function of the valve or structure.

Biliary Tract

47420 Choledochotomy or choledochostomy with exploration, drainage, or removal of calculus, with or without cholecystotomy; without transduodenal sphincterotomy or sphincteroplasty

47425 with transduodenal sphincterotomy or sphincteroplasty

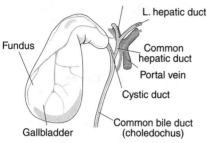

Explanation

The physician explores the common bile duct, removing calculus, draining purulent matter, and/or constructing a new duct. The physician exposes the common bile duct within the portal triad through a subcostal or upper midline incision. The common bile duct is incised, explored, and drained. The common bile duct is closed with interrupted sutures primarily or around a drainage tube (choledochostomy). If placed, the drainage tube is brought out through the skin at a site separate from the incision. The abdominal incision is closed. Report 47425 if this procedure is performed with transduodenal sphincterotomy or sphincteroplasty.

Coding Tips

Intraoperative biliary endoscopy is reported with 47550, when performed. These procedures can also be performed endoscopically by means of endoscopic cholangiopancreatography (ERCP). For ERCP with endoscopic removal of stones (calculus), see 43264; with endoscopic retrograde destruction (lithotripsy) of stones, see 43265; with sphincterotomy/papillotomy, see 43262.

ICD-10-CM Diagnostic Codes

C23	Malignant neoplasm of gallbladder
C24.0	Malignant neoplasm of extrahepatic bile duct
C24.1	Malignant neoplasm of ampulla of Vater
C24.8	Malignant neoplasm of overlapping sites of biliary tract
K80.32	Calculus of bile duct with acute cholangitis without obstruction
K80.33	Calculus of bile duct with acute cholangitis with obstruction
K80.34	Calculus of bile duct with chronic cholangitis without obstruction
K80.35	Calculus of bile duct with chronic cholangitis with obstruction
K80.36	Calculus of bile duct with acute and chronic cholangitis without obstruction
K80.37	Calculus of bile duct with acute and chronic cholangitis with obstruction
K80.42	Calculus of bile duct with acute cholecystitis without obstruction
K80.43	Calculus of bile duct with acute cholecystitis with obstruction
K80.44	Calculus of bile duct with chronic cholecystitis without obstruction
K80.45	Calculus of bile duct with chronic cholecystitis with obstruction
K80.46	Calculus of bile duct with acute and chronic cholecystitis without obstruction
K80.47	Calculus of bile duct with acute and chronic cholecystitis with obstruction
K80.50	Calculus of bile duct without cholangitis or cholecystitis without obstruction
K80.51	Calculus of bile duct without cholangitis or cholecystitis with obstruction
K80.62	Calculus of gallbladder and bile duct with acute cholecystitis without obstruction
K80.63	Calculus of gallbladder and bile duct with acute cholecystitis with obstruction
K80.64	Calculus of gallbladder and bile duct with chronic cholecystitis without obstruction
K80.65	Calculus of gallbladder and bile duct with chronic cholecystitis with obstruction
K80.66	Calculus of gallbladder and bile duct with acute and chronic cholecystitis without obstruction
K80.67	Calculus of gallbladder and bile duct with acute and chronic cholecystitis with obstruction
K80.70	Calculus of gallbladder and bile duct without cholecystitis without obstruction
K80.71	Calculus of gallbladder and bile duct without cholecystitis with obstruction
K80.80	Other cholelithiasis without obstruction
K80.81	Other cholelithiasis with obstruction
K81.0	Acute cholecystitis
K81.1	Chronic cholecystitis
K81.2	Acute cholecystitis with chronic cholecystitis
K83.01	Primary sclerosing cholangitis
K83.09	Other cholangitis
K83.1	Obstruction of bile duct
K83.2	Perforation of bile duct
K83.3	Fistula of bile duct
K83.4	Spasm of sphincter of Oddi
K83.5	Biliary cyst
K83.8	Other specified diseases of biliary tract
K85.00	Idiopathic acute pancreatitis without necrosis or infection
K85.01	Idiopathic acute pancreatitis with uninfected necrosis
K85.02	Idiopathic acute pancreatitis with infected necrosis
K85.10	Biliary acute pancreatitis without necrosis or infection
K85.11	Biliary acute pancreatitis with uninfected necrosis
K85.12	Biliary acute pancreatitis with infected necrosis
K85.20	Alcohol induced acute pancreatitis without necrosis or infection
K85.21	Alcohol induced acute pancreatitis with uninfected necrosis
K85.22	Alcohol induced acute pancreatitis with infected necrosis
K85.30	Drug induced acute pancreatitis without necrosis or infection
K85.31	Drug induced acute pancreatitis with uninfected necrosis
K85.32	Drug induced acute pancreatitis with infected necrosis
K85.80	Other acute pancreatitis without necrosis or infection
K85.81	Other acute pancreatitis with uninfected necrosis
K85.82	Other acute pancreatitis with infected necrosis
K86.0	Alcohol-induced chronic pancreatitis
K86.1	Other chronic pancreatitis

AMA: **47420** 2014,Jan,11 **47425** 2014,Jan,11

Biliary Tract

Relative Value Units/Medicare Edits

Non-Facility RVU	Work	PE	MP	Total
47420	22.03	12.3	5.18	39.51
47425	22.31	12.83	5.47	40.61
Facility RVU	**Work**	**PE**	**MP**	**Total**
47420	22.03	12.3	5.18	39.51
47425	22.31	12.83	5.47	40.61

	FUD	Status	MUE	Modifiers				IOM Reference
47420	90	A	1(2)	51	N/A	62*	80	None
47425	90	A	1(2)	51	N/A	62*	80	

* with documentation

Terms To Know

acute. Sudden, severe.

calcification. Normal process of calcium salts deposition in bone. Calcification can also occur abnormally in fibroconnective soft tissues.

calculus. Abnormal, stone-like concretion of calcium, cholesterol, mineral salts, or other substances that forms in any part of the body.

cholecystitis. Inflammation of the gallbladder. Acute cholecystitis is most often the result of an obstruction at the outlet of the gallbladder, with consequent edema and congestion that can progress to serious cases of gangrene and perforation. Chronic cholecystitis is a mild symptomatic inflammation of the gallbladder that continues over a long period. Acute and chronic forms may also occur together.

choledochotomy. Surgical incision into the common bile duct for exploration or for the removal of stones.

chronic. Persistent, continuing, or recurring.

drainage. Releasing, taking, or letting out fluids and/or gases from a body part.

pancreatitis. Inflammation of the pancreas that may be acute or chronic, symptomatic or asymptomatic, due to the autodigestion of pancreatic tissue by its own enzymes that have escaped into the pancreas, most often as a result of alcoholism or biliary tract disease such as calculi in the pancreatic duct.

sphincteroplasty. Surgical repair done to correct, augment, or improve the muscular function of a sphincter, such as the anus or intestines.

47460

47460 Transduodenal sphincterotomy or sphincteroplasty, with or without transduodenal extraction of calculus (separate procedure)

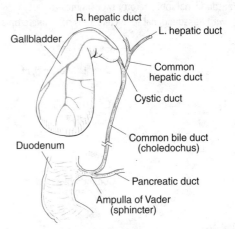

The common bile duct and the main pancreatic duct usually converge and enter the duodenum through a sphincter known as the ampulla of Vater

Explanation

The physician performs a transduodenal sphincterotomy or sphincteroplasty and may repair the duodenal sphincter or remove a stone, as needed. The physician exposes the second portion of the duodenum via a subcostal or upper midline incision through skin, fascia, and muscle. The duodenum is opened using a longitudinal incision. The ampulla of Vater is identified and an incision is made in the ampulla at the two o'clock position. The common bile duct mucosa may be reapproximated to the duodenal mucosa and the duodenum transversely closed with interrupted sutures. Stones may be removed. The abdominal incision is closed.

Coding Tips

This separate procedure by definition is usually a component of a more complex service and is not identified separately. When performed alone or with other unrelated procedures/services it may be reported. If performed alone, list the code; if performed with other procedures/services, list the code and append modifier 59 or an X{EPSU} modifier. When this procedure is combined with choledochotomy or choledochostomy, report 47425 instead. This procedure can also be performed endoscopically by means of endoscopic cholangiopancreatography (ERCP). For ERCP with endoscopic removal of stones (calculus), see 43264; with endoscopic retrograde destruction (lithotripsy) of stones, see 43265; with sphincterotomy/papillotomy, see 43262.

ICD-10-CM Diagnostic Codes

C24.0	Malignant neoplasm of extrahepatic bile duct
C24.1	Malignant neoplasm of ampulla of Vater
K80.32	Calculus of bile duct with acute cholangitis without obstruction
K80.33	Calculus of bile duct with acute cholangitis with obstruction
K80.34	Calculus of bile duct with chronic cholangitis without obstruction
K80.35	Calculus of bile duct with chronic cholangitis with obstruction
K80.36	Calculus of bile duct with acute and chronic cholangitis without obstruction
K80.37	Calculus of bile duct with acute and chronic cholangitis with obstruction
K80.42	Calculus of bile duct with acute cholecystitis without obstruction
K80.43	Calculus of bile duct with acute cholecystitis with obstruction

K80.44	Calculus of bile duct with chronic cholecystitis without obstruction
K80.45	Calculus of bile duct with chronic cholecystitis with obstruction
K80.46	Calculus of bile duct with acute and chronic cholecystitis without obstruction
K80.47	Calculus of bile duct with acute and chronic cholecystitis with obstruction
K80.50	Calculus of bile duct without cholangitis or cholecystitis without obstruction
K80.51	Calculus of bile duct without cholangitis or cholecystitis with obstruction
K80.62	Calculus of gallbladder and bile duct with acute cholecystitis without obstruction
K80.63	Calculus of gallbladder and bile duct with acute cholecystitis with obstruction
K80.64	Calculus of gallbladder and bile duct with chronic cholecystitis without obstruction
K80.65	Calculus of gallbladder and bile duct with chronic cholecystitis with obstruction
K80.66	Calculus of gallbladder and bile duct with acute and chronic cholecystitis without obstruction
K80.67	Calculus of gallbladder and bile duct with acute and chronic cholecystitis with obstruction
K80.70	Calculus of gallbladder and bile duct without cholecystitis without obstruction
K80.71	Calculus of gallbladder and bile duct without cholecystitis with obstruction
K81.0	Acute cholecystitis
K81.1	Chronic cholecystitis
K81.2	Acute cholecystitis with chronic cholecystitis
K83.01	Primary sclerosing cholangitis
K83.09	Other cholangitis
K83.1	Obstruction of bile duct
K83.2	Perforation of bile duct
K83.3	Fistula of bile duct
K83.4	Spasm of sphincter of Oddi
K83.5	Biliary cyst
K83.8	Other specified diseases of biliary tract
K85.00	Idiopathic acute pancreatitis without necrosis or infection
K85.01	Idiopathic acute pancreatitis with uninfected necrosis
K85.02	Idiopathic acute pancreatitis with infected necrosis
K85.10	Biliary acute pancreatitis without necrosis or infection
K85.11	Biliary acute pancreatitis with uninfected necrosis
K85.12	Biliary acute pancreatitis with infected necrosis
K85.20	Alcohol induced acute pancreatitis without necrosis or infection
K85.21	Alcohol induced acute pancreatitis with uninfected necrosis
K85.22	Alcohol induced acute pancreatitis with infected necrosis
K85.30	Drug induced acute pancreatitis without necrosis or infection
K85.31	Drug induced acute pancreatitis with uninfected necrosis
K85.32	Drug induced acute pancreatitis with infected necrosis
K85.80	Other acute pancreatitis without necrosis or infection
K85.81	Other acute pancreatitis with uninfected necrosis
K85.82	Other acute pancreatitis with infected necrosis
K86.0	Alcohol-induced chronic pancreatitis
K86.1	Other chronic pancreatitis

K86.2	Cyst of pancreas
K86.3	Pseudocyst of pancreas
K90.3	Pancreatic steatorrhea

AMA: 47460 2014,Jan,11

Relative Value Units/Medicare Edits

Non-Facility RVU	Work	PE	MP	Total
47460	20.52	12.18	5.0	37.7
Facility RVU	**Work**	**PE**	**MP**	**Total**
47460	20.52	12.18	5.0	37.7

	FUD	Status	MUE	Modifiers				IOM Reference
47460	90	A	1(2)	51	N/A	62*	80	None

* with documentation

Terms To Know

ampulla of Vater. Tubular structure with flask-like dilation where the common bile and pancreatic ducts join before emptying into the duodenum.

anomaly. Irregularity in the structure or position of an organ or tissue.

calculus. Abnormal, stone-like concretion of calcium, cholesterol, mineral salts, or other substances that forms in any part of the body.

chronic. Persistent, continuing, or recurring.

duodenum. First portion of the small intestine connected to the stomach at the pylorus and extending to the jejunum.

extraction. Removal of a tooth and tooth fragments from the alveolus.

jaundice. Increased bilirubin and deposits of bile pigment in the skin and sclera, causing a yellow tint.

malignant neoplasm. Any cancerous tumor or lesion exhibiting uncontrolled tissue growth that can progressively invade other parts of the body with its disease-generating cells.

sphincteroplasty. Surgical repair done to correct, augment, or improve the muscular function of a sphincter, such as the anus or intestines.

47480

47480 Cholecystotomy or cholecystostomy, open, with exploration, drainage, or removal of calculus (separate procedure)

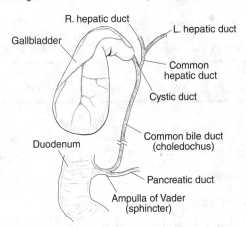

The common bile duct and the main pancreatic duct usually converge and enter the duodenum through a sphincter known as the ampulla of Vater

Explanation

The physician performs an open cholecystotomy or cholecystostomy with exploration, drainage, or removal of calculus. The physician exposes the gallbladder through a subcostal or upper midline incision. The gallbladder is incised, explored, and may be drained. Calculi may be removed. The gallbladder is closed with interrupted sutures primarily or around a drainage tube. If placed, the drainage tube is brought out through the skin at a site separate from the incision. The abdominal incision is closed.

Coding Tips

This separate procedure by definition is usually a component of a more complex service and is not identified separately. When performed alone or with other unrelated procedures/services it may be reported. If performed alone, list the code; if performed with other procedures/services, list the code and append modifier 59 or an X{EPSU} modifier. For percutaneous cholecystostomy, report 47490. This procedure can also be performed endoscopically by means of endoscopic cholangiopancreatography (ERCP). For ERCP with endoscopic removal of stones (calculus), see 43264; with endoscopic retrograde destruction (lithotripsy) of stones, see 43265; with sphincterotomy/papillotomy, see 43262.

ICD-10-CM Diagnostic Codes

C23	Malignant neoplasm of gallbladder
K80.00	Calculus of gallbladder with acute cholecystitis without obstruction
K80.01	Calculus of gallbladder with acute cholecystitis with obstruction
K80.10	Calculus of gallbladder with chronic cholecystitis without obstruction
K80.11	Calculus of gallbladder with chronic cholecystitis with obstruction
K80.12	Calculus of gallbladder with acute and chronic cholecystitis without obstruction
K80.13	Calculus of gallbladder with acute and chronic cholecystitis with obstruction
K80.18	Calculus of gallbladder with other cholecystitis without obstruction
K80.19	Calculus of gallbladder with other cholecystitis with obstruction
K80.20	Calculus of gallbladder without cholecystitis without obstruction
K80.21	Calculus of gallbladder without cholecystitis with obstruction
K80.62	Calculus of gallbladder and bile duct with acute cholecystitis without obstruction
K80.63	Calculus of gallbladder and bile duct with acute cholecystitis with obstruction
K80.64	Calculus of gallbladder and bile duct with chronic cholecystitis without obstruction
K80.65	Calculus of gallbladder and bile duct with chronic cholecystitis with obstruction
K80.66	Calculus of gallbladder and bile duct with acute and chronic cholecystitis without obstruction
K80.67	Calculus of gallbladder and bile duct with acute and chronic cholecystitis with obstruction
K80.70	Calculus of gallbladder and bile duct without cholecystitis without obstruction
K80.71	Calculus of gallbladder and bile duct without cholecystitis with obstruction
K80.80	Other cholelithiasis without obstruction
K80.81	Other cholelithiasis with obstruction
K81.0	Acute cholecystitis
K81.1	Chronic cholecystitis
K81.2	Acute cholecystitis with chronic cholecystitis
K82.0	Obstruction of gallbladder
K82.1	Hydrops of gallbladder
K82.2	Perforation of gallbladder
K82.3	Fistula of gallbladder
K82.4	Cholesterolosis of gallbladder
K82.8	Other specified diseases of gallbladder
K87	Disorders of gallbladder, biliary tract and pancreas in diseases classified elsewhere

AMA: **47480** 2018,Jan,8; 2017,Jan,8; 2016,Jan,13; 2015,Jan,16

Relative Value Units/Medicare Edits

Non-Facility RVU	Work	PE	MP	Total
47480	13.25	9.75	3.1	26.1
Facility RVU	**Work**	**PE**	**MP**	**Total**
47480	13.25	9.75	3.1	26.1

	FUD	Status	MUE	Modifiers				IOM Reference
47480	90	A	1(2)	51	N/A	62*	80	None

* with documentation

47490

47490 Cholecystostomy, percutaneous, complete procedure, including imaging guidance, catheter placement, cholecystogram when performed, and radiological supervision and interpretation

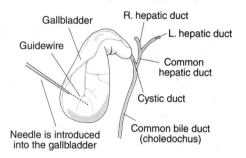

Needle is introduced into the gallbladder

The gallbladder is accessed percutaneously

Explanation

The physician inserts a tube into the gallbladder to allow drainage through the skin. The physician uses ultrasound guidance to place a subcostal drainage tube into the gallbladder. The physician places a needle between the ribs into the gallbladder. The needle position is checked by aspiration. A guidewire is passed through the needle. A catheter is passed over the wire into the biliary tree. The wire is removed and the tube is left in place. This code reports the complete procedure and includes placement of the catheter under image guidance, a cholecystogram if performed, and radiological supervision and interpretation.

Coding Tips

Do not report 47490 with 47531, 47532, 75989, 76942, 77002, 77012, or 77021. Radiological supervision and interpretation is included in the code descriptor. For open cholecystotomy or cholecystostomy, see 47480.

ICD-10-CM Diagnostic Codes

C23	Malignant neoplasm of gallbladder
K80.00	Calculus of gallbladder with acute cholecystitis without obstruction
K80.01	Calculus of gallbladder with acute cholecystitis with obstruction
K80.10	Calculus of gallbladder with chronic cholecystitis without obstruction
K80.11	Calculus of gallbladder with chronic cholecystitis with obstruction
K80.12	Calculus of gallbladder with acute and chronic cholecystitis without obstruction
K80.13	Calculus of gallbladder with acute and chronic cholecystitis with obstruction
K80.18	Calculus of gallbladder with other cholecystitis without obstruction
K80.19	Calculus of gallbladder with other cholecystitis with obstruction
K80.20	Calculus of gallbladder without cholecystitis without obstruction
K80.21	Calculus of gallbladder without cholecystitis with obstruction
K80.62	Calculus of gallbladder and bile duct with acute cholecystitis without obstruction
K80.63	Calculus of gallbladder and bile duct with acute cholecystitis with obstruction
K80.64	Calculus of gallbladder and bile duct with chronic cholecystitis without obstruction
K80.65	Calculus of gallbladder and bile duct with chronic cholecystitis with obstruction
K80.66	Calculus of gallbladder and bile duct with acute and chronic cholecystitis without obstruction
K80.67	Calculus of gallbladder and bile duct with acute and chronic cholecystitis with obstruction
K80.70	Calculus of gallbladder and bile duct without cholecystitis without obstruction
K80.71	Calculus of gallbladder and bile duct without cholecystitis with obstruction
K80.80	Other cholelithiasis without obstruction
K80.81	Other cholelithiasis with obstruction
K81.0	Acute cholecystitis
K81.1	Chronic cholecystitis
K81.2	Acute cholecystitis with chronic cholecystitis
K82.0	Obstruction of gallbladder
K82.1	Hydrops of gallbladder
K82.2	Perforation of gallbladder
K82.3	Fistula of gallbladder
K82.4	Cholesterolosis of gallbladder
K82.8	Other specified diseases of gallbladder
K87	Disorders of gallbladder, biliary tract and pancreas in diseases classified elsewhere

AMA: **47490** 2018,Jan,8; 2017,Jan,8; 2016,Jan,13; 2015,Jan,16; 2015,Dec,3

Relative Value Units/Medicare Edits

Non-Facility RVU	Work	PE	MP	Total
47490	4.76	4.55	0.42	9.73
Facility RVU	**Work**	**PE**	**MP**	**Total**
47490	4.76	4.55	0.42	9.73

	FUD	Status	MUE	Modifiers				IOM Reference
47490	10	A	1(2)	51	N/A	N/A	N/A	None

* with documentation

Biliary Tract

47531-47532

47531 Injection procedure for cholangiography, percutaneous, complete diagnostic procedure including imaging guidance (eg, ultrasound and/or fluoroscopy) and all associated radiological supervision and interpretation; existing access

47532 new access (eg, percutaneous transhepatic cholangiogram)

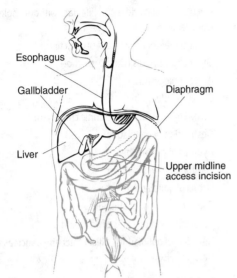

Percutaneous access for cholangiography injection

Explanation

A radiographic medium is injected into the common bile duct, gallbladder, and/or liver for diagnostic purposes. The physician inserts a needle between the ribs into the lumen of the common bile duct and checks positioning by aspiration. Radiographic dye is injected. The needle is removed. This procedure includes imaging guidance and all radiological supervision and interpretation. Report 47531 when the service is performed through an existing access, such as a T-tube. Report 47532 when the service is performed via a new access.

Coding Tips

These codes include contrast material injections. Note that 47532 also includes needle or catheter access of the biliary system. Do not report 47531–47532 in addition to 47490 or 47533–47541 when procedures are performed percutaneously through the same access site. For cholangiography performed intraoperatively, see 74300–74301.

ICD-10-CM Diagnostic Codes

C22.0	Liver cell carcinoma
C22.1	Intrahepatic bile duct carcinoma
C22.2	Hepatoblastoma
C22.3	Angiosarcoma of liver
C22.4	Other sarcomas of liver
C22.7	Other specified carcinomas of liver
C23	Malignant neoplasm of gallbladder
C24.0	Malignant neoplasm of extrahepatic bile duct
C24.1	Malignant neoplasm of ampulla of Vater
C25.3	Malignant neoplasm of pancreatic duct
D01.5	Carcinoma in situ of liver, gallbladder and bile ducts
D01.7	Carcinoma in situ of other specified digestive organs
D13.4	Benign neoplasm of liver

K74.3	Primary biliary cirrhosis
K74.4	Secondary biliary cirrhosis
K80.00	Calculus of gallbladder with acute cholecystitis without obstruction
K80.01	Calculus of gallbladder with acute cholecystitis with obstruction
K80.10	Calculus of gallbladder with chronic cholecystitis without obstruction
K80.11	Calculus of gallbladder with chronic cholecystitis with obstruction
K80.12	Calculus of gallbladder with acute and chronic cholecystitis without obstruction
K80.13	Calculus of gallbladder with acute and chronic cholecystitis with obstruction
K80.18	Calculus of gallbladder with other cholecystitis without obstruction
K80.20	Calculus of gallbladder without cholecystitis without obstruction
K80.21	Calculus of gallbladder without cholecystitis with obstruction
K80.33	Calculus of bile duct with acute cholangitis with obstruction
K80.34	Calculus of bile duct with chronic cholangitis without obstruction
K80.35	Calculus of bile duct with chronic cholangitis with obstruction
K80.36	Calculus of bile duct with acute and chronic cholangitis without obstruction
K80.37	Calculus of bile duct with acute and chronic cholangitis with obstruction
K80.42	Calculus of bile duct with acute cholecystitis without obstruction
K80.43	Calculus of bile duct with acute cholecystitis with obstruction
K80.44	Calculus of bile duct with chronic cholecystitis without obstruction
K80.45	Calculus of bile duct with chronic cholecystitis with obstruction
K80.46	Calculus of bile duct with acute and chronic cholecystitis without obstruction
K80.47	Calculus of bile duct with acute and chronic cholecystitis with obstruction
K80.50	Calculus of bile duct without cholangitis or cholecystitis without obstruction
K80.51	Calculus of bile duct without cholangitis or cholecystitis with obstruction
K80.62	Calculus of gallbladder and bile duct with acute cholecystitis without obstruction
K80.63	Calculus of gallbladder and bile duct with acute cholecystitis with obstruction
K80.64	Calculus of gallbladder and bile duct with chronic cholecystitis without obstruction
K80.65	Calculus of gallbladder and bile duct with chronic cholecystitis with obstruction
K80.66	Calculus of gallbladder and bile duct with acute and chronic cholecystitis without obstruction
K80.67	Calculus of gallbladder and bile duct with acute and chronic cholecystitis with obstruction
K80.70	Calculus of gallbladder and bile duct without cholecystitis without obstruction
K80.71	Calculus of gallbladder and bile duct without cholecystitis with obstruction
K80.80	Other cholelithiasis without obstruction
K80.81	Other cholelithiasis with obstruction
K81.0	Acute cholecystitis
K81.1	Chronic cholecystitis

Biliary Tract

K81.2	Acute cholecystitis with chronic cholecystitis
K82.0	Obstruction of gallbladder
K82.1	Hydrops of gallbladder
K82.2	Perforation of gallbladder
K82.3	Fistula of gallbladder
K82.4	Cholesterolosis of gallbladder
K82.8	Other specified diseases of gallbladder
K83.01	Primary sclerosing cholangitis
K83.09	Other cholangitis
K83.1	Obstruction of bile duct
K83.2	Perforation of bile duct
K83.3	Fistula of bile duct
K83.4	Spasm of sphincter of Oddi
K83.5	Biliary cyst
K86.0	Alcohol-induced chronic pancreatitis
K86.1	Other chronic pancreatitis
K86.2	Cyst of pancreas
K86.3	Pseudocyst of pancreas
K86.81	Exocrine pancreatic insufficiency
K86.89	Other specified diseases of pancreas
K91.5	Postcholecystectomy syndrome
Q44.0	Agenesis, aplasia and hypoplasia of gallbladder
Q44.1	Other congenital malformations of gallbladder
Q44.2	Atresia of bile ducts
Q44.3	Congenital stenosis and stricture of bile ducts
Q44.4	Choledochal cyst
Q44.5	Other congenital malformations of bile ducts
R74.8	Abnormal levels of other serum enzymes
R94.5	Abnormal results of liver function studies

AMA: **47531** 2018,Jan,8; 2017,Jan,8; 2015,Dec,3 **47532** 2018,Jan,8; 2017,Jan,8; 2015,Dec,3

Relative Value Units/Medicare Edits

Non-Facility RVU	Work	PE	MP	Total
47531	1.3	11.26	0.13	12.69
47532	4.25	21.37	0.42	26.04
Facility RVU	Work	PE	MP	Total
47531	1.3	0.62	0.13	2.05
47532	4.25	1.49	0.42	6.16

	FUD	Status	MUE	Modifiers				IOM Reference
47531	0	A	2(3)	51	N/A	N/A	N/A	None
47532	0	A	1(3)	51	N/A	N/A	N/A	

* with documentation

47533-47534

47533 Placement of biliary drainage catheter, percutaneous, including diagnostic cholangiography when performed, imaging guidance (eg, ultrasound and/or fluoroscopy), and all associated radiological supervision and interpretation; external

47534   internal-external

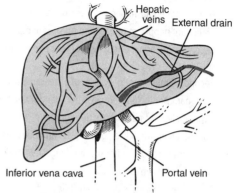

Biliary external drainage catheter

Explanation

In 47533, the physician introduces a catheter into the liver to drain fluid using ultrasound and/or fluoroscopy to guide the process. The puncture site on the right side of the body is incised, the needle inserted between the ribs, advanced into the liver, and into the bile duct. Contrast medium is injected to visualize the intrahepatic bile ducts. A guidewire is inserted and advanced to the point of obstruction through an optimal duct permitting access and drainage. A catheter is threaded over the guidewire and dilators may be used to enlarge the opening and the tract from the skin to the bile duct. The drainage catheter is inserted and positioned above the point of the obstruction and secured to the skin. All of the bile drains out of the body through the catheter and into a collection bag. Occasionally, the use of two separate catheters is necessary to drain the right and left biliary duct systems. In 47534, the physician introduces a catheter into the liver to drain fluid internally and externally, usually on patients with inoperable bile duct obstruction. The procedure is the same as in the external procedure except that a drainage catheter is inserted and positioned so that openings for drainage are both above and below the obstruction and secured in place. This allows bile to flow to an external drainage system as well as into the duodenum (internal). Codes 47533-47534 include diagnostic cholangiography (when performed), imaging guidance (fluoroscopy), as well as all associated radiological supervision and interpretation.

Coding Tips

These codes include catheter placement, removal and replacement, and/or removal, as well as stent placement. Report 47533 and 47534 once for each catheter or stent inserted. Do not report 47533–47534 with 47531-47532 or 47544 or in addition to 47540 for the same percutaneous access.

ICD-10-CM Diagnostic Codes

C22.0	Liver cell carcinoma
C22.1	Intrahepatic bile duct carcinoma
C22.2	Hepatoblastoma
C22.3	Angiosarcoma of liver
C22.4	Other sarcomas of liver
C22.7	Other specified carcinomas of liver
C23	Malignant neoplasm of gallbladder

C24.0	Malignant neoplasm of extrahepatic bile duct
C24.1	Malignant neoplasm of ampulla of Vater
C24.8	Malignant neoplasm of overlapping sites of biliary tract
C25.0	Malignant neoplasm of head of pancreas
C25.1	Malignant neoplasm of body of pancreas
C25.2	Malignant neoplasm of tail of pancreas
C25.3	Malignant neoplasm of pancreatic duct
C25.4	Malignant neoplasm of endocrine pancreas
C25.7	Malignant neoplasm of other parts of pancreas
C25.8	Malignant neoplasm of overlapping sites of pancreas
C78.7	Secondary malignant neoplasm of liver and intrahepatic bile duct
C78.89	Secondary malignant neoplasm of other digestive organs
C7A.1	Malignant poorly differentiated neuroendocrine tumors
C7A.8	Other malignant neuroendocrine tumors
D01.5	Carcinoma in situ of liver, gallbladder and bile ducts
D01.7	Carcinoma in situ of other specified digestive organs
D13.4	Benign neoplasm of liver
D13.5	Benign neoplasm of extrahepatic bile ducts
D13.6	Benign neoplasm of pancreas
D37.6	Neoplasm of uncertain behavior of liver, gallbladder and bile ducts
K74.3	Primary biliary cirrhosis
K74.4	Secondary biliary cirrhosis
K80.00	Calculus of gallbladder with acute cholecystitis without obstruction
K80.01	Calculus of gallbladder with acute cholecystitis with obstruction
K80.10	Calculus of gallbladder with chronic cholecystitis without obstruction
K80.11	Calculus of gallbladder with chronic cholecystitis with obstruction
K80.12	Calculus of gallbladder with acute and chronic cholecystitis without obstruction
K80.13	Calculus of gallbladder with acute and chronic cholecystitis with obstruction
K80.18	Calculus of gallbladder with other cholecystitis without obstruction
K80.19	Calculus of gallbladder with other cholecystitis with obstruction
K80.20	Calculus of gallbladder without cholecystitis without obstruction
K80.21	Calculus of gallbladder without cholecystitis with obstruction
K80.32	Calculus of bile duct with acute cholangitis without obstruction
K80.33	Calculus of bile duct with acute cholangitis with obstruction
K80.34	Calculus of bile duct with chronic cholangitis without obstruction
K80.35	Calculus of bile duct with chronic cholangitis with obstruction
K80.36	Calculus of bile duct with acute and chronic cholangitis without obstruction
K80.37	Calculus of bile duct with acute and chronic cholangitis with obstruction
K80.42	Calculus of bile duct with acute cholecystitis without obstruction
K80.43	Calculus of bile duct with acute cholecystitis with obstruction
K80.44	Calculus of bile duct with chronic cholecystitis without obstruction
K80.45	Calculus of bile duct with chronic cholecystitis with obstruction
K80.46	Calculus of bile duct with acute and chronic cholecystitis without obstruction
K80.47	Calculus of bile duct with acute and chronic cholecystitis with obstruction
K80.50	Calculus of bile duct without cholangitis or cholecystitis without obstruction
K80.51	Calculus of bile duct without cholangitis or cholecystitis with obstruction
K80.62	Calculus of gallbladder and bile duct with acute cholecystitis without obstruction
K80.63	Calculus of gallbladder and bile duct with acute cholecystitis with obstruction
K80.64	Calculus of gallbladder and bile duct with chronic cholecystitis without obstruction
K80.65	Calculus of gallbladder and bile duct with chronic cholecystitis with obstruction
K80.66	Calculus of gallbladder and bile duct with acute and chronic cholecystitis without obstruction
K80.67	Calculus of gallbladder and bile duct with acute and chronic cholecystitis with obstruction
K80.70	Calculus of gallbladder and bile duct without cholecystitis without obstruction
K80.71	Calculus of gallbladder and bile duct without cholecystitis with obstruction
K80.80	Other cholelithiasis without obstruction
K80.81	Other cholelithiasis with obstruction
K81.0	Acute cholecystitis
K81.1	Chronic cholecystitis
K81.2	Acute cholecystitis with chronic cholecystitis
K82.0	Obstruction of gallbladder
K82.1	Hydrops of gallbladder
K82.2	Perforation of gallbladder
K82.3	Fistula of gallbladder
K82.4	Cholesterolosis of gallbladder
K82.8	Other specified diseases of gallbladder
K83.01	Primary sclerosing cholangitis
K83.09	Other cholangitis
K83.1	Obstruction of bile duct
K83.2	Perforation of bile duct
K83.3	Fistula of bile duct
K83.4	Spasm of sphincter of Oddi
K83.5	Biliary cyst
K86.0	Alcohol-induced chronic pancreatitis
Q44.0	Agenesis, aplasia and hypoplasia of gallbladder
Q44.1	Other congenital malformations of gallbladder
Q44.2	Atresia of bile ducts
Q44.3	Congenital stenosis and stricture of bile ducts
R94.5	Abnormal results of liver function studies
T86.41	Liver transplant rejection
T86.42	Liver transplant failure
T86.43	Liver transplant infection

AMA: 47533 2018,Jan,8; 2017,Jan,8; 2015,Dec,3 47534 2018,Jan,8; 2017,Jan,8; 2015,Dec,3

Relative Value Units/Medicare Edits

Non-Facility RVU	Work	PE	MP	Total
47533	5.38	31.52	0.48	37.38
47534	7.6	33.18	0.65	41.43
Facility RVU	Work	PE	MP	Total
47533	5.38	1.79	0.48	7.65
47534	7.6	2.42	0.65	10.67

	FUD	Status	MUE	Modifiers				IOM Reference
47533	0	A	1(3)	51	N/A	N/A	N/A	None
47534	0	A	2(3)	51	N/A	N/A	N/A	

* with documentation

Terms To Know

calculus. Abnormal, stone-like concretion of calcium, cholesterol, mineral salts, or other substances that forms in any part of the body.

cholecystitis. Inflammation of the gallbladder. Acute cholecystitis is most often the result of an obstruction at the outlet of the gallbladder, with consequent edema and congestion that can progress to serious cases of gangrene and perforation. Chronic cholecystitis is a mild symptomatic inflammation of the gallbladder that continues over a long period. Acute and chronic forms may also occur together.

cholesterolosis of gallbladder. Accumulation of cholesterol deposits within the tissues of the gallbladder.

contrast material. Any internally administered substance that has a different opacity from soft tissue on radiography or computed tomograph; includes barium, used to opacify parts of the gastrointestinal tract; water-soluble iodinated compounds, used to opacify blood vessels or the genitourinary tract; may refer to air occurring naturally or introduced into the body; also, paramagnetic substances used in magnetic resonance imaging. Substances may also be documented as contrast agent or contrast medium.

guidewire. Flexible metal instrument designed to lead another instrument in its proper course.

percutaneous. Through the skin.

47535-47536

47535 Conversion of external biliary drainage catheter to internal-external biliary drainage catheter, percutaneous, including diagnostic cholangiography when performed, imaging guidance (eg, fluoroscopy), and all associated radiological supervision and interpretation

47536 Exchange of biliary drainage catheter (eg, external, internal-external, or conversion of internal-external to external only), percutaneous, including diagnostic cholangiography when performed, imaging guidance (eg, fluoroscopy), and all associated radiological supervision and interpretation

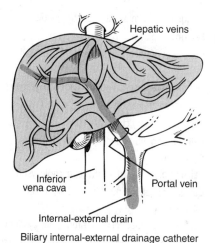

Biliary internal-external drainage catheter

Explanation

In 47535, the physician performs a percutaneous conversion from an external biliary drainage catheter to internal-external. In 47536, the physician performs a percutaneous exchange, such as external, internal-external, or conversion of internal-external to external only. Report 47537 for the removal of a biliary drainage catheter. Codes 47535-47536 include diagnostic cholangiography (when performed), imaging guidance (fluoroscopy), as well as all associated radiological supervision and interpretation.

Coding Tips

Report 47535 once for each catheter conversion. Code 47536 includes the exchange of one catheter; for more than one catheter exchange, append modifier 59 to each additional procedure. Do not report 47535–47536 with 47531-47532 or 47536 or in addition to 47538 when performed through the same access site.

ICD-10-CM Diagnostic Codes

C22.0	Liver cell carcinoma
C22.1	Intrahepatic bile duct carcinoma
C22.2	Hepatoblastoma
C22.3	Angiosarcoma of liver
C22.4	Other sarcomas of liver
C22.7	Other specified carcinomas of liver
C23	Malignant neoplasm of gallbladder
C24.0	Malignant neoplasm of extrahepatic bile duct
C24.1	Malignant neoplasm of ampulla of Vater
C25.0	Malignant neoplasm of head of pancreas
C25.1	Malignant neoplasm of body of pancreas
C25.2	Malignant neoplasm of tail of pancreas

Biliary Tract

C25.3	Malignant neoplasm of pancreatic duct
C25.4	Malignant neoplasm of endocrine pancreas
C25.7	Malignant neoplasm of other parts of pancreas
C78.7	Secondary malignant neoplasm of liver and intrahepatic bile duct
C78.89	Secondary malignant neoplasm of other digestive organs
C7A.1	Malignant poorly differentiated neuroendocrine tumors
C7A.8	Other malignant neuroendocrine tumors
C7B.8	Other secondary neuroendocrine tumors
D01.5	Carcinoma in situ of liver, gallbladder and bile ducts
D01.7	Carcinoma in situ of other specified digestive organs
D13.4	Benign neoplasm of liver
D13.5	Benign neoplasm of extrahepatic bile ducts
D13.6	Benign neoplasm of pancreas
D37.6	Neoplasm of uncertain behavior of liver, gallbladder and bile ducts
D49.0	Neoplasm of unspecified behavior of digestive system
K74.3	Primary biliary cirrhosis
K74.4	Secondary biliary cirrhosis
K80.00	Calculus of gallbladder with acute cholecystitis without obstruction
K80.01	Calculus of gallbladder with acute cholecystitis with obstruction
K80.10	Calculus of gallbladder with chronic cholecystitis without obstruction
K80.11	Calculus of gallbladder with chronic cholecystitis with obstruction
K80.12	Calculus of gallbladder with acute and chronic cholecystitis without obstruction
K80.13	Calculus of gallbladder with acute and chronic cholecystitis with obstruction
K80.18	Calculus of gallbladder with other cholecystitis without obstruction
K80.19	Calculus of gallbladder with other cholecystitis with obstruction
K80.20	Calculus of gallbladder without cholecystitis without obstruction
K80.21	Calculus of gallbladder without cholecystitis with obstruction
K80.32	Calculus of bile duct with acute cholangitis without obstruction
K80.33	Calculus of bile duct with acute cholangitis with obstruction
K80.34	Calculus of bile duct with chronic cholangitis without obstruction
K80.35	Calculus of bile duct with chronic cholangitis with obstruction
K80.36	Calculus of bile duct with acute and chronic cholangitis without obstruction
K80.37	Calculus of bile duct with acute and chronic cholangitis with obstruction
K80.42	Calculus of bile duct with acute cholecystitis without obstruction
K80.43	Calculus of bile duct with acute cholecystitis with obstruction
K80.44	Calculus of bile duct with chronic cholecystitis without obstruction
K80.45	Calculus of bile duct with chronic cholecystitis with obstruction
K80.46	Calculus of bile duct with acute and chronic cholecystitis without obstruction
K80.47	Calculus of bile duct with acute and chronic cholecystitis with obstruction
K80.50	Calculus of bile duct without cholangitis or cholecystitis without obstruction
K80.51	Calculus of bile duct without cholangitis or cholecystitis with obstruction

K80.62	Calculus of gallbladder and bile duct with acute cholecystitis without obstruction
K80.63	Calculus of gallbladder and bile duct with acute cholecystitis with obstruction
K80.64	Calculus of gallbladder and bile duct with chronic cholecystitis without obstruction
K80.65	Calculus of gallbladder and bile duct with chronic cholecystitis with obstruction
K80.66	Calculus of gallbladder and bile duct with acute and chronic cholecystitis without obstruction
K80.67	Calculus of gallbladder and bile duct with acute and chronic cholecystitis with obstruction
K80.70	Calculus of gallbladder and bile duct without cholecystitis without obstruction
K80.71	Calculus of gallbladder and bile duct without cholecystitis with obstruction
K80.80	Other cholelithiasis without obstruction
K80.81	Other cholelithiasis with obstruction
K81.0	Acute cholecystitis
K81.1	Chronic cholecystitis
K81.2	Acute cholecystitis with chronic cholecystitis
K82.0	Obstruction of gallbladder
K82.1	Hydrops of gallbladder
K82.2	Perforation of gallbladder
K82.3	Fistula of gallbladder
K82.4	Cholesterolosis of gallbladder
K82.8	Other specified diseases of gallbladder
K83.01	Primary sclerosing cholangitis
K83.09	Other cholangitis
K83.1	Obstruction of bile duct
K83.2	Perforation of bile duct
K83.3	Fistula of bile duct
K83.4	Spasm of sphincter of Oddi
K83.5	Biliary cyst
K86.0	Alcohol-induced chronic pancreatitis
K86.1	Other chronic pancreatitis
K91.5	Postcholecystectomy syndrome
Q44.0	Agenesis, aplasia and hypoplasia of gallbladder
Q44.1	Other congenital malformations of gallbladder
Q44.2	Atresia of bile ducts
Q44.3	Congenital stenosis and stricture of bile ducts
Q44.4	Choledochal cyst
Q44.5	Other congenital malformations of bile ducts
T85.510A	Breakdown (mechanical) of bile duct prosthesis, initial encounter
T85.520A	Displacement of bile duct prosthesis, initial encounter
T85.590A	Other mechanical complication of bile duct prosthesis, initial encounter
T86.41	Liver transplant rejection
T86.42	Liver transplant failure
T86.43	Liver transplant infection

AMA: **47535** 2018,Jan,8; 2017,Jan,8; 2015,Dec,3 **47536** 2018,Jan,8; 2017,Jan,8; 2015,Dec,3

Relative Value Units/Medicare Edits

Non-Facility RVU	Work	PE	MP	Total
47535	3.95	24.6	0.34	28.89
47536	2.61	17.79	0.23	20.63
Facility RVU	Work	PE	MP	Total
47535	3.95	1.35	0.34	5.64
47536	2.61	0.96	0.23	3.8

	FUD	Status	MUE	Modifiers				IOM Reference
47535	0	A	1(3)	51	N/A	N/A	N/A	None
47536	0	A	2(3)	51	N/A	N/A	N/A	

* with documentation

Terms To Know

calculus. Abnormal, stone-like concretion of calcium, cholesterol, mineral salts, or other substances that forms in any part of the body.

cholangitis. Inflammation of the bile ducts.

cirrhosis. Disease of the liver that has the characteristics of intertwining band of fibrous tissue that divides the parenchyma into micro- and macronodular areas, which cause the liver to stop functioning over time.

supervision and interpretation. Radiology services that usually contain an invasive component and are reported by the radiologist for supervision of the procedure and the personnel involved with performing the examination, reading the film, and preparing the written report.

47537

47537 Removal of biliary drainage catheter, percutaneous, requiring fluoroscopic guidance (eg, with concurrent indwelling biliary stents), including diagnostic cholangiography when performed, imaging guidance (eg, fluoroscopy), and all associated radiological supervision and interpretation

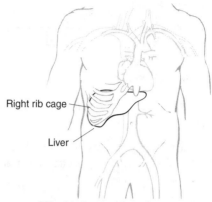

Right rib cage

Liver

Biliary drainage catheter is removed under fluoroscopic guidance

Explanation

The physician removes a biliary drainage catheter. This code includes diagnostic cholangiography (when performed), imaging guidance (fluoroscopy), as well as all associated radiological supervision and interpretation.

Coding Tips

Do not report 47537 with 47538 when performed through the same access site. Report 47537 once for each catheter removal. When fluoroscopic guidance is not required for removal, report the appropriate level of E/M service (99202–99215, 99217–99226, or 99231–99233) according to the service provided. Do not report 47537 with 47531-47532.

ICD-10-CM Diagnostic Codes

T85.510A	Breakdown (mechanical) of bile duct prosthesis, initial encounter
T85.520A	Displacement of bile duct prosthesis, initial encounter
T85.590A	Other mechanical complication of bile duct prosthesis, initial encounter
T85.79XA	Infection and inflammatory reaction due to other internal prosthetic devices, implants and grafts, initial encounter
T85.818A	Embolism due to other internal prosthetic devices, implants and grafts, initial encounter
T85.828A	Fibrosis due to other internal prosthetic devices, implants and grafts, initial encounter
T85.838A	Hemorrhage due to other internal prosthetic devices, implants and grafts, initial encounter
T85.848A	Pain due to other internal prosthetic devices, implants and grafts, initial encounter
T85.858A	Stenosis due to other internal prosthetic devices, implants and grafts, initial encounter
T85.868A	Thrombosis due to other internal prosthetic devices, implants and grafts, initial encounter
T85.898A	Other specified complication of other internal prosthetic devices, implants and grafts, initial encounter
Z48.03	Encounter for change or removal of drains

Biliary Tract

Relative Value Units/Medicare Edits

Non-Facility RVU	Work	PE	MP	Total
47537	1.84	12.71	0.16	14.71
Facility RVU	**Work**	**PE**	**MP**	**Total**
47537	1.84	0.77	0.16	2.77

	FUD	Status	MUE	Modifiers				IOM Reference
47537	0	A	1(3)	51	N/A	N/A	N/A	None

* with documentation

Terms To Know

catheter. Flexible tube inserted into an area of the body for introducing or withdrawing fluid.

fluoroscopy. Radiology technique that allows visual examination of part of the body or a function of an organ using a device that projects an x-ray image on a fluorescent screen.

stent. Tube to provide support in a body cavity or lumen.

supervision and interpretation. Radiology services that usually contain an invasive component and are reported by the radiologist for supervision of the procedure and the personnel involved with performing the examination, reading the film, and preparing the written report.

47538-47540

47538 Placement of stent(s) into a bile duct, percutaneous, including diagnostic cholangiography, imaging guidance (eg, fluoroscopy and/or ultrasound), balloon dilation, catheter exchange(s) and catheter removal(s) when performed, and all associated radiological supervision and interpretation; existing access

47539 new access, without placement of separate biliary drainage catheter

47540 new access, with placement of separate biliary drainage catheter (eg, external or internal-external)

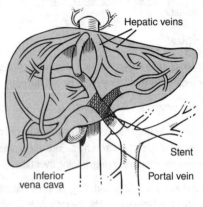

Biliary stent

Explanation

The physician inserts a thin needle through the skin and into the liver and injects contrast material for x-rays in order to diagnose and treat obstructions impacting the flow of bile from the liver to the gastrointestinal (GI) tract. Once the stricture or obstruction is identified, the physician places an introducer sheath into the biliary system. Under ultrasonic or fluoroscopic guidance, a stent delivery system is placed within a narrow section of the bile duct in order to keep the duct patent. Stents may be comprised of metallic mesh or plastic tubing. A balloon-tipped catheter may be required to achieve adequate expansion of the narrow duct. The stent may be a self-expandable stent, which means it opens by itself once deployed, or balloon expandable, meaning a balloon is required in order to open the stent. When a balloon expandable stent is used, the stent is generally placed over a balloon tipped catheter because once the balloon is expanded the catheter pushes the stent into place against the duct wall. Once the balloon tipped catheter is deflated and removed, the stent stays in place and functions similarly to a scaffold for the duct. A hilar malignancy may create an obstruction within both hepatic ducts and require the use of a bilateral stent. Report 47538 when this procedure is performed via an existing access site; 47539 when performed via a new access site without placement of separate biliary drainage catheters; and 47540 when performed via a new access site with placement of separate biliary drainage catheters (external or internal-external). The use of imaging, diagnostic cholangiography, balloon dilation, and/or the exchange or removal of catheters, as well as all supervision and interpretation, is included in these procedures, when performed.

Coding Tips

These codes should only be reported once per surgical encounter when two or more ductal segments are bridged using the same percutaneous access site or if one or more stents are placed in the same bile duct. However, these codes can be reported more than once per session in cases where specific conditions have been met as described in the Introduction contained in the Biliary Tract subsection of CPT. Do not report 47538–47540 in addition to

Biliary Tract

47531-47532, 43277, 47542, 47555, or 47556 for the same lesion in the same surgical session. Do not report 47538 in addition to 47536–47537 when performed percutaneously through the same access site. Do not report 47540 in addition to 47531–47534 when performed percutaneously through the same access site.

ICD-10-CM Diagnostic Codes

C22.0	Liver cell carcinoma
C22.1	Intrahepatic bile duct carcinoma
C22.2	Hepatoblastoma
C22.3	Angiosarcoma of liver
C22.4	Other sarcomas of liver
C22.7	Other specified carcinomas of liver
C23	Malignant neoplasm of gallbladder
C24.0	Malignant neoplasm of extrahepatic bile duct
C24.1	Malignant neoplasm of ampulla of Vater
C24.8	Malignant neoplasm of overlapping sites of biliary tract
C25.0	Malignant neoplasm of head of pancreas
C25.1	Malignant neoplasm of body of pancreas
C25.2	Malignant neoplasm of tail of pancreas
C25.3	Malignant neoplasm of pancreatic duct
C25.4	Malignant neoplasm of endocrine pancreas
C25.7	Malignant neoplasm of other parts of pancreas
C25.8	Malignant neoplasm of overlapping sites of pancreas
C78.7	Secondary malignant neoplasm of liver and intrahepatic bile duct
C78.89	Secondary malignant neoplasm of other digestive organs
C7A.1	Malignant poorly differentiated neuroendocrine tumors
C7A.8	Other malignant neuroendocrine tumors
C7B.8	Other secondary neuroendocrine tumors
D01.5	Carcinoma in situ of liver, gallbladder and bile ducts
D01.7	Carcinoma in situ of other specified digestive organs
D13.4	Benign neoplasm of liver
D13.5	Benign neoplasm of extrahepatic bile ducts
D13.6	Benign neoplasm of pancreas
D37.6	Neoplasm of uncertain behavior of liver, gallbladder and bile ducts
K65.3	Choleperitonitis
K80.01	Calculus of gallbladder with acute cholecystitis with obstruction
K80.11	Calculus of gallbladder with chronic cholecystitis with obstruction
K80.12	Calculus of gallbladder with acute and chronic cholecystitis without obstruction
K80.13	Calculus of gallbladder with acute and chronic cholecystitis with obstruction
K80.18	Calculus of gallbladder with other cholecystitis without obstruction
K80.19	Calculus of gallbladder with other cholecystitis with obstruction
K80.21	Calculus of gallbladder without cholecystitis with obstruction
K80.32	Calculus of bile duct with acute cholangitis without obstruction
K80.33	Calculus of bile duct with acute cholangitis with obstruction
K80.35	Calculus of bile duct with chronic cholangitis with obstruction
K80.36	Calculus of bile duct with acute and chronic cholangitis without obstruction
K80.37	Calculus of bile duct with acute and chronic cholangitis with obstruction
K80.43	Calculus of bile duct with acute cholecystitis with obstruction
K80.45	Calculus of bile duct with chronic cholecystitis with obstruction
K80.46	Calculus of bile duct with acute and chronic cholecystitis without obstruction
K80.47	Calculus of bile duct with acute and chronic cholecystitis with obstruction
K80.50	Calculus of bile duct without cholangitis or cholecystitis without obstruction
K80.51	Calculus of bile duct without cholangitis or cholecystitis with obstruction
K80.63	Calculus of gallbladder and bile duct with acute cholecystitis with obstruction
K80.64	Calculus of gallbladder and bile duct with chronic cholecystitis without obstruction
K80.65	Calculus of gallbladder and bile duct with chronic cholecystitis with obstruction
K80.66	Calculus of gallbladder and bile duct with acute and chronic cholecystitis without obstruction
K80.67	Calculus of gallbladder and bile duct with acute and chronic cholecystitis with obstruction
K80.70	Calculus of gallbladder and bile duct without cholecystitis without obstruction
K80.71	Calculus of gallbladder and bile duct without cholecystitis with obstruction
K80.80	Other cholelithiasis without obstruction
K80.81	Other cholelithiasis with obstruction
K81.0	Acute cholecystitis
K81.1	Chronic cholecystitis
K81.2	Acute cholecystitis with chronic cholecystitis
K82.0	Obstruction of gallbladder
K82.8	Other specified diseases of gallbladder
K83.01	Primary sclerosing cholangitis
K83.09	Other cholangitis
K83.1	Obstruction of bile duct
K83.5	Biliary cyst
K83.8	Other specified diseases of biliary tract
K85.10	Biliary acute pancreatitis without necrosis or infection
K85.11	Biliary acute pancreatitis with uninfected necrosis
K85.12	Biliary acute pancreatitis with infected necrosis
K86.0	Alcohol-induced chronic pancreatitis
K86.1	Other chronic pancreatitis
K91.5	Postcholecystectomy syndrome
K91.89	Other postprocedural complications and disorders of digestive system
Q44.0	Agenesis, aplasia and hypoplasia of gallbladder
Q44.1	Other congenital malformations of gallbladder
Q44.2	Atresia of bile ducts
Q44.3	Congenital stenosis and stricture of bile ducts
Q44.4	Choledochal cyst
Q44.5	Other congenital malformations of bile ducts

AMA: **47538** 2018,Jan,8; 2017,Jan,8; 2016,Mar,10; 2015,Dec,3 **47539** 2018,Jan,8; 2017,Jan,8; 2016,Mar,10; 2015,Dec,3 **47540** 2018,Jan,8; 2017,Jan,8; 2016,Mar,10; 2015,Dec,3

Biliary Tract

Relative Value Units/Medicare Edits

Non-Facility RVU	Work	PE	MP	Total
47538	4.75	120.85	0.43	126.03
47539	8.75	128.69	0.82	138.26
47540	9.03	131.53	0.8	141.36
Facility RVU	Work	PE	MP	Total
47538	4.75	1.62	0.43	6.8
47539	8.75	2.55	0.82	12.12
47540	9.03	2.84	0.8	12.67

	FUD	Status	MUE	Modifiers				IOM Reference
47538	0	A	2(3)	51	N/A	N/A	N/A	None
47539	0	A	2(3)	51	N/A	N/A	N/A	
47540	0	A	2(3)	51	N/A	N/A	N/A	

* with documentation

Terms To Know

balloon catheter. Any catheter equipped with an inflatable balloon at the end to hold it in place in a body cavity or to be used for dilation of a vessel lumen.

diagnostic procedures. Procedure performed on a patient to obtain information to assess the medical condition of the patient or to identify a disease and to determine the nature and severity of an illness or injury.

obstruction. Blockage that prevents normal function of the valve or structure.

percutaneous. Through the skin.

stent. Tube to provide support in a body cavity or lumen.

47541

47541   Placement of access through the biliary tree and into small bowel to assist with an endoscopic biliary procedure (eg, rendezvous procedure), percutaneous, including diagnostic cholangiography when performed, imaging guidance (eg, ultrasound and/or fluoroscopy), and all associated radiological supervision and interpretation, new access

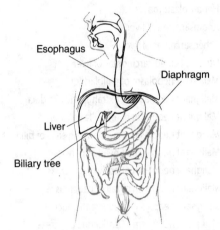

Access is placed from biliary tree into the small bowel

Explanation

Placement of access through the biliary tree and into the small bowel is performed to assist in an endoscopic biliary procedure, such as rendezvous. The physician inserts a needle through the skin and liver moving it into the bile duct for a biliary drainage procedure. For stent placement, a drainage tube is typically placed prior to stent insertion. If this fails to resolve the obstruction, the physician inserts a guidewire and the tube is removed. A sheath is placed over the guidewire and a stent delivery system is placed within the narrow section. Tissue samples and stone removal may be performed via this access. This code includes all imaging guidance. Report this code if the access is new.

Coding Tips

It is inappropriate to report this code when there is an existing catheter access. Do not report 47541 with 47531–47540.

ICD-10-CM Diagnostic Codes

This code is not identified as an add-on code by CPT® but is performed at the same time as another primary procedure. Refer to the corresponding primary procedure code for ICD-10-CM diagnosis code links.

AMA: 47541 2018,Jan,8; 2017,Jan,8; 2015,Dec,3

Relative Value Units/Medicare Edits

Non-Facility RVU	Work	PE	MP	Total
47541	6.75	29.2	0.64	36.59
Facility RVU	Work	PE	MP	Total
47541	6.75	2.22	0.64	9.61

	FUD	Status	MUE	Modifiers				IOM Reference
47541	0	A	1(3)	51	N/A	N/A	N/A	None

* with documentation

Coding Companion for General Surgery/Gastroenterology

47542

+ **47542** Balloon dilation of biliary duct(s) or of ampulla (sphincteroplasty), percutaneous, including imaging guidance (eg, fluoroscopy), and all associated radiological supervision and interpretation, each duct (List separately in addition to code for primary procedure)

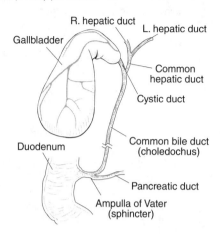

Balloon dilation of biliary duct or ampulla

Explanation

Percutaneous balloon dilation of a biliary duct or repair of the ampulla is most often required to widen a stricture or remove stones. The repair is done due to damage caused by the stricture, stone, or by the dilation itself. The provider inserts a needle through the skin and into the biliary duct and the needle is advanced through the stricture, allowing for insertion of a balloon catheter. A guidewire is inserted over the needle into the biliary duct and the needle is removed. The balloon is placed over the guidewire. Under imaging guidance, the balloon is filled with saline in order to stretch the vessel. The size of inflation and continuity depend on the patient's diagnosis and dispensation. Once the procedure is complete, the instruments are removed and simple closure of the access site is performed.

Coding Tips

Report 47542 in addition to 47531–47537 or 47541. This code should be reported with modifier 59 for subsequent dilations but only once regardless of how many additional ducts are dilated. For endoscopic balloon dilation, see 43277 and 47555–47556. Do not report 47542 with 43262, 43277, 47538–47540, or 47555–47556. Do not report 47542 in addition to 47544 if a balloon is employed for the removal of calculus, debris, or sludge in lieu of dilation.

ICD-10-CM Diagnostic Codes

This/these CPT code(s) are add-on code(s). See the primary procedure code that this code is performed with for your ICD-10-CM code selections.

AMA: **47542** 2018,Jan,8; 2017,Jan,8; 2015,Dec,3

Relative Value Units/Medicare Edits

Non-Facility RVU	Work	PE	MP	Total
47542	2.85	12.52	0.25	15.62
Facility RVU	**Work**	**PE**	**MP**	**Total**
47542	2.85	0.82	0.25	3.92

	FUD	Status	MUE	Modifiers				IOM Reference
47542	N/A	A	2(3)	N/A	N/A	N/A	N/A	None

* with documentation

Terms To Know

dilation. Artificial increase in the diameter of an opening or lumen made by medication or by instrumentation.

guidewire. Flexible metal instrument designed to lead another instrument in its proper course.

sphincteroplasty. Surgical repair done to correct, augment, or improve the muscular function of a sphincter, such as the anus or intestines.

stricture. Narrowing of an anatomical structure.

supervision and interpretation. Radiology services that usually contain an invasive component and are reported by the radiologist for supervision of the procedure and the personnel involved with performing the examination, reading the film, and preparing the written report.

47543

+ **47543** Endoluminal biopsy(ies) of biliary tree, percutaneous, any method(s) (eg, brush, forceps, and/or needle), including imaging guidance (eg, fluoroscopy), and all associated radiological supervision and interpretation, single or multiple (List separately in addition to code for primary procedure)

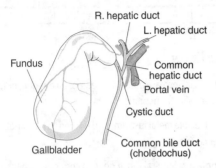

Percutaneous endoluminal biopsies
are taken of the biliary tree

Explanation

Endoluminal surgery, such as a biopsy, is performed in a hollow organ (biliary tree, stomach, etc.) using common surgical techniques. Because of the nature of these procedures, they must be performed under endoscopic control and, ideally, performed via natural orifices. The physician performs a percutaneous, endoluminal biopsy of the biliary tree by brush or forceps catheters or needle using real-time imaging (ultrasound, fluoroscopy), and the specimen is deposited on a glass slide. Smears are made from the biopsy specimen, which may be used for immediate analysis (e.g., Diff-Quik) or fixed in ethanol for immunohistochemical stains. If possible, the use of an on-site cytopathologist or cytotechnologist ensures an immediate interpretation of the sample. The use of ultrasound is particularly helpful to identify small lesions that may move during respiration. Fluoroscopy is often used in conjunction with percutaneous transhepatic biliary drainage (PTBD) as a means to access the biliary tract for the purposes of conducting endoluminal biopsy.

Coding Tips

Report 47543 in addition to 47531–47540. This code should be reported once per surgical encounter. For endoscopic biopsy, see 43261 or 47553; endoscopic brushings, see 43260 or 47552.

ICD-10-CM Diagnostic Codes

This/these CPT code(s) are add-on code(s). See the primary procedure code that this code is performed with for your ICD-10-CM code selections.

AMA: 47543 2018,Jan,8; 2017,Jan,8; 2015,Dec,3

Relative Value Units/Medicare Edits

Non-Facility RVU	Work	PE	MP	Total
47543	3.0	9.7	0.26	12.96
Facility RVU	**Work**	**PE**	**MP**	**Total**
47543	3.0	0.89	0.26	4.15

	FUD	Status	MUE	Modifiers				IOM Reference
47543	N/A	A	1(3)	N/A	N/A	N/A	N/A	None

* with documentation

47544

+ **47544** Removal of calculi/debris from biliary duct(s) and/or gallbladder, percutaneous, including destruction of calculi by any method (eg, mechanical, electrohydraulic, lithotripsy) when performed, imaging guidance (eg, fluoroscopy), and all associated radiological supervision and interpretation (List separately in addition to code for primary procedure)

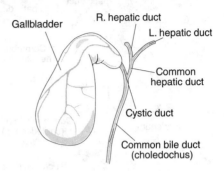

Calculi or debris are removed from
biliary ducts and/or gallbladder

Explanation

The physician removes a stone from the biliary duct after previous surgery. The common bile duct is approached by placing a scope into the tract through a previously placed drainage tube (T-tube). Manipulating basket or snare tools through the scope, the physician removes the stone(s). This code reports only the radiological supervision and interpretation required in performing this procedure.

Coding Tips

Report 47544 in addition to 47531–47540. If no calculi or debris is found, this code should not be reported, regardless of whether a device was deployed. For endoscopic removal of calculi, see 43264 or 47554; endoscopic destruction of calculi, see 43265. Do not report 47544 with 43264 or 47554. Do not report 47544 in addition to 47531–47543 for the removal of incidental debris.

ICD-10-CM Diagnostic Codes

This/these CPT code(s) are add-on code(s). See the primary procedure code that this code is performed with for your ICD-10-CM code selections.

AMA: 47544 2018,Jan,8; 2017,Jan,8; 2015,Dec,3

Relative Value Units/Medicare Edits

Non-Facility RVU	Work	PE	MP	Total
47544	3.28	24.66	0.3	28.24
Facility RVU	**Work**	**PE**	**MP**	**Total**
47544	3.28	0.93	0.3	4.51

	FUD	Status	MUE	Modifiers				IOM Reference
47544	N/A	A	1(3)	N/A	N/A	N/A	N/A	None

* with documentation

Biliary Tract

47550

+ **47550** Biliary endoscopy, intraoperative (choledochoscopy) (List separately in addition to code for primary procedure)

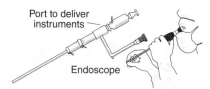

Port to deliver instruments

Endoscope

Examination using rigid endoscope

Explanation

The physician performs a biliary endoscopy during the same surgical session as other biliary procedures. The physician advances an endoscope through the previously made abdominal incision. With the endoscope the physician is able to directly visualize portions of the biliary tract, which may be filled with contrast medium for identifying the common bile duct, biliary tree and gall bladder (including areas of abnormality, stricture, or obstruction) under separately reportable fluoroscopy.

Coding Tips

This procedure is reported when performed intraoperatively. For other biliary endoscopy, see 47552–47556.

ICD-10-CM Diagnostic Codes

This/these CPT code(s) are add-on code(s). See the primary procedure code that this code is performed with for your ICD-10-CM code selections.

AMA: **47550** 2014,Jan,11

Relative Value Units/Medicare Edits

Non-Facility RVU	Work	PE	MP	Total
47550	3.02	1.13	0.71	4.86
Facility RVU	**Work**	**PE**	**MP**	**Total**
47550	3.02	1.13	0.71	4.86

	FUD	Status	MUE	Modifiers				IOM Reference
47550	N/A	A	1(3)	N/A	N/A	62*	80	None

* with documentation

Terms To Know

contrast material. Radiopaque substance placed into the body to enable a system or body structure to be visualized, such as nonionic and low osmolar contrast media (LOCM), ionic and high osmolar contrast media (HOCM), barium, and gadolinium.

fluoroscopy. Radiology technique that allows visual examination of part of the body or a function of an organ using a device that projects an x-ray image on a fluorescent screen.

obstruction. Blockage that prevents normal function of the valve or structure.

stricture. Narrowing of an anatomical structure.

47552-47553

47552 Biliary endoscopy, percutaneous via T-tube or other tract; diagnostic, with collection of specimen(s) by brushing and/or washing, when performed (separate procedure)
47553   with biopsy, single or multiple

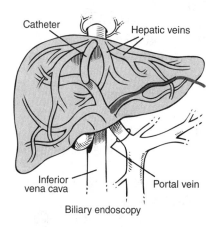

Catheter

Hepatic veins

Inferior vena cava

Portal vein

Biliary endoscopy

Explanation

The physician makes a small incision in the abdominal wall. The physician advances an endoscope through an opening in the abdominal wall or through a T-tube inserted through the abdominal wall into the common bile duct. With the endoscope, the physician is able to directly visualize portions of the biliary tract, which may be filled with contrast medium for identifying the common bile duct, biliary tree, and gallbladder (including areas of abnormality, stricture, or obstruction) under separately reportable fluoroscopy. In 47552, the physician may collect specimens by brushing and/or washing. In 47553, the physician advances biopsy forceps along the tract or T-tube to obtain single or multiple biopsies under direct endoscopic visualization or with the use of fluoroscopy. The endoscope is removed. The T-tube is withdrawn and the defect in the common bile duct is sutured closed. The tract, peritoneum, and abdominal wall are closed with layered sutures.

Coding Tips

Note that 47552, a separate procedure by definition, is usually a component of a more complex service and is not identified separately. When performed alone or with other unrelated procedures/services it may be reported. If performed alone, list the code; if performed with other procedures/services, list the code and append modifier 59 or an X{EPSU} modifier.

ICD-10-CM Diagnostic Codes

C23	Malignant neoplasm of gallbladder
C24.0	Malignant neoplasm of extrahepatic bile duct
C24.1	Malignant neoplasm of ampulla of Vater
C24.8	Malignant neoplasm of overlapping sites of biliary tract
C78.7	Secondary malignant neoplasm of liver and intrahepatic bile duct
C7B.8	Other secondary neuroendocrine tumors
D01.5	Carcinoma in situ of liver, gallbladder and bile ducts
D13.5	Benign neoplasm of extrahepatic bile ducts
D37.6	Neoplasm of uncertain behavior of liver, gallbladder and bile ducts
K74.3	Primary biliary cirrhosis
K74.4	Secondary biliary cirrhosis
K80.80	Other cholelithiasis without obstruction

Biliary Tract

K81.0	Acute cholecystitis
K81.1	Chronic cholecystitis
K81.2	Acute cholecystitis with chronic cholecystitis
K82.0	Obstruction of gallbladder
K82.1	Hydrops of gallbladder
K82.2	Perforation of gallbladder
K82.3	Fistula of gallbladder
K82.4	Cholesterolosis of gallbladder
K82.8	Other specified diseases of gallbladder
K83.01	Primary sclerosing cholangitis
K83.09	Other cholangitis
K83.1	Obstruction of bile duct
K83.2	Perforation of bile duct
K83.3	Fistula of bile duct
K83.4	Spasm of sphincter of Oddi
K83.5	Biliary cyst
K83.8	Other specified diseases of biliary tract
Q44.2	Atresia of bile ducts
Q44.3	Congenital stenosis and stricture of bile ducts
Q44.4	Choledochal cyst
Q44.5	Other congenital malformations of bile ducts

AMA: **47552** 2018,Jan,8; 2017,Jan,8; 2016,Jan,13; 2015,Jan,16; 2015,Dec,3
47553 2018,Jan,8; 2017,Jan,8; 2016,Jan,13; 2015,Jan,16; 2015,Dec,3

Relative Value Units/Medicare Edits

Non-Facility RVU	Work	PE	MP	Total
47552	6.03	1.32	0.59	7.94
47553	6.34	1.02	0.63	7.99
Facility RVU	**Work**	**PE**	**MP**	**Total**
47552	6.03	1.32	0.59	7.94
47553	6.34	1.02	0.63	7.99

	FUD	Status	MUE	Modifiers				IOM Reference
47552	0	A	1(3)	51	N/A	62*	N/A	None
47553	0	A	1(2)	51	N/A	N/A	N/A	

* with documentation

Terms To Know

biopsy. Tissue or fluid removed for diagnostic purposes through analysis of the cells in the biopsy material.

cirrhosis. Disease of the liver that has the characteristics of intertwining band of fibrous tissue that divides the parenchyma into micro- and macronodular areas, which cause the liver to stop functioning over time.

fluoroscopy. Radiology technique that allows visual examination of part of the body or a function of an organ using a device that projects an x-ray image on a fluorescent screen.

47554

47554 Biliary endoscopy, percutaneous via T-tube or other tract; with removal of calculus/calculi

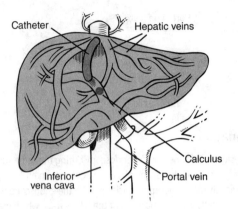

Biliary calculus

Explanation

The physician makes a small incision in the abdomen. The physician advances an endoscope through an opening in the abdominal wall or through a T-tube inserted through the abdominal wall into the common bile duct. With the endoscope, the physician is able to directly visualize portions of the biliary tract, which may be filled with contrast medium for identifying the common bile duct, biliary tree, and gallbladder (including areas of abnormality, stricture, or obstruction) under separately reportable fluoroscopy. Calculi are identified and removed. The endoscope is removed. The T-tube is withdrawn and the defect in the common bile duct is sutured closed. The tract, peritoneum, and abdominal wall are closed using a layered technique.

Coding Tips

For ERCP, with removal of calculi/debris from biliary or pancreatic ducts, see 43264.

ICD-10-CM Diagnostic Codes

K80.00	Calculus of gallbladder with acute cholecystitis without obstruction
K80.01	Calculus of gallbladder with acute cholecystitis with obstruction
K80.10	Calculus of gallbladder with chronic cholecystitis without obstruction
K80.11	Calculus of gallbladder with chronic cholecystitis with obstruction
K80.12	Calculus of gallbladder with acute and chronic cholecystitis without obstruction
K80.13	Calculus of gallbladder with acute and chronic cholecystitis with obstruction
K80.18	Calculus of gallbladder with other cholecystitis without obstruction
K80.19	Calculus of gallbladder with other cholecystitis with obstruction
K80.20	Calculus of gallbladder without cholecystitis without obstruction
K80.21	Calculus of gallbladder without cholecystitis with obstruction
K80.32	Calculus of bile duct with acute cholangitis without obstruction
K80.33	Calculus of bile duct with acute cholangitis with obstruction
K80.34	Calculus of bile duct with chronic cholangitis without obstruction
K80.35	Calculus of bile duct with chronic cholangitis with obstruction
K80.36	Calculus of bile duct with acute and chronic cholangitis without obstruction

K80.37	Calculus of bile duct with acute and chronic cholangitis with obstruction
K80.42	Calculus of bile duct with acute cholecystitis without obstruction
K80.43	Calculus of bile duct with acute cholecystitis with obstruction
K80.44	Calculus of bile duct with chronic cholecystitis without obstruction
K80.45	Calculus of bile duct with chronic cholecystitis with obstruction
K80.46	Calculus of bile duct with acute and chronic cholecystitis without obstruction
K80.47	Calculus of bile duct with acute and chronic cholecystitis with obstruction
K80.50	Calculus of bile duct without cholangitis or cholecystitis without obstruction
K80.51	Calculus of bile duct without cholangitis or cholecystitis with obstruction
K80.62	Calculus of gallbladder and bile duct with acute cholecystitis without obstruction
K80.63	Calculus of gallbladder and bile duct with acute cholecystitis with obstruction
K80.64	Calculus of gallbladder and bile duct with chronic cholecystitis without obstruction
K80.65	Calculus of gallbladder and bile duct with chronic cholecystitis with obstruction
K80.66	Calculus of gallbladder and bile duct with acute and chronic cholecystitis without obstruction
K80.67	Calculus of gallbladder and bile duct with acute and chronic cholecystitis with obstruction
K80.70	Calculus of gallbladder and bile duct without cholecystitis without obstruction
K80.71	Calculus of gallbladder and bile duct without cholecystitis with obstruction
K80.81	Other cholelithiasis with obstruction

AMA: **47554** 2018,Jan,8; 2017,Jan,8; 2016,Jan,13; 2015,Jan,16; 2015,Dec,3

Relative Value Units/Medicare Edits

Non-Facility RVU	Work	PE	MP	Total
47554	9.05	3.91	2.22	15.18
Facility RVU	Work	PE	MP	Total
47554	9.05	3.91	2.22	15.18

	FUD	Status	MUE	Modifiers				IOM Reference
47554	0	A	1(3)	51	N/A	62*	N/A	None

* with documentation

47555-47556

47555 Biliary endoscopy, percutaneous via T-tube or other tract; with dilation of biliary duct stricture(s) without stent

47556 with dilation of biliary duct stricture(s) with stent

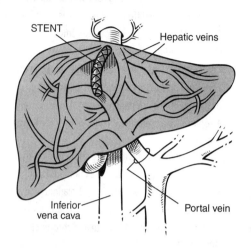

STENT
Hepatic veins
Inferior vena cava
Portal vein

Explanation

The physician makes a small incision in the abdomen. The physician advances an endoscope through an opening in the abdominal wall or through a T-tube inserted through the abdominal wall into the common bile duct. With the endoscope, the physician is able to directly visualize portions of the biliary tract, which may be filled with contrast medium for identifying the common bile duct, biliary tree, and gallbladder (including areas of abnormality, stricture, or obstruction) under fluoroscopy. The physician advances a balloon-tipped catheter through the tract or T-tube so that it is above the site of the duct stricture, inflates the balloon, and draws it back through the site of stricture to achieve dilation. This procedure may be repeated until optimal dilation is obtained. The endoscope is removed and the tract, peritoneum, and abdominal wall are approximated. The T-tube is withdrawn and the common bile duct is sutured closed. The abdomen is sutured closed. In 47556, the physician places a stent to prevent future stricture before the endoscope is withdrawn.

Coding Tips

For ERCP services, see 43260–43278, 74328–74330, and 74363. Imaging guidance, when performed, is reported with 74363.

ICD-10-CM Diagnostic Codes

C22.0	Liver cell carcinoma
C22.1	Intrahepatic bile duct carcinoma
C22.2	Hepatoblastoma
C22.3	Angiosarcoma of liver
C22.4	Other sarcomas of liver
C22.7	Other specified carcinomas of liver
C23	Malignant neoplasm of gallbladder
C24.0	Malignant neoplasm of extrahepatic bile duct
C24.1	Malignant neoplasm of ampulla of Vater
C24.8	Malignant neoplasm of overlapping sites of biliary tract
C25.0	Malignant neoplasm of head of pancreas
C25.1	Malignant neoplasm of body of pancreas
C25.2	Malignant neoplasm of tail of pancreas
C25.3	Malignant neoplasm of pancreatic duct

Biliary Tract

C25.4	Malignant neoplasm of endocrine pancreas
C25.7	Malignant neoplasm of other parts of pancreas
C25.8	Malignant neoplasm of overlapping sites of pancreas
C78.7	Secondary malignant neoplasm of liver and intrahepatic bile duct
C78.89	Secondary malignant neoplasm of other digestive organs
C7A.1	Malignant poorly differentiated neuroendocrine tumors
C7A.8	Other malignant neuroendocrine tumors
C7B.8	Other secondary neuroendocrine tumors
D01.5	Carcinoma in situ of liver, gallbladder and bile ducts
D13.5	Benign neoplasm of extrahepatic bile ducts
D13.6	Benign neoplasm of pancreas
D37.6	Neoplasm of uncertain behavior of liver, gallbladder and bile ducts
K80.32	Calculus of bile duct with acute cholangitis without obstruction
K80.33	Calculus of bile duct with acute cholangitis with obstruction
K80.34	Calculus of bile duct with chronic cholangitis without obstruction
K80.35	Calculus of bile duct with chronic cholangitis with obstruction
K80.36	Calculus of bile duct with acute and chronic cholangitis without obstruction
K80.37	Calculus of bile duct with acute and chronic cholangitis with obstruction
K80.43	Calculus of bile duct with acute cholecystitis with obstruction
K80.45	Calculus of bile duct with chronic cholecystitis with obstruction
K80.47	Calculus of bile duct with acute and chronic cholecystitis with obstruction
K80.50	Calculus of bile duct without cholangitis or cholecystitis without obstruction
K80.51	Calculus of bile duct without cholangitis or cholecystitis with obstruction
K80.63	Calculus of gallbladder and bile duct with acute cholecystitis with obstruction
K80.65	Calculus of gallbladder and bile duct with chronic cholecystitis with obstruction
K80.67	Calculus of gallbladder and bile duct with acute and chronic cholecystitis with obstruction
K80.71	Calculus of gallbladder and bile duct without cholecystitis with obstruction
K80.81	Other cholelithiasis with obstruction
K83.01	Primary sclerosing cholangitis
K83.09	Other cholangitis
K83.1	Obstruction of bile duct
K83.5	Biliary cyst
K83.8	Other specified diseases of biliary tract
K86.81	Exocrine pancreatic insufficiency
K86.89	Other specified diseases of pancreas
K87	Disorders of gallbladder, biliary tract and pancreas in diseases classified elsewhere
K91.5	Postcholecystectomy syndrome
K91.86	Retained cholelithiasis following cholecystectomy
K91.89	Other postprocedural complications and disorders of digestive system
Q44.2	Atresia of bile ducts
Q44.3	Congenital stenosis and stricture of bile ducts
Q44.4	Choledochal cyst

Q44.5	Other congenital malformations of bile ducts
S36.13XA	Injury of bile duct, initial encounter

AMA: **47555** 2018,Jan,8; 2017,Jan,8; 2016,Jan,13; 2015,Jan,16; 2015,Dec,3
47556 2018,Jan,8; 2017,Jan,8; 2016,Jan,13; 2015,Jan,16; 2015,Dec,3

Relative Value Units/Medicare Edits

Non-Facility RVU	Work	PE	MP	Total
47555	7.55	1.22	0.74	9.51
47556	8.55	1.38	0.84	10.77
Facility RVU	Work	PE	MP	Total
47555	7.55	1.22	0.74	9.51
47556	8.55	1.38	0.84	10.77

	FUD	Status	MUE	Modifiers				IOM Reference
47555	0	A	1(2)	51	N/A	N/A	N/A	None
47556	0	A	1(2)	51	N/A	N/A	N/A	

* with documentation

Terms To Know

balloon catheter. Any catheter equipped with an inflatable balloon at the end to hold it in place in a body cavity or to be used for dilation of a vessel lumen.

dilation. Artificial increase in the diameter of an opening or lumen made by medication or by instrumentation.

ERCP. Endoscopic retrograde cholangiopancreatography. Examination of the hepatobiliary system and gallbladder performed through a flexible fiberoptic endoscope.

fluoroscopy. Radiology technique that allows visual examination of part of the body or a function of an organ using a device that projects an x-ray image on a fluorescent screen.

obstruction. Blockage that prevents normal function of the valve or structure.

percutaneous. Through the skin.

stent. Tube to provide support in a body cavity or lumen.

stricture. Narrowing of an anatomical structure.

47562-47564

47562 Laparoscopy, surgical; cholecystectomy
47563 Laparoscopy, surgical; cholecystectomy with cholangiography
47564 cholecystectomy with exploration of common duct

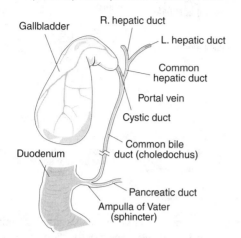

The gallbladder is removed in a laparoscopic surgical session

Explanation

The physician removes the gallbladder through a laparoscope. The physician makes a 1.0-centimeter infraumbilical incision through which a trocar is inserted. Pneumoperitoneum is achieved by insufflating the abdominal cavity with carbon dioxide. A fiberoptic laparoscope fitted with a camera and light source is inserted through the trocar. Other incisions are made on the right side of the abdomen and in the subxiphoid area to allow other instruments or an additional light source to be passed into the abdomen. The tip of the gallbladder is mobilized and placed in traction. The Hartmann's pouch (junction of the cystic duct and gallbladder neck) is identified. Tissue is dissected free from around the area for exposure of Calot's triangle (formed by the cystic artery, and cystic and common bile ducts). Clips are applied to the proximal area of the cystic duct and artery (close to the gallbladder) and the cystic duct and artery are cut. In 47563, a contrast study is also obtained through the cystic duct. In 47564, a contrast study of the bile ducts is usually obtained through the cystic duct. The common bile duct may be explored with a small choledochoscope through the cystic duct or a separate incision may be made in the common bile duct. The common duct is visualized with a choledochoscope and stones may be extracted from the duct with a variety of instruments. If an incision was made in the common bile duct, this is usually closed with sutures over a T-tube that is brought out through the abdominal wall. The cystic duct and artery are divided. The gallbladder is removed through the trocar site. A drain is usually placed below the liver and brought out through the abdominal wall. The trocars are removed and the incisions are closed.

Coding Tips

Surgical laparoscopy always includes diagnostic laparoscopy. For intraoperative cholangiography radiological supervision and interpretation, see 74300-74301; percutaneous cholangiography, see 47531-47532.

ICD-10-CM Diagnostic Codes

C23	Malignant neoplasm of gallbladder
K56.3	Gallstone ileus
K74.3	Primary biliary cirrhosis
K74.4	Secondary biliary cirrhosis

K80.00	Calculus of gallbladder with acute cholecystitis without obstruction
K80.01	Calculus of gallbladder with acute cholecystitis with obstruction
K80.10	Calculus of gallbladder with chronic cholecystitis without obstruction
K80.11	Calculus of gallbladder with chronic cholecystitis with obstruction
K80.12	Calculus of gallbladder with acute and chronic cholecystitis without obstruction
K80.13	Calculus of gallbladder with acute and chronic cholecystitis with obstruction
K80.18	Calculus of gallbladder with other cholecystitis without obstruction
K80.19	Calculus of gallbladder with other cholecystitis with obstruction
K80.20	Calculus of gallbladder without cholecystitis without obstruction
K80.21	Calculus of gallbladder without cholecystitis with obstruction
K80.32	Calculus of bile duct with acute cholangitis without obstruction
K80.33	Calculus of bile duct with acute cholangitis with obstruction
K80.34	Calculus of bile duct with chronic cholangitis without obstruction
K80.35	Calculus of bile duct with chronic cholangitis with obstruction
K80.36	Calculus of bile duct with acute and chronic cholangitis without obstruction
K80.37	Calculus of bile duct with acute and chronic cholangitis with obstruction
K80.42	Calculus of bile duct with acute cholecystitis without obstruction
K80.43	Calculus of bile duct with acute cholecystitis with obstruction
K80.44	Calculus of bile duct with chronic cholecystitis without obstruction
K80.45	Calculus of bile duct with chronic cholecystitis with obstruction
K80.46	Calculus of bile duct with acute and chronic cholecystitis without obstruction
K80.47	Calculus of bile duct with acute and chronic cholecystitis with obstruction
K80.50	Calculus of bile duct without cholangitis or cholecystitis without obstruction
K80.51	Calculus of bile duct without cholangitis or cholecystitis with obstruction
K80.62	Calculus of gallbladder and bile duct with acute cholecystitis without obstruction
K80.63	Calculus of gallbladder and bile duct with acute cholecystitis with obstruction
K80.64	Calculus of gallbladder and bile duct with chronic cholecystitis without obstruction
K80.65	Calculus of gallbladder and bile duct with chronic cholecystitis with obstruction
K80.66	Calculus of gallbladder and bile duct with acute and chronic cholecystitis without obstruction
K80.67	Calculus of gallbladder and bile duct with acute and chronic cholecystitis with obstruction
K80.70	Calculus of gallbladder and bile duct without cholecystitis without obstruction
K80.71	Calculus of gallbladder and bile duct without cholecystitis with obstruction
K80.80	Other cholelithiasis without obstruction
K80.81	Other cholelithiasis with obstruction
K81.0	Acute cholecystitis
K81.1	Chronic cholecystitis

K81.2	Acute cholecystitis with chronic cholecystitis
K82.0	Obstruction of gallbladder
K82.1	Hydrops of gallbladder
K82.2	Perforation of gallbladder
K82.3	Fistula of gallbladder
K82.4	Cholesterolosis of gallbladder
K82.A1	Gangrene of gallbladder in cholecystitis
K82.A2	Perforation of gallbladder in cholecystitis
K83.01	Primary sclerosing cholangitis
K83.09	Other cholangitis
K83.1	Obstruction of bile duct
K83.2	Perforation of bile duct
K83.3	Fistula of bile duct
K83.4	Spasm of sphincter of Oddi
K83.5	Biliary cyst
K85.10	Biliary acute pancreatitis without necrosis or infection
K85.11	Biliary acute pancreatitis with uninfected necrosis
K85.12	Biliary acute pancreatitis with infected necrosis
K85.20	Alcohol induced acute pancreatitis without necrosis or infection
K85.21	Alcohol induced acute pancreatitis with uninfected necrosis
K85.22	Alcohol induced acute pancreatitis with infected necrosis
K85.30	Drug induced acute pancreatitis without necrosis or infection
K85.31	Drug induced acute pancreatitis with uninfected necrosis
K85.32	Drug induced acute pancreatitis with infected necrosis
K85.80	Other acute pancreatitis without necrosis or infection
K85.81	Other acute pancreatitis with uninfected necrosis
K85.82	Other acute pancreatitis with infected necrosis
R10.11	Right upper quadrant pain

AMA: 47562 2020,Aug,14; 2018,Jan,8; 2017,Jan,8; 2016,Jan,13; 2015,Jan,16 **47563** 2019,Mar,10; 2018,Jan,8; 2017,Jan,8; 2016,Jan,13; 2015,Jan,16 **47564** 2018,Jan,8; 2017,Jan,8; 2016,Jan,13; 2015,Jan,16

Relative Value Units/Medicare Edits

Non-Facility RVU	Work	PE	MP	Total
47562	10.47	6.54	2.53	19.54
47563	11.47	7.04	2.75	21.26
47564	18.0	10.73	4.36	33.09
Facility RVU	Work	PE	MP	Total
47562	10.47	6.54	2.53	19.54
47563	11.47	7.04	2.75	21.26
47564	18.0	10.73	4.36	33.09

	FUD	Status	MUE	Modifiers				IOM Reference
47562	90	A	1(2)	51	N/A	62*	80	None
47563	90	A	1(2)	51	N/A	62*	80	
47564	90	A	1(2)	51	N/A	62*	80	

* with documentation

47570

47570 Laparoscopy, surgical; cholecystoenterostomy

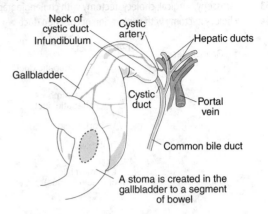

A stoma is created in the gallbladder to a segment of bowel

Explanation

Through the laparoscope the physician performs an anastomosis between the gallbladder and small bowel (cholecystoenterostomy). The physician places a trocar at the umbilicus and insufflates the abdominal cavity. The laparoscope is placed through the umbilical port and additional trocars are placed into the abdominal cavity. The gallbladder and a proximal loop of small bowel are identified and mobilized. An anastomosis is created between the gallbladder and loop or limb of proximal small bowel with staples or sutures. The trocars are removed and the incisions are closed.

Coding Tips

Surgical laparoscopy always includes diagnostic laparoscopy. For direct cholecystoenterostomy, see 47720; with gastroenterostomy, see 47721; with Roux-en-Y, see 47740; with Roux-en-Y with gastroenterostomy, see 47741.

ICD-10-CM Diagnostic Codes

C22.1	Intrahepatic bile duct carcinoma
C23	Malignant neoplasm of gallbladder
C24.0	Malignant neoplasm of extrahepatic bile duct
C24.1	Malignant neoplasm of ampulla of Vater
C24.8	Malignant neoplasm of overlapping sites of biliary tract
C25.0	Malignant neoplasm of head of pancreas
C25.1	Malignant neoplasm of body of pancreas
C25.2	Malignant neoplasm of tail of pancreas
C25.3	Malignant neoplasm of pancreatic duct
C25.4	Malignant neoplasm of endocrine pancreas
C25.7	Malignant neoplasm of other parts of pancreas
C25.8	Malignant neoplasm of overlapping sites of pancreas
C78.7	Secondary malignant neoplasm of liver and intrahepatic bile duct
C78.89	Secondary malignant neoplasm of other digestive organs
C7A.1	Malignant poorly differentiated neuroendocrine tumors
C7A.8	Other malignant neuroendocrine tumors
D01.5	Carcinoma in situ of liver, gallbladder and bile ducts
D13.4	Benign neoplasm of liver
D13.5	Benign neoplasm of extrahepatic bile ducts
D37.6	Neoplasm of uncertain behavior of liver, gallbladder and bile ducts
K56.3	Gallstone ileus

K74.3	Primary biliary cirrhosis
K74.4	Secondary biliary cirrhosis
K74.69	Other cirrhosis of liver
K80.80	Other cholelithiasis without obstruction
K80.81	Other cholelithiasis with obstruction
K81.0	Acute cholecystitis
K81.1	Chronic cholecystitis
K81.2	Acute cholecystitis with chronic cholecystitis
K82.0	Obstruction of gallbladder
K82.1	Hydrops of gallbladder
K82.2	Perforation of gallbladder
K82.3	Fistula of gallbladder
K82.4	Cholesterolosis of gallbladder
K82.8	Other specified diseases of gallbladder
K83.01	Primary sclerosing cholangitis
K83.09	Other cholangitis
K83.1	Obstruction of bile duct
K83.2	Perforation of bile duct
K83.3	Fistula of bile duct
K83.4	Spasm of sphincter of Oddi
K83.5	Biliary cyst
K83.8	Other specified diseases of biliary tract
K85.12	Biliary acute pancreatitis with infected necrosis
K85.20	Alcohol induced acute pancreatitis without necrosis or infection
K85.21	Alcohol induced acute pancreatitis with uninfected necrosis
K85.32	Drug induced acute pancreatitis with infected necrosis
K85.82	Other acute pancreatitis with infected necrosis
K86.0	Alcohol-induced chronic pancreatitis
K86.1	Other chronic pancreatitis
K86.2	Cyst of pancreas
K86.3	Pseudocyst of pancreas
K87	Disorders of gallbladder, biliary tract and pancreas in diseases classified elsewhere

AMA: 47570 2018,Jan,8; 2017,Jan,8; 2016,Jan,13; 2015,Jan,16

Relative Value Units/Medicare Edits

Non-Facility RVU	Work	PE	MP	Total
47570	12.56	7.36	3.08	23.0
Facility RVU	**Work**	**PE**	**MP**	**Total**
47570	12.56	7.36	3.08	23.0

	FUD	Status	MUE	Modifiers				IOM Reference
47570	90	A	1(2)	51	N/A	62*	80	None

* with documentation

47600 Cholecystectomy;
47605   with cholangiography

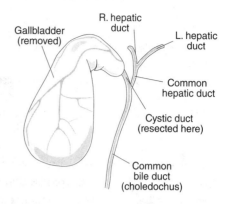

Explanation

The physician removes the gallbladder by open incision. The patient is placed in the supine position and general anesthesia is administered. The physician makes a 6-inch incision into the abdomen on the right side. There are two approaches for open cholecystectomy: retrograde and antegrade, with the more common being retrograde, and discussed here. Incision into the anterior rectus sheath is performed following the length of incision with division of the muscles. An incision is then made into the posterior rectus sheath and peritoneum to open the abdomen. A retractor may be placed to allow adequate inspection of the liver and gallbladder. Inspection and palpation of the liver and gallbladder are performed. A clamp is used to grab and lift the dome of the gallbladder. If adhesions are present between the gallbladder and colon or duodenum, they are lysed by sharp dissection or use of electrocautery. The retrograde technique removes the gallbladder starting at the top and working down from the fundus toward the porta hepatis. The visceral peritoneum is cut at 1 cm from the liver and the clamp holds the fundus of the gallbladder at which time, the physician continues the incision along the gallbladder running parallel to the liver. Once the gallbladder is mobilized from the liver bed, dissection within Calot's triangle is performed and division of the cystic duct and artery are performed with ligation (suture, staple, and clip). At this point, the small veins may be present requiring division and/or ligation in order to completely remove the gallbladder. The incision is closed with layered sutures. The entire procedure can take up to two hours and inpatient hospitalization of two to three days with full recovery at about four to six weeks. Report 47605 if this is performed with a cholangiography.

Coding Tips

For laparoscopic cholecystectomy (any method), see 47562; with cholangiography, see 47563.

ICD-10-CM Diagnostic Codes

C23	Malignant neoplasm of gallbladder
C24.0	Malignant neoplasm of extrahepatic bile duct
C24.1	Malignant neoplasm of ampulla of Vater
C24.8	Malignant neoplasm of overlapping sites of biliary tract
C78.7	Secondary malignant neoplasm of liver and intrahepatic bile duct
D01.5	Carcinoma in situ of liver, gallbladder and bile ducts
D13.5	Benign neoplasm of extrahepatic bile ducts
D37.6	Neoplasm of uncertain behavior of liver, gallbladder and bile ducts

Biliary Tract

K56.3	Gallstone ileus
K80.00	Calculus of gallbladder with acute cholecystitis without obstruction
K80.01	Calculus of gallbladder with acute cholecystitis with obstruction
K80.10	Calculus of gallbladder with chronic cholecystitis without obstruction
K80.11	Calculus of gallbladder with chronic cholecystitis with obstruction
K80.12	Calculus of gallbladder with acute and chronic cholecystitis without obstruction
K80.13	Calculus of gallbladder with acute and chronic cholecystitis with obstruction
K80.18	Calculus of gallbladder with other cholecystitis without obstruction
K80.19	Calculus of gallbladder with other cholecystitis with obstruction
K80.20	Calculus of gallbladder without cholecystitis without obstruction
K80.21	Calculus of gallbladder without cholecystitis with obstruction
K80.62	Calculus of gallbladder and bile duct with acute cholecystitis without obstruction
K80.63	Calculus of gallbladder and bile duct with acute cholecystitis with obstruction
K80.64	Calculus of gallbladder and bile duct with chronic cholecystitis without obstruction
K80.65	Calculus of gallbladder and bile duct with chronic cholecystitis with obstruction
K80.66	Calculus of gallbladder and bile duct with acute and chronic cholecystitis without obstruction
K80.67	Calculus of gallbladder and bile duct with acute and chronic cholecystitis with obstruction
K80.70	Calculus of gallbladder and bile duct without cholecystitis without obstruction
K80.71	Calculus of gallbladder and bile duct without cholecystitis with obstruction
K80.80	Other cholelithiasis without obstruction
K80.81	Other cholelithiasis with obstruction
K81.0	Acute cholecystitis
K81.1	Chronic cholecystitis
K81.2	Acute cholecystitis with chronic cholecystitis
K82.0	Obstruction of gallbladder
K82.1	Hydrops of gallbladder
K82.2	Perforation of gallbladder
K82.3	Fistula of gallbladder
K82.4	Cholesterolosis of gallbladder
K82.8	Other specified diseases of gallbladder
K83.8	Other specified diseases of biliary tract
K85.00	Idiopathic acute pancreatitis without necrosis or infection
K85.01	Idiopathic acute pancreatitis with uninfected necrosis
K85.02	Idiopathic acute pancreatitis with infected necrosis
K85.10	Biliary acute pancreatitis without necrosis or infection
K85.11	Biliary acute pancreatitis with uninfected necrosis
K85.12	Biliary acute pancreatitis with infected necrosis
K85.20	Alcohol induced acute pancreatitis without necrosis or infection
K85.21	Alcohol induced acute pancreatitis with uninfected necrosis
K85.22	Alcohol induced acute pancreatitis with infected necrosis
K85.30	Drug induced acute pancreatitis without necrosis or infection
K85.31	Drug induced acute pancreatitis with uninfected necrosis

K85.32	Drug induced acute pancreatitis with infected necrosis
K85.80	Other acute pancreatitis without necrosis or infection
K85.81	Other acute pancreatitis with uninfected necrosis
K85.82	Other acute pancreatitis with infected necrosis
K87	Disorders of gallbladder, biliary tract and pancreas in diseases classified elsewhere
R10.11	Right upper quadrant pain
R19.01	Right upper quadrant abdominal swelling, mass and lump
S36.122A	Contusion of gallbladder, initial encounter
S36.123A	Laceration of gallbladder, initial encounter
S36.128A	Other injury of gallbladder, initial encounter
S36.13XA	Injury of bile duct, initial encounter

AMA: **47600** 2018,Jan,8; 2017,Jan,8; 2016,Jan,13; 2015,Jan,16 **47605** 2018,Jan,8; 2017,Jan,8; 2016,Jan,13; 2015,Jan,16

Relative Value Units/Medicare Edits

Non-Facility RVU	Work	PE	MP	Total
47600	17.48	10.02	4.14	31.64
47605	18.48	10.45	4.42	33.35
Facility RVU	**Work**	**PE**	**MP**	**Total**
47600	17.48	10.02	4.14	31.64
47605	18.48	10.45	4.42	33.35

	FUD	Status	MUE	Modifiers				IOM Reference
47600	90	A	1(2)	51	N/A	62*	80	None
47605	90	A	1(2)	51	N/A	62*	80	

* with documentation

Terms To Know

calculus. Abnormal, stone-like concretion of calcium, cholesterol, mineral salts, or other substances that forms in any part of the body.

cholecystectomy. Surgical removal of the gallbladder and its contents. Cholecystectomy may be performed by an open incision into the abdominal cavity or laparoscopically via instruments inserted through small incisions into the peritoneum for video-controlled imaging.

cholecystitis. Inflammation of the gallbladder. Acute cholecystitis is most often the result of an obstruction at the outlet of the gallbladder, with consequent edema and congestion that can progress to serious cases of gangrene and perforation. Chronic cholecystitis is a mild symptomatic inflammation of the gallbladder that continues over a long period. Acute and chronic forms may also occur together.

electrocautery. Division or cutting of tissue using high-frequency electrical current to produce heat, which destroys cells.

Biliary Tract

47610-47620

47610 Cholecystectomy with exploration of common duct;
47612   with choledochoenterostomy
47620   with transduodenal sphincterotomy or sphincteroplasty, with or without cholangiography

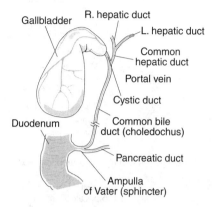

Explanation

The physician removes the gallbladder and explores the common duct. The physician exposes the liver and gallbladder via a right subcostal incision. The cystic duct and cystic artery are ligated and the gallbladder removed using electrocautery. The common bile duct is exposed in the portal triad, incised, and the stones removed. The common bile duct is closed and the abdominal incision is closed with sutures. Report 47612 if this procedure is performed with choledochoenterostomy, establishment of communication between the intestine and the common bile duct; report 47620 if this procedure is performed with transduodenal sphincterotomy or sphincteroplasty, with or without cholangiography.

Coding Tips

Intraoperative biliary endoscopy is reported 47550, when performed. For laparoscopic cholecystectomy with exploration of common duct, see 47564.

ICD-10-CM Diagnostic Codes

C22.1	Intrahepatic bile duct carcinoma
C23	Malignant neoplasm of gallbladder
C24.0	Malignant neoplasm of extrahepatic bile duct
C24.1	Malignant neoplasm of ampulla of Vater
C24.8	Malignant neoplasm of overlapping sites of biliary tract
C25.3	Malignant neoplasm of pancreatic duct
C25.4	Malignant neoplasm of endocrine pancreas
C78.7	Secondary malignant neoplasm of liver and intrahepatic bile duct
C78.89	Secondary malignant neoplasm of other digestive organs
D01.5	Carcinoma in situ of liver, gallbladder and bile ducts
D13.5	Benign neoplasm of extrahepatic bile ducts
D37.6	Neoplasm of uncertain behavior of liver, gallbladder and bile ducts
K56.3	Gallstone ileus
K80.00	Calculus of gallbladder with acute cholecystitis without obstruction
K80.01	Calculus of gallbladder with acute cholecystitis with obstruction
K80.10	Calculus of gallbladder with chronic cholecystitis without obstruction
K80.11	Calculus of gallbladder with chronic cholecystitis with obstruction
K80.12	Calculus of gallbladder with acute and chronic cholecystitis without obstruction
K80.13	Calculus of gallbladder with acute and chronic cholecystitis with obstruction
K80.18	Calculus of gallbladder with other cholecystitis without obstruction
K80.19	Calculus of gallbladder with other cholecystitis with obstruction
K80.20	Calculus of gallbladder without cholecystitis without obstruction
K80.21	Calculus of gallbladder without cholecystitis with obstruction
K80.32	Calculus of bile duct with acute cholangitis without obstruction
K80.33	Calculus of bile duct with acute cholangitis with obstruction
K80.34	Calculus of bile duct with chronic cholangitis without obstruction
K80.35	Calculus of bile duct with chronic cholangitis with obstruction
K80.36	Calculus of bile duct with acute and chronic cholangitis without obstruction
K80.37	Calculus of bile duct with acute and chronic cholangitis with obstruction
K80.42	Calculus of bile duct with acute cholecystitis without obstruction
K80.43	Calculus of bile duct with acute cholecystitis with obstruction
K80.44	Calculus of bile duct with chronic cholecystitis without obstruction
K80.45	Calculus of bile duct with chronic cholecystitis with obstruction
K80.46	Calculus of bile duct with acute and chronic cholecystitis without obstruction
K80.47	Calculus of bile duct with acute and chronic cholecystitis with obstruction
K80.50	Calculus of bile duct without cholangitis or cholecystitis without obstruction
K80.51	Calculus of bile duct without cholangitis or cholecystitis with obstruction
K80.62	Calculus of gallbladder and bile duct with acute cholecystitis without obstruction
K80.63	Calculus of gallbladder and bile duct with acute cholecystitis with obstruction
K80.64	Calculus of gallbladder and bile duct with chronic cholecystitis without obstruction
K80.65	Calculus of gallbladder and bile duct with chronic cholecystitis with obstruction
K80.66	Calculus of gallbladder and bile duct with acute and chronic cholecystitis without obstruction
K80.67	Calculus of gallbladder and bile duct with acute and chronic cholecystitis with obstruction
K80.70	Calculus of gallbladder and bile duct without cholecystitis without obstruction
K80.71	Calculus of gallbladder and bile duct without cholecystitis with obstruction
K80.80	Other cholelithiasis without obstruction
K80.81	Other cholelithiasis with obstruction
K81.0	Acute cholecystitis
K81.1	Chronic cholecystitis
K81.2	Acute cholecystitis with chronic cholecystitis
K82.0	Obstruction of gallbladder
K82.1	Hydrops of gallbladder
K82.2	Perforation of gallbladder

Biliary Tract

K82.3	Fistula of gallbladder
K82.4	Cholesterolosis of gallbladder
K82.8	Other specified diseases of gallbladder
K82.A1	Gangrene of gallbladder in cholecystitis
K82.A2	Perforation of gallbladder in cholecystitis
K83.01	Primary sclerosing cholangitis
K83.09	Other cholangitis
K83.1	Obstruction of bile duct
K83.2	Perforation of bile duct
K83.3	Fistula of bile duct
K83.4	Spasm of sphincter of Oddi
K83.5	Biliary cyst
K83.8	Other specified diseases of biliary tract
K85.02	Idiopathic acute pancreatitis with infected necrosis
K85.21	Alcohol induced acute pancreatitis with uninfected necrosis
K85.32	Drug induced acute pancreatitis with infected necrosis
K85.81	Other acute pancreatitis with uninfected necrosis
R10.0	Acute abdomen
R10.11	Right upper quadrant pain
R19.01	Right upper quadrant abdominal swelling, mass and lump
S36.122A	Contusion of gallbladder, initial encounter
S36.123A	Laceration of gallbladder, initial encounter
S36.128A	Other injury of gallbladder, initial encounter
S36.13XA	Injury of bile duct, initial encounter

AMA: 47610 2018,Jan,8; 2017,Jan,8; 2016,Jan,13; 2015,Jan,16

Relative Value Units/Medicare Edits

Non-Facility RVU	Work	PE	MP	Total
47610	20.92	11.17	5.01	37.1
47612	21.21	11.41	5.18	37.8
47620	23.07	12.11	5.63	40.81
Facility RVU	**Work**	**PE**	**MP**	**Total**
47610	20.92	11.17	5.01	37.1
47612	21.21	11.41	5.18	37.8
47620	23.07	12.11	5.63	40.81

	FUD	Status	MUE		Modifiers			IOM Reference
47610	90	A	1(2)	51	N/A	62*	80	None
47612	90	A	1(2)	51	N/A	62*	80	
47620	90	A	1(2)	51	N/A	62*	80	

* with documentation

47700

47700 Exploration for congenital atresia of bile ducts, without repair, with or without liver biopsy, with or without cholangiography

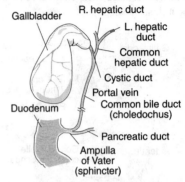

This surgery is usually performed very early in life

Atresia is the congenital failure of the biliary tract to develop lumina

Explanation

The physician explores a congenital atresia of the bile ducts without making a repair, with or without liver biopsy, with or without cholangiography. The physician uses an upper midline abdominal incision to expose the liver, gallbladder, and bile ducts. Inspection and evaluation of the gallbladder, common bile ducts, and duodenum is carried out to determine the status of the bile ducts. A tissue sample may be removed. Cholangiography may be performed. A biliary drainage tube may be placed.

Coding Tips

Liver biopsy and cholangiography, if performed, are included in this procedure and should not be reported separately. Do not append modifier 63 to 47700 as the description or nature of the procedure includes infants up to 4 kg.

ICD-10-CM Diagnostic Codes

Q44.2   Atresia of bile ducts

AMA: 47700 2014,Jan,11

Relative Value Units/Medicare Edits

Non-Facility RVU	Work	PE	MP	Total
47700	16.5	10.95	4.03	31.48
Facility RVU	**Work**	**PE**	**MP**	**Total**
47700	16.5	10.95	4.03	31.48

	FUD	Status	MUE		Modifiers			IOM Reference
47700	90	A	1(2)	51	N/A	62*	80	None

* with documentation

47711-47712

47711 Excision of bile duct tumor, with or without primary repair of bile duct; extrahepatic
47712 intrahepatic

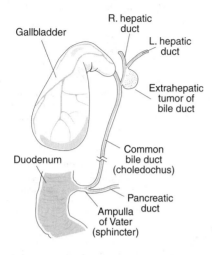

Explanation

The physician performs excision of an extrahepatic bile duct tumor and reconstructs bile duct drainage. The physician makes an abdominal incision and explores the abdomen. The bile duct is dissected from surrounding structures and the tumor is identified and mobilized. The tumor is excised with a margin of normal bile duct tissue proximal and distal to the tumor. An anastomosis is usually created between the proximal end of the bile duct and a loop of small bowel to allow biliary drainage. The distal end of the bile duct is oversewn. The incision is closed. In 44712, an intrahepatic bile duct tumor is excised and reconstruction of the bile duct drainage is performed. Through an abdominal excision, the physician isolates the distal bile duct. The tumor is identified and dissection is continued proximally along the bile duct into the parenchyma of the liver beyond the tumor onto the left and right hepatic ducts. The tumor is excised with a normal margin of bile duct or hepatic duct proximal and distal to the tumor. An anastomosis is created between the proximal bile duct or left and right hepatic ducts and a limb of small bowel to allow biliary drainage. The distal end of the bile duct is oversewn. The incision is closed.

Coding Tips

For anastomosis of the biliary ducts and the gastrointestinal tract, see 47760–47785. Reconstruction of the extrahepatic ducts with end-to-end anastomosis is reported with 47800.

ICD-10-CM Diagnostic Codes

C22.1	Intrahepatic bile duct carcinoma
C24.0	Malignant neoplasm of extrahepatic bile duct
C24.1	Malignant neoplasm of ampulla of Vater
C24.8	Malignant neoplasm of overlapping sites of biliary tract
C78.7	Secondary malignant neoplasm of liver and intrahepatic bile duct
C78.89	Secondary malignant neoplasm of other digestive organs
C7A.1	Malignant poorly differentiated neuroendocrine tumors
D01.5	Carcinoma in situ of liver, gallbladder and bile ducts
D13.5	Benign neoplasm of extrahepatic bile ducts

D37.6	Neoplasm of uncertain behavior of liver, gallbladder and bile ducts
K83.5	Biliary cyst
K83.8	Other specified diseases of biliary tract
K87	Disorders of gallbladder, biliary tract and pancreas in diseases classified elsewhere

AMA: 47711 2014,Jan,11 **47712** 2014,Jan,11

Relative Value Units/Medicare Edits

Non-Facility RVU	Work	PE	MP	Total
47711	25.9	14.04	6.14	46.08
47712	33.72	17.22	8.25	59.19
Facility RVU	**Work**	**PE**	**MP**	**Total**
47711	25.9	14.04	6.14	46.08
47712	33.72	17.22	8.25	59.19

	FUD	Status	MUE	Modifiers				IOM Reference
47711	90	A	1(2)	51	N/A	62*	80	None
47712	90	A	1(2)	51	N/A	62*	80	

* with documentation

Terms To Know

ampulla of Vater. Tubular structure with flask-like dilation where the common bile and pancreatic ducts join before emptying into the duodenum.

anastomosis. Surgically created connection between ducts, blood vessels, or bowel segments to allow flow from one to the other.

carcinoma in situ. Malignancy that arises from the cells of the vessel, gland, or organ of origin that remains confined to that site or has not invaded neighboring tissue.

exploration. Examination for diagnostic purposes.

hepatic portal vein. Blood vessel that delivers unoxygenated blood from the gastrointestinal tract, spleen, pancreas, and gallbladder to the liver.

malignant. Any condition tending to progress toward death, specifically an invasive tumor with a loss of cellular differentiation that has the ability to spread or metastasize to other body areas.

neoplasm. New abnormal growth, tumor.

proximal. Located closest to a specified reference point, usually the midline or trunk.

reconstruction. Recreating, restoring, or rebuilding a body part or organ.

Biliary Tract

47715

47715   Excision of choledochal cyst

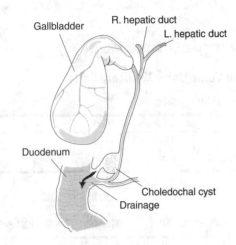

Gallbladder
R. hepatic duct
L. hepatic duct
Duodenum
Choledochal cyst
Drainage

Explanation

The physician excises a cyst in the common bile duct. The physician exposes the liver and gallbladder via an upper midline or subcostal incision made through skin, fascia, and muscle. The cyst is exposed and excised and the defect of the biliary system is repaired. The abdominal incision is closed with layered sutures.

Coding Tips

For an excision of a bile duct tumor, see 47711–47712.

ICD-10-CM Diagnostic Codes

Q44.4   Choledochal cyst

AMA: 47715 2018,Jan,8; 2017,Jan,8; 2016,Jan,13; 2015,Jan,16

Relative Value Units/Medicare Edits

Non-Facility RVU	Work	PE	MP	Total
47715	21.55	12.71	5.25	39.51
Facility RVU	**Work**	**PE**	**MP**	**Total**
47715	21.55	12.71	5.25	39.51

	FUD	Status	MUE	Modifiers				IOM Reference
47715	90	A	1(2)	51	N/A	62*	80	None

* with documentation

47720-47741

47720   Cholecystoenterostomy; direct
47721   with gastroenterostomy
47740   Roux-en-Y
47741   Roux-en-Y with gastroenterostomy

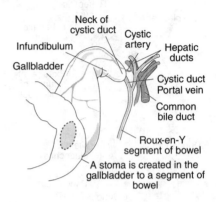

Neck of cystic duct
Cystic artery
Infundibulum
Hepatic ducts
Gallbladder
Cystic duct
Portal vein
Common bile duct
Roux-en-Y segment of bowel
A stoma is created in the gallbladder to a segment of bowel

Explanation

The physician performs a cholecystoenterostomy, in which a communication is made between the gallbladder and an artificial anus or fistula in the abdominal wall. The physician exposes the liver and gallbladder via an upper midline or subcostal incision. The cyst is opened and connected to the small intestine for drainage. The abdominal incision is closed. Report 47721 if this procedure is performed with gastroenterostomy; report 47740 if this procedure is performed with Roux-en-Y; and report 47741 if this procedure is performed with Roux-en-Y with gastroenterostomy.

Coding Tips

For laparoscopic cholecystoenterostomy, see 47570. For anastomosis of the biliary ducts and the gastrointestinal tract, see 47760–47785.

ICD-10-CM Diagnostic Codes

C22.1	Intrahepatic bile duct carcinoma
C23	Malignant neoplasm of gallbladder
C24.0	Malignant neoplasm of extrahepatic bile duct
C24.1	Malignant neoplasm of ampulla of Vater
C24.8	Malignant neoplasm of overlapping sites of biliary tract
C25.0	Malignant neoplasm of head of pancreas
C25.1	Malignant neoplasm of body of pancreas
C25.2	Malignant neoplasm of tail of pancreas
C25.3	Malignant neoplasm of pancreatic duct
C25.4	Malignant neoplasm of endocrine pancreas
C25.7	Malignant neoplasm of other parts of pancreas
C25.8	Malignant neoplasm of overlapping sites of pancreas
C78.7	Secondary malignant neoplasm of liver and intrahepatic bile duct
C78.89	Secondary malignant neoplasm of other digestive organs
C7A.1	Malignant poorly differentiated neuroendocrine tumors
C7A.8	Other malignant neuroendocrine tumors
D01.5	Carcinoma in situ of liver, gallbladder and bile ducts
D13.4	Benign neoplasm of liver
D13.5	Benign neoplasm of extrahepatic bile ducts
D37.6	Neoplasm of uncertain behavior of liver, gallbladder and bile ducts

Biliary Tract

K56.3	Gallstone ileus	
K74.3	Primary biliary cirrhosis	
K74.4	Secondary biliary cirrhosis	
K74.69	Other cirrhosis of liver	
K80.80	Other cholelithiasis without obstruction	
K80.81	Other cholelithiasis with obstruction	
K81.0	Acute cholecystitis	
K81.1	Chronic cholecystitis	
K81.2	Acute cholecystitis with chronic cholecystitis	
K82.0	Obstruction of gallbladder	
K82.1	Hydrops of gallbladder	
K82.2	Perforation of gallbladder	
K82.3	Fistula of gallbladder	
K82.4	Cholesterolosis of gallbladder	
K82.8	Other specified diseases of gallbladder	
K83.01	Primary sclerosing cholangitis	
K83.09	Other cholangitis	
K83.1	Obstruction of bile duct	
K83.2	Perforation of bile duct	
K83.3	Fistula of bile duct	
K83.4	Spasm of sphincter of Oddi	
K83.5	Biliary cyst	
K83.8	Other specified diseases of biliary tract	
K85.00	Idiopathic acute pancreatitis without necrosis or infection	
K85.01	Idiopathic acute pancreatitis with uninfected necrosis	
K85.02	Idiopathic acute pancreatitis with infected necrosis	
K85.10	Biliary acute pancreatitis without necrosis or infection	
K85.11	Biliary acute pancreatitis with uninfected necrosis	
K85.12	Biliary acute pancreatitis with infected necrosis	
K85.20	Alcohol induced acute pancreatitis without necrosis or infection	
K85.21	Alcohol induced acute pancreatitis with uninfected necrosis	
K85.22	Alcohol induced acute pancreatitis with infected necrosis	
K85.30	Drug induced acute pancreatitis without necrosis or infection	
K85.31	Drug induced acute pancreatitis with uninfected necrosis	
K85.32	Drug induced acute pancreatitis with infected necrosis	
K85.80	Other acute pancreatitis without necrosis or infection	
K85.81	Other acute pancreatitis with uninfected necrosis	
K85.82	Other acute pancreatitis with infected necrosis	
K86.0	Alcohol-induced chronic pancreatitis	
K86.1	Other chronic pancreatitis	
K86.2	Cyst of pancreas	
K86.3	Pseudocyst of pancreas	
K87	Disorders of gallbladder, biliary tract and pancreas in diseases classified elsewhere	

AMA: **47720** 2018,Jan,8; 2017,Jan,8; 2016,Jan,13; 2015,Jan,16

Relative Value Units/Medicare Edits

Non-Facility RVU	Work	PE	MP	Total
47720	18.34	11.52	4.49	34.35
47721	21.99	12.87	5.38	40.24
47740	21.23	12.59	5.19	39.01
47741	24.21	13.7	5.93	43.84
Facility RVU	Work	PE	MP	Total
47720	18.34	11.52	4.49	34.35
47721	21.99	12.87	5.38	40.24
47740	21.23	12.59	5.19	39.01
47741	24.21	13.7	5.93	43.84

	FUD	Status	MUE	Modifiers				IOM Reference
47720	90	A	1(2)	51	N/A	62*	80	None
47721	90	A	1(2)	51	N/A	62*	80	
47740	90	A	1(2)	51	N/A	62*	80	
47741	90	A	1(2)	51	N/A	62*	80	

* with documentation

Terms To Know

calculus. Abnormal, stone-like concretion of calcium, cholesterol, mineral salts, or other substances that forms in any part of the body.

closure. Repairing an incision or wound by suture or other means.

cyst. Elevated encapsulated mass containing fluid, semisolid, or solid material with a membranous lining.

drain. Device that creates a channel to allow fluid from a cavity, wound, or infected area to exit the body.

jaundice. Increased bilirubin and deposits of bile pigment in the skin and sclera, causing a yellow tint.

malignant. Any condition tending to progress toward death, specifically an invasive tumor with a loss of cellular differentiation that has the ability to spread or metastasize to other body areas.

neoplasm. New abnormal growth, tumor.

obstruction. Blockage that prevents normal function of the valve or structure.

Roux-en-Y anastomosis. Y-shaped attachment of the distal end of a divided small intestine segment to the stomach, esophagus, biliary tract, or other structure with anastomosis of the proximal end to the side of the small intestine further down for reflux-free drainage.

stoma. Opening created in the abdominal wall from an internal organ or structure for diversion of waste elimination, drainage, and access.

Biliary Tract

47760-47765

47760 Anastomosis, of extrahepatic biliary ducts and gastrointestinal tract
47765 Anastomosis, of intrahepatic ducts and gastrointestinal tract

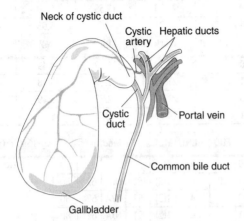

A connection between the hepatic
ducts (near the top of the hepatic tree)
and a segment of bowel is performed

Explanation

The physician performs an anastomosis between an extrahepatic biliary duct and the small bowel. The physician makes an abdominal incision and explores the abdomen. The extrahepatic biliary duct is divided and anastomosis is formed between an extrahepatic biliary duct and the small bowel with sutures or staples (end-to-side). The incision is closed in layers. Report 47765 for an intrahepatic biliary duct.

Coding Tips

For excision of a bile duct tumor, with or without primary repair of bile duct, see 47711–47712. For anastomosis with Roux-en-Y reconstruction, see 47780 and 47785.

ICD-10-CM Diagnostic Codes

C22.1	Intrahepatic bile duct carcinoma
C23	Malignant neoplasm of gallbladder
C24.0	Malignant neoplasm of extrahepatic bile duct
C24.1	Malignant neoplasm of ampulla of Vater
C24.8	Malignant neoplasm of overlapping sites of biliary tract
C78.7	Secondary malignant neoplasm of liver and intrahepatic bile duct
C78.89	Secondary malignant neoplasm of other digestive organs
C7A.1	Malignant poorly differentiated neuroendocrine tumors
C7A.8	Other malignant neuroendocrine tumors
D01.5	Carcinoma in situ of liver, gallbladder and bile ducts
D13.5	Benign neoplasm of extrahepatic bile ducts
K83.01	Primary sclerosing cholangitis
K83.09	Other cholangitis
K83.1	Obstruction of bile duct
K83.2	Perforation of bile duct
K83.3	Fistula of bile duct
K83.4	Spasm of sphincter of Oddi
K83.5	Biliary cyst
K83.8	Other specified diseases of biliary tract

K87	Disorders of gallbladder, biliary tract and pancreas in diseases classified elsewhere
Q44.2	Atresia of bile ducts
Q44.3	Congenital stenosis and stricture of bile ducts
Q44.5	Other congenital malformations of bile ducts

AMA: 47760 2014,Jan,11 **47765** 2014,Jan,11

Relative Value Units/Medicare Edits

Non-Facility RVU	Work	PE	MP	Total
47760	38.32	19.22	9.02	66.56
47765	52.19	24.85	12.77	89.81
Facility RVU	**Work**	**PE**	**MP**	**Total**
47760	38.32	19.22	9.02	66.56
47765	52.19	24.85	12.77	89.81

	FUD	Status	MUE	Modifiers				IOM Reference
47760	90	A	1(2)	51	N/A	62*	80	None
47765	90	A	1(2)	51	N/A	62*	80	

* with documentation

Terms To Know

anastomosis. Surgically created connection between ducts, blood vessels, or bowel segments to allow flow from one to the other.

benign. Mild or nonmalignant in nature.

exploration. Examination for diagnostic purposes.

incision. Act of cutting into tissue or an organ.

malignant. Any condition tending to progress toward death, specifically an invasive tumor with a loss of cellular differentiation that has the ability to spread or metastasize to other body areas.

neoplasm. New abnormal growth, tumor.

obstruction. Blockage that prevents normal function of the valve or structure.

suture. Numerous stitching techniques employed in wound closure.

buried suture. Continuous or interrupted suture placed under the skin for a layered closure.

continuous suture. Running stitch with tension evenly distributed across a single strand to provide a leakproof closure line.

interrupted suture. Series of single stitches with tension isolated at each stitch, in which all stitches are not affected if one becomes loose, and the isolated sutures cannot act as a wick to transport an infection.

purse-string suture. Continuous suture placed around a tubular structure and tightened, to reduce or close the lumen.

retention suture. Secondary stitching that bridges the primary suture, providing support for the primary repair; a plastic or rubber bolster may be placed over the primary repair and under the retention sutures.

Biliary Tract

47780-47785

47780 Anastomosis, Roux-en-Y, of extrahepatic biliary ducts and gastrointestinal tract

47785 Anastomosis, Roux-en-Y, of intrahepatic biliary ducts and gastrointestinal tract

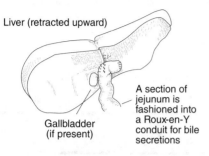

Liver (retracted upward)

Gallbladder (if present)

A section of jejunum is fashioned into a Roux-en-Y conduit for bile secretions

The hepatic biliary ducts near the top of the biliary tree are anastomosed into a Roux-en-Y segment of bowel

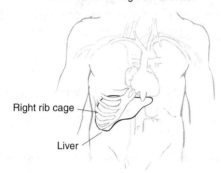

Right rib cage

Liver

Explanation

In 47780, the physician performs an anastomosis between a limb of small bowel (Roux-en-Y) and the gallbladder and stomach. The physician makes an abdominal incision and explores the abdomen. The proximal small bowel is divided and anastomoses are formed between the distal limb of jejunum and the gallbladder and the stomach with sutures or staples. The proximal end of bowel is approximated to the limb of jejunum distal to the gallbladder and stomach anastomoses. This procedure is usually performed for a mass obstructing the bile duct and stomach. The incision is closed. In 47785, the anastomosis is between a limb of small bowel (Roux-en-Y) and the intrahepatic biliary ducts. The bile duct is isolated and dissection is carried proximally along the duct into the liver parenchyma exposing the intrahepatic biliary ducts. The bile duct is divided or excised. The proximal small bowel is divided and an anastomosis is created between the distal limb of jejunum and the intrahepatic biliary ducts with sutures. The distal bile duct is oversewn. The proximal end of bowel is approximated to the limb of jejunum distal to the bile duct anastomosis. The incision is closed.

Coding Tips

For excision of a bile duct tumor, with or without primary repair of the bile duct, see 47711–47712. For anastomosis without Roux-en-Y reconstruction, see 47760–47765.

ICD-10-CM Diagnostic Codes

C22.1	Intrahepatic bile duct carcinoma
C23	Malignant neoplasm of gallbladder
C24.0	Malignant neoplasm of extrahepatic bile duct
C24.1	Malignant neoplasm of ampulla of Vater
C24.8	Malignant neoplasm of overlapping sites of biliary tract
C78.7	Secondary malignant neoplasm of liver and intrahepatic bile duct
C78.89	Secondary malignant neoplasm of other digestive organs
C7A.1	Malignant poorly differentiated neuroendocrine tumors
C7A.8	Other malignant neuroendocrine tumors
D01.5	Carcinoma in situ of liver, gallbladder and bile ducts
D13.5	Benign neoplasm of extrahepatic bile ducts
K83.01	Primary sclerosing cholangitis
K83.09	Other cholangitis
K83.1	Obstruction of bile duct
K83.2	Perforation of bile duct
K83.3	Fistula of bile duct
K83.4	Spasm of sphincter of Oddi
K83.5	Biliary cyst
K83.8	Other specified diseases of biliary tract
K87	Disorders of gallbladder, biliary tract and pancreas in diseases classified elsewhere
Q44.2	Atresia of bile ducts
Q44.3	Congenital stenosis and stricture of bile ducts
Q44.5	Other congenital malformations of bile ducts

AMA: 47780 2014,Jan,11 **47785** 2014,Jan,11

Relative Value Units/Medicare Edits

Non-Facility RVU	Work	PE	MP	Total
47780	42.32	20.66	10.14	73.12
47785	56.19	26.11	13.3	95.6
Facility RVU	Work	PE	MP	Total
47780	42.32	20.66	10.14	73.12
47785	56.19	26.11	13.3	95.6

	FUD	Status	MUE	Modifiers				IOM Reference
47780	90	A	1(2)	51	N/A	62*	80	None
47785	90	A	1(2)	51	N/A	62*	80	

* with documentation

Terms To Know

anastomosis. Surgically created connection between ducts, blood vessels, or bowel segments to allow flow from one to the other.

dissect. Cut apart or separate tissue for surgical purposes or for visual or microscopic study.

malignant. Any condition tending to progress toward death, specifically an invasive tumor with a loss of cellular differentiation that has the ability to spread or metastasize to other body areas.

obstruction. Blockage that prevents normal function of the valve or structure.

Roux-en-Y anastomosis. Y-shaped attachment of the distal end of a divided small intestine segment to the stomach, esophagus, biliary tract, or other structure with anastomosis of the proximal end to the side of the small intestine further down for reflux-free drainage.

Biliary Tract

47800

47800   Reconstruction, plastic, of extrahepatic biliary ducts with end-to-end anastomosis

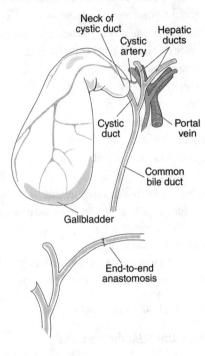

Neck of cystic duct

Cystic artery

Hepatic ducts

Cystic duct

Portal vein

Common bile duct

Gallbladder

End-to-end anastomosis

Explanation

The physician reconstructs the biliary ducts through anastomosis. The physician exposes the liver and gallbladder via an upper midline or subcostal incision made via skin, fascia, and muscle. The abnormal biliary tree is excised and the resected ends are reconnected. The incision is closed with layered sutures.

Coding Tips

For excision of a bile duct tumor, with or without primary repair of the bile duct, see 47711–47712. For anastomosis without Roux-en-Y, see 47760 and 47765; with, see 47780 and 47785.

ICD-10-CM Diagnostic Codes

C22.1	Intrahepatic bile duct carcinoma
C24.0	Malignant neoplasm of extrahepatic bile duct
C24.1	Malignant neoplasm of ampulla of Vater
C24.8	Malignant neoplasm of overlapping sites of biliary tract
C78.7	Secondary malignant neoplasm of liver and intrahepatic bile duct
C78.89	Secondary malignant neoplasm of other digestive organs
C7A.1	Malignant poorly differentiated neuroendocrine tumors
C7A.8	Other malignant neuroendocrine tumors
D01.5	Carcinoma in situ of liver, gallbladder and bile ducts
D13.5	Benign neoplasm of extrahepatic bile ducts
K83.01	Primary sclerosing cholangitis
K83.09	Other cholangitis
K83.1	Obstruction of bile duct
K83.2	Perforation of bile duct
K83.3	Fistula of bile duct
K83.4	Spasm of sphincter of Oddi
K83.5	Biliary cyst
K83.8	Other specified diseases of biliary tract
K87	Disorders of gallbladder, biliary tract and pancreas in diseases classified elsewhere
Q44.2	Atresia of bile ducts
Q44.3	Congenital stenosis and stricture of bile ducts
Q44.5	Other congenital malformations of bile ducts
S36.13XA	Injury of bile duct, initial encounter

AMA: 47800 2014,Jan,11

Relative Value Units/Medicare Edits

Non-Facility RVU	Work	PE	MP	Total
47800	26.17	14.12	5.9	46.19
Facility RVU	**Work**	**PE**	**MP**	**Total**
47800	26.17	14.12	5.9	46.19

	FUD	Status	MUE	Modifiers				IOM Reference
47800	90	A	1(2)	51	N/A	62*	80	None

* with documentation

Terms To Know

anastomosis. Surgically created connection between ducts, blood vessels, or bowel segments to allow flow from one to the other.

benign. Mild or nonmalignant in nature.

closure. Repairing an incision or wound by suture or other means.

excision. Surgical removal of an organ or tissue.

fascia. Fibrous sheet or band of tissue that envelops organs, muscles, and groupings of muscles.

incision. Act of cutting into tissue or an organ.

malignant. Any condition tending to progress toward death, specifically an invasive tumor with a loss of cellular differentiation that has the ability to spread or metastasize to other body areas.

neoplasm. New abnormal growth, tumor.

obstruction. Blockage that prevents normal function of the valve or structure.

reconstruction. Recreating, restoring, or rebuilding a body part or organ.

resect. Cutting out or removing a portion or all of a bone, organ, or other structure.

skin. Outer protective covering of the body composed of the epidermis and dermis, situated above the subcutaneous tissues.

Biliary Tract

47801

47801 Placement of choledochal stent

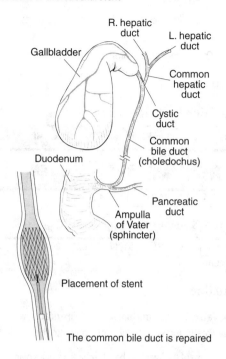

Placement of stent

The common bile duct is repaired

Explanation

The physician inserts a stent into the bile duct. The physician makes a small incision overlying the bile duct. Using an endoscope or percutaneous choledochostomy tube, a catheter and stent are placed to bridge a narrowing in the common bile duct. The scope or tube is removed and the incision closed.

Coding Tips

For cholangiopancreatography (ERCP) with endoscopic retrograde insertion or stent into the bile or pancreatic duct, see 43274; removal and/or replacement of stent, see 43275–43276. For biliary endoscopy, percutaneous via T-tube or other tract with dilation of biliary duct strictures with stent placement, see 47556.

ICD-10-CM Diagnostic Codes

C22.1	Intrahepatic bile duct carcinoma
C24.0	Malignant neoplasm of extrahepatic bile duct
C24.1	Malignant neoplasm of ampulla of Vater
C24.8	Malignant neoplasm of overlapping sites of biliary tract
C78.7	Secondary malignant neoplasm of liver and intrahepatic bile duct
C78.89	Secondary malignant neoplasm of other digestive organs
C7A.1	Malignant poorly differentiated neuroendocrine tumors
C7A.8	Other malignant neuroendocrine tumors
D01.5	Carcinoma in situ of liver, gallbladder and bile ducts
D13.5	Benign neoplasm of extrahepatic bile ducts
K83.01	Primary sclerosing cholangitis
K83.09	Other cholangitis
K83.1	Obstruction of bile duct
K83.2	Perforation of bile duct
K83.3	Fistula of bile duct
K83.4	Spasm of sphincter of Oddi
K83.5	Biliary cyst
K83.8	Other specified diseases of biliary tract
K87	Disorders of gallbladder, biliary tract and pancreas in diseases classified elsewhere
Q44.2	Atresia of bile ducts
Q44.3	Congenital stenosis and stricture of bile ducts
Q44.5	Other congenital malformations of bile ducts

AMA: 47801 2018,Jan,8; 2017,Jan,8; 2016,Jan,13; 2015,Jan,16

Relative Value Units/Medicare Edits

Non-Facility RVU	Work	PE	MP	Total
47801	17.6	11.25	4.32	33.17
Facility RVU	**Work**	**PE**	**MP**	**Total**
47801	17.6	11.25	4.32	33.17

	FUD	Status	MUE	Modifiers				IOM Reference
47801	90	A	1(3)	51	N/A	62*	80	None

* with documentation

Terms To Know

ampulla of Vater. Tubular structure with flask-like dilation where the common bile and pancreatic ducts join before emptying into the duodenum.

benign. Mild or nonmalignant in nature.

catheter. Flexible tube inserted into an area of the body for introducing or withdrawing fluid.

duodenum. First portion of the small intestine connected to the stomach at the pylorus and extending to the jejunum.

endoscopy. Visual inspection of the body using a fiberoptic scope.

hepatic portal vein. Blood vessel that delivers unoxygenated blood from the gastrointestinal tract, spleen, pancreas, and gallbladder to the liver.

incision. Act of cutting into tissue or an organ.

malignant. Any condition tending to progress toward death, specifically an invasive tumor with a loss of cellular differentiation that has the ability to spread or metastasize to other body areas.

neoplasm. New abnormal growth, tumor.

obstruction. Blockage that prevents normal function of the valve or structure.

percutaneous. Through the skin.

stent. Tube to provide support in a body cavity or lumen.

tube. Long, hollow cylindrical instrument or body structure.

Biliary Tract

47802

47802   U-tube hepaticoenterostomy

R. hepatic duct
L. hepatic duct
Gallbladder
Common hepatic duct
Cystic duct
Common bile duct (choledochus)
Duodenum
Pancreatic duct
Ampulla of Vater (sphincter)

A tube is introduced from an upper hepatic duct to a segment of bowel

To intestine

Explanation

The physician establishes a communication between the hepatic ducts and the intestine. The physician exposes the liver and gallbladder via an upper midline or subcostal incision. A Silastic tube is connected between the biliary tree and the intestine for drainage of the biliary obstruction. The abdominal incision is closed.

Coding Tips

For portoenterostomy (Kasai procedure), see 47701.

ICD-10-CM Diagnostic Codes

C22.1	Intrahepatic bile duct carcinoma
C24.0	Malignant neoplasm of extrahepatic bile duct
C24.1	Malignant neoplasm of ampulla of Vater
C24.8	Malignant neoplasm of overlapping sites of biliary tract
C78.7	Secondary malignant neoplasm of liver and intrahepatic bile duct
C78.89	Secondary malignant neoplasm of other digestive organs
C7A.1	Malignant poorly differentiated neuroendocrine tumors
C7A.8	Other malignant neuroendocrine tumors
D01.5	Carcinoma in situ of liver, gallbladder and bile ducts
D13.5	Benign neoplasm of extrahepatic bile ducts
K83.01	Primary sclerosing cholangitis
K83.09	Other cholangitis
K83.1	Obstruction of bile duct
K83.2	Perforation of bile duct
K83.3	Fistula of bile duct
K83.4	Spasm of sphincter of Oddi
K83.5	Biliary cyst

K83.8	Other specified diseases of biliary tract
K87	Disorders of gallbladder, biliary tract and pancreas in diseases classified elsewhere
Q44.2	Atresia of bile ducts
Q44.3	Congenital stenosis and stricture of bile ducts
Q44.4	Choledochal cyst
Q44.5	Other congenital malformations of bile ducts

AMA: 47802 2014,Jan,11

Relative Value Units/Medicare Edits

Non-Facility RVU	Work	PE	MP	Total
47802	24.93	14.29	6.1	45.32
Facility RVU	**Work**	**PE**	**MP**	**Total**
47802	24.93	14.29	6.1	45.32

	FUD	Status	MUE	Modifiers				IOM Reference
47802	90	A	1(2)	51	N/A	62*	80	None

* with documentation

Terms To Know

ampulla of Vater. Tubular structure with flask-like dilation where the common bile and pancreatic ducts join before emptying into the duodenum.

cirrhosis. Disease of the liver that has the characteristics of intertwining band of fibrous tissue that divides the parenchyma into micro- and macronodular areas, which cause the liver to stop functioning over time.

closure. Repairing an incision or wound by suture or other means.

drain. Device that creates a channel to allow fluid from a cavity, wound, or infected area to exit the body.

duodenum. First portion of the small intestine connected to the stomach at the pylorus and extending to the jejunum.

incision. Act of cutting into tissue or an organ.

malignant. Any condition tending to progress toward death, specifically an invasive tumor with a loss of cellular differentiation that has the ability to spread or metastasize to other body areas.

neoplasm. New abnormal growth, tumor.

obstruction. Blockage that prevents normal function of the valve or structure.

secondary. Second in order of occurrence or importance, or appearing during the course of another disease or condition.

tube. Long, hollow cylindrical instrument or body structure.

Biliary Tract

47900

47900 Suture of extrahepatic biliary duct for pre-existing injury (separate procedure)

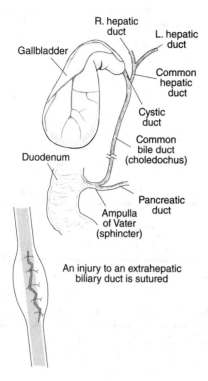

R. hepatic duct
L. hepatic duct
Gallbladder
Common hepatic duct
Cystic duct
Common bile duct (choledochus)
Duodenum
Pancreatic duct
Ampulla of Vater (sphincter)

An injury to an extrahepatic biliary duct is sutured

Explanation

The physician performs suture closure of a biliary duct injury. The physician makes an abdominal incision. The bile duct is dissected from surrounding structures and the injury of the duct is identified. The duct injury is closed with sutures. A drain is usually placed and brought out through the abdominal wall. The incision is closed.

Coding Tips

This separate procedure by definition is usually a component of a more complex service and is not identified separately. When performed alone or with other unrelated procedures/services it may be reported. If performed alone, list the code; if performed with other procedures/services, list the code and append modifier 59 or an X{EPSU} modifier.

ICD-10-CM Diagnostic Codes

S36.13XA   Injury of bile duct, initial encounter

AMA: 47900 2014,Jan,11

Relative Value Units/Medicare Edits

Non-Facility RVU	Work	PE	MP	Total
47900	22.44	12.56	5.21	40.21
Facility RVU	**Work**	**PE**	**MP**	**Total**
47900	22.44	12.56	5.21	40.21

	FUD	Status	MUE	Modifiers				IOM Reference
47900	90	A	1(2)	51	N/A	62*	80	None

* with documentation

48000-48001

48000 Placement of drains, peripancreatic, for acute pancreatitis;
48001 with cholecystostomy, gastrostomy, and jejunostomy

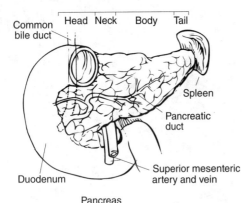

Pancreas

Explanation

The physician places peripancreatic drains for acute pancreatitis. The physician makes an upper transverse abdominal incision. The transverse colon and small intestines are retracted to reveal the underlying pancreas. Necrotic pancreatic tissue may be resected. Drains are placed circumferentially around the pancreas, sutured secure, and anchored through the abdominal wall. The upper transverse abdominal incision is closed with sutures. Report 48001 when placement of the drains is performed with cholecystostomy, gastrostomy, and jejunostomy. Through an abdominal incision the pancreas is exposed, necrotic pancreatic tissue may be debrided, and drains are placed around the pancreas. The gallbladder is identified and a tube is sutured into the gallbladder and brought out through the abdominal wall. An incision is made in the anterior gastric wall and a tube is sutured into the stomach and brought out through the anterior abdominal wall. An incision is made in a proximal segment of jejunum and a tube is sutured into the jejunum and brought out through the anterior abdominal wall. The abdominal incision is closed.

Coding Tips

For resection or debridement of the pancreas and peripancreatic tissue for acute necrotizing pancreatitis, see 48105.

ICD-10-CM Diagnostic Codes

B25.2	Cytomegaloviral pancreatitis
K85.00	Idiopathic acute pancreatitis without necrosis or infection
K85.01	Idiopathic acute pancreatitis with uninfected necrosis
K85.02	Idiopathic acute pancreatitis with infected necrosis
K85.10	Biliary acute pancreatitis without necrosis or infection
K85.11	Biliary acute pancreatitis with uninfected necrosis
K85.12	Biliary acute pancreatitis with infected necrosis
K85.20	Alcohol induced acute pancreatitis without necrosis or infection
K85.21	Alcohol induced acute pancreatitis with uninfected necrosis
K85.22	Alcohol induced acute pancreatitis with infected necrosis
K85.30	Drug induced acute pancreatitis without necrosis or infection
K85.31	Drug induced acute pancreatitis with uninfected necrosis
K85.32	Drug induced acute pancreatitis with infected necrosis
K85.80	Other acute pancreatitis without necrosis or infection
K85.81	Other acute pancreatitis with uninfected necrosis
K85.82	Other acute pancreatitis with infected necrosis
K86.81	Exocrine pancreatic insufficiency
K86.89	Other specified diseases of pancreas
K87	Disorders of gallbladder, biliary tract and pancreas in diseases classified elsewhere
T81.41XA	Infection following a procedure, superficial incisional surgical site, initial encounter
T81.42XA	Infection following a procedure, deep incisional surgical site, initial encounter
T81.43XA	Infection following a procedure, organ and space surgical site, initial encounter
T81.44XA	Sepsis following a procedure, initial encounter
T81.49XA	Infection following a procedure, other surgical site, initial encounter

AMA: 48000 2014,Jan,11 **48001** 2014,Jan,11

Relative Value Units/Medicare Edits

Non-Facility RVU	Work	PE	MP	Total
48000	31.95	15.99	7.81	55.75
48001	39.69	18.87	9.72	68.28
Facility RVU	**Work**	**PE**	**MP**	**Total**
48000	31.95	15.99	7.81	55.75
48001	39.69	18.87	9.72	68.28

	FUD	Status	MUE	Modifiers				IOM Reference
48000	90	A	1(2)	51	N/A	62*	80	None
48001	90	A	1(2)	51	N/A	62*	80	

* with documentation

Terms To Know

acute. Sudden, severe.

drain. Device that creates a channel to allow fluid from a cavity, wound, or infected area to exit the body.

gastrostomy. Temporary or permanent artificial opening made in the stomach for gastrointestinal decompression or to provide nutrition when not maintained by other methods.

idiopathic. Having no known cause.

jejunostomy. Permanent, surgical opening into the jejunum, the part of the small intestine between the duodenum and ileum, through the abdominal wall, often used for placing a feeding tube.

pancreatitis. Inflammation of the pancreas that may be acute or chronic, symptomatic or asymptomatic, due to the autodigestion of pancreatic tissue by its own enzymes that have escaped into the pancreas, most often as a result of alcoholism or biliary tract disease such as calculi in the pancreatic duct.

transverse. Crosswise at right angles to the long axis of a structure or part.

Pancreas

48020

48020   Removal of pancreatic calculus

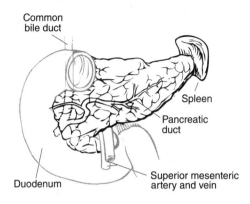

Common bile duct

Spleen

Pancreatic duct

Duodenum

Superior mesenteric artery and vein

A calculus (stone) is surgically removed from the pancreas

Explanation

The physician removes a stone from the pancreas. The physician exposes the pancreas via an upper midline incision through skin, fascia, and muscle. The pancreatic duct is opened and calculus removed. The pancreatic duct is connected directly to the small bowel for drainage. The abdominal incision is closed.

Coding Tips

This procedure can also be performed endoscopically. For endoscopic retrograde cholangiopancreatography (ERCP) with removal of stones from pancreatic ducts, see 43264; with destruction (lithotripsy) of stones, see 43265.

ICD-10-CM Diagnostic Codes

K86.81	Exocrine pancreatic insufficiency
K86.89	Other specified diseases of pancreas
K87	Disorders of gallbladder, biliary tract and pancreas in diseases classified elsewhere

AMA: 48020 2014,Jan,11

Relative Value Units/Medicare Edits

Non-Facility RVU	Work	PE	MP	Total
48020	19.09	11.23	4.67	34.99
Facility RVU	Work	PE	MP	Total
48020	19.09	11.23	4.67	34.99

	FUD	Status	MUE	Modifiers				IOM Reference
48020	90	A	1(3)	51	N/A	62*	80	None

* with documentation

48100-48102

48100   Biopsy of pancreas, open (eg, fine needle aspiration, needle core biopsy, wedge biopsy)
48102   Biopsy of pancreas, percutaneous needle

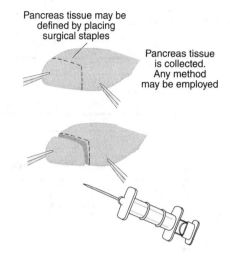

Pancreas tissue may be defined by placing surgical staples

Pancreas tissue is collected. Any method may be employed

Explanation

In 48100, the physician obtains a biopsy of the pancreas. The physician makes a midline epigastric incision and retracts the skin and underlying tissues laterally. The physician approaches the pancreas through the lesser sac of the omental bursa. The pancreas is palpated, the lesion is identified, and a biopsy is obtained by various methods, such as fine needle aspiration or needle core or wedge biopsy. Bleeding is controlled and the lesser sac is closed. Tissues are reapproximated to the anatomical position and the incision is sutured in layers. In 48102, a biopsy needle is passed through the skin of the upper abdomen under separately reportable computerized tomography guidance. The pancreatic lesion is removed and the specimen is sent for pathology examination (reported separately).

Coding Tips

For cholangiopancreatography (ERCP) with biopsy, see 43261. Radiological supervision and interpretation is reported with 76942, 77002, 77012, and 77021, when performed. For fine needle aspiration, see 10004–10012 and 10021; evaluation of aspirate, see 88172–88173.

ICD-10-CM Diagnostic Codes

C25.0	Malignant neoplasm of head of pancreas
C25.1	Malignant neoplasm of body of pancreas
C25.2	Malignant neoplasm of tail of pancreas
C25.3	Malignant neoplasm of pancreatic duct
C25.4	Malignant neoplasm of endocrine pancreas
C25.7	Malignant neoplasm of other parts of pancreas
C25.8	Malignant neoplasm of overlapping sites of pancreas
C78.89	Secondary malignant neoplasm of other digestive organs
C7A.1	Malignant poorly differentiated neuroendocrine tumors
C7A.8	Other malignant neuroendocrine tumors
D01.7	Carcinoma in situ of other specified digestive organs
D13.6	Benign neoplasm of pancreas
D13.7	Benign neoplasm of endocrine pancreas
D37.8	Neoplasm of uncertain behavior of other specified digestive organs

Pancreas

K86.81   Exocrine pancreatic insufficiency
K86.89   Other specified diseases of pancreas
K87   Disorders of gallbladder, biliary tract and pancreas in diseases classified elsewhere

AMA: **48102** 2019,Apr,4

Relative Value Units/Medicare Edits

Non-Facility RVU	Work	PE	MP	Total
48100	14.46	8.35	3.28	26.09
48102	4.7	10.86	0.42	15.98
Facility RVU	**Work**	**PE**	**MP**	**Total**
48100	14.46	8.35	3.28	26.09
48102	4.7	1.75	0.42	6.87

	FUD	Status	MUE	Modifiers				IOM Reference
48100	90	A	1(3)	51	N/A	62*	80	None
48102	10	A	1(3)	51	N/A	N/A	N/A	

* with documentation

Terms To Know

fine needle aspiration biopsy. Insertion of a fine-gauge needle attached to a syringe into a tissue mass for the suctioned withdrawal of cells used for diagnostic study.

pancreatitis. Inflammation of the pancreas that may be acute or chronic, symptomatic or asymptomatic, due to the autodigestion of pancreatic tissue by its own enzymes that have escaped into the pancreas, most often as a result of alcoholism or biliary tract disease such as calculi in the pancreatic duct.

puncture aspiration. Use of a knife or needle to pierce a fluid-filled cavity and then withdraw the fluid using a syringe or suction device.

specimen. Tissue cells or sample of fluid taken for analysis, pathologic examination, and diagnosis.

wedge excision. Surgical removal of a section of tissue that is thick at one edge and tapers to a thin edge.

48105

48105   Resection or debridement of pancreas and peripancreatic tissue for acute necrotizing pancreatitis

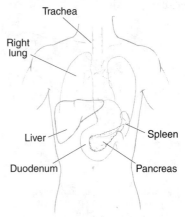

The pancreas secretes insulin and glucagon, which regulates glucose, lipid, and protein metabolism

Explanation

The physician performs resection and debridement of the pancreas for necrotizing pancreatitis. The physician makes an abdominal incision. The pancreas is exposed and necrotic areas of the pancreas and peripancreatic tissue are debrided. Drains are usually placed around the pancreas. The incision is closed.

Coding Tips

For placement of drains, see 48000 and 48001. For an excision of a lesion of the pancreas, see 48120.

ICD-10-CM Diagnostic Codes

B25.2	Cytomegaloviral pancreatitis
K85.00	Idiopathic acute pancreatitis without necrosis or infection
K85.01	Idiopathic acute pancreatitis with uninfected necrosis
K85.02	Idiopathic acute pancreatitis with infected necrosis
K85.10	Biliary acute pancreatitis without necrosis or infection
K85.11	Biliary acute pancreatitis with uninfected necrosis
K85.12	Biliary acute pancreatitis with infected necrosis
K85.20	Alcohol induced acute pancreatitis without necrosis or infection
K85.21	Alcohol induced acute pancreatitis with uninfected necrosis
K85.22	Alcohol induced acute pancreatitis with infected necrosis
K85.30	Drug induced acute pancreatitis without necrosis or infection
K85.31	Drug induced acute pancreatitis with uninfected necrosis
K85.32	Drug induced acute pancreatitis with infected necrosis
K85.80	Other acute pancreatitis without necrosis or infection
K85.81	Other acute pancreatitis with uninfected necrosis
K85.82	Other acute pancreatitis with infected necrosis
K86.81	Exocrine pancreatic insufficiency
K86.89	Other specified diseases of pancreas
K87	Disorders of gallbladder, biliary tract and pancreas in diseases classified elsewhere

AMA: **48105** 2014,Jan,11

Relative Value Units/Medicare Edits

Non-Facility RVU	Work	PE	MP	Total
48105	49.26	23.6	11.04	83.9
Facility RVU	Work	PE	MP	Total
48105	49.26	23.6	11.04	83.9

	FUD	Status	MUE	Modifiers				IOM Reference
48105	90	A	1(2)	51	N/A	62*	80	None

* with documentation

Terms To Know

cytomegalovirus. Herpes virus that infects directly through mucous membrane contact, tissue transplant, or blood transfusion, producing enlarged, infected cells containing inclusion bodies.

debridement. Removal of dead or contaminated tissue and foreign matter from a wound.

necrosis. Death of cells or tissue within a living organ or structure.

necrotic. Pathological condition of death occurring in a group of cells or tissues within a living part or organism.

pancreatitis. Inflammation of the pancreas that may be acute or chronic, symptomatic or asymptomatic, due to the autodigestion of pancreatic tissue by its own enzymes that have escaped into the pancreas, most often as a result of alcoholism or biliary tract disease such as calculi in the pancreatic duct.

resection. Surgical removal of a part or all of an organ or body part.

48120

48120   Excision of lesion of pancreas (eg, cyst, adenoma)

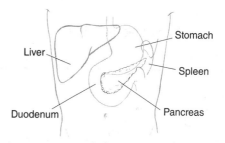

A lesion on the pancreas is removed

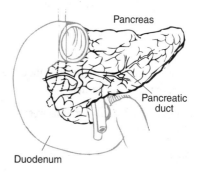

Explanation

The physician excises a lesion of the pancreas. The physician makes a midline epigastric incision and retracts the skin and underlying tissues laterally. The physician approaches the pancreas through the lesser sac of the omental bursa or the through the transverse mesocolon. The pancreas is palpated, the lesion is identified and excised. Bleeding is controlled, and the lesser sac is closed. Tissues are reapproximated to anatomical position, and the incision is sutured in layers.

Coding Tips

A biopsy is not reported separately when performed at the time of excision of a lesion. For endoscopic retrograde cholangiopancreatography (ERCP) with ablation of tumors, polyps, or other lesions, see 43278.

ICD-10-CM Diagnostic Codes

C25.0	Malignant neoplasm of head of pancreas
C25.1	Malignant neoplasm of body of pancreas
C25.2	Malignant neoplasm of tail of pancreas
C25.3	Malignant neoplasm of pancreatic duct
C25.4	Malignant neoplasm of endocrine pancreas
C25.7	Malignant neoplasm of other parts of pancreas
C25.8	Malignant neoplasm of overlapping sites of pancreas
C78.89	Secondary malignant neoplasm of other digestive organs
D01.7	Carcinoma in situ of other specified digestive organs
D13.6	Benign neoplasm of pancreas
D13.7	Benign neoplasm of endocrine pancreas
D37.8	Neoplasm of uncertain behavior of other specified digestive organs
K86.2	Cyst of pancreas
K86.3	Pseudocyst of pancreas
K86.81	Exocrine pancreatic insufficiency

Pancreas

| K86.89 | Other specified diseases of pancreas |
| K87 | Disorders of gallbladder, biliary tract and pancreas in diseases classified elsewhere |

AMA: 48120 2014,Jan,11

Relative Value Units/Medicare Edits

Non-Facility RVU	Work	PE	MP	Total
48120	18.41	9.95	4.39	32.75
Facility RVU	Work	PE	MP	Total
48120	18.41	9.95	4.39	32.75

	FUD	Status	MUE	Modifiers				IOM Reference
48120	90	A	1(3)	51	N/A	62*	80	None

* with documentation

Terms To Know

adenoma. Epithelial tumor, often benign, in which the cells are derived from glandular tissue or have a glandular structure.

bursa. Cavity or sac containing fluid that occurs between articulating surfaces and serves to reduce friction from moving parts.

cyst. Elevated encapsulated mass containing fluid, semisolid, or solid material with a membranous lining.

excision. Surgical removal of an organ or tissue.

lesion. Area of damaged tissue that has lost continuity or function, due to disease or trauma.

mesentery. Two layers of peritoneum that fold to surround the organs and attach to the abdominal wall.

mesocolon. Mesentery.

tissue. Group of similar cells with a similar function that form definite structures and organs. Tissue types include epithelial tissue, muscle tissue, connective tissue, and nervous tissue.

transverse. Crosswise at right angles to the long axis of a structure or part.

48140-48145

48140 Pancreatectomy, distal subtotal, with or without splenectomy; without pancreaticojejunostomy
48145   with pancreaticojejunostomy

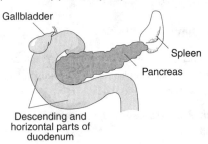

A portion of the distal pancreas is resected, the spleen may be removed, and a pancreaticojejunostomy may also be performed

Explanation

The physician removes the distal portion of the pancreas, with or without removing the spleen and jejunum. The physician makes a midline epigastric incision and retracts the skin and underlying tissues laterally. The physician approaches the pancreas through the lesser sac of the omental bursa or the through the transverse mesocolon. The pancreas is identified and freed from attachments. If the blood supply to the distal pancreas also supplies the spleen, the spleen is sacrificed in the resection. The pancreas is transected, and the distal portion is removed, with or without the spleen. In 48140, the pancreatic duct is not obstructed, permitting free drainage of pancreatic enzymes. In 48145, the duct flow is obstructed and a jejunal loop is brought up to create a fistula for enzyme flow to the digestive tract. Bleeding is controlled, and the lesser sac is closed. Tissues are reapproximated to anatomical position, and the incision is sutured in layers.

Coding Tips

For pancreatectomy, distal, near-total with preservation of the duodenum (Child-type procedure), see 48146; proximal subtotal with total duodenectomy, partial gastrectomy, choledochoenterostomy and gastrojejunostomy (Whipple-type procedure) with pancreatojejunostomy, see 48150; without pancreatojejunostomy, see 48152; proximal subtotal with near-total duodenectomy, choledochoenterostomy and duodenojejunostomy (pylorus-sparing, Whipple-type procedure), with pancreatojejunostomy, see 48153; without pancreatojejunostomy, see 48154.

ICD-10-CM Diagnostic Codes

C25.0	Malignant neoplasm of head of pancreas
C25.1	Malignant neoplasm of body of pancreas
C25.2	Malignant neoplasm of tail of pancreas
C25.3	Malignant neoplasm of pancreatic duct
C25.4	Malignant neoplasm of endocrine pancreas
C25.7	Malignant neoplasm of other parts of pancreas
C25.8	Malignant neoplasm of overlapping sites of pancreas
C78.89	Secondary malignant neoplasm of other digestive organs
C7A.1	Malignant poorly differentiated neuroendocrine tumors
C7A.8	Other malignant neuroendocrine tumors
D01.7	Carcinoma in situ of other specified digestive organs
D13.6	Benign neoplasm of pancreas

D13.7	Benign neoplasm of endocrine pancreas	
D37.8	Neoplasm of uncertain behavior of other specified digestive organs	
K86.0	Alcohol-induced chronic pancreatitis	
K86.1	Other chronic pancreatitis	
K86.81	Exocrine pancreatic insufficiency	
K86.89	Other specified diseases of pancreas	
S36.250A	Moderate laceration of head of pancreas, initial encounter	
S36.251A	Moderate laceration of body of pancreas, initial encounter	
S36.252A	Moderate laceration of tail of pancreas, initial encounter	
S36.260A	Major laceration of head of pancreas, initial encounter	
S36.261A	Major laceration of body of pancreas, initial encounter	
S36.262A	Major laceration of tail of pancreas, initial encounter	
S36.290A	Other injury of head of pancreas, initial encounter	
S36.291A	Other injury of body of pancreas, initial encounter	
S36.292A	Other injury of tail of pancreas, initial encounter	

AMA: **48140** 2018,Jan,8; 2017,Jul,10

Relative Value Units/Medicare Edits

Non-Facility RVU	Work	PE	MP	Total
48140	26.32	13.66	6.22	46.2
48145	27.39	14.3	6.69	48.38
Facility RVU	Work	PE	MP	Total
48140	26.32	13.66	6.22	46.2
48145	27.39	14.3	6.69	48.38

	FUD	Status	MUE	Modifiers				IOM Reference
48140	90	A	1(2)	51	N/A	62*	80	None
48145	90	A	1(2)	51	N/A	62*	80	

* with documentation

Terms To Know

pancreatitis. Inflammation of the pancreas that may be acute or chronic, symptomatic or asymptomatic, due to the autodigestion of pancreatic tissue by its own enzymes that have escaped into the pancreas, most often as a result of alcoholism or biliary tract disease such as calculi in the pancreatic duct.

48146

48146	Pancreatectomy, distal, near-total with preservation of duodenum (Child-type procedure)

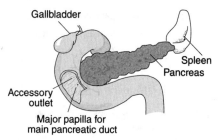

Nearly the entire pancreas is resected

Explanation

The physician performs a near-total pancreatectomy. The physician makes an abdominal incision. The pancreas is exposed and the body and tail of the pancreas are mobilized. The pancreas is transected at the junction of the head and body of the pancreas over the superior mesenteric vessels. The distal pancreas is removed. Frequently the spleen is removed with the distal pancreas. The end of the proximal pancreas is closed with staples or sutures. Drains are usually placed in the pancreatic bed. The incision is closed.

Coding Tips

For pancreatectomy, distal, subtotal with or without splenectomy; without pancreaticojejunostomy, see 48140; with pancreaticojejunostomy, see 48145; proximal subtotal with total duodenectomy, partial gastrectomy, choledochoenterostomy and gastrojejunostomy (Whipple-type procedure) with pancreatojejunostomy, see 48150; without pancreatojejunostomy, see 48152; proximal subtotal with near-total duodenectomy, choledochoenterostomy and duodenojejunostomy (pylorus-sparing, Whipple-type procedure), with pancreatojejunostomy, see 48153; without pancreatojejunostomy, see 48154.

ICD-10-CM Diagnostic Codes

C25.0	Malignant neoplasm of head of pancreas
C25.1	Malignant neoplasm of body of pancreas
C25.2	Malignant neoplasm of tail of pancreas
C25.3	Malignant neoplasm of pancreatic duct
C25.4	Malignant neoplasm of endocrine pancreas
C25.7	Malignant neoplasm of other parts of pancreas
C25.8	Malignant neoplasm of overlapping sites of pancreas
C7A.1	Malignant poorly differentiated neuroendocrine tumors
C7A.8	Other malignant neuroendocrine tumors
D01.7	Carcinoma in situ of other specified digestive organs
D13.6	Benign neoplasm of pancreas
D13.7	Benign neoplasm of endocrine pancreas
D37.8	Neoplasm of uncertain behavior of other specified digestive organs
K86.0	Alcohol-induced chronic pancreatitis
K86.1	Other chronic pancreatitis
K86.81	Exocrine pancreatic insufficiency
K86.89	Other specified diseases of pancreas
S36.250A	Moderate laceration of head of pancreas, initial encounter
S36.251A	Moderate laceration of body of pancreas, initial encounter

Pancreas

S36.252A	Moderate laceration of tail of pancreas, initial encounter
S36.260A	Major laceration of head of pancreas, initial encounter
S36.261A	Major laceration of body of pancreas, initial encounter
S36.262A	Major laceration of tail of pancreas, initial encounter
S36.290A	Other injury of head of pancreas, initial encounter
S36.291A	Other injury of body of pancreas, initial encounter
S36.292A	Other injury of tail of pancreas, initial encounter

AMA: 48146 2014,Jan,11

Relative Value Units/Medicare Edits

Non-Facility RVU	Work	PE	MP	Total
48146	30.6	17.89	7.48	55.97
Facility RVU	Work	PE	MP	Total
48146	30.6	17.89	7.48	55.97

	FUD	Status	MUE	Modifiers				IOM Reference
48146	90	A	1(2)	51	N/A	62*	80	None

* with documentation

Terms To Know

distal. Located farther away from a specified reference point or the trunk.

drain. Device that creates a channel to allow fluid from a cavity, wound, or infected area to exit the body.

neoplasm. New abnormal growth, tumor.

pancreatitis. Inflammation of the pancreas that may be acute or chronic, symptomatic or asymptomatic, due to the autodigestion of pancreatic tissue by its own enzymes that have escaped into the pancreas, most often as a result of alcoholism or biliary tract disease such as calculi in the pancreatic duct.

proximal. Located closest to a specified reference point, usually the midline or trunk.

spleen. Largest organ of the lymph system located in the upper left side of the abdomen that disintegrates red blood cells and releases hemoglobin; rids the body of worn-out, damaged red blood cells and platelets; produces plasma cells and lymphocytes; and has other functions not fully understood.

48148

48148   Excision of ampulla of Vater

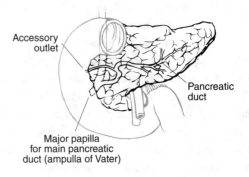

Accessory outlet

Pancreatic duct

Major papilla for main pancreatic duct (ampulla of Vater)

Explanation

The physician excises the ampulla of Vater, a saccular dilation of liver and/or pancreas. The physician exposes the duodenum and pancreas via an upper midline abdominal incision. The duodenum is opened with a longitudinal incision. The ampulla of Vater is exposed and the abnormality is excised. The common bile duct and duodenal mucosa are re-approximated as needed. The duodenum is closed with transverse interrupted sutures. The abdominal incision is closed.

Coding Tips

For pancreatectomy, distal, subtotal with or without splenectomy; without pancreaticojejunostomy, see 48140; with pancreaticojejunostomy, see 48145; distal, near-total with preservation of the duodenum (Child-type procedure), see 48146; proximal subtotal with total duodenectomy, partial gastrectomy, choledochoenterostomy and gastrojejunostomy (Whipple-type procedure), with pancreatojejunostomy, see 48150; without pancreatojejunostomy, see 48152; proximal subtotal with near-total duodenectomy, choledochoenterostomy and duodenojejunostomy (pylorus-sparing, Whipple-type procedure), with pancreatojejunostomy, see 48153; without pancreatojejunostomy, see 48154. For pancreatectomy, total, see 48155. For pancreatectomy, total or subtotal, with autologous transplantation of pancreas or pancreatic islets, see 48160.

ICD-10-CM Diagnostic Codes

C24.1	Malignant neoplasm of ampulla of Vater
C78.89	Secondary malignant neoplasm of other digestive organs
D01.5	Carcinoma in situ of liver, gallbladder and bile ducts
D13.5	Benign neoplasm of extrahepatic bile ducts
D37.6	Neoplasm of uncertain behavior of liver, gallbladder and bile ducts
D49.0	Neoplasm of unspecified behavior of digestive system

AMA: 48148 2014,Jan,11

Relative Value Units/Medicare Edits

Non-Facility RVU	Work	PE	MP	Total
48148	20.39	11.71	4.98	37.08
Facility RVU	Work	PE	MP	Total
48148	20.39	11.71	4.98	37.08

	FUD	Status	MUE	Modifiers				IOM Reference
48148	90	A	1(2)	51	N/A	62*	80	None

* with documentation

Terms To Know

ampulla of Vater. Tubular structure with flask-like dilation where the common bile and pancreatic ducts join before emptying into the duodenum.

benign. Mild or nonmalignant in nature.

carcinoma in situ. Malignancy that arises from the cells of the vessel, gland, or organ of origin that remains confined to that site or has not invaded neighboring tissue.

closure. Repairing an incision or wound by suture or other means.

duodenum. First portion of the small intestine connected to the stomach at the pylorus and extending to the jejunum.

excision. Surgical removal of an organ or tissue.

incision. Act of cutting into tissue or an organ.

malignant. Any condition tending to progress toward death, specifically an invasive tumor with a loss of cellular differentiation that has the ability to spread or metastasize to other body areas.

neoplasm. New abnormal growth, tumor.

secondary. Second in order of occurrence or importance, or appearing during the course of another disease or condition.

transverse. Crosswise at right angles to the long axis of a structure or part.

48150-48152

48150 Pancreatectomy, proximal subtotal with total duodenectomy, partial gastrectomy, choledochoenterostomy and gastrojejunostomy (Whipple-type procedure); with pancreatojejunostomy
48152   without pancreatojejunostomy

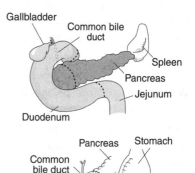

Explanation

The physician performs excision of the proximal pancreas, duodenum, distal bile duct and distal stomach with reconstruction (Whipple procedure) but with pancreatojejunostomy. The physician makes an abdominal incision and explores the abdomen. The duodenum, proximal pancreas, and bile duct are mobilized. The distal bile duct, distal stomach, and distal duodenum are divided. The pancreas is transected at the junction of the head and body and the pancreatic head, duodenum, distal stomach, and distal bile duct are removed en bloc. The anatomy is reconstructed by performing sequential anastomoses between the proximal jejunum and the distal bile duct and distal stomach. The edge of the remaining distal pancreas is closed with sutures or staples. The incision is closed. In 48152, the same procedure is done without pancreatojejunostomy.

Coding Tips

For pancreatectomy, distal, subtotal with or without splenectomy; without pancreaticojejunostomy, see 48140; with pancreaticojejunostomy, see 48145; distal, near-total with preservation of the duodenum (Child-type procedure), see 48146; proximal subtotal with near-total duodenectomy, choledochoenterostomy and duodenojejunostomy (pylorus-sparing, Whipple-type procedure), with pancreatojejunostomy, see 48153; without pancreatojejunostomy, see 48154.

ICD-10-CM Diagnostic Codes

C25.0	Malignant neoplasm of head of pancreas
C25.1	Malignant neoplasm of body of pancreas
C25.2	Malignant neoplasm of tail of pancreas
C25.3	Malignant neoplasm of pancreatic duct
C25.4	Malignant neoplasm of endocrine pancreas
C25.7	Malignant neoplasm of other parts of pancreas
C25.8	Malignant neoplasm of overlapping sites of pancreas
C78.89	Secondary malignant neoplasm of other digestive organs
C7A.1	Malignant poorly differentiated neuroendocrine tumors
C7A.8	Other malignant neuroendocrine tumors
D01.7	Carcinoma in situ of other specified digestive organs

Pancreas

● New ▲ Revised + Add On ★ Telemedicine AMA: CPT Assist [Resequenced] ☑ Laterality

D13.6	Benign neoplasm of pancreas
D13.7	Benign neoplasm of endocrine pancreas
D3A.010	Benign carcinoid tumor of the duodenum
K86.1	Other chronic pancreatitis
K86.81	Exocrine pancreatic insufficiency
K86.89	Other specified diseases of pancreas
K92.89	Other specified diseases of the digestive system
S36.240A	Minor laceration of head of pancreas, initial encounter
S36.241A	Minor laceration of body of pancreas, initial encounter
S36.242A	Minor laceration of tail of pancreas, initial encounter
S36.250A	Moderate laceration of head of pancreas, initial encounter
S36.251A	Moderate laceration of body of pancreas, initial encounter
S36.252A	Moderate laceration of tail of pancreas, initial encounter
S36.260A	Major laceration of head of pancreas, initial encounter
S36.261A	Major laceration of body of pancreas, initial encounter
S36.262A	Major laceration of tail of pancreas, initial encounter
S36.290A	Other injury of head of pancreas, initial encounter
S36.291A	Other injury of body of pancreas, initial encounter
S36.292A	Other injury of tail of pancreas, initial encounter

AMA: **48150** 2020,Jun,14; 2018,Jan,8; 2017,Jan,8; 2016,Jan,13; 2015,Dec,16

Relative Value Units/Medicare Edits

Non-Facility RVU	Work	PE	MP	Total
48150	52.84	26.64	12.6	92.08
48152	48.65	25.11	11.89	85.65
Facility RVU	Work	PE	MP	Total
48150	52.84	26.64	12.6	92.08
48152	48.65	25.11	11.89	85.65

	FUD	Status	MUE	Modifiers				IOM Reference
48150	90	A	1(2)	51	N/A	62*	80	None
48152	90	A	1(2)	51	N/A	62*	80	

* with documentation

Terms To Know

distal. Located farther away from a specified reference point or the trunk.

proximal. Located closest to a specified reference point, usually the midline or trunk.

Whipple procedure. Pancreaticoduodenectomy (removal of gallbladder, part of the duodenum, and the head of the pancreas) performed to treat pancreatic cancer or chronic pancreatitis.

48153-48154

48153	Pancreatectomy, proximal subtotal with near-total duodenectomy, choledochoenterostomy and duodenojejunostomy (pylorus-sparing, Whipple-type procedure); with pancreatojejunostomy
48154	without pancreatojejunostomy

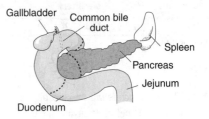

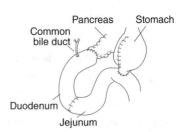

Explanation

The physician performs excision of the proximal pancreas, duodenum, and distal bile duct with reconstruction (pylorus preserving Whipple procedure). The physician makes an abdominal incision and explores the abdomen. The duodenum, proximal pancreas, and bile duct are mobilized. The distal bile duct and distal duodenum are divided. The proximal duodenum is divided just distal to the pylorus. The pancreas is transected at the junction of the head and body and the proximal pancreas, duodenum and distal bile duct are removed en bloc. The anatomy is reconstructed by performing sequential anastomoses between the proximal jejunum and the remaining pancreatic tail, distal bile duct, and pylorus. The incision is closed. In 48154, the same procedure is performed, without the pancreatojejunostomy.

Coding Tips

For pancreatectomy, distal, subtotal with or without splenectomy; without pancreaticojejunostomy, see 48140; with pancreaticojejunostomy, see 48145; proximal subtotal with total duodenectomy, partial gastrectomy, choledochoenterostomy and gastrojejunostomy (Whipple-type procedure) with pancreatojejunostomy, see 48150; without pancreatojejunostomy, see 48152.

ICD-10-CM Diagnostic Codes

C24.8	Malignant neoplasm of overlapping sites of biliary tract
C25.0	Malignant neoplasm of head of pancreas
C25.1	Malignant neoplasm of body of pancreas
C25.2	Malignant neoplasm of tail of pancreas
C25.3	Malignant neoplasm of pancreatic duct
C25.4	Malignant neoplasm of endocrine pancreas
C25.7	Malignant neoplasm of other parts of pancreas
C25.8	Malignant neoplasm of overlapping sites of pancreas
C78.89	Secondary malignant neoplasm of other digestive organs
C7A.1	Malignant poorly differentiated neuroendocrine tumors
C7A.8	Other malignant neuroendocrine tumors
D01.7	Carcinoma in situ of other specified digestive organs

Pancreas

D13.6	Benign neoplasm of pancreas	
D13.7	Benign neoplasm of endocrine pancreas	
K86.0	Alcohol-induced chronic pancreatitis	
K86.1	Other chronic pancreatitis	
K86.81	Exocrine pancreatic insufficiency	
K86.89	Other specified diseases of pancreas	
K87	Disorders of gallbladder, biliary tract and pancreas in diseases classified elsewhere	
K92.89	Other specified diseases of the digestive system	
S36.240A	Minor laceration of head of pancreas, initial encounter	
S36.241A	Minor laceration of body of pancreas, initial encounter	
S36.242A	Minor laceration of tail of pancreas, initial encounter	
S36.250A	Moderate laceration of head of pancreas, initial encounter	
S36.251A	Moderate laceration of body of pancreas, initial encounter	
S36.252A	Moderate laceration of tail of pancreas, initial encounter	
S36.260A	Major laceration of head of pancreas, initial encounter	
S36.261A	Major laceration of body of pancreas, initial encounter	
S36.262A	Major laceration of tail of pancreas, initial encounter	
S36.290A	Other injury of head of pancreas, initial encounter	
S36.291A	Other injury of body of pancreas, initial encounter	
S36.292A	Other injury of tail of pancreas, initial encounter	

AMA: **48153** 2014,Jan,11 **48154** 2014,Jan,11

Relative Value Units/Medicare Edits

Non-Facility RVU	Work	PE	MP	Total
48153	52.79	26.37	12.64	91.8
48154	48.88	25.19	11.96	86.03
Facility RVU	**Work**	**PE**	**MP**	**Total**
48153	52.79	26.37	12.64	91.8
48154	48.88	25.19	11.96	86.03

	FUD	Status	MUE	Modifiers				IOM Reference
48153	90	A	1(2)	51	N/A	62*	80	None
48154	90	A	1(2)	51	N/A	62*	80	

* with documentation

Terms To Know

anastomosis. Surgically created connection between ducts, blood vessels, or bowel segments to allow flow from one to the other.

pancreatitis. Inflammation of the pancreas that may be acute or chronic, symptomatic or asymptomatic, due to the autodigestion of pancreatic tissue by its own enzymes that have escaped into the pancreas, most often as a result of alcoholism or biliary tract disease such as calculi in the pancreatic duct.

48155-48160

48155 Pancreatectomy, total
48160 Pancreatectomy, total or subtotal, with autologous transplantation of pancreas or pancreatic islet cells

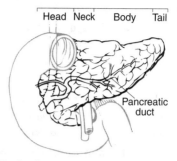

Regional components of the pancreas

Explanation

The physician removes all or part of the pancreas. The physician makes a midline epigastric incision and retracts the skin and underlying tissues laterally. The physician approaches the pancreas through the lesser sac of the omental bursa or the through the transverse mesocolon. The pancreas is identified and freed from attachments. In 48155, the pancreas is removed. In 48160, all or part of the pancreas is removed and pancreatic islet cells are transplanted into the abdominal tissue. Blood vessels are ligated and the affected pancreas is removed. Bleeding is controlled, and the lesser sac is closed. Tissues are reapproximated to anatomical position, and the incision is sutured in layers.

Coding Tips

Code 48160 includes autologous transplantation of pancreas or pancreatic islets. For pancreatectomy, distal subtotal, see 48140–48145. For pancreatectomy, distal, near-total, see 48146. For proximal subtotal pancreatectomy, see 48153–48154. For transplantation of pancreatic allograft, see 48554. Medicare and some other payers may require HCPCS Level II code G0341 be reported for this service. For pancreatic islet cell transplantation performed using portal vein catheterization and infusion, see 0584T-0586T.

ICD-10-CM Diagnostic Codes

C25.0	Malignant neoplasm of head of pancreas
C25.1	Malignant neoplasm of body of pancreas
C25.2	Malignant neoplasm of tail of pancreas
C25.3	Malignant neoplasm of pancreatic duct
C25.4	Malignant neoplasm of endocrine pancreas
C25.7	Malignant neoplasm of other parts of pancreas
C25.8	Malignant neoplasm of overlapping sites of pancreas
C78.89	Secondary malignant neoplasm of other digestive organs
C7A.1	Malignant poorly differentiated neuroendocrine tumors
C7A.8	Other malignant neuroendocrine tumors
D01.7	Carcinoma in situ of other specified digestive organs
D13.6	Benign neoplasm of pancreas
D13.7	Benign neoplasm of endocrine pancreas
K86.0	Alcohol-induced chronic pancreatitis
K86.1	Other chronic pancreatitis
K86.81	Exocrine pancreatic insufficiency
K86.89	Other specified diseases of pancreas

Pancreas

K87	Disorders of gallbladder, biliary tract and pancreas in diseases classified elsewhere
K92.89	Other specified diseases of the digestive system
S36.240A	Minor laceration of head of pancreas, initial encounter
S36.241A	Minor laceration of body of pancreas, initial encounter
S36.242A	Minor laceration of tail of pancreas, initial encounter
S36.250A	Moderate laceration of head of pancreas, initial encounter
S36.251A	Moderate laceration of body of pancreas, initial encounter
S36.252A	Moderate laceration of tail of pancreas, initial encounter
S36.260A	Major laceration of head of pancreas, initial encounter
S36.261A	Major laceration of body of pancreas, initial encounter
S36.262A	Major laceration of tail of pancreas, initial encounter
S36.290A	Other injury of head of pancreas, initial encounter
S36.291A	Other injury of body of pancreas, initial encounter
S36.292A	Other injury of tail of pancreas, initial encounter

AMA: 48155 2014,Jan,11 **48160** 2014,Jan,11

Relative Value Units/Medicare Edits

Non-Facility RVU	Work	PE	MP	Total
48155	29.45	17.57	6.9	53.92
48160	0.0	0.0	0.0	0.0
Facility RVU	Work	PE	MP	Total
48155	29.45	17.57	6.9	53.92
48160	0.0	0.0	0.0	0.0

	FUD	Status	MUE	Modifiers				IOM Reference
48155	90	A	1(2)	51	N/A	62*	80	100-03,260.3
48160	N/A	N	0(3)	N/A	N/A	N/A	N/A	

* with documentation

48400

+ **48400** Injection procedure for intraoperative pancreatography (List separately in addition to code for primary procedure)

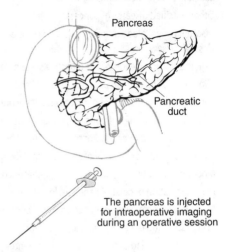

The pancreas is injected for intraoperative imaging during an operative session

Explanation

The physician performs a contrast study of the pancreatic duct. The physician makes an abdominal incision. The pancreas is exposed and may be mobilized by dissecting it from its retroperitoneal attachments. A separately reported pancreatogram may be obtained by injecting contrast into the common bile duct thus filling the pancreatic duct in a retrograde fashion and a radiograph obtained. Alternately, the duodenum may be opened and the pancreatic duct injected directly, or the tail of the pancreas may be transected and the pancreatic duct injected directly with contrast and a radiograph obtained. The duodenum is closed or the pancreatic tail is sutured closed. The incision is closed.

Coding Tips

For radiological supervision and interpretation, see 74300–74301.

ICD-10-CM Diagnostic Codes

This/these CPT code(s) are add-on code(s). See the primary procedure code that this code is performed with for your ICD-10-CM code selections.

AMA: 48400 2018,Jan,8; 2017,Jan,8; 2016,Jan,13; 2015,Jan,16

Relative Value Units/Medicare Edits

Non-Facility RVU	Work	PE	MP	Total
48400	1.95	0.73	0.47	3.15
Facility RVU	Work	PE	MP	Total
48400	1.95	0.73	0.47	3.15

	FUD	Status	MUE	Modifiers				IOM Reference
48400	N/A	A	1(3)	N/A	N/A	N/A	80*	None

* with documentation

48500

48500   Marsupialization of pancreatic cyst

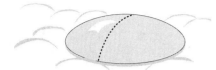

A cyst of the pancreas is identified and approached
surgically. The roof of the cyst is incised

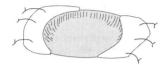

The roof edges are reflected back and sutured
to the sides, creating a pouch (marsupialization)

Explanation

The physician marsupializes a pancreatic cyst. The physician approaches the pancreas through a midline abdominal incision and retracts the skin and underlying tissues laterally. The physician approaches the pancreas through the lesser sac of the omental bursa or the through the transverse mesocolon. The cyst is located, and the anterior cyst wall is incised. The cut edges of the cyst are sutured to the skin edges establishing a pouch of what was formally an enclosed cyst. The remainder of the operative site is sutured in layers.

Coding Tips

For excision of a lesion of the pancreas (cyst, adenoma), see 48120. For external drainage of a pseudocyst, see 48510. For percutaneous, image-guided drainage of a pancreatic pseudocyst, via catheter, see 49405. For internal anastomosis of a pancreatic cyst to the gastrointestinal tract, see 48520 and 48540.

ICD-10-CM Diagnostic Codes

K86.2   Cyst of pancreas
K86.3   Pseudocyst of pancreas
Q45.2   Congenital pancreatic cyst

AMA: **48500** 2014,Jan,11

Relative Value Units/Medicare Edits

Non-Facility RVU	Work	PE	MP	Total
48500	18.16	11.6	4.43	34.19
Facility RVU	Work	PE	MP	Total
48500	18.16	11.6	4.43	34.19

	FUD	Status	MUE	Modifiers				IOM Reference
48500	90	A	1(3)	51	N/A	62*	80	None

* with documentation

48510

48510   External drainage, pseudocyst of pancreas, open

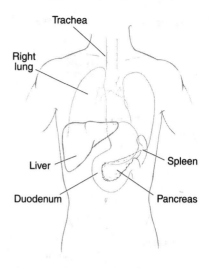

Explanation

The physician externally drains a pancreatic cyst. The physician approaches the pancreas through a midline abdominal incision. The physician locates the cyst through an incision and approaches the pancreas through the lesser sac of the omental bursa or the through the transverse mesocolon. Once the drain is placed, the adjacent tissues are returned to anatomic position and the operative site is sutured in layers.

Coding Tips

For excision of a lesion of the pancreas (cyst, adenoma), see 48120. For marsupialization of a cyst of the pancreas, see 48500. For internal anastomosis of a pancreatic cyst to the gastrointestinal tract, see 48520 and 48540. For percutaneous, image-guided drainage of a pancreatic pseudocyst, via catheter, see 49405.

ICD-10-CM Diagnostic Codes

K86.2   Cyst of pancreas
K86.3   Pseudocyst of pancreas
Q45.2   Congenital pancreatic cyst

AMA: **48510** 2014,Jan,11

Relative Value Units/Medicare Edits

Non-Facility RVU	Work	PE	MP	Total
48510	17.19	11.24	4.21	32.64
Facility RVU	Work	PE	MP	Total
48510	17.19	11.24	4.21	32.64

	FUD	Status	MUE	Modifiers				IOM Reference
48510	90	A	1(3)	51	N/A	62*	80	None

* with documentation

Pancreas

48520

48520   Internal anastomosis of pancreatic cyst to gastrointestinal tract; direct

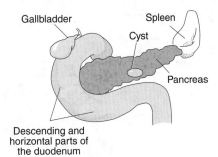

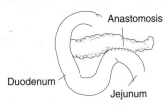

Explanation

The physician creates an internal anastomosis of a pancreatic cyst to a portion of the gastrointestinal tract. The physician approaches the pancreas through a midline abdominal incision and retracts the skin and underlying tissues laterally. The physician approaches the pancreas through the lesser sac of the omental bursa or the through the transverse mesocolon. The cyst is located. The physician approximates the stomach wall or a loop of duodenum or jejunum and incises it. The anterior cyst wall is incised and the cyst edges are approximated with the cut edges of the gastrointestinal tract and sutured. The cyst is decompressed through the drainage tract. The surrounding tissues are returned to anatomic position and the operative site is sutured in layers.

Coding Tips

For excision of a lesion of the pancreas (cyst, adenoma), see 48120. For external drainage of a pseudocyst, see 48510. For marsupialization of a cyst of the pancreas, see 48500. For internal anastomosis of a pancreatic cyst to the gastrointestinal tract with Roux-en-Y, see 48540. For percutaneous, image-guided drainage of a pancreatic pseudocyst, via catheter, see 49405.

ICD-10-CM Diagnostic Codes

K86.2   Cyst of pancreas

K86.3   Pseudocyst of pancreas

Q45.2   Congenital pancreatic cyst

AMA: 48520 2014,Jan,11

Relative Value Units/Medicare Edits

Non-Facility RVU	Work	PE	MP	Total
48520	18.15	10.07	4.43	32.65
Facility RVU	Work	PE	MP	Total
48520	18.15	10.07	4.43	32.65

	FUD	Status	MUE	Modifiers				IOM Reference
48520	90	A	1(3)	51	N/A	62*	80	None

* with documentation

48540

48540   Internal anastomosis of pancreatic cyst to gastrointestinal tract; Roux-en-Y

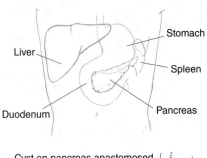

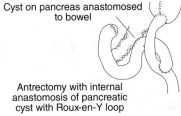

Antrectomy with internal anastomosis of pancreatic cyst with Roux-en-Y loop

Explanation

The physician creates a Roux-en-Y anastomosis to drain enzymes from the pancreatic duct. The physician approaches the pancreas through a midline abdominal incision and retracts the skin and underlying tissues laterally. The physician approaches the pancreas through the lesser sac of the omental bursa or the through the transverse mesocolon. The physician divides a loop of small intestine (usually the jejunum) and implants the distal end into the stomach or duodenum. The proximal end is anastomosed distal to the first anastomosis to prevent reflux. The pancreatic duct is fistulized to the proximal end to create a drain to the gastrointestinal tract for pancreatic enzymes. The surrounding tissues are returned to anatomic position and the operative site is sutured in layers.

Coding Tips

For excision of a lesion of the pancreas (cyst, adenoma), see 48120. For external drainage of a pseudocyst, see 48510. For marsupialization of a cyst of the pancreas, see 48500. For internal anastomosis of a pancreatic cyst to the gastrointestinal tract, direct, see 48520. For percutaneous, image-guided drainage of a pancreatic pseudocyst, via catheter, see 49405.

ICD-10-CM Diagnostic Codes

K86.2   Cyst of pancreas

K86.3   Pseudocyst of pancreas

Q45.2   Congenital pancreatic cyst

AMA: 48540 2014,Jan,11

Pancreas

Relative Value Units/Medicare Edits

Non-Facility RVU	Work	PE	MP	Total
48540	21.94	11.48	5.38	38.8
Facility RVU	Work	PE	MP	Total
48540	21.94	11.48	5.38	38.8

	FUD	Status	MUE	Modifiers				IOM Reference
48540	90	A	1(3)	51	N/A	62*	80	None

* with documentation

Terms To Know

anomaly. Irregularity in the structure or position of an organ or tissue.

bursa. Cavity or sac containing fluid that occurs between articulating surfaces and serves to reduce friction from moving parts. An anatomical structure frequently referenced in orthopedic notes as it may become diseased or need removal.

chronic. Persistent, continuing, or recurring.

congenital. Present at birth, occurring through heredity or an influence during gestation up to the moment of birth.

cyst. Elevated encapsulated mass containing fluid, semisolid, or solid material with a membranous lining.

debridement. Removal of dead or contaminated tissue and foreign matter from a wound.

distal. Located farther away from a specified reference point or the trunk.

drain. Device that creates a channel to allow fluid from a cavity, wound, or infected area to exit the body.

duodenum. First portion of the small intestine connected to the stomach at the pylorus and extending to the jejunum.

jejunum. Highly vascular upper two-fifths of the small intestine, extending from the duodenum to the ileum.

omentum. Fold of peritoneal tissue suspended between the stomach and neighboring visceral organs of the abdominal cavity.

pancreatitis. Inflammation of the pancreas that may be acute or chronic, symptomatic or asymptomatic, due to the autodigestion of pancreatic tissue by its own enzymes that have escaped into the pancreas, most often as a result of alcoholism or biliary tract disease such as calculi in the pancreatic duct.

proximal. Located closest to a specified reference point, usually the midline or trunk.

pseudocyst. Enlarged, abnormal cavity resembling a cyst but without epithelial lining; a complication of acute pancreatitis, fluid and dead cell debris that collect within the walls of the pancreas.

Roux-en-Y anastomosis. Y-shaped attachment of the distal end of a divided small intestine segment to the stomach, esophagus, biliary tract, or other structure with anastomosis of the proximal end to the side of the small intestine further down for reflux-free drainage.

48545-48547

48545 Pancreatorrhaphy for injury
48547 Duodenal exclusion with gastrojejunostomy for pancreatic injury

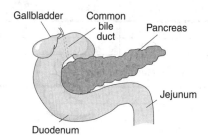

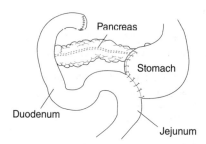

Explanation

In 48545, the physician repairs a pancreatic injury (pancreatorrhaphy). The physician makes an abdominal incision and the abdomen is explored. The pancreas is exposed and the pancreatic injury is identified and repaired with sutures. A peripancreatic drain is usually placed. The incision is closed. In 48547, the physician performs duodenal exclusion and gastrojejunostomy for a pancreatic injury. The physician makes an abdominal incision and explores the abdomen. The pancreas is exposed and an injury in the duodenum or pancreas may be closed with sutures. An incision is made in the stomach (gastrotomy). The natural opening from the stomach to the duodenum is closed with sutures or staples. A limb of proximal small bowel is brought up to the stomach and an anastomosis is performed (gastrojejunostomy) at the site of the gastrotomy. The abdominal incision is closed.

Coding Tips

When these codes are performed with another separately identifiable procedure, the highest dollar value code is listed as the primary procedure and subsequent procedures are appended with modifier 51.

ICD-10-CM Diagnostic Codes

S36.240A	Minor laceration of head of pancreas, initial encounter
S36.241A	Minor laceration of body of pancreas, initial encounter
S36.242A	Minor laceration of tail of pancreas, initial encounter
S36.250A	Moderate laceration of head of pancreas, initial encounter
S36.251A	Moderate laceration of body of pancreas, initial encounter
S36.252A	Moderate laceration of tail of pancreas, initial encounter
S36.260A	Major laceration of head of pancreas, initial encounter
S36.261A	Major laceration of body of pancreas, initial encounter
S36.262A	Major laceration of tail of pancreas, initial encounter
S36.290A	Other injury of head of pancreas, initial encounter
S36.291A	Other injury of body of pancreas, initial encounter
S36.292A	Other injury of tail of pancreas, initial encounter

AMA: 48545 2014,Jan,11 **48547** 2014,Jan,11

Pancreas

Relative Value Units/Medicare Edits

Non-Facility RVU	Work	PE	MP	Total
48545	22.23	12.25	5.46	39.94
48547	30.38	15.27	7.44	53.09
Facility RVU	**Work**	**PE**	**MP**	**Total**
48545	22.23	12.25	5.46	39.94
48547	30.38	15.27	7.44	53.09

	FUD	Status	MUE	Modifiers				IOM Reference
48545	90	A	1(3)	51	N/A	62*	80	None
48547	90	A	1(2)	51	N/A	62*	80	

* with documentation

Terms To Know

anastomosis. Surgically created connection between ducts, blood vessels, or bowel segments to allow flow from one to the other.

duodenum. First portion of the small intestine connected to the stomach at the pylorus and extending to the jejunum.

exploration. Examination for diagnostic purposes.

incision. Act of cutting into tissue or an organ.

jejunum. Highly vascular upper two-fifths of the small intestine, extending from the duodenum to the ileum.

small intestine. First portion of intestine connecting to the pylorus at the proximal end and consisting of the duodenum, jejunum, and ileum.

48548

48548   Pancreaticojejunostomy, side-to-side anastomosis (Puestow-type operation)

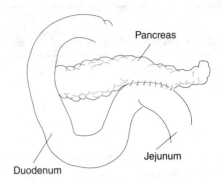

The pancreas is anastomosed in
a side-to-side fashion to the jejunum

Explanation

The physician creates a pancreaticojejunostomy to drain pancreatic enzymes through a side-to-side anastomosis. The physician makes a midline epigastric incision and retracts the skin and underlying tissues laterally. The physician approaches the pancreas through the lesser sac of the omental bursa or through the transverse mesocolon. A jejunal loop is brought up to create a fistula for enzyme flow to the digestive tract. Bleeding is controlled and the lesser sac is closed. Tissues are reapproximated to the anatomical position and the incision is sutured in layers.

Coding Tips

For pancreatectomy with pancreaticojejunostomy, see 48145, 48150, and 48153.

ICD-10-CM Diagnostic Codes

C25.0	Malignant neoplasm of head of pancreas
C25.1	Malignant neoplasm of body of pancreas
C25.2	Malignant neoplasm of tail of pancreas
C25.3	Malignant neoplasm of pancreatic duct
C25.4	Malignant neoplasm of endocrine pancreas
C25.7	Malignant neoplasm of other parts of pancreas
C25.8	Malignant neoplasm of overlapping sites of pancreas
C7A.1	Malignant poorly differentiated neuroendocrine tumors
C7A.8	Other malignant neuroendocrine tumors
K31.5	Obstruction of duodenum
K83.1	Obstruction of bile duct
K86.0	Alcohol-induced chronic pancreatitis
K86.1	Other chronic pancreatitis
K86.2	Cyst of pancreas
K86.3	Pseudocyst of pancreas
K86.81	Exocrine pancreatic insufficiency
K86.89	Other specified diseases of pancreas
K87	Disorders of gallbladder, biliary tract and pancreas in diseases classified elsewhere

AMA: **48548** 2014,Jan,11

Relative Value Units/Medicare Edits

Non-Facility RVU	Work	PE	MP	Total
48548	28.09	14.57	6.87	49.53
Facility RVU	Work	PE	MP	Total
48548	28.09	14.57	6.87	49.53

	FUD	Status	MUE	Modifiers				IOM Reference
48548	90	A	1(2)	51	N/A	62*	80	None

* with documentation

Terms To Know

anastomosis. Surgically created connection between ducts, blood vessels, or bowel segments to allow flow from one to the other.

cyst. Elevated encapsulated mass containing fluid, semisolid, or solid material with a membranous lining.

duodenum. First portion of the small intestine connected to the stomach at the pylorus and extending to the jejunum.

jejunum. Highly vascular upper two-fifths of the small intestine, extending from the duodenum to the ileum.

omentum. Fold of peritoneal tissue suspended between the stomach and neighboring visceral organs of the abdominal cavity.

pancreatitis. Inflammation of the pancreas that may be acute or chronic, symptomatic or asymptomatic, due to the autodigestion of pancreatic tissue by its own enzymes that have escaped into the pancreas, most often as a result of alcoholism or biliary tract disease such as calculi in the pancreatic duct.

pseudocyst. Enlarged, abnormal cavity resembling a cyst but without epithelial lining; a complication of acute pancreatitis, fluid and dead cell debris that collect within the walls of the pancreas.

48551

48551 Backbench standard preparation of cadaver donor pancreas allograft prior to transplantation, including dissection of allograft from surrounding soft tissues, splenectomy, duodenotomy, ligation of bile duct, ligation of mesenteric vessels, and Y-graft arterial anastomoses from iliac artery to superior mesenteric artery and to splenic artery

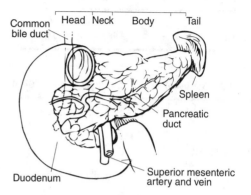

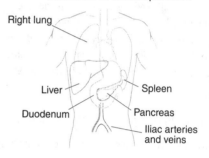

The pancreas and iliac arteries and veins are removed and prepared on the backbench for allotransplantation

Explanation

The physician performs a standard backbench preparation of a cadaver donor pancreas. Backbench or back table preparation refers to procedures performed on the donor organ following procurement to prepare the donor organ for transplant. In a separately reportable procedure, the physician removes the pancreas in conjunction with the thoracic organs, liver, and spleen from a cadaver donor. One pair of donor iliac arteries and vein are also procured for use in back table reconstruction procedures. Backbench procedures on the pancreas are accomplished at very cold temperatures to prevent the organ from deteriorating. Considerable back table preparation is required to prepare the pancreas for the transplant procedure. First, the pancreas is separated from the thoracic organs and liver. The spleen is removed by tying the individual vessels with 2-0 silk ligatures. The surrounding soft tissues are dissected from the pancreas allograft. The duodenal segment of bowel attached to the head of the pancreas is mobilized and shortened to allow for transplantation. The bile duct is ligated. Since the pancreas receives blood flow from two arteries, the superior mesenteric artery and the splenic artery, the arteries must be combined into one to allow anastomosis of the blood vessels in the transplant recipient. The physician performs a bypass graft from the previously procured iliac artery. The bypass graft consists of Y-graft arterial anastomoses of the internal iliac artery to the splenic artery and the external iliac artery to the superior mesenteric artery.

Coding Tips

Do not report 48551 with 35531, 35563, 35685, 38100–38102, 44010, 44820, 44850, 47460, 47550–47556, 48100–48120, or 48545.

Pancreas

ICD-10-CM Diagnostic Codes

The application of this code is too broad to adequately present ICD-10-CM diagnostic code links here. Refer to your ICD-10-CM book.

AMA: 48551 2014,Jan,11

Relative Value Units/Medicare Edits

Non-Facility RVU	Work	PE	MP	Total
48551	0.0	0.0	0.0	0.0
Facility RVU	Work	PE	MP	Total
48551	0.0	0.0	0.0	0.0

	FUD	Status	MUE	Modifiers				IOM Reference
48551	N/A	C	1(2)	51	N/A	62*	80	None

* with documentation

Terms To Know

allograft. Graft from one individual to another of the same species.

anastomosis. Surgically created connection between ducts, blood vessels, or bowel segments to allow flow from one to the other.

backbench preparation. Procedures performed on a donor organ following procurement to prepare the organ for transplant into the recipient. Excess fat and other tissue may be removed, the organ may be perfused, and vital arteries may be sized, repaired, or modified to fit the patient. These procedures are done on a back table in the operating room before transplantation can begin.

cadaver. Dead body.

dissection. Separating by cutting tissue or body structures apart.

donor. Person from whom tissues or organs are removed for transplantation.

reconstruction. Recreating, restoring, or rebuilding a body part or organ.

transplant. Insertion of an organ or tissue from one person or site into another.

48552

48552   Backbench reconstruction of cadaver donor pancreas allograft prior to transplantation, venous anastomosis, each

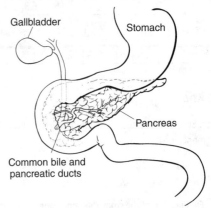

A backbench reconstruction of a donor pancreas from a cadaver is performed in preparation for transplant

Explanation

The physician performs a backbench venous reconstruction of a cadaver donor pancreas allograft. Backbench or back table refers to procedures performed on the donor organ following procurement to prepare the donor organ for transplant. Backbench procedures on the pancreas are accomplished at very cold temperatures to prevent the organ from deteriorating. The physician dissects the portal vein. Venous anastomosis of the portal vein is required when there is not sufficient length or when there are anatomic variations in the donor organ. Previously procured iliac vein segments are fashioned and anastomosed as required to provide for systemic and portal drainage. More than one anastomosis may be required to accomplish this. Code 48552 is reported for each anastomosis.

Coding Tips

Do not report 48552 with 35531, 35563, 35685, 38100–38102, 44010, 44820, 44850, 47460, 47550–47556, 48100–48120, or 48545.

ICD-10-CM Diagnostic Codes

The application of this code is too broad to adequately present ICD-10-CM diagnostic code links here. Refer to your ICD-10-CM book.

AMA: 48552 2014,Jan,11

Relative Value Units/Medicare Edits

Non-Facility RVU	Work	PE	MP	Total
48552	4.3	1.6	1.04	6.94
Facility RVU	Work	PE	MP	Total
48552	4.3	1.6	1.04	6.94

	FUD	Status	MUE	Modifiers				IOM Reference
48552	N/A	A	2(3)	51	N/A	62*	80	None

* with documentation

49000

49000 Exploratory laparotomy, exploratory celiotomy with or without biopsy(s) (separate procedure)

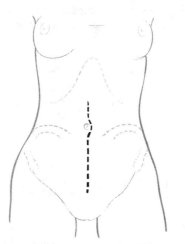

Typical incision for laparotomy

Explanation

To explore the intra-abdominal organs and structures, the physician makes a large incision extending from just above the pubic hairline to the rib cage. The abdominal cavity is opened for a systematic examination of all organs. The physician may take tissue samples of any or all intra-abdominal organs for diagnosis. The incision is closed with sutures.

Coding Tips

This separate procedure by definition is usually a component of a more complex service and is not identified separately. When performed alone or with other unrelated procedures/services it may be reported. If performed alone, list the code; if performed with other procedures/services, list the code and append modifier 59 or an X{EPSU} modifier. To report wound exploration due to a penetrating trauma without laparotomy, see 20102. For reopening of a recent laparotomy, see 49002. For exploration of the retroperitoneal area with or without biopsy, see 49010.

ICD-10-CM Diagnostic Codes

The application of this code is too broad to adequately present ICD-10-CM diagnostic code links here. Refer to your ICD-10-CM book.

AMA: **49000** 2020,Jan,6; 2019,Dec,5; 2018,Jan,8; 2017,Jan,8; 2017,Dec,3; 2016,Jan,13; 2015,Jan,16

Relative Value Units/Medicare Edits

Non-Facility RVU	Work	PE	MP	Total
49000	12.54	7.33	2.82	22.69
Facility RVU	Work	PE	MP	Total
49000	12.54	7.33	2.82	22.69

	FUD	Status	MUE	Modifiers				IOM Reference
49000	90	A	1(2)	51	N/A	62*	80	None

* with documentation

49002

49002 Reopening of recent laparotomy

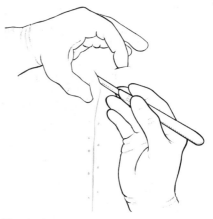

The site of a previous laparotomy is reopened

Explanation

The physician reopens the incision of a recent laparotomy before the incision has fully healed to control bleeding, remove packing, or drain a postoperative infection.

Coding Tips

For re-exploration of a hepatic wound for removal of packing, see 47362. For re-exploration of a pelvic wound to remove preperitoneal pelvic packing, see 49014.

ICD-10-CM Diagnostic Codes

The application of this code is too broad to adequately present ICD-10-CM diagnostic code links here. Refer to your ICD-10-CM book.

AMA: **49002** 2020,Jan,6; 2018,Jan,8; 2017,Jan,8; 2016,Jan,13; 2015,Jan,16

Relative Value Units/Medicare Edits

Non-Facility RVU	Work	PE	MP	Total
49002	17.63	9.17	4.02	30.82
Facility RVU	Work	PE	MP	Total
49002	17.63	9.17	4.02	30.82

	FUD	Status	MUE	Modifiers				IOM Reference
49002	90	A	1(3)	51	N/A	62*	80	None

* with documentation

49010

| 49010 | Exploration, retroperitoneal area with or without biopsy(s) (separate procedure) |

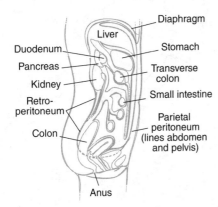

The retroperitoneal area can generally be defined as the posterior wall of the abdominal cavity

Explanation

The physician explores the retroperitoneum and may obtain sample tissue for separately reportable diagnostic testing. The physician may approach the retroperitoneum through a flank or an abdominal incision. The surface of the retroperitoneum is inspected and any area of interest of the retroperitoneum may be opened and the retroperitoneum explored. Tissues may be sampled. The incision is closed.

Coding Tips

This separate procedure by definition is usually a component of a more complex service and is not identified separately. When performed alone or with other unrelated procedures/services it may be reported. If performed alone, list the code; if performed with other procedures/services, list the code and append modifier 59 or an X{EPSU} modifier. To report wound exploration due to a penetrating trauma without laparotomy, see 20102.

ICD-10-CM Diagnostic Codes

The application of this code is too broad to adequately present ICD-10-CM diagnostic code links here. Refer to your ICD-10-CM book.

AMA: 49010 2020,Jan,6; 2019,Dec,5

Relative Value Units/Medicare Edits

Non-Facility RVU	Work	PE	MP	Total
49010	16.06	7.59	3.54	27.19
Facility RVU	Work	PE	MP	Total
49010	16.06	7.59	3.54	27.19

	FUD	Status	MUE	Modifiers				IOM Reference
49010	90	A	1(3)	51	N/A	62*	80	None

* with documentation

49013-49014

| 49013 | Preperitoneal pelvic packing for hemorrhage associated with pelvic trauma, including local exploration |
| 49014 | Re-exploration of pelvic wound with removal of preperitoneal pelvic packing, including repacking, when performed |

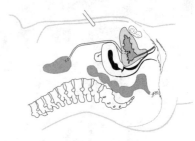

Preperitoneal pelvic packing is placed or removed with re-exploration of pelvic wound

Explanation

In 49013, the physician performs local exploration and preperitoneal pelvic packing (PPP) for hemorrhage associated with pelvic trauma. This type of hemorrhage is often from venous or bony sources and not amenable to correction by angioembolization, which is effective in controlling hemorrhages from arterial sources. The physician makes a 6 to 8 cm vertical midline incision from the pubic symphysis extending upwards, through skin and subcutaneous tissue to fascia. The fascia is incised in the midline and the preperitoneal space is entered. The physician retracts the bladder to permit the placement of surgical laparotomy pads. Because of lack of visibility due to the amount of hemorrhage in the pelvic space, rapid packing is necessary. The first laparotomy pad is pressed down onto the sacrum using a blunt instrument, followed by six to nine pads to complete the packing and tamponade. If a laparotomy is necessary, a separate incision may be made that extends from the xiphoid to just below the umbilicus in order to keep abdominal and pelvic spaces separate for adequate tamponade to be achieved. Utilizing a running suture at the fascial level, the physician closes the pelvic packing incision. In 49014, the physician performs re-exploration of the pelvic wound. The previously placed preperitoneal pelvic packing is removed and, if the physician deems it necessary, the wound is repacked.

Coding Tips

For drainage of a peritoneal abscess or localized peritonitis, by catheter, percutaneously, see 49406; transvaginally or transrectally, see 49407. For wound exploration due to a penetrating trauma without laparotomy, see 20102.

ICD-10-CM Diagnostic Codes

K91.841	Postprocedural hemorrhage of a digestive system organ or structure following other procedure
S31.610A	Laceration without foreign body of abdominal wall, right upper quadrant with penetration into peritoneal cavity, initial encounter ☑
S31.612A	Laceration without foreign body of abdominal wall, epigastric region with penetration into peritoneal cavity, initial encounter
S31.613A	Laceration without foreign body of abdominal wall, right lower quadrant with penetration into peritoneal cavity, initial encounter ☑
S31.615A	Laceration without foreign body of abdominal wall, periumbilic region with penetration into peritoneal cavity, initial encounter

S31.620A	Laceration with foreign body of abdominal wall, right upper quadrant with penetration into peritoneal cavity, initial encounter ☑
S31.622A	Laceration with foreign body of abdominal wall, epigastric region with penetration into peritoneal cavity, initial encounter
S31.623A	Laceration with foreign body of abdominal wall, right lower quadrant with penetration into peritoneal cavity, initial encounter ☑
S31.625A	Laceration with foreign body of abdominal wall, periumbilic region with penetration into peritoneal cavity, initial encounter
S31.630A	Puncture wound without foreign body of abdominal wall, right upper quadrant with penetration into peritoneal cavity, initial encounter ☑
S31.632A	Puncture wound without foreign body of abdominal wall, epigastric region with penetration into peritoneal cavity, initial encounter
S31.633A	Puncture wound without foreign body of abdominal wall, right lower quadrant with penetration into peritoneal cavity, initial encounter ☑
S31.635A	Puncture wound without foreign body of abdominal wall, periumbilic region with penetration into peritoneal cavity, initial encounter
S31.640A	Puncture wound with foreign body of abdominal wall, right upper quadrant with penetration into peritoneal cavity, initial encounter ☑
S31.642A	Puncture wound with foreign body of abdominal wall, epigastric region with penetration into peritoneal cavity, initial encounter
S31.643A	Puncture wound with foreign body of abdominal wall, right lower quadrant with penetration into peritoneal cavity, initial encounter ☑
S31.645A	Puncture wound with foreign body of abdominal wall, periumbilic region with penetration into peritoneal cavity, initial encounter
S31.650A	Open bite of abdominal wall, right upper quadrant with penetration into peritoneal cavity, initial encounter ☑
S31.652A	Open bite of abdominal wall, epigastric region with penetration into peritoneal cavity, initial encounter
S31.653A	Open bite of abdominal wall, right lower quadrant with penetration into peritoneal cavity, initial encounter ☑
S31.655A	Open bite of abdominal wall, periumbilic region with penetration into peritoneal cavity, initial encounter

AMA: **49013** 2020,Jan,6 **49014** 2020,Jan,6

Relative Value Units/Medicare Edits

Non-Facility RVU	Work	PE	MP	Total
49013	8.35	2.95	1.43	12.73
49014	6.73	2.65	1.15	10.53
Facility RVU	**Work**	**PE**	**MP**	**Total**
49013	8.35	2.95	1.43	12.73
49014	6.73	2.65	1.15	10.53

	FUD	Status	MUE	Modifiers				IOM Reference
49013	0	A	1(2)	51	N/A	N/A	N/A	None
49014	0	A	1(3)	51	N/A	N/A	N/A	
* with documentation								

49020

| 49020 | Drainage of peritoneal abscess or localized peritonitis, exclusive of appendiceal abscess, open |

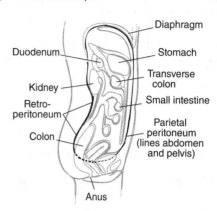

Explanation

The physician makes an open abdominal or flank incision (laparotomy) to gain access to the peritoneal cavity. The peritoneum is explored and the abscess or isolated area of peritoneal inflammation is identified. The abscess is incised and drained and inflamed peritoneal tissue may be excised. The abscess and surrounding peritoneal cavity may be irrigated. A drain may be placed whereby a separate abdominal incision is made and the drain is drawn through it and sutured in place. The physician may completely reapproximate the abdominal incision or leave a portion of the incision open to allow for further drainage. Specimens taken during the procedure are typically sent to microbiology for identification and to determine antibiotic suitability. If a drain is placed, it is removed at a later date.

Coding Tips

For drainage of a peritoneal abscess or localized peritonitis, by catheter, percutaneously, see 49406; transvaginally or transrectally, see 49407.

ICD-10-CM Diagnostic Codes

K65.1	Peritoneal abscess
K65.2	Spontaneous bacterial peritonitis
K65.3	Choleperitonitis
K65.4	Sclerosing mesenteritis
K65.8	Other peritonitis
K66.1	Hemoperitoneum
K66.8	Other specified disorders of peritoneum
K67	Disorders of peritoneum in infectious diseases classified elsewhere
K68.11	Postprocedural retroperitoneal abscess
K68.12	Psoas muscle abscess
K68.19	Other retroperitoneal abscess
K68.9	Other disorders of retroperitoneum

AMA: **49020** 2014,Jan,11

Relative Value Units/Medicare Edits

Non-Facility RVU	Work	PE	MP	Total
49020	26.67	14.38	5.99	47.04
Facility RVU	Work	PE	MP	Total
49020	26.67	14.38	5.99	47.04

	FUD	Status	MUE	Modifiers				IOM Reference
49020	90	A	2(3)	51	N/A	N/A	80	None

* with documentation

Terms To Know

abscess. Circumscribed collection of pus resulting from bacteria, frequently associated with swelling and other signs of inflammation.

drainage. Releasing, taking, or letting out fluids and/or gases from a body part.

inflammation. Cytologic and chemical reactions that occur in affected blood vessels and adjacent tissues in response to injury or abnormal stimulation from a physical, chemical, or biologic agent.

irrigation. To wash out or cleanse a body cavity, wound, or tissue with water or other fluid.

laparotomy. Incision through the flank or abdomen for therapeutic or diagnostic purposes.

peritoneal cavity. Space between the lining of the abdominal wall, or parietal peritoneum, and the surface layer of the abdominal organs, or visceral peritoneum. It contains a thin, watery fluid that keeps the peritoneal surfaces moist.

peritonitis. Inflammation and infection within the peritoneal cavity, the space between the membrane lining the abdominopelvic walls and covering the internal organs.

specimen. Tissue cells or sample of fluid taken for analysis, pathologic examination, and diagnosis.

49040

49040   Drainage of subdiaphragmatic or subphrenic abscess, open

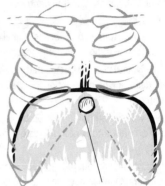

The lungs and most thoracic structures lie entirely above the diaphragm

The esophagus runs the length of the thorax and emerges through the diaphragm

The diaphragm is the muscular wall separating the thorax and its structures from the abdomen below

Explanation

The physician drains a subdiaphragmatic or subphrenic abscess. The physician makes an abdominal incision and the abdomen is explored. The abscess beneath the diaphragm is identified and the abscess cavity is opened and drained. Irrigation of the cavity is usually performed. A drain is usually placed into the abscess cavity and brought out through the abdominal wall. The incision is closed. The superficial portion of the incision may be packed open to allow drainage.

Coding Tips

Drainage of abscess codes are defined by site (appendiceal, peritoneal, subdiaphragmatic, subphrenic, retroperitoneal) and by the nature of the procedure (open, percutaneous). For drainage of an appendiceal abscess, see 44900. For drainage of a retroperitoneal abscess, see 49060. For percutaneous image-guided drainage of a subdiaphragmatic or subphrenic abscess via catheter, see 49406.

ICD-10-CM Diagnostic Codes

K65.1   Peritoneal abscess

AMA: **49040** 2014,Jan,11

Relative Value Units/Medicare Edits

Non-Facility RVU	Work	PE	MP	Total
49040	16.52	9.35	3.84	29.71
Facility RVU	Work	PE	MP	Total
49040	16.52	9.35	3.84	29.71

	FUD	Status	MUE	Modifiers				IOM Reference
49040	90	A	2(3)	51	N/A	62*	80	None

* with documentation

49060

49060   Drainage of retroperitoneal abscess, open

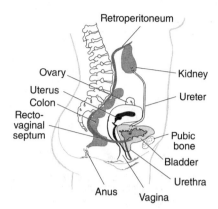

The retroperitoneal area can generally be defined as the posterior wall of the abdominal cavity

Explanation

The physician drains a retroperitoneal abscess. The physician makes an abdominal or flank incision. The abscess is identified and the retroperitoneal space is entered. The abscess cavity is opened and drained. Irrigation of the cavity is usually performed. A drain is usually placed in the abscess cavity and brought out through the abdominal wall. The incision is closed. The superficial portion of the incision may be packed open to allow drainage.

Coding Tips

Drainage of abscess codes are defined by site (appendiceal, peritoneal, subdiaphragmatic, subphrenic, retroperitoneal) and by the nature of the procedure (open, percutaneous). For drainage of an appendiceal abscess, see 44900. For drainage of a subdiaphragmatic or subphrenic abscess, see 49040. For laparoscopic drainage, see 49323. For image-guided percutaneous drainage of a retroperitoneal abscess via catheter, see 49406; transvaginally or transrectally, see 49407.

ICD-10-CM Diagnostic Codes

K68.11   Postprocedural retroperitoneal abscess
K68.12   Psoas muscle abscess
K68.19   Other retroperitoneal abscess

AMA: **49060** 2018,Jan,8; 2017,Jan,8; 2016,Jan,13; 2015,Jan,16

Relative Value Units/Medicare Edits

Non-Facility RVU	Work	PE	MP	Total
49060	18.53	9.81	4.04	32.38
Facility RVU	**Work**	**PE**	**MP**	**Total**
49060	18.53	9.81	4.04	32.38

	FUD	Status	MUE	Modifiers				IOM Reference
49060	90	A	2(3)	51	N/A	62*	N/A	None

* with documentation

49062

49062   Drainage of extraperitoneal lymphocele to peritoneal cavity, open

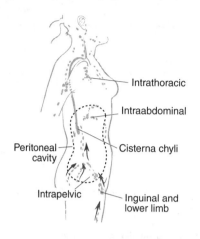

Explanation

The physician drains a lymphocele to the peritoneal cavity. The physician creates an opening in a lymphatic swelling or cavity (lymphocele) located outside the abdominopelvic walls to drain the material contained within to a cavity of the peritoneum. Irrigation of the lymphocele is performed. The incision is sutured closed. For radiological supervision and interpretation, see 75989.

Coding Tips

Placement of a drainage catheter is included and should not be reported separately. For laparoscopic drainage of a lymphocele to the peritoneal cavity, see 49323. For image-guided percutaneous drainage of a peritoneal or retroperitoneal lymphocele via catheter, see 49406.

ICD-10-CM Diagnostic Codes

I89.8	Other specified noninfective disorders of lymphatic vessels and lymph nodes
K91.89	Other postprocedural complications and disorders of digestive system
N99.89	Other postprocedural complications and disorders of genitourinary system
T81.89XA	Other complications of procedures, not elsewhere classified, initial encounter
T86.13	Kidney transplant infection
T86.19	Other complication of kidney transplant
T86.852	Intestine transplant infection
T86.858	Other complications of intestine transplant
T88.8XXA	Other specified complications of surgical and medical care, not elsewhere classified, initial encounter
Z48.22	Encounter for aftercare following kidney transplant

AMA: **49062** 2018,Jan,8; 2017,Jan,8; 2016,Jan,13; 2015,Jan,16

Abdomen/Digestive

Relative Value Units/Medicare Edits

Non-Facility RVU	Work	PE	MP	Total
49062	12.22	7.55	2.98	22.75
Facility RVU	Work	PE	MP	Total
49062	12.22	7.55	2.98	22.75

	FUD	Status	MUE	Modifiers				IOM Reference
49062	90	A	1(3)	51	N/A	62*	80	None

* with documentation

Terms To Know

catheter. Flexible tube inserted into an area of the body for introducing or withdrawing fluid.

drain. Device that creates a channel to allow fluid from a cavity, wound, or infected area to exit the body.

incision. Act of cutting into tissue or an organ.

irrigation. To wash out or cleanse a body cavity, wound, or tissue with water or other fluid.

laparoscopy. Direct visualization of the peritoneal cavity, outer fallopian tubes, uterus, and ovaries utilizing a laparoscope, a thin, flexible fiberoptic tube.

lymph. Clear, sometimes yellow fluid that flows through the tissues in the body, through the lymphatic system, and into the blood stream.

lymphocele. Cyst that contains lymph.

omentum. Fold of peritoneal tissue suspended between the stomach and neighboring visceral organs of the abdominal cavity.

peritoneal cavity. Space between the lining of the abdominal wall, or parietal peritoneum, and the surface layer of the abdominal organs, or visceral peritoneum. It contains a thin, watery fluid that keeps the peritoneal surfaces moist.

49082-49083

49082 Abdominal paracentesis (diagnostic or therapeutic); without imaging guidance
49083 with imaging guidance

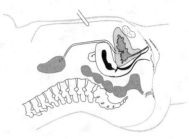

The peritoneum is accessed by a nick incision and a catheter is introduced into the cavity

Explanation

The physician inserts a needle or catheter into the abdominal cavity and withdraws and drains fluid for diagnostic or therapeutic purposes. The needle or catheter is removed at the completion of the procedure. Report 49082 if imaging guidance is not used and 49083 if imaging guidance is used.

Coding Tips

Code 49083 includes imaging guidance. Peritoneal lavage with imaging guidance, when performed, is reported with 49084. For image-guided, percutaneous drainage of a retroperitoneal abscess via catheter, see 49406. Do not report 49083 with 76942, 77002, 77012, or 77021.

ICD-10-CM Diagnostic Codes

A18.31	Tuberculous peritonitis
A52.74	Syphilis of liver and other viscera
K65.0	Generalized (acute) peritonitis
K65.2	Spontaneous bacterial peritonitis
K65.3	Choleperitonitis
K65.4	Sclerosing mesenteritis
K65.8	Other peritonitis
K66.1	Hemoperitoneum
K66.8	Other specified disorders of peritoneum
K70.11	Alcoholic hepatitis with ascites 🄰
K70.31	Alcoholic cirrhosis of liver with ascites 🄰
K71.51	Toxic liver disease with chronic active hepatitis with ascites
K74.3	Primary biliary cirrhosis
K74.4	Secondary biliary cirrhosis
K76.89	Other specified diseases of liver
K85.00	Idiopathic acute pancreatitis without necrosis or infection
K85.01	Idiopathic acute pancreatitis with uninfected necrosis
K85.02	Idiopathic acute pancreatitis with infected necrosis
K85.10	Biliary acute pancreatitis without necrosis or infection
K85.11	Biliary acute pancreatitis with uninfected necrosis
K85.12	Biliary acute pancreatitis with infected necrosis
K85.20	Alcohol induced acute pancreatitis without necrosis or infection
K85.21	Alcohol induced acute pancreatitis with uninfected necrosis
K85.22	Alcohol induced acute pancreatitis with infected necrosis
K85.30	Drug induced acute pancreatitis without necrosis or infection
K85.31	Drug induced acute pancreatitis with uninfected necrosis

K85.32	Drug induced acute pancreatitis with infected necrosis
K85.80	Other acute pancreatitis without necrosis or infection
K85.81	Other acute pancreatitis with uninfected necrosis
K85.82	Other acute pancreatitis with infected necrosis
K86.0	Alcohol-induced chronic pancreatitis
K86.1	Other chronic pancreatitis
K86.81	Exocrine pancreatic insufficiency
K86.89	Other specified diseases of pancreas
R18.0	Malignant ascites
R18.8	Other ascites
S36.81XA	Injury of peritoneum, initial encounter
S36.892A	Contusion of other intra-abdominal organs, initial encounter
S36.893A	Laceration of other intra-abdominal organs, initial encounter
S36.898A	Other injury of other intra-abdominal organs, initial encounter
T79.A3XA	Traumatic compartment syndrome of abdomen, initial encounter
T79.A9XA	Traumatic compartment syndrome of other sites, initial encounter

AMA: **49082** 2018,Jan,8; 2017,Jan,8; 2016,Jan,13; 2015,Jan,16 **49083** 2018,Jan,8; 2017,Jan,8; 2016,Jan,13; 2015,Jan,16

Relative Value Units/Medicare Edits

Non-Facility RVU	Work	PE	MP	Total
49082	1.24	5.06	0.17	6.47
49083	2.0	6.9	0.17	9.07
Facility RVU	Work	PE	MP	Total
49082	1.24	0.72	0.17	2.13
49083	2.0	0.91	0.17	3.08

	FUD	Status	MUE	Modifiers				IOM Reference
49082	0	A	1(3)	51	N/A	N/A	N/A	None
49083	0	A	2(3)	51	N/A	N/A	N/A	

* with documentation

Terms To Know

imaging. Radiologic means of producing pictures for clinical study of the internal structures and functions of the body, such as x-ray, ultrasound, magnetic resonance, or positron emission tomography.

paracentesis. Surgical puncture of a body cavity with a specialized needle or hollow tubing to aspirate fluid for diagnostic or therapeutic reasons.

therapeutic. Act meant to alleviate a medical or mental condition.

49084

49084 Peritoneal lavage, including imaging guidance, when performed

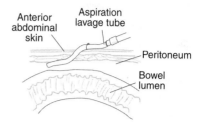

Anterior abdominal skin / Aspiration lavage tube / Peritoneum / Bowel lumen

The peritoneum is accessed by a nick incision and a catheter is introduced into the cavity

Explanation

Peritoneal lavage is usually performed to determine the presence and/or extent of internal bleeding within the peritoneum. The physician makes a small incision to insert a catheter into the abdominal cavity. Fluids are infused into the cavity and subsequently aspirated for diagnostic testing. The catheter is removed at the completion of the procedure and the incision is closed.

Coding Tips

Imaging is included in this procedure and should not be reported separately. For image-guided, percutaneous drainage of a retroperitoneal abscess via catheter, see 49406. Do not report 49084 with 76942, 77002, 77012, or 77021.

ICD-10-CM Diagnostic Codes

A18.31	Tuberculous peritonitis
A52.74	Syphilis of liver and other viscera
C22.0	Liver cell carcinoma
C22.1	Intrahepatic bile duct carcinoma
C22.2	Hepatoblastoma
C22.3	Angiosarcoma of liver
C22.4	Other sarcomas of liver
C22.7	Other specified carcinomas of liver
C78.6	Secondary malignant neoplasm of retroperitoneum and peritoneum
E87.2	Acidosis
E87.79	Other fluid overload
E87.8	Other disorders of electrolyte and fluid balance, not elsewhere classified
I81	Portal vein thrombosis
I89.8	Other specified noninfective disorders of lymphatic vessels and lymph nodes
K56.51	Intestinal adhesions [bands], with partial obstruction
K56.52	Intestinal adhesions [bands] with complete obstruction
K56.690	Other partial intestinal obstruction
K56.691	Other complete intestinal obstruction
K65.0	Generalized (acute) peritonitis
K65.1	Peritoneal abscess
K65.2	Spontaneous bacterial peritonitis
K65.3	Choleperitonitis
K65.4	Sclerosing mesenteritis
K65.8	Other peritonitis
K66.1	Hemoperitoneum

K66.8	Other specified disorders of peritoneum
K67	Disorders of peritoneum in infectious diseases classified elsewhere
K70.11	Alcoholic hepatitis with ascites 🅐
K70.31	Alcoholic cirrhosis of liver with ascites 🅐
K70.40	Alcoholic hepatic failure without coma 🅐
K70.41	Alcoholic hepatic failure with coma 🅐
K71.51	Toxic liver disease with chronic active hepatitis with ascites
K72.00	Acute and subacute hepatic failure without coma
K72.01	Acute and subacute hepatic failure with coma
K72.10	Chronic hepatic failure without coma
K72.11	Chronic hepatic failure with coma
K74.3	Primary biliary cirrhosis
K74.4	Secondary biliary cirrhosis
K74.69	Other cirrhosis of liver
K75.89	Other specified inflammatory liver diseases
K76.89	Other specified diseases of liver
K85.00	Idiopathic acute pancreatitis without necrosis or infection
K85.01	Idiopathic acute pancreatitis with uninfected necrosis
K85.02	Idiopathic acute pancreatitis with infected necrosis
K85.10	Biliary acute pancreatitis without necrosis or infection
K85.11	Biliary acute pancreatitis with uninfected necrosis
K85.12	Biliary acute pancreatitis with infected necrosis
K85.20	Alcohol induced acute pancreatitis without necrosis or infection
K85.21	Alcohol induced acute pancreatitis with uninfected necrosis
K85.22	Alcohol induced acute pancreatitis with infected necrosis
K85.30	Drug induced acute pancreatitis without necrosis or infection
K85.31	Drug induced acute pancreatitis with uninfected necrosis
K85.32	Drug induced acute pancreatitis with infected necrosis
K85.80	Other acute pancreatitis without necrosis or infection
K85.81	Other acute pancreatitis with uninfected necrosis
K85.82	Other acute pancreatitis with infected necrosis
K86.0	Alcohol-induced chronic pancreatitis
K86.1	Other chronic pancreatitis
K86.81	Exocrine pancreatic insufficiency
K86.89	Other specified diseases of pancreas
K87	Disorders of gallbladder, biliary tract and pancreas in diseases classified elsewhere
N18.1	Chronic kidney disease, stage 1
N18.2	Chronic kidney disease, stage 2 (mild)
N18.31	Chronic kidney disease, stage 3a
N18.32	Chronic kidney disease, stage 3b
N18.4	Chronic kidney disease, stage 4 (severe)
N18.5	Chronic kidney disease, stage 5
N18.6	End stage renal disease
N25.89	Other disorders resulting from impaired renal tubular function
R18.0	Malignant ascites
R18.8	Other ascites
S36.81XA	Injury of peritoneum, initial encounter
S36.892A	Contusion of other intra-abdominal organs, initial encounter
S36.893A	Laceration of other intra-abdominal organs, initial encounter
S36.898A	Other injury of other intra-abdominal organs, initial encounter
T79.A3XA	Traumatic compartment syndrome of abdomen, initial encounter
T79.A9XA	Traumatic compartment syndrome of other sites, initial encounter

AMA: 49084 2018,Jan,8; 2017,Jan,8; 2016,Jan,13; 2015,Jan,16

Relative Value Units/Medicare Edits

Non-Facility RVU	Work	PE	MP	Total
49084	2.0	0.75	0.42	3.17
Facility RVU	Work	PE	MP	Total
49084	2.0	0.75	0.42	3.17

	FUD	Status	MUE	Modifiers				IOM Reference
49084	0	A	1(3)	51	N/A	N/A	N/A	None

* with documentation

Terms To Know

ascites. Abnormal accumulation of free fluid in the abdominal cavity, causing distention and tightness in addition to shortness of breath as the fluid accumulates. Ascites is usually an underlying disorder and can be a manifestation of any number of diseases.

aspiration. Drawing fluid out by suction.

catheter. Flexible tube inserted into an area of the body for introducing or withdrawing fluid.

hemorrhage. Internal or external bleeding with loss of significant amounts of blood.

imaging. Radiologic means of producing pictures for clinical study of the internal structures and functions of the body, such as x-ray, ultrasound, magnetic resonance, or positron emission tomography.

lavage. Washing.

peritoneal cavity. Space between the lining of the abdominal wall, or parietal peritoneum, and the surface layer of the abdominal organs, or visceral peritoneum. It contains a thin, watery fluid that keeps the peritoneal surfaces moist.

49180

49180 Biopsy, abdominal or retroperitoneal mass, percutaneous needle

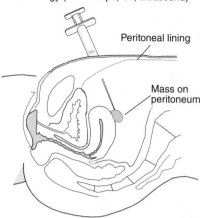

Biopsy needle guided to mass with aid
of radiology (fluoroscope, CT, ultrasound)

Peritoneal lining

Mass on
peritoneum

Explanation

Using radiological supervision, the physician locates the mass within or immediately outside the peritoneal lining of the abdominal cavity. A biopsy needle is passed into the mass, a tissue sample is removed, and the needle is withdrawn. This may be repeated several times. No incision is necessary.

Coding Tips

Imaging guidance is reported with 76942, 77002, 77012, and 77021, when performed. For fine needle aspiration, see 10004–10012 and 10021. For evaluation of aspirate, see 88172–88173.

ICD-10-CM Diagnostic Codes

C48.0	Malignant neoplasm of retroperitoneum
C76.2	Malignant neoplasm of abdomen
C77.2	Secondary and unspecified malignant neoplasm of intra-abdominal lymph nodes
C78.6	Secondary malignant neoplasm of retroperitoneum and peritoneum
C7A.1	Malignant poorly differentiated neuroendocrine tumors
D20.0	Benign neoplasm of soft tissue of retroperitoneum
D48.3	Neoplasm of uncertain behavior of retroperitoneum
D48.4	Neoplasm of uncertain behavior of peritoneum
D48.7	Neoplasm of uncertain behavior of other specified sites
D49.89	Neoplasm of unspecified behavior of other specified sites
R10.817	Generalized abdominal tenderness
R10.827	Generalized rebound abdominal tenderness
R16.0	Hepatomegaly, not elsewhere classified
R19.01	Right upper quadrant abdominal swelling, mass and lump
R19.02	Left upper quadrant abdominal swelling, mass and lump
R19.03	Right lower quadrant abdominal swelling, mass and lump
R19.04	Left lower quadrant abdominal swelling, mass and lump
R19.05	Periumbilic swelling, mass or lump
R19.06	Epigastric swelling, mass or lump
R19.07	Generalized intra-abdominal and pelvic swelling, mass and lump
R19.09	Other intra-abdominal and pelvic swelling, mass and lump
R59.0	Localized enlarged lymph nodes
R59.1	Generalized enlarged lymph nodes

AMA: 49180 2019,Feb,8; 2019,Apr,4; 2018,Jan,8; 2017,Jan,8; 2016,Jan,13; 2015,Jan,16

Relative Value Units/Medicare Edits

Non-Facility RVU	Work	PE	MP	Total
49180	1.73	3.26	0.15	5.14
Facility RVU	**Work**	**PE**	**MP**	**Total**
49180	1.73	0.55	0.15	2.43

	FUD	Status	MUE	Modifiers				IOM Reference
49180	0	A	2(3)	51	N/A	N/A	N/A	None

* with documentation

Terms To Know

biopsy. Tissue or fluid removed for diagnostic purposes through analysis of the cells in the biopsy material.

fluoroscopy. Radiology technique that allows visual examination of part of the body or a function of an organ using a device that projects an x-ray image on a fluorescent screen.

imaging. Radiologic means of producing pictures for clinical study of the internal structures and functions of the body, such as x-ray, ultrasound, magnetic resonance, or positron emission tomography.

percutaneous. Through the skin.

retroperitoneal. Located behind the peritoneum, the membrane that lines the abdominopelvic walls and forms a covering for the internal organs.

49185

49185 Sclerotherapy of a fluid collection (eg, lymphocele, cyst, or seroma), percutaneous, including contrast injection(s), sclerosant injection(s), diagnostic study, imaging guidance (eg, ultrasound, fluoroscopy) and radiological supervision and interpretation when performed

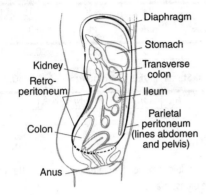

Fluid collection is treated with sclerotherapy

Explanation

Sclerotherapy is the therapeutic use of sclerosing agents (e.g., ethanol, povidone-iodine, tetracycline, doxycycline, bleomycin, talc, or fibrin glue) to systematically destroy undesired fluid collections such as cysts, lymphoceles, or seromas. This procedure is usually performed with the patient under moderate conscious sedation and involves a minimally invasive, percutaneous approach; depending on the size of the cyst or lymphocele, treatment may involve catheter drainage by gravity for approximately one day with subsequent administration of a sclerosing agent, such as ethanol, into the fluid collection under fluoroscopic guidance. For larger fluid collections, a catheter is placed using ultrasound or fluoroscopy and ethanol is administered via the catheter daily until the fluid collection has been reduced. The process involves percutaneous placement of a catheter over a guidewire into the area of fluid collection where the catheter is left in place and the sclerosing agent(s) is administered via the catheter as the patient remains in the supine position. The patient may be asked to change positions after the sclerosing agent has been injected in order to allow the entire area where the fluid collection is located to have contact with the sclerosing agent. Drainage of the sclerosing agent may take between 15 minutes and one hour depending on the agent used. Occasionally, depending on the size of the fluid collection, two catheters may be used. Aspirated fluid from the lymphocele, seroma, or cyst is sent for histopathology. The catheter is removed.

Coding Tips

Note that 49185 includes imaging guidance (i.e. fluoroscopy), contrast injections, sclerosant injection, diagnostic study, and radiological supervision and interpretation, when performed. When multiple lesions are treated on the same calendar date, and require a separate access, append modifier 59 to each additional lesion. When multiple lesions are treated using a single access, this code should be reported only one time. When an existing catheter is exchanged before or after the injection of a sclerosant, see 49423 and 75984. For sclerosing of veins or endovenous ablation of veins, see 36468–36479. For sclerotherapy of a lymphatic or vascular malformation, see 37241. For access or drainage, with a needle, see 10160 or 50390; with a catheter, see 10030, 49405–49407, or 50390. Do not report 49185 with 49424 or 76080.

ICD-10-CM Diagnostic Codes

B67.0	Echinococcus granulosus infection of liver
B67.5	Echinococcus multilocularis infection of liver
B67.99	Other echinococcosis
E04.1	Nontoxic single thyroid nodule
I89.8	Other specified noninfective disorders of lymphatic vessels and lymph nodes
K86.2	Cyst of pancreas
L05.01	Pilonidal cyst with abscess
L05.91	Pilonidal cyst without abscess
L72.0	Epidermal cyst
L72.2	Steatocystoma multiplex
L72.3	Sebaceous cyst
L72.8	Other follicular cysts of the skin and subcutaneous tissue
M27.49	Other cysts of jaw
M67.411	Ganglion, right shoulder ☑
M67.412	Ganglion, left shoulder ☑
M67.421	Ganglion, right elbow ☑
M67.422	Ganglion, left elbow ☑
M67.431	Ganglion, right wrist ☑
M67.432	Ganglion, left wrist ☑
M67.441	Ganglion, right hand ☑
M67.442	Ganglion, left hand ☑
M67.451	Ganglion, right hip ☑
M67.452	Ganglion, left hip ☑
M67.461	Ganglion, right knee ☑
M67.462	Ganglion, left knee ☑
M67.471	Ganglion, right ankle and foot ☑
M67.472	Ganglion, left ankle and foot ☑
M67.48	Ganglion, other site
M67.49	Ganglion, multiple sites
M71.21	Synovial cyst of popliteal space [Baker], right knee ☑
M71.22	Synovial cyst of popliteal space [Baker], left knee ☑
M79.81	Nontraumatic hematoma of soft tissue
M85.511	Aneurysmal bone cyst, right shoulder ☑
M85.512	Aneurysmal bone cyst, left shoulder ☑
M85.521	Aneurysmal bone cyst, right upper arm ☑
M85.522	Aneurysmal bone cyst, left upper arm ☑
M85.531	Aneurysmal bone cyst, right forearm ☑
M85.532	Aneurysmal bone cyst, left forearm ☑
M85.541	Aneurysmal bone cyst, right hand ☑
M85.542	Aneurysmal bone cyst, left hand ☑
M85.551	Aneurysmal bone cyst, right thigh ☑
M85.552	Aneurysmal bone cyst, left thigh ☑
M85.561	Aneurysmal bone cyst, right lower leg ☑
M85.562	Aneurysmal bone cyst, left lower leg ☑
M85.571	Aneurysmal bone cyst, right ankle and foot ☑
M85.572	Aneurysmal bone cyst, left ankle and foot ☑
M85.58	Aneurysmal bone cyst, other site
M85.59	Aneurysmal bone cyst, multiple sites
N83.01	Follicular cyst of right ovary ♀ ☑
N83.02	Follicular cyst of left ovary ♀ ☑
N83.11	Corpus luteum cyst of right ovary ♀ ☑
N83.12	Corpus luteum cyst of left ovary ♀ ☑
N83.291	Other ovarian cyst, right side ♀ ☑
N83.292	Other ovarian cyst, left side ♀ ☑

Q44.6	Cystic disease of liver	
Q45.2	Congenital pancreatic cyst	
T79.2XXA	Traumatic secondary and recurrent hemorrhage and seroma, initial encounter	

AMA: **49185** 2018,Jan,8; 2017,Jan,8; 2016,Mar,10

Relative Value Units/Medicare Edits

Non-Facility RVU	Work	PE	MP	Total
49185	2.35	35.74	0.22	38.31
Facility RVU	Work	PE	MP	Total
49185	2.35	0.87	0.22	3.44

	FUD	Status	MUE	Modifiers				IOM Reference
49185	0	A	2(3)	N/A	N/A	N/A	N/A	None

* with documentation

Terms To Know

cyst. Elevated encapsulated mass containing fluid, semisolid, or solid material with a membranous lining.

lymphocele. Cyst that contains lymph.

percutaneous. Through the skin.

sclerotherapy. Injection of a chemical agent that will irritate, inflame, and cause fibrosis in a vein, eventually obliterating hemorrhoids or varicose veins.

seroma. Swelling caused by the collection of serum, or clear fluid, in the tissues.

supervision and interpretation. Radiology services that usually contain an invasive component and are reported by the radiologist for supervision of the procedure and the personnel involved with performing the examination, reading the film, and preparing the written report.

49203-49205

49203	Excision or destruction, open, intra-abdominal tumors, cysts or endometriomas, 1 or more peritoneal, mesenteric, or retroperitoneal primary or secondary tumors; largest tumor 5 cm diameter or less
49204	largest tumor 5.1-10.0 cm diameter
49205	largest tumor greater than 10.0 cm diameter

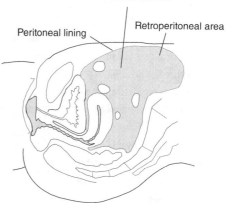

Area of tumors, cysts, and endometriomas

Peritoneal lining

Retroperitoneal area

Explanation

The physician removes or destroys intraabdominal tumors, cysts, or endometriomas (displaced endometrial tissue) or primary or secondary mesenteric, peritoneal, or retroperitoneal tumors. The physician makes a large incision extending from just above the pubic hairline to the rib cage. The growths are removed using a laser, electric cautery, or a scalpel. The incision is closed with sutures. Report 49203 when the diameter of the largest tumor is 5 cm or smaller, 49204 when the diameter is 5.1 to 10 cm, and 49205 when the diameter is larger than 10 cm.

Coding Tips

Do not report these codes with 38770, 38780, 49000, 49010, 49215, 50010, 50205, 50225, 50236, 50250, 50290, 58920, 58925, 58940, 58943, 58951-58954, 58956-58958, or 58960. The following codes may be reported with 49203–49205, when performed: partial or total nephrectomy, see 50220 or 50240; colectomy, see 44140; small bowel resection, see 44120; and vena caval resection with reconstruction, see 37799.

ICD-10-CM Diagnostic Codes

C45.1	Mesothelioma of peritoneum
C48.0	Malignant neoplasm of retroperitoneum
C48.1	Malignant neoplasm of specified parts of peritoneum
C48.8	Malignant neoplasm of overlapping sites of retroperitoneum and peritoneum
C49.4	Malignant neoplasm of connective and soft tissue of abdomen
C49.5	Malignant neoplasm of connective and soft tissue of pelvis
C56.1	Malignant neoplasm of right ovary ♀ ☑
C56.2	Malignant neoplasm of left ovary ♀ ☑
C56.3	Malignant neoplasm of bilateral ovaries ♀ ☑
C57.11	Malignant neoplasm of right broad ligament ♀ ☑
C57.12	Malignant neoplasm of left broad ligament ♀ ☑
C57.21	Malignant neoplasm of right round ligament ♀ ☑
C57.22	Malignant neoplasm of left round ligament ♀ ☑

C57.3	Malignant neoplasm of parametrium ♀
C76.2	Malignant neoplasm of abdomen
C78.6	Secondary malignant neoplasm of retroperitoneum and peritoneum
C7A.1	Malignant poorly differentiated neuroendocrine tumors
C7A.8	Other malignant neuroendocrine tumors
C7B.04	Secondary carcinoid tumors of peritoneum
D18.03	Hemangioma of intra-abdominal structures
D19.1	Benign neoplasm of mesothelial tissue of peritoneum
D20.0	Benign neoplasm of soft tissue of retroperitoneum
D20.1	Benign neoplasm of soft tissue of peritoneum
D48.4	Neoplasm of uncertain behavior of peritoneum
D49.0	Neoplasm of unspecified behavior of digestive system
K66.8	Other specified disorders of peritoneum
K68.9	Other disorders of retroperitoneum
N73.6	Female pelvic peritoneal adhesions (postinfective) ♀
N80.0	Endometriosis of uterus ♀
N80.1	Endometriosis of ovary ♀
N80.2	Endometriosis of fallopian tube ♀
N80.3	Endometriosis of pelvic peritoneum ♀
N80.5	Endometriosis of intestine ♀
N80.8	Other endometriosis ♀
N83.01	Follicular cyst of right ovary ♀ ☑
N83.02	Follicular cyst of left ovary ♀ ☑
N83.291	Other ovarian cyst, right side ♀ ☑
N83.292	Other ovarian cyst, left side ♀ ☑

AMA: 49203 2018,Jan,8; 2017,Jan,8; 2016,Jan,13; 2015,Jan,16 **49204** 2018,Jan,8; 2017,Jan,8; 2016,Jan,13; 2015,Jan,16 **49205** 2018,Jan,8; 2017,Jan,8; 2016,Jan,13; 2015,Jan,16

Relative Value Units/Medicare Edits

Non-Facility RVU	Work	PE	MP	Total
49203	20.13	10.81	4.22	35.16
49204	26.13	13.27	5.33	44.73
49205	30.13	14.99	6.2	51.32
Facility RVU	Work	PE	MP	Total
49203	20.13	10.81	4.22	35.16
49204	26.13	13.27	5.33	44.73
49205	30.13	14.99	6.2	51.32

	FUD	Status	MUE	Modifiers				IOM Reference
49203	90	A	1(2)	51	N/A	62*	80	None
49204	90	A	1(2)	51	N/A	62*	80	
49205	90	A	1(2)	51	N/A	62*	80	

* with documentation

49215

49215   Excision of presacral or sacrococcygeal tumor

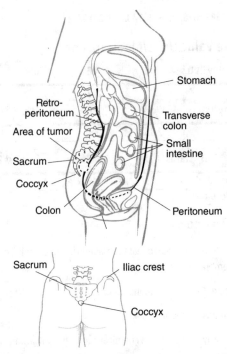

A tumor in the sacrococcygeal region is excised. Access may be abdominal or dorsal

Explanation

The physician performs resection of a presacral or sacrococcygeal tumor. The physician makes an abdominal incision and explores the abdomen. The tumor is identified and the rectum is mobilized from the sacrum to expose the tumor. The tumor is dissected free of surrounding structures and removed. Alternately, the tumor may be approached posteriorly through an incision between the sacrum and coccyx. The coccyx is removed, the rectum is mobilized from the sacrum and the tumor is dissected from surrounding structures and removed. A portion of the sacrum may be excised en bloc with the tumor. The incision is closed.

Coding Tips

Do not append modifier 63 to 49215 as the description or nature of the procedure includes infants up to 4 kg.

ICD-10-CM Diagnostic Codes

C41.4	Malignant neoplasm of pelvic bones, sacrum and coccyx
D16.8	Benign neoplasm of pelvic bones, sacrum and coccyx
D49.2	Neoplasm of unspecified behavior of bone, soft tissue, and skin

AMA: 49215 2014,Jan,11

Relative Value Units/Medicare Edits

Non-Facility RVU	Work	PE	MP	Total
49215	37.81	19.72	7.84	65.37
Facility RVU	Work	PE	MP	Total
49215	37.81	19.72	7.84	65.37

	FUD	Status	MUE	Modifiers				IOM Reference
49215	90	A	1(2)	51	N/A	62*	80	None

* with documentation

Terms To Know

coccyx. Lowest extremity of the vertebral column, formed by the fusion of three to five rudimentary vertebral segments under the sacrum.

en bloc. In total.

resection. Surgical removal of a part or all of an organ or body part.

sacrum. Lower portion of the spine composed of five fused vertebrae designated as S1-S5.

tumor. Pathological swelling or enlargement; a neoplastic growth of uncontrolled, abnormal multiplication of cells.

49255

49255   Omentectomy, epiploectomy, resection of omentum (separate procedure)

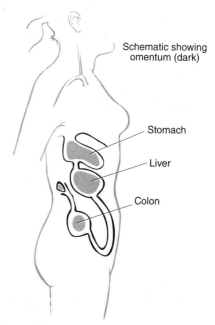

Schematic showing omentum (dark)

Stomach

Liver

Colon

The omentum is resected in a separate surgical procedure

Explanation

The physician performs resection of the omentum or epiploectomy. The physician makes an abdominal incision and the abdomen is explored. The omentum is mobilized from the stomach and colon, divided from its blood supply, and removed. One or more epiploica of the colon may be removed. The incision is closed.

Coding Tips

This separate procedure by definition is usually a component of a more complex service and is not identified separately. When performed alone or with other unrelated procedures/services it may be reported. If performed alone, list the code; if performed with other procedures/services, list the code and append modifier 59 or an X{EPSU} modifier. For umbilectomy, omphalectomy, see 49250.

ICD-10-CM Diagnostic Codes

C45.7	Mesothelioma of other sites
C47.4	Malignant neoplasm of peripheral nerves of abdomen
C48.1	Malignant neoplasm of specified parts of peritoneum
C49.4	Malignant neoplasm of connective and soft tissue of abdomen
C76.2	Malignant neoplasm of abdomen
C77.2	Secondary and unspecified malignant neoplasm of intra-abdominal lymph nodes
C78.4	Secondary malignant neoplasm of small intestine
C78.5	Secondary malignant neoplasm of large intestine and rectum
C78.6	Secondary malignant neoplasm of retroperitoneum and peritoneum
C78.7	Secondary malignant neoplasm of liver and intrahepatic bile duct
C78.89	Secondary malignant neoplasm of other digestive organs

C79.89	Secondary malignant neoplasm of other specified sites
C7A.098	Malignant carcinoid tumors of other sites
C7A.1	Malignant poorly differentiated neuroendocrine tumors
C7A.8	Other malignant neuroendocrine tumors
C7B.01	Secondary carcinoid tumors of distant lymph nodes
C7B.02	Secondary carcinoid tumors of liver
C7B.04	Secondary carcinoid tumors of peritoneum
D19.1	Benign neoplasm of mesothelial tissue of peritoneum
D20.0	Benign neoplasm of soft tissue of retroperitoneum
D20.1	Benign neoplasm of soft tissue of peritoneum
D3A.098	Benign carcinoid tumors of other sites
D48.1	Neoplasm of uncertain behavior of connective and other soft tissue
D48.2	Neoplasm of uncertain behavior of peripheral nerves and autonomic nervous system
D48.3	Neoplasm of uncertain behavior of retroperitoneum
D48.4	Neoplasm of uncertain behavior of peritoneum
D49.0	Neoplasm of unspecified behavior of digestive system
D49.89	Neoplasm of unspecified behavior of other specified sites
K65.0	Generalized (acute) peritonitis
K65.1	Peritoneal abscess
K65.2	Spontaneous bacterial peritonitis

AMA: **49255** 2018,Mar,11; 2018,Jan,8; 2017,Jan,8; 2016,Jan,13; 2015,Jan,16

Relative Value Units/Medicare Edits

Non-Facility RVU	Work	PE	MP	Total
49255	12.56	8.14	2.59	23.29
Facility RVU	Work	PE	MP	Total
49255	12.56	8.14	2.59	23.29

	FUD	Status	MUE	Modifiers				IOM Reference
49255	90	A	1(2)	51	N/A	62*	80	None

* with documentation

Terms To Know

disseminated. Spread over an extensive area.

epiploic. Of or relating to the omentum, as in epiploic fat.

exploration. Examination for diagnostic purposes.

omentum. Fold of peritoneal tissue suspended between the stomach and neighboring visceral organs of the abdominal cavity.

resection. Surgical removal of a part or all of an organ or body part.

49320

49320 Laparoscopy, abdomen, peritoneum, and omentum, diagnostic, with or without collection of specimen(s) by brushing or washing (separate procedure)

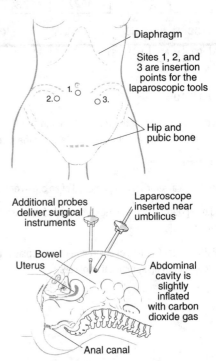

Sites 1, 2, and 3 are insertion points for the laparoscopic tools

Diaphragm

Hip and pubic bone

Additional probes deliver surgical instruments

Laparoscope inserted near umbilicus

Bowel Uterus

Abdominal cavity is slightly inflated with carbon dioxide gas

Anal canal

Explanation

The physician makes a 1.0-centimeter incision in the umbilicus through which the abdomen is inflated and a fiberoptic laparoscope is inserted. Other incisions are also made through which trocars can be passed into the abdominal cavity to deliver instruments, a video camera, and when needed an additional light source. The physician manipulates the tools so that the pelvic organs, peritoneum, abdomen, and omentum can be viewed through the laparoscope and/or video monitor. Biopsy from any or all of the areas observed are obtained by brushing the surface and collecting the cells or by washing (bathing) the area with a saline solution, and suctioning out the cell rich solution. When the procedure is complete, the laparoscope, instruments, and light source are removed and the incisions are closed with sutures. If biopsy of pelvic organs is performed, the physician may also insert an instrument through the vagina to grasp the cervix and pass another instrument through the cervix, into the uterus to manipulate the uterus.

Coding Tips

This separate procedure by definition is usually a component of a more complex service and is not identified separately. When performed alone or with other unrelated procedures/services it may be reported. If performed alone, list the code; if performed with other procedures/services, list the code and append modifier 59 or an X{EPSU} modifier. For exploratory laparotomy (open approach), exploratory celiotomy, with or without biopsies, see 49000.

ICD-10-CM Diagnostic Codes

The application of this code is too broad to adequately present ICD-10-CM diagnostic code links here. Refer to your ICD-10-CM book.

AMA: **49320** 2018,Jan,8; 2017,Jan,8; 2017,Apr,7; 2016,Jan,13; 2015,Jan,16; 2015,Dec,16

Relative Value Units/Medicare Edits

Non-Facility RVU	Work	PE	MP	Total
49320	5.14	3.42	1.15	9.71
Facility RVU	Work	PE	MP	Total
49320	5.14	3.42	1.15	9.71

	FUD	Status	MUE	Modifiers				IOM Reference
49320	10	A	1(3)	51	N/A	N/A	80	None

* with documentation

Terms To Know

carcinoma in situ. Malignancy that arises from the cells of the vessel, gland, or organ of origin that remains confined to that site or has not invaded neighboring tissue.

insufflation. Blowing air or gas into a body cavity.

laparoscopy. Direct visualization of the peritoneal cavity, outer fallopian tubes, uterus, and ovaries utilizing a laparoscope, a thin, flexible fiberoptic tube.

omentum. Fold of peritoneal tissue suspended between the stomach and neighboring visceral organs of the abdominal cavity.

peritoneum. Strong, continuous membrane that forms the lining of the abdominal and pelvic cavity. The parietal peritoneum, or outer layer, is attached to the abdominopelvic walls and the visceral peritoneum, or inner layer, surrounds the organs inside the abdominal cavity.

49321

49321   Laparoscopy, surgical; with biopsy (single or multiple)

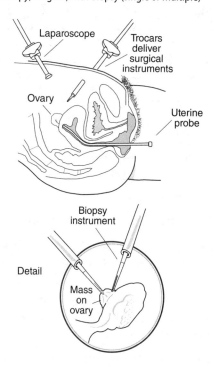

Explanation

The physician makes a 1.0 centimeter incision in the umbilicus through which the abdomen is inflated and a fiberoptic laparoscope is inserted. Other incisions are also made through which trocars can be passed into the abdominal cavity to deliver instruments, a video camera, and, when needed, an additional light source. The physician manipulates the tools so that the pelvic organs, peritoneum, abdomen, and omentum can be viewed through the laparoscope and/or video monitor. Biopsy from any or all of the areas observed are obtained by grasping a sample with a biopsy forceps that is capable of "biting off" small pieces of tissue. When the procedure is complete, the laparoscope, instruments, and light source are removed and the incisions are closed with sutures. If a biopsy of female pelvic organs is performed, the physician may also insert an instrument through the vagina to grasp the cervix and pass another instrument through the cervix and into the uterus to manipulate the uterus.

Coding Tips

Surgical laparoscopy always includes diagnostic laparoscopy. To report a diagnostic laparoscopy (peritoneoscopy), see 49320. For laparoscopic aspiration (single or multiple), see 49322. For exploratory laparotomy, exploratory celiotomy, with or without biopsies, see 49000.

ICD-10-CM Diagnostic Codes

The application of this code is too broad to adequately present ICD-10-CM diagnostic code links here. Refer to your ICD-10-CM book.

AMA: **49321** 2018,Jan,8; 2018,Aug,10; 2017,Jan,8; 2016,Jan,13; 2015,Jan,16

Relative Value Units/Medicare Edits

Non-Facility RVU	Work	PE	MP	Total
49321	5.44	3.57	1.18	10.19
Facility RVU	Work	PE	MP	Total
49321	5.44	3.57	1.18	10.19

	FUD	Status	MUE	Modifiers				IOM Reference
49321	10	A	1(2)	51	N/A	62	80	None

* with documentation

Terms To Know

benign. Mild or nonmalignant in nature.

biopsy. Tissue or fluid removed for diagnostic purposes through analysis of the cells in the biopsy material.

forceps. Tool used for grasping or compressing tissue.

laparoscopy. Direct visualization of the peritoneal cavity, outer fallopian tubes, uterus, and ovaries utilizing a laparoscope, a thin, flexible fiberoptic tube.

malignant. Any condition tending to progress toward death, specifically an invasive tumor with a loss of cellular differentiation that has the ability to spread or metastasize to other body areas.

neoplasm. New abnormal growth, tumor.

omentum. Fold of peritoneal tissue suspended between the stomach and neighboring visceral organs of the abdominal cavity.

peritoneum. Strong, continuous membrane that forms the lining of the abdominal and pelvic cavity. The parietal peritoneum, or outer layer, is attached to the abdominopelvic walls and the visceral peritoneum, or inner layer, surrounds the organs inside the abdominal cavity.

trocar. Cannula or a sharp pointed instrument used to puncture and aspirate fluid from cavities.

umbilicus. Depression or scar left in the middle of the abdomen marking where the umbilical cord was attached in utero.

49322

49322   Laparoscopy, surgical; with aspiration of cavity or cyst (eg, ovarian cyst) (single or multiple)

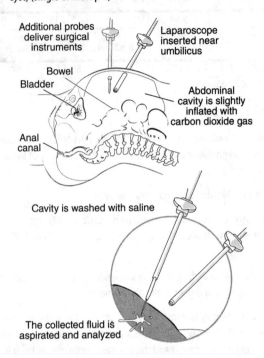

Additional probes deliver surgical instruments

Laparoscope inserted near umbilicus

Bowel
Bladder

Abdominal cavity is slightly inflated with carbon dioxide gas

Anal canal

Cavity is washed with saline

The collected fluid is aspirated and analyzed

Explanation

The physician makes a 1.0-centimeter incision in the umbilicus through which the abdomen is inflated and a fiberoptic laparoscope is inserted. A second incision is made directly below the umbilicus, just above the pubic hairline, through which a trocar can be passed into the abdominal cavity to deliver instruments. The physician manipulates the tools to view the pelvic organs through the laparoscope. An additional incision may be needed for a second light source. Once the biopsy site is viewed through the laparoscope, a 5.0-centimeter incision is made just above the site. Through this incision, the physician uses an aspirating probe to aspirate a cavity or cyst or to collect fluid for culture. The instruments are removed and the incisions are sutured.

Coding Tips

Surgical laparoscopy always includes diagnostic laparoscopy. To report a diagnostic laparoscopy (peritoneoscopy), see 49320. For laparoscopic fulguration or excision of lesions of the ovary, pelvic viscera, or peritoneal surface by any method, see 58662. For laparoscopic retroperitoneal lymph node sampling, single or multiple, see 38570–38572.

ICD-10-CM Diagnostic Codes

N70.01	Acute salpingitis ♀
N70.02	Acute oophoritis ♀
N70.03	Acute salpingitis and oophoritis ♀
N70.11	Chronic salpingitis ♀
N70.12	Chronic oophoritis ♀
N70.13	Chronic salpingitis and oophoritis ♀
N73.0	Acute parametritis and pelvic cellulitis ♀
N73.1	Chronic parametritis and pelvic cellulitis ♀
N73.4	Female chronic pelvic peritonitis ♀
N73.8	Other specified female pelvic inflammatory diseases ♀

N74	Female pelvic inflammatory disorders in diseases classified elsewhere ♀
N83.01	Follicular cyst of right ovary ♀ ☑
N83.02	Follicular cyst of left ovary ♀ ☑
N83.11	Corpus luteum cyst of right ovary ♀ ☑
N83.12	Corpus luteum cyst of left ovary ♀ ☑
N83.291	Other ovarian cyst, right side ♀ ☑
N83.292	Other ovarian cyst, left side ♀ ☑
N83.6	Hematosalpinx ♀

AMA: 49322 2018,Jan,8; 2017,Jan,8; 2016,Jan,13; 2015,Jan,16

Relative Value Units/Medicare Edits

Non-Facility RVU	Work	PE	MP	Total
49322	6.01	3.73	1.34	11.08
Facility RVU	**Work**	**PE**	**MP**	**Total**
49322	6.01	3.73	1.34	11.08

	FUD	Status	MUE	Modifiers				IOM Reference
49322	10	A	1(2)	51	N/A	62	80	None

* with documentation

Terms To Know

aspiration. Drawing fluid out by suction.

cyst. Elevated encapsulated mass containing fluid, semisolid, or solid material with a membranous lining.

laparoscopy. Direct visualization of the peritoneal cavity, outer fallopian tubes, uterus, and ovaries utilizing a laparoscope, a thin, flexible fiberoptic tube.

trocar. Cannula or a sharp pointed instrument used to puncture and aspirate fluid from cavities.

49323

49323 Laparoscopy, surgical; with drainage of lymphocele to peritoneal cavity

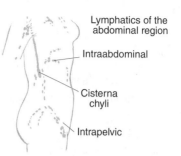

A lymphocele is drained to the peritoneal cavity by surgical laparoscopy

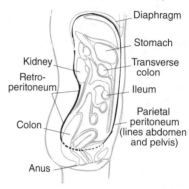

Explanation

The physician drains a lymphocele to the peritoneal cavity. With the patient under anesthesia, the physician places a trocar at the umbilicus into the abdominal or retroperitoneal space and insufflates the abdominal cavity. The physician places a laparoscope through the umbilical incision and additional trocars are placed into the abdomen. The lymphocele is identified and instruments are passed through to open and drain the lymphocele. The trocars are removed and the incisions are closed with sutures.

Coding Tips

Surgical laparoscopy always includes diagnostic laparoscopy. For diagnostic laparoscopy (peritoneoscopy), see 49320; with aspiration (single or multiple), see 49322. For open drainage of a retroperitoneal abscess, see 49060; open drainage of a lymphocele to the peritoneal cavity, see 49062.

ICD-10-CM Diagnostic Codes

C19	Malignant neoplasm of rectosigmoid junction
C54.1	Malignant neoplasm of endometrium ♀
C54.2	Malignant neoplasm of myometrium ♀
C54.3	Malignant neoplasm of fundus uteri ♀
C56.1	Malignant neoplasm of right ovary ♀ ☑
C56.2	Malignant neoplasm of left ovary ♀ ☑
C61	Malignant neoplasm of prostate ♂
C80.2	Malignant neoplasm associated with transplanted organ
C82.03	Follicular lymphoma grade I, intra-abdominal lymph nodes
C82.13	Follicular lymphoma grade II, intra-abdominal lymph nodes
C82.33	Follicular lymphoma grade IIIa, intra-abdominal lymph nodes
C82.43	Follicular lymphoma grade IIIb, intra-abdominal lymph nodes
C82.53	Diffuse follicle center lymphoma, intra-abdominal lymph nodes

C82.63	Cutaneous follicle center lymphoma, intra-abdominal lymph nodes
C82.83	Other types of follicular lymphoma, intra-abdominal lymph nodes
C83.53	Lymphoblastic (diffuse) lymphoma, intra-abdominal lymph nodes
C84.Z3	Other mature T/NK-cell lymphomas, intra-abdominal lymph nodes
C85.23	Mediastinal (thymic) large B-cell lymphoma, intra-abdominal lymph nodes
C85.83	Other specified types of non-Hodgkin lymphoma, intra-abdominal lymph nodes
D89.41	Monoclonal mast cell activation syndrome
D89.42	Idiopathic mast cell activation syndrome
D89.43	Secondary mast cell activation
D89.49	Other mast cell activation disorder
D89.810	Acute graft-versus-host disease
D89.811	Chronic graft-versus-host disease
D89.812	Acute on chronic graft-versus-host disease
I88.1	Chronic lymphadenitis, except mesenteric
I89.8	Other specified noninfective disorders of lymphatic vessels and lymph nodes
L04.1	Acute lymphadenitis of trunk
R22.2	Localized swelling, mass and lump, trunk
R59.0	Localized enlarged lymph nodes
R59.1	Generalized enlarged lymph nodes
T86.11	Kidney transplant rejection
T86.12	Kidney transplant failure
T86.13	Kidney transplant infection
T86.19	Other complication of kidney transplant
Z48.22	Encounter for aftercare following kidney transplant

AMA: **49323** 2018,Jan,8; 2017,Jan,8; 2016,Jan,13; 2015,Jan,16

Relative Value Units/Medicare Edits

Non-Facility RVU	Work	PE	MP	Total
49323	10.23	6.27	2.22	18.72
Facility RVU	**Work**	**PE**	**MP**	**Total**
49323	10.23	6.27	2.22	18.72

	FUD	Status	MUE	Modifiers				IOM Reference
49323	90	A	1(2)	51	N/A	62	80	None

* with documentation

49324-49325

| 49324 | Laparoscopy, surgical; with insertion of tunneled intraperitoneal catheter |
| 49325 | with revision of previously placed intraperitoneal cannula or catheter, with removal of intraluminal obstructive material if performed |

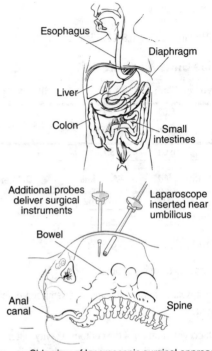

Side view of laparoscopic surgical approach

Explanation

A permanent intraperitoneal catheter is inserted laparoscopically using a tunneling technique. The physician makes a 1 cm incision in the umbilicus through which the abdomen is inflated and a fiberoptic laparoscope is inserted. Other incisions are also made through which trocars can be passed into the abdominal cavity to deliver additional instruments. The physician manipulates the tools so that the pelvic organs, peritoneum, abdomen, and omentum can be viewed through the laparoscope and/or video monitor. Using various tunneling techniques, the physician inserts the intraperitoneal catheter, positioning the tip inside the peritoneal cavity. A separately reportable subcutaneous extension of the catheter with a remote chest exit site may also be performed. If the physician is revising an intraperitoneal catheter, the catheter is inspected and freed of occlusion or blockage. When either procedure is complete, the laparoscope and other instruments are removed and the incisions are closed with sutures. Report 49324 for the tunneled insertion of an intraperitoneal cannula or catheter and 49325 for its revision.

Coding Tips

Surgical laparoscopy always includes diagnostic laparoscopy. For diagnostic laparoscopy (peritoneoscopy), see 49320. Report subcutaneous extension of intraperitoneal catheter with remote chest exit site (49435) with 49324, when performed. For open insertion of a tunneled intraperitoneal catheter, see 49421. When omentopexy is performed with these codes, report with 49326.

ICD-10-CM Diagnostic Codes

| N18.6 | End stage renal disease |
| R18.0 | Malignant ascites |

R18.8	Other ascites
T85.611A	Breakdown (mechanical) of intraperitoneal dialysis catheter, initial encounter
T85.691A	Other mechanical complication of intraperitoneal dialysis catheter, initial encounter

AMA: **49324** 2014,Jan,11 **49325** 2014,Jan,11

Relative Value Units/Medicare Edits

Non-Facility RVU	Work	PE	MP	Total
49324	6.32	3.67	1.51	11.5
49325	6.82	3.82	1.63	12.27
Facility RVU	**Work**	**PE**	**MP**	**Total**
49324	6.32	3.67	1.51	11.5
49325	6.82	3.82	1.63	12.27

	FUD	Status	MUE	Modifiers				IOM Reference
49324	10	A	1(2)	51	N/A	62	80	None
49325	10	A	1(2)	51	N/A	62	80	

* with documentation

Terms To Know

cannula. Tube inserted into a blood vessel, duct, or body cavity to facilitate passage.

catheter. Flexible tube inserted into an area of the body for introducing or withdrawing fluid.

obstruction. Blockage that prevents normal function of the valve or structure.

revision. Reordering or rearrangement of tissue to suit a particular need or function.

49326

+ 49326 Laparoscopy, surgical; with omentopexy (omental tacking procedure) (List separately in addition to code for primary procedure)

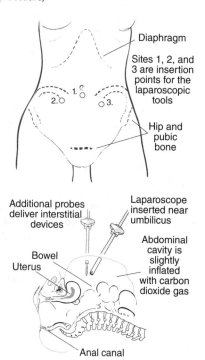

- Diaphragm
- Sites 1, 2, and 3 are insertion points for the laparoscopic tools
- Hip and pubic bone
- Additional probes deliver interstitial devices
- Laparoscope inserted near umbilicus
- Abdominal cavity is slightly inflated with carbon dioxide gas
- Bowel
- Uterus
- Anal canal

Explanation

Omentum is a strong and highly vascularized serous membrane in the abdomen. The physician makes a 1 cm incision in the umbilicus through which the abdomen is inflated and a fiberoptic laparoscope is inserted. Other incisions are also made through which trocars can be passed into the abdominal cavity to deliver instruments, a video camera, and, when needed, an additional light source. The physician manipulates the tools so the pelvic organs, peritoneum, abdomen, and omentum can be viewed through the laparoscope and/or video monitor. The physician isolates the omentum at the stomach and intestine and may cut, suture, or plicate omental tissue to achieve the desired effect. When the procedure is complete, the laparoscope, instruments, and light source are removed and the incisions are closed with sutures.

Coding Tips

Report 49326 in addition to 49324–49325. Surgical laparoscopy always includes diagnostic laparoscopy. To report a diagnostic laparoscopy (peritoneoscopy), see 49320.

ICD-10-CM Diagnostic Codes

This/these CPT code(s) are add-on code(s). See the primary procedure code that this code is performed with for your ICD-10-CM code selections.

AMA: **49326** 2014,Jan,11

● New   ▲ Revised   + Add On   ★ Telemedicine   AMA: CPT Assist   [Resequenced]   ☑ Laterality   © 2021 Optum360, LLC

Relative Value Units/Medicare Edits

Non-Facility RVU	Work	PE	MP	Total
49326	3.5	1.22	0.84	5.56
Facility RVU	Work	PE	MP	Total
49326	3.5	1.22	0.84	5.56

	FUD	Status	MUE	Modifiers				IOM Reference
49326	N/A	A	1(2)	N/A	N/A	62*	80	None

* with documentation

Terms To Know

laparoscope. Endoscopic instrument placed through the peritoneum to visualize the abdominal cavity internally.

omentum. Fold of peritoneal tissue suspended between the stomach and neighboring visceral organs of the abdominal cavity.

peritoneum. Strong, continuous membrane that forms the lining of the abdominal and pelvic cavity. The parietal peritoneum, or outer layer, is attached to the abdominopelvic walls and the visceral peritoneum, or inner layer, surrounds the organs inside the abdominal cavity.

plication. Surgical technique involving folding, tucking, or pleating to reduce the size of a hollow structure or organ.

49327

+ 49327 Laparoscopy, surgical; with placement of interstitial device(s) for radiation therapy guidance (eg, fiducial markers, dosimeter), intra-abdominal, intrapelvic, and/or retroperitoneum, including imaging guidance, if performed, single or multiple (List separately in addition to code for primary procedure)

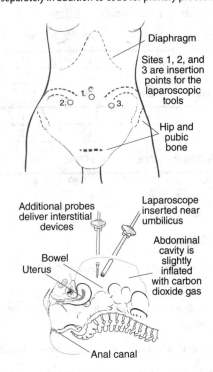

Explanation

The physician makes a 1 cm incision in the umbilicus through which the abdomen is inflated and a fiberoptic laparoscope is inserted. Other incisions are also made through which trocars can be passed into the abdominal cavity to deliver instruments, a video camera, and, when needed, an additional light source. The physician manipulates the tools so that the pelvic organs, peritoneum, abdomen, and omentum can be viewed through the laparoscope and/or video monitor. In conjunction with other laparoscopic abdominal, pelvic, or retroperitoneal procedures that are performed concurrently, and using image guidance if necessary, the physician places one or more interstitial devices such as gold seeds (fiducial markers) for radiation therapy guidance or a dosimeter to gauge the amount of radiation received into the targeted soft tissue tumor. Allowing for precision in targeting radiation and/or for measuring the radiation doses received, a fiducial marker is visible by ultrasound and fluoroscopy and permits accurate triangulation of the tissue to be treated. A capsule dosimeter relays radiation dose information so that the clinical team can monitor for any deviation between the radiation plan and the actual radiation received. When the procedure is complete, the laparoscope, instruments, and light source are removed and the incisions are closed with sutures.

Coding Tips

Report 49327 with laparoscopic abdominal, pelvic, or retroperitoneal procedures, when performed at the same operative session. To report placement of interstitial devices for intra-abdominal, intrapelvic, and/or retroperitoneal radiation therapy guidance at the same time as an open procedure, see 49412; percutaneous, see 49411.

ICD-10-CM Diagnostic Codes

This/these CPT code(s) are add-on code(s). See the primary procedure code that this code is performed with for your ICD-10-CM code selections.

AMA: 49327 2014,Jan,11

Relative Value Units/Medicare Edits

Non-Facility RVU	Work	PE	MP	Total
49327	2.38	0.89	0.59	3.86
Facility RVU	Work	PE	MP	Total
49327	2.38	0.89	0.59	3.86

	FUD	Status	MUE	Modifiers				IOM Reference
49327	N/A	A	1(2)	N/A	N/A	62*	80	None

* with documentation

Terms To Know

imaging. Radiologic means of producing pictures for clinical study of the internal structures and functions of the body, such as x-ray, ultrasound, magnetic resonance, or positron emission tomography.

interstitial. Within the small spaces or gaps occurring in tissue or organs.

laparoscopy. Direct visualization of the peritoneal cavity, outer fallopian tubes, uterus, and ovaries utilizing a laparoscope, a thin, flexible fiberoptic tube.

trocar. Cannula or a sharp pointed instrument used to puncture and aspirate fluid from cavities.

49400

49400	Injection of air or contrast into peritoneal cavity (separate procedure)

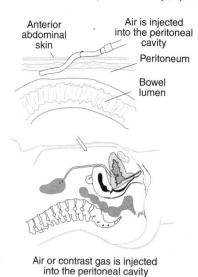

Anterior abdominal skin

Air is injected into the peritoneal cavity

Peritoneum

Bowel lumen

Air or contrast gas is injected into the peritoneal cavity

Explanation

The physician injects air contrast into the peritoneal cavity. The physician inserts a needle or catheter into the peritoneal cavity and injects air as a diagnostic procedure. An x-ray is usually obtained to define the pattern of air in the abdomen. The needle or catheter is removed at the completion of the procedure.

Coding Tips

Radiological supervision and interpretation is reported with 74190, when performed. For peritoneal drainage or lavage, open or percutaneous, see 49406, 49020, 49040, or 49082-49084. Surgical trays, A4550, are not separately reimbursed by Medicare; however, other third-party payers may cover them. Check with the specific payer to determine coverage.

ICD-10-CM Diagnostic Codes

The application of this code is too broad to adequately present ICD-10-CM diagnostic code links here. Refer to your ICD-10-CM book.

AMA: 49400 2018,Jan,8; 2017,Jan,8; 2016,Jan,13; 2015,Jan,16

Relative Value Units/Medicare Edits

Non-Facility RVU	Work	PE	MP	Total
49400	1.88	2.32	0.2	4.4
Facility RVU	Work	PE	MP	Total
49400	1.88	0.57	0.2	2.65

	FUD	Status	MUE	Modifiers				IOM Reference
49400	0	A	1(3)	51	N/A	N/A	N/A	None

* with documentation

49402

49402   Removal of peritoneal foreign body from peritoneal cavity

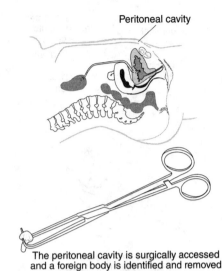

Peritoneal cavity

The peritoneal cavity is surgically accessed
and a foreign body is identified and removed

Explanation

The physician removes a foreign body from the abdominal cavity. The physician makes an abdominal incision and explores the abdominal cavity. The foreign body is identified and removed. The incision is closed.

Coding Tips

For lysis of intestinal adhesions, see 44005.

ICD-10-CM Diagnostic Codes

S31.620A   Laceration with foreign body of abdominal wall, right upper quadrant with penetration into peritoneal cavity, initial encounter ☑

S31.621A   Laceration with foreign body of abdominal wall, left upper quadrant with penetration into peritoneal cavity, initial encounter ☑

S31.622A   Laceration with foreign body of abdominal wall, epigastric region with penetration into peritoneal cavity, initial encounter

S31.623A   Laceration with foreign body of abdominal wall, right lower quadrant with penetration into peritoneal cavity, initial encounter ☑

S31.624A   Laceration with foreign body of abdominal wall, left lower quadrant with penetration into peritoneal cavity, initial encounter ☑

S31.625A   Laceration with foreign body of abdominal wall, periumbilic region with penetration into peritoneal cavity, initial encounter

S31.640A   Puncture wound with foreign body of abdominal wall, right upper quadrant with penetration into peritoneal cavity, initial encounter ☑

S31.641A   Puncture wound with foreign body of abdominal wall, left upper quadrant with penetration into peritoneal cavity, initial encounter ☑

S31.642A   Puncture wound with foreign body of abdominal wall, epigastric region with penetration into peritoneal cavity, initial encounter

S31.643A   Puncture wound with foreign body of abdominal wall, right lower quadrant with penetration into peritoneal cavity, initial encounter ☑

S31.644A   Puncture wound with foreign body of abdominal wall, left lower quadrant with penetration into peritoneal cavity, initial encounter ☑

S31.645A   Puncture wound with foreign body of abdominal wall, periumbilic region with penetration into peritoneal cavity, initial encounter

AMA: **49402** 2014,Jan,11

Relative Value Units/Medicare Edits

Non-Facility RVU	Work	PE	MP	Total
49402	14.09	7.93	3.24	25.26
Facility RVU	Work	PE	MP	Total
49402	14.09	7.93	3.24	25.26

	FUD	Status	MUE	Modifiers				IOM Reference
49402	90	A	1(3)	51	N/A	62*	N/A	None

* with documentation

Terms To Know

closure. Repairing an incision or wound by suture or other means.

exploration. Examination for diagnostic purposes.

foreign body. Any object or substance found in an organ and tissue that does not belong under normal circumstances.

incision. Act of cutting into tissue or an organ.

peritoneal cavity. Space between the lining of the abdominal wall, or parietal peritoneum, and the surface layer of the abdominal organs, or visceral peritoneum. It contains a thin, watery fluid that keeps the peritoneal surfaces moist.

removal. Process of moving out of or away from, or the fact of being removed.

49405

49405 Image-guided fluid collection drainage by catheter (eg, abscess, hematoma, seroma, lymphocele, cyst); visceral (eg, kidney, liver, spleen, lung/mediastinum), percutaneous

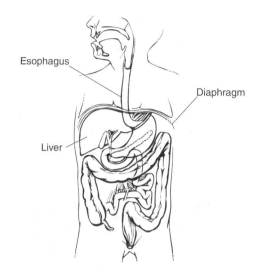

Percutaneous drainage of visceral organ abscess, hematoma, seroma, or lymphocele using image guidance

Explanation

A fluid collection in the visceral organs (kidney, liver, spleen, lung, mediastinum, etc.), such as a hematoma, seroma, abscess, lymphocele, or cyst, is drained using a catheter. The area over the affected organ is cleansed and local anesthesia is administered. Imaging is performed to assist in the insertion of a needle or guidewire into the fluid collection. Small tissue samples may be collected from the site for pathological examination. A catheter is inserted to drain and collect the fluid for analysis. The catheter is removed. More imaging may be performed to ensure hemostasis. A bandage is applied. In some cases, the catheter may be attached to a bag to allow for further drainage over the course of days.

Coding Tips

This code should be reported for each individual collection drained using a separate catheter. For open drainage of an abscess or a cyst via hepatotomy, see 47010; via pneumonostomy, see 32200; open external drainage of a pseudocyst of the pancreas, see 48510; open drainage of perirenal or renal abscess, see 50020. For percutaneous cholecystostomy, see 47490; pleural drainage, see 32556–32557. For thoracentesis without imaging, see 32554; with imaging guidance, see 32555. Do not report 49405 with 75989, 76942, 77002–77003, 77012, or 77021.

ICD-10-CM Diagnostic Codes

A06.4	Amebic liver abscess
A06.5	Amebic lung abscess
D73.3	Abscess of spleen
D73.4	Cyst of spleen
D78.21	Postprocedural hemorrhage of the spleen following a procedure on the spleen
D78.22	Postprocedural hemorrhage of the spleen following other procedure
D78.31	Postprocedural hematoma of the spleen following a procedure on the spleen
D78.32	Postprocedural hematoma of the spleen following other procedure
D78.33	Postprocedural seroma of the spleen following a procedure on the spleen
D78.34	Postprocedural seroma of the spleen following other procedure
I97.610	Postprocedural hemorrhage of a circulatory system organ or structure following a cardiac catheterization
I97.611	Postprocedural hemorrhage of a circulatory system organ or structure following cardiac bypass
I97.618	Postprocedural hemorrhage of a circulatory system organ or structure following other circulatory system procedure
I97.622	Postprocedural seroma of a circulatory system organ or structure following other procedure
I97.630	Postprocedural hematoma of a circulatory system organ or structure following a cardiac catheterization
I97.631	Postprocedural hematoma of a circulatory system organ or structure following cardiac bypass
I97.638	Postprocedural hematoma of a circulatory system organ or structure following other circulatory system procedure
J85.1	Abscess of lung with pneumonia
J85.2	Abscess of lung without pneumonia
J85.3	Abscess of mediastinum
J95.830	Postprocedural hemorrhage of a respiratory system organ or structure following a respiratory system procedure
J95.831	Postprocedural hemorrhage of a respiratory system organ or structure following other procedure
J95.860	Postprocedural hematoma of a respiratory system organ or structure following a respiratory system procedure
J95.861	Postprocedural hematoma of a respiratory system organ or structure following other procedure
J95.862	Postprocedural seroma of a respiratory system organ or structure following a respiratory system procedure
K65.1	Peritoneal abscess
K68.11	Postprocedural retroperitoneal abscess
K68.12	Psoas muscle abscess
K68.19	Other retroperitoneal abscess
K75.0	Abscess of liver
K81.0	Acute cholecystitis
K85.02	Idiopathic acute pancreatitis with infected necrosis
K85.10	Biliary acute pancreatitis without necrosis or infection
K85.20	Alcohol induced acute pancreatitis without necrosis or infection
K85.21	Alcohol induced acute pancreatitis with uninfected necrosis
K85.30	Drug induced acute pancreatitis without necrosis or infection
K85.82	Other acute pancreatitis with infected necrosis
K91.840	Postprocedural hemorrhage of a digestive system organ or structure following a digestive system procedure
K91.841	Postprocedural hemorrhage of a digestive system organ or structure following other procedure
K91.871	Postprocedural hematoma of a digestive system organ or structure following other procedure
K91.872	Postprocedural seroma of a digestive system organ or structure following a digestive system procedure
K91.873	Postprocedural seroma of a digestive system organ or structure following other procedure
N15.1	Renal and perinephric abscess

N34.0	Urethral abscess	
N41.2	Abscess of prostate 🅐 ♂	
N99.820	Postprocedural hemorrhage of a genitourinary system organ or structure following a genitourinary system procedure	
N99.821	Postprocedural hemorrhage of a genitourinary system organ or structure following other procedure	

AMA: 49405 2020,Feb,13; 2018,Jan,8; 2017,Jan,8; 2016,Jan,13; 2015,Jan,16

Relative Value Units/Medicare Edits

Non-Facility RVU	Work	PE	MP	Total
49405	4.0	22.98	0.34	27.32
Facility RVU	Work	PE	MP	Total
49405	4.0	1.32	0.34	5.66

	FUD	Status	MUE	Modifiers				IOM Reference
49405	0	A	2(3)	51	N/A	N/A	N/A	None

* with documentation

Terms To Know

abscess. Circumscribed collection of pus resulting from bacteria, frequently associated with swelling and other signs of inflammation.

hematoma. Tumor-like collection of blood in some part of the body caused by a break in a blood vessel wall, usually as a result of trauma.

lymphocele. Cyst that contains lymph.

seroma. Swelling caused by the collection of serum, or clear fluid, in the tissues.

49406

49406	Image-guided fluid collection drainage by catheter (eg, abscess, hematoma, seroma, lymphocele, cyst); peritoneal or retroperitoneal, percutaneous

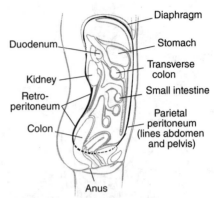

Percutaneous drainage of peritoneal or retroperitoneal abscess, hematoma, seroma, or lymphocele using image guidance

Explanation

A fluid collection in the peritoneum or retroperitoneum, such as a hematoma, a seroma, an abscess, a lymphocele, or a cyst, is drained using a catheter. The area over the affected site is cleansed and local anesthesia is administered. Imaging is performed to assist in the insertion of a needle or guidewire into the fluid collection. Small tissue samples may be collected from the site for pathological examination. A catheter is inserted to drain and collect the fluid for analysis and is then removed. More imaging may be performed to ensure hemostasis. A bandage is applied. In some cases, the catheter may be attached to a bag to allow for further drainage over the course of days.

Coding Tips

This code should be reported for each individual collection drained using a separate catheter. To report percutaneous insertion of a tunneled intraperitoneal catheter without a subcutaneous port, see 49418. For percutaneous paracentesis, see 49082–49083. For open drainage of an abscess, appendiceal, see 44900; peritoneal, see 49020; subdiaphragmatic or subphrenic, see 49040; retroperitoneal, see 49060; extraperitoneal to peritoneal cavity, see 49062; peritoneal lavage, see 49084; perirenal or renal, see 50020; and ovarian, see 58805 or 58822. For transvaginal or transrectal image-guided drainage of a peritoneal or retroperitoneal abscess, see 49407; transrectal drainage of a pelvic abscess, see 45000. Do not report 49406 with 75989, 76942, 77002–77003, 77012, or 77021.

ICD-10-CM Diagnostic Codes

K35.20	Acute appendicitis with generalized peritonitis, without abscess
K35.21	Acute appendicitis with generalized peritonitis, with abscess
K35.30	Acute appendicitis with localized peritonitis, without perforation or gangrene
K35.31	Acute appendicitis with localized peritonitis and gangrene, without perforation
K35.32	Acute appendicitis with perforation and localized peritonitis, without abscess
K35.33	Acute appendicitis with perforation and localized peritonitis, with abscess
K65.1	Peritoneal abscess
K68.11	Postprocedural retroperitoneal abscess

AMA: **49406** 2020,Feb,13; 2018,Jan,8; 2017,Jan,8; 2016,Jan,13; 2015,Jan,16

Relative Value Units/Medicare Edits

Non-Facility RVU	Work	PE	MP	Total
49406	4.0	22.99	0.34	27.33
Facility RVU	**Work**	**PE**	**MP**	**Total**
49406	4.0	1.32	0.34	5.66

	FUD	Status	MUE	Modifiers				IOM Reference
49406	0	A	2(3)	51	N/A	N/A	N/A	None

* with documentation

Terms To Know

abscess. Circumscribed collection of pus resulting from bacteria, frequently associated with swelling and other signs of inflammation.

cyst. Elevated encapsulated mass containing fluid, semisolid, or solid material with a membranous lining.

drainage. Releasing, taking, or letting out fluids and/or gases from a body part.

hematoma. Tumor-like collection of blood in some part of the body caused by a break in a blood vessel wall, usually as a result of trauma.

imaging. Radiologic means of producing pictures for clinical study of the internal structures and functions of the body, such as x-ray, ultrasound, magnetic resonance, or positron emission tomography.

lymphocele. Cyst that contains lymph.

percutaneous. Through the skin.

seroma. Swelling caused by the collection of serum, or clear fluid, in the tissues.

49407

49407   Image-guided fluid collection drainage by catheter (eg, abscess, hematoma, seroma, lymphocele, cyst); peritoneal or retroperitoneal, transvaginal or transrectal

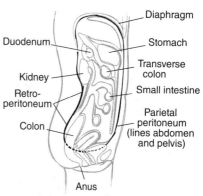

Transrectal or transvaginal approach is used to drain abscess, hematoma, seroma, or lymphocele using image guidance

Explanation

A fluid collection in the peritoneum or retroperitoneum, such as a hematoma, a seroma, an abscess, a lymphocele, or a cyst, is drained via a vaginal or rectal approach. An intracavitary probe is used to create access through the rectal or vaginal wall. Imaging is performed to assist in the insertion of a needle or guidewire into the fluid collection. Small tissue samples may be collected from the site for pathological examination. A catheter is inserted to drain and collect the fluid for analysis and is then removed. In some cases, the catheter may be attached to a bag to allow for further drainage over the course of days.

Coding Tips

This code should be reported for each individual collection drained using a separate catheter. For open drainage of an abscess, transvaginal or transrectal, pelvic, see 45000; ovarian cyst, see 58800; ovarian abscess, see 58820. For peritoneal drainage or lavage, open or percutaneous, see 49020, 49040, or 49082. For percutaneous drainage of the abdominal wall soft tissue, by catheter, see 10030. Do not report 49407 with 75989, 76942, 77002–77003, 77012, or 77021.

ICD-10-CM Diagnostic Codes

K65.1	Peritoneal abscess
K68.11	Postprocedural retroperitoneal abscess
K68.19	Other retroperitoneal abscess

AMA: **49407** 2018,Jan,8; 2017,Jan,8; 2016,Jan,13; 2015,Jan,16

Relative Value Units/Medicare Edits

Non-Facility RVU	Work	PE	MP	Total
49407	4.25	18.03	0.42	22.7
Facility RVU	**Work**	**PE**	**MP**	**Total**
49407	4.25	1.36	0.42	6.03

	FUD	Status	MUE	Modifiers				IOM Reference
49407	0	A	1(3)	51	N/A	N/A	N/A	None

* with documentation

49411

49411 Placement of interstitial device(s) for radiation therapy guidance (eg, fiducial markers, dosimeter), percutaneous, intra-abdominal, intra-pelvic (except prostate), and/or retroperitoneum, single or multiple

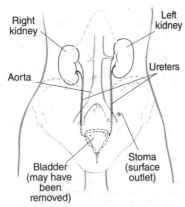

Right kidney
Left kidney
Aorta
Ureters
Bladder (may have been removed)
Stoma (surface outlet)

One or more interstitial devices may be percutaneously placed in the intra-abdominal or intra-pelvic areas or the retroperitoneum

Explanation

The physician places one or more interstitial devices such as gold seeds (fiducial markers) for radiation therapy guidance or a dosimeter to gauge the amount of radiation received. Implanted percutaneously in and/or around an intra-abdominal, intra-pelvic (excluding prostate), and/or retroperitoneal soft tissue tumor, these act as radiographic landmarks to define the position of the target lesion. Under CT or other image guidance, the physician injects a small capsule or seed into the targeted tissue using a needle injection device. Allowing for precision in targeting radiation and/or for measuring the radiation doses received, an injected fiducial marker is visible by ultrasound and fluoroscopy and permits accurate triangulation of the tissue to be treated. An injected capsule dosimeter relays radiation dose information so that the clinical team can monitor for any deviation between the radiation plan and the actual radiation received.

Coding Tips

For imaging guidance, see 76942, 77002, 77012, or 77021. Supply of the device is reported separately. For percutaneous placement of interstitial device for intra-thoracic radiation therapy guidance, see 32553.

ICD-10-CM Diagnostic Codes

The application of this code is too broad to adequately present ICD-10-CM diagnostic code links here. Refer to your ICD-10-CM book.

AMA: 49411 2018,Jan,8; 2017,Jan,8; 2016,Jun,3; 2016,Jan,13; 2015,Jan,16

Relative Value Units/Medicare Edits

Non-Facility RVU	Work	PE	MP	Total
49411	3.57	10.88	0.3	14.75
Facility RVU	Work	PE	MP	Total
49411	3.57	1.45	0.3	5.32

	FUD	Status	MUE	Modifiers				IOM Reference
49411	0	A	1(2)	51	N/A	N/A	80*	None

* with documentation

49412

+ 49412 Placement of interstitial device(s) for radiation therapy guidance (eg, fiducial markers, dosimeter), open, intra-abdominal, intrapelvic, and/or retroperitoneum, including image guidance, if performed, single or multiple (List separately in addition to code for primary procedure)

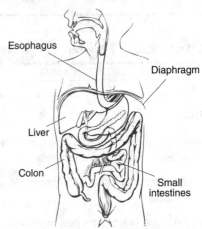

Esophagus
Diaphragm
Liver
Colon
Small intestines

Interstitial devices are placed into the abdomen, pelvis, or retroperitoneum

Explanation

The physician places one or more interstitial devices such as gold seeds (fiducial markers) for radiation therapy guidance or a dosimeter to gauge the amount of radiation received into a targeted intra-abdominal, intrapelvic, or retroperitoneal soft tissue tumor. Implanted in conjunction with an open abdominal, pelvic, or retroperitoneal procedure performed concurrently, these act as radiographic landmarks to define the position of the target lesion. Using image guidance if necessary, the physician places a small capsule or seed into the targeted tissue. Allowing for precision in targeting radiation and/or for measuring the radiation doses received, a fiducial marker is visible by ultrasound and fluoroscopy and permits accurate triangulation of the tissue to be treated. A capsule dosimeter relays radiation dose information so that the clinical team can monitor for any deviation between the radiation plan and the actual radiation received. When the procedures are complete, the incisions are closed with sutures.

Coding Tips

Report 49412 with open abdominal, pelvic, or retroperitoneal procedures, when performed at the same operative session. For placement of interstitial devices for intra-abdominal, intrapelvic, and/or retroperitoneal radiation therapy guidance at the same time as a laparoscopic procedure, see 49327; percutaneous, see 49411.

ICD-10-CM Diagnostic Codes

This/these CPT code(s) are add-on code(s). See the primary procedure code that this code is performed with for your ICD-10-CM code selections.

AMA: 49412 2014,Jan,11

Relative Value Units/Medicare Edits

Non-Facility RVU	Work	PE	MP	Total
49412	1.5	0.56	0.37	2.43
Facility RVU	Work	PE	MP	Total
49412	1.5	0.56	0.37	2.43

	FUD	Status	MUE	Modifiers				IOM Reference
49412	N/A	A	1(2)	N/A	N/A	62*	80*	None

* with documentation

Terms To Know

dosimetry. Component in the administration of radiation oncology therapy in which a radiation dose is calculated to a specific site, including implant or beam orientation and exposure, isodose strengths, tissue inhomogeneities, and volume.

fluoroscopy. Radiology technique that allows visual examination of part of the body or a function of an organ using a device that projects an x-ray image on a fluorescent screen.

interstitial radiation. Radioactive source placed into the tissue being treated.

percutaneous. Through the skin.

retroperitoneal. Located behind the peritoneum, the membrane that lines the abdominopelvic walls and forms a covering for the internal organs.

49418

49418   Insertion of tunneled intraperitoneal catheter (eg, dialysis, intraperitoneal chemotherapy instillation, management of ascites), complete procedure, including imaging guidance, catheter placement, contrast injection when performed, and radiological supervision and interpretation, percutaneous

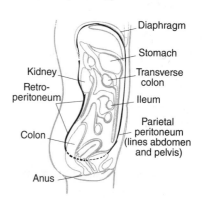

Explanation

The physician places a tunneled intraperitoneal catheter for drainage, dialysis, or chemotherapy instillation using a percutaneous approach. The physician makes a small abdominal incision, opens the peritoneum (the double-layered sac covering the internal organs and lining the abdominopelvic walls), and inserts the catheter into the cavity. The proximal end of the catheter is tunneled subcutaneously away from the initial incision and brought out through the skin. The incision is closed. Alternately, the physician may percutaneously insert the catheter over a wire placed through a needle inserted into the peritoneal cavity. This code reports the complete procedure and includes placement of the catheter under imaging guidance, contrast injection if performed, and radiological supervision and interpretation.

Coding Tips

For insertion of a tunneled intraperitoneal catheter, with subcutaneous port, see, 49419; removal, see 49422.

ICD-10-CM Diagnostic Codes

C16.0	Malignant neoplasm of cardia
C16.1	Malignant neoplasm of fundus of stomach
C16.2	Malignant neoplasm of body of stomach
C16.3	Malignant neoplasm of pyloric antrum
C16.4	Malignant neoplasm of pylorus
C22.0	Liver cell carcinoma
C22.2	Hepatoblastoma
C22.3	Angiosarcoma of liver
C22.4	Other sarcomas of liver
C22.7	Other specified carcinomas of liver
C45.1	Mesothelioma of peritoneum
C48.0	Malignant neoplasm of retroperitoneum
C48.1	Malignant neoplasm of specified parts of peritoneum
C78.6	Secondary malignant neoplasm of retroperitoneum and peritoneum
C78.7	Secondary malignant neoplasm of liver and intrahepatic bile duct
C79.61	Secondary malignant neoplasm of right ovary ♀ ☑
C79.62	Secondary malignant neoplasm of left ovary ♀ ☑

C7A.092	Malignant carcinoid tumor of the stomach	
C7B.02	Secondary carcinoid tumors of liver	
E08.22	Diabetes mellitus due to underlying condition with diabetic chronic kidney disease	
E09.21	Drug or chemical induced diabetes mellitus with diabetic nephropathy	
E09.22	Drug or chemical induced diabetes mellitus with diabetic chronic kidney disease	
E09.29	Drug or chemical induced diabetes mellitus with other diabetic kidney complication	
E13.21	Other specified diabetes mellitus with diabetic nephropathy	
E13.22	Other specified diabetes mellitus with diabetic chronic kidney disease	
M35.04	Sjögren syndrome with tubulo-interstitial nephropathy	
M35.0A	Sjögren syndrome with glomerular disease	
N01.A	Rapidly progressive nephritic syndrome with C3 glomerulonephritis	
N03.A	Chronic nephritic syndrome with C3 glomerulonephritis	
N18.31	Chronic kidney disease, stage 3a	
N18.32	Chronic kidney disease, stage 3b	
N18.4	Chronic kidney disease, stage 4 (severe)	
N18.5	Chronic kidney disease, stage 5	
N18.6	End stage renal disease	
R18.0	Malignant ascites	

AMA: 49418 2014,Jan,11

Relative Value Units/Medicare Edits

Non-Facility RVU	Work	PE	MP	Total
49418	3.96	29.31	0.39	33.66
Facility RVU	**Work**	**PE**	**MP**	**Total**
49418	3.96	1.5	0.39	5.85

	FUD	Status	MUE	Modifiers				IOM Reference
49418	0	A	1(3)	51	N/A	N/A	80*	None

* with documentation

49419

49419	Insertion of tunneled intraperitoneal catheter, with subcutaneous port (ie, totally implantable)

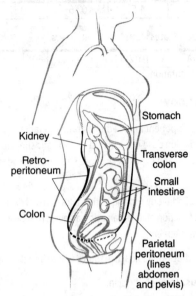

A permanent catheter is placed within the peritoneal cavity and a subcutaneous reservoir is implanted

Explanation

The physician inserts a tunneled intraperitoneal catheter with subcutaneous reservoir (port) for continuous drug infusion of substances such as insulin, morphine, or chemotherapeutic agents. In the case of a totally implantable, intraperitoneal insulin delivery system, the pump reservoir is inserted under general or local anesthesia into a surgically prepared pocket in the subcutaneous fat of the lower or mid-left abdomen. The infusion line catheter from the pump is placed inside the peritoneal cavity using a tunneling technique with the tip free moving.

Coding Tips

For removal of a tunneled intraperitoneal catheter, see 49422. Removal of a non-tunneled catheter is reported with the appropriate E/M code. For open placement of a tunneled catheter for dialysis, see 49421. For percutaneous insertion of a tunneled catheter without a port, see 49418.

ICD-10-CM Diagnostic Codes

C16.0	Malignant neoplasm of cardia
C16.1	Malignant neoplasm of fundus of stomach
C16.2	Malignant neoplasm of body of stomach
C16.3	Malignant neoplasm of pyloric antrum
C16.4	Malignant neoplasm of pylorus
C16.8	Malignant neoplasm of overlapping sites of stomach
C22.0	Liver cell carcinoma
C22.2	Hepatoblastoma
C22.3	Angiosarcoma of liver
C22.4	Other sarcomas of liver
C45.1	Mesothelioma of peritoneum
C48.0	Malignant neoplasm of retroperitoneum
C48.1	Malignant neoplasm of specified parts of peritoneum

C48.8	Malignant neoplasm of overlapping sites of retroperitoneum and peritoneum
C54.0	Malignant neoplasm of isthmus uteri ♀
C54.1	Malignant neoplasm of endometrium ♀
C54.2	Malignant neoplasm of myometrium ♀
C54.3	Malignant neoplasm of fundus uteri ♀
C54.8	Malignant neoplasm of overlapping sites of corpus uteri ♀
C56.1	Malignant neoplasm of right ovary ♀ ☑
C56.2	Malignant neoplasm of left ovary ♀ ☑
C56.3	Malignant neoplasm of bilateral ovaries ♀ ☑
C57.01	Malignant neoplasm of right fallopian tube ♀ ☑
C57.02	Malignant neoplasm of left fallopian tube ♀ ☑
C57.21	Malignant neoplasm of right round ligament ♀ ☑
C57.22	Malignant neoplasm of left round ligament ♀ ☑
C57.7	Malignant neoplasm of other specified female genital organs ♀
C57.8	Malignant neoplasm of overlapping sites of female genital organs ♀
C78.6	Secondary malignant neoplasm of retroperitoneum and peritoneum
C79.61	Secondary malignant neoplasm of right ovary ♀ ☑
C79.62	Secondary malignant neoplasm of left ovary ♀ ☑
C79.63	Secondary malignant neoplasm of bilateral ovaries ♀ ☑
C7A.092	Malignant carcinoid tumor of the stomach
C7B.02	Secondary carcinoid tumors of liver
E08.22	Diabetes mellitus due to underlying condition with diabetic chronic kidney disease
E09.21	Drug or chemical induced diabetes mellitus with diabetic nephropathy
E09.22	Drug or chemical induced diabetes mellitus with diabetic chronic kidney disease
E09.29	Drug or chemical induced diabetes mellitus with other diabetic kidney complication
E10.21	Type 1 diabetes mellitus with diabetic nephropathy
E11.21	Type 2 diabetes mellitus with diabetic nephropathy
E11.29	Type 2 diabetes mellitus with other diabetic kidney complication
E13.21	Other specified diabetes mellitus with diabetic nephropathy
E13.22	Other specified diabetes mellitus with diabetic chronic kidney disease
E13.29	Other specified diabetes mellitus with other diabetic kidney complication
M35.04	Sjögren syndrome with tubulo-interstitial nephropathy
M35.0A	Sjögren syndrome with glomerular disease
N01.A	Rapidly progressive nephritic syndrome with C3 glomerulonephritis
N03.A	Chronic nephritic syndrome with C3 glomerulonephritis
N18.31	Chronic kidney disease, stage 3a
N18.32	Chronic kidney disease, stage 3b
N18.4	Chronic kidney disease, stage 4 (severe)
N18.5	Chronic kidney disease, stage 5
N18.6	End stage renal disease

AMA: **49419** 2014,Jan,11

Relative Value Units/Medicare Edits

Non-Facility RVU	Work	PE	MP	Total
49419	7.08	4.25	1.29	12.62
Facility RVU	Work	PE	MP	Total
49419	7.08	4.25	1.29	12.62

	FUD	Status	MUE	Modifiers				IOM Reference
49419	90	A	1(2)	51	N/A	N/A	N/A	None

* with documentation

Terms To Know

catheter. Flexible tube inserted into an area of the body for introducing or withdrawing fluid.

chemotherapeutic. Treatment for systemic or localized disease that employs a drug or chemical agent, usually designed to treat cancerous conditions.

infusion. Introduction of a therapeutic fluid, other than blood, into the bloodstream.

intraperitoneal. Within the cavity or space created by the double-layered sac that lines the abdominopelvic walls and forms a covering for the internal organs.

reservoir. Space or body cavity for storage of liquid.

49421

49421 Insertion of tunneled intraperitoneal catheter for dialysis, open

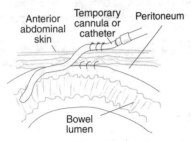

Anterior abdominal skin

Temporary cannula or catheter

Peritoneum

Bowel lumen

An intraperitoneal cannula or catheter
is placed for drainage or dialysis

Explanation

The physician places a tunneled intraperitoneal catheter for dialysis using an open technique. The physician makes a small abdominal incision, opens the peritoneum (the double-layered sac covering the internal organs and lining the abdominopelvic walls), and inserts the catheter into the cavity. The proximal end of the catheter is tunneled subcutaneously away from the initial incision and brought out through the skin. The incision is closed. A separately reportable subcutaneous extension of the intraperitoneal catheter with a remote chest exit site may also be performed at this time.

Coding Tips

For laparoscopic insertion of a tunneled intraperitoneal catheter, see 49324. To report the insertion of a tunneled intraperitoneal catheter, with subcutaneous port, see 49419. Subcutaneous extension of intraperitoneal catheter with remote chest exit site (49435) is reported with 49421, when performed. For removal of a non-tunneled catheter, report the appropriate E/M code; tunneled intraperitoneal catheter, see 49422.

ICD-10-CM Diagnostic Codes

B52.0	Plasmodium malariae malaria with nephropathy
E08.21	Diabetes mellitus due to underlying condition with diabetic nephropathy
E08.22	Diabetes mellitus due to underlying condition with diabetic chronic kidney disease
E08.29	Diabetes mellitus due to underlying condition with other diabetic kidney complication
E09.21	Drug or chemical induced diabetes mellitus with diabetic nephropathy
E09.22	Drug or chemical induced diabetes mellitus with diabetic chronic kidney disease
E09.29	Drug or chemical induced diabetes mellitus with other diabetic kidney complication
E10.21	Type 1 diabetes mellitus with diabetic nephropathy
E10.22	Type 1 diabetes mellitus with diabetic chronic kidney disease
E10.29	Type 1 diabetes mellitus with other diabetic kidney complication
E11.21	Type 2 diabetes mellitus with diabetic nephropathy
E11.22	Type 2 diabetes mellitus with diabetic chronic kidney disease
E11.29	Type 2 diabetes mellitus with other diabetic kidney complication
E13.21	Other specified diabetes mellitus with diabetic nephropathy
E13.22	Other specified diabetes mellitus with diabetic chronic kidney disease
E13.29	Other specified diabetes mellitus with other diabetic kidney complication
M32.15	Tubulo-interstitial nephropathy in systemic lupus erythematosus
M35.04	Sjögren syndrome with tubulo-interstitial nephropathy
M35.0A	Sjögren syndrome with glomerular disease
N01.A	Rapidly progressive nephritic syndrome with C3 glomerulonephritis
N03.A	Chronic nephritic syndrome with C3 glomerulonephritis
N08	Glomerular disorders in diseases classified elsewhere
N17.0	Acute kidney failure with tubular necrosis
N17.1	Acute kidney failure with acute cortical necrosis
N17.2	Acute kidney failure with medullary necrosis
N17.8	Other acute kidney failure
N18.1	Chronic kidney disease, stage 1
N18.2	Chronic kidney disease, stage 2 (mild)
N18.31	Chronic kidney disease, stage 3a
N18.32	Chronic kidney disease, stage 3b
N18.4	Chronic kidney disease, stage 4 (severe)
N18.5	Chronic kidney disease, stage 5
N18.6	End stage renal disease

AMA: **49421** 2018,Jan,8; 2017,Jan,8; 2016,Jan,13; 2015,Jan,16

Relative Value Units/Medicare Edits

Non-Facility RVU	Work	PE	MP	Total
49421	4.21	1.53	0.96	6.7
Facility RVU	**Work**	**PE**	**MP**	**Total**
49421	4.21	1.53	0.96	6.7

	FUD	Status	MUE	Modifiers				IOM Reference
49421	0	A	1(2)	51	N/A	N/A	N/A	None

* with documentation

Terms To Know

catheter. Flexible tube inserted into an area of the body for introducing or withdrawing fluid.

intraperitoneal. Within the cavity or space created by the double-layered sac that lines the abdominopelvic walls and forms a covering for the internal organs.

49422

49422   Removal of tunneled intraperitoneal catheter

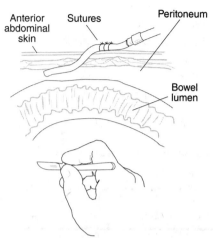

Tissues immediately surrounding the placement
are incised and the catheter or cannula is
removed and closure is accomplished

Explanation

The physician removes a tunneled intraperitoneal catheter. The physician
makes an incision over the insertion site of the catheter. The catheter is
dissected free of surrounding scar tissue, transected, and removed from the
peritoneal insertion site and skin exit site. The incision at the insertion site of
the catheter is closed. The skin exit site is left open to allow drainage.

Coding Tips

When this procedure is performed with another separately identifiable
procedure, the highest dollar value code is listed as the primary procedure
and subsequent procedures are appended with modifier 51. For removal of
a non-tunneled catheter, report the appropriate E/M code. For insertion of a
tunneled intraperitoneal catheter for dialysis, open, see 49421; laparoscopic,
see 49324. percutaneous, complete procedure, see 49418.

ICD-10-CM Diagnostic Codes

T85.611A	Breakdown (mechanical) of intraperitoneal dialysis catheter, initial encounter
T85.621A	Displacement of intraperitoneal dialysis catheter, initial encounter
T85.631A	Leakage of intraperitoneal dialysis catheter, initial encounter
T85.691A	Other mechanical complication of intraperitoneal dialysis catheter, initial encounter
T85.71XA	Infection and inflammatory reaction due to peritoneal dialysis catheter, initial encounter
Z49.02	Encounter for fitting and adjustment of peritoneal dialysis catheter
Z49.32	Encounter for adequacy testing for peritoneal dialysis

AMA: **49422** 2014,Jan,11

Relative Value Units/Medicare Edits

Non-Facility RVU	Work	PE	MP	Total
49422	4.0	1.62	0.91	6.53
Facility RVU	**Work**	**PE**	**MP**	**Total**
49422	4.0	1.62	0.91	6.53

	FUD	Status	MUE	Modifiers				IOM Reference
49422	0	A	1(2)	51	N/A	N/A	N/A	None

* with documentation

Terms To Know

cannula. Tube inserted into a blood vessel, duct, or body cavity to facilitate
passage.

catheter. Flexible tube inserted into an area of the body for introducing or
withdrawing fluid.

complication. Condition arising after the beginning of observation and
treatment that modifies the course of the patient's illness or the medical care
required, or an undesired result or misadventure in medical care.

drain. Device that creates a channel to allow fluid from a cavity, wound, or
infected area to exit the body.

embolism. Obstruction of a blood vessel resulting from a clot or foreign
substance.

peritoneum. Strong, continuous membrane that forms the lining of the
abdominal and pelvic cavity. The parietal peritoneum, or outer layer, is attached
to the abdominopelvic walls and the visceral peritoneum, or inner layer,
surrounds the organs inside the abdominal cavity.

stenosis. Narrowing or constriction of a passage.

thrombosis. Condition arising from the presence or formation of blood clots
within a blood vessel that may cause vascular obstruction and insufficient
oxygenation.

49423

49423 Exchange of previously placed abscess or cyst drainage catheter under radiological guidance (separate procedure)

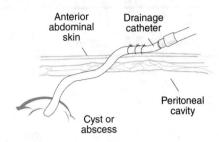

A previously placed drainage catheter is replaced under radiological guidance

Explanation

The physician exchanges a previously placed drainage catheter. The physician locates the drainage catheter and removes sutures that may be holding it in place. The drainage catheter is removed. With the use of fluoroscopy, the physician places a new drainage catheter and may elect to use a catheter guidewire to assist in this maneuver. Once placed and found to be patent, the new drainage catheter may be sutured in place. For radiological supervision and interpretation, see 75984.

Coding Tips

Code 49423 is a replacement procedure. It should not be reported at the time of the original percutaneous or open drainage. For initial insertion of a catheter, see 49419 and 49421. This separate procedure by definition is usually a component of a more complex service and is not identified separately. When performed alone or with other unrelated procedures/services it may be reported. If performed alone, list the code; if performed with other procedures/services, list the code and append modifier 59 or an X{EPSU} modifier.

ICD-10-CM Diagnostic Codes

K35.31	Acute appendicitis with localized peritonitis and gangrene, without perforation
K35.33	Acute appendicitis with perforation and localized peritonitis, with abscess
K50.014	Crohn's disease of small intestine with abscess
K50.114	Crohn's disease of large intestine with abscess
K50.814	Crohn's disease of both small and large intestine with abscess
K51.014	Ulcerative (chronic) pancolitis with abscess
K51.214	Ulcerative (chronic) proctitis with abscess
K51.314	Ulcerative (chronic) rectosigmoiditis with abscess
K51.414	Inflammatory polyps of colon with abscess
K51.514	Left sided colitis with abscess
K51.814	Other ulcerative colitis with abscess
K57.00	Diverticulitis of small intestine with perforation and abscess without bleeding
K57.01	Diverticulitis of small intestine with perforation and abscess with bleeding
K57.20	Diverticulitis of large intestine with perforation and abscess without bleeding
K57.21	Diverticulitis of large intestine with perforation and abscess with bleeding
K57.40	Diverticulitis of both small and large intestine with perforation and abscess without bleeding
K57.41	Diverticulitis of both small and large intestine with perforation and abscess with bleeding
K63.0	Abscess of intestine
K65.1	Peritoneal abscess
K68.11	Postprocedural retroperitoneal abscess
K68.12	Psoas muscle abscess
K68.19	Other retroperitoneal abscess
N15.1	Renal and perinephric abscess

AMA: **49423** 2018,Jan,8; 2017,Jan,8; 2016,Jan,13; 2015,Jan,16

Relative Value Units/Medicare Edits

Non-Facility RVU	Work	PE	MP	Total
49423	1.46	17.03	0.13	18.62
Facility RVU	**Work**	**PE**	**MP**	**Total**
49423	1.46	0.46	0.13	2.05

	FUD	Status	MUE	Modifiers				IOM Reference
49423	0	A	2(3)	51	N/A	N/A	80*	None

* with documentation

Terms To Know

catheter. Flexible tube inserted into an area of the body for introducing or withdrawing fluid.

cyst. Elevated encapsulated mass containing fluid, semisolid, or solid material with a membranous lining.

fluoroscopy. Radiology technique that allows visual examination of part of the body or a function of an organ using a device that projects an x-ray image on a fluorescent screen.

peritonitis. Inflammation and infection within the peritoneal cavity, the space between the membrane lining the abdominopelvic walls and covering the internal organs.

suppurative. Forming pus.

49425

49425 Insertion of peritoneal-venous shunt

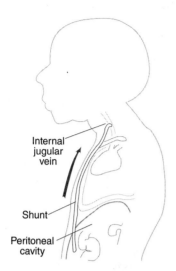

A shunt is prepared and inserted
from the peritoneal cavity to a major vein

Explanation

The physician places a peritoneal-venous shunt. The physician makes a small lateral upper abdominal incision. Dissection is carried through the abdominal wall layers, the peritoneum is entered, and the peritoneal end of the catheter is inserted into the peritoneal cavity and sutured into place. A subcutaneous tunnel is created from the abdominal incision up to the neck and the catheter is pulled through the tunnel into the neck. A counter incision is made in the neck over the internal jugular vein and the venous end of the catheter is inserted into the jugular vein. The incisions are closed.

Coding Tips

When 49425 is performed with another separately identifiable procedure, the highest dollar value code is listed as the primary procedure and subsequent procedures are appended with modifier 51. For a shunt patency test, see 78291. For percutaneous insertion of a tunneled catheter, see 49418.

ICD-10-CM Diagnostic Codes

K70.11	Alcoholic hepatitis with ascites ▲
K70.31	Alcoholic cirrhosis of liver with ascites ▲
K71.51	Toxic liver disease with chronic active hepatitis with ascites
R18.0	Malignant ascites
R18.8	Other ascites

AMA: 49425 2014,Jan,11

Relative Value Units/Medicare Edits

Non-Facility RVU	Work	PE	MP	Total
49425	12.22	6.52	1.99	20.73
Facility RVU	**Work**	**PE**	**MP**	**Total**
49425	12.22	6.52	1.99	20.73

	FUD	Status	MUE	Modifiers				IOM Reference
49425	90	A	1(2)	51	N/A	62*	80	None

* with documentation

49426

49426 Revision of peritoneal-venous shunt

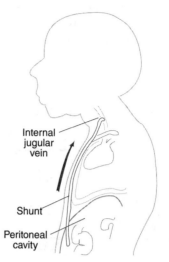

A revision of a peritoneal-venous shunt is performed

Explanation

The physician performs revision of a peritoneal-venous shunt. The physician may remove the shunt by incisions over the venous and peritoneal insertion sites with a subcutaneous tunnel is created from the abdominal incision up to the neck and the catheter is pulled through the tunnel into the neck. A counter incision is made in the neck over the internal jugular vein and the venous end of the catheter is inserted into the jugular vein. Alternately, the physician may make an incision over the dysfunctional end of the shunt and replace that portion of the shunt and insert it back into the peritoneal cavity or jugular vein. The incisions are closed.

Coding Tips

For a shunt patency test, see 78291. For insertion of a peritoneal-venous shunt, see 49425. For ligation of a peritoneal-venous shunt, see 49428. For removal of a peritoneal-venous shunt, see 49429.

ICD-10-CM Diagnostic Codes

T85.618A	Breakdown (mechanical) of other specified internal prosthetic devices, implants and grafts, initial encounter
T85.628A	Displacement of other specified internal prosthetic devices, implants and grafts, initial encounter
T85.638A	Leakage of other specified internal prosthetic devices, implants and grafts, initial encounter
T85.698A	Other mechanical complication of other specified internal prosthetic devices, implants and grafts, initial encounter
T85.79XA	Infection and inflammatory reaction due to other internal prosthetic devices, implants and grafts, initial encounter
T85.818A	Embolism due to other internal prosthetic devices, implants and grafts, initial encounter
T85.828A	Fibrosis due to other internal prosthetic devices, implants and grafts, initial encounter
T85.838A	Hemorrhage due to other internal prosthetic devices, implants and grafts, initial encounter
T85.848A	Pain due to other internal prosthetic devices, implants and grafts, initial encounter

T85.858A	Stenosis due to other internal prosthetic devices, implants and grafts, initial encounter
T85.868A	Thrombosis due to other internal prosthetic devices, implants and grafts, initial encounter
T85.898A	Other specified complication of other internal prosthetic devices, implants and grafts, initial encounter
Z45.89	Encounter for adjustment and management of other implanted devices

AMA: **49426** 2014,Jan,11

Relative Value Units/Medicare Edits

Non-Facility RVU	Work	PE	MP	Total
49426	10.41	6.89	2.54	19.84
Facility RVU	**Work**	**PE**	**MP**	**Total**
49426	10.41	6.89	2.54	19.84

	FUD	Status	MUE	Modifiers				IOM Reference
49426	90	A	1(3)	51	N/A	N/A	N/A	None

* with documentation

Terms To Know

ascites. Abnormal accumulation of free fluid in the abdominal cavity, causing distention and tightness in addition to shortness of breath as the fluid accumulates. Ascites is usually an underlying disorder and can be a manifestation of any number of diseases.

catheter. Flexible tube inserted into an area of the body for introducing or withdrawing fluid.

dysfunction. Abnormal or impaired function of an organ, part, or system.

jugular vein. Two pairs of veins on either side of the neck that open into the subclavian, sending blood from the head and neck to the heart.

patency. State of a tube-like structure or conduit being open and unobstructed.

peritoneal cavity. Space between the lining of the abdominal wall, or parietal peritoneum, and the surface layer of the abdominal organs, or visceral peritoneum. It contains a thin, watery fluid that keeps the peritoneal surfaces moist.

peritoneum. Strong, continuous membrane that forms the lining of the abdominal and pelvic cavity. The parietal peritoneum, or outer layer, is attached to the abdominopelvic walls and the visceral peritoneum, or inner layer, surrounds the organs inside the abdominal cavity.

revision. Reordering or rearrangement of tissue to suit a particular need or function.

shunt. Surgically created passage between blood vessels or other natural passages, such as an arteriovenous anastomosis, to divert or bypass blood flow from the normal channel.

49427

| 49427 | Injection procedure (eg, contrast media) for evaluation of previously placed peritoneal-venous shunt |

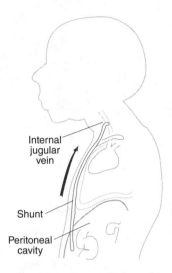

Internal jugular vein

Shunt

Peritoneal cavity

An injection procedure is performed

Explanation

The physician injects contrast into a peritoneo-venous shunt. The physician injects contrast material through the skin into the reservoir of the peritoneo-venous shunt. Radiography is used to visualize the flow of contrast through the shunt into the peritoneal and venous ends for evaluation.

Coding Tips

Radiological supervision and interpretation is reported with 75809 or 78291, when performed. For insertion of a peritoneal-venous shunt, see 49425; revision, see 49426; ligation, see 49428; removal, see 49429.

ICD-10-CM Diagnostic Codes

T85.618A	Breakdown (mechanical) of other specified internal prosthetic devices, implants and grafts, initial encounter
T85.628A	Displacement of other specified internal prosthetic devices, implants and grafts, initial encounter
T85.638A	Leakage of other specified internal prosthetic devices, implants and grafts, initial encounter
T85.698A	Other mechanical complication of other specified internal prosthetic devices, implants and grafts, initial encounter
T85.79XA	Infection and inflammatory reaction due to other internal prosthetic devices, implants and grafts, initial encounter
T85.818A	Embolism due to other internal prosthetic devices, implants and grafts, initial encounter
T85.828A	Fibrosis due to other internal prosthetic devices, implants and grafts, initial encounter
T85.838A	Hemorrhage due to other internal prosthetic devices, implants and grafts, initial encounter
T85.848A	Pain due to other internal prosthetic devices, implants and grafts, initial encounter
T85.858A	Stenosis due to other internal prosthetic devices, implants and grafts, initial encounter
T85.868A	Thrombosis due to other internal prosthetic devices, implants and grafts, initial encounter

T85.898A   Other specified complication of other internal prosthetic devices, implants and grafts, initial encounter

AMA: 49427 2014,Jan,11

Relative Value Units/Medicare Edits

Non-Facility RVU	Work	PE	MP	Total
49427	0.89	0.14	0.09	1.12
Facility RVU	**Work**	**PE**	**MP**	**Total**
49427	0.89	0.14	0.09	1.12

	FUD	Status	MUE	Modifiers				IOM Reference
49427	0	A	1(3)	51	N/A	N/A	80*	None

* with documentation

Terms To Know

contrast material. Any internally administered substance that has a different opacity from soft tissue on radiography or computed tomograph; includes barium, used to opacify parts of the gastrointestinal tract; water-soluble iodinated compounds, used to opacify blood vessels or the genitourinary tract; may refer to air occurring naturally or introduced into the body; also, paramagnetic substances used in magnetic resonance imaging. Substances may also be documented as contrast agent or contrast medium.

reservoir. Space or body cavity for storage of liquid.

shunt. Surgically created passage between blood vessels or other natural passages, such as an arteriovenous anastomosis, to divert or bypass blood flow from the normal channel.

49428

49428   Ligation of peritoneal-venous shunt

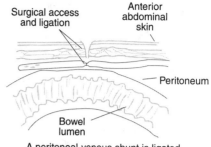

A peritoneal-venous shunt is ligated. Access is usually by incising the skin over the percutaneous tunnel

Explanation

The physician performs ligation of a previously placed peritoneo-venous shunt. The physician makes an incision over the path of the shunt. The shunt tubing under the incision is isolated and ligated with sutures. The incision is closed.

Coding Tips

For revision of a peritoneal-venous shunt, see 49426. For an injection procedure for evaluation of a previously placed peritoneal-venous shunt, see 49427. For removal of a peritoneal-venous shunt, see 49429.

ICD-10-CM Diagnostic Codes

T85.618A	Breakdown (mechanical) of other specified internal prosthetic devices, implants and grafts, initial encounter
T85.638A	Leakage of other specified internal prosthetic devices, implants and grafts, initial encounter
T85.698A	Other mechanical complication of other specified internal prosthetic devices, implants and grafts, initial encounter
T85.838A	Hemorrhage due to other internal prosthetic devices, implants and grafts, initial encounter
T85.898A	Other specified complication of other internal prosthetic devices, implants and grafts, initial encounter
Z45.89	Encounter for adjustment and management of other implanted devices

AMA: 49428 2014,Jan,11

Relative Value Units/Medicare Edits

Non-Facility RVU	Work	PE	MP	Total
49428	6.87	4.23	1.67	12.77
Facility RVU	**Work**	**PE**	**MP**	**Total**
49428	6.87	4.23	1.67	12.77

	FUD	Status	MUE	Modifiers				IOM Reference
49428	10	A	1(2)	51	N/A	N/A	N/A	None

* with documentation

49429

49429   Removal of peritoneal-venous shunt

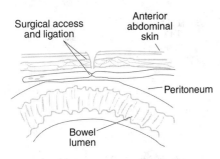

Surgical access and ligation

Anterior abdominal skin

Peritoneum

Bowel lumen

Access is usually by incising the skin over the percutaneous tunnel

Explanation

The physician performs removal of a peritoneal venous shunt. An incision is made over the abdominal insertion site of the shunt. The shunt is dissected from surrounding scar tissue and removed from the abdominal cavity. The fascia and peritoneum of the abdominal insertion site is closed. Usually the venous end of the catheter can be removed by placing traction on the shunt through the abdominal incision and pulling it through the subcutaneous tunnel. If necessary a second incision is made over the venous insertion site and the catheter removed from the jugular vein. The incisions are closed.

Coding Tips

For revision of a peritoneal-venous shunt, see 49426. For an injection procedure for evaluation of a previously placed peritoneal-venous shunt, see 49427. For ligation of a peritoneal-venous shunt, see 49428.

ICD-10-CM Diagnostic Codes

T85.618A	Breakdown (mechanical) of other specified internal prosthetic devices, implants and grafts, initial encounter
T85.628A	Displacement of other specified internal prosthetic devices, implants and grafts, initial encounter
T85.638A	Leakage of other specified internal prosthetic devices, implants and grafts, initial encounter
T85.698A	Other mechanical complication of other specified internal prosthetic devices, implants and grafts, initial encounter
T85.79XA	Infection and inflammatory reaction due to other internal prosthetic devices, implants and grafts, initial encounter
T85.818A	Embolism due to other internal prosthetic devices, implants and grafts, initial encounter
T85.828A	Fibrosis due to other internal prosthetic devices, implants and grafts, initial encounter
T85.838A	Hemorrhage due to other internal prosthetic devices, implants and grafts, initial encounter
T85.848A	Pain due to other internal prosthetic devices, implants and grafts, initial encounter
T85.858A	Stenosis due to other internal prosthetic devices, implants and grafts, initial encounter
T85.868A	Thrombosis due to other internal prosthetic devices, implants and grafts, initial encounter
T85.898A	Other specified complication of other internal prosthetic devices, implants and grafts, initial encounter

AMA: 49429 2014,Jan,11

Relative Value Units/Medicare Edits

Non-Facility RVU	Work	PE	MP	Total
49429	7.44	4.32	1.82	13.58
Facility RVU	**Work**	**PE**	**MP**	**Total**
49429	7.44	4.32	1.82	13.58

	FUD	Status	MUE	Modifiers				IOM Reference
49429	10	A	1(2)	51	N/A	N/A	N/A	None

* with documentation

Terms To Know

ascites. Abnormal accumulation of free fluid in the abdominal cavity, causing distention and tightness in addition to shortness of breath as the fluid accumulates. Ascites is usually an underlying disorder and can be a manifestation of any number of diseases.

complication. Condition arising after the beginning of observation and treatment that modifies the course of the patient's illness or the medical care required, or an undesired result or misadventure in medical care.

dissection. Separating by cutting tissue or body structures apart.

fascia. Fibrous sheet or band of tissue that envelops organs, muscles, and groupings of muscles.

infection. Presence of microorganisms in body tissues that may result in cellular damage.

peritoneal cavity. Space between the lining of the abdominal wall, or parietal peritoneum, and the surface layer of the abdominal organs, or visceral peritoneum. It contains a thin, watery fluid that keeps the peritoneal surfaces moist.

peritoneum. Strong, continuous membrane that forms the lining of the abdominal and pelvic cavity. The parietal peritoneum, or outer layer, is attached to the abdominopelvic walls and the visceral peritoneum, or inner layer, surrounds the organs inside the abdominal cavity.

shunt. Surgically created passage between blood vessels or other natural passages, such as an arteriovenous anastomosis, to divert or bypass blood flow from the normal channel.

49435

+ **49435** Insertion of subcutaneous extension to intraperitoneal cannula or catheter with remote chest exit site (List separately in addition to code for primary procedure)

The catheter is extended and exits the chest

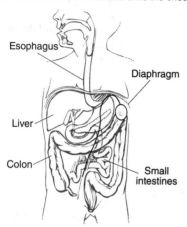

Explanation

A permanent, subcutaneous intraperitoneal catheter is lengthened with an extension and brought to the surface of the skin during the primary procedure in which a catheter/cannula is established. In the primary procedure, the physician makes a small abdominal incision, opens the peritoneum, and establishes the cannula. In 49435, the physician fits an extension to the cannula and tunnels subcutaneously to accommodate the extension. The physician makes a separate incision in the chest as an exit site for the extension. The extension is brought out through the skin and may be attached to the drug delivery system. The operative incision is closed.

Coding Tips

Report 49435 in addition to 49324 or 49421.

ICD-10-CM Diagnostic Codes

This/these CPT code(s) are add-on code(s). See the primary procedure code that this code is performed with for your ICD-10-CM code selections.

AMA: 49435 2014,Jan,11

Relative Value Units/Medicare Edits

Non-Facility RVU	Work	PE	MP	Total
49435	2.25	0.72	0.54	3.51
Facility RVU	Work	PE	MP	Total
49435	2.25	0.72	0.54	3.51

	FUD	Status	MUE	Modifiers				IOM Reference
49435	N/A	A	1(2)	N/A	N/A	62*	80	None

* with documentation

49436

49436 Delayed creation of exit site from embedded subcutaneous segment of intraperitoneal cannula or catheter

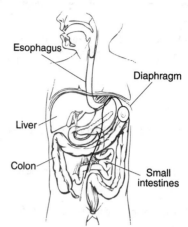

An exit site for the intraperitoneal catheter is created

Explanation

A previously implanted, permanent subcutaneous intraperitoneal catheter is brought to the surface of the skin. The physician makes a small abdominal incision, opens the peritoneum, and locates the end of the existing intraperitoneal cannula. An extension may be fitted to the existing cannula. The physician makes a separate incision as an exit site for the cannula. The cannula is brought out through the skin and may be attached to the drug delivery system. The operative incision is closed.

Coding Tips

For laparoscopic insertion of an intraperitoneal catheter, see 49324; revision with removal of intraluminal obstructive material if performed, see 49325; with omentopexy, see 49326.

ICD-10-CM Diagnostic Codes

T81.41XA	Infection following a procedure, superficial incisional surgical site, initial encounter
T81.42XA	Infection following a procedure, deep incisional surgical site, initial encounter
T82.818A	Embolism due to vascular prosthetic devices, implants and grafts, initial encounter
T82.828A	Fibrosis due to vascular prosthetic devices, implants and grafts, initial encounter
T82.838A	Hemorrhage due to vascular prosthetic devices, implants and grafts, initial encounter
T82.848A	Pain due to vascular prosthetic devices, implants and grafts, initial encounter
T82.858A	Stenosis of other vascular prosthetic devices, implants and grafts, initial encounter
T82.868A	Thrombosis due to vascular prosthetic devices, implants and grafts, initial encounter
T82.898A	Other specified complication of vascular prosthetic devices, implants and grafts, initial encounter

AMA: 49436 2014,Jan,11

Relative Value Units/Medicare Edits

Non-Facility RVU	Work	PE	MP	Total
49436	2.72	2.19	0.65	5.56
Facility RVU	Work	PE	MP	Total
49436	2.72	2.19	0.65	5.56

	FUD	Status	MUE	Modifiers				IOM Reference
49436	10	A	1(2)	51	N/A	62*	80	None

* with documentation

Terms To Know

cannula. Tube inserted into a blood vessel, duct, or body cavity to facilitate passage.

catheter. Flexible tube inserted into an area of the body for introducing or withdrawing fluid.

embolism. Obstruction of a blood vessel resulting from a clot or foreign substance.

fibrosis. Formation of fibrous tissue as part of the restorative process.

peritoneal cavity. Space between the lining of the abdominal wall, or parietal peritoneum, and the surface layer of the abdominal organs, or visceral peritoneum. It contains a thin, watery fluid that keeps the peritoneal surfaces moist.

subcutaneous. Below the skin.

thrombosis. Condition arising from the presence or formation of blood clots within a blood vessel that may cause vascular obstruction and insufficient oxygenation.

49440-49442

49440 Insertion of gastrostomy tube, percutaneous, under fluoroscopic guidance including contrast injection(s), image documentation and report

49441 Insertion of duodenostomy or jejunostomy tube, percutaneous, under fluoroscopic guidance including contrast injection(s), image documentation and report

49442 Insertion of cecostomy or other colonic tube, percutaneous, under fluoroscopic guidance including contrast injection(s), image documentation and report

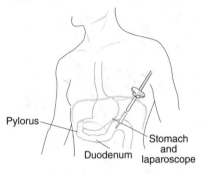

A gastrostomy, duodenostomy, jejunostomy, or cecostomy tube is inserted percutaneously

Explanation

The physician inserts a gastrostomy tube (49440), duodenostomy or jejunostomy tube (49441) or a cecostomy or other colonic tube (49442) via percutaneous (under the skin) approach using fluoroscopic guidance. Percutaneous image-guided gastrostomy or enterostomy procedures may be indicated for patients who have an impaired swallowing mechanism, mechanical obstruction of the upper GI tract due to malignancy, or those with aberrant upper GI anatomy. Particularly in patients who have undergone gastrectomy or gastric pull-up, the jejunum or duodenum is often a viable site for percutaneous feeding tube placement. Following administration of any necessary sedation and/or contrast materials, nasogastric or orogastric intubation is performed under fluoroscopic guidance and the stomach is insufflated. The skin and subcutaneous tissues overlying the stomach are anesthetized with lidocaine. In 49440, via a subcostal (below the ribs) approach and fluoroscopic guidance, the physician inserts a 7 cm, 18-gauge needle in the area of the horizontal portion of the greater curvature. A guidewire is passed through the needle and the needle is withdrawn. A dilator is introduced over the wire and the tract is dilated. The physician places a self-retaining loop catheter into the stomach and injects a small amount of contrast material in order to confirm placement. A loop-locking suture is tied and nasogastric or orogastric tubes are removed. Antiseptic ointment and sterile dressings are applied. In 49441, the physician identifies a suitable site for puncture of the duodenum or jejunum and a needle is inserted percutaneously. When the contrast material can be aspirated from the needle, a guidewire is inserted under fluoroscopic guidance. The tract is dilated and an appropriate catheter is inserted and secured to the skin with a stoma device. Nasogastric or orogastric tubes are removed. Antiseptic ointment and sterile dressings are applied. In 49442, the physician inserts a silicone catheter into the rectum and a retention balloon is filled with air after identification of the gallbladder, liver, and urinary bladder by ultrasound. The abdomen is prepared and draped in sterile fashion and appropriate anesthesia is administered. The colon is inflated with air via the rectal catheter and the physician assesses the position of the cecum to determine the appropriate tract site. The physician makes a small incision in the skin and inserts a puncture needle through the skin and soft tissues. Under fluoroscopic guidance, the needle is advanced into the cecum and contrast is injected to confirm the needle's position. Still using fluoroscopic guidance, a guidewire is advanced through the needle and positions the retention sutures. The physician removes the needle and clamps the sutures. A dilator is introduced over the wire, followed by an appropriately sized catheter. The catheter is locked and the physician confirms placement with contrast. The locked portion of the catheter is pulled against the cecum's anterior wall, where the retention sutures are anchored. Antiseptic ointment and sterile dressings are applied. These codes include image documentation and report.

Coding Tips

For conversion to a gastrojejunostomy tube at the time of initial gastrostomy tube placement, report 49440 in addition to 49446.

ICD-10-CM Diagnostic Codes

C15.3	Malignant neoplasm of upper third of esophagus
C15.4	Malignant neoplasm of middle third of esophagus
C15.5	Malignant neoplasm of lower third of esophagus
C16.0	Malignant neoplasm of cardia
C16.1	Malignant neoplasm of fundus of stomach
C16.2	Malignant neoplasm of body of stomach
C16.3	Malignant neoplasm of pyloric antrum
C16.4	Malignant neoplasm of pylorus
C18.0	Malignant neoplasm of cecum
C18.2	Malignant neoplasm of ascending colon
C18.3	Malignant neoplasm of hepatic flexure
C18.4	Malignant neoplasm of transverse colon
C18.5	Malignant neoplasm of splenic flexure
C18.6	Malignant neoplasm of descending colon
C18.7	Malignant neoplasm of sigmoid colon
C7A.092	Malignant carcinoid tumor of the stomach
D01.1	Carcinoma in situ of rectosigmoid junction
D12.7	Benign neoplasm of rectosigmoid junction
D37.8	Neoplasm of uncertain behavior of other specified digestive organs
E03.5	Myxedema coma
E08.11	Diabetes mellitus due to underlying condition with ketoacidosis with coma
E08.641	Diabetes mellitus due to underlying condition with hypoglycemia with coma
E09.11	Drug or chemical induced diabetes mellitus with ketoacidosis with coma
E09.641	Drug or chemical induced diabetes mellitus with hypoglycemia with coma
E10.11	Type 1 diabetes mellitus with ketoacidosis with coma
E10.641	Type 1 diabetes mellitus with hypoglycemia with coma
E10.65	Type 1 diabetes mellitus with hyperglycemia
E11.01	Type 2 diabetes mellitus with hyperosmolarity with coma
E11.641	Type 2 diabetes mellitus with hypoglycemia with coma
E41	Nutritional marasmus
G12.21	Amyotrophic lateral sclerosis ▲
G93.1	Anoxic brain damage, not elsewhere classified
K20.0	Eosinophilic esophagitis
K22.10	Ulcer of esophagus without bleeding
K22.11	Ulcer of esophagus with bleeding
K22.2	Esophageal obstruction
K22.3	Perforation of esophagus
K22.4	Dyskinesia of esophagus
K22.5	Diverticulum of esophagus, acquired
K22.6	Gastro-esophageal laceration-hemorrhage syndrome
K22.710	Barrett's esophagus with low grade dysplasia
K22.711	Barrett's esophagus with high grade dysplasia
K56.51	Intestinal adhesions [bands], with partial obstruction
K56.52	Intestinal adhesions [bands] with complete obstruction
K56.690	Other partial intestinal obstruction
K56.691	Other complete intestinal obstruction
K91.31	Postprocedural partial intestinal obstruction
K91.32	Postprocedural complete intestinal obstruction
Q39.0	Atresia of esophagus without fistula
Q39.1	Atresia of esophagus with tracheo-esophageal fistula
Q39.2	Congenital tracheo-esophageal fistula without atresia
Q39.3	Congenital stenosis and stricture of esophagus
Q39.4	Esophageal web
R13.0	Aphagia
R13.12	Dysphagia, oropharyngeal phase
R40.2111	Coma scale, eyes open, never, in the field [EMT or ambulance]
R40.2113	Coma scale, eyes open, never, at hospital admission
R40.2123	Coma scale, eyes open, to pain, at hospital admission
R40.2211	Coma scale, best verbal response, none, in the field [EMT or ambulance]
R40.2214	Coma scale, best verbal response, none, 24 hours or more after hospital admission
R40.2221	Coma scale, best verbal response, incomprehensible words, in the field [EMT or ambulance]
R40.2223	Coma scale, best verbal response, incomprehensible words, at hospital admission
R40.2224	Coma scale, best verbal response, incomprehensible words, 24 hours or more after hospital admission
R40.2311	Coma scale, best motor response, none, in the field [EMT or ambulance]
R40.2314	Coma scale, best motor response, none, 24 hours or more after hospital admission
R40.2322	Coma scale, best motor response, extension, at arrival to emergency department
R40.2323	Coma scale, best motor response, extension, at hospital admission
R40.2341	Coma scale, best motor response, flexion withdrawal, in the field [EMT or ambulance]
R40.2343	Coma scale, best motor response, flexion withdrawal, at hospital admission
R40.2344	Coma scale, best motor response, flexion withdrawal, 24 hours or more after hospital admission
R62.51	Failure to thrive (child) ▣
R62.7	Adult failure to thrive ▲
R63.0	Anorexia
R63.32	Pediatric feeding disorder, chronic ▣
R63.39	Other feeding difficulties

AMA: **49440** 2018,Jan,8; 2017,Jan,8; 2016,Jan,13; 2015,Jan,16 **49441** 2018,Jan,8; 2017,Jan,8; 2016,Jan,13; 2015,Jan,16 **49442** 2018,Jan,8; 2017,Jan,8; 2016,Jan,13; 2015,Jan,16

Relative Value Units/Medicare Edits

Non-Facility RVU	Work	PE	MP	Total
49440	3.93	22.9	0.37	27.2
49441	4.52	25.82	0.54	30.88
49442	3.75	21.85	0.3	25.9
Facility RVU	Work	PE	MP	Total
49440	3.93	1.59	0.37	5.89
49441	4.52	1.88	0.54	6.94
49442	3.75	1.92	0.3	5.97

	FUD	Status	MUE	Modifiers				IOM Reference
49440	10	A	1(3)	51	N/A	N/A	80*	None
49441	10	A	1(3)	51	N/A	N/A	80*	
49442	10	A	1(3)	51	N/A	N/A	80*	

* with documentation

Terms To Know

contrast material. Any internally administered substance that has a different opacity from soft tissue on radiography or computed tomograph; includes barium, used to opacify parts of the gastrointestinal tract; water-soluble iodinated compounds, used to opacify blood vessels or the genitourinary tract; may refer to air occurring naturally or introduced into the body; also, paramagnetic substances used in magnetic resonance imaging. Substances may also be documented as contrast agent or contrast medium.

fluoroscopy. Radiology technique that allows visual examination of part of the body or a function of an organ using a device that projects an x-ray image on a fluorescent screen.

percutaneous. Through the skin.

49446

49446 Conversion of gastrostomy tube to gastro-jejunostomy tube, percutaneous, under fluoroscopic guidance including contrast injection(s), image documentation and report

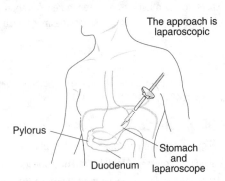

Gastrostomy tube is converted to gastrojejunostomy tube

Explanation

The physician converts a gastrostomy tube to a gastrojejunostomy tube via percutaneous (under the skin) approach using fluoroscopic guidance. Following administration of any necessary sedation and contrast materials, the physician advances a jejunostomy tube through the previously placed gastrostomy tube into the proximal jejunum. This code includes contrast injections, image documentation, and report.

Coding Tips

For conversion to a gastrojejunostomy tube at the time of initial gastrostomy tube placement, report this code with 49440.

ICD-10-CM Diagnostic Codes

C15.3	Malignant neoplasm of upper third of esophagus
C15.4	Malignant neoplasm of middle third of esophagus
C15.8	Malignant neoplasm of overlapping sites of esophagus
C16.0	Malignant neoplasm of cardia
C16.1	Malignant neoplasm of fundus of stomach
C16.2	Malignant neoplasm of body of stomach
C16.3	Malignant neoplasm of pyloric antrum
C16.4	Malignant neoplasm of pylorus
C7A.092	Malignant carcinoid tumor of the stomach
D37.8	Neoplasm of uncertain behavior of other specified digestive organs
E03.5	Myxedema coma
E08.11	Diabetes mellitus due to underlying condition with ketoacidosis with coma
E08.641	Diabetes mellitus due to underlying condition with hypoglycemia with coma
E09.11	Drug or chemical induced diabetes mellitus with ketoacidosis with coma
E09.641	Drug or chemical induced diabetes mellitus with hypoglycemia with coma
E10.11	Type 1 diabetes mellitus with ketoacidosis with coma
E10.641	Type 1 diabetes mellitus with hypoglycemia with coma
E11.01	Type 2 diabetes mellitus with hyperosmolarity with coma
E11.641	Type 2 diabetes mellitus with hypoglycemia with coma
E13.11	Other specified diabetes mellitus with ketoacidosis with coma

E13.641	Other specified diabetes mellitus with hypoglycemia with coma
G20	Parkinson's disease
G35	Multiple sclerosis
K20.0	Eosinophilic esophagitis
K22.11	Ulcer of esophagus with bleeding
K22.2	Esophageal obstruction
K22.3	Perforation of esophagus
K22.4	Dyskinesia of esophagus
K22.5	Diverticulum of esophagus, acquired
K22.6	Gastro-esophageal laceration-hemorrhage syndrome
K22.70	Barrett's esophagus without dysplasia
K22.710	Barrett's esophagus with low grade dysplasia
K22.711	Barrett's esophagus with high grade dysplasia
K94.22	Gastrostomy infection
K94.23	Gastrostomy malfunction
K94.29	Other complications of gastrostomy
Q39.0	Atresia of esophagus without fistula
Q39.1	Atresia of esophagus with tracheo-esophageal fistula
Q39.2	Congenital tracheo-esophageal fistula without atresia
Q39.3	Congenital stenosis and stricture of esophagus
Q39.4	Esophageal web
R40.2111	Coma scale, eyes open, never, in the field [EMT or ambulance]
R40.2113	Coma scale, eyes open, never, at hospital admission
R40.2114	Coma scale, eyes open, never, 24 hours or more after hospital admission
R40.2121	Coma scale, eyes open, to pain, in the field [EMT or ambulance]
R40.2122	Coma scale, eyes open, to pain, at arrival to emergency department
R40.2123	Coma scale, eyes open, to pain, at hospital admission
R40.2211	Coma scale, best verbal response, none, in the field [EMT or ambulance]
R40.2212	Coma scale, best verbal response, none, at arrival to emergency department
R40.2213	Coma scale, best verbal response, none, at hospital admission
R40.2214	Coma scale, best verbal response, none, 24 hours or more after hospital admission
R40.2221	Coma scale, best verbal response, incomprehensible words, in the field [EMT or ambulance]
R40.2222	Coma scale, best verbal response, incomprehensible words, at arrival to emergency department
R40.2311	Coma scale, best motor response, none, in the field [EMT or ambulance]
R40.2314	Coma scale, best motor response, none, 24 hours or more after hospital admission
R40.2321	Coma scale, best motor response, extension, in the field [EMT or ambulance]
R40.2322	Coma scale, best motor response, extension, at arrival to emergency department
R40.2344	Coma scale, best motor response, flexion withdrawal, 24 hours or more after hospital admission
R62.7	Adult failure to thrive ◮
R63.32	Pediatric feeding disorder, chronic ◪
R63.39	Other feeding difficulties

AMA: 49446 2018,Jan,8; 2017,Jan,8; 2016,Jan,13; 2015,Jan,16

Relative Value Units/Medicare Edits

Non-Facility RVU	Work	PE	MP	Total
49446	3.06	22.87	0.26	26.19
Facility RVU	**Work**	**PE**	**MP**	**Total**
49446	3.06	0.93	0.26	4.25

	FUD	Status	MUE	Modifiers				IOM Reference
49446	0	A	1(2)	51	N/A	N/A	80*	None

* with documentation

Terms To Know

fluoroscopy. Radiology technique that allows visual examination of part of the body or a function of an organ using a device that projects an x-ray image on a fluorescent screen.

gastrojejunostomy. Surgical creation of an opening from the stomach to the jejunum.

gastrostomy. Temporary or permanent artificial opening made in the stomach for gastrointestinal decompression or to provide nutrition when not maintained by other methods.

percutaneous. Through the skin.

49450-49452

49450 Replacement of gastrostomy or cecostomy (or other colonic) tube, percutaneous, under fluoroscopic guidance including contrast injection(s), image documentation and report

49451 Replacement of duodenostomy or jejunostomy tube, percutaneous, under fluoroscopic guidance including contrast injection(s), image documentation and report

49452 Replacement of gastro-jejunostomy tube, percutaneous, under fluoroscopic guidance including contrast injection(s), image documentation and report

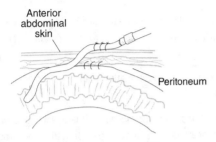

A gastrostomy, cecostomy, duodenostomy, jejunostomy, or gastrojejunostomy tube is replaced

Explanation

In 49450, the physician replaces an existing gastrostomy, cecostomy, or other colonic tube via percutaneous (under the skin) approach using fluoroscopic guidance and contrast monitoring. The existing tube is removed and the replacement is placed percutaneously via the existing tract. Contrast injection allows for correct positioning to be visualized with fluoroscopic images displayed on a screen. In 49451, the physician replaces an existing duodenostomy or jejunostomy tube via percutaneous (under the skin) approach using fluoroscopic guidance and contrast monitoring. The existing tube is removed and the replacement is placed percutaneously through the abdominal wall via the existing tract. Contrast injection allows for correct positioning to be visualized with fluoroscopic images displayed on a screen. In 49452, the physician replaces an existing gastrojejunostomy tube via percutaneous (under the skin) approach using fluoroscopic guidance and contrast monitoring. The existing tube is removed and the replacement is placed percutaneously through the abdominal wall via the existing tract. Contrast injection allows for correct positioning to be visualized with fluoroscopic images displayed on a screen. In order for these codes to be reported, the new tube must be placed via the existing percutaneous access site. These procedures include contrast injection, image documentation, and report.

Coding Tips

Replacement of a gastrostomy or cecostomy tube, see 49450; duodenostomy or jejunostomy tube, see 49451; gastrojejunostomy tube, see 49452.

ICD-10-CM Diagnostic Codes

K94.01	Colostomy hemorrhage
K94.02	Colostomy infection
K94.03	Colostomy malfunction
K94.09	Other complications of colostomy
K94.11	Enterostomy hemorrhage
K94.12	Enterostomy infection
K94.13	Enterostomy malfunction
K94.19	Other complications of enterostomy
K94.21	Gastrostomy hemorrhage
K94.22	Gastrostomy infection
K94.23	Gastrostomy malfunction
K94.29	Other complications of gastrostomy
L02.211	Cutaneous abscess of abdominal wall
L02.213	Cutaneous abscess of chest wall
L02.214	Cutaneous abscess of groin
L02.215	Cutaneous abscess of perineum
L02.216	Cutaneous abscess of umbilicus
L03.311	Cellulitis of abdominal wall
L03.313	Cellulitis of chest wall
L03.314	Cellulitis of groin
L03.315	Cellulitis of perineum
L03.316	Cellulitis of umbilicus
L03.321	Acute lymphangitis of abdominal wall
L03.323	Acute lymphangitis of chest wall
L03.324	Acute lymphangitis of groin
L03.325	Acute lymphangitis of perineum
L03.326	Acute lymphangitis of umbilicus
Z43.1	Encounter for attention to gastrostomy
Z43.2	Encounter for attention to ileostomy
Z43.3	Encounter for attention to colostomy
Z43.4	Encounter for attention to other artificial openings of digestive tract
Z46.59	Encounter for fitting and adjustment of other gastrointestinal appliance and device

AMA: **49450** 2019,Feb,5; 2018,Jan,8; 2017,Jan,8; 2016,Jan,13; 2015,Jan,16 **49451** 2018,Jan,8; 2017,Jan,8; 2016,Jan,13; 2015,Jan,16 **49452** 2018,Jan,8; 2017,Jan,8; 2016,Jan,13; 2015,Jan,16

Relative Value Units/Medicare Edits

Non-Facility RVU	Work	PE	MP	Total
49450	1.36	18.02	0.13	19.51
49451	1.84	18.99	0.17	21.0
49452	2.86	22.43	0.25	25.54
Facility RVU	Work	PE	MP	Total
49450	1.36	0.42	0.13	1.91
49451	1.84	0.56	0.17	2.57
49452	2.86	0.86	0.25	3.97

	FUD	Status	MUE	Modifiers				IOM Reference
49450	0	A	1(3)	51	N/A	N/A	80*	None
49451	0	A	1(3)	51	N/A	N/A	80*	
49452	0	A	1(3)	51	N/A	N/A	80*	

* with documentation

49460

49460 Mechanical removal of obstructive material from gastrostomy, duodenostomy, jejunostomy, gastro-jejunostomy, or cecostomy (or other colonic) tube, any method, under fluoroscopic guidance including contrast injection(s), if performed, image documentation and report

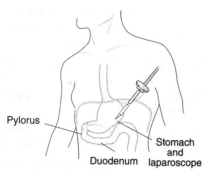

Pylorus

Stomach and laparoscope

Duodenum

Obstructions are mechanically removed

Explanation

The physician mechanically removes obstructive material from an existing tube (gastrostomy, duodenostomy, jejunostomy, gastrojejunostomy, or cecostomy) by any method. Fluoroscopic guidance and contrast imaging may be utilized. This procedure includes image documentation and report.

Coding Tips

Do not report 49460 with 49450–49452 and 49465.

ICD-10-CM Diagnostic Codes

K31.89	Other diseases of stomach and duodenum
K94.01	Colostomy hemorrhage
K94.09	Other complications of colostomy
K94.11	Enterostomy hemorrhage
K94.19	Other complications of enterostomy
K94.21	Gastrostomy hemorrhage
K94.22	Gastrostomy infection
K94.23	Gastrostomy malfunction
K94.29	Other complications of gastrostomy
L02.211	Cutaneous abscess of abdominal wall
L02.212	Cutaneous abscess of back [any part, except buttock]
L02.213	Cutaneous abscess of chest wall
L02.215	Cutaneous abscess of perineum
L02.216	Cutaneous abscess of umbilicus
L03.311	Cellulitis of abdominal wall
L03.313	Cellulitis of chest wall
L03.315	Cellulitis of perineum
L03.316	Cellulitis of umbilicus
L03.321	Acute lymphangitis of abdominal wall
L03.322	Acute lymphangitis of back [any part except buttock]
L03.323	Acute lymphangitis of chest wall
L03.324	Acute lymphangitis of groin
L03.325	Acute lymphangitis of perineum
L03.326	Acute lymphangitis of umbilicus
T85.510A	Breakdown (mechanical) of bile duct prosthesis, initial encounter
T85.511A	Breakdown (mechanical) of esophageal anti-reflux device, initial encounter
T85.518A	Breakdown (mechanical) of other gastrointestinal prosthetic devices, implants and grafts, initial encounter
T85.520A	Displacement of bile duct prosthesis, initial encounter
T85.521A	Displacement of esophageal anti-reflux device, initial encounter
T85.528A	Displacement of other gastrointestinal prosthetic devices, implants and grafts, initial encounter
T85.590A	Other mechanical complication of bile duct prosthesis, initial encounter
T85.591A	Other mechanical complication of esophageal anti-reflux device, initial encounter
T85.598A	Other mechanical complication of other gastrointestinal prosthetic devices, implants and grafts, initial encounter
T85.618A	Breakdown (mechanical) of other specified internal prosthetic devices, implants and grafts, initial encounter
T85.692A	Other mechanical complication of permanent sutures, initial encounter
T85.698A	Other mechanical complication of other specified internal prosthetic devices, implants and grafts, initial encounter
Z43.1	Encounter for attention to gastrostomy
Z43.2	Encounter for attention to ileostomy

AMA: **49460** 2018,Jan,8; 2017,Jan,8; 2016,Jan,13; 2015,Jan,16

Relative Value Units/Medicare Edits

Non-Facility RVU	Work	PE	MP	Total
49460	0.96	20.74	0.11	21.81
Facility RVU	**Work**	**PE**	**MP**	**Total**
49460	0.96	0.35	0.11	1.42

	FUD	Status	MUE	Modifiers				IOM Reference
49460	0	A	1(3)	51	N/A	N/A	80*	None

* with documentation

49465

49465 Contrast injection(s) for radiological evaluation of existing gastrostomy, duodenostomy, jejunostomy, gastro-jejunostomy, or cecostomy (or other colonic) tube, from a percutaneous approach including image documentation and report

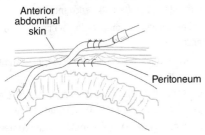

Contrast media is injected into
the tube for radiology evaluation

Explanation

The physician injects contrast via a percutaneous approach for the radiological evaluation of existing tubes (gastrostomy, duodenostomy, jejunostomy, gastrojejunostomy, or cecostomy). Image documentation and report are included in this procedure.

Coding Tips

Do not report 49465 with 49450–49460.

ICD-10-CM Diagnostic Codes

K31.89	Other diseases of stomach and duodenum
K94.01	Colostomy hemorrhage
K94.09	Other complications of colostomy
K94.11	Enterostomy hemorrhage
K94.19	Other complications of enterostomy
K94.21	Gastrostomy hemorrhage
K94.22	Gastrostomy infection
K94.23	Gastrostomy malfunction
K94.29	Other complications of gastrostomy
L02.211	Cutaneous abscess of abdominal wall
L02.212	Cutaneous abscess of back [any part, except buttock]
L02.213	Cutaneous abscess of chest wall
L02.214	Cutaneous abscess of groin
L02.215	Cutaneous abscess of perineum
L02.216	Cutaneous abscess of umbilicus
L03.311	Cellulitis of abdominal wall
L03.312	Cellulitis of back [any part except buttock]
L03.313	Cellulitis of chest wall
L03.314	Cellulitis of groin
L03.315	Cellulitis of perineum
L03.316	Cellulitis of umbilicus
L03.321	Acute lymphangitis of abdominal wall
L03.322	Acute lymphangitis of back [any part except buttock]
L03.323	Acute lymphangitis of chest wall
L03.324	Acute lymphangitis of groin
L03.325	Acute lymphangitis of perineum
L03.326	Acute lymphangitis of umbilicus

T85.318A	Breakdown (mechanical) of other ocular prosthetic devices, implants and grafts, initial encounter
T85.510A	Breakdown (mechanical) of bile duct prosthesis, initial encounter
T85.511A	Breakdown (mechanical) of esophageal anti-reflux device, initial encounter
T85.518A	Breakdown (mechanical) of other gastrointestinal prosthetic devices, implants and grafts, initial encounter
T85.520A	Displacement of bile duct prosthesis, initial encounter
T85.521A	Displacement of esophageal anti-reflux device, initial encounter
T85.528A	Displacement of other gastrointestinal prosthetic devices, implants and grafts, initial encounter
T85.590A	Other mechanical complication of bile duct prosthesis, initial encounter
T85.591A	Other mechanical complication of esophageal anti-reflux device, initial encounter
T85.598A	Other mechanical complication of other gastrointestinal prosthetic devices, implants and grafts, initial encounter
T85.618A	Breakdown (mechanical) of other specified internal prosthetic devices, implants and grafts, initial encounter
T85.692A	Other mechanical complication of permanent sutures, initial encounter
T85.698A	Other mechanical complication of other specified internal prosthetic devices, implants and grafts, initial encounter
Z43.1	Encounter for attention to gastrostomy
Z43.2	Encounter for attention to ileostomy

AMA: **49465** 2018,Jan,8; 2017,Jan,8; 2016,Jan,13; 2015,Jan,16

Relative Value Units/Medicare Edits

Non-Facility RVU	Work	PE	MP	Total
49465	0.62	3.69	0.05	4.36
Facility RVU	**Work**	**PE**	**MP**	**Total**
49465	0.62	0.22	0.05	0.89

	FUD	Status	MUE	Modifiers				IOM Reference
49465	0	A	1(3)	51	N/A	N/A	80*	None

* with documentation

49491-49492

49491 Repair, initial inguinal hernia, preterm infant (younger than 37 weeks gestation at birth), performed from birth up to 50 weeks postconception age, with or without hydrocelectomy; reducible

49492 incarcerated or strangulated

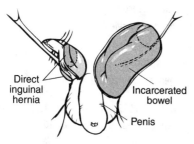

Direct inguinal hernia
Incarcerated bowel
Penis

An initial inguinal hernia is repaired on a preterm infant

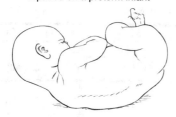

Explanation

The physician repairs an initial, reducible, inguinal hernia in a preterm infant (less than 37 weeks gestation at birth), performed up to 50 weeks postconceptual age, with or without hydrocelectomy. The physician dissects in the preperitoneal plane to present the hernia ring. The physician applies manual pressure to the inguinal region from outside while trying to dissect the hernia sac to reduce the hernia. If that fails, which can occur when there is a discrepancy in size of the hernia compared to its contents, the physician enlarges the hernia ring by an electrocautery incision in a ventral direction. The incision is made in a ventromedial direction for medial hernias and a ventrolateral direction for lateral hernias. The hernia is reduced using pleural insufflation of carbon dioxide. If a hydrocele is present, it is incised and drained. The hernia defect is repaired by suture and reinforced by staples or mesh. Report 49492 if, in the case of an incarcerated or strangulated hernia, the physician empties the contents of the hernia sac, places the contents in the lower abdomen, and repairs the hernia defect by suture.

Coding Tips

These are unilateral procedures. If performed bilaterally, report the procedure once with modifier 50 appended. Modifier 50 identifies a procedure performed identically on the opposite side of the body (mirror image). Do not append modifier 63 to 49491–49492 as the description or nature of the procedure includes infants up to 4 kg.

ICD-10-CM Diagnostic Codes

K40.00	Bilateral inguinal hernia, with obstruction, without gangrene, not specified as recurrent
K40.10	Bilateral inguinal hernia, with gangrene, not specified as recurrent
K40.20	Bilateral inguinal hernia, without obstruction or gangrene, not specified as recurrent
K40.30	Unilateral inguinal hernia, with obstruction, without gangrene, not specified as recurrent
K40.40	Unilateral inguinal hernia, with gangrene, not specified as recurrent
K40.90	Unilateral inguinal hernia, without obstruction or gangrene, not specified as recurrent
N43.0	Encysted hydrocele ♂
N43.1	Infected hydrocele ♂
N43.2	Other hydrocele ♂
P83.5	Congenital hydrocele ♂

AMA: 49491 2018,Jan,8; 2017,Jan,8; 2016,Jan,13; 2015,Jan,16 **49492** 2018,Jan,8; 2017,Jan,8; 2016,Jan,13; 2015,Jan,16

Relative Value Units/Medicare Edits

Non-Facility RVU	Work	PE	MP	Total
49491	12.53	8.05	3.07	23.65
49492	15.43	9.22	3.77	28.42
Facility RVU	**Work**	**PE**	**MP**	**Total**
49491	12.53	8.05	3.07	23.65
49492	15.43	9.22	3.77	28.42

	FUD	Status	MUE	Modifiers				IOM Reference
49491	90	A	1(2)	51	50	62*	80	None
49492	90	A	1(2)	51	50	62*	80	

* with documentation

Terms To Know

hydrocele. Serous fluid that collects in the tunica vaginalis, the spermatic cord, or the canal of Nuck. Hydroceles may be congenital, due to a defect in the tunica vaginalis, or secondary, due to fluid accumulation, injury, infection, or radiotherapy.

insufflation. Blowing air or gas into a body cavity.

reducible hernia. Protrusion of tissue through the wall of another structure that can be manually returned to the correct anatomical position.

ot49495 Repair, initial inguinal hernia, full term infant younger than age 6 months, or preterm infant older than 50 weeks postconception age and younger than age 6 months at the time of surgery, with or without hydrocelectomy; reducible

ot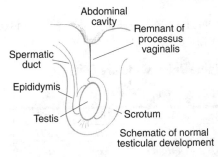

ot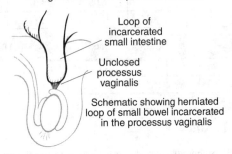

otSchematic showing herniated loop of small bowel incarcerated in the processus vaginalis

otThe physician repairs an initial, reducible, inguinal hernia in a full-term infant under age 6 months, or a preterm infant over 50 weeks postconceptual age and under 6 months at the time of surgery, with or without hydrocelectomy. The physician dissects in the preperitoneal plane to present the hernia ring. The physician applies manual pressure to the inguinal region from outside while trying to dissect the hernia sac to reduce the hernia. If that fails, which can occur when there is a discrepancy in size of the hernia compared to its contents, the physician enlarges the hernia ring by an electrocautery incision in a ventral direction. The incision is made in a ventromedial direction for medial hernias and a ventrolateral direction for lateral hernias. The hernia is reduced using pleural insufflation of carbon dioxide. If a hydrocele is present, it is incised and drained. The hernia defect is repaired by suture and reinforced by staples or mesh. Report 49496 if, in the case of an incarcerated or strangulated hernia, the physician empties the contents of the hernia sac, places the contents in the lower abdomen, and repairs the hernia defect by suture.

otThese are unilateral procedures. If performed bilaterally, report the procedure once with modifier 50 appended. Modifier 50 identifies a procedure performed identically on the opposite side of the body (mirror image). Do not append modifier 63 to 49495–49496 as the description or nature of the procedure includes infants up to 4 kg.

otK40.00 Bilateral inguinal hernia, with obstruction, without gangrene, not specified as recurrent
otK40.20 Bilateral inguinal hernia, without obstruction or gangrene, not specified as recurrent
otK40.30 Unilateral inguinal hernia, with obstruction, without gangrene, not specified as recurrent
otK40.90 Unilateral inguinal hernia, without obstruction or gangrene, not specified as recurrent

ot**AMA: 49495** 2018,Jan,8; 2017,Jan,8; 2016,Jan,13; 2015,Jan,16 **49496** 2018,Jan,8; 2017,Jan,8; 2016,Jan,13; 2015,Jan,16

ot| Non-Facility RVU | Work | PE | MP | Total |
ot| 49495 | 6.2 | 4.42 | 1.51 | 12.13 |
ot| 49496 | 9.42 | 6.51 | 2.29 | 18.22 |
ot| Facility RVU | Work | PE | MP | Total |
ot| 49495 | 6.2 | 4.42 | 1.51 | 12.13 |
ot| 49496 | 9.42 | 6.51 | 2.29 | 18.22 |

ot| | FUD | Status | MUE | Modifiers | | | | IOM Reference |
ot| 49495 | 90 | A | 1(2) | 51 | 50 | 62* | 80 | None |
ot| 49496 | 90 | A | 1(2) | 51 | 50 | 62* | 80 | |

ot**hydrocele.** Serous fluid that collects in the tunica vaginalis, the spermatic cord, or the canal of Nuck. Hydroceles may be congenital, due to a defect in the tunica vaginalis, or secondary, due to fluid accumulation, injury, infection, or radiotherapy.

ot**inguinal hernia.** Loop of intestine that protrudes through the abdominal peritoneum into the inguinal canal.

ot**strangulated.** Constricted and congested area, typically in an intestine, caused by herniation that results in compromised blood supply to that area.

49500-49501

49500 Repair initial inguinal hernia, age 6 months to younger than 5 years, with or without hydrocelectomy; reducible
49501   incarcerated or strangulated

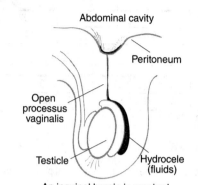

An inguinal hernia is repaired

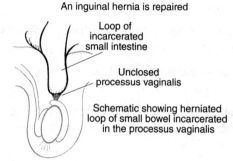

Schematic showing herniated loop of small bowel incarcerated in the processus vaginalis

Explanation

The physician repairs an inguinal hernia in a child between six months and 5 years of age. The physician makes a groin incision. The hernia sac is identified and dissected free of surrounding structures. In 49500, the hernia sac is ligated and resected. In 49501, the hernia sac is opened and the contents of the sac are examined. If the hernia contents are viable, the hernia is reduced and the sac ligated and resected. If a hydrocele is present, it is incised and drained. The groin incision is closed.

Coding Tips

These are unilateral procedures. If performed bilaterally, report the procedure once with modifier 50 appended. Modifier 50 identifies a procedure performed identically on the opposite side of the body (mirror image). For repair of an inguinal hernia, younger than 6 months, see 49495–49496; age 5 years and older, see 49505–49507.

ICD-10-CM Diagnostic Codes

K40.00	Bilateral inguinal hernia, with obstruction, without gangrene, not specified as recurrent
K40.10	Bilateral inguinal hernia, with gangrene, not specified as recurrent
K40.20	Bilateral inguinal hernia, without obstruction or gangrene, not specified as recurrent
K40.30	Unilateral inguinal hernia, with obstruction, without gangrene, not specified as recurrent
K40.40	Unilateral inguinal hernia, with gangrene, not specified as recurrent
K40.90	Unilateral inguinal hernia, without obstruction or gangrene, not specified as recurrent
N43.0	Encysted hydrocele ♂
N43.1	Infected hydrocele ♂
N43.2	Other hydrocele ♂
P83.5	Congenital hydrocele ♂

AMA: 49500 2018,Jan,8; 2017,Jan,8; 2016,Jan,13; 2015,Jan,16 **49501** 2018,Jan,8; 2017,Jan,8; 2016,Jan,13; 2015,Jan,16

Relative Value Units/Medicare Edits

Non-Facility RVU	Work	PE	MP	Total
49500	5.84	5.03	1.44	12.31
49501	9.36	6.33	2.29	17.98
Facility RVU	**Work**	**PE**	**MP**	**Total**
49500	5.84	5.03	1.44	12.31
49501	9.36	6.33	2.29	17.98

	FUD	Status	MUE	Modifiers				IOM Reference
49500	90	A	1(2)	51	50	62*	80	None
49501	90	A	1(2)	51	50	62*	80	

* with documentation

Terms To Know

congenital. Present at birth, occurring through heredity or an influence during gestation up to the moment of birth.

gangrene. Death of tissue, usually resulting from a loss of vascular supply, followed by a bacterial attack or onset of disease.

hydrocele. Serous fluid that collects in the tunica vaginalis, the spermatic cord, or the canal of Nuck. Hydroceles may be congenital, due to a defect in the tunica vaginalis, or secondary, due to fluid accumulation, injury, infection, or radiotherapy.

ligate. To tie off a blood vessel or duct with a suture or a soft, thin wire (ligature wire).

obstruction. Blockage that prevents normal function of the valve or structure.

resect. Cutting out or removing a portion or all of a bone, organ, or other structure.

49505-49507

49505 Repair initial inguinal hernia, age 5 years or older; reducible
49507 incarcerated or strangulated

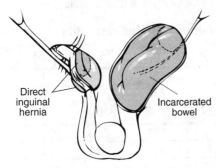

Direct
inguinal
hernia

Incarcerated
bowel

An inguinal hernia is repaired

Explanation

The physician repairs an inguinal hernia in a patient age 5 and older. The physician makes a groin incision. The hernia sac is identified and dissected free of surrounding structures. In 49505, the hernia sac is ligated and resected. In 49507, the physician repairs an incarcerated inguinal hernia. The hernia sac is opened and the contents of the sac are examined. If the hernia contents are viable, the hernia is reduced and the sac is ligated and resected. The groin incision is closed.

Coding Tips

These are unilateral procedures. If performed bilaterally, report the procedure once with modifier 50 appended. Modifier 50 identifies a procedure performed identically on the opposite side of the body (mirror image). Simple orchiectomy is reported separately, see 54520. Excision of hydrocele or spermatocele is reported separately, see 54840 or 55040. For repair of an inguinal hernia, 6 months and younger, see 49495–49496; age 6 months to younger than 5 years, see 49500–49501.

ICD-10-CM Diagnostic Codes

K40.00	Bilateral inguinal hernia, with obstruction, without gangrene, not specified as recurrent
K40.10	Bilateral inguinal hernia, with gangrene, not specified as recurrent
K40.20	Bilateral inguinal hernia, without obstruction or gangrene, not specified as recurrent
K40.30	Unilateral inguinal hernia, with obstruction, without gangrene, not specified as recurrent
K40.40	Unilateral inguinal hernia, with gangrene, not specified as recurrent
K40.90	Unilateral inguinal hernia, without obstruction or gangrene, not specified as recurrent

AMA: 49505 2018,Jan,8; 2017,Jan,8; 2016,Jan,13; 2015,Jan,16 **49507** 2018,Jan,8; 2017,Jan,8; 2016,Jan,13; 2015,Jan,16

Relative Value Units/Medicare Edits

Non-Facility RVU	Work	PE	MP	Total
49505	7.96	5.6	1.92	15.48
49507	9.09	6.12	2.16	17.37
Facility RVU	**Work**	**PE**	**MP**	**Total**
49505	7.96	5.6	1.92	15.48
49507	9.09	6.12	2.16	17.37

	FUD	Status	MUE	Modifiers				IOM Reference
49505	90	A	1(2)	51	50	62*	80	None
49507	90	A	1(2)	51	50	62*	80	

* with documentation

Terms To Know

dissect. Cut apart or separate tissue for surgical purposes or for visual or microscopic study.

gangrene. Death of tissue, usually resulting from a loss of vascular supply, followed by a bacterial attack or onset of disease.

inguinal hernia. Loop of intestine that protrudes through the abdominal peritoneum into the inguinal canal.

orchiectomy. Surgical removal of one or both testicles via a scrotal or groin incision, indicated in cases of cancer, traumatic injury, and sex reassignment surgery.

reducible hernia. Protrusion of tissue through the wall of another structure that can be manually returned to the correct anatomical position.

spermatocele. Noncancerous accumulation of fluid and dead sperm cells normally located at the head of the epididymis that exhibits itself as a hard, smooth scrotal mass and does not normally require treatment unless it becomes enlarged or causes pain.

strangulated. Constricted and congested area, typically in an intestine, caused by herniation that results in compromised blood supply to that area.

49520-49521

49520   Repair recurrent inguinal hernia, any age; reducible
49521   incarcerated or strangulated

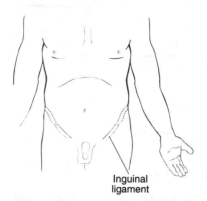

An inguinal hernia is repaired in a patient

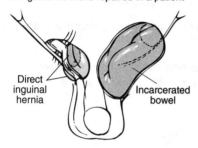

Explanation

The physician repairs a recurrent inguinal hernia. The physician makes a groin incision. Dissection is continued through scar tissue and the spermatic cord and the hernia sac are identified and dissected from surrounding structures. In 49520, the hernia sac may be ligated and resected. In 49521, the physician repairs an incarcerated recurrent inguinal hernia. The hernia sac is opened and the contents of the sac are examined. If the hernia contents are viable, the hernia is reduced and the sac ligated and resected. The incision is closed.

Coding Tips

Hernia repairs are defined by age (younger than 6 months, 6 months to 5 years, age 5 years and older), type (inguinal, femoral, incisional, ventral, epigastric, umbilical, spigelian), whether or not the hernia has been previously repaired (initial, recurrent), and clinical presentation (reducible, incarcerated, strangulated, sliding). These are unilateral procedures. If performed bilaterally, report the procedure once with modifier 50 appended. Modifier 50 identifies a procedure performed identically on the opposite side of the body (mirror image). For repair of an initial inguinal hernia, see 49491–49507.

ICD-10-CM Diagnostic Codes

K40.01	Bilateral inguinal hernia, with obstruction, without gangrene, recurrent
K40.11	Bilateral inguinal hernia, with gangrene, recurrent
K40.21	Bilateral inguinal hernia, without obstruction or gangrene, recurrent
K40.31	Unilateral inguinal hernia, with obstruction, without gangrene, recurrent
K40.41	Unilateral inguinal hernia, with gangrene, recurrent
K40.91	Unilateral inguinal hernia, without obstruction or gangrene, recurrent

AMA: **49520** 2018,Jan,8; 2017,Jan,8; 2016,Jan,13; 2015,Jan,16 **49521** 2018,Jan,8; 2017,Jan,8; 2016,Jan,13; 2015,Jan,16

Relative Value Units/Medicare Edits

Non-Facility RVU	Work	PE	MP	Total
49520	9.99	6.35	2.4	18.74
49521	11.48	7.0	2.74	21.22
Facility RVU	Work	PE	MP	Total
49520	9.99	6.35	2.4	18.74
49521	11.48	7.0	2.74	21.22

	FUD	Status	MUE	Modifiers				IOM Reference
49520	90	A	1(2)	51	50	62*	80	None
49521	90	A	1(2)	51	50	62*	80	

* with documentation

Terms To Know

absorbable sutures. Strands used for suture or repair of tissue prepared from collagen or a synthetic polymer and capable of being absorbed by tissue over time.

ligate. To tie off a blood vessel or duct with a suture or a soft, thin wire (ligature wire).

nonabsorbable sutures. Strands of natural or synthetic material that resist absorption into living tissue and are removed once healing is under way. Nonabsorbable sutures are commonly used to close skin wounds and repair tendons or collagenous tissue. Examples include surgical silk, surgical cotton, linen, stainless steel, surgical nylon, polyester fiber, polybutester (Novofil), polyethylene (Dermalene), and polypropylene (Prolene, Surilene).

reducible hernia. Protrusion of tissue through the wall of another structure that can be manually returned to the correct anatomical position.

resect. Cutting out or removing a portion or all of a bone, organ, or other structure.

spermatic cord. Structure of the male reproductive organs that consists of the ductus deferens, testicular artery, nerves, and veins that drain the testes.

49525

49525   Repair inguinal hernia, sliding, any age

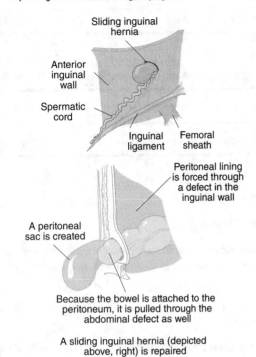

Sliding inguinal hernia

Anterior inguinal wall

Spermatic cord

Inguinal ligament

Femoral sheath

Peritoneal lining is forced through a defect in the inguinal wall

A peritoneal sac is created

Because the bowel is attached to the peritoneum, it is pulled through the abdominal defect as well

A sliding inguinal hernia (depicted above, right) is repaired

Relative Value Units/Medicare Edits

Non-Facility RVU	Work	PE	MP	Total
49525	8.93	5.94	2.12	16.99
Facility RVU	Work	PE	MP	Total
49525	8.93	5.94	2.12	16.99

	FUD	Status	MUE	Modifiers				IOM Reference
49525	90	A	1(2)	51	50	62*	80	None

* with documentation

Terms To Know

dissection. Separating by cutting tissue or body structures apart.

gangrene. Death of tissue, usually resulting from a loss of vascular supply, followed by a bacterial attack or onset of disease.

inguinal hernia. Loop of intestine that protrudes through the abdominal peritoneum into the inguinal canal.

resect. Cutting out or removing a portion or all of a bone, organ, or other structure.

viscera. Large interior organs enclosed within a cavity, generally referring to the abdominal organs.

Explanation

The physician repairs a sliding inguinal hernia. The physician makes a groin incision. The hernia sac is identified and dissected from surrounding structures. The hernia sac is opened and the abdominal viscera attached to the sac are dissected away from the sac if possible. The hernia contents are reduced and the hernia sac is closed and a portion of the sac may be resected. The incision is closed.

Coding Tips

Hernia repairs are defined by age (younger than 6 months, 6 months to 5 years, age 5 years and older), type (inguinal, femoral, incisional, ventral, epigastric, umbilical, spigelian), whether or not the hernia has been previously repaired (initial, recurrent), and clinical presentation (reducible, incarcerated, strangulated, sliding). This is a unilateral procedure. If performed bilaterally, report the procedure once with modifier 50 appended. Modifier 50 identifies a procedure performed identically on the opposite side of the body (mirror image). For incarcerated or strangulated inguinal hernia repair, see 49492, 49496, 49501, 49507, and 49521.

ICD-10-CM Diagnostic Codes

K40.20	Bilateral inguinal hernia, without obstruction or gangrene, not specified as recurrent
K40.21	Bilateral inguinal hernia, without obstruction or gangrene, recurrent
K40.90	Unilateral inguinal hernia, without obstruction or gangrene, not specified as recurrent
K40.91	Unilateral inguinal hernia, without obstruction or gangrene, recurrent

AMA: 49525 2018,Jan,8; 2017,Jan,8; 2016,Jan,13; 2015,Jan,16

49540

49540   Repair lumbar hernia

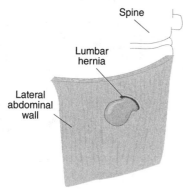

A hernia of the lateral abdominal wall, the so-called
lumbar hernia, is surgically accessed and repaired

Explanation

The physician repairs a lumbar hernia. The physician makes an incision
posteriorly over the hernia. The hernia sac is identified and dissected from
surrounding structures to expose the fascial defect. The hernia is reduced and
the hernia sac may be resected. The fascial defect is closed with sutures. The
incision is closed.

Coding Tips

Hernia repairs are defined by age (younger than 6 months, 6 months to 5
years, age 5 years and older), type (inguinal, femoral, incisional, ventral,
epigastric, umbilical, spigelian), whether or not the hernia has been previously
repaired (initial, recurrent), and clinical presentation (reducible, incarcerated,
strangulated, sliding). This is a unilateral procedure. If performed bilaterally,
report the procedure once with modifier 50 appended. Modifier 50 identifies
a procedure performed identically on the opposite side of the body (mirror
image).

ICD-10-CM Diagnostic Codes

K45.0	Other specified abdominal hernia with obstruction, without gangrene
K45.1	Other specified abdominal hernia with gangrene
K45.8	Other specified abdominal hernia without obstruction or gangrene

AMA: **49540** 2018,Jan,8; 2017,Jan,8; 2016,Jan,13; 2015,Jan,16

Relative Value Units/Medicare Edits

Non-Facility RVU	Work	PE	MP	Total
49540	10.74	6.86	2.57	20.17
Facility RVU	**Work**	**PE**	**MP**	**Total**
49540	10.74	6.86	2.57	20.17

	FUD	Status	MUE	Modifiers				IOM Reference
49540	90	A	1(2)	51	50	62*	80	None

* with documentation

49550-49553

49550   Repair initial femoral hernia, any age; reducible
49553   incarcerated or strangulated

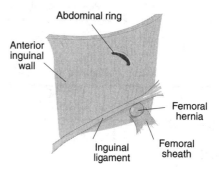

An initial femoral hernia is repaired

Explanation

The physician repairs a femoral hernia (49550) or an incarcerated femoral
hernia (49553). The physician makes a femoral or groin incision. The hernia
sac is identified and dissected from surrounding structures. The femoral defect
is closed with a prosthetic patch or sutures by plicating the fascia and muscles
to cover the defect. In 49553, the hernia sac is opened and the contents of the
sac are examined. If the contents of the hernia are viable, the hernia is reduced
and the hernia sac is closed and may be resected. The femoral defect is closed
with sutures by plicating the fascia and muscles to cover the defect. The
incisions are closed.

Coding Tips

Hernia repairs are defined by age (younger than 6 months, 6 months to 5
years, age 5 years and older), type (inguinal, femoral, incisional, ventral,
epigastric, umbilical, spigelian), whether or not the hernia has been previously
repaired (initial, recurrent), and clinical presentation (reducible, incarcerated,
strangulated, sliding). These are unilateral procedures. If performed bilaterally,
report the procedure once with modifier 50 appended. Modifier 50 identifies
a procedure performed identically on the opposite side of the body (mirror
image). For repair of a recurrent femoral hernia, see 49555 and 49557.

ICD-10-CM Diagnostic Codes

K41.10	Bilateral femoral hernia, with gangrene, not specified as recurrent
K41.20	Bilateral femoral hernia, without obstruction or gangrene, not specified as recurrent
K41.30	Unilateral femoral hernia, with obstruction, without gangrene, not specified as recurrent
K41.40	Unilateral femoral hernia, with gangrene, not specified as recurrent
K41.90	Unilateral femoral hernia, without obstruction or gangrene, not specified as recurrent

AMA: **49550** 2018,Jan,8; 2017,Jan,8; 2016,Jan,13; 2015,Jan,16 **49553**
2018,Jan,8; 2017,Jan,8; 2016,Jan,13; 2015,Jan,16

Relative Value Units/Medicare Edits

Non-Facility RVU	Work	PE	MP	Total
49550	8.99	5.95	2.15	17.09
49553	9.92	6.44	2.36	18.72
Facility RVU	Work	PE	MP	Total
49550	8.99	5.95	2.15	17.09
49553	9.92	6.44	2.36	18.72

	FUD	Status	MUE	Modifiers				IOM Reference
49550	90	A	1(2)	51	50	62*	80	None
49553	90	A	1(2)	51	50	62*	80	

* with documentation

Terms To Know

defect. Imperfection, flaw, or absence.

dissection. Separating by cutting tissue or body structures apart.

fascia. Fibrous sheet or band of tissue that envelops organs, muscles, and groupings of muscles.

gangrene. Death of tissue, usually resulting from a loss of vascular supply, followed by a bacterial attack or onset of disease.

hernia. Protrusion of a body structure through tissue.

incision. Act of cutting into tissue or an organ.

mesh. Synthetic fabric used as a prosthetic patch in hernia repair.

obstruction. Blockage that prevents normal function of the valve or structure.

plication. Surgical technique involving folding, tucking, or pleating to reduce the size of a hollow structure or organ.

reducible hernia. Protrusion of tissue through the wall of another structure that can be manually returned to the correct anatomical position.

resect. Cutting out or removing a portion or all of a bone, organ, or other structure.

strangulated. Constricted and congested area, typically in an intestine, caused by herniation that results in compromised blood supply to that area.

49555-49557

49555 Repair recurrent femoral hernia; reducible
49557   incarcerated or strangulated

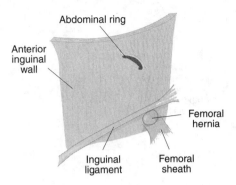

The femoral hernia that has been surgically treated in the past recurs

Explanation

The physician repairs a recurrent femoral hernia (49555) or an incarcerated recurrent femoral hernia (49557). The physician makes a groin or femoral incision. Dissection is continued through scar tissue and the hernia sac is identified and dissected from surrounding structures. The hernia sac is reduced and may be resected. The femoral defect is closed with sutures by plicating the fascia and muscles to cover the defect. In 49557, the hernia sac is opened and the contents of the sac are examined. If the hernia contents are viable, the hernia is reduced and the hernia sac is closed and may be resected. The femoral defect is closed with sutures by plicating fascia and muscle to cover the defect. The incisions are closed.

Coding Tips

Hernia repairs are defined by age (younger than 6 months, 6 months to 5 years, age 5 years and older), type (inguinal, femoral, incisional, ventral, epigastric, umbilical, spigelian), whether or not the hernia has been previously repaired (initial, recurrent), and clinical presentation (reducible, incarcerated, strangulated, sliding). These are unilateral procedures. If performed bilaterally, report the procedure once with modifier 50 appended. Modifier 50 identifies a procedure performed identically on the opposite side of the body (mirror image). For repair of an initial femoral hernia, see 49550 and 49553.

ICD-10-CM Diagnostic Codes

K41.01	Bilateral femoral hernia, with obstruction, without gangrene, recurrent
K41.11	Bilateral femoral hernia, with gangrene, recurrent
K41.21	Bilateral femoral hernia, without obstruction or gangrene, recurrent
K41.31	Unilateral femoral hernia, with obstruction, without gangrene, recurrent
K41.41	Unilateral femoral hernia, with gangrene, recurrent
K41.91	Unilateral femoral hernia, without obstruction or gangrene, recurrent

AMA: **49555** 2018,Jan,8; 2017,Jan,8; 2016,Jan,13; 2015,Jan,16 **49557** 2018,Jan,8; 2017,Jan,8; 2016,Jan,13; 2015,Jan,16

Relative Value Units/Medicare Edits

Non-Facility RVU	Work	PE	MP	Total
49555	9.39	6.21	2.27	17.87
49557	11.62	7.03	2.74	21.39
Facility RVU	Work	PE	MP	Total
49555	9.39	6.21	2.27	17.87
49557	11.62	7.03	2.74	21.39

	FUD	Status	MUE	Modifiers				IOM Reference
49555	90	A	1(2)	51	50	62*	80	None
49557	90	A	1(2)	51	50	62*	80	

* with documentation

Terms To Know

closure. Repairing an incision or wound by suture or other means.

defect. Imperfection, flaw, or absence.

dissection. Separating by cutting tissue or body structures apart.

fascia. Fibrous sheet or band of tissue that envelops organs, muscles, and groupings of muscles.

gangrene. Death of tissue, usually resulting from a loss of vascular supply, followed by a bacterial attack or onset of disease.

hernia. Protrusion of a body structure through tissue.

incision. Act of cutting into tissue or an organ.

obstruction. Blockage that prevents normal function of the valve or structure.

plication. Surgical technique involving folding, tucking, or pleating to reduce the size of a hollow structure or organ.

reducible hernia. Protrusion of tissue through the wall of another structure that can be manually returned to the correct anatomical position.

scar tissue. Fibrous connective tissue that forms around a wounded area or injury, composed mainly of fibroblasts or collagenous fibers.

strangulated. Constricted and congested area, typically in an intestine, caused by herniation that results in compromised blood supply to that area.

49560-49561

49560   Repair initial incisional or ventral hernia; reducible
49561   incarcerated or strangulated

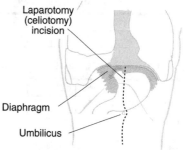

Laparotomy (celiotomy) incision

Diaphragm

Umbilicus

A ventral hernia is one that occurs on the abdominal wall other than the groin region

Explanation

The physician repairs an incisional or ventral (49560) or incarcerated incisional (49561) hernia. The physician makes an incision over the hernia. Dissection is continued through scar tissue and the hernia sac is identified and dissected from surrounding structures. The fascial defect is identified circumferentially. The hernia is reduced and the hernia sac may be resected. The hernia defect is closed with sutures. In 49561, the hernia sac is opened and the contents of the sac are examined. If the contents of the hernia sac are viable, the hernia is reduced and the hernia sac is closed and may be resected. The hernia defect is closed with sutures. The incisions are closed.

Coding Tips

Hernia repairs are defined by age (younger than 6 months, 6 months to 5 years, age 5 years and older), type (inguinal, femoral, incisional, ventral, epigastric, umbilical, spigelian), whether the hernia has been previously repaired (initial, recurrent), and clinical presentation (reducible, incarcerated, strangulated, sliding). These are unilateral procedures. If performed bilaterally, report the procedure once with modifier 50 appended. Modifier 50 identifies a procedure performed identically on the opposite side of the body (mirror image). The use of mesh or other prosthesis is reported separately, see 49568. For repair of a recurrent incisional or ventral hernia, see 49565 and 49566.

ICD-10-CM Diagnostic Codes

K43.0	Incisional hernia with obstruction, without gangrene
K43.1	Incisional hernia with gangrene
K43.2	Incisional hernia without obstruction or gangrene
K43.6	Other and unspecified ventral hernia with obstruction, without gangrene
K43.7	Other and unspecified ventral hernia with gangrene
K43.9	Ventral hernia without obstruction or gangrene

AMA: 49560 2019,Nov,14; 2018,Jan,8; 2017,Jan,8; 2016,Jan,13; 2015,Jan,16 **49561** 2019,Nov,14; 2018,Mar,11; 2018,Jul,14; 2018,Jan,8; 2017,Jan,8; 2016,Jan,13; 2015,Jan,16

Relative Value Units/Medicare Edits

Non-Facility RVU	Work	PE	MP	Total
49560	11.92	7.11	2.79	21.82
49561	15.38	8.45	3.64	27.47
Facility RVU	Work	PE	MP	Total
49560	11.92	7.11	2.79	21.82
49561	15.38	8.45	3.64	27.47

	FUD	Status	MUE	Modifiers				IOM Reference
49560	90	A	2(3)	51	50	62*	80	None
49561	90	A	1(3)	51	50	62*	80	

* with documentation

Terms To Know

dissection. Separating by cutting tissue or body structures apart.

gangrene. Death of tissue, usually resulting from a loss of vascular supply, followed by a bacterial attack or onset of disease.

hernia. Protrusion of a body structure through tissue.

incision. Act of cutting into tissue or an organ.

mesh. Synthetic fabric used as a prosthetic patch in hernia repair.

reducible hernia. Protrusion of tissue through the wall of another structure that can be manually returned to the correct anatomical position.

reduction. Correction of a fracture, dislocation, or hernia to the correct place and alignment, manually or by surgery.

resection. Surgical removal of a part or all of an organ or body part.

strangulated. Constricted and congested area, typically in an intestine, caused by herniation that results in compromised blood supply to that area.

49565-49566

49565 Repair recurrent incisional or ventral hernia; reducible
49566   incarcerated or strangulated

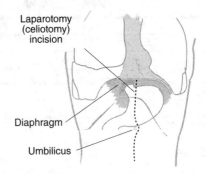

A ventral hernia is one that occurs on the abdominal wall other than the groin region

Explanation

The physician repairs a recurrent incisional or ventral (49565) or incarcerated recurrent incisional (49566) hernia. The physician makes an incision over the hernia. Dissection is continued through scar tissue and the hernia sac is identified and dissected from surrounding structures. The fascial defect is identified circumferentially. The hernia is reduced and the sac may be resected. The hernia defect is closed with sutures. In 49566, the hernia sac is opened and the contents of the sac are examined. If the contents of the hernia sac are viable, the hernia is reduced and the hernia sac is closed and may be resected. The hernia defect is closed with sutures. The incisions are closed.

Coding Tips

Hernia repairs are defined by age (younger than 6 months, 6 months to 5 years, age 5 years and older), type (inguinal, femoral, incisional, ventral, epigastric, umbilical, spigelian), whether the hernia has been previously repaired (initial, recurrent), and clinical presentation (reducible, incarcerated, strangulated, sliding). These are unilateral procedures. If performed bilaterally, report the procedure once with modifier 50 appended. Modifier 50 identifies a procedure performed identically on the opposite side of the body (mirror image). The use of mesh or other prosthesis is reported separately, see 49568. For repair of an initial incisional or ventral hernia, see 49560 and 49561.

ICD-10-CM Diagnostic Codes

K43.0	Incisional hernia with obstruction, without gangrene
K43.1	Incisional hernia with gangrene
K43.2	Incisional hernia without obstruction or gangrene

AMA: 49565 2019,Nov,14; 2018,Jan,8; 2017,Jan,8; 2016,Jan,13; 2015,Jan,16
49566 2019,Nov,14; 2018,Jan,8; 2017,Jan,8; 2016,Jan,13; 2015,Jan,16

Relative Value Units/Medicare Edits

Non-Facility RVU	Work	PE	MP	Total
49565	12.37	7.46	2.9	22.73
49566	15.53	8.51	3.68	27.72
Facility RVU	Work	PE	MP	Total
49565	12.37	7.46	2.9	22.73
49566	15.53	8.51	3.68	27.72

	FUD	Status	MUE	Modifiers				IOM Reference
49565	90	A	2(3)	51	50	62*	80	None
49566	90	A	2(3)	51	50	62*	80	

* with documentation

Terms To Know

dissection. Separating by cutting tissue or body structures apart.

gangrene. Death of tissue, usually resulting from a loss of vascular supply, followed by a bacterial attack or onset of disease.

hernia. Protrusion of a body structure through tissue.

incision. Act of cutting into tissue or an organ.

mesh. Synthetic fabric used as a prosthetic patch in hernia repair.

reducible hernia. Protrusion of tissue through the wall of another structure that can be manually returned to the correct anatomical position.

reduction. Correction of a fracture, dislocation, or hernia to the correct place and alignment, manually or by surgery.

resection. Surgical removal of a part or all of an organ or body part.

strangulated. Constricted and congested area, typically in an intestine, caused by herniation that results in compromised blood supply to that area.

49568

+ 49568 Implantation of mesh or other prosthesis for open incisional or ventral hernia repair or mesh for closure of debridement for necrotizing soft tissue infection (List separately in addition to code for the incisional or ventral hernia repair)

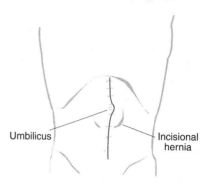

Umbilicus   Incisional hernia

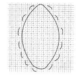

In some instances, a piece of synthetic mesh is placed under the fascial layer to provide support to the area

Synthetic mesh

Explanation

The physician implants mesh for an open incisional or ventral hernia repair or for closure of debridement for a necrotizing soft tissue infection. The defect is closed with mesh or some other prosthetic material. The incision is closed.

Coding Tips

Report 49568 in addition to 11004–11006 or 49560–49566. When mesh or a prosthesis is implanted at the time of an incisional or a ventral hernia repair, report 49568 in addition to the primary procedure code. Code 49568 should be reported twice when performed bilaterally. Do not report with modifier 50 per CPT guidelines. Medicare may still require the use of modifier 50.

ICD-10-CM Diagnostic Codes

A48.0	Gas gangrene
A48.52	Wound botulism
A48.8	Other specified bacterial diseases
B95.0	Streptococcus, group A, as the cause of diseases classified elsewhere
B95.1	Streptococcus, group B, as the cause of diseases classified elsewhere
B95.2	Enterococcus as the cause of diseases classified elsewhere
B95.3	Streptococcus pneumoniae as the cause of diseases classified elsewhere
B95.4	Other streptococcus as the cause of diseases classified elsewhere
B95.61	Methicillin susceptible Staphylococcus aureus infection as the cause of diseases classified elsewhere
B95.62	Methicillin resistant Staphylococcus aureus infection as the cause of diseases classified elsewhere
B95.7	Other staphylococcus as the cause of diseases classified elsewhere
B96.1	Klebsiella pneumoniae [K. pneumoniae] as the cause of diseases classified elsewhere

B96.21	Shiga toxin-producing Escherichia coli [E. coli] [STEC] O157 as the cause of diseases classified elsewhere
B96.22	Other specified Shiga toxin-producing Escherichia coli [E. coli] [STEC] as the cause of diseases classified elsewhere
B96.29	Other Escherichia coli [E. coli] as the cause of diseases classified elsewhere
B96.4	Proteus (mirabilis) (morganii) as the cause of diseases classified elsewhere
B96.5	Pseudomonas (aeruginosa) (mallei) (pseudomallei) as the cause of diseases classified elsewhere
B96.6	Bacteroides fragilis [B. fragilis] as the cause of diseases classified elsewhere
B96.7	Clostridium perfringens [C. perfringens] as the cause of diseases classified elsewhere
B96.82	Vibrio vulnificus as the cause of diseases classified elsewhere
B96.89	Other specified bacterial agents as the cause of diseases classified elsewhere
I96	Gangrene, not elsewhere classified
K43.0	Incisional hernia with obstruction, without gangrene
K43.1	Incisional hernia with gangrene
K43.2	Incisional hernia without obstruction or gangrene
K43.6	Other and unspecified ventral hernia with obstruction, without gangrene
K43.7	Other and unspecified ventral hernia with gangrene
K43.9	Ventral hernia without obstruction or gangrene
M72.6	Necrotizing fasciitis
N49.3	Fournier gangrene ♂
T81.42XA	Infection following a procedure, deep incisional surgical site, initial encounter
T81.43XA	Infection following a procedure, organ and space surgical site, initial encounter
T81.44XA	Sepsis following a procedure, initial encounter
T81.49XA	Infection following a procedure, other surgical site, initial encounter

AMA: **49568** 2019,Nov,14; 2018,Jan,8; 2017,Jan,8; 2016,Jan,13; 2015,Jan,16

Relative Value Units/Medicare Edits

Non-Facility RVU	Work	PE	MP	Total
49568	4.88	1.82	1.15	7.85
Facility RVU	Work	PE	MP	Total
49568	4.88	1.82	1.15	7.85

	FUD	Status	MUE	Modifiers				IOM Reference
49568	N/A	A	2(3)	N/A	N/A	62*	80	None

* with documentation

49570-49572

49570	Repair epigastric hernia (eg, preperitoneal fat); reducible (separate procedure)
49572	incarcerated or strangulated

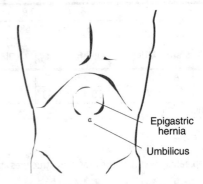

An epigastric hernia is categorized as ventral and occurs in a fascial defect just above the umbilicus

Explanation

The physician repairs an epigastric (49570) or incarcerated epigastric (49572) hernia. The physician makes an incision over the hernia. The hernia sac is identified and dissected from surrounding structures. The fascial defect is identified circumferentially. The hernia is reduced and the hernia sac may be resected. The hernia defect is closed with sutures. In 49572, the hernia sac is opened and the contents of the sac are examined. If the contents of the hernia are viable, the hernia is reduced and the hernia sac may be resected. The hernia defect is closed with sutures. The incisions are closed.

Coding Tips

Hernia repairs are defined by age (younger than 6 months, 6 months to 5 years, age 5 years and older), type (inguinal, femoral, incisional, ventral, epigastric, umbilical, spigelian), whether the hernia has been previously repaired (initial, recurrent), and clinical presentation (reducible, incarcerated, strangulated, sliding). Note that 49570 is a separate procedure by definition and is usually a component of a more complex service and is not identified separately. When performed alone or with other unrelated procedures/services it may be reported. If performed alone, list the code; if performed with other procedures/services, list the code and append modifier 59 or an X{EPSU} modifier. These are unilateral procedures. If performed bilaterally, report the procedure once with modifier 50 appended. Modifier 50 identifies a procedure performed identically on the opposite side of the body (mirror image).

ICD-10-CM Diagnostic Codes

K42.0	Umbilical hernia with obstruction, without gangrene
K42.1	Umbilical hernia with gangrene
K42.9	Umbilical hernia without obstruction or gangrene

AMA: **49570** 2018,Jan,8; 2017,Jan,8; 2016,Jan,13; 2015,Jan,16 **49572** 2018,Jan,8; 2017,Jan,8; 2016,Jan,13; 2015,Jan,16

Relative Value Units/Medicare Edits

Non-Facility RVU	Work	PE	MP	Total
49570	6.05	4.93	1.46	12.44
49572	7.87	5.6	1.9	15.37
Facility RVU	Work	PE	MP	Total
49570	6.05	4.93	1.46	12.44
49572	7.87	5.6	1.9	15.37

	FUD	Status	MUE	Modifiers				IOM Reference
49570	90	A	1(3)	51	50	62*	80	None
49572	90	A	1(3)	51	50	62*	80	

* with documentation

Terms To Know

absorbable sutures. Strands used for suture or repair of tissue prepared from collagen or a synthetic polymer and capable of being absorbed by tissue over time.

epigastric hernia. Protrusion of a section of the intestine, omentum, or other structure through a fascial defect opening in the abdominal wall just above the umbilicus.

nonabsorbable sutures. Strands of natural or synthetic material that resist absorption into living tissue and are removed once healing is under way. Nonabsorbable sutures are commonly used to close skin wounds and repair tendons or collagenous tissue.

reducible hernia. Protrusion of tissue through the wall of another structure that can be manually returned to the correct anatomical position.

strangulated. Constricted and congested area, typically in an intestine, caused by herniation that results in compromised blood supply to that area.

suture. Numerous stitching techniques employed in wound closure.

buried suture. Continuous or interrupted suture placed under the skin for a layered closure.

continuous suture. Running stitch with tension evenly distributed across a single strand to provide a leakproof closure line.

interrupted suture. Series of single stitches with tension isolated at each stitch, in which all stitches are not affected if one becomes loose, and the isolated sutures cannot act as a wick to transport an infection.

purse-string suture. Continuous suture placed around a tubular structure and tightened, to reduce or close the lumen.

retention suture. Secondary stitching that bridges the primary suture, providing support for the primary repair; a plastic or rubber bolster may be placed over the primary repair and under the retention sutures.

49580-49587

49580	Repair umbilical hernia, younger than age 5 years; reducible
49582	incarcerated or strangulated
49585	Repair umbilical hernia, age 5 years or older; reducible
49587	incarcerated or strangulated

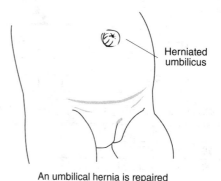

Herniated umbilicus

An umbilical hernia is repaired

Explanation

The physician repairs an umbilical (49580) or incarcerated umbilical (49582) hernia in a child younger than 5 years of age. The physician makes an umbilical incision. The hernia sac and fascial defect are identified and dissected from surrounding structures. The hernia sac is reduced and may be resected. In 49582, the hernia sac is opened and the contents of the sac are examined. If the contents of the hernia sac are viable, the hernia is reduced and the hernia sac may be resected. The hernia defect is closed with sutures. The incisions are closed. For patients 5 years of age or older, report 49585 for an umbilical hernia repair and 49587 for an incarcerated umbilical hernia repair.

Coding Tips

Hernia repairs are defined by age (younger than 6 months, 6 months to 5 years, age 5 years and older), type (inguinal, femoral, incisional, ventral, epigastric, umbilical, spigelian), whether the hernia has been previously repaired (initial, recurrent), and clinical presentation (reducible, incarcerated, strangulated, sliding). These are unilateral procedures. If performed bilaterally, report the procedure once with modifier 50 appended. Modifier 50 identifies a procedure performed identically on the opposite side of the body (mirror image).

ICD-10-CM Diagnostic Codes

K42.0	Umbilical hernia with obstruction, without gangrene
K42.1	Umbilical hernia with gangrene
K42.9	Umbilical hernia without obstruction or gangrene

AMA: **49580** 2018,Jan,8; 2017,Jan,8; 2016,Jan,13; 2015,Jan,16 **49582** 2018,Jan,8; 2017,Jan,8; 2016,Jan,13; 2015,Jan,16 **49585** 2018,Jan,8; 2017,Jan,8; 2016,Jan,13; 2015,Jan,16 **49587** 2018,Jan,8; 2017,Jan,8; 2016,Jan,13; 2015,Jan,16

Relative Value Units/Medicare Edits

Non-Facility RVU	Work	PE	MP	Total
49580	4.47	4.42	1.1	9.99
49582	7.13	5.5	1.74	14.37
49585	6.59	5.1	1.56	13.25
49587	7.08	5.37	1.69	14.14
Facility RVU	Work	PE	MP	Total
49580	4.47	4.42	1.1	9.99
49582	7.13	5.5	1.74	14.37
49585	6.59	5.1	1.56	13.25
49587	7.08	5.37	1.69	14.14

	FUD	Status	MUE	Modifiers				IOM Reference
49580	90	A	1(2)	51	N/A	62*	80	None
49582	90	A	1(2)	51	N/A	62*	80	
49585	90	A	1(2)	51	N/A	62*	80	
49587	90	A	1(2)	51	N/A	62*	80	

* with documentation

Terms To Know

absorbable sutures. Strands used for suture or repair of tissue prepared from collagen or a synthetic polymer and capable of being absorbed by tissue over time.

dissection. Separating by cutting tissue or body structures apart.

fascia. Fibrous sheet or band of tissue that envelops organs, muscles, and groupings of muscles.

gangrene. Death of tissue, usually resulting from a loss of vascular supply, followed by a bacterial attack or onset of disease.

hernia. Protrusion of a body structure through tissue.

nonabsorbable sutures. Strands of natural or synthetic material that resist absorption into living tissue and are removed once healing is under way. Nonabsorbable sutures are commonly used to close skin wounds and repair tendons or collagenous tissue.

reducible hernia. Protrusion of tissue through the wall of another structure that can be manually returned to the correct anatomical position.

reduction. Correction of a fracture, dislocation, or hernia to the correct place and alignment, manually or by surgery.

resection. Surgical removal of a part or all of an organ or body part.

strangulated. Constricted and congested area, typically in an intestine, caused by herniation that results in compromised blood supply to that area.

49590

49590   Repair spigelian hernia

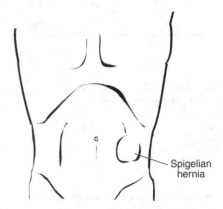

Spigelian hernias occur along the potentially weak lateral border of the rectus abdominis muscle

Explanation

The physician repairs a spigelian hernia. The physician makes an incision over the hernia. The hernia sac and fascial defect are identified and dissected from surrounding structures. The hernia is reduced and the hernia sac may be resected. The hernia defect is closed with a prosthetic patch or by plicating layers of muscle and fascia over the defect with sutures. The incision is closed.

Coding Tips

Hernia repairs are defined by age (younger than 6 months, 6 months to 5 years, age 5 years and older), type (inguinal, femoral, incisional, ventral, epigastric, umbilical, spigelian), whether the hernia has been previously repaired (initial, recurrent), and clinical presentation (reducible, incarcerated, strangulated, sliding). This is a unilateral procedure. If performed bilaterally, report the procedure once with modifier 50 appended. Modifier 50 identifies a procedure performed identically on the opposite side of the body (mirror image). For repair of an initial incisional or ventral hernia, reducible, see 49560; incarcerated or strangulated, see 49561; recurrent, reducible, see 49565; incarcerated or strangulated, see 49566.

ICD-10-CM Diagnostic Codes

K43.6	Other and unspecified ventral hernia with obstruction, without gangrene
K43.7	Other and unspecified ventral hernia with gangrene
K43.9	Ventral hernia without obstruction or gangrene

AMA: **49590** 2018,Jan,8; 2017,Jan,8; 2016,Jan,13; 2015,Jan,16

Relative Value Units/Medicare Edits

Non-Facility RVU	Work	PE	MP	Total
49590	8.9	5.98	2.14	17.02
Facility RVU	Work	PE	MP	Total
49590	8.9	5.98	2.14	17.02

	FUD	Status	MUE	Modifiers				IOM Reference
49590	90	A	1(2)	51	50	62*	80	None

* with documentation

49600

49600 Repair of small omphalocele, with primary closure

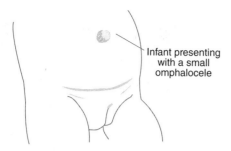

Surgical repair of a small omphalocele

Explanation

The physician repairs a small omphalocele. The physician identifies the omphalocele and dissects the peritoneal sac from the umbilicus and the abdominal wall defect. The peritoneal sac is reduced and the abdominal wall defect is closed with sutures. The umbilicus is reconstructed and the skin is loosely closed.

Coding Tips

For repair of a large omphalocele or gastroschisis, see 49605 and 49606. For repair of an omphalocele (Gross type operation), see 49610 and 49611. Do not append modifier 63 to 49600 as the description or nature of the procedure includes infants up to 4 kg.

ICD-10-CM Diagnostic Codes

Q79.2   Exomphalos

Q79.59   Other congenital malformations of abdominal wall

AMA: 49600 2018,Jan,8; 2017,Jan,8; 2016,Jan,13; 2015,Jan,16

Relative Value Units/Medicare Edits

Non-Facility RVU	Work	PE	MP	Total
49600	11.55	7.41	2.81	21.77
Facility RVU	**Work**	**PE**	**MP**	**Total**
49600	11.55	7.41	2.81	21.77

	FUD	Status	MUE	Modifiers				IOM Reference
49600	90	A	1(2)	51	N/A	62*	80	None

* with documentation

Terms To Know

omphalocele. Congenital protrusion of the intestine through a defect in the abdominal wall at the umbilicus. Repair usually requires a series of surgical procedures to complete, unless the omphalocele is small.

49605-49606

49605 Repair of large omphalocele or gastroschisis; with or without prosthesis
49606   with removal of prosthesis, final reduction and closure, in operating room

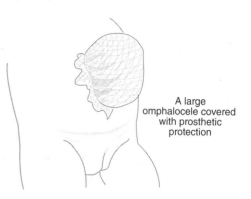

A large omphalocele covered with prosthetic protection

Explanation

In 49605, the physician repairs a large omphalocele or gastroschisis. The peritoneal sac of the omphalocele is dissected from the umbilicus and surrounding structures and reduced or the herniated contents of the gastroschisis are reduced into the abdominal cavity if possible. The abdominal wall defect is identified. If possible the abdominal wall defect is closed with sutures and the umbilicus is reconstructed. If the defect is too large or if the herniated contents cannot be reduced a prosthetic material is used to create a patch or silo that is sutured over the defect to close the defect and accommodate the herniated contents. In 49606, the physician removes a previously placed prosthesis and closes an omphalocele or gastroschisis. The physician removes the previously placed prosthetic material covering the abdominal wall defect. The herniated contents are reduced and the edges of the defect are identified. The abdominal wall defect is closed with sutures. The umbilicus is reconstructed with skin flaps if possible. The remainder of the skin incision is usually left open to allow drainage.

Coding Tips

For repair of a small omphalocele, see 49600. For repair of an omphalocele (Gross type operation), see 49610 and 49611. Do not append modifier 63 to 49605–49606 as the description or nature of the procedure includes infants up to 4 kg.

ICD-10-CM Diagnostic Codes

Q79.2   Exomphalos

Q79.3   Gastroschisis

AMA: 49605 2018,Jan,8; 2017,Jan,8; 2016,Jan,13; 2015,Jan,16 **49606** 2018,Jan,8; 2017,Jan,8; 2016,Jan,13; 2015,Jan,16

Relative Value Units/Medicare Edits

Non-Facility RVU	Work	PE	MP	Total
49605	87.09	37.0	21.31	145.4
49606	19.0	9.96	4.62	33.58
Facility RVU	Work	PE	MP	Total
49605	87.09	37.0	21.31	145.4
49606	19.0	9.96	4.62	33.58

	FUD	Status	MUE	Modifiers				IOM Reference
49605	90	A	1(2)	51	N/A	62*	80	None
49606	90	A	1(2)	51	N/A	62*	80	

* with documentation

Terms To Know

anomaly. Irregularity in the structure or position of an organ or tissue.

congenital. Present at birth, occurring through heredity or an influence during gestation up to the moment of birth.

dissect. Cut apart or separate tissue for surgical purposes or for visual or microscopic study.

drain. Device that creates a channel to allow fluid from a cavity, wound, or infected area to exit the body.

gastroschisis. Congenital anomaly of the abdominal wall in which a fissure remains open, typically resulting in herniation of the small intestine and part of the large intestine.

hernia. Protrusion of a body structure through tissue.

mesh. Synthetic fabric used as a prosthetic patch in hernia repair.

omphalocele. Congenital protrusion of the intestine through a defect in the abdominal wall at the umbilicus. Repair usually requires a series of surgical procedures to complete, unless the omphalocele is small.

prosthesis. Man-made substitute for a missing body part.

umbilicus. Depression or scar left in the middle of the abdomen marking where the umbilical cord was attached in utero.

49610-49611

49610	Repair of omphalocele (Gross type operation); first stage
49611	second stage

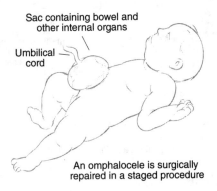

Sac containing bowel and other internal organs

Umbilical cord

An omphalocele is surgically repaired in a staged procedure

Explanation

In 49610, the physician performs the first stage of an omphalocele repair (Gross type operation). The physician identifies the omphalocele. Skin flaps are widely mobilized around the omphalocele and the skin flaps are closed over the intact omphalocele with sutures. The abdominal wall defect is not addressed. In 49611, the physician performs the second stage of an omphalocele repair (Gross type operation). The physician makes an incision in the previously closed skin over the omphalocele. Skin flaps are mobilized off the omphalocele and the peritoneal sac of the omphalocele is dissected from the abdominal wall defect. The abdominal wall defect is closed with sutures. The skin flaps are closed over the repair thus closing the incision.

Coding Tips

For repair of a small omphalocele, see 49600. For repair of a large omphalocele or gastroschisis, see 49605 and 49606. For diaphragmatic or hiatal hernia repair, see 39503 and 43332. Do not append modifier 63 to 49610–49611 as the description or nature of the procedure includes infants up to 4 kg.

ICD-10-CM Diagnostic Codes

Q79.2	Exomphalos

AMA: 49610 2018,Jan,8; 2017,Jan,8; 2016,Jan,13; 2015,Jan,16 **49611** 2018,Jan,8; 2017,Jan,8; 2016,Jan,13; 2015,Jan,16

Relative Value Units/Medicare Edits

Non-Facility RVU	Work	PE	MP	Total
49610	10.91	6.96	2.66	20.53
49611	9.34	6.49	2.28	18.11
Facility RVU	Work	PE	MP	Total
49610	10.91	6.96	2.66	20.53
49611	9.34	6.49	2.28	18.11

	FUD	Status	MUE	Modifiers				IOM Reference
49610	90	A	1(2)	51	N/A	62*	80	None
49611	90	A	1(2)	51	N/A	62*	80	

* with documentation

49650-49651

49650 Laparoscopy, surgical; repair initial inguinal hernia
49651 repair recurrent inguinal hernia

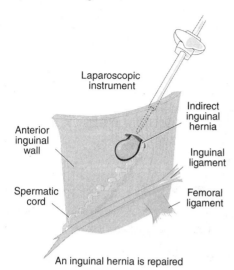

Laparoscopic instrument
Indirect inguinal hernia
Anterior inguinal wall
Inguinal ligament
Spermatic cord
Femoral ligament

An inguinal hernia is repaired

Explanation

The physician performs laparoscopic repair of an initial (49650) or recurrent (49651) inguinal hernia. The physician places a trocar at the umbilicus and insufflates the abdominal or retroperitoneal cavity. The laparoscope is placed through the umbilical port and additional trocars are placed into the peritoneal or retroperitoneal space. The hernia sac is identified and reduced into the abdominal cavity. A sheet of mesh is placed into the abdominal or retroperitoneal cavity and stapled into place on the pubis and abdominal wall covering the hernial defect. The trocars are removed, and the incisions are closed.

Coding Tips

Surgical laparoscopy always includes diagnostic laparoscopy. For diagnostic laparoscopy only, see 49320. For inguinal hernia repair via an open approach, see 49491–49525. These are unilateral procedures. If performed bilaterally, report the procedure once with modifier 50 appended. Modifier 50 identifies a procedure performed identically on the opposite side of the body (mirror image).

ICD-10-CM Diagnostic Codes

K40.00	Bilateral inguinal hernia, with obstruction, without gangrene, not specified as recurrent
K40.01	Bilateral inguinal hernia, with obstruction, without gangrene, recurrent
K40.10	Bilateral inguinal hernia, with gangrene, not specified as recurrent
K40.11	Bilateral inguinal hernia, with gangrene, recurrent
K40.20	Bilateral inguinal hernia, without obstruction or gangrene, not specified as recurrent
K40.21	Bilateral inguinal hernia, without obstruction or gangrene, recurrent
K40.30	Unilateral inguinal hernia, with obstruction, without gangrene, not specified as recurrent
K40.40	Unilateral inguinal hernia, with gangrene, not specified as recurrent
K40.41	Unilateral inguinal hernia, with gangrene, recurrent
K40.90	Unilateral inguinal hernia, without obstruction or gangrene, not specified as recurrent
K40.91	Unilateral inguinal hernia, without obstruction or gangrene, recurrent

AMA: 49650 2018,Jan,8; 2017,Jan,8; 2016,Jan,13; 2015,Jan,16 **49651** 2018,Jan,8; 2017,Jan,8; 2016,Jan,13; 2015,Jan,16

Relative Value Units/Medicare Edits

Non-Facility RVU	Work	PE	MP	Total
49650	6.36	4.91	1.52	12.79
49651	8.38	6.28	1.99	16.65
Facility RVU	**Work**	**PE**	**MP**	**Total**
49650	6.36	4.91	1.52	12.79
49651	8.38	6.28	1.99	16.65

	FUD	Status	MUE	Modifiers				IOM Reference
49650	90	A	1(2)	51	50	62*	80	None
49651	90	A	1(2)	51	50	62*	80	

* with documentation

Terms To Know

insufflation. Blowing air or gas into a body cavity.

laparoscopy. Direct visualization of the peritoneal cavity, outer fallopian tubes, uterus, and ovaries utilizing a laparoscope, a thin, flexible fiberoptic tube.

peritoneal. Space between the lining of the abdominal wall, or parietal peritoneum, and the surface layer of the abdominal organs, or visceral peritoneum. It contains a thin, watery fluid that keeps the peritoneal surfaces moist.

retroperitoneal. Located behind the peritoneum, the membrane that lines the abdominopelvic walls and forms a covering for the internal organs.

trocar. Cannula or a sharp pointed instrument used to puncture and aspirate fluid from cavities.

umbilicus. Depression or scar left in the middle of the abdomen marking where the umbilical cord was attached in utero.

wound repair. Surgical closure of a wound is divided into three categories: simple, intermediate, and complex. *simple repair:* Surgical closure of a superficial wound, requiring single layer suturing of the skin epidermis, dermis, or subcutaneous tissue. *intermediate repair:* Surgical closure of a wound requiring closure of one or more of the deeper subcutaneous tissue and non-muscle fascia layers in addition to suturing the skin; contaminated wounds with single layer closure that need extensive cleaning or foreign body removal. *complex repair:* Repair of wounds requiring more than layered closure (debridement, scar revision, stents, retention sutures).

49652-49653

49652   Laparoscopy, surgical, repair, ventral, umbilical, spigelian or epigastric hernia (includes mesh insertion, when performed); reducible

49653   incarcerated or strangulated

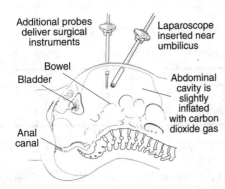

Ventral, umbilical, spigelian, or epigastric hernias are repaired after spigelian

Explanation

The physician performs laparoscopic repair of a ventral, lateral ventral (spigelian), umbilical, or epigastric hernia. Code 49652 reports repair of a reducible hernia; 49653 reports repair of a hernia that is incarcerated or strangulated. The physician places a trocar at the umbilicus and insufflates the abdominal or retroperitoneal cavity. The laparoscope is placed through the umbilical port and additional trocars are placed into the peritoneal or retroperitoneal space. The hernia sac is identified and reduced into the abdominal cavity. A sheet of mesh is often placed into the abdominal or retroperitoneal cavity and stapled into place on the pubis and abdominal wall covering the hernial defect. The trocars are removed, and the incisions are closed. These codes include the insertion of mesh, when performed.

Coding Tips

Surgical laparoscopy always includes diagnostic laparoscopy; the diagnostic laparoscopy should not be reported separately. Do not report these codes with 44180 or 49568.

ICD-10-CM Diagnostic Codes

K42.0	Umbilical hernia with obstruction, without gangrene
K42.1	Umbilical hernia with gangrene
K42.9	Umbilical hernia without obstruction or gangrene
K43.6	Other and unspecified ventral hernia with obstruction, without gangrene
K43.7	Other and unspecified ventral hernia with gangrene
K43.9	Ventral hernia without obstruction or gangrene

AMA: **49652** 2014,Jan,11 **49653** 2014,Jan,11

Relative Value Units/Medicare Edits

Non-Facility RVU	Work	PE	MP	Total
49652	11.92	7.26	2.85	22.03
49653	14.94	9.02	3.6	27.56
Facility RVU	**Work**	**PE**	**MP**	**Total**
49652	11.92	7.26	2.85	22.03
49653	14.94	9.02	3.6	27.56

	FUD	Status	MUE	Modifiers				IOM Reference
49652	90	A	2(3)	51	50	62*	80	None
49653	90	A	2(3)	51	50	62*	80	

* with documentation

Terms To Know

dissection. Separating by cutting tissue or body structures apart.

gangrene. Death of tissue, usually resulting from a loss of vascular supply, followed by a bacterial attack or onset of disease.

hernia. Protrusion of a body structure through tissue.

incision. Act of cutting into tissue or an organ.

mesh. Synthetic fabric used as a prosthetic patch in hernia repair.

reducible hernia. Protrusion of tissue through the wall of another structure that can be manually returned to the correct anatomical position.

strangulated. Constricted and congested area, typically in an intestine, caused by herniation that results in compromised blood supply to that area.

49654-49655

49654   Laparoscopy, surgical, repair, incisional hernia (includes mesh insertion, when performed); reducible

49655   incarcerated or strangulated

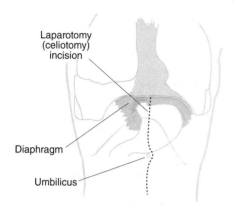

Old surgical incisions are common areas of herniation

Explanation

The physician performs laparoscopic repair of an incisional hernia. The physician places a trocar at the umbilicus and insufflates the abdominal or retroperitoneal cavity. The laparoscope is placed through the umbilical port, and additional trocars are placed into the peritoneal or retroperitoneal space. The hernia sac is identified and reduced into the abdominal cavity. A sheet of mesh is often placed into the abdominal or retroperitoneal cavity and stapled into place on the pubis and abdominal wall covering the hernial defect. The trocars are removed, and the incisions are closed. Report code 49654 for repair of an initial reducible hernia. Report 49655 for an initial incarcerated or strangulated hernia. These codes include the insertion of mesh, when performed.

Coding Tips

Surgical laparoscopy always includes diagnostic laparoscopy; the diagnostic laparoscopy should not be reported separately. Do not report these codes with 44180 or 49568.

ICD-10-CM Diagnostic Codes

K43.0   Incisional hernia with obstruction, without gangrene
K43.1   Incisional hernia with gangrene
K43.2   Incisional hernia without obstruction or gangrene

AMA: **49654** 2018,Jan,7 **49655** 2018,Jan,7

Relative Value Units/Medicare Edits

Non-Facility RVU	Work	PE	MP	Total
49654	13.76	7.95	3.28	24.99
49655	16.84	9.73	4.03	30.6
Facility RVU	**Work**	**PE**	**MP**	**Total**
49654	13.76	7.95	3.28	24.99
49655	16.84	9.73	4.03	30.6

	FUD	Status	MUE	Modifiers				IOM Reference
49654	90	A	1(3)	51	50	62*	80	None
49655	90	A	1(3)	51	50	62*	80	
* with documentation								

49656-49657

49656   Laparoscopy, surgical, repair, recurrent incisional hernia (includes mesh insertion, when performed); reducible

49657   incarcerated or strangulated

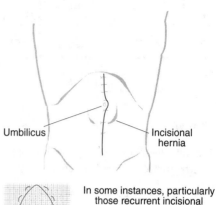

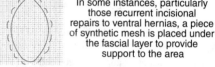

In some instances, particularly those recurrent incisional repairs to ventral hernias, a piece of synthetic mesh is placed under the fascial layer to provide support to the area

Synthetic mesh

Explanation

The physician performs laparoscopic repair of an incisional hernia. The physician places a trocar at the umbilicus and insufflates the abdominal or retroperitoneal cavity. The laparoscope is placed through the umbilical port, and additional trocars are placed into the peritoneal or retroperitoneal space. The hernia sac is identified and reduced into the abdominal cavity. A sheet of mesh is often placed into the abdominal or retroperitoneal cavity and stapled into place on the pubis and abdominal wall covering the hernial defect. The trocars are removed, and the incisions are closed. Report 49656 for repair of a recurrent reducible hernia. Report 49657 for repair of a recurrent incarcerated or strangulated hernia. These codes include the insertion of mesh, when performed.

Coding Tips

Surgical laparoscopy always includes diagnostic laparoscopy; the diagnostic laparoscopy should not be reported separately. Do not report these codes with 44180 or 49568.

ICD-10-CM Diagnostic Codes

K43.0   Incisional hernia with obstruction, without gangrene
K43.1   Incisional hernia with gangrene
K43.2   Incisional hernia without obstruction or gangrene

AMA: **49656** 2014,Jan,11 **49657** 2014,Jan,11

Relative Value Units/Medicare Edits

Non-Facility RVU	Work	PE	MP	Total
49656	15.08	8.43	3.61	27.12
49657	22.11	11.62	5.29	39.02
Facility RVU	**Work**	**PE**	**MP**	**Total**
49656	15.08	8.43	3.61	27.12
49657	22.11	11.62	5.29	39.02

	FUD	Status	MUE	Modifiers				IOM Reference
49656	90	A	1(3)	51	50	62*	80	None
49657	90	A	1(3)	51	50	62*	80	

* with documentation

Terms To Know

gangrene. Death of tissue, usually resulting from a loss of vascular supply, followed by a bacterial attack or onset of disease.

hernia. Protrusion of a body structure through tissue.

laparoscopic. Minimally invasive procedure used for intraabdominal inspection; surgery that uses an endoscopic instrument inserted through small access incisions into the peritoneum for video-controlled imaging.

mesh. Synthetic fabric used as a prosthetic patch in hernia repair.

reducible hernia. Protrusion of tissue through the wall of another structure that can be manually returned to the correct anatomical position.

strangulated. Constricted and congested area, typically in an intestine, caused by herniation that results in compromised blood supply to that area.

49900

49900   Suture, secondary, of abdominal wall for evisceration or dehiscence

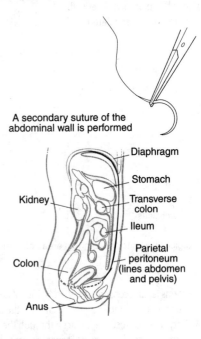

A secondary suture of the abdominal wall is performed

Explanation

The physician performs a secondary closure of the abdominal wall for dehiscence or evisceration. The physician completely opens the former incision and removes the remaining sutures. Necrotic fascia is debrided to viable tissue. Any eviscerated abdominal contents are reduced into the abdominal cavity. The abdominal wall is closed with sutures.

Coding Tips

For debridement of abdominal wall, report 11042 or 11043. For secondary closure of a surgical wound or dehiscence, extensive or complicated, see 13160. Suture of a ruptured diaphragm is reported with codes 39540 and 39541.

ICD-10-CM Diagnostic Codes

O90.0	Disruption of cesarean delivery wound Ⓜ ♀
T81.31XA	Disruption of external operation (surgical) wound, not elsewhere classified, initial encounter
T81.32XA	Disruption of internal operation (surgical) wound, not elsewhere classified, initial encounter
T81.33XA	Disruption of traumatic injury wound repair, initial encounter

AMA: 49900 2018,Jan,8; 2017,Jan,8; 2016,Jan,13; 2015,Jan,16

Relative Value Units/Medicare Edits

Non-Facility RVU	Work	PE	MP	Total
49900	12.41	8.93	2.8	24.14
Facility RVU	**Work**	**PE**	**MP**	**Total**
49900	12.41	8.93	2.8	24.14

	FUD	Status	MUE	Modifiers				IOM Reference
49900	90	A	1(3)	51	N/A	62*	80	None

* with documentation

49904-49906

49904   Omental flap, extra-abdominal (eg, for reconstruction of sternal and chest wall defects)

+   49905   Omental flap, intra-abdominal (List separately in addition to code for primary procedure)

49906   Free omental flap with microvascular anastomosis

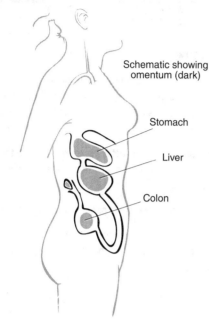

Schematic showing omentum (dark)

Stomach

Liver

Colon

A flap of omentum is used in an extra-abdominal repair, such as of the chest wall

Explanation

The physician mobilizes an omental flap for reconstruction of a defect. The surgical recipient site of the flap is prepared. An upper abdominal transverse or midline incision is made. A laparotomy and manual exploration of the abdominal cavity is done first and the omentum and transverse colon are delivered from the cavity. The omentum is dissected from the transverse colon from left to right and small vessels are ligated. When completely separated from the transverse colon, the omentum is dissected from the stomach with careful clamping, division, and ligation of vessels. The omentum is fully mobilized and pedicled on the right or left gastroepiploic vessel, depending on the purpose. More incisions and tunneling may be necessary to bring the flap into its new location to fill a defect. The flap may be used as a pedicled transposition flap or a free microvascular transfer flap. Report 49904 when the flap is transpositioned to repair an extra-abdominal defect, such as chest wounds after radiation and mastectomy or lower extremity trauma wounds. Report 49905 when the omental flap is repositioned to repair a defect intra-abdominally. Report 49906 when the omentum is used as a free vascularized transfer flap to repair defects such as hemifacial atrophy. Microvascular anastomosis is performed to maintain blood flow to the omental flap. The abdominal incision is closed. If a separate split-thickness skin graft is required for omental coverage, it is done immediately and applied directly over the omentum and a dressing is applied.

Coding Tips

Note that 49904 includes harvest and transfer. If a second surgeon harvests the omental flap, the two surgeons should report 49904 as co-surgeons using modifier 62. Do not report 49905 with 47700. Use of an operating microscope (69990) is included in 49906 and is not reported separately.

ICD-10-CM Diagnostic Codes

S21.111A	Laceration without foreign body of right front wall of thorax without penetration into thoracic cavity, initial encounter
S21.112A	Laceration without foreign body of left front wall of thorax without penetration into thoracic cavity, initial encounter
S21.121A	Laceration with foreign body of right front wall of thorax without penetration into thoracic cavity, initial encounter
S21.122A	Laceration with foreign body of left front wall of thorax without penetration into thoracic cavity, initial encounter
S21.131A	Puncture wound without foreign body of right front wall of thorax without penetration into thoracic cavity, initial encounter
S21.132A	Puncture wound without foreign body of left front wall of thorax without penetration into thoracic cavity, initial encounter
S21.141A	Puncture wound with foreign body of right front wall of thorax without penetration into thoracic cavity, initial encounter
S21.142A	Puncture wound with foreign body of left front wall of thorax without penetration into thoracic cavity, initial encounter
S21.151A	Open bite of right front wall of thorax without penetration into thoracic cavity, initial encounter
S21.152A	Open bite of left front wall of thorax without penetration into thoracic cavity, initial encounter
S28.1XXA	Traumatic amputation (partial) of part of thorax, except breast, initial encounter
S29.021A	Laceration of muscle and tendon of front wall of thorax, initial encounter
T21.31XA	Burn of third degree of chest wall, initial encounter
T21.71XA	Corrosion of third degree of chest wall, initial encounter
T81.31XA	Disruption of external operation (surgical) wound, not elsewhere classified, initial encounter
T81.32XA	Disruption of internal operation (surgical) wound, not elsewhere classified, initial encounter
T81.33XA	Disruption of traumatic injury wound repair, initial encounter
T81.89XA	Other complications of procedures, not elsewhere classified, initial encounter

AMA: **49905** 2020,Feb,13; 2018,Jan,8; 2017,Jan,8; 2016,Jan,13; 2015,Jan,16 **49906** 2019,Dec,5; 2018,Jan,8; 2017,Jan,8; 2016,Jan,13; 2016,Feb,12; 2015,Jan,16

Relative Value Units/Medicare Edits

Non-Facility RVU	Work	PE	MP	Total
49904	22.35	14.07	4.59	41.01
49905	6.54	2.4	1.43	10.37
49906	0.0	0.0	0.0	0.0
Facility RVU	Work	PE	MP	Total
49904	22.35	14.07	4.59	41.01
49905	6.54	2.4	1.43	10.37
49906	0.0	0.0	0.0	0.0

	FUD	Status	MUE	Modifiers				IOM Reference
49904	90	A	1(3)	51	N/A	62*	N/A	None
49905	N/A	A	1(3)	N/A	N/A	62	80	
49906	90	C	1(3)	51	N/A	62*	N/A	

* with documentation

55920

55920 Placement of needles or catheters into pelvic organs and/or genitalia (except prostate) for subsequent interstitial radioelement application

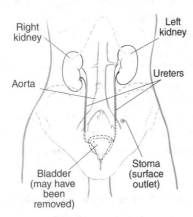

Needles or catheters are placed in the genitalia or pelvic organs

Explanation

The physician places needles or catheters into the pelvic organs and/or genitalia, excluding the prostate, for subsequent interstitial radioelement application. The radioactive isotopes that are introduced subsequently, such as iodine-125 or palladium-103, are contained within tiny seeds that are left in place to deliver radiation over a period of months. They do not cause any harm after becoming inert. This method provides radiation to the prescribed body area while minimizing exposure to normal tissue.

Coding Tips

For placement of needles or catheters into the prostate, see 55875. For insertion of uterine tandems and/or vaginal ovoids for clinical brachytherapy, see 57155. For insertion of Heyman capsules for clinical brachytherapy, see 58346.

ICD-10-CM Diagnostic Codes

C20	Malignant neoplasm of rectum
C21.1	Malignant neoplasm of anal canal
C49.A3	Gastrointestinal stromal tumor of small intestine
C49.A5	Gastrointestinal stromal tumor of rectum
C56.1	Malignant neoplasm of right ovary ♀ ☑
C56.2	Malignant neoplasm of left ovary ♀ ☑
C56.3	Malignant neoplasm of bilateral ovaries ♀ ☑
C62.01	Malignant neoplasm of undescended right testis ♂ ☑
C62.02	Malignant neoplasm of undescended left testis ♂ ☑
C62.11	Malignant neoplasm of descended right testis ♂ ☑
C62.12	Malignant neoplasm of descended left testis ♂ ☑
C7A.026	Malignant carcinoid tumor of the rectum
D01.2	Carcinoma in situ of rectum
D01.3	Carcinoma in situ of anus and anal canal

AMA: 55920 2018,Jan,8; 2017,Jan,8; 2016,Jan,13; 2015,Jan,16

Relative Value Units/Medicare Edits

Non-Facility RVU	Work	PE	MP	Total
55920	8.31	4.29	0.68	13.28
Facility RVU	**Work**	**PE**	**MP**	**Total**
55920	8.31	4.29	0.68	13.28

	FUD	Status	MUE	Modifiers				IOM Reference
55920	0	A	1(2)	51	N/A	N/A	80*	None

* with documentation

Terms To Know

carcinoid tumor. Specific type of slow-growing neuroendocrine tumors. Carcinoid tumors occur most commonly in the hormone producing cells of the gastrointestinal tracts and can also occur in the pancreas, testes, ovaries, or lungs.

carcinoma in situ. Malignancy that arises from the cells of the vessel, gland, or organ of origin that remains confined to that site or has not invaded neighboring tissue.

interstitial. Within the small spaces or gaps occurring in tissue or organs.

radioelement. Any element that emits particle or electromagnetic radiations from nuclear disintegration, occurring naturally in any element with an atomic number above 83.

60000

60000 Incision and drainage of thyroglossal duct cyst, infected

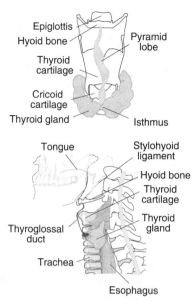

Cysts can occur anywhere along the remnant of the thyroglossal duct

Explanation

The physician incises and drains an infected thyroglossal (also called thyrolingual) cyst in the neck caused by incomplete closure or persistence of the embryonic thyroglossal duct between the developing thyroid and the back of the tongue. After the physician incises the cyst and drains the infected fluid, the wound may be irrigated with normal saline and a drainage system inserted. The drainage tubes may be stitched in place. A collection unit applies gentle suction to collect fluid from the incision site.

Coding Tips

For excision of a thyroglossal duct cyst or sinus, see 60280; recurrent, see 60281.

ICD-10-CM Diagnostic Codes

Q89.2   Congenital malformations of other endocrine glands

AMA: 60000 2014,Jan,11

Relative Value Units/Medicare Edits

Non-Facility RVU	Work	PE	MP	Total
60000	1.81	3.22	0.25	5.28
Facility RVU	Work	PE	MP	Total
60000	1.81	2.43	0.25	4.49

	FUD	Status	MUE	Modifiers				IOM Reference
60000	10	A	1(3)	51	N/A	N/A	80*	None

* with documentation

Terms To Know

thyroglossal duct. Embryonic duct at the front of the neck, which becomes the pyramidal lobe of the thyroid gland with obliteration of the remaining duct, but may form a cyst or sinus in adulthood if it persists.

60100

60100 Biopsy thyroid, percutaneous core needle

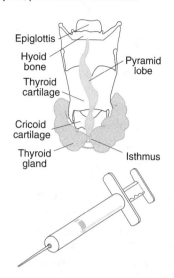

The thyroid gland is biopsied percutaneously using a biopsy needle. A section of tissue is withdrawn

Explanation

The physician removes tissue from the thyroid for examination. The physician localizes the area to be biopsied by palpation or separately reportable ultrasound. A large, hollow, bore needle is passed through skin and muscle, into the thyroid. The tissue is removed and sent for separately reportable analysis.

Coding Tips

Imaging guidance is reported with 76942, 77002, 77012, or 77021, when performed. For fine needle aspiration, see 10004–10012 and 10021; aspirate evaluation, see 88172–88173.

ICD-10-CM Diagnostic Codes

C73	Malignant neoplasm of thyroid gland
C79.89	Secondary malignant neoplasm of other specified sites
D09.3	Carcinoma in situ of thyroid and other endocrine glands
D09.8	Carcinoma in situ of other specified sites
D34	Benign neoplasm of thyroid gland
D44.0	Neoplasm of uncertain behavior of thyroid gland
E01.0	Iodine-deficiency related diffuse (endemic) goiter
E01.1	Iodine-deficiency related multinodular (endemic) goiter
E04.0	Nontoxic diffuse goiter
E04.1	Nontoxic single thyroid nodule
E04.2	Nontoxic multinodular goiter
E04.8	Other specified nontoxic goiter
E05.10	Thyrotoxicosis with toxic single thyroid nodule without thyrotoxic crisis or storm
E05.11	Thyrotoxicosis with toxic single thyroid nodule with thyrotoxic crisis or storm
E05.20	Thyrotoxicosis with toxic multinodular goiter without thyrotoxic crisis or storm
E05.21	Thyrotoxicosis with toxic multinodular goiter with thyrotoxic crisis or storm

E05.30	Thyrotoxicosis from ectopic thyroid tissue without thyrotoxic crisis or storm
E05.31	Thyrotoxicosis from ectopic thyroid tissue with thyrotoxic crisis or storm
E06.0	Acute thyroiditis
E06.1	Subacute thyroiditis
E06.2	Chronic thyroiditis with transient thyrotoxicosis
E06.3	Autoimmune thyroiditis
E06.4	Drug-induced thyroiditis
E06.5	Other chronic thyroiditis
E07.89	Other specified disorders of thyroid
O90.5	Postpartum thyroiditis M ♀
O99.281	Endocrine, nutritional and metabolic diseases complicating pregnancy, first trimester M ♀
O99.282	Endocrine, nutritional and metabolic diseases complicating pregnancy, second trimester M ♀
O99.283	Endocrine, nutritional and metabolic diseases complicating pregnancy, third trimester M ♀
O99.284	Endocrine, nutritional and metabolic diseases complicating childbirth M ♀
O99.285	Endocrine, nutritional and metabolic diseases complicating the puerperium M ♀
Q89.2	Congenital malformations of other endocrine glands
R94.6	Abnormal results of thyroid function studies
R94.7	Abnormal results of other endocrine function studies

AMA: 60100 2019,Apr,4; 2018,Jan,8; 2017,Jan,8; 2016,Jan,13; 2015,Jan,16

Relative Value Units/Medicare Edits

Non-Facility RVU	Work	PE	MP	Total
60100	1.56	1.54	0.15	3.25
Facility RVU	Work	PE	MP	Total
60100	1.56	0.54	0.15	2.25

	FUD	Status	MUE	Modifiers				IOM Reference
60100	0	A	3(3)	51	N/A	N/A	N/A	None

* with documentation

Terms To Know

core biopsy. Large-bore biopsy needle is inserted into a mass and a core of tissue is removed for diagnostic study.

goiter. Abnormal enlargement of the thyroid gland commonly caused by a deficiency of dietary iodine.

thyroid. Endocrine gland located in the front of the lower neck composed of two lobes on either side of the trachea, responsible for secreting and storing the thyroid hormones that regulate metabolism.

thyroiditis. Inflammation of the thyroid gland.

60200

60200	Excision of cyst or adenoma of thyroid, or transection of isthmus

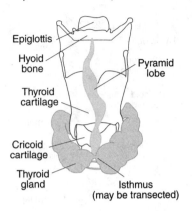

Explanation

The physician removes a cyst or adenoma from a thyroid or transects the isthmus. The physician exposes the thyroid via a transverse cervical incision in the skin line. The platysmas are divided and the strap muscles separated in the midline. The thyroid mass is identified. Blood supply to and from the lesion is controlled and the mass is locally excised. The skin and platysmas are closed.

Coding Tips

For excision of a thyroglossal duct cyst and sinus, see 60280; recurrent, see 60281. For percutaneous core needle thyroid biopsy, see 60100. For partial thyroidectomy, unilateral, with or without isthmusectomy, see 60210; with contralateral subtotal lobectomy, including isthmusectomy, see 60212.

ICD-10-CM Diagnostic Codes

D34	Benign neoplasm of thyroid gland
D44.0	Neoplasm of uncertain behavior of thyroid gland
D44.2	Neoplasm of uncertain behavior of parathyroid gland
E01.0	Iodine-deficiency related diffuse (endemic) goiter
E01.1	Iodine-deficiency related multinodular (endemic) goiter
E01.2	Iodine-deficiency related (endemic) goiter, unspecified
E04.0	Nontoxic diffuse goiter
E04.1	Nontoxic single thyroid nodule
E04.2	Nontoxic multinodular goiter
E04.8	Other specified nontoxic goiter
E05.10	Thyrotoxicosis with toxic single thyroid nodule without thyrotoxic crisis or storm
E05.11	Thyrotoxicosis with toxic single thyroid nodule with thyrotoxic crisis or storm
E05.20	Thyrotoxicosis with toxic multinodular goiter without thyrotoxic crisis or storm
E05.21	Thyrotoxicosis with toxic multinodular goiter with thyrotoxic crisis or storm
E05.30	Thyrotoxicosis from ectopic thyroid tissue without thyrotoxic crisis or storm
E05.31	Thyrotoxicosis from ectopic thyroid tissue with thyrotoxic crisis or storm
E06.0	Acute thyroiditis
E06.1	Subacute thyroiditis
E06.2	Chronic thyroiditis with transient thyrotoxicosis

Thyroid

E06.3	Autoimmune thyroiditis
E06.4	Drug-induced thyroiditis
E06.5	Other chronic thyroiditis
E07.89	Other specified disorders of thyroid
O90.5	Postpartum thyroiditis Ⓜ ♀

AMA: 60200 2018,Jan,8; 2017,Jan,8; 2016,Jan,13; 2015,Jan,16

Relative Value Units/Medicare Edits

Non-Facility RVU	Work	PE	MP	Total
60200	10.02	7.66	1.91	19.59
Facility RVU	Work	PE	MP	Total
60200	10.02	7.66	1.91	19.59

	FUD	Status	MUE	Modifiers				IOM Reference
60200	90	A	2(3)	51	N/A	62*	80	None

* with documentation

Terms To Know

cyst. Elevated encapsulated mass containing fluid, semisolid, or solid material with a membranous lining.

goiter. Abnormal enlargement of the thyroid gland commonly caused by a deficiency of dietary iodine.

platysma. Muscle originating from the neck region attached to the mandible that opens the jaw.

transection. Transverse dissection; to cut across a long axis; cross section.

transverse. Crosswise at right angles to the long axis of a structure or part.

60210-60212

60210 Partial thyroid lobectomy, unilateral; with or without isthmusectomy
60212   with contralateral subtotal lobectomy, including isthmusectomy

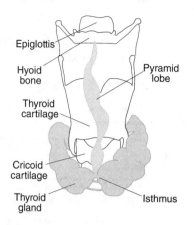

Explanation

The physician removes part of a thyroid lobe, with or without an isthmusectomy. The physician exposes the thyroid via a transverse cervical incision in the skin line. The platysmas are divided and the strap muscles separated in the midline. The superior and inferior thyroid vessels are divided in the area for resection. The thyroid parenchyma is divided and dissected with cautery dissection. The skin and platysmas are closed. Report 60212 when a contralateral subtotal lobectomy, including isthmusectomy is also performed.

Coding Tips

Parathyroid autotransplantation is reported with 60512, when performed. When this procedure is performed with total thyroid lobectomy, see 60220; contralateral subtotal lobectomy, with isthmusectomy, see 60225.

ICD-10-CM Diagnostic Codes

C73	Malignant neoplasm of thyroid gland
C79.89	Secondary malignant neoplasm of other specified sites
D09.3	Carcinoma in situ of thyroid and other endocrine glands
D09.8	Carcinoma in situ of other specified sites
D34	Benign neoplasm of thyroid gland
D44.0	Neoplasm of uncertain behavior of thyroid gland
D44.2	Neoplasm of uncertain behavior of parathyroid gland
D49.7	Neoplasm of unspecified behavior of endocrine glands and other parts of nervous system
E01.0	Iodine-deficiency related diffuse (endemic) goiter
E01.1	Iodine-deficiency related multinodular (endemic) goiter
E04.0	Nontoxic diffuse goiter
E04.1	Nontoxic single thyroid nodule
E04.2	Nontoxic multinodular goiter
E04.8	Other specified nontoxic goiter
E05.00	Thyrotoxicosis with diffuse goiter without thyrotoxic crisis or storm
E05.01	Thyrotoxicosis with diffuse goiter with thyrotoxic crisis or storm
E05.10	Thyrotoxicosis with toxic single thyroid nodule without thyrotoxic crisis or storm
E05.11	Thyrotoxicosis with toxic single thyroid nodule with thyrotoxic crisis or storm

E05.20	Thyrotoxicosis with toxic multinodular goiter without thyrotoxic crisis or storm
E05.21	Thyrotoxicosis with toxic multinodular goiter with thyrotoxic crisis or storm
E05.30	Thyrotoxicosis from ectopic thyroid tissue without thyrotoxic crisis or storm

AMA: 60210 2018,Jan,8; 2017,Jan,8; 2016,Jan,13; 2015,Jan,16 **60212** 2018,Jan,8; 2017,Jan,8; 2016,Jan,13; 2015,Jan,16

Relative Value Units/Medicare Edits

Non-Facility RVU	Work	PE	MP	Total
60210	11.23	7.37	2.17	20.77
60212	16.43	9.96	4.02	30.41
Facility RVU	**Work**	**PE**	**MP**	**Total**
60210	11.23	7.37	2.17	20.77
60212	16.43	9.96	4.02	30.41

	FUD	Status	MUE	Modifiers				IOM Reference
60210	90	A	1(2)	51	N/A	62*	80	100-04,12,40.7
60212	90	A	1(2)	51	N/A	62*	80	

* with documentation

Terms To Know

contralateral. Located on, or affecting, the opposite side of the body, usually as it relates to a bilateral body part.

isthmusectomy. Excision of the isthmus glandulae thyroideae; the connecting tissue between the two thyroid lobes.

platysma. Muscle originating from the neck region attached to the mandible that opens the jaw.

thyroid. Endocrine gland located in the front of the lower neck composed of two lobes on either side of the trachea, responsible for secreting and storing the thyroid hormones that regulate metabolism.

thyrotoxicosis. Excessive quantities of hormones from the thyroid gland caused by overproduction or loss of storage ability.

60220-60225

| 60220 | Total thyroid lobectomy, unilateral; with or without isthmusectomy |
| 60225 | with contralateral subtotal lobectomy, including isthmusectomy |

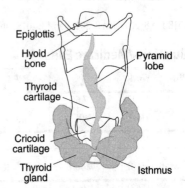

Epiglottis
Hyoid bone
Pyramid lobe
Thyroid cartilage
Cricoid cartilage
Thyroid gland
Isthmus

Thyroid anatomy is variable; about 40 percent of people exhibit some portion of a pyramid lobe extending from the isthmus

Explanation

The physician removes all of a thyroid lobe, with or without isthmusectomy. The physician exposes the thyroid via a transverse cervical incision in the skin line. The platysmas are divided and the strap muscles separated in the midline. The thyroid lobe to be excised is isolated and superior and inferior thyroid vessels serving that lobe are ligated. Parathyroid glands are preserved. The thyroid gland is divided in the midline of the isthmus over the anterior trachea. The thyroid lobe is resected. The platysmas and skin are closed. Report 60225 if performed with contralateral subtotal lobectomy, including isthmusectomy.

Coding Tips

Parathyroid autotransplantation is reported with 60512, when performed. For removal of thyroid tissue following previous removal of the thyroid, see 60260. For parathyroidectomy or exploration of the parathyroid, see 60500; re-exploration, see 60502; with mediastinal exploration, sternal split or transthoracic approach, see 60505.

ICD-10-CM Diagnostic Codes

C73	Malignant neoplasm of thyroid gland
C79.89	Secondary malignant neoplasm of other specified sites
D09.3	Carcinoma in situ of thyroid and other endocrine glands
D09.8	Carcinoma in situ of other specified sites
D34	Benign neoplasm of thyroid gland
D44.0	Neoplasm of uncertain behavior of thyroid gland
E01.0	Iodine-deficiency related diffuse (endemic) goiter
E01.1	Iodine-deficiency related multinodular (endemic) goiter
E04.0	Nontoxic diffuse goiter
E04.1	Nontoxic single thyroid nodule
E04.2	Nontoxic multinodular goiter
E04.8	Other specified nontoxic goiter
E05.00	Thyrotoxicosis with diffuse goiter without thyrotoxic crisis or storm
E05.01	Thyrotoxicosis with diffuse goiter with thyrotoxic crisis or storm
E05.10	Thyrotoxicosis with toxic single thyroid nodule without thyrotoxic crisis or storm
E05.11	Thyrotoxicosis with toxic single thyroid nodule with thyrotoxic crisis or storm

E05.20	Thyrotoxicosis with toxic multinodular goiter without thyrotoxic crisis or storm	
E05.21	Thyrotoxicosis with toxic multinodular goiter with thyrotoxic crisis or storm	
E05.30	Thyrotoxicosis from ectopic thyroid tissue without thyrotoxic crisis or storm	
E05.31	Thyrotoxicosis from ectopic thyroid tissue with thyrotoxic crisis or storm	

AMA: 60220 2020,Aug,14; 2018,Jan,8; 2017,Jan,8; 2016,Jan,13; 2015,Jan,16
60225 2018,Jan,8; 2017,Jan,8; 2016,Jan,13; 2015,Jan,16

Relative Value Units/Medicare Edits

Non-Facility RVU	Work	PE	MP	Total
60220	11.19	7.47	2.05	20.71
60225	14.79	9.89	2.66	27.34
Facility RVU	**Work**	**PE**	**MP**	**Total**
60220	11.19	7.47	2.05	20.71
60225	14.79	9.89	2.66	27.34

	FUD	Status	MUE	Modifiers				IOM Reference
60220	90	A	1(3)	51	N/A	62*	80	100-04,12,40.7
60225	90	A	1(2)	51	N/A	62*	80	

* with documentation

Terms To Know

contralateral. Located on, or affecting, the opposite side of the body, usually as it relates to a bilateral body part.

isthmusectomy. Excision of the isthmus glandulae thyroideae; the connecting tissue between the two thyroid lobes.

lobectomy. Excision of a lobe of an organ such as the liver, thyroid, lung, or brain.

60240

60240 Thyroidectomy, total or complete

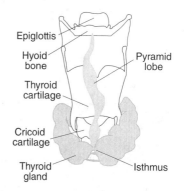

Epiglottis
Hyoid bone
Pyramid lobe
Thyroid cartilage
Cricoid cartilage
Thyroid gland
Isthmus

Both lobes of the thyroid gland are removed along with any tissues associated with the isthmus

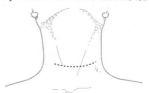

Typical incision for total thyroidectomy

Explanation

The physician removes all of the thyroid. The physician exposes the thyroid via a transverse cervical incision in the skin line. The platysmas are divided and the strap muscles separated in the midline. The thyroid gland is mobilized and the superior and inferior thyroid vessels are ligated. The parathyroid glands are preserved and the thyroid is resected free of the trachea and removed. The platysmas and skin are closed.

Coding Tips

Parathyroid autotransplantation is reported with 60512, when performed. For total or subtotal thyroidectomy for malignancy, with limited neck dissection, see 60252; with radical neck dissection, see 60254. For thyroidectomy including substernal thyroid gland, sternal split or transthoracic approach, see 60270; cervical approach, see 60271. For parathyroidectomy or exploration of parathyroids, see 60500; re-exploration, see 60502.

ICD-10-CM Diagnostic Codes

C73	Malignant neoplasm of thyroid gland
C79.89	Secondary malignant neoplasm of other specified sites
D09.3	Carcinoma in situ of thyroid and other endocrine glands
D34	Benign neoplasm of thyroid gland
D44.2	Neoplasm of uncertain behavior of parathyroid gland
E01.0	Iodine-deficiency related diffuse (endemic) goiter
E01.1	Iodine-deficiency related multinodular (endemic) goiter
E04.0	Nontoxic diffuse goiter
E04.2	Nontoxic multinodular goiter
E04.8	Other specified nontoxic goiter
E05.00	Thyrotoxicosis with diffuse goiter without thyrotoxic crisis or storm
E05.01	Thyrotoxicosis with diffuse goiter with thyrotoxic crisis or storm
E05.10	Thyrotoxicosis with toxic single thyroid nodule without thyrotoxic crisis or storm

Thyroid

E05.11	Thyrotoxicosis with toxic single thyroid nodule with thyrotoxic crisis or storm
E05.20	Thyrotoxicosis with toxic multinodular goiter without thyrotoxic crisis or storm
E05.30	Thyrotoxicosis from ectopic thyroid tissue without thyrotoxic crisis or storm

AMA: 60240 2018,Jan,8; 2017,Jan,8; 2016,Jan,13; 2015,Jan,16

Relative Value Units/Medicare Edits

Non-Facility RVU	Work	PE	MP	Total
60240	15.04	8.97	2.9	26.91
Facility RVU	**Work**	**PE**	**MP**	**Total**
60240	15.04	8.97	2.9	26.91

	FUD	Status	MUE	Modifiers				IOM Reference
60240	90	A	1(2)	51	N/A	62*	80	None

* with documentation

Terms To Know

goiter. Abnormal enlargement of the thyroid gland commonly caused by a deficiency of dietary iodine.

ligation. Tying off a blood vessel or duct with a suture or a soft, thin wire.

platysma. Muscle originating from the neck region attached to the mandible that opens the jaw.

resection. Surgical removal of a part or all of an organ or body part.

thyroidectomy. Partial or complete removal of the thyroid gland.

thyrotoxicosis. Excessive quantities of hormones from the thyroid gland caused by overproduction or loss of storage ability.

total thyroidectomy. Excision of both lobes.

transverse. Crosswise at right angles to the long axis of a structure or part.

60252-60254

| 60252 | Thyroidectomy, total or subtotal for malignancy; with limited neck dissection |
| 60254 | with radical neck dissection |

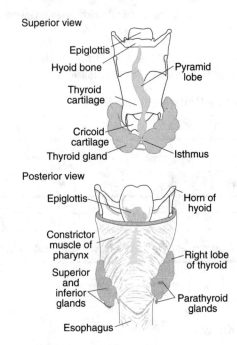

Explanation

The physician removes a malignant thyroid and some lymph nodes. The physician exposes the thyroid via a transverse cervical incision in the skin line. The platysmas are divided and the strap muscles separated in the midline. The thyroid gland is mobilized and the superior and inferior thyroid vessels are ligated. The parathyroid glands are preserved and the thyroid is resected free of the trachea and removed. All enlarged lymph nodes are identified and excised. The platysmas and skin are closed. Report 60254 if a radical neck dissection is included in the procedure.

Coding Tips

Parathyroid autotransplantation is reported with 60512, when performed. For percutaneous needle core thyroid biopsy, see 60100. For unilateral partial thyroidectomy, see 60210–60212. For total or complete thyroidectomy, other than malignancy, see 60240.

ICD-10-CM Diagnostic Codes

C73	Malignant neoplasm of thyroid gland
C79.89	Secondary malignant neoplasm of other specified sites
D09.3	Carcinoma in situ of thyroid and other endocrine glands

AMA: 60252 2018,Jan,8; 2017,Jan,8; 2016,Jan,13; 2015,Jan,16 **60254** 2018,Jan,8; 2017,Jan,8; 2016,Jan,13; 2015,Jan,16

Relative Value Units/Medicare Edits

Non-Facility RVU	Work	PE	MP	Total
60252	22.01	12.47	4.23	38.71
60254	28.42	15.25	4.99	48.66
Facility RVU	Work	PE	MP	Total
60252	22.01	12.47	4.23	38.71
60254	28.42	15.25	4.99	48.66

	FUD	Status	MUE	Modifiers				IOM Reference
60252	90	A	1(2)	51	N/A	62*	80	None
60254	90	A	1(2)	51	N/A	62*	80	

* with documentation

Terms To Know

carcinoma in situ. Malignancy that arises from the cells of the vessel, gland, or organ of origin that remains confined to that site or has not invaded neighboring tissue.

dissect. Cut apart or separate tissue for surgical purposes or for visual or microscopic study.

ligation. Tying off a blood vessel or duct with a suture or a soft, thin wire.

lymph nodes. Bean-shaped structures along the lymphatic vessels that intercept and destroy foreign materials in the tissue and bloodstream.

malignant. Any condition tending to progress toward death, specifically an invasive tumor with a loss of cellular differentiation that has the ability to spread or metastasize to other body areas.

neoplasm. New abnormal growth, tumor.

platysma. Muscle originating from the neck region attached to the mandible that opens the jaw.

resection. Surgical removal of a part or all of an organ or body part.

secondary. Second in order of occurrence or importance, or appearing during the course of another disease or condition.

thyroidectomy. Partial or complete removal of the thyroid gland.

total thyroidectomy. Excision of both lobes.

transverse. Crosswise at right angles to the long axis of a structure or part.

60260

60260   Thyroidectomy, removal of all remaining thyroid tissue following previous removal of a portion of thyroid

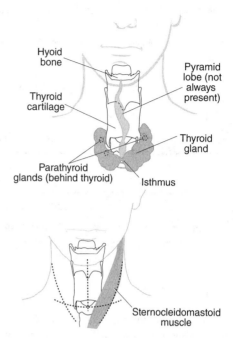

Common incisions for neck dissection

Explanation

The physician removes thyroid tissue remaining following a partial thyroidectomy. The physician enters through the previous incision scar. The platysmas and scar tissue are divided and the strap muscles are divided in the midline. While preserving the parathyroid glands, all the remaining scar tissue is resected. The platysmas and skin are closed.

Coding Tips

This is a unilateral procedure. If performed bilaterally, some payers require that the service be reported twice with modifier 50 appended to the second code while others require identification of the service only once with modifier 50 appended. Check with individual payers. Modifier 50 identifies a procedure performed identically on the opposite side of the body (mirror image). Parathyroid autotransplantation is reported with 60512, when performed. For partial lobectomy, see 60210–60212. For total thyroid lobectomy, see 60220–60225. For total or complete thyroidectomy, other than malignancy, see 60240. For total or subtotal thyroidectomy for malignancy, see 60252–60254.

ICD-10-CM Diagnostic Codes

C73	Malignant neoplasm of thyroid gland
C79.89	Secondary malignant neoplasm of other specified sites
D09.3	Carcinoma in situ of thyroid and other endocrine glands
D09.8	Carcinoma in situ of other specified sites
D44.0	Neoplasm of uncertain behavior of thyroid gland
E01.0	Iodine-deficiency related diffuse (endemic) goiter
E04.0	Nontoxic diffuse goiter
E04.8	Other specified nontoxic goiter
E05.00	Thyrotoxicosis with diffuse goiter without thyrotoxic crisis or storm

E05.01	Thyrotoxicosis with diffuse goiter with thyrotoxic crisis or storm
E05.10	Thyrotoxicosis with toxic single thyroid nodule without thyrotoxic crisis or storm
E05.11	Thyrotoxicosis with toxic single thyroid nodule with thyrotoxic crisis or storm
E05.20	Thyrotoxicosis with toxic multinodular goiter without thyrotoxic crisis or storm
E05.30	Thyrotoxicosis from ectopic thyroid tissue without thyrotoxic crisis or storm

AMA: 60260 2018,Jan,8; 2017,Jan,8; 2016,Jan,13; 2015,Jan,16

Relative Value Units/Medicare Edits

Non-Facility RVU	Work	PE	MP	Total
60260	18.26	10.33	3.31	31.9
Facility RVU	**Work**	**PE**	**MP**	**Total**
60260	18.26	10.33	3.31	31.9

	FUD	Status	MUE	Modifiers				IOM Reference
60260	90	A	1(2)	51	50	62*	80	None

* with documentation

Terms To Know

carcinoma in situ. Malignancy that arises from the cells of the vessel, gland, or organ of origin that remains confined to that site or has not invaded neighboring tissue.

closure. Repairing an incision or wound by suture or other means.

hyoid bone. Single, U-shaped bone palpable in the neck above the larynx and below the mandible (lower jaw) with various muscles attached but not articulating with any other bone.

incision. Act of cutting into tissue or an organ.

malignant. Any condition tending to progress toward death, specifically an invasive tumor with a loss of cellular differentiation that has the ability to spread or metastasize to other body areas.

neoplasm. New abnormal growth, tumor.

platysma. Muscle originating from the neck region attached to the mandible that opens the jaw.

resection. Surgical removal of a part or all of an organ or body part.

scar tissue. Fibrous connective tissue that forms around a wounded area or injury, composed mainly of fibroblasts or collagenous fibers.

secondary. Second in order of occurrence or importance, or appearing during the course of another disease or condition.

sternocleidomastoid. Large superficial muscle that passes obliquely across the anterolateral neck, originating at the sternum and clavicle and inserting at the mastoid process of the temporal bone.

thyroidectomy. Partial or complete removal of the thyroid gland.

60270-60271

| 60270 | Thyroidectomy, including substernal thyroid; sternal split or transthoracic approach |
| 60271 | cervical approach |

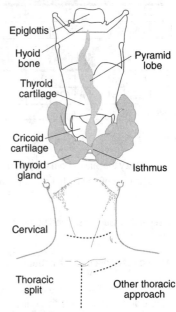

The anatomy of the thyroid varies greatly and in some patients a significant portion, even an entire lobe, may occur in the thoracic region

Explanation

The physician removes the thyroid, including the substernal thyroid gland. The physician exposes the thyroid via sternal split/transthoracic approach in 60270 or via a transverse cervical incision in the skin line in 60271. The platysmas are divided and the strap muscles separated in the midline. The thyroid gland is mobilized and the superior and inferior thyroid vessels are ligated. The parathyroid glands are preserved and the thyroid is resected free of the trachea and removed. Any substernal thyroid is bluntly dissected. Upper sternal incision may be necessary for complete excision of substernal thyroid. The platysmas and skin are closed. Report 60271 for cervical approach.

Coding Tips

When these codes are performed with another separately identifiable procedure, the highest dollar value code is listed as the primary procedure and subsequent procedures are appended with modifier 51. Parathyroidectomy or exploration of the parathyroid, with mediastinal exploration, sternal split or transthoracic approach, is reported with 60505. Parathyroid autotransplantation is reported with 60512, when performed.

ICD-10-CM Diagnostic Codes

C73	Malignant neoplasm of thyroid gland
C79.89	Secondary malignant neoplasm of other specified sites
D09.3	Carcinoma in situ of thyroid and other endocrine glands
D09.8	Carcinoma in situ of other specified sites
D34	Benign neoplasm of thyroid gland
D44.0	Neoplasm of uncertain behavior of thyroid gland
E01.0	Iodine-deficiency related diffuse (endemic) goiter
E04.0	Nontoxic diffuse goiter
E04.1	Nontoxic single thyroid nodule

E04.2	Nontoxic multinodular goiter
E04.8	Other specified nontoxic goiter
E05.00	Thyrotoxicosis with diffuse goiter without thyrotoxic crisis or storm
E05.01	Thyrotoxicosis with diffuse goiter with thyrotoxic crisis or storm
E05.10	Thyrotoxicosis with toxic single thyroid nodule without thyrotoxic crisis or storm
E05.11	Thyrotoxicosis with toxic single thyroid nodule with thyrotoxic crisis or storm
E05.20	Thyrotoxicosis with toxic multinodular goiter without thyrotoxic crisis or storm
E05.21	Thyrotoxicosis with toxic multinodular goiter with thyrotoxic crisis or storm
E05.30	Thyrotoxicosis from ectopic thyroid tissue without thyrotoxic crisis or storm

AMA: 60270 2018,Jan,8; 2017,Jan,8; 2016,Jan,13; 2015,Jan,16 **60271** 2020,Aug,14; 2018,Jan,8; 2017,Jan,8; 2016,Jan,13; 2015,Jan,16

Relative Value Units/Medicare Edits

Non-Facility RVU	Work	PE	MP	Total
60270	23.2	12.34	4.5	40.04
60271	17.62	10.02	3.27	30.91
Facility RVU	Work	PE	MP	Total
60270	23.2	12.34	4.5	40.04
60271	17.62	10.02	3.27	30.91

	FUD	Status	MUE	Modifiers				IOM Reference
60270	90	A	1(2)	51	N/A	62*	80	None
60271	90	A	1(2)	51	N/A	62*	80	

* with documentation

Terms To Know

closure. Repairing an incision or wound by suture or other means.

dissect. Cut apart or separate tissue for surgical purposes or for visual or microscopic study.

goiter. Abnormal enlargement of the thyroid gland commonly caused by a deficiency of dietary iodine.

ligation. Tying off a blood vessel or duct with a suture or a soft, thin wire.

platysma. Muscle originating from the neck region attached to the mandible that opens the jaw.

resection. Surgical removal of a part or all of an organ or body part.

thyroidectomy. Partial or complete removal of the thyroid gland.

thyrotoxicosis. Excessive quantities of hormones from the thyroid gland caused by overproduction or loss of storage ability.

total thyroidectomy. Excision of both lobes.

transverse. Crosswise at right angles to the long axis of a structure or part.

60280-60281

| 60280 | Excision of thyroglossal duct cyst or sinus; |
| 60281 | recurrent |

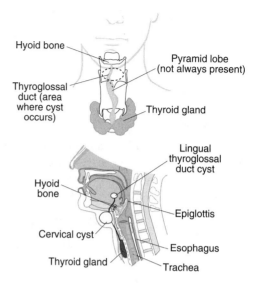

Explanation

The physician excises a thyroglossal duct cyst or sinus. The physician circumferentially incises the skin around the cyst or sinus and extends the incision along the tract to its origin. The midpart of the hyoid bone is excised. The wound is packed and allowed to heal by secondary intention. Report 60281 if thyroglossal duct cyst or sinus is recurrent.

Coding Tips

For incision and drainage of an infected thyroglossal cyst, see 60000. For aspiration and/or injection of a thyroid cyst, see 60300. For excision of a thyroid cyst or adenoma or transection of isthmus, see 60200. For diagnostic thyroid ultrasonography, see 76536.

ICD-10-CM Diagnostic Codes

| Q89.2 | Congenital malformations of other endocrine glands |

AMA: 60280 2014,Jan,11 **60281** 2014,Jan,11

Relative Value Units/Medicare Edits

Non-Facility RVU	Work	PE	MP	Total
60280	6.16	6.08	0.91	13.15
60281	8.82	7.24	1.21	17.27
Facility RVU	Work	PE	MP	Total
60280	6.16	6.08	0.91	13.15
60281	8.82	7.24	1.21	17.27

	FUD	Status	MUE	Modifiers				IOM Reference
60280	90	A	1(3)	51	N/A	62*	80	None
60281	90	A	1(3)	51	N/A	62*	80	

* with documentation

60300

60300   Aspiration and/or injection, thyroid cyst

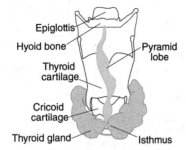

A cyst of the thyroid is aspirated and/or injected

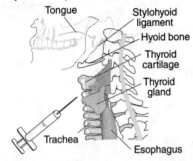

Using anatomical landmarks and/or ultrasound, a
cyst of the thyroid gland is injected and/or aspirated

Explanation

The physician aspirates or injects a thyroid cyst. The physician localizes the
thyroid cyst by palpation or separately reportable ultrasound. A needle is
passed through the skin into the cyst. The cyst is aspirated and tissue captured
is sent for separately reportable analysis, or the cyst is injected with therapeutic
or diagnostic matter.

Coding Tips

For excision of a thyroid cyst or adenoma or transection of isthmus, see 60200.
For fine needle aspiration, see 10004–10012 and 10021. Imaging guidance is
reported with 76942 or 77012, when performed. For diagnostic thyroid
ultrasonography, see 76536.

ICD-10-CM Diagnostic Codes

E04.1   Nontoxic single thyroid nodule

AMA: 60300 2014,Jan,11

Relative Value Units/Medicare Edits

Non-Facility RVU	Work	PE	MP	Total
60300	0.97	2.23	0.1	3.3
Facility RVU	Work	PE	MP	Total
60300	0.97	0.36	0.1	1.43

	FUD	Status	MUE	Modifiers				IOM Reference
60300	0	A	2(3)	51	N/A	N/A	N/A	None

* with documentation

60500	Parathyroidectomy or exploration of parathyroid(s);	
60502	re-exploration	
60505	with mediastinal exploration, sternal split or transthoracic approach	

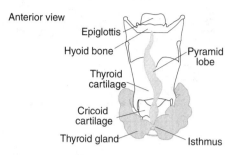

Anterior view

Epiglottis
Hyoid bone
Pyramid lobe
Thyroid cartilage
Cricoid cartilage
Thyroid gland
Isthmus

Posterior view

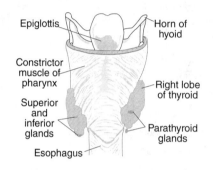

Epiglottis
Horn of hyoid
Constrictor muscle of pharynx
Right lobe of thyroid
Superior and inferior glands
Parathyroid glands
Esophagus

Explanation

The physician removes or explores the parathyroids, glands adjacent to the thyroids. The physician exposes the thyroid via a transverse cervical incision in the skin line (60500), a previous excision (60502) for re-exploration, or a sternal split or transthoracic approach with exploration of the mediastinum (60505). The platysmas are divided and the strap muscles separated in the midline. The parathyroid glands are identified and tissue is excised for separately reportable pathological examination. The parathyroid may be removed; usually a port remains following excision. The platysmas and skin are closed.

Coding Tips

For thyroidectomy with sternal split or transthoracic approach, see 60270; cervical approach, see 60271. Parathyroid autotransplantation is reported with 60512, when performed.

ICD-10-CM Diagnostic Codes

C75.0	Malignant neoplasm of parathyroid gland
D09.3	Carcinoma in situ of thyroid and other endocrine glands
D35.1	Benign neoplasm of parathyroid gland
D44.2	Neoplasm of uncertain behavior of parathyroid gland
D49.7	Neoplasm of unspecified behavior of endocrine glands and other parts of nervous system
E20.0	Idiopathic hypoparathyroidism
E20.1	Pseudohypoparathyroidism
E20.8	Other hypoparathyroidism
E21.0	Primary hyperparathyroidism
E21.1	Secondary hyperparathyroidism, not elsewhere classified
E21.2	Other hyperparathyroidism
E83.51	Hypocalcemia
E83.52	Hypercalcemia
N25.81	Secondary hyperparathyroidism of renal origin

AMA: **60500** 2018,Jan,8; 2017,Jan,8; 2016,Jan,13; 2015,Jan,16 **60502** 2018,Jan,8; 2017,Jan,8; 2016,Jan,13; 2015,Jan,16 **60505** 2018,Jan,8; 2017,Jan,8; 2016,Jan,13; 2015,Jan,16

Relative Value Units/Medicare Edits

Non-Facility RVU	Work	PE	MP	Total
60500	15.6	9.64	3.25	28.49
60502	21.15	12.51	4.49	38.15
60505	23.06	13.43	4.39	40.88
Facility RVU	**Work**	**PE**	**MP**	**Total**
60500	15.6	9.64	3.25	28.49
60502	21.15	12.51	4.49	38.15
60505	23.06	13.43	4.39	40.88

	FUD	Status	MUE	Modifiers				IOM Reference
60500	90	A	1(2)	51	N/A	62*	80	None
60502	90	A	1(3)	51	N/A	62*	80	
60505	90	A	1(3)	51	N/A	62*	80	

* with documentation

Terms To Know

exploration. Examination for diagnostic purposes.

hypercalcemia. Abnormally high levels of calcium in the blood, resulting in symptoms of muscle weakness, fatigue, nausea, depression, and constipation.

malignant neoplasm. Any cancerous tumor or lesion exhibiting uncontrolled tissue growth that can progressively invade other parts of the body with its disease-generating cells.

platysma. Muscle originating from the neck region attached to the mandible that opens the jaw.

transverse. Crosswise at right angles to the long axis of a structure or part.

Parathyroid

60520-60522

60520 Thymectomy, partial or total; transcervical approach (separate procedure)

60521 sternal split or transthoracic approach, without radical mediastinal dissection (separate procedure)

60522 sternal split or transthoracic approach, with radical mediastinal dissection (separate procedure)

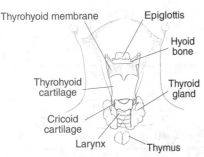

The thymus is removed, either partially or in total. A radical dissection of the mediastinum may be performed

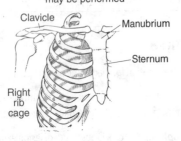

Explanation

The physician removes part or all of the thymus gland. The physician exposes the thymus via a cervical incision in the skin line in 60520. The sternum is retracted and strap muscles separated. The superior lobe of the thymus is separated from the inferior aspect of the thyroid. The blood supply to the thymus is divided and the thymus is dissected free from the pericardium and removed. The incision is closed. Report 60521 if performed with a sternal split or transthoracic approach without radical mediastinal dissection; report 60522 if performed with a sternal split or transthoracic approach, with radical mediastinal dissection.

Coding Tips

These separate procedures by definition are usually a component of a more complex service and are not identified separately. When performed alone or with other unrelated procedures/services they may be reported. If performed alone, list the code; if performed with other procedures/services, list the code and append modifier 59 or an X{EPSU} modifier. Report thoracoscopic (VATS) thymectomy with code 32673.

ICD-10-CM Diagnostic Codes

C37	Malignant neoplasm of thymus
C7A.091	Malignant carcinoid tumor of the thymus
D15.0	Benign neoplasm of thymus
D38.4	Neoplasm of uncertain behavior of thymus
D3A.091	Benign carcinoid tumor of the thymus
D49.7	Neoplasm of unspecified behavior of endocrine glands and other parts of nervous system
D49.89	Neoplasm of unspecified behavior of other specified sites

G70.01	Myasthenia gravis with (acute) exacerbation
Q89.2	Congenital malformations of other endocrine glands

AMA: **60520** 2019,Mar,10 **60521** 2018,Jan,8; 2017,Jan,8; 2016,Jan,13; 2015,Jan,16

Relative Value Units/Medicare Edits

Non-Facility RVU	Work	PE	MP	Total
60520	17.16	9.81	3.84	30.81
60521	19.18	9.29	4.38	32.85
60522	23.48	11.24	5.33	40.05
Facility RVU	Work	PE	MP	Total
60520	17.16	9.81	3.84	30.81
60521	19.18	9.29	4.38	32.85
60522	23.48	11.24	5.33	40.05

	FUD	Status	MUE	Modifiers				IOM Reference
60520	90	A	1(2)	51	N/A	62*	80	None
60521	90	A	1(2)	51	N/A	62*	80	
60522	90	A	1(2)	51	N/A	62*	80	

* with documentation

Terms To Know

epiglottis. Lid-like cartilaginous tissue that covers the entrance to the larynx and blocks food from entering the trachea.

lymph nodes. Bean-shaped structures along the lymphatic vessels that intercept and destroy foreign materials in the tissue and bloodstream.

myasthenia gravis. Autoimmune neuromuscular disorder caused by antibodies to the acetylcholine receptors at the neuromuscular junction, interfering with proper binding of the neurotransmitter from the neuron to the target muscle, causing muscle weakness, fatigue, and exhaustion, without pain or atrophy.

pericardium. Thin and slippery case in which the heart lies that is lined with fluid so that the heart is free to pulse and move as it beats.

radical. Extensive surgery.

thymus. Lymphoid organ located in the front of the upper mediastinum, composed of two symmetrical pyramid-shaped lobes, that is the site where T-lymphocytes are produced.

60540-60545

60540 Adrenalectomy, partial or complete, or exploration of adrenal gland with or without biopsy, transabdominal, lumbar or dorsal (separate procedure);

60545 with excision of adjacent retroperitoneal tumor

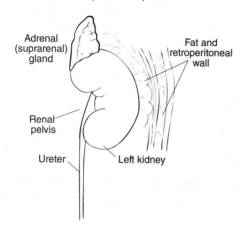

Adrenal (suprarenal) gland

Fat and retroperitoneal wall

Renal pelvis

Ureter

Left kidney

Explanation

The physician removes part or all of the adrenal gland with or without biopsy. The physician exposes the adrenal gland via an upper anterior midline abdominal or posterior incision. The retroperitoneal space is explored. The capsule of the kidney is incised and the adrenal capsule is opened. Blood supply to the adrenal gland is ligated and the gland is removed. The physician may remove tissue from the site for separately reportable pathological study. The physician closes the incision with sutures. Report 60545 if this procedure is performed with excision of an adjacent retroperitoneal tumor.

Coding Tips

These separate procedures by definition are usually a component of a more complex service and are not identified separately. When performed alone or with other unrelated procedures/services they may be reported. If performed alone, list the code; if performed with other procedures/services, list the code and append modifier 59 or an X{EPSU} modifier. Code 60540 is a unilateral procedure. If performed bilaterally, some payers require that the service be reported twice with modifier 50 appended to the second code while others require identification of the service only once with modifier 50 appended. Check with individual payers. Modifier 50 identifies a procedure performed identically on the opposite side of the body (mirror image). Do not report these codes with 50323. For excision of remote or disseminated pheochromocytoma, see 49203–49205. For a laparoscopic approach, see 60650.

ICD-10-CM Diagnostic Codes

C74.01	Malignant neoplasm of cortex of right adrenal gland ☑
C74.02	Malignant neoplasm of cortex of left adrenal gland ☑
C74.11	Malignant neoplasm of medulla of right adrenal gland ☑
C74.12	Malignant neoplasm of medulla of left adrenal gland ☑
C79.71	Secondary malignant neoplasm of right adrenal gland ☑
C79.72	Secondary malignant neoplasm of left adrenal gland ☑
D09.3	Carcinoma in situ of thyroid and other endocrine glands
D35.01	Benign neoplasm of right adrenal gland ☑
D35.02	Benign neoplasm of left adrenal gland ☑
D44.11	Neoplasm of uncertain behavior of right adrenal gland ☑
D44.12	Neoplasm of uncertain behavior of left adrenal gland ☑
D49.7	Neoplasm of unspecified behavior of endocrine glands and other parts of nervous system
E24.3	Ectopic ACTH syndrome
E24.8	Other Cushing's syndrome
E25.0	Congenital adrenogenital disorders associated with enzyme deficiency
E26.01	Conn's syndrome
E26.02	Glucocorticoid-remediable aldosteronism
E26.09	Other primary hyperaldosteronism
E27.0	Other adrenocortical overactivity
E27.1	Primary adrenocortical insufficiency
E27.2	Addisonian crisis
E27.3	Drug-induced adrenocortical insufficiency
E27.49	Other adrenocortical insufficiency
E27.5	Adrenomedullary hyperfunction
E27.8	Other specified disorders of adrenal gland

AMA: 60540 2014,Jan,11 **60545** 2014,Jan,11

Relative Value Units/Medicare Edits

Non-Facility RVU	Work	PE	MP	Total
60540	18.02	10.01	3.6	31.63
60545	20.93	11.22	4.43	36.58
Facility RVU	Work	PE	MP	Total
60540	18.02	10.01	3.6	31.63
60545	20.93	11.22	4.43	36.58

	FUD	Status	MUE	Modifiers				IOM Reference
60540	90	A	1(2)	51	50	62*	80	None
60545	90	A	1(2)	51	50	62*	80	

* with documentation

Terms To Know

adrenal gland. Specialized group of secretory cells located above the kidneys that produce hormones that regulate the metabolism, maintain fluid balance, and control blood pressure. The adrenal glands also produce slight amounts of androgens, estrogens, and progesterone.

adrenogenital disorders. Congenital or acquired disorders of the genitals due to adrenal dysfunction.

hyperaldosteronism. Oversecretion of aldosterone causing electrolyte balance problems, fluid retention, and hypertension.

tumor. Pathological swelling or enlargement; a neoplastic growth of uncontrolled, abnormal multiplication of cells.

Parathyroid

60600-60605

60600 Excision of carotid body tumor; without excision of carotid artery
60605　　with excision of carotid artery

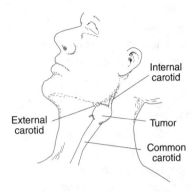

Schematic showing tumor at
bifurcation of carotid artery

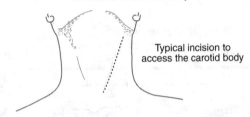

Typical incision to
access the carotid body

Explanation

This physician removes a tumor from a small epithelioid structure (carotid body) just above the bifurcation of the carotid. The physician exposes the carotid body via an incision anterior to the sternocleidomastoid. After dissection down to the carotid sheath, the vein is retracted and the carotid bifurcation exposed. The blood supply to the tumor is ligated and the tumor resected. The incision is closed. Report 60605 if the carotid body tumor excision is performed with excision of the carotid artery.

Coding Tips

When these codes are performed with another separately identifiable procedure, the highest dollar value code is listed as the primary procedure and subsequent procedures are appended with modifier 51.

ICD-10-CM Diagnostic Codes

C75.4	Malignant neoplasm of carotid body
C79.89	Secondary malignant neoplasm of other specified sites
D35.5	Benign neoplasm of carotid body
D44.6	Neoplasm of uncertain behavior of carotid body
D49.7	Neoplasm of unspecified behavior of endocrine glands and other parts of nervous system

AMA: **60605** 2018,Sep,9; 2017,Sep,13; 2016,Sep,8; 2016,Oct,10; 2016,Nov,8; 2016,Jul,10

Relative Value Units/Medicare Edits

Non-Facility RVU	Work	PE	MP	Total
60600	25.09	9.33	5.4	39.82
60605	31.96	8.56	7.73	48.25
Facility RVU	**Work**	**PE**	**MP**	**Total**
60600	25.09	9.33	5.4	39.82
60605	31.96	8.56	7.73	48.25

	FUD	Status	MUE	Modifiers				IOM Reference
60600	90	A	1(3)	51	N/A	62*	80	100-03,20.18
60605	90	A	1(3)	51	N/A	62*	80	

* with documentation

Terms To Know

benign. Mild or nonmalignant in nature.

bifurcated. Having two branches or divisions, such as the left pulmonary veins that split off from the left atrium to carry oxygenated blood away from the heart.

carotid bodies. Small, oval nodules of highly neurovascular structure located at the fork of the carotid arteries. The carotid bodies monitor the oxygen content of the blood and help regulate respiration, blood pressure, and heart rate in response to changes in hydrogen and carbon dioxide levels.

carotid body tumor. Benign growth that forms at the fork of the common carotid artery causing symptoms such as dizziness due to its effect on carotid body functions.

dissection. Separating by cutting tissue or body structures apart.

epithelial tissue. Cells arranged in sheets that cover internal and external body surfaces that can absorb, protect, and/or secrete and includes the protective covering for external surfaces (skin), absorptive linings for internal surfaces such as the intestine, and secreting structures such as salivary or sweat glands.

ligation. Tying off a blood vessel or duct with a suture or a soft, thin wire.

malignant neoplasm. Any cancerous tumor or lesion exhibiting uncontrolled tissue growth that can progressively invade other parts of the body with its disease-generating cells.

resection. Surgical removal of a part or all of an organ or body part.

retraction. Act of holding tissue or a structure back away from its normal position or the field of interest.

secondary. Second in order of occurrence or importance, or appearing during the course of another disease or condition.

sternocleidomastoid. Large superficial muscle that passes obliquely across the anterolateral neck, originating at the sternum and clavicle and inserting at the mastoid process of the temporal bone.

tumor. Pathological swelling or enlargement; a neoplastic growth of uncontrolled, abnormal multiplication of cells.

Parathyroid

60650

60650 Laparoscopy, surgical, with adrenalectomy, partial or complete, or exploration of adrenal gland with or without biopsy, transabdominal, lumbar or dorsal

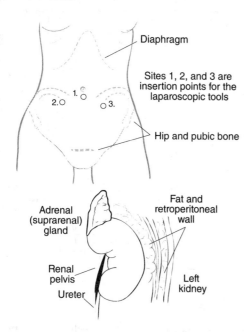

Explanation

The physician performs a laparoscopic excision (removal) of the adrenal gland, or performs and laparoscopic exploration of the adrenal gland through the abdomen or back. In the abdominal approach, a trocar is placed at the level of the umbilicus and the abdomen is insufflated. The laparoscope is placed through the umbilical port and additional trocars are placed into the abdominal cavity as needed. In the back approach, the trocar is placed at the back proximal to the retroperitoneal space superior to the kidney, adjacent to the adrenal gland. The physician uses the laparoscope fitted with a fiberoptic camera and/or an operating tool to explore, biopsy, or removal of all or part of the adrenal gland. The abdomen is the deflated, the trocars are removed and the incisions are closed with sutures.

Coding Tips

Surgical laparoscopy always includes diagnostic laparoscopy. Diagnostic laparoscopy alone is reported with 49320. For open approach, see 60540–60545.

ICD-10-CM Diagnostic Codes

C74.01	Malignant neoplasm of cortex of right adrenal gland ☑
C74.02	Malignant neoplasm of cortex of left adrenal gland ☑
C74.11	Malignant neoplasm of medulla of right adrenal gland ☑
C74.12	Malignant neoplasm of medulla of left adrenal gland ☑
C79.71	Secondary malignant neoplasm of right adrenal gland ☑
C79.72	Secondary malignant neoplasm of left adrenal gland ☑
D09.3	Carcinoma in situ of thyroid and other endocrine glands
D35.01	Benign neoplasm of right adrenal gland ☑
D35.02	Benign neoplasm of left adrenal gland ☑
D44.11	Neoplasm of uncertain behavior of right adrenal gland ☑
D44.12	Neoplasm of uncertain behavior of left adrenal gland ☑

D49.7	Neoplasm of unspecified behavior of endocrine glands and other parts of nervous system
E24.0	Pituitary-dependent Cushing's disease
E24.3	Ectopic ACTH syndrome
E24.8	Other Cushing's syndrome
E25.0	Congenital adrenogenital disorders associated with enzyme deficiency
E26.01	Conn's syndrome
E26.02	Glucocorticoid-remediable aldosteronism
E26.09	Other primary hyperaldosteronism
E27.0	Other adrenocortical overactivity
E27.1	Primary adrenocortical insufficiency
E27.2	Addisonian crisis
E27.3	Drug-induced adrenocortical insufficiency
E27.49	Other adrenocortical insufficiency
E27.5	Adrenomedullary hyperfunction
E27.8	Other specified disorders of adrenal gland

AMA: **60650** 2018,Jan,8; 2017,Jan,8; 2016,Jan,13; 2015,Jan,16

Relative Value Units/Medicare Edits

Non-Facility RVU	Work	PE	MP	Total
60650	20.73	10.12	4.18	35.03
Facility RVU	**Work**	**PE**	**MP**	**Total**
60650	20.73	10.12	4.18	35.03

	FUD	Status	MUE	Modifiers				IOM Reference
60650	90	A	1(2)	51	50	62*	80	None

* with documentation

Terms To Know

adrenal gland. Specialized group of secretory cells located above the kidneys that produce hormones that regulate the metabolism, maintain fluid balance, and control blood pressure. The adrenal glands also produce slight amounts of androgens, estrogens, and progesterone.

adrenogenital disorders. Congenital or acquired disorders of the genitals due to adrenal dysfunction.

corticoadrenal insufficiency. Underproduction of the adrenal hormones, aldosterone and cortisol, causing low blood pressure, weight loss, weakness, and anemia.

hyperaldosteronism. Oversecretion of aldosterone causing electrolyte balance problems, fluid retention, and hypertension.

64486-64489

AMA: **64486** 2018,Jan,8; 2017,Jan,8; 2016,Jan,13; 2015,Jun,3 **64487** 2018,Jan,8; 2017,Jan,8; 2016,Jan,13; 2015,Jun,3 **64488** 2018,Jan,8; 2017,Jan,8; 2016,Jan,13; 2015,Jun,3 **64489** 2018,Jan,8; 2017,Jan,8; 2016,Jan,13; 2015,Jun,3

64486	Transversus abdominis plane (TAP) block (abdominal plane block, rectus sheath block) unilateral; by injection(s) (includes imaging guidance, when performed)		
64487		by continuous infusion(s) (includes imaging guidance, when performed)	
64488	Transversus abdominis plane (TAP) block (abdominal plane block, rectus sheath block) bilateral; by injections (includes imaging guidance, when performed)		
64489		by continuous infusions (includes imaging guidance, when performed)	

Relative Value Units/Medicare Edits

Non-Facility RVU	Work	PE	MP	Total
64486	1.27	1.98	0.11	3.36
64487	1.48	4.57	0.13	6.18
64488	1.6	2.41	0.13	4.14
64489	1.8	7.92	0.15	9.87

Facility RVU	Work	PE	MP	Total
64486	1.27	0.25	0.11	1.63
64487	1.48	0.27	0.13	1.88
64488	1.6	0.29	0.13	2.02
64489	1.8	0.32	0.15	2.27

	FUD	Status	MUE	Modifiers				IOM Reference
64486	0	A	1(3)	51	50	N/A	N/A	None
64487	0	A	1(2)	51	50	N/A	N/A	
64488	0	A	1(3)	51	N/A	N/A	N/A	
64489	0	A	1(2)	51	N/A	N/A	N/A	

* with documentation

Terms To Know

analgesia. Absence of a normal sense of pain without loss of consciousness.

catheter. Flexible tube inserted into an area of the body for introducing or withdrawing fluid.

imaging. Radiologic means of producing pictures for clinical study of the internal structures and functions of the body, such as x-ray, ultrasound, magnetic resonance, or positron emission tomography.

infusion. Introduction of a therapeutic fluid, other than blood, into the bloodstream.

injection. Forcing a liquid substance into a body part such as a joint or muscle.

local anesthesia. Induced loss of feeling or sensation restricted to a certain area of the body, including topical, local tissue infiltration, field block, or nerve block methods.

transverse. Crosswise at right angles to the long axis of a structure or part.

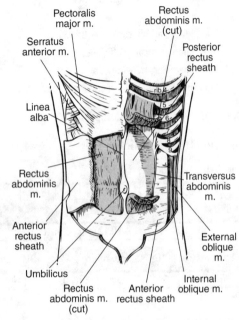

Pectoralis major m.
Rectus abdominis m. (cut)
Serratus anterior m.
Posterior rectus sheath
rib 4
5
6
Linea alba
Rectus abdominis m.
Transversus abdominis m.
Anterior rectus sheath
External oblique m.
Umbilicus
Internal oblique m.
Rectus abdominis m. (cut)
Anterior rectus sheath

Anterior abdominal wall muscles

Explanation

The transversus abdominis plane (TAP) block is a relatively new regional anesthesia technique with a high margin of safety and is technically simple to perform. The physician injects a local anesthetic in the space between the aponeurosis of the internal oblique and transversus abdominis muscles to anesthetize the nerves that supply the anterior abdominal wall (T6–L1) for postoperative pain control in a wide variety of abdominal procedures, including large bowel resection, open/laparoscopic appendectomy, cesarean section, total abdominal hysterectomy, laparoscopic cholecystectomy, open prostatectomy, renal transplant surgery, abdominoplasty with/without flank liposuction, iliac crest bone graft, and inguinal hernia repairs. This technique is also useful for procedures in which epidural analgesia is contraindicated (e.g., anticoagulated patients). For prolonged analgesia, continuous infusions via a catheter may also be performed. Imaging guidance, when performed, is included in these services. Report 64486 for a unilateral TAP, by injection; 64487 for a unilateral TAP, continuous infusion; 64488 for a bilateral TAP, by injection; and 64489 for a bilateral TAP, continuous infusion.

Coding Tips

For injection of an anesthetic agent or steroid, transforaminal epidural, with imaging guidance, see 64479–64480 and 64483–64484.

ICD-10-CM Diagnostic Codes

G89.18	Other acute postprocedural pain
G89.28	Other chronic postprocedural pain

Extracranial Nerves

64590

64590 Insertion or replacement of peripheral or gastric neurostimulator pulse generator or receiver, direct or inductive coupling

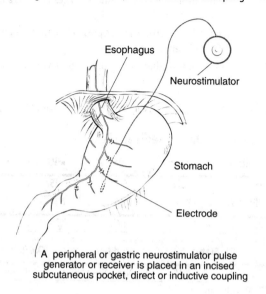

Esophagus

Neurostimulator

Stomach

Electrode

A peripheral or gastric neurostimulator pulse generator or receiver is placed in an incised subcutaneous pocket, direct or inductive coupling

Explanation

The physician inserts or replaces a peripheral or gastric neurostimulator pulse generator or receiver into a subcutaneous pocket. Peripheral neurostimulators are used to transmit electrical impulses to nerves outside of the brain or spinal cord, such as the sacral nerve to help the bladder muscles contract and treat cases of urinary incontinence or retention, or for pain relief. Gastric neurostimulators transmit electrical impulses in the same way, to treat nausea and vomiting in patients with gastroparesis. The physician selects a location site, usually the abdominal area, and incises the skin. Using blunt dissection, the physician creates a pocket for the generator or receiver. The unit is connected to a previously placed electrode, which is separately implanted to stimulate the target nerve. After ensuring that the device is functioning, the generator or receiver is sutured into place within its subcutaneous pocket.

Coding Tips

For revision or removal of peripheral or gastric neurostimulator pulse generator or receiver, see 64595; peripheral neurostimulator electrodes, see 64585. Do not report 64590 with 64595.

ICD-10-CM Diagnostic Codes

K31.84	Gastroparesis
T85.111A	Breakdown (mechanical) of implanted electronic neurostimulator of peripheral nerve electrode (lead), initial encounter
T85.113A	Breakdown (mechanical) of implanted electronic neurostimulator, generator, initial encounter
T85.121A	Displacement of implanted electronic neurostimulator of peripheral nerve electrode (lead), initial encounter
T85.123A	Displacement of implanted electronic neurostimulator, generator, initial encounter
T85.191A	Other mechanical complication of implanted electronic neurostimulator of peripheral nerve electrode (lead), initial encounter
T85.193A	Other mechanical complication of implanted electronic neurostimulator, generator, initial encounter
T85.628A	Displacement of other specified internal prosthetic devices, implants and grafts, initial encounter
T85.638A	Leakage of other specified internal prosthetic devices, implants and grafts, initial encounter
T85.732A	Infection and inflammatory reaction due to implanted electronic neurostimulator of peripheral nerve, electrode (lead), initial encounter
T85.738A	Infection and inflammatory reaction due to other nervous system device, implant or graft, initial encounter
T85.79XA	Infection and inflammatory reaction due to other internal prosthetic devices, implants and grafts, initial encounter
T85.830A	Hemorrhage due to nervous system prosthetic devices, implants and grafts, initial encounter
T85.840A	Pain due to nervous system prosthetic devices, implants and grafts, initial encounter
T85.848A	Pain due to other internal prosthetic devices, implants and grafts, initial encounter

AMA: 64590 2019,Feb,6; 2018,Jan,8; 2018,Aug,10; 2017,Jan,8; 2017,Dec,13; 2016,Jan,13; 2015,Jan,13; 2015,Jan,16

Relative Value Units/Medicare Edits

Non-Facility RVU	Work	PE	MP	Total
64590	2.45	5.24	0.34	8.03
Facility RVU	**Work**	**PE**	**MP**	**Total**
64590	2.45	1.92	0.34	4.71

	FUD	Status	MUE	Modifiers				IOM Reference
64590	10	A	1(3)	51	N/A	62*	N/A	100-04,32,40.1

* with documentation

Terms To Know

gastroparesis. Delay in the emptying of food from the stomach into the small bowel due to a degree of paralysis in the muscles lining the stomach wall.

incontinence. Inability to control urination or defecation.

peripheral. Outside of a structure or organ.

subcutaneous pocket. Small space created under the skin in a suitable location for holding an implantable device, such as the pulse generator of a pacemaker or cardioverter defibrillator.

64595

64595   Revision or removal of peripheral or gastric neurostimulator pulse generator or receiver

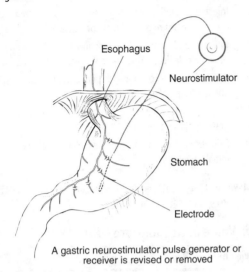

Esophagus

Neurostimulator

Stomach

Electrode

A gastric neurostimulator pulse generator or receiver is revised or removed

Explanation

The physician revises or removes a peripheral or gastric neurostimulator pulse generator or receiver with or without replacement. The placement incision is reopened, and tissues are dissected to the transmitter pocket. If the procedure is performed because the device is malfunctioning, the unit is checked and repairs are made. If the device is no longer required, it is removed. The incision is closed in layered sutures. This code applies to both simple and complex neurostimulators and includes test stimulations and electronic analysis.

Coding Tips

For revision or removal of peripheral neurostimulator electrodes, see 64585. Do not report 64595 with 64590.

ICD-10-CM Diagnostic Codes

T85.111A	Breakdown (mechanical) of implanted electronic neurostimulator of peripheral nerve electrode (lead), initial encounter
T85.113A	Breakdown (mechanical) of implanted electronic neurostimulator, generator, initial encounter
T85.121A	Displacement of implanted electronic neurostimulator of peripheral nerve electrode (lead), initial encounter
T85.123A	Displacement of implanted electronic neurostimulator, generator, initial encounter
T85.191A	Other mechanical complication of implanted electronic neurostimulator of peripheral nerve electrode (lead), initial encounter
T85.193A	Other mechanical complication of implanted electronic neurostimulator, generator, initial encounter
T85.628A	Displacement of other specified internal prosthetic devices, implants and grafts, initial encounter
T85.638A	Leakage of other specified internal prosthetic devices, implants and grafts, initial encounter
T85.732A	Infection and inflammatory reaction due to implanted electronic neurostimulator of peripheral nerve, electrode (lead), initial encounter
T85.738A	Infection and inflammatory reaction due to other nervous system device, implant or graft, initial encounter
T85.79XA	Infection and inflammatory reaction due to other internal prosthetic devices, implants and grafts, initial encounter
T85.840A	Pain due to nervous system prosthetic devices, implants and grafts, initial encounter
T85.848A	Pain due to other internal prosthetic devices, implants and grafts, initial encounter
T85.850A	Stenosis due to nervous system prosthetic devices, implants and grafts, initial encounter
T85.858A	Stenosis due to other internal prosthetic devices, implants and grafts, initial encounter

AMA: 64595 2019,Feb,6; 2018,Jan,8; 2017,Jan,8; 2016,Jan,13; 2015,Jan,16

Relative Value Units/Medicare Edits

Non-Facility RVU	Work	PE	MP	Total
64595	1.78	5.14	0.25	7.17
Facility RVU	**Work**	**PE**	**MP**	**Total**
64595	1.78	1.69	0.25	3.72

	FUD	Status	MUE	Modifiers			IOM Reference
64595	10	A	1(3)	51	N/A	N/A	N/A	None

* with documentation

Terms To Know

embolism. Obstruction of a blood vessel resulting from a clot or foreign substance.

fibrosis. Formation of fibrous tissue as part of the restorative process.

pulse generator. Circuit used to generate pulses. Pulse generators contain the battery, the electronic circuit, and the connector in a hermetically sealed encasement. Pulse generators may be temporary transcutaneous or placed in a subcutaneous pocket.

Extracranial Nerves

64646-64647

64646 Chemodenervation of trunk muscle(s); 1-5 muscle(s)
64647 6 or more muscles

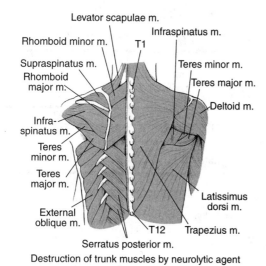
Destruction of trunk muscles by neurolytic agent

Levator scapulae m.
Infraspinatus m.
Rhomboid minor m.
T1
Supraspinatus m.
Teres minor m.
Rhomboid major m.
Teres major m.
Deltoid m.
Infra-spinatus m.
Teres minor m.
Teres major m.
Latissimus dorsi m.
External oblique m.
T12
Trapezius m.
Serratus posterior m.

Explanation

The physician administers a neurotoxin to paralyze dysfunctional muscle tissue in the trunk, including the erector spinae, rectus abdominis, oblique, and paraspinal muscles. Chemodenervation works by introducing a substance used to block the transfer of chemicals at the presynaptic membrane. Botulinum toxin type A (BTX-A, Botox®), phenol (sometimes combined with botulinum toxin type A), and/or ethyl alcohol may be used. The physician identifies the nerve(s) or muscle endplate(s) by direct surgical exposure or through the insertion of an electromyographic needle into the muscle. A small amount of the selected agent is injected into nerve(s) or muscle endplate(s), inducing muscle paralysis. The duration of the effect is variable, usually one to 12 months when phenol or alcohol is used and three to four months when BTX-A is used. BTX-A is dose-dependent and reversible secondary to the regeneration process. Gradually, blocked nerves form new neuromuscular junctions resulting in the return of muscle function. Report 64646 when one to five muscles are treated and 64647 when six or more muscles are treated.

Coding Tips

These codes should only be reported one time per session. If needle electromyography or muscle electrical stimulation is used for guidance in addition to chemodenervation, see 95873–95874. Only one form of guidance may be reported for each chemodenervation performed on the trunk.

ICD-10-CM Diagnostic Codes

G24.1	Genetic torsion dystonia
G24.2	Idiopathic nonfamilial dystonia
G24.8	Other dystonia
G25.89	Other specified extrapyramidal and movement disorders
G35	Multiple sclerosis
G80.0	Spastic quadriplegic cerebral palsy
G80.1	Spastic diplegic cerebral palsy
G80.2	Spastic hemiplegic cerebral palsy
G80.3	Athetoid cerebral palsy
G80.8	Other cerebral palsy
G81.11	Spastic hemiplegia affecting right dominant side ☑
G81.12	Spastic hemiplegia affecting left dominant side ☑
G81.13	Spastic hemiplegia affecting right nondominant side ☑
G81.14	Spastic hemiplegia affecting left nondominant side ☑
G83.81	Brown-Sequard syndrome
G83.82	Anterior cord syndrome
G83.83	Posterior cord syndrome
G83.89	Other specified paralytic syndromes

AMA: **64646** 2019,Apr,9; 2018,Jan,8; 2017,Jan,8; 2016,Jan,13; 2015,Jan,16
64647 2019,Apr,9; 2018,Jan,8; 2017,Jan,8; 2016,Jan,13; 2015,Jan,16

Relative Value Units/Medicare Edits

Non-Facility RVU	Work	PE	MP	Total
64646	1.8	2.39	0.43	4.62
64647	2.11	2.63	0.54	5.28
Facility RVU	**Work**	**PE**	**MP**	**Total**
64646	1.8	1.16	0.43	3.39
64647	2.11	1.27	0.54	3.92

	FUD	Status	MUE	Modifiers				IOM Reference
64646	0	A	1(2)	51	N/A	N/A	N/A	None
64647	0	A	1(2)	51	N/A	N/A	N/A	

* with documentation

Terms To Know

Botox. Trademark preparation of onabotulinumtoxin A or botulinum toxin type A.

chemodenervation. Chemical destruction of nerves. A substance, for example, Botox, is used to temporarily inhibit the transfer of chemicals at the presynaptic membrane, blocking the neuromuscular junctions.

dystonia. Condition characterized by irregular elasticity of muscle tissue.

electromyography. Test that measures muscle response to nerve stimulation determining if muscle weakness is present and if it is related to the muscles themselves or a problem with the nerves that supply the muscles.

injection. Forcing a liquid substance into a body part such as a joint or muscle.

multiple sclerosis. Disorder affecting the central nervous system by decreasing the nerve function and causing inflammation of the nerve covering.

myalgia. Pain in the muscles.

neurolytic. Destruction of nerve tissue.

neuromuscular junction. Nerve synapse at the meeting point between the terminal end of a nerve (motor neuron) and a muscle fiber.

Extracranial Nerves

64719-64721

64719 Neuroplasty and/or transposition; ulnar nerve at wrist
64721 median nerve at carpal tunnel

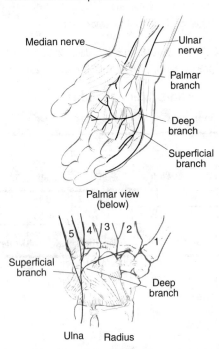

Median nerve
Ulnar nerve
Palmar branch
Deep branch
Superficial branch

Palmar view
(below)

Superficial branch
Deep branch

Ulna   Radius

Explanation

The physician decompresses or transposes a portion of the ulnar or median nerve to restore feeling to the hand. The physician makes a horizontal incision in the wrist at the metacarpal joints and locates the nerve. In 64719, the ulnar nerve is located and freed. In 64721, the median nerve is decompressed by freeing the nerve inside the carpal tunnel. Soft tissues are resected and the nerve is freed from the underlying bed. Care is taken to ensure tension is released and the incision is sutured in layers.

Coding Tips

Neuroplasty includes external neurolysis and transposition. For internal neurolysis requiring the use of an operating microscope, report 64727 in addition to the code for the primary procedure. For carpel tunnel release performed endoscopically, see 29848.

ICD-10-CM Diagnostic Codes

G56.01	Carpal tunnel syndrome, right upper limb ☑
G56.02	Carpal tunnel syndrome, left upper limb ☑
G56.21	Lesion of ulnar nerve, right upper limb ☑
G56.22	Lesion of ulnar nerve, left upper limb ☑
M79.641	Pain in right hand ☑
M79.642	Pain in left hand ☑
M79.644	Pain in right finger(s) ☑
M79.645	Pain in left finger(s) ☑
S64.01XA	Injury of ulnar nerve at wrist and hand level of right arm, initial encounter ☑
S64.02XA	Injury of ulnar nerve at wrist and hand level of left arm, initial encounter ☑
S64.11XA	Injury of median nerve at wrist and hand level of right arm, initial encounter ☑
S64.12XA	Injury of median nerve at wrist and hand level of left arm, initial encounter ☑

AMA: **64719** 2018,Jan,8; 2017,Jan,8; 2016,Jan,13; 2015,Jan,16 **64721** 2018,Jan,8; 2017,Jan,8; 2016,Jan,13; 2015,Jul,10; 2015,Jan,16

Relative Value Units/Medicare Edits

Non-Facility RVU	Work	PE	MP	Total
64719	4.97	6.09	0.92	11.98
64721	4.97	7.12	0.96	13.05
Facility RVU	**Work**	**PE**	**MP**	**Total**
64719	4.97	6.09	0.92	11.98
64721	4.97	6.9	0.96	12.83

	FUD	Status	MUE	Modifiers				IOM Reference
64719	90	A	1(2)	51	50	N/A	N/A	None
64721	90	A	1(2)	51	50	N/A	N/A	

* with documentation

Terms To Know

carpal tunnel syndrome. Swelling and inflammation in the tendons or bursa surrounding the median nerve caused by repetitive activity. The resulting compression on the nerve causes pain, numbness, and tingling especially to the palm, index, middle finger, and thumb.

closure. Repairing an incision or wound by suture or other means.

decompression. Release of pressure.

ganglion. Fluid-filled, benign cyst appearing on a tendon sheath or aponeurosis, frequently connecting to an underlying joint.

mononeuritis. Inflammation of one nerve.

polyneuropathy. Disease process of severe inflammation of multiple nerves.

resection. Surgical removal of a part or all of an organ or body part.

scar tissue. Fibrous connective tissue that forms around a wounded area or injury, composed mainly of fibroblasts or collagenous fibers.

soft tissue. Nonepithelial tissues outside of the skeleton that includes subcutaneous adipose tissue, fibrous tissue, fascia, muscles, blood and lymph vessels, and peripheral nervous system tissue.

transposition. Removal or exchange from one side to another; change of position from one place to another.

64755-64760

64755 Transection or avulsion of; vagus nerves limited to proximal stomach (selective proximal vagotomy, proximal gastric vagotomy, parietal cell vagotomy, supra- or highly selective vagotomy)

64760 vagus nerve (vagotomy), abdominal

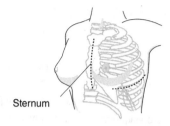

Sternum

Access is by thoracotomy

Trunks of vagus nerve govern gastric functions

Esophagus

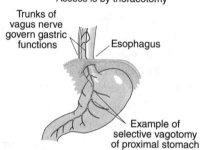

Example of selective vagotomy of proximal stomach

Branches of the vagus nerve serving the proximal stomach are transected or avulsed

Explanation

The physician transects or removes a portion of the vagus nerve. The vagus nerves supplies parasympathetic fibers to the heart and gastrointestinal tract. In 64755, the physician makes a vertical midline epigastric incision and locates specific branches of the vagus nerve responsible for acid production in the stomach. In 64760, the physician makes a vertical midline epigastric incision and locates the vagus nerve. After locating the nerve or nerve branches, the physician transects them. The incision is sutured in layers.

Coding Tips

For injection of an anesthetic agent, vagus nerve, see 64408. For vagotomy including pyloroplasty, with or without gastrostomy, truncal or selective, see 43640; parietal cell (highly selective), see 43641. For laparoscopic transection of the vagus nerve, truncal, see 43651; selective or highly selective, see 43652. For vagotomy when performed with partial distal gastrectomy, see 43635.

ICD-10-CM Diagnostic Codes

K22.10	Ulcer of esophagus without bleeding
K22.11	Ulcer of esophagus with bleeding
K22.70	Barrett's esophagus without dysplasia
K22.710	Barrett's esophagus with low grade dysplasia
K22.711	Barrett's esophagus with high grade dysplasia
K25.4	Chronic or unspecified gastric ulcer with hemorrhage
K25.5	Chronic or unspecified gastric ulcer with perforation
K25.6	Chronic or unspecified gastric ulcer with both hemorrhage and perforation
K25.7	Chronic gastric ulcer without hemorrhage or perforation
K26.4	Chronic or unspecified duodenal ulcer with hemorrhage
K26.5	Chronic or unspecified duodenal ulcer with perforation
K26.6	Chronic or unspecified duodenal ulcer with both hemorrhage and perforation
K26.7	Chronic duodenal ulcer without hemorrhage or perforation
K27.4	Chronic or unspecified peptic ulcer, site unspecified, with hemorrhage
K27.5	Chronic or unspecified peptic ulcer, site unspecified, with perforation
K27.6	Chronic or unspecified peptic ulcer, site unspecified, with both hemorrhage and perforation
K27.7	Chronic peptic ulcer, site unspecified, without hemorrhage or perforation
K28.4	Chronic or unspecified gastrojejunal ulcer with hemorrhage
K28.5	Chronic or unspecified gastrojejunal ulcer with perforation
K28.6	Chronic or unspecified gastrojejunal ulcer with both hemorrhage and perforation
K28.7	Chronic gastrojejunal ulcer without hemorrhage or perforation

AMA: 64755 2018,Jan,8; 2017,Jan,8; 2016,Jan,13; 2015,Jan,16 **64760** 2018,Jan,8; 2017,Jan,8; 2016,Jan,13; 2015,Jan,16

Relative Value Units/Medicare Edits

Non-Facility RVU	Work	PE	MP	Total
64755	15.05	8.56	3.7	27.31
64760	7.59	5.93	1.85	15.37
Facility RVU	**Work**	**PE**	**MP**	**Total**
64755	15.05	8.56	3.7	27.31
64760	7.59	5.93	1.85	15.37

	FUD	Status	MUE	Modifiers			IOM Reference
64755	90	A	1(2)	51	N/A	62*	80	None
64760	90	A	1(2)	51	N/A	62*	80	

* with documentation

Terms To Know

avulsion. Forcible tearing away of a part, by surgical means or traumatic injury.

fistula. Abnormal tube-like passage between two body cavities or organs or from an organ to the outside surface.

motility. Capability of independent, spontaneous movement.

transection. Transverse dissection; to cut across a long axis; cross section.

vagotomy. Division of the vagus nerves, interrupting impulses resulting in lower gastric acid production and hastening gastric emptying. Used in the treatment of chronic gastric, pyloric, and duodenal ulcers that can cause severe pain and difficulties in eating and sleeping.

Extracranial Nerves

91010-91013

91010   Esophageal motility (manometric study of the esophagus and/or gastroesophageal junction) study with interpretation and report;

+   91013   with stimulation or perfusion (eg, stimulant, acid or alkali perfusion) (List separately in addition to code for primary procedure)

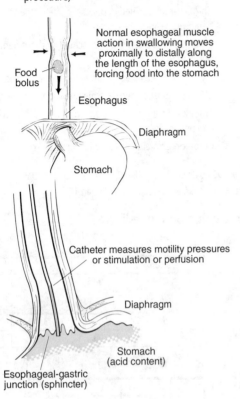

Normal esophageal muscle action in swallowing moves proximally to distally along the length of the esophagus, forcing food into the stomach

Food bolus

Esophagus

Diaphragm

Stomach

Catheter measures motility pressures or stimulation or perfusion

Diaphragm

Stomach (acid content)

Esophageal-gastric junction (sphincter)

Explanation

Esophageal motility studies using a manometer are performed to measure the competency of the lower esophageal sphincter and the muscles of the esophagus. The physician inserts a thin tube with pressure sensors (also called a manometer) into the patient's nose or mouth and down into the stomach to perform an esophageal motility study. In 91010, the muscles of the esophagus and/or the gastroesophageal junction, which propel food and water into the stomach, are studied to measure the pressure of the contraction waves and diagnose abnormalities in the esophageal muscles that affect swallowing. The tube is slowly withdrawn and stopped at different points along the esophagus. The patient is directed to swallow a little amount of water at each stopping point and the contraction wave pressure and swallowing action are measured and graphed. Report 91013 in addition to the motility study code when the motility study is combined with stimulation and/or acid or alkali perfusion. This type of study may be administered to attempt to replicate the type of chest pain a patient has been experiencing by diagnosing the pain as noncardiac, due to esophageal reflux. Using a second catheter inserted through the nares, a probe is placed in the distal esophagus and the perfusion substances are introduced. Commonly, these substances consist of hydrochloric acid and an alternate saline control solution infused one after the other, without the patient being aware of the identity of the solution. The symptoms of chest pain are recorded as the patient identifies them. The patient is again directed to swallow at given intervals in order to record additional pressure measurements. The catheter is removed and the information saved for interpretation.

Coding Tips

Report 91013 in addition to 91010. Report 91013 once per session. For esophageal motility studies with high-resolution esophageal pressure topography, see 91299. For esophagoscopy procedures, see 43180–43232; esophagogastroduodenoscopy, see 43210, 43233, 43235–43259, 43266, and 43270; endoscopy, small intestine, see 44360–44379; and endoscopy, stomal, see 44380–44408.

ICD-10-CM Diagnostic Codes

K20.80	Other esophagitis without bleeding
K20.81	Other esophagitis with bleeding
K21.00	Gastro-esophageal reflux disease with esophagitis, without bleeding
K21.01	Gastro-esophageal reflux disease with esophagitis, with bleeding
K21.9	Gastro-esophageal reflux disease without esophagitis
K22.0	Achalasia of cardia
K22.10	Ulcer of esophagus without bleeding
K22.11	Ulcer of esophagus with bleeding
K22.2	Esophageal obstruction
K22.4	Dyskinesia of esophagus
K22.5	Diverticulum of esophagus, acquired
K22.70	Barrett's esophagus without dysplasia
K22.710	Barrett's esophagus with low grade dysplasia
K22.711	Barrett's esophagus with high grade dysplasia
K22.81	Esophageal polyp
K22.82	Esophagogastric junction polyp
K22.89	Other specified disease of esophagus
R12	Heartburn
R13.11	Dysphagia, oral phase
R13.12	Dysphagia, oropharyngeal phase
R13.13	Dysphagia, pharyngeal phase
R13.14	Dysphagia, pharyngoesophageal phase
R13.19	Other dysphagia

AMA: **91010** 2018,Feb,11 **91013** 2018,Feb,11

Relative Value Units/Medicare Edits

Non-Facility RVU	Work	PE	MP	Total
91010	1.28	5.17	0.07	6.52
91013	0.18	0.59	0.01	0.78
Facility RVU	**Work**	**PE**	**MP**	**Total**
91010	1.28	5.17	0.07	6.52
91013	0.18	0.59	0.01	0.78

	FUD	Status	MUE	Modifiers				IOM Reference
91010	0	A	1(2)	N/A	N/A	N/A	80*	100-03,100.4
91013	N/A	A	1(3)	N/A	N/A	N/A	80*	

* with documentation

Medicine

91020

91020 Gastric motility (manometric) studies

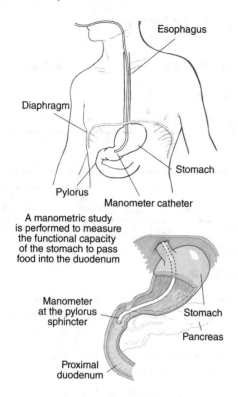

A manometric study is performed to measure the functional capacity of the stomach to pass food into the duodenum

Explanation

The physician inserts a tube with sensors into the patient's nose or mouth and down into the stomach to perform a gastric motility study. The muscles of the stomach and the gastroduodenal junction, which propel food and water into the first part of the small intestines, are studied to measure the pressure of the contraction waves and diagnose abnormalities in the muscle that affect digestion. Sensors on the tube measure the amount of pressure generated by the stomach muscles as food is moved into the small intestine. The tighter the muscles contract around the tube, the greater pressure that is sensed. The data is recorded for computer analysis.

Coding Tips

For a duodenal motility (manometric) study, see 91022. Fluoroscopy is reported with 76000, when performed. For a diagnostic esophagogastroduodenoscopy, see 43235. Do not report 91020 with 91112.

ICD-10-CM Diagnostic Codes

K30	Functional dyspepsia
K31.0	Acute dilatation of stomach
K31.1	Adult hypertrophic pyloric stenosis ◪
K31.2	Hourglass stricture and stenosis of stomach
K31.3	Pylorospasm, not elsewhere classified
K31.4	Gastric diverticulum
K31.84	Gastroparesis
K31.89	Other diseases of stomach and duodenum
K59.01	Slow transit constipation
K59.02	Outlet dysfunction constipation
K59.09	Other constipation
K59.81	Ogilvie syndrome

K92.81	Gastrointestinal mucositis (ulcerative)
R11.0	Nausea
R11.11	Vomiting without nausea
R11.12	Projectile vomiting

AMA: 91020 2018,Jan,8; 2018,Feb,11; 2017,Jan,8; 2016,Jan,13; 2015,Jan,16

Relative Value Units/Medicare Edits

Non-Facility RVU	Work	PE	MP	Total
91020	1.44	6.76	0.07	8.27
Facility RVU	**Work**	**PE**	**MP**	**Total**
91020	1.44	6.76	0.07	8.27

	FUD	Status	MUE	Modifiers				IOM Reference
91020	0	A	1(2)	N/A	N/A	N/A	80*	100-03,100.4

* with documentation

Terms To Know

achalasia. Failure of the smooth muscles within the gastrointestinal tract to relax at points of junction; most commonly referring to the esophagogastric sphincter's failure to relax when swallowing.

digestion. Mechanical, chemical, and enzymatic process converting ingested food into a substance that can be used for synthesis of tissues or release of energy.

dyspepsia. Epigastric discomfort after eating, due to impaired digestive function.

manometric. Pertaining to pressure, as measured in a meter.

motility. Capability of independent, spontaneous movement.

Ogilvie's syndrome. Colonic obstruction with symptoms of persistent contraction of intestinal musculature, caused by a defect in the sympathetic nerve supply.

stenosis. Narrowing or constriction of a passage.

stricture. Narrowing of an anatomical structure.

Medicine

91022

91022 Duodenal motility (manometric) study

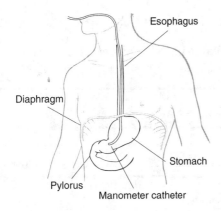

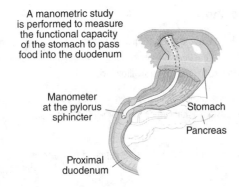

A manometric study is performed to measure the functional capacity of the stomach to pass food into the duodenum

Explanation

The physician inserts a tube with sensors into the patient's nose or mouth and down into the duodenum to perform a duodenal motility study. The muscles of the duodenum and the gastroduodenal junction, which propel food and water into the first part of the small intestines, are studied to measure the pressure of the contraction waves and diagnose abnormalities in the muscle that affect digestion. Sensors on the tube measure the amount of pressure generated by the duodenal muscles as food is moved into the small intestine. The tighter the muscles contract around the tube, the greater pressure that is sensed. The data is recorded for computer analysis.

Coding Tips

For a gastric motility study, see 91020. Fluoroscopy is reported with 76000, when performed. For diagnostic esophagogastroduodenoscopy, see 43235. Do not report 91022 with 91112.

ICD-10-CM Diagnostic Codes

K30	Functional dyspepsia
K31.0	Acute dilatation of stomach
K31.1	Adult hypertrophic pyloric stenosis ▲
K31.2	Hourglass stricture and stenosis of stomach
K31.3	Pylorospasm, not elsewhere classified
K31.4	Gastric diverticulum
K31.5	Obstruction of duodenum
K31.84	Gastroparesis
K31.89	Other diseases of stomach and duodenum
K59.01	Slow transit constipation
K59.02	Outlet dysfunction constipation
K59.04	Chronic idiopathic constipation
K59.09	Other constipation
K92.81	Gastrointestinal mucositis (ulcerative)
R11.0	Nausea
R11.11	Vomiting without nausea
R11.12	Projectile vomiting

AMA: 91022 2018,Jan,8; 2018,Feb,11; 2017,Jan,8; 2016,Jan,13; 2015,Jan,16

Relative Value Units/Medicare Edits

Non-Facility RVU	Work	PE	MP	Total
91022	1.44	3.64	0.06	5.14
Facility RVU	**Work**	**PE**	**MP**	**Total**
91022	1.44	3.64	0.06	5.14

	FUD	Status	MUE	Modifiers				IOM Reference
91022	0	A	1(2)	N/A	N/A	N/A	80*	None

* with documentation

Terms To Know

achalasia. Failure of the smooth muscles within the gastrointestinal tract to relax at points of junction; most commonly referring to the esophagogastric sphincter's failure to relax when swallowing.

duodenum. First portion of the small intestine connected to the stomach at the pylorus and extending to the jejunum.

dyskinesia of esophagus. Difficult or impaired voluntary muscle movement of the esophagus.

dyspepsia. Epigastric discomfort after eating, due to impaired digestive function.

ileus. Persistent obstruction of the intestines.

manometric. Pertaining to pressure, as measured in a meter.

motility. Capability of independent, spontaneous movement.

Medicine

91030

91030   Esophagus, acid perfusion (Bernstein) test for esophagitis

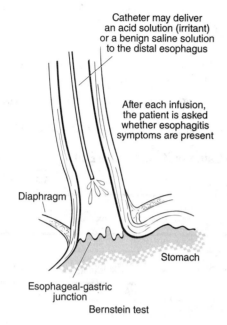

Catheter may deliver an acid solution (irritant) or a benign saline solution to the distal esophagus

After each infusion, the patient is asked whether esophagitis symptoms are present

Diaphragm

Stomach

Esophageal-gastric junction

Bernstein test

Explanation

This code reports a provocative acid perfusion study, also called a Bernstein test, performed on the esophagus, not in conjunction with a motility test. The acid perfusion test is done to try and replicate atypical chest pain the patient has been experiencing and aid in diagnosing the pain as non-cardiac, or due to esophageal reflux/esophagitis. Both hydrochloric acid and an alternate saline control solution are infused one after the other via a nasogastric tube, without the patient being aware of the identity of the solution. The symptoms of chest pain are recorded as the patient identifies them.

Coding Tips

For esophagoscopy, see 43180 and 43191–43232. For an esophagogastroduodenoscopy, see 43210, 43233, 43235–43259, 43266, and 43270.

ICD-10-CM Diagnostic Codes

K20.80	Other esophagitis without bleeding
K20.81	Other esophagitis with bleeding
K21.00	Gastro-esophageal reflux disease with esophagitis, without bleeding
K21.01	Gastro-esophageal reflux disease with esophagitis, with bleeding
K21.9	Gastro-esophageal reflux disease without esophagitis
K22.0	Achalasia of cardia
K22.4	Dyskinesia of esophagus
K22.5	Diverticulum of esophagus, acquired
K22.70	Barrett's esophagus without dysplasia
K22.710	Barrett's esophagus with low grade dysplasia
K22.711	Barrett's esophagus with high grade dysplasia
K22.81	Esophageal polyp
K22.82	Esophagogastric junction polyp
K22.89	Other specified disease of esophagus
R07.89	Other chest pain
R12	Heartburn
R13.11	Dysphagia, oral phase
R13.12	Dysphagia, oropharyngeal phase
R13.13	Dysphagia, pharyngeal phase
R13.14	Dysphagia, pharyngoesophageal phase
R13.19	Other dysphagia

AMA: **91030** 2018,Feb,11

Relative Value Units/Medicare Edits

Non-Facility RVU	Work	PE	MP	Total
91030	0.91	3.37	0.06	4.34
Facility RVU	**Work**	**PE**	**MP**	**Total**
91030	0.91	3.37	0.06	4.34

	FUD	Status	MUE	Modifiers				IOM Reference
91030	0	A	1(2)	N/A	N/A	N/A	80*	None

* with documentation

Terms To Know

achalasia. Failure of the smooth muscles within the gastrointestinal tract to relax at points of junction; most commonly referring to the esophagogastric sphincter's failure to relax when swallowing.

acute. Sudden, severe. Documentation and reporting of an acute condition is important to establishing medical necessity.

Barrett's esophagus. Complication of gastroesophageal reflux disease causing peptic ulcer and stricture in the lower part of the esophagus due to columnar epithelial cells from the lining of the stomach and intestine replacing the natural esophageal lining made of normal squamous cell epithelium. Barrett's esophagus is linked to an elevated risk of esophageal cancer, and is sometimes followed by esophageal adenocarcinoma.

Bernstein test. Acid perfusion test used to differentiate substernal chest pain due to gastroesophageal reflux disease (GERD).

dyskinesia of esophagus. Difficult or impaired voluntary muscle movement of the esophagus.

dysphagia. Difficulty and pain upon swallowing.

esophagitis. Inflammation of the esophagus.

esophagus. Muscular tube that carries swallowed liquids and foods from the pharynx to the stomach.

fistula. Abnormal tube-like passage between two body cavities or organs or from an organ to the outside surface.

reflux. Return or backward flow.

Medicine

91065

91065 Breath hydrogen or methane test (eg, for detection of lactase deficiency, fructose intolerance, bacterial overgrowth, or oro-cecal gastrointestinal transit)

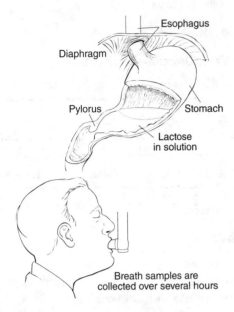

Breath samples are collected over several hours

Explanation

The hydrogen or methane breath test uses a measurement of these gases in the breath to test for a number of conditions that cause gastrointestinal symptoms. It can be used to diagnose lactase deficiency, fructose intolerance, bacterial overgrowth, or orocecal gastrointestinal (rapid) transit. Bacteria produce gases when they are exposed to unabsorbed food. Regardless of the condition causing the excessive production of gas, some is absorbed into the blood flowing through the wall of the intestine and colon. The blood travels to the lungs where it is released and exhaled in the breath where it can be measured. Prior to hydrogen or methane breath testing, a special diet may be required and individuals must fast for at least 12 hours. At the start of the test, a sample breath is taken. The individual blows into and fills a balloon with a breath of air. The concentration of hydrogen or methane from the sample breath is removed from the balloon and measured. The individual ingests a small amount of the test sugar (lactose, fructose, lactulose). Samples of breath are collected and analyzed every 15 minutes for three to five hours.

Coding Tips

This code should be reported only one time per administered challenge. For H. pylori breath testing, nonradioactive (C-13) isotope, see 83013; radioactive (C-14) isotope, see 78268. Placement of an esophageal tamponade tube to manage variceal bleeding is reported with 43460; long intestinal Miller-Abbott tube, see 44500. For abdominal paracentesis, see 49082-49084; with instillation of medication, see 96440 or 96446.

ICD-10-CM Diagnostic Codes

E72.52	Trimethylaminuria
E73.0	Congenital lactase deficiency
E73.1	Secondary lactase deficiency
E73.8	Other lactose intolerance
E74.21	Galactosemia
E74.29	Other disorders of galactose metabolism
E74.31	Sucrase-isomaltase deficiency
E74.39	Other disorders of intestinal carbohydrate absorption
E74.4	Disorders of pyruvate metabolism and gluconeogenesis
E74.810	Glucose transporter protein type 1 deficiency
E74.818	Other disorders of glucose transport
E77.1	Defects in glycoprotein degradation
K31.84	Gastroparesis
K90.41	Non-celiac gluten sensitivity
K90.49	Malabsorption due to intolerance, not elsewhere classified
K90.89	Other intestinal malabsorption
K91.2	Postsurgical malabsorption, not elsewhere classified

AMA: 91065 2018,Jan,8; 2018,Feb,11; 2017,Jan,8; 2016,Jan,13; 2015,Jan,16

Relative Value Units/Medicare Edits

Non-Facility RVU	Work	PE	MP	Total
91065	0.2	2.48	0.02	2.7
Facility RVU	**Work**	**PE**	**MP**	**Total**
91065	0.2	2.48	0.02	2.7

	FUD	Status	MUE	Modifiers				IOM Reference
91065	0	A	2(2)	N/A	N/A	N/A	80*	100-03,100.5

* with documentation

Terms To Know

detection. Search for presence of a tissue or material.

galactosemia. Congenital disorder marked by the inability to metabolize galactose due to a missing enzyme.

malabsorption. Body's inability to absorb a substance or nutrient, usually occurring in the small intestine.

metabolism. Combination of processes occurring in any living organism to produce and maintain organized building blocks (anabolism) and to break down food substances into usable, available energy (catabolism).

Medicine

91110-91111

91110 Gastrointestinal tract imaging, intraluminal (eg, capsule endoscopy), esophagus through ileum, with interpretation and report
91111 Gastrointestinal tract imaging, intraluminal (eg, capsule endoscopy), esophagus with interpretation and report

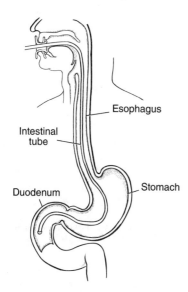

An intestinal bleeding tube is passed, positioned, and a site monitored

Explanation

Gastrointestinal (GI) tract imaging from inside the lumen of the intestinal tract is done in a noninvasive manner by capsule endoscopy. The patient is required to fast for 10 hours before the procedure. The patient swallows the endoscopic capsule with a glass of water. Color video images from inside the GI tract are recorded as the natural peristaltic movement passes the capsule smoothly and painlessly through the system. Sensors are secured to the patient's abdomen and worn like a belt around the waist, allowing data from the capsule to transmit to a data recorder while the patient goes about daily ambulatory activities. After eight hours, the patient returns the equipment for processing at the computer workstation. The images are reviewed, interpreted, and a report is prepared. Report 91110 when the imaging includes the esophagus through the ileum. Report 91111 when the imaging is of the esophagus only.

Coding Tips

These procedures have both a technical and professional component. To report only the professional component, append modifier 26; technical component, append modifier TC. To report the complete procedure (i.e., both the professional and technical components), submit without a modifier. Visualization of the esophagus, stomach, duodenum, ileum, colon is not reported separately. Report modifier 52 if the ileum is not visualized. Do not report 91110–91111 with 91113, 0651T, or each other. Measurement of gastrointestinal tract transit times or pressure via a wireless capsule is reported with 91112.

ICD-10-CM Diagnostic Codes

C15.3	Malignant neoplasm of upper third of esophagus
C15.4	Malignant neoplasm of middle third of esophagus
C15.5	Malignant neoplasm of lower third of esophagus
C17.0	Malignant neoplasm of duodenum
C17.1	Malignant neoplasm of jejunum
C17.2	Malignant neoplasm of ileum
C49.A1	Gastrointestinal stromal tumor of esophagus
C49.A2	Gastrointestinal stromal tumor of stomach
C49.A3	Gastrointestinal stromal tumor of small intestine
D00.1	Carcinoma in situ of esophagus
D00.2	Carcinoma in situ of stomach
D13.0	Benign neoplasm of esophagus
D13.1	Benign neoplasm of stomach
D13.2	Benign neoplasm of duodenum
D50.0	Iron deficiency anemia secondary to blood loss (chronic)
E44.0	Moderate protein-calorie malnutrition
I78.0	Hereditary hemorrhagic telangiectasia
I85.00	Esophageal varices without bleeding
I85.01	Esophageal varices with bleeding
K20.80	Other esophagitis without bleeding
K20.81	Other esophagitis with bleeding
K21.00	Gastro-esophageal reflux disease with esophagitis, without bleeding
K21.01	Gastro-esophageal reflux disease with esophagitis, with bleeding
K21.9	Gastro-esophageal reflux disease without esophagitis
K22.0	Achalasia of cardia
K22.2	Esophageal obstruction
K22.4	Dyskinesia of esophagus
K22.5	Diverticulum of esophagus, acquired
K22.6	Gastro-esophageal laceration-hemorrhage syndrome
K22.81	Esophageal polyp
K22.82	Esophagogastric junction polyp
K22.89	Other specified disease of esophagus
K50.00	Crohn's disease of small intestine without complications
K50.011	Crohn's disease of small intestine with rectal bleeding
K50.012	Crohn's disease of small intestine with intestinal obstruction
K50.013	Crohn's disease of small intestine with fistula
K50.014	Crohn's disease of small intestine with abscess
K50.812	Crohn's disease of both small and large intestine with intestinal obstruction
K50.813	Crohn's disease of both small and large intestine with fistula
K55.011	Focal (segmental) acute (reversible) ischemia of small intestine
K55.012	Diffuse acute (reversible) ischemia of small intestine
K56.0	Paralytic ileus
K56.1	Intussusception
K56.2	Volvulus
K56.3	Gallstone ileus
K56.41	Fecal impaction
K56.51	Intestinal adhesions [bands], with partial obstruction
K56.52	Intestinal adhesions [bands] with complete obstruction
K56.690	Other partial intestinal obstruction
K56.691	Other complete intestinal obstruction
K58.0	Irritable bowel syndrome with diarrhea
K59.01	Slow transit constipation
K59.02	Outlet dysfunction constipation
K63.0	Abscess of intestine
K63.1	Perforation of intestine (nontraumatic)
K63.2	Fistula of intestine

Medicine

K63.3	Ulcer of intestine
K63.81	Dieulafoy lesion of intestine
K92.0	Hematemesis
K92.1	Melena
K92.81	Gastrointestinal mucositis (ulcerative)
M35.08	Sjögren syndrome with gastrointestinal involvement
Q39.4	Esophageal web
R62.7	Adult failure to thrive ▲
R63.4	Abnormal weight loss
R63.6	Underweight

AMA: 91110 2018,Jan,8; 2018,Feb,11; 2017,Jan,8; 2016,Jan,13; 2015,Jan,16
91111 2018,Jan,8; 2018,Feb,11; 2017,Jan,8; 2016,Jan,13; 2015,Jan,16

Relative Value Units/Medicare Edits

Non-Facility RVU	Work	PE	MP	Total
91110	2.49	22.79	0.1	25.38
91111	1.0	26.74	0.05	27.79
Facility RVU	Work	PE	MP	Total
91110	2.49	22.79	0.1	25.38
91111	1.0	26.74	0.05	27.79

	FUD	Status	MUE	Modifiers				IOM Reference
91110	N/A	A	1(2)	N/A	N/A	N/A	80*	None
91111	N/A	A	1(2)	N/A	N/A	N/A	80*	

* with documentation

[91113]

● **91113** Gastrointestinal tract imaging, intraluminal (eg, capsule endoscopy), colon, with interpretation and report

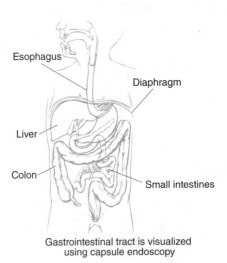

Gastrointestinal tract is visualized
using capsule endoscopy

Explanation

Colon capsule endoscopy (CCE) is a noninvasive and painless ingestible capsule technique that allows exploration of the colon without the need for sedation and gas insufflation. Imaging of the colon is performed from inside via a very small camera. This camera is encased in a capsule that is swallowed by the patient. As this capsule/camera travels through the colon, many images are captured and delivered to a recorder worn outside the body by the patient. This form of endoscopy allows a visual of areas within the colon that may not otherwise be observed using standard endoscopy. This can aid in detection of cancer, polyps, and other GI tract disorders, as well as helping to evaluate GI bleeds and other obscure symptoms. The images are reviewed, interpreted, and a report is prepared.

Coding Tips

Do not report 91113 with 91110 or 91111. Visualization of the esophagus, stomach, duodenum, and/or ileum is not reported separately, when performed with this procedure.

ICD-10-CM Diagnostic Codes

C18.2	Malignant neoplasm of ascending colon
C18.6	Malignant neoplasm of descending colon
C18.7	Malignant neoplasm of sigmoid colon
K50.111	Crohn's disease of large intestine with rectal bleeding
K50.112	Crohn's disease of large intestine with intestinal obstruction
K50.113	Crohn's disease of large intestine with fistula
K50.114	Crohn's disease of large intestine with abscess
K50.118	Crohn's disease of large intestine with other complication
K50.811	Crohn's disease of both small and large intestine with rectal bleeding
K50.812	Crohn's disease of both small and large intestine with intestinal obstruction
K50.813	Crohn's disease of both small and large intestine with fistula
K50.814	Crohn's disease of both small and large intestine with abscess
K51.011	Ulcerative (chronic) pancolitis with rectal bleeding

K51.012	Ulcerative (chronic) pancolitis with intestinal obstruction
K51.013	Ulcerative (chronic) pancolitis with fistula
K51.014	Ulcerative (chronic) pancolitis with abscess
K51.411	Inflammatory polyps of colon with rectal bleeding
K51.412	Inflammatory polyps of colon with intestinal obstruction
K51.413	Inflammatory polyps of colon with fistula
K51.414	Inflammatory polyps of colon with abscess
K51.511	Left sided colitis with rectal bleeding
K51.512	Left sided colitis with intestinal obstruction
K51.513	Left sided colitis with fistula
K51.514	Left sided colitis with abscess
K52.21	Food protein-induced enterocolitis syndrome
K52.22	Food protein-induced enteropathy
K52.82	Eosinophilic colitis

Relative Value Units/Medicare Edits

Non-Facility RVU	Work	PE	MP	Total
91113				
Facility RVU	Work	PE	MP	Total
91113				

	FUD	Status	MUE	Modifiers				IOM Reference
91113	N/A		-	N/A	N/A	N/A	N/A	None

* with documentation

Terms To Know

Crohn's disease. Chronic inflammation of the gastrointestinal tract characterized by chronic granulomatous disease, most commonly affecting the intestines and the terminal ileum.

imaging. Radiologic means of producing pictures for clinical study of the internal structures and functions of the body, such as x-ray, ultrasound, magnetic resonance, or positron emission tomography.

insufflation. Blowing air or gas into a body cavity.

interpretation. Professional health care provider's review of data with a written or verbal opinion.

malignant neoplasm. Any cancerous tumor or lesion exhibiting uncontrolled tissue growth that can progressively invade other parts of the body with its disease-generating cells.

polyp. Small growth on a stalk-like attachment projecting from a mucous membrane.

91112

91112 Gastrointestinal transit and pressure measurement, stomach through colon, wireless capsule, with interpretation and report

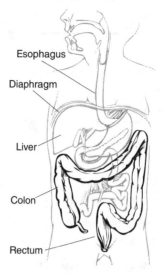

Capsule is used to map digestive tract and pressure measurements stomach to rectum

Explanation

Gastrointestinal (GI) transit and pressure measurement are performed via wireless capsule. The patient swallows the capsule with a glass of water. Pressure, pH, and temperature are recorded as the natural peristaltic movement passes the capsule smoothly and painlessly through the system. This information is used to calculate regional transit times, including gastric emptying time, small bowel transit time, colonic transit time, combined small/large bowel transit time, whole gut transit time, pressure contraction patterns from the antrum and duodenum, and motility indices. The data is transmitted from the capsule to a data recorder, worn like a belt around the patient's waist or around the neck, while the patient goes about daily ambulatory activities. The equipment is brought to the provider for processing at the computer workstation. The images are reviewed, interpreted, and a report is prepared.

Coding Tips

Do not report this code with 83986, 91020, 91022, or 91117.

ICD-10-CM Diagnostic Codes

K59.01	Slow transit constipation
K59.02	Outlet dysfunction constipation
K59.03	Drug induced constipation
K59.04	Chronic idiopathic constipation
K59.09	Other constipation
K59.31	Toxic megacolon
K59.39	Other megacolon
K59.81	Ogilvie syndrome
R15.0	Incomplete defecation
R15.2	Fecal urgency
R15.9	Full incontinence of feces
R19.2	Visible peristalsis
R19.4	Change in bowel habit

Medicine

R19.8   Other specified symptoms and signs involving the digestive system and abdomen

AMA: **91112** 2018,Jan,8; 2018,Feb,11; 2017,Jan,8; 2016,Jan,13; 2015,Jan,16

Relative Value Units/Medicare Edits

Non-Facility RVU	Work	PE	MP	Total
91112	2.1	47.04	0.07	49.21
Facility RVU	**Work**	**PE**	**MP**	**Total**
91112	2.1	47.04	0.07	49.21

	FUD	Status	MUE	Modifiers				IOM Reference
91112	N/A	A	1(3)	N/A	N/A	N/A	80*	None

* with documentation

Terms To Know

antrum. Chamber or cavity, typically with a small opening.

duodenum. First portion of the small intestine connected to the stomach at the pylorus and extending to the jejunum.

interpretation. Professional health care provider's review of data with a written or verbal opinion.

motility. Capability of independent, spontaneous movement.

Ogilvie's syndrome. Colonic obstruction with symptoms of persistent contraction of intestinal musculature, caused by a defect in the sympathetic nerve supply.

peristalsis. Smooth muscle action of automatic contractions that propel substances through the body, such as urine into the bladder and food through the digestive tract.

small intestine. First portion of intestine connecting to the pylorus at the proximal end and consisting of the duodenum, jejunum, and ileum.

91117

91117   Colon motility (manometric) study, minimum 6 hours continuous recording (including provocation tests, eg, meal, intracolonic balloon distension, pharmacologic agents, if performed), with interpretation and report

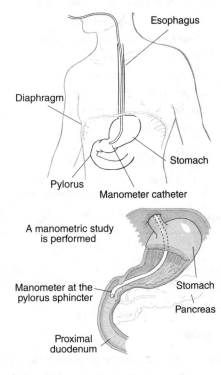

A manometric study is performed

Explanation

Colonic motility is measured using various manometric techniques. In one method, a manometric catheter is positioned endoscopically and clipped to the colonic mucosa. A minimum of six hours of continuous recording ensues. Any provocation tests performed are included, as is the interpretation and report.

Coding Tips

Do not report 91117 with 91120 or 91122. For wireless capsule pressure measurements, see 91112.

ICD-10-CM Diagnostic Codes

K59.01	Slow transit constipation
K59.02	Outlet dysfunction constipation
K59.03	Drug induced constipation
K59.04	Chronic idiopathic constipation
K59.09	Other constipation
K59.81	Ogilvie syndrome
R15.0	Incomplete defecation
R15.2	Fecal urgency
R15.9	Full incontinence of feces
R19.4	Change in bowel habit
R19.8	Other specified symptoms and signs involving the digestive system and abdomen

AMA: **91117** 2018,Jan,8; 2018,Feb,11; 2017,Jan,8; 2016,Jan,13; 2015,Jan,16

Medicine

Relative Value Units/Medicare Edits

Non-Facility RVU	Work	PE	MP	Total
91117	2.45	1.36	0.15	3.96
Facility RVU	Work	PE	MP	Total
91117	2.45	1.36	0.15	3.96

	FUD	Status	MUE	Modifiers				IOM Reference
91117	0	A	1(2)	N/A	N/A	N/A	80*	None

* with documentation

Terms To Know

catheter. Flexible tube inserted into an area of the body for introducing or withdrawing fluid.

constipation. Infrequent or incomplete and difficult bowel movements.

endoscopy. Visual inspection of the body using a fiberoptic scope.

manometric. Pertaining to pressure, as measured in a meter.

motility. Capability of independent, spontaneous movement.

mucosa. Moist tissue lining the mouth (buccal mucosa), stomach (gastric mucosa), intestines, and respiratory tract.

Ogilvie's syndrome. Colonic obstruction with symptoms of persistent contraction of intestinal musculature, caused by a defect in the sympathetic nerve supply.

pharmacological agent. Drug used to produce a chemical effect.

91120

91120   Rectal sensation, tone, and compliance test (ie, response to graded balloon distention)

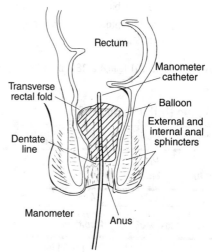

A manometer catheter with balloon is inserted into the anorectal area to measure muscular functions of the distal tract

Explanation

The physician performs a rectal sensation tone and compliance test using graded balloon distention to evaluate anorectal pathology. Tone tests for relaxation or rigidity in the rectum. Compliance tests the distensibility of the rectum. Sensation tests for fullness and discomfort upon distention. The patient is asked to empty his or her bowels. The patient is placed in left lateral decubitus position with the head lowered 20 degrees. The physician inserts a two-lumen catheter containing a cylindrical bag into the rectum. One lumen is used to inflate the bag; the other is used to measure pressure within the bag. With the distal end of the bag 5 cm from the anal verge, the bag is inflated with air. Inflation is slowly increased and sensation, tone, and compliance monitored. The balloon is deflated when the patient experiences discomfort and urgency lasting more than 30 seconds.

Coding Tips

Biofeedback training is reported with 90912-90913. For anorectal manometry, see 91122. Do not report 91120 with 91117.

ICD-10-CM Diagnostic Codes

A18.32	Tuberculous enteritis
F45.8	Other somatoform disorders
K52.21	Food protein-induced enterocolitis syndrome
K52.22	Food protein-induced enteropathy
K52.29	Other allergic and dietetic gastroenteritis and colitis
K59.01	Slow transit constipation
K59.02	Outlet dysfunction constipation
K59.03	Drug induced constipation
K59.04	Chronic idiopathic constipation
K59.09	Other constipation
K59.1	Functional diarrhea
K62.4	Stenosis of anus and rectum
K83.8	Other specified diseases of biliary tract

Medicine

K91.89	Other postprocedural complications and disorders of digestive system
R15.0	Incomplete defecation
R15.2	Fecal urgency
R15.9	Full incontinence of feces
R19.4	Change in bowel habit
R19.8	Other specified symptoms and signs involving the digestive system and abdomen

AMA: 91120 2020,Jun,13; 2018,Jan,8; 2018,Feb,11; 2017,Jan,8; 2016,Jan,13; 2015,Jan,16

Relative Value Units/Medicare Edits

Non-Facility RVU	Work	PE	MP	Total
91120	0.97	14.68	0.06	15.71
Facility RVU	Work	PE	MP	Total
91120	0.97	14.68	0.06	15.71

	FUD	Status	MUE	Modifiers				IOM Reference
91120	N/A	A	1(2)	N/A	N/A	N/A	80*	None

* with documentation

Terms To Know

catheter. Flexible tube inserted into an area of the body for introducing or withdrawing fluid.

decubitus. Patient lying on the side.

distal. Located farther away from a specified reference point or the trunk.

distention. Enlarged or expanded due to pressure from inside.

stenosis. Narrowing or constriction of a passage.

tuberculosis. Bacterial infection that typically spreads by inhalation of an airborne agent that usually attacks the lungs, but may also affect other organs.

91122

91122   Anorectal manometry

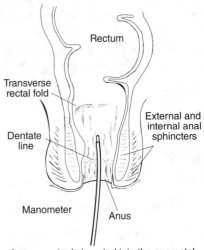

A manometer is inserted into the anorectal area to measure muscular functions of the distal tract

Explanation

The physician performs anorectal manometry to help in diagnosing constipation and/or incontinence due to myotonic dysfunction or suspected cases of Hirschsprung's Disease. Hirschsprung's Disease is a congenital absence of ganglion nerve cells in the plexus that innervates the colon and/or rectum to relax the internal anorectal sphincter in response to rectal distension. A manometry probe is advanced into the rectum after a digital exam. The probe is slowly withdrawn, taking continuous pressure measurements until the high pressure area of the anal sphincters is located. With the patient relaxed, the "basal anal pressure" is recorded, and highest pressures are recorded as the patient performs a maximum squeeze. The manometry catheter is inserted again with a rectal balloon that is slowly inflated to the patient's first sensation of fullness and the volume is recorded. The anal sphincter response to the rectal distention is also recorded. Another manometry technique using a 3 balloon apparatus may also be employed in which pressure measurements are taken as the external, middle, and internal rectal balloons are inflated and deflated to note threshold levels and sphincter responses.

Coding Tips

For rectal sensation, tone, and compliance testing, see 91120. Do not report 91122 with 91117.

ICD-10-CM Diagnostic Codes

A18.32	Tuberculous enteritis
F45.8	Other somatoform disorders
K52.21	Food protein-induced enterocolitis syndrome
K52.22	Food protein-induced enteropathy
K52.29	Other allergic and dietetic gastroenteritis and colitis
K59.01	Slow transit constipation
K59.02	Outlet dysfunction constipation
K59.03	Drug induced constipation
K59.04	Chronic idiopathic constipation
K59.09	Other constipation
K59.1	Functional diarrhea
K59.4	Anal spasm

Medicine

K62.4	Stenosis of anus and rectum
K83.8	Other specified diseases of biliary tract
K91.89	Other postprocedural complications and disorders of digestive system
R15.0	Incomplete defecation
R15.2	Fecal urgency
R15.9	Full incontinence of feces
R19.4	Change in bowel habit
R19.8	Other specified symptoms and signs involving the digestive system and abdomen

AMA: 91122 2018,Feb,11

Relative Value Units/Medicare Edits

Non-Facility RVU	Work	PE	MP	Total
91122	1.77	6.11	0.11	7.99
Facility RVU	**Work**	**PE**	**MP**	**Total**
91122	1.77	6.11	0.11	7.99

	FUD	Status	MUE	Modifiers				IOM Reference
91122	0	A	1(2)	N/A	N/A	N/A	80*	None

* with documentation

Terms To Know

incontinence. Inability to control urination or defecation.

manometric. Pertaining to pressure, as measured in a meter.

motility. Capability of independent, spontaneous movement.

rectal. Pertaining to the rectum, the end portion of the large intestine.

spasm. Involuntary muscle contraction.

stenosis. Narrowing or constriction of a passage.

tube. Long, hollow cylindrical instrument or body structure.

91132-91133

91132	Electrogastrography, diagnostic, transcutaneous;
91133	with provocative testing

Explanation

In electrogastrography (EGG), electrodes are placed on the skin over the stomach at a specific distance from each other and attached to a recording computer. The electrical activity initiated by the distal two-thirds of the stomach (gastric electrical activity - GEA) is recorded and analyzed by the computer. Report 91132 when diagnostic electrogastrography is performed alone. Report 91133 when diagnostic EGG is performed in conjunction with the administration of a drug in an attempt to manipulate conditions and provoke a measurable abnormality.

Coding Tips

For gastrointestinal radiologic procedures, see 74210–74363.

ICD-10-CM Diagnostic Codes

K22.6	Gastro-esophageal laceration-hemorrhage syndrome
K25.0	Acute gastric ulcer with hemorrhage
K25.1	Acute gastric ulcer with perforation
K25.2	Acute gastric ulcer with both hemorrhage and perforation
K25.3	Acute gastric ulcer without hemorrhage or perforation
K25.4	Chronic or unspecified gastric ulcer with hemorrhage
K25.5	Chronic or unspecified gastric ulcer with perforation
K25.6	Chronic or unspecified gastric ulcer with both hemorrhage and perforation
K25.7	Chronic gastric ulcer without hemorrhage or perforation
K28.0	Acute gastrojejunal ulcer with hemorrhage
K28.1	Acute gastrojejunal ulcer with perforation
K28.2	Acute gastrojejunal ulcer with both hemorrhage and perforation
K28.3	Acute gastrojejunal ulcer without hemorrhage or perforation
K28.5	Chronic or unspecified gastrojejunal ulcer with perforation
K28.6	Chronic or unspecified gastrojejunal ulcer with both hemorrhage and perforation
K28.7	Chronic gastrojejunal ulcer without hemorrhage or perforation
K29.00	Acute gastritis without bleeding
K29.01	Acute gastritis with bleeding
K29.20	Alcoholic gastritis without bleeding
K29.21	Alcoholic gastritis with bleeding
K29.30	Chronic superficial gastritis without bleeding
K29.31	Chronic superficial gastritis with bleeding
K29.40	Chronic atrophic gastritis without bleeding
K29.41	Chronic atrophic gastritis with bleeding
K29.60	Other gastritis without bleeding
K29.61	Other gastritis with bleeding
K30	Functional dyspepsia
K31.0	Acute dilatation of stomach
K31.1	Adult hypertrophic pyloric stenosis 🅰
K31.2	Hourglass stricture and stenosis of stomach
K31.3	Pylorospasm, not elsewhere classified
K31.4	Gastric diverticulum
K31.6	Fistula of stomach and duodenum

Medicine

K31.811	Angiodysplasia of stomach and duodenum with bleeding
K31.819	Angiodysplasia of stomach and duodenum without bleeding
K31.82	Dieulafoy lesion (hemorrhagic) of stomach and duodenum
K31.83	Achlorhydria
K31.84	Gastroparesis
K92.81	Gastrointestinal mucositis (ulcerative)

AMA: **91132** 2018,Feb,11 **91133** 2018,Feb,11

Relative Value Units/Medicare Edits

Non-Facility RVU	Work	PE	MP	Total
91132	0.52	11.72	0.03	12.27
91133	0.66	12.25	0.03	12.94
Facility RVU	**Work**	**PE**	**MP**	**Total**
91132	0.52	11.72	0.03	12.27
91133	0.66	12.25	0.03	12.94

	FUD	Status	MUE	Modifiers				IOM Reference
91132	N/A	A	1(3)	N/A	N/A	N/A	80*	None
91133	N/A	A	1(3)	N/A	N/A	N/A	80*	

* with documentation

Terms To Know

diagnostic procedures. Procedure performed on a patient to obtain information to assess the medical condition of the patient or to identify a disease and to determine the nature and severity of an illness or injury.

electrode. Electric terminal specialized for a particular electrochemical reaction that acts as a medium between a body surface and another instrument, commonly termed a lead.

91200

91200 Liver elastography, mechanically induced shear wave (eg, vibration), without imaging, with interpretation and report

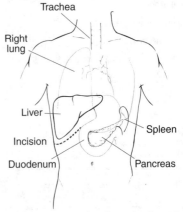

Shear wave is measured to determine liver elasticity

Explanation

Liver elastography is a noninvasive procedure for assessing liver stiffness beneficial in determining the amount of fibrosis and scarring of the liver due to damage and may also be used to survey any disorder advancement and help evaluate ongoing therapy. A probe is applied to the skin between the ribs focusing on the liver. The shear wave is mechanically generated causing the probe to discharge pulses that meet the shear wave and bounce back to the probe. This process allows the shear wave to be measured, which leads to values for liver stiffness. This code indicates no imaging; however, interpretation and report is required.

Coding Tips

Interpretation and report are included in this service and are not reported separately. Coverage of this procedure varies by payer. Check with the payer for specific coverage guidelines.

ICD-10-CM Diagnostic Codes

K70.0	Alcoholic fatty liver △
K70.2	Alcoholic fibrosis and sclerosis of liver △
K70.30	Alcoholic cirrhosis of liver without ascites △
K70.31	Alcoholic cirrhosis of liver with ascites △
K71.7	Toxic liver disease with fibrosis and cirrhosis of liver
K74.01	Hepatic fibrosis, early fibrosis
K74.02	Hepatic fibrosis, advanced fibrosis
K74.2	Hepatic fibrosis with hepatic sclerosis
K74.3	Primary biliary cirrhosis
K74.4	Secondary biliary cirrhosis
K74.69	Other cirrhosis of liver
K76.0	Fatty (change of) liver, not elsewhere classified

AMA: **91200** 2019,Aug,3; 2018,Jan,8; 2018,Feb,11; 2017,Oct,9

Medicine

Relative Value Units/Medicare Edits

Non-Facility RVU	Work	PE	MP	Total
91200	0.21	0.71	0.02	0.94
Facility RVU	Work	PE	MP	Total
91200	0.21	0.71	0.02	0.94

	FUD	Status	MUE	Modifiers				IOM Reference
91200	N/A	A	1(2)	N/A	N/A	N/A	80*	None

* with documentation

Terms To Know

ascites. Abnormal accumulation of free fluid in the abdominal cavity, causing distention and tightness in addition to shortness of breath as the fluid accumulates. Ascites is usually an underlying disorder and can be a manifestation of any number of diseases.

cirrhosis. Disease of the liver that has the characteristics of intertwining band of fibrous tissue that divides the parenchyma into micro- and macronodular areas, which cause the liver to stop functioning over time.

fibrosis. Formation of fibrous tissue as part of the restorative process.

interpretation. Professional health care provider's review of data with a written or verbal opinion.

scar tissue. Fibrous connective tissue that forms around a wounded area or injury, composed mainly of fibroblasts or collagenous fibers.

95980-95982

95980 Electronic analysis of implanted neurostimulator pulse generator system (eg, rate, pulse amplitude and duration, configuration of wave form, battery status, electrode selectability, output modulation, cycling, impedance and patient measurements) gastric neurostimulator pulse generator/transmitter; intraoperative, with programming

95981 subsequent, without reprogramming

95982 subsequent, with reprogramming

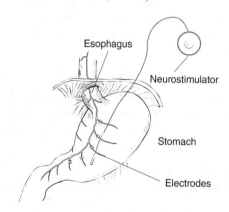

Explanation

The physician tests a gastric neurostimulator pulse generator to verify that it is functioning properly. Functions that may be tested include rate, pulse amplitude and duration, configuration of waveform, battery status, electrode selectability, output modulation, cycling, impedance, and patient measurement. This code reports intraoperative testing with programming of the device. Report 95981 for subsequent testing without reprogramming of device; with reprogramming, see 95982.

Coding Tips

For implantation of neurostimulator electrodes, see 43647 and 43881; revision or removal, see 43648 and 43882. For laparoscopic implantation, revision, or removal of gastric neurostimulator electrodes, lesser curvature (morbid obesity), see 43659. For insertion of a gastric neurostimulator pulse generator, see 64590; revision or removal, see 64595. For intraoperative or subsequent analysis, with programming when appropriate, of vagus nerve trunk stimulator used for blocking therapy (morbid obesity), see 0312T or 0317T.

ICD-10-CM Diagnostic Codes

E66.01	Morbid (severe) obesity due to excess calories
K31.84	Gastroparesis
K31.89	Other diseases of stomach and duodenum
T85.111A	Breakdown (mechanical) of implanted electronic neurostimulator of peripheral nerve electrode (lead), initial encounter
T85.121A	Displacement of implanted electronic neurostimulator of peripheral nerve electrode (lead), initial encounter
T85.191A	Other mechanical complication of implanted electronic neurostimulator of peripheral nerve electrode (lead), initial encounter
T85.732A	Infection and inflammatory reaction due to implanted electronic neurostimulator of peripheral nerve, electrode (lead), initial encounter
T85.810A	Embolism due to nervous system prosthetic devices, implants and grafts, initial encounter

Medicine

T85.820A	Fibrosis due to nervous system prosthetic devices, implants and grafts, initial encounter
T85.830A	Hemorrhage due to nervous system prosthetic devices, implants and grafts, initial encounter
T85.840A	Pain due to nervous system prosthetic devices, implants and grafts, initial encounter
Z45.89	Encounter for adjustment and management of other implanted devices
Z46.89	Encounter for fitting and adjustment of other specified devices

AMA: **95980** 2018,Jan,8; 2018,Feb,11; 2017,Jan,8; 2016,Jul,7; 2016,Jan,13; 2015,Jan,16 **95981** 2018,Jan,8; 2018,Feb,11; 2017,Jan,8; 2016,Jul,7; 2016,Jan,13; 2015,Jan,16 **95982** 2018,Jan,8; 2018,Feb,11; 2017,Jan,8; 2016,Jul,7; 2016,Jan,13; 2015,Jan,16

Relative Value Units/Medicare Edits

Non-Facility RVU	Work	PE	MP	Total
95980	0.8	0.35	0.17	1.32
95981	0.3	0.73	0.05	1.08
95982	0.65	0.93	0.13	1.71
Facility RVU	Work	PE	MP	Total
95980	0.8	0.35	0.17	1.32
95981	0.3	0.17	0.05	0.52
95982	0.65	0.31	0.13	1.09

	FUD	Status	MUE	Modifiers				IOM Reference
95980	N/A	A	1(3)	N/A	N/A	N/A	80*	None
95981	N/A	A	1(3)	N/A	N/A	N/A	80*	
95982	N/A	A	1(3)	N/A	N/A	N/A	80*	

* with documentation

Terms To Know

analysis. Study of body fluid, tissue, section, or parts.

body mass index. Tool for calculating weight appropriateness in adults categorized as underweight (below 18.5), normal (18.5-24.9), overweight (25.0-29.9) and obese (30.0 and over). May be used as an indicator for bariatric procedures.

gastroparesis. Delay in the emptying of food from the stomach into the small bowel due to a degree of paralysis in the muscles lining the stomach wall.

pulse generator. Circuit used to generate pulses. Pulse generators contain the battery, the electronic circuit, and the connector in a hermetically sealed encasement. Pulse generators may be temporary transcutaneous or placed in a subcutaneous pocket.

Medicine

G0104, G0106, G0122

G0104 Colorectal cancer screening; flexible sigmoidoscopy
G0106 Colorectal cancer screening; alternative to G0104, screening sigmoidoscopy, barium enema
G0122 Colorectal cancer screening; barium enema

Explanation

In G0104, a flexible sigmoidoscopy is performed for colorectal cancer screening. After the patient's bowel has been prepped, the physician inserts the flexible sigmoidoscope through the anus and advances the scope into the sigmoid colon. The lumen of the sigmoid colon and rectum are visualized and brushings or washings may be obtained. The sigmoidoscope is withdrawn. In G0106, a colorectal screening for cancer is performed via barium enema as an alternative to a screening sigmoidoscopy (G0104). Both G0106 and G0122 are a radiological exam of the large intestine carried out after the administration of a barium enema to instill the contrast medium into the colon. Fluoroscopy and x-rays are used to observe the images as the contrast fills the colon and helps the physician to diagnose cancer, even colitis, and other diseases. After the patient has emptied the colon, more films are taken.

Coding Tips

Medicare covers a flexible sigmoidoscopy for screening of colorectal cancer once every four years for patients 50 years of age or older.

ICD-10-CM Diagnostic Codes

K51.00	Ulcerative (chronic) pancolitis without complications
K51.011	Ulcerative (chronic) pancolitis with rectal bleeding
K51.012	Ulcerative (chronic) pancolitis with intestinal obstruction
K51.013	Ulcerative (chronic) pancolitis with fistula
K51.014	Ulcerative (chronic) pancolitis with abscess
K51.018	Ulcerative (chronic) pancolitis with other complication
K51.20	Ulcerative (chronic) proctitis without complications
K51.211	Ulcerative (chronic) proctitis with rectal bleeding
K51.212	Ulcerative (chronic) proctitis with intestinal obstruction
K51.213	Ulcerative (chronic) proctitis with fistula
K51.214	Ulcerative (chronic) proctitis with abscess
K51.218	Ulcerative (chronic) proctitis with other complication
K51.30	Ulcerative (chronic) rectosigmoiditis without complications
K51.311	Ulcerative (chronic) rectosigmoiditis with rectal bleeding
K51.312	Ulcerative (chronic) rectosigmoiditis with intestinal obstruction
K51.313	Ulcerative (chronic) rectosigmoiditis with fistula
K51.314	Ulcerative (chronic) rectosigmoiditis with abscess
K51.318	Ulcerative (chronic) rectosigmoiditis with other complication
K51.40	Inflammatory polyps of colon without complications
K51.411	Inflammatory polyps of colon with rectal bleeding
K51.412	Inflammatory polyps of colon with intestinal obstruction
K51.413	Inflammatory polyps of colon with fistula
K51.414	Inflammatory polyps of colon with abscess
K51.418	Inflammatory polyps of colon with other complication
K51.50	Left sided colitis without complications
K51.511	Left sided colitis with rectal bleeding
K51.512	Left sided colitis with intestinal obstruction
K51.513	Left sided colitis with fistula
K51.514	Left sided colitis with abscess
K51.518	Left sided colitis with other complication
K51.80	Other ulcerative colitis without complications
K51.811	Other ulcerative colitis with rectal bleeding
K51.812	Other ulcerative colitis with intestinal obstruction
K51.813	Other ulcerative colitis with fistula
K51.814	Other ulcerative colitis with abscess
K51.818	Other ulcerative colitis with other complication
K52.0	Gastroenteritis and colitis due to radiation
K52.1	Toxic gastroenteritis and colitis
K52.21	Food protein-induced enterocolitis syndrome
K52.22	Food protein-induced enteropathy
K52.29	Other allergic and dietetic gastroenteritis and colitis
K52.3	Indeterminate colitis
K52.81	Eosinophilic gastritis or gastroenteritis
K52.82	Eosinophilic colitis
K52.831	Collagenous colitis
K52.832	Lymphocytic colitis
K52.838	Other microscopic colitis
K52.89	Other specified noninfective gastroenteritis and colitis
K55.031	Focal (segmental) acute (reversible) ischemia of large intestine
K55.032	Diffuse acute (reversible) ischemia of large intestine
K55.041	Focal (segmental) acute infarction of large intestine
K55.042	Diffuse acute infarction of large intestine
K55.1	Chronic vascular disorders of intestine
Z12.11	Encounter for screening for malignant neoplasm of colon
Z12.12	Encounter for screening for malignant neoplasm of rectum

Relative Value Units/Medicare Edits

Non-Facility RVU	Work	PE	MP	Total
G0104	0.84	4.65	0.11	5.6
G0106	1.26	5.41	0.06	6.73
G0122	0.99	8.76	0.07	9.82

Facility RVU	Work	PE	MP	Total
G0104	0.84	0.67	0.11	1.62
G0106	1.26	5.41	0.06	6.73
G0122	0.99	8.76	0.07	9.82

	FUD	Status	MUE	Modifiers				IOM Reference
G0104	0	A	1(2)	51	N/A	N/A	N/A	None
G0106	N/A	A	1(2)	N/A	N/A	N/A	80*	
G0122	N/A	N	0(3)	N/A	N/A	N/A	N/A	

* with documentation

Terms To Know

barium enema. Radiology exam for viewing the intestine that utilizes a suspension of barium sulfate, a chalk-like substance that appears white on x-ray, to delineate the lining of the colon and rectum. The barium is administered via the rectum and held inside the colon while x-rays are taken. Barium enema may also be performed therapeutically in order to relieve intussusception or intestinal obstructions.

colitis. Inflammation of the colon, caused by an infection or external influences such as laxatives, radiation, or antibiotics.

HCPCS

G0105 Colorectal cancer screening; colonoscopy on individual at high risk
G0120 Colorectal cancer screening; alternative to G0105, screening colonoscopy, barium enema
G0121 Colorectal cancer screening; colonoscopy on individual not meeting criteria for high risk

Explanation

In G0105, a colonoscopy is performed on a high-risk patient for colorectal cancer screening. A high-risk patient is one with ulcerative enteritis or a history of malignant neoplasm of the lower gastrointestinal tract. After the patient's bowel has been prepped, the physician inserts the colonoscope through the anus and advances the scope through the colon past the splenic flexure. The lumen of the colon and rectum is visualized. Brushings or washings may be obtained. The colonoscope is withdrawn. In G0120, a colorectal screening for cancer is performed via barium enema as an alternative to a screening colonoscopy on a high-risk individual (G0105). This is a radiological exam of the large intestine carried out after the administration of a barium enema to instill the contrast medium into the colon. Fluoroscopy and x-rays are used to observe the images as the contrast fills the colon and helps the physician to diagnose cancer, even colitis, and other diseases. After the patient has emptied the colon, more films are taken. In G0121, a colonoscopy is performed for colorectal cancer screening on a patient who does not meet high-risk criteria. This would be a patient without a diagnosis of ulcerative enteritis or without a history of malignant neoplasm of the lower gastrointestinal tract.

Coding Tips

Medicare covers a screening colonoscopy for patients at average risk for colorectal cancer every 10 years, or for patients at high risk for colorectal cancer every three years. A high-risk patient is identified as a patient with a personal or family history of colorectal cancer or certain types of polyps, family history of hereditary colorectal cancer, or personal history of inflammatory bowel disease.

ICD-10-CM Diagnostic Codes

K51.00	Ulcerative (chronic) pancolitis without complications
K51.011	Ulcerative (chronic) pancolitis with rectal bleeding
K51.012	Ulcerative (chronic) pancolitis with intestinal obstruction
K51.013	Ulcerative (chronic) pancolitis with fistula
K51.014	Ulcerative (chronic) pancolitis with abscess
K51.018	Ulcerative (chronic) pancolitis with other complication
K51.20	Ulcerative (chronic) proctitis without complications
K51.211	Ulcerative (chronic) proctitis with rectal bleeding
K51.212	Ulcerative (chronic) proctitis with intestinal obstruction
K51.213	Ulcerative (chronic) proctitis with fistula
K51.214	Ulcerative (chronic) proctitis with abscess
K51.218	Ulcerative (chronic) proctitis with other complication
K51.30	Ulcerative (chronic) rectosigmoiditis without complications
K51.311	Ulcerative (chronic) rectosigmoiditis with rectal bleeding
K51.312	Ulcerative (chronic) rectosigmoiditis with intestinal obstruction
K51.313	Ulcerative (chronic) rectosigmoiditis with fistula
K51.314	Ulcerative (chronic) rectosigmoiditis with abscess
K51.318	Ulcerative (chronic) rectosigmoiditis with other complication
K51.40	Inflammatory polyps of colon without complications
K51.411	Inflammatory polyps of colon with rectal bleeding
K51.412	Inflammatory polyps of colon with intestinal obstruction
K51.413	Inflammatory polyps of colon with fistula
K51.414	Inflammatory polyps of colon with abscess
K51.418	Inflammatory polyps of colon with other complication
K51.50	Left sided colitis without complications
K51.511	Left sided colitis with rectal bleeding
K51.512	Left sided colitis with intestinal obstruction
K51.513	Left sided colitis with fistula
K51.514	Left sided colitis with abscess
K51.518	Left sided colitis with other complication
K51.80	Other ulcerative colitis without complications
K51.811	Other ulcerative colitis with rectal bleeding
K51.812	Other ulcerative colitis with intestinal obstruction
K51.813	Other ulcerative colitis with fistula
K51.814	Other ulcerative colitis with abscess
K51.818	Other ulcerative colitis with other complication
K52.0	Gastroenteritis and colitis due to radiation
K52.1	Toxic gastroenteritis and colitis
K52.21	Food protein-induced enterocolitis syndrome
K52.22	Food protein-induced enteropathy
K52.29	Other allergic and dietetic gastroenteritis and colitis
K52.3	Indeterminate colitis
K52.81	Eosinophilic gastritis or gastroenteritis
K52.82	Eosinophilic colitis
K52.831	Collagenous colitis
K52.832	Lymphocytic colitis
K52.838	Other microscopic colitis
K52.89	Other specified noninfective gastroenteritis and colitis
K55.031	Focal (segmental) acute (reversible) ischemia of large intestine
K55.032	Diffuse acute (reversible) ischemia of large intestine
K55.039	Acute (reversible) ischemia of large intestine, extent unspecified
K55.041	Focal (segmental) acute infarction of large intestine
K55.042	Diffuse acute infarction of large intestine
K55.1	Chronic vascular disorders of intestine
Z12.11	Encounter for screening for malignant neoplasm of colon
Z12.12	Encounter for screening for malignant neoplasm of rectum
Z80.0	Family history of malignant neoplasm of digestive organs
Z83.71	Family history of colonic polyps
Z86.010	Personal history of colonic polyps

Relative Value Units/Medicare Edits

Non-Facility RVU	Work	PE	MP	Total
G0105	3.26	6.56	0.41	10.23
G0120	1.26	5.41	0.06	6.73
G0121	3.26	6.56	0.42	10.24
Facility RVU	**Work**	**PE**	**MP**	**Total**
G0105	3.26	1.73	0.41	5.4
G0120	1.26	5.41	0.06	6.73
G0121	3.26	1.73	0.42	5.41

	FUD	Status	MUE	Modifiers				IOM Reference
G0105	0	A	1(2)	51	N/A	N/A	N/A	None
G0120	N/A	A	1(2)	N/A	N/A	N/A	80*	
G0121	0	A	1(2)	51	N/A	N/A	N/A	

* with documentation

Terms To Know

barium enema. Radiology exam for viewing the intestine that utilizes a suspension of barium sulfate, a chalk-like substance that appears white on x-ray, to delineate the lining of the colon and rectum. The barium is administered via the rectum and held inside the colon while x-rays are taken. Barium enema may also be performed therapeutically in order to relieve intussusception or intestinal obstructions.

pancolitis. Severe form of ulcerative colitis, where inflammation affects the entire colon. May be caused by infection or external influences such as laxatives, radiation, or antibiotics.

polyp. Small growth on a stalk-like attachment projecting from a mucous membrane.

screening test. Exam or study used by a physician to identify abnormalities, regardless of whether the patient exhibits symptoms.

G0166

G0166 External counterpulsation, per treatment session

Explanation

External counterpulsation is a therapy for relieving angina and is also beneficial for congestive heart failure patients. The treatment increases blood flow into the arteries and decreases the workload of the heart. The therapy is believed to work by stimulating the growth of new blood vessels around the arteries in the heart that are blocked. The patient has compressive cuffs wrapped around his/her calves and upper and lower thighs. The cuffs inflate when the heart is filling with blood and deflate when the heart is ejecting blood. Treatment sessions last one hour and are usually for a period of five times a week for seven weeks. This code reports one treatment session.

Coding Tips

Per Medicare, a full course of treatment usually consists of 35 one-hour sessions, which may be offered once or twice daily, usually five days per week.

ICD-10-CM Diagnostic Codes

I20.0	Unstable angina
I20.1	Angina pectoris with documented spasm
I20.8	Other forms of angina pectoris
I50.1	Left ventricular failure, unspecified
I50.21	Acute systolic (congestive) heart failure
I50.22	Chronic systolic (congestive) heart failure
I50.23	Acute on chronic systolic (congestive) heart failure
I50.31	Acute diastolic (congestive) heart failure
I50.32	Chronic diastolic (congestive) heart failure
I50.33	Acute on chronic diastolic (congestive) heart failure
I50.41	Acute combined systolic (congestive) and diastolic (congestive) heart failure
I50.42	Chronic combined systolic (congestive) and diastolic (congestive) heart failure
I50.43	Acute on chronic combined systolic (congestive) and diastolic (congestive) heart failure

Relative Value Units/Medicare Edits

Non-Facility RVU	Work	PE	MP	Total
G0166	0.0	3.35	0.04	3.39
Facility RVU	**Work**	**PE**	**MP**	**Total**
G0166	0.0	3.35	0.04	3.39

	FUD	Status	MUE	Modifiers				IOM Reference
G0166	N/A	A	2(3)	N/A	N/A	N/A	N/A	None

* with documentation

G0168

G0168 Wound closure utilizing tissue adhesive(s) only

Explanation

Wound closure done by using tissue adhesive only, not any kind of suturing or stapling, is reported with this code. Tissue adhesives, such as Dermabond, are materials that are applied directly to the skin or tissue of an open wound to hold the margins closed for healing.

Coding Tips

Code G0168 is reported when a Medicare patient undergoes a superficial repair or closure using tissue adhesive only. This includes instances where sutures have been used for the repair of deeper layers and tissue adhesive is used to close the superficial layer. Payment for this service is at the discretion of the contractor.

ICD-10-CM Diagnostic Codes

S00.01XA	Abrasion of scalp, initial encounter
S00.511A	Abrasion of lip, initial encounter
S00.571A	Other superficial bite of lip, initial encounter
S00.81XA	Abrasion of other part of head, initial encounter
S01.01XA	Laceration without foreign body of scalp, initial encounter
S01.03XA	Puncture wound without foreign body of scalp, initial encounter
S01.05XA	Open bite of scalp, initial encounter
S01.111A	Laceration without foreign body of right eyelid and periocular area, initial encounter ☑
S01.121A	Laceration with foreign body of right eyelid and periocular area, initial encounter ☑
S01.131A	Puncture wound without foreign body of right eyelid and periocular area, initial encounter ☑
S01.141A	Puncture wound with foreign body of right eyelid and periocular area, initial encounter ☑
S01.21XA	Laceration without foreign body of nose, initial encounter
S01.23XA	Puncture wound without foreign body of nose, initial encounter
S01.25XA	Open bite of nose, initial encounter
S01.311A	Laceration without foreign body of right ear, initial encounter ☑
S01.312A	Laceration without foreign body of left ear, initial encounter ☑
S01.331A	Puncture wound without foreign body of right ear, initial encounter ☑
S01.332A	Puncture wound without foreign body of left ear, initial encounter ☑
S01.351A	Open bite of right ear, initial encounter ☑
S01.352A	Open bite of left ear, initial encounter ☑
S01.411A	Laceration without foreign body of right cheek and temporomandibular area, initial encounter ☑
S01.412A	Laceration without foreign body of left cheek and temporomandibular area, initial encounter ☑
S01.431A	Puncture wound without foreign body of right cheek and temporomandibular area, initial encounter ☑
S01.432A	Puncture wound without foreign body of left cheek and temporomandibular area, initial encounter ☑
S01.451A	Open bite of right cheek and temporomandibular area, initial encounter ☑
S01.452A	Open bite of left cheek and temporomandibular area, initial encounter ☑
S01.511A	Laceration without foreign body of lip, initial encounter
S01.531A	Puncture wound without foreign body of lip, initial encounter
S01.532A	Puncture wound without foreign body of oral cavity, initial encounter
S01.551A	Open bite of lip, initial encounter

Relative Value Units/Medicare Edits

Non-Facility RVU	Work	PE	MP	Total
G0168	0.31	3.2	0.05	3.56
Facility RVU	**Work**	**PE**	**MP**	**Total**
G0168	0.31	0.08	0.05	0.44

	FUD	Status	MUE	Modifiers				IOM Reference
G0168	0	A	2(3)	51	N/A	N/A	N/A	None

* with documentation

Terms To Know

closure. Repairing an incision or wound by suture or other means.

HCPCS Level II. Healthcare Common Procedure Coding System Level II. National coding system, developed by CMS, that contains alphanumeric codes for physician and nonphysician services not included in the CPT coding system. HCPCS Level II covers such things as ambulance services, durable medical equipment, and orthotic and prosthetic devices.

suture. Numerous stitching techniques employed in wound closure.

buried suture. Continuous or interrupted suture placed under the skin for a layered closure.

continuous suture. Running stitch with tension evenly distributed across a single strand to provide a leakproof closure line.

interrupted suture. Series of single stitches with tension isolated at each stitch, in which all stitches are not affected if one becomes loose, and the isolated sutures cannot act as a wick to transport an infection.

purse-string suture. Continuous suture placed around a tubular structure and tightened, to reduce or close the lumen.

retention suture. Secondary stitching that bridges the primary suture, providing support for the primary repair; a plastic or rubber bolster may be placed over the primary repair and under the retention sutures.

G0281-G0283

G0281 Electrical stimulation, (unattended), to one or more areas, for chronic Stage III and Stage IV pressure ulcers, arterial ulcers, diabetic ulcers, and venous stasis ulcers not demonstrating measurable signs of healing after 30 days of conventional care, as part of a therapy plan of care

G0282 Electrical stimulation, (unattended), to one or more areas, for wound care other than described in G0281

G0283 Electrical stimulation (unattended), to one or more areas for indication(s) other than wound care, as part of a therapy plan of care

Explanation

Electrical stimulation is the use of electric current that mimics the body's own natural bioelectric system's current when injured or impaired, and jumpstarts or accelerates the healing process by attracting the body's repair cells, changing cell membrane permeability and hence cellular secretion, and orientating cell structures. A current is generated between the skin and inner tissues when there is a break in the skin. The current is kept flowing until the open skin defect is repaired. There may be different types of electricity used, controlled by different electrical sources. A moist wound environment is required for capacitively coupled electrical stimulation, which involves using a surface electrode pad in wet contact (capacitively coupled) with the external skin surface and/or wound bed. Two electrodes are required to complete the electric circuit and are usually placed over a wet conductive medium in the wound bed and on the skin away from the wound. One of the most safe and effective wavelengths used is monophasic twin peaked high voltage pulsed current (HVPC), allowing for selection of polarity, variation in pulse rates, and very short pulse duration. Significant changes in tissue pH and temperature are avoided, which is good for healing. Codes G0281 and G0282 are reported for wound care. Code G0283 is reported for purposes other than wound care, such as nerve stimulation, pain reduction, and muscle contraction.

Coding Tips

Medicare covers G0281 and G0282 for the treatment of chronic stage III or stage IV pressure ulcers, arterial ulcers, diabetic ulcers, and venous stasis ulcers only. In addition, the use of electrical stimulation will only be covered by Medicare after appropriate standard wound care has been tried for at least 30 days and there are no measurable signs of healing. If electrical stimulation is being used, wounds must be evaluated periodically by the treating physician but no less than every 30 days. Continued treatment with electrical stimulation is not covered if measurable signs of healing have not been demonstrated within any 30-day period of treatment. Additionally, electrical stimulation must be discontinued when the wound demonstrates a 100 percent epithelialized wound bed. Electrical stimulation for non-wound purposes (G0283) must be documented in the patient record. Third-party payers may not separately reimburse for this service. Check with the payer for their specific guidelines.

ICD-10-CM Diagnostic Codes

I70.238	Atherosclerosis of native arteries of right leg with ulceration of other part of lower leg ▲ ☑
I70.434	Atherosclerosis of autologous vein bypass graft(s) of the right leg with ulceration of heel and midfoot ▲ ☑
I70.443	Atherosclerosis of autologous vein bypass graft(s) of the left leg with ulceration of ankle ▲ ☑
I70.45	Atherosclerosis of autologous vein bypass graft(s) of other extremity with ulceration ▲
I70.541	Atherosclerosis of nonautologous biological bypass graft(s) of the left leg with ulceration of thigh ▲ ☑
I70.542	Atherosclerosis of nonautologous biological bypass graft(s) of the left leg with ulceration of calf ▲ ☑
I70.544	Atherosclerosis of nonautologous biological bypass graft(s) of the left leg with ulceration of heel and midfoot ▲ ☑
I70.55	Atherosclerosis of nonautologous biological bypass graft(s) of other extremity with ulceration ▲
I70.631	Atherosclerosis of nonbiological bypass graft(s) of the right leg with ulceration of thigh ▲ ☑
I70.632	Atherosclerosis of nonbiological bypass graft(s) of the right leg with ulceration of calf ▲ ☑
I70.633	Atherosclerosis of nonbiological bypass graft(s) of the right leg with ulceration of ankle ▲ ☑
I70.643	Atherosclerosis of nonbiological bypass graft(s) of the left leg with ulceration of ankle ▲ ☑
I70.644	Atherosclerosis of nonbiological bypass graft(s) of the left leg with ulceration of heel and midfoot ▲ ☑
L89.013	Pressure ulcer of right elbow, stage 3 ☑
L89.014	Pressure ulcer of right elbow, stage 4 ☑
L89.024	Pressure ulcer of left elbow, stage 4 ☑
L89.113	Pressure ulcer of right upper back, stage 3 ☑
L89.114	Pressure ulcer of right upper back, stage 4 ☑
L89.116	Pressure-induced deep tissue damage of right upper back ☑
L89.124	Pressure ulcer of left upper back, stage 4 ☑
L89.133	Pressure ulcer of right lower back, stage 3 ☑
L89.134	Pressure ulcer of right lower back, stage 4 ☑
L89.136	Pressure-induced deep tissue damage of right lower back ☑
L89.213	Pressure ulcer of right hip, stage 3 ☑
L89.214	Pressure ulcer of right hip, stage 4 ☑
L89.316	Pressure-induced deep tissue damage of right buttock ☑
L89.324	Pressure ulcer of left buttock, stage 4 ☑
L89.516	Pressure-induced deep tissue damage of right ankle ☑
L89.524	Pressure ulcer of left ankle, stage 4 ☑
L89.613	Pressure ulcer of right heel, stage 3 ☑
L89.614	Pressure ulcer of right heel, stage 4 ☑
L97.111	Non-pressure chronic ulcer of right thigh limited to breakdown of skin ☑
L97.112	Non-pressure chronic ulcer of right thigh with fat layer exposed ☑
L97.123	Non-pressure chronic ulcer of left thigh with necrosis of muscle ☑
L97.124	Non-pressure chronic ulcer of left thigh with necrosis of bone ☑
L97.211	Non-pressure chronic ulcer of right calf limited to breakdown of skin ☑
L97.212	Non-pressure chronic ulcer of right calf with fat layer exposed ☑
L97.223	Non-pressure chronic ulcer of left calf with necrosis of muscle ☑
L97.224	Non-pressure chronic ulcer of left calf with necrosis of bone ☑
L97.311	Non-pressure chronic ulcer of right ankle limited to breakdown of skin ☑
L97.312	Non-pressure chronic ulcer of right ankle with fat layer exposed ☑
L97.313	Non-pressure chronic ulcer of right ankle with necrosis of muscle ☑
L97.314	Non-pressure chronic ulcer of right ankle with necrosis of bone ☑
L97.321	Non-pressure chronic ulcer of left ankle limited to breakdown of skin ☑

L97.322	Non-pressure chronic ulcer of left ankle with fat layer exposed ☑	
L97.413	Non-pressure chronic ulcer of right heel and midfoot with necrosis of muscle ☑	
L97.414	Non-pressure chronic ulcer of right heel and midfoot with necrosis of bone ☑	
L97.421	Non-pressure chronic ulcer of left heel and midfoot limited to breakdown of skin ☑	
L97.422	Non-pressure chronic ulcer of left heel and midfoot with fat layer exposed ☑	
L98.411	Non-pressure chronic ulcer of buttock limited to breakdown of skin	
L98.412	Non-pressure chronic ulcer of buttock with fat layer exposed	
L98.413	Non-pressure chronic ulcer of buttock with necrosis of muscle	
L98.421	Non-pressure chronic ulcer of back limited to breakdown of skin	
L98.424	Non-pressure chronic ulcer of back with necrosis of bone	

Relative Value Units/Medicare Edits

Non-Facility RVU	Work	PE	MP	Total
G0281	0.18	0.19	0.01	0.38
G0282	0.0	0.0	0.0	0.0
G0283	0.18	0.19	0.01	0.38
Facility RVU	Work	PE	MP	Total
G0281	0.18	0.19	0.01	0.38
G0282	0.0	0.0	0.0	0.0
G0283	0.18	0.19	0.01	0.38

	FUD	Status	MUE	Modifiers				IOM Reference
G0281	N/A	A	1(3)	N/A	N/A	N/A	80*	100-04,32,11.1
G0282	N/A	N	0(3)	N/A	N/A	N/A	N/A	
G0283	N/A	A	1(3)	N/A	N/A	N/A	80*	

* with documentation

Terms To Know

atherosclerosis. Buildup of yellowish plaques composed of cholesterol and lipoid material within the arteries.

pressure ulcers. Progressively eroding skin lesion produced by inflamed necrotic tissue as it sloughs off, caused by continual pressure impeding blood circulation, especially over bony areas, when a patient lies still for too long without changing position.

G0329

G0329 Electromagnetic therapy, to one or more areas for chronic Stage III and Stage IV pressure ulcers, arterial ulcers, diabetic ulcers and venous stasis ulcers not demonstrating measurable signs of healing after 30 days of conventional care as part of a therapy plan of care

Explanation

Electromagnetic therapy is a distinct form of treatment using application of electromagnetic fields rather than direct electrical current. Electromagnetic therapy is used for wound treatment for stage III and/or stage IV pressure ulcers, arterial ulcers, diabetic ulcers, and venous stasis ulcers. Electromagnetic therapy is only considered appropriate after standard wound therapy has been tried for a minimum of 30 days with documentation showing no measurable signs of healing.

Coding Tips

Medicare covers this service for the treatment of chronic stage III or stage IV pressure ulcers, arterial ulcers, diabetic ulcers, and venous stasis ulcers only. Electromagnetic therapy is not covered as an initial treatment modality. The use of electromagnetic therapy is only covered after appropriate standard wound care has been tried for at least 30 days and there are no measurable signs of healing. If electromagnetic therapy is being used, wounds must be evaluated periodically by the treating physician but no less than every 30 days. Continued treatment with electromagnetic therapy is not covered if measurable signs of healing have not been demonstrated within any 30-day period of treatment. Additionally, electromagnetic therapy must be discontinued when the wound demonstrates a 100 percent epithelialized wound bed. Third-party payers may not reimburse separately for this service. Check with payers for specific guidelines.

ICD-10-CM Diagnostic Codes

I70.232	Atherosclerosis of native arteries of right leg with ulceration of calf 🅰 ☑	
I70.233	Atherosclerosis of native arteries of right leg with ulceration of ankle 🅰 ☑	
I70.234	Atherosclerosis of native arteries of right leg with ulceration of heel and midfoot 🅰 ☑	
I70.235	Atherosclerosis of native arteries of right leg with ulceration of other part of foot 🅰 ☑	
I70.238	Atherosclerosis of native arteries of right leg with ulceration of other part of lower leg 🅰 ☑	
I70.242	Atherosclerosis of native arteries of left leg with ulceration of calf 🅰 ☑	
I70.243	Atherosclerosis of native arteries of left leg with ulceration of ankle 🅰 ☑	
I70.244	Atherosclerosis of native arteries of left leg with ulceration of heel and midfoot 🅰 ☑	
I70.245	Atherosclerosis of native arteries of left leg with ulceration of other part of foot 🅰 ☑	
I70.332	Atherosclerosis of unspecified type of bypass graft(s) of the right leg with ulceration of calf 🅰 ☑	
I70.333	Atherosclerosis of unspecified type of bypass graft(s) of the right leg with ulceration of ankle 🅰 ☑	
I70.334	Atherosclerosis of unspecified type of bypass graft(s) of the right leg with ulceration of heel and midfoot 🅰 ☑	
I70.335	Atherosclerosis of unspecified type of bypass graft(s) of the right leg with ulceration of other part of foot 🅰 ☑	

I70.338	Atherosclerosis of unspecified type of bypass graft(s) of the right leg with ulceration of other part of lower leg 🄰 ☑
I70.342	Atherosclerosis of unspecified type of bypass graft(s) of the left leg with ulceration of calf 🄰 ☑
I70.343	Atherosclerosis of unspecified type of bypass graft(s) of the left leg with ulceration of ankle 🄰 ☑
I70.344	Atherosclerosis of unspecified type of bypass graft(s) of the left leg with ulceration of heel and midfoot 🄰 ☑
I70.348	Atherosclerosis of unspecified type of bypass graft(s) of the left leg with ulceration of other part of lower leg 🄰 ☑
I70.432	Atherosclerosis of autologous vein bypass graft(s) of the right leg with ulceration of calf 🄰 ☑
I70.433	Atherosclerosis of autologous vein bypass graft(s) of the right leg with ulceration of ankle 🄰 ☑
I70.434	Atherosclerosis of autologous vein bypass graft(s) of the right leg with ulceration of heel and midfoot 🄰 ☑
I70.435	Atherosclerosis of autologous vein bypass graft(s) of the right leg with ulceration of other part of foot 🄰 ☑
I70.442	Atherosclerosis of autologous vein bypass graft(s) of the left leg with ulceration of calf 🄰 ☑
I70.443	Atherosclerosis of autologous vein bypass graft(s) of the left leg with ulceration of ankle 🄰 ☑
I70.444	Atherosclerosis of autologous vein bypass graft(s) of the left leg with ulceration of heel and midfoot 🄰 ☑
I70.445	Atherosclerosis of autologous vein bypass graft(s) of the left leg with ulceration of other part of foot 🄰 ☑
I70.532	Atherosclerosis of nonautologous biological bypass graft(s) of the right leg with ulceration of calf 🄰 ☑
I70.533	Atherosclerosis of nonautologous biological bypass graft(s) of the right leg with ulceration of ankle 🄰 ☑
I70.534	Atherosclerosis of nonautologous biological bypass graft(s) of the right leg with ulceration of heel and midfoot 🄰 ☑
I70.535	Atherosclerosis of nonautologous biological bypass graft(s) of the right leg with ulceration of other part of foot 🄰 ☑
I70.542	Atherosclerosis of nonautologous biological bypass graft(s) of the left leg with ulceration of calf 🄰 ☑
I70.543	Atherosclerosis of nonautologous biological bypass graft(s) of the left leg with ulceration of ankle 🄰 ☑
I70.544	Atherosclerosis of nonautologous biological bypass graft(s) of the left leg with ulceration of heel and midfoot 🄰 ☑
I70.545	Atherosclerosis of nonautologous biological bypass graft(s) of the left leg with ulceration of other part of foot 🄰 ☑
I70.55	Atherosclerosis of nonautologous biological bypass graft(s) of other extremity with ulceration 🄰
I70.632	Atherosclerosis of nonbiological bypass graft(s) of the right leg with ulceration of calf 🄰 ☑
I70.633	Atherosclerosis of nonbiological bypass graft(s) of the right leg with ulceration of ankle 🄰 ☑
I70.634	Atherosclerosis of nonbiological bypass graft(s) of the right leg with ulceration of heel and midfoot 🄰 ☑
I70.635	Atherosclerosis of nonbiological bypass graft(s) of the right leg with ulceration of other part of foot 🄰 ☑
I70.642	Atherosclerosis of nonbiological bypass graft(s) of the left leg with ulceration of calf 🄰 ☑
I70.643	Atherosclerosis of nonbiological bypass graft(s) of the left leg with ulceration of ankle 🄰 ☑
I70.644	Atherosclerosis of nonbiological bypass graft(s) of the left leg with ulceration of heel and midfoot 🄰 ☑
I70.645	Atherosclerosis of nonbiological bypass graft(s) of the left leg with ulceration of other part of foot 🄰 ☑
I70.732	Atherosclerosis of other type of bypass graft(s) of the right leg with ulceration of calf 🄰 ☑
I70.733	Atherosclerosis of other type of bypass graft(s) of the right leg with ulceration of ankle 🄰 ☑
I70.734	Atherosclerosis of other type of bypass graft(s) of the right leg with ulceration of heel and midfoot 🄰 ☑
I70.735	Atherosclerosis of other type of bypass graft(s) of the right leg with ulceration of other part of foot 🄰 ☑
I70.742	Atherosclerosis of other type of bypass graft(s) of the left leg with ulceration of calf 🄰 ☑
I70.743	Atherosclerosis of other type of bypass graft(s) of the left leg with ulceration of ankle 🄰 ☑
I70.744	Atherosclerosis of other type of bypass graft(s) of the left leg with ulceration of heel and midfoot 🄰 ☑
I70.745	Atherosclerosis of other type of bypass graft(s) of the left leg with ulceration of other part of foot 🄰 ☑
L89.513	Pressure ulcer of right ankle, stage 3 ☑
L89.514	Pressure ulcer of right ankle, stage 4 ☑
L89.516	Pressure-induced deep tissue damage of right ankle ☑
L89.523	Pressure ulcer of left ankle, stage 3 ☑
L89.524	Pressure ulcer of left ankle, stage 4 ☑
L89.526	Pressure-induced deep tissue damage of left ankle ☑
L89.613	Pressure ulcer of right heel, stage 3 ☑
L89.614	Pressure ulcer of right heel, stage 4 ☑
L89.616	Pressure-induced deep tissue damage of right heel ☑
L89.623	Pressure ulcer of left heel, stage 3 ☑
L89.624	Pressure ulcer of left heel, stage 4 ☑
L89.626	Pressure-induced deep tissue damage of left heel ☑

Relative Value Units/Medicare Edits

Non-Facility RVU	Work	PE	MP	Total
G0329	0.06	0.25	0.01	0.32
Facility RVU	**Work**	**PE**	**MP**	**Total**
G0329	0.06	0.25	0.01	0.32

	FUD	Status	MUE	Modifiers				IOM Reference
G0329	N/A	A	1(3)	N/A	N/A	N/A	80*	100-04,32,11.2

* with documentation

Terms To Know

atherosclerosis. Buildup of yellowish plaques composed of cholesterol and lipoid material within the arteries.

pressure ulcers. Progressively eroding skin lesion produced by inflamed necrotic tissue as it sloughs off, caused by continual pressure impeding blood circulation, especially over bony areas, when a patient lies still for too long without changing position.

HCPCS

G0341-G0343

G0341 Percutaneous islet cell transplant, includes portal vein catheterization and infusion
G0342 Laparoscopy for islet cell transplant, includes portal vein catheterization and infusion
G0343 Laparotomy for islet cell transplant, includes portal vein catheterization and infusion

Explanation

Islets cells are found in clusters throughout the pancreas and can be taken from an organ donor and transferred into the pancreas of the patient. Once transplanted, the cells can take over the task of destroyed cells. For example, diabetic Type I patients have a pancreas that no longer makes insulin and must take insulin daily. Once implanted, the islet cells, which contain beta cells, begin to make insulin. Each approach requires access to the portal vein, commonly via a transhepatic approach.

Coding Tips

Medicare covers transplantation of pancreatic islet cells, the insulin producing cells of the pancreas. Coverage includes the costs of acquisition and delivery of the pancreatic islet cells, as well as clinically necessary inpatient and outpatient medical care and immunosuppressants. Partial pancreatic tissue transplantation or islet cell transplantation performed outside the context of a clinical trial is not covered by Medicare. Third-party payers may not reimburse this code and may require the use of the appropriate CPT procedure code. Check with the payer for specific guidelines.

ICD-10-CM Diagnostic Codes

E10.10	Type 1 diabetes mellitus with ketoacidosis without coma
E10.11	Type 1 diabetes mellitus with ketoacidosis with coma
E10.21	Type 1 diabetes mellitus with diabetic nephropathy
E10.22	Type 1 diabetes mellitus with diabetic chronic kidney disease
E10.29	Type 1 diabetes mellitus with other diabetic kidney complication
E10.311	Type 1 diabetes mellitus with unspecified diabetic retinopathy with macular edema
E10.319	Type 1 diabetes mellitus with unspecified diabetic retinopathy without macular edema
E10.36	Type 1 diabetes mellitus with diabetic cataract
E10.39	Type 1 diabetes mellitus with other diabetic ophthalmic complication
E10.41	Type 1 diabetes mellitus with diabetic mononeuropathy
E10.42	Type 1 diabetes mellitus with diabetic polyneuropathy
E10.43	Type 1 diabetes mellitus with diabetic autonomic (poly)neuropathy
E10.44	Type 1 diabetes mellitus with diabetic amyotrophy
E10.49	Type 1 diabetes mellitus with other diabetic neurological complication
E10.51	Type 1 diabetes mellitus with diabetic peripheral angiopathy without gangrene
E10.52	Type 1 diabetes mellitus with diabetic peripheral angiopathy with gangrene
E10.59	Type 1 diabetes mellitus with other circulatory complications
E10.610	Type 1 diabetes mellitus with diabetic neuropathic arthropathy
E10.618	Type 1 diabetes mellitus with other diabetic arthropathy
E10.620	Type 1 diabetes mellitus with diabetic dermatitis
E10.621	Type 1 diabetes mellitus with foot ulcer
E10.622	Type 1 diabetes mellitus with other skin ulcer
E10.628	Type 1 diabetes mellitus with other skin complications
E10.630	Type 1 diabetes mellitus with periodontal disease
E10.638	Type 1 diabetes mellitus with other oral complications
E10.641	Type 1 diabetes mellitus with hypoglycemia with coma
E10.649	Type 1 diabetes mellitus with hypoglycemia without coma
E10.65	Type 1 diabetes mellitus with hyperglycemia
E10.69	Type 1 diabetes mellitus with other specified complication
E10.9	Type 1 diabetes mellitus without complications

Relative Value Units/Medicare Edits

Non-Facility RVU	Work	PE	MP	Total
G0341	6.98	55.49	0.56	63.03
G0342	11.92	6.91	0.95	19.78
G0343	19.85	11.99	4.84	36.68
Facility RVU	Work	PE	MP	Total
G0341	6.98	2.86	0.56	10.4
G0342	11.92	6.91	0.95	19.78
G0343	19.85	11.99	4.84	36.68

	FUD	Status	MUE	Modifiers				IOM Reference
G0341	0	A	1(2)	51	N/A	62*	80*	100-04,32,70
G0342	90	A	1(2)	51	N/A	62*	80	
G0343	90	A	1(2)	51	N/A	62*	80	

* with documentation

Terms To Know

catheterization. Use or insertion of a tubular device into a duct, blood vessel, hollow organ, or body cavity for injecting or withdrawing fluids for diagnostic or therapeutic purposes.

infusion. Introduction of a therapeutic fluid, other than blood, into the bloodstream.

islet cell. Islet of Langerhans, hormone producing pancreatic cells.

laparotomy. Incision through the flank or abdomen for therapeutic or diagnostic purposes.

G0455

G0455 Preparation with instillation of fecal microbiota by any method, including assessment of donor specimen

Explanation

Fecal microbiota transplantation (FMT) is the process of instilling fecal matter from a donor to a patient to treat a Clostridium difficile (C. diff) infection, most commonly. The donor stool is thinned using a normal saline solution and filtered for use in a nasogastric tube or an enema application. This code includes the screening protocol of the donor specimen for C. diff and other enteric bacterial pathogens and any ova or parasites.

Coding Tips

Third-party payers may not reimburse this code and may require the use of CPT code 44705. Check with the payer for specific guidelines.

ICD-10-CM Diagnostic Codes

A04.71	Enterocolitis due to Clostridium difficile, recurrent
A04.72	Enterocolitis due to Clostridium difficile, not specified as recurrent
K51.00	Ulcerative (chronic) pancolitis without complications
K51.011	Ulcerative (chronic) pancolitis with rectal bleeding
K51.012	Ulcerative (chronic) pancolitis with intestinal obstruction
K51.013	Ulcerative (chronic) pancolitis with fistula
K51.014	Ulcerative (chronic) pancolitis with abscess
K51.018	Ulcerative (chronic) pancolitis with other complication
K51.80	Other ulcerative colitis without complications
K51.811	Other ulcerative colitis with rectal bleeding
K51.812	Other ulcerative colitis with intestinal obstruction
K51.813	Other ulcerative colitis with fistula
K51.814	Other ulcerative colitis with abscess
K51.818	Other ulcerative colitis with other complication
K58.0	Irritable bowel syndrome with diarrhea
K59.01	Slow transit constipation
K59.02	Outlet dysfunction constipation
K59.09	Other constipation

Relative Value Units/Medicare Edits

Non-Facility RVU	Work	PE	MP	Total
G0455	1.34	2.31	0.14	3.79

Facility RVU	Work	PE	MP	Total
G0455	1.34	0.6	0.14	2.08

	FUD	Status	MUE	Modifiers				IOM Reference
G0455	0	A	1(2)	N/A	N/A	N/A	80*	None

* with documentation

[99091]

99091 Collection and interpretation of physiologic data (eg, ECG, blood pressure, glucose monitoring) digitally stored and/or transmitted by the patient and/or caregiver to the physician or other qualified health care professional, qualified by education, training, licensure/regulation (when applicable) requiring a minimum of 30 minutes of time, each 30 days

Explanation

A physician or other qualified health care professional collects and interprets physiologic data. The data (e.g., blood pressure) is stored digitally and may be transmitted by the patient and/or the caregiver to the provider. The report should contain the time it took the provider to acquire the physiologic data, review and interpret the data, and modify any care plan due to the additional data acquisition. A minimum of 30 minutes every 30 days must be spent in the collection and interpretation of data to report this service.

Relative Value Units/Medicare Edits

Non-Facility RVU	Work	PE	MP	Total
99091	1.1	0.47	0.06	1.63
Facility RVU	**Work**	**PE**	**MP**	**Total**
99091	1.1	0.47	0.06	1.63

[99457, 99458]

99457 Remote physiologic monitoring treatment management services, clinical staff/physician/other qualified health care professional time in a calendar month requiring interactive communication with the patient/caregiver during the month; first 20 minutes

+ 99458 Remote physiologic monitoring treatment management services, clinical staff/physician/other qualified health care professional time in a calendar month requiring interactive communication with the patient/caregiver during the month; each additional 20 minutes (List separately in addition to code for primary procedure)

Explanation

The provider or clinical staff utilizes the results obtained from an FDA-defined remote patient physiologic monitoring (RPM) device to oversee the patient's treatment plan. The device is ordered by a physician or other qualified health care provider and used by the patient for the purposes of collecting, monitoring, and reporting health-related data, including, but not limited to, weight, blood pressure, or pulse oximetry. This technology allows for the gathering of health data from the patient in one location and the electronic transmission of that data to a provider in a different location for review and subsequent recommendations, particularly in patients with ongoing and/or chronic disease processes. Report these codes to identify time spent managing care when the patient or the practice does not meet requirements for reporting a more specific service. These codes may be reported simultaneously with chronic care management, transitional care management, and behavioral health integration services. Time involved in performing this service should remain separate and distinct from other services and does not count toward the required time for both services in a single month. Live and interactive communication with the patient and/or caregiver is required. Report 99457 for the first 20 minutes of clinician time per calendar month and 99458 for each additional 20 minutes.

Relative Value Units/Medicare Edits

Non-Facility RVU	Work	PE	MP	Total
99457	0.61	0.81	0.04	1.46
99458	0.61	0.53	0.04	1.18
Facility RVU	**Work**	**PE**	**MP**	**Total**
99457	0.61	0.26	0.04	0.91
99458	0.61	0.26	0.04	0.91

76981-76983

76981 Ultrasound, elastography; parenchyma (eg, organ)

76982 first target lesion

+ 76983 each additional target lesion (List separately in addition to code for primary procedure)

Explanation

Ultrasound elastography (USE), also known as sonoelastography, is a noninvasive imaging technique that can be used to measure and depict relative tissue stiffness (shear wave) or displacement (strain) in response to an imparted force. Although the most common clinical application for USE is for chronic liver disease, tumor identification using this imaging modality is also effective since tumors are usually stiffer, or less elastic, than the surrounding soft tissue. The ultrasound technician takes a normal image followed by an image while pushing down or compressing the organ area. This happens multiple times and the images are generated in real time by using algorithms to give a clearer picture of the motion of the tissue being imaged. Report 76981 for imaging of an organ; 76982 for the initial target lesion; and 76983 for each additional target lesion.

Relative Value Units/Medicare Edits

Non-Facility RVU	Work	PE	MP	Total
76981	0.59	2.5	0.05	3.14
76982	0.59	2.28	0.05	2.92
76983	0.5	1.31	0.02	1.83
Facility RVU	**Work**	**PE**	**MP**	**Total**
76981	0.59	2.5	0.05	3.14
76982	0.59	2.28	0.05	2.92
76983	0.5	1.31	0.02	1.83

77001

+ 77001 Fluoroscopic guidance for central venous access device placement, replacement (catheter only or complete), or removal (includes fluoroscopic guidance for vascular access and catheter manipulation, any necessary contrast injections through access site or catheter with related venography radiologic supervision and interpretation, and radiographic documentation of final catheter position) (List separately in addition to code for primary procedure)

Explanation

This code reports the fluoroscopic guidance for placement, replacement, or removal of a central venous access device (CVAD) to be used in conjunction with the code for the procedure. For example, a tunneled, centrally inserted CVAD is inserted without subcutaneous port or pump. The site over the access vein (e.g., subclavian, jugular) is injected with local anesthesia and punctured with a needle or accessed by cutdown approach. A guidewire is inserted. A subcutaneous tunnel is created using a blunt pair of forceps or sharp tunneling tools over the clavicle from the anterior chest wall to the venotomy site, which is dilated to the right size. The catheter is passed through this tunnel over the guidewire and into the target vein. Fluoroscopy is used throughout the procedure to guide catheter placement and to check the positioning of the catheter tip.

This code includes any contrast injections done through the access site or through the catheter with the necessary corresponding radiological supervision and interpretation of the venography, and the radiographic check of final catheter position.

Relative Value Units/Medicare Edits

Non-Facility RVU	Work	PE	MP	Total
77001	0.38	2.58	0.05	3.01
Facility RVU	Work	PE	MP	Total
77001	0.38	2.58	0.05	3.01

77002

+ **77002** Fluoroscopic guidance for needle placement (eg, biopsy, aspiration, injection, localization device) (List separately in addition to code for primary procedure)

Explanation

Fluoroscopic guidance produces x-ray images shown on a screen to assist in visualization of the anatomy, instrument insertion, and/or contrast. This code is specifically reported when utilized for needle biopsy or fine needle aspiration. A cutting biopsy or fine needle is inserted into the target area and the position reaffirmed by fluoroscopy. This is done for an internal mass or lesion that has been positively identified by other diagnostic imaging performed earlier.

Relative Value Units/Medicare Edits

Non-Facility RVU	Work	PE	MP	Total
77002	0.54	2.82	0.05	3.41
Facility RVU	Work	PE	MP	Total
77002	0.54	2.82	0.05	3.41

77011

77011 Computed tomography guidance for stereotactic localization

Explanation

For stereotactic localization, a movable arm holding a needle is guided by computerized tomography (CT) to locate the lesion from different angles at different fixed points. The CT images tell the computer where the coordinates are to correctly align the needle.

Relative Value Units/Medicare Edits

Non-Facility RVU	Work	PE	MP	Total
77011	1.21	5.59	0.1	6.9
Facility RVU	Work	PE	MP	Total
77011	1.21	5.59	0.1	6.9

80051

80051 Electrolyte panel This panel must include the following: Carbon dioxide (bicarbonate) (82374) Chloride (82435) Potassium (84132) Sodium (84295)

Explanation

An electrolyte panel includes the following tests: carbon dioxide (82374), chloride (82435), potassium (84132), and sodium (84295). Blood specimen is obtained by venipuncture. See specific codes for additional information about the listed tests.

Relative Value Units/Medicare Edits

Non-Facility RVU	Work	PE	MP	Total
80051	0.0	0.0	0.0	0.0
Facility RVU	Work	PE	MP	Total
80051	0.0	0.0	0.0	0.0

80061

80061 Lipid panel This panel must include the following: Cholesterol, serum, total (82465) Lipoprotein, direct measurement, high density cholesterol (HDL cholesterol) (83718) Triglycerides (84478)

Explanation

A lipid panel includes the following tests: total serum cholesterol (82465), high-density cholesterol (HDL cholesterol) by direct measurement (83718), and triglycerides (84478). Blood specimen is obtained by venipuncture. See specific codes for additional information about the listed tests.

Relative Value Units/Medicare Edits

Non-Facility RVU	Work	PE	MP	Total
80061	0.0	0.0	0.0	0.0
Facility RVU	Work	PE	MP	Total
80061	0.0	0.0	0.0	0.0

81000

81000 Urinalysis, by dip stick or tablet reagent for bilirubin, glucose, hemoglobin, ketones, leukocytes, nitrite, pH, protein, specific gravity, urobilinogen, any number of these constituents; non-automated, with microscopy

Explanation

This type of test may be ordered by the brand name product and the analytes tested. Although screens are considered to show the presence of an analyte (qualitative), some newer products are semi-quantitative. Many are plastic strips that contain sites impregnated with chemicals that react with urine when the strip is dipped into a specimen. The result is a color change that is compared against a standardized chart. Most strips will test for numerous analytes, as well as for pH and specific gravity. Tablets work in a similar fashion. A drop of urine is placed on the tablet and a chemical reaction causes a color change that is compared to a standard chart. Usually only a single analyte is under consideration, per tablet. Code 81000 involves a manual (nonautomated) test and includes a microscopic examination. Microscopy involves examination of the urine sediments or solids. The urine is first centrifuged in a graduated tube to concentrate the sediments. Samples (either wet or dry) are examined, usually under both high and low power, and abnormal constituents are noted. These may include a wide range of biological abnormalities, such as blood cells, casts, and bacteria, as well as chemical anomalies, such as crystals.

Relative Value Units/Medicare Edits

Non-Facility RVU	Work	PE	MP	Total
81000	0.0	0.0	0.0	0.0
Facility RVU	Work	PE	MP	Total
81000	0.0	0.0	0.0	0.0

Appendix

81001

81001 Urinalysis, by dip stick or tablet reagent for bilirubin, glucose, hemoglobin, ketones, leukocytes, nitrite, pH, protein, specific gravity, urobilinogen, any number of these constituents; automated, with microscopy

Explanation

This type of test may be ordered by the type of processor used and the analytes tested. The testing methodology is similar to the manual strips, except that the color change caused by the chemical reaction with urine is processed and read mechanically. The strip is exposed to the urine sample and is mechanically fed through a processor that reads the colors emitted by the reaction. The unit will be calibrated according to international standards and readings have a high degree of accuracy. The result may be displayed on a monitor, but is always printed or recorded in some form. Code 81001 also includes a microscopy. Microscopy involves examination of the urine sediments or solids. The urine is first centrifuged in a graduated tube to concentrate the sediments. Samples (either wet or dry) are examined, usually under both high and low power, and abnormal constituents are noted. These may include a wide range of biological abnormalities, such as blood cells, casts, and bacteria, as well as chemical anomalies, such as crystals.

Relative Value Units/Medicare Edits

Non-Facility RVU	Work	PE	MP	Total
81001	0.0	0.0	0.0	0.0
Facility RVU	Work	PE	MP	Total
81001	0.0	0.0	0.0	0.0

81002

81002 Urinalysis, by dip stick or tablet reagent for bilirubin, glucose, hemoglobin, ketones, leukocytes, nitrite, pH, protein, specific gravity, urobilinogen, any number of these constituents; non-automated, without microscopy

Explanation

This type of test may be ordered by the brand name product and the analytes tested. Although usually considered screens to show the presence of an analyte (qualitative), some newer products are semi-quantitative. Many are plastic strips that contain sites impregnated with chemicals that react with urine when the strip is dipped into a specimen. The result is a color change that is compared against a standardized chart. Most strips will test for numerous analytes, as well as for pH and specific gravity. Tablets work in a similar fashion. A drop of urine is placed on the tablet and a chemical reaction causes a color change that is compared to a standard chart. Usually only a single analyte is under consideration per tablet, however. Code 81002 does not include a microscopic examination of the urine sample or its components.

Relative Value Units/Medicare Edits

Non-Facility RVU	Work	PE	MP	Total
81002	0.0	0.0	0.0	0.0
Facility RVU	Work	PE	MP	Total
81002	0.0	0.0	0.0	0.0

81003

81003 Urinalysis, by dip stick or tablet reagent for bilirubin, glucose, hemoglobin, ketones, leukocytes, nitrite, pH, protein, specific gravity, urobilinogen, any number of these constituents; automated, without microscopy

Explanation

This type of test may be ordered by the type of processor used and the analytes tested. The testing methodology is similar to the manual strips, except that the color change caused by the chemical reaction with urine is processed and read mechanically. The strip is exposed to the urine sample and is mechanically fed through a processor that reads the colors emitted by the reaction. The unit will be calibrated according to international standards and readings have a high degree of accuracy. The result may be displayed on a monitor, but is always printed or recorded in some form. Code 81003 does not include a microscopic examination of the urine sample or its components.

Relative Value Units/Medicare Edits

Non-Facility RVU	Work	PE	MP	Total
81003	0.0	0.0	0.0	0.0
Facility RVU	Work	PE	MP	Total
81003	0.0	0.0	0.0	0.0

81007

81007 Urinalysis; bacteriuria screen, except by culture or dipstick

Explanation

This type of test may be ordered by the brand name of the commercial kit used and the bacteria that the kit screens for. Human urine is normally free of bacteria. However, bacteria can easily be introduced upon voiding. In addition, specimens containing any amount of pathological bacteria can have the organisms rapidly multiply after collection. For this reason, specimens are often examined shortly after collection. Method includes any method except culture or dipstick. The test is often performed by commercial kit. The type of kit used should be specified in the report.

Relative Value Units/Medicare Edits

Non-Facility RVU	Work	PE	MP	Total
81007	0.0	0.0	0.0	0.0
Facility RVU	Work	PE	MP	Total
81007	0.0	0.0	0.0	0.0

82040

82040 Albumin; serum, plasma or whole blood

Explanation

This test measures the concentration of albumin in serum, plasma, or whole blood. It is often used to determine nutritional status, renal disease, and other chronic diseases, particularly those involving the kidneys or liver. A blood sample is typically drawn from a vein in the hand or forearm. The skin over the vein is cleaned with an antiseptic, and a tourniquet is wrapped around the upper arm to enlarge the lower arm veins by restricting the blood flow. A thin needle is inserted into the vein, the tourniquet is removed, and blood flows from the vein through the needle and is collected into a vial or syringe. The needle is withdrawn and the puncture site covered to prevent bleeding. The blood sample is sent to the laboratory for testing.

Relative Value Units/Medicare Edits

Non-Facility RVU	Work	PE	MP	Total
82040	0.0	0.0	0.0	0.0
Facility RVU	Work	PE	MP	Total
82040	0.0	0.0	0.0	0.0

Appendix

82150

82150   Amylase

Explanation

Serum amylase is elevated in acute pancreatitis and is, therefore, a common test when abdominal pain, epigastric tenderness, nausea, and vomiting are present. There are multiple methods of testing for amylase.

Relative Value Units/Medicare Edits

Non-Facility RVU	Work	PE	MP	Total
82150	0.0	0.0	0.0	0.0
Facility RVU	Work	PE	MP	Total
82150	0.0	0.0	0.0	0.0

82247-82248

82247   Bilirubin; total
82248   direct

Explanation

Bilirubin is a bile pigment formed by the breakdown of hemoglobin during both normal and abnormal erythrocyte destruction. Direct (conjugated) bilirubin is that portion of the bilirubin that has been taken up by the liver cells to form bilirubin diglucuronide. Indirect (unconjugated) bilirubin is that portion of the bilirubin that has not been taken up by the liver cells. Total bilirubin is the sum of direct and indirect bilirubin present in the specimen. Blood is obtained by venipuncture. Method is diazotization. Spectrophotometry may be used in neonates six weeks or younger. Report 82247 for total bilirubin. Report 82248 for direct bilirubin.

Relative Value Units/Medicare Edits

Non-Facility RVU	Work	PE	MP	Total
82247	0.0	0.0	0.0	0.0
82248	0.0	0.0	0.0	0.0
Facility RVU	Work	PE	MP	Total
82247	0.0	0.0	0.0	0.0
82248	0.0	0.0	0.0	0.0

82270

82270   Blood, occult, by peroxidase activity (eg, guaiac), qualitative; feces, consecutive collected specimens with single determination, for colorectal neoplasm screening (ie, patient was provided 3 cards or single triple card for consecutive collection)

Explanation

This test may be requested as a screening guaiac, screening stool guaiac, or by a variety of brand names. The patient is instructed to obtain three consecutive stool specimens and send the kit to a lab or physician office for performance of the test. The method is peroxidase activity. This test reports the presence (qualitative analysis) of blood in the stool, but does not quantify the amount. This code is used to report the service when performed as colorectal neoplasm screening.

Relative Value Units/Medicare Edits

Non-Facility RVU	Work	PE	MP	Total
82270	0.0	0.0	0.0	0.0
Facility RVU	Work	PE	MP	Total
82270	0.0	0.0	0.0	0.0

82274

82274   Blood, occult, by fecal hemoglobin determination by immunoassay, qualitative, feces, 1-3 simultaneous determinations

Explanation

Fecal sample is dispersed in a diluent with antibodies for hemoglobin antigen to form a complex of antibody and antigen. A complex of antibody and antigen is separated from the specimen and exposed to a second antibody for the hemoglobin antigen. A sample from the first complex is bound to a solid carrier, and a sample from the second antibody exposure is labeled with a detection agent to determine the presence of hemoglobin antigen in the original fecal specimen. This code requires one to three consecutive stool samples, which must be obtained from separate bowel movements, and each sample must be placed in a sterile, leakproof container with a screw-cap lid for transport to the laboratory.

Relative Value Units/Medicare Edits

Non-Facility RVU	Work	PE	MP	Total
82274	0.0	0.0	0.0	0.0
Facility RVU	Work	PE	MP	Total
82274	0.0	0.0	0.0	0.0

82465

82465   Cholesterol, serum or whole blood, total

Explanation

Cholesterol level is a risk indicator for atherosclerosis and myocardial infarction. Blood specimen is obtained by venipuncture. Method is enzymatic. This test reports total cholesterol in serum or whole blood.

Relative Value Units/Medicare Edits

Non-Facility RVU	Work	PE	MP	Total
82465	0.0	0.0	0.0	0.0
Facility RVU	Work	PE	MP	Total
82465	0.0	0.0	0.0	0.0

82948

82948   Glucose; blood, reagent strip

Explanation

This test is used to monitor disorders of carbohydrate metabolism. Blood specimen is obtained by finger stick. A drop of blood is placed on the reagent strip for a specified amount of time. When the prescribed amount of time has elapsed, the strip is blotted and the reagent strip is compared to a color chart. Method is reagent strip with visual comparison.

Relative Value Units/Medicare Edits

Non-Facility RVU	Work	PE	MP	Total
82948	0.0	0.0	0.0	0.0
Facility RVU	Work	PE	MP	Total
82948	0.0	0.0	0.0	0.0

83718

83718   Lipoprotein, direct measurement; high density cholesterol (HDL cholesterol)

Appendix

Explanation

This test may be requested as HDL, HDLC, or HDL cholesterol. Lipoproteins are compounds composed of lipids bound to proteins, which are transported through the blood. High-density lipoprotein (HDL) is frequently referred to as "good cholesterol," or "friendly lipid," as it is responsible for decreasing plaque deposits in blood vessels. High levels of HDL decrease the risk of premature coronary artery disease. This code reports direct measurement only, normally performed using an enzymatic or precipitation method.

Relative Value Units/Medicare Edits

Non-Facility RVU	Work	PE	MP	Total
83718	0.0	0.0	0.0	0.0
Facility RVU	Work	PE	MP	Total
83718	0.0	0.0	0.0	0.0

83719

83719   Lipoprotein, direct measurement; VLDL cholesterol

Explanation

This test measures VLDL, the lipoprotein that carries triglycerides in the blood. The test is useful to determine a patient's risk of arteriosclerotic occlusive disease, as well as other cholesterol-related disorders. The method used is electrophoresis and may first involve ultracentrifugation.

Relative Value Units/Medicare Edits

Non-Facility RVU	Work	PE	MP	Total
83719	0.0	0.0	0.0	0.0
Facility RVU	Work	PE	MP	Total
83719	0.0	0.0	0.0	0.0

83721

83721   Lipoprotein, direct measurement; LDL cholesterol

Explanation

This test may also be referred to as LDL-C. It measures the amount of low-density lipoprotein (LDL), also known as "bad cholesterol." The test is useful to determine the patient's risk of coronary heart disease (CHD), among other disorders. Method may be by precipitation procedure with results derived by the Friedewald formula.

Relative Value Units/Medicare Edits

Non-Facility RVU	Work	PE	MP	Total
83721	0.0	0.0	0.0	0.0
Facility RVU	Work	PE	MP	Total
83721	0.0	0.0	0.0	0.0

83722

83722   Lipoprotein, direct measurement; small dense LDL cholesterol

Explanation

This test may be ordered as sd-LDL. It measures the heavier, small dense LDL, the lipoprotein that carries triglycerides in the blood. This test is useful in determining a patient's risk for arteriosclerotic occlusive disease, as well as other cholesterol-related disorders. Specimen is serum. The method used is automated colorimetry.

Relative Value Units/Medicare Edits

Non-Facility RVU	Work	PE	MP	Total
83722	0.0	0.0	0.0	0.0
Facility RVU	Work	PE	MP	Total
83722	0.0	0.0	0.0	0.0

84132

84132   Potassium; serum, plasma or whole blood

Explanation

This test may be requested as K or K+. Potassium is the major electrolyte found in intracellular fluids. Potassium influences skeletal and cardiac muscle activity. Very small fluctuations outside the normal range may cause significant health risk, including muscle weakness and cardiac arrhythmias. Blood specimen is serum, plasma, or whole blood. Methods include atomic absorption spectrometry (AAS), ion-selective electrode (ISE), and flame emission spectroscopy (FES).

Relative Value Units/Medicare Edits

Non-Facility RVU	Work	PE	MP	Total
84132	0.0	0.0	0.0	0.0
Facility RVU	Work	PE	MP	Total
84132	0.0	0.0	0.0	0.0

84525

84525   Urea nitrogen; semiquantitative (eg, reagent strip test)

Explanation

This test may also be ordered as a BUN. This test may provide useful information regarding carbohydrate metabolism (diabetes), kidney function, and acid-base balance. The specimen type is plasma. Method is reagent strip.

Relative Value Units/Medicare Edits

Non-Facility RVU	Work	PE	MP	Total
84525	0.0	0.0	0.0	0.0
Facility RVU	Work	PE	MP	Total
84525	0.0	0.0	0.0	0.0

85002

85002   Bleeding time

Explanation

This test may be ordered as a bleeding time or as an Ivy bleeding time. A small, superficial wound is nicked in the patient's forearm. Essentially, the amount of time it takes for the wound to stop bleeding is recorded at bedside. The Ivy bleeding time test is one standardized method. All methods are manual or point of care. A bleeding time is a rough measure of platelet (thrombocyte) function. The test is often performed on a preoperative patient.

Relative Value Units/Medicare Edits

Non-Facility RVU	Work	PE	MP	Total
85002	0.0	0.0	0.0	0.0
Facility RVU	Work	PE	MP	Total
85002	0.0	0.0	0.0	0.0

85004

85004   Blood count; automated differential WBC count

Appendix

Explanation

This test may be ordered as a blood count with automated differential. The specimen is whole blood. Method is automated cell counter. The blood count typically includes a measurement of normal cell constituents including white blood cells or leukocytes, red blood cells, and platelets. In addition, this test includes a differential count of the white blood cells or "diff" in which the following leukocytes are differentiated and counted automatically: neutrophils or granulocytes, lymphocytes, monocytes, eosinophils, and basophils.

Relative Value Units/Medicare Edits

Non-Facility RVU	Work	PE	MP	Total
85004	0.0	0.0	0.0	0.0
Facility RVU	Work	PE	MP	Total
85004	0.0	0.0	0.0	0.0

85007-85008

85007   Blood count; blood smear, microscopic examination with manual differential WBC count

85008   blood smear, microscopic examination without manual differential WBC count

Explanation

These tests may be ordered as a manual blood smear examination, RBC smear, peripheral blood smear, or RBC morphology without differential parameters in 85008 and with manual WBC differential in 85007. The specimen is whole blood. The method is manual testing. A blood smear is prepared and microscopically examined for the presence of normal cell constituents, including white blood cells, red blood cells, and platelets. In 85008, the white blood cell and platelet or thrombocyte counts are estimated and red cell morphology is commented on if abnormal. In 85007, a manual differential of white blood cells is included in which the following leukocytes are differentiated: neutrophils or granulocytes, lymphocytes, monocytes, eosinophils, and basophils.

Relative Value Units/Medicare Edits

Non-Facility RVU	Work	PE	MP	Total
85007	0.0	0.0	0.0	0.0
85008	0.0	0.0	0.0	0.0
Facility RVU	Work	PE	MP	Total
85007	0.0	0.0	0.0	0.0
85008	0.0	0.0	0.0	0.0

85013

85013   Blood count; spun microhematocrit

Explanation

This test may be ordered as a microhematocrit, a spun microhematocrit, or a "spun crit." The specimen (whole blood) is by finger stick or heel stick in infants. The sample is placed in a tube and into a microcentrifuge device. The vials can be read manually against a chart for the volume of packed red cells or a digital reader in the centrifuge device. A spun microhematocrit only reports the volume of packed red cells. It is typically performed at sites where limited testing is available, the patient is a very difficult blood draw, or on infants.

Relative Value Units/Medicare Edits

Non-Facility RVU	Work	PE	MP	Total
85013	0.0	0.0	0.0	0.0
Facility RVU	Work	PE	MP	Total
85013	0.0	0.0	0.0	0.0

85014

85014   Blood count; hematocrit (Hct)

Explanation

This test may be ordered as a hematocrit, Hmt, or Hct. The specimen is whole blood. Method is automated cell counter. The hematocrit or volume of packed red cells (VPRC) in the blood sample is calculated by multiplying the red blood cell count or RBC times the mean corpuscular volume or MCV.

Relative Value Units/Medicare Edits

Non-Facility RVU	Work	PE	MP	Total
85014	0.0	0.0	0.0	0.0
Facility RVU	Work	PE	MP	Total
85014	0.0	0.0	0.0	0.0

85018

85018   Blood count; hemoglobin (Hgb)

Explanation

This test may be ordered as hemoglobin, Hgb, or hemoglobin concentration. The specimen is whole blood. Method is usually automated cell counter but a manual method is seen in labs with a limited test menu and blood bank drawing stations. Hemoglobin is an index of the oxygen-carrying capacity of the blood.

Relative Value Units/Medicare Edits

Non-Facility RVU	Work	PE	MP	Total
85018	0.0	0.0	0.0	0.0
Facility RVU	Work	PE	MP	Total
85018	0.0	0.0	0.0	0.0

85651

85651   Sedimentation rate, erythrocyte; non-automated

Explanation

This test may be ordered as an erythrocyte sedimentation rate (ESR), a Westergren sedimentation rate, Wintrobe sedimentation rate, or simply as a "sed rate." The specimen is whole blood. This test is a non-specific screening test for a number of diseases including anemia, disorders of protein production such as multiple myeloma, other conditions that alter the size and/or shape of red cells or erythrocytes, and to screen diseases that cause an increase or decrease in the amount of protein in the plasma. Further studies are often launched by ESR results. The method is manual. A variety of procedures have been used over time to study sedimentation rate. A common one performed manually is the Westergren tube.

Relative Value Units/Medicare Edits

Non-Facility RVU	Work	PE	MP	Total
85651	0.0	0.0	0.0	0.0
Facility RVU	Work	PE	MP	Total
85651	0.0	0.0	0.0	0.0

86318

86318   Immunoassay for infectious agent antibody(ies), qualitative or semiquantitative, single-step method (eg, reagent strip);

Explanation

This code may be requested as a single step qualitative or semi-quantitative immunoassay to identify the presence of specific infectious agent antibodies.

Specimen is serum. Method is immunoassay. Single step methods frequently use a reagent strip for the specific antibody.

Relative Value Units/Medicare Edits

Non-Facility RVU	Work	PE	MP	Total
86318	0.0	0.0	0.0	0.0
Facility RVU	Work	PE	MP	Total
86318	0.0	0.0	0.0	0.0

87086-87088

87086 Culture, bacterial; quantitative colony count, urine
87088 with isolation and presumptive identification of each isolate, urine

Explanation

These codes report the performance of a urine bacterial culture with a calibrated inoculating device so that a colony count accurately correlates with the number of organisms in the urine. In 87088, isolation and presumptive identification of bacteria recovered from the sample is done by means of identifying colony morphology, subculturing organisms to selective media and the performance of a gram stain or other simple test to identify bacteria to the genus level. There are several automated systems that detect the presence of bacteria using colorimetric, radiometric, or spectrophotometric means. In 87086, quantified colony count numbers within the urine sample are measured.

Relative Value Units/Medicare Edits

Non-Facility RVU	Work	PE	MP	Total
87086	0.0	0.0	0.0	0.0
87088	0.0	0.0	0.0	0.0
Facility RVU	Work	PE	MP	Total
87086	0.0	0.0	0.0	0.0
87088	0.0	0.0	0.0	0.0

88375

88375 Optical endomicroscopic image(s), interpretation and report, real-time or referred, each endoscopic session

Explanation

The images captured using an optical endomicroscope during endoscopy are reviewed, interpreted, and a report is generated. The endomicroscope uses laser light to magnify the cells of the mucosa in order to identify the histopathology without a biopsy. This service can be performed during the procedure (real time) or at a later time. This code is reported per endoscopic procedure, not per image.

Relative Value Units/Medicare Edits

Non-Facility RVU	Work	PE	MP	Total
88375	0.91	0.45	0.05	1.41
Facility RVU	Work	PE	MP	Total
88375	0.91	0.45	0.05	1.41

90389

90389 Tetanus immune globulin (TIg), human, for intramuscular use

Explanation

This code identifies a tetanus immune globulin (TIg), human, for intramuscular use. This immune globulin is a passive immunization agent that gives protection against tetanus and is obtained from donated, pooled human plasma. Passive immunity is achieved for a short period as the antibodies received through the

immune globulin are circulated through the body. The recipient's immune system is not stimulated to build its own antibodies. Report this code with the appropriate administration code.

Relative Value Units/Medicare Edits

Non-Facility RVU	Work	PE	MP	Total
90389	0.0	0.0	0.0	0.0
Facility RVU	Work	PE	MP	Total
90389	0.0	0.0	0.0	0.0

91034

91034 Esophagus, gastroesophageal reflux test; with nasal catheter pH electrode(s) placement, recording, analysis and interpretation

Explanation

The physician performs a gastroesophageal reflux test using esophageal pH electrode placement and recording. This procedure evaluates the proper functioning of the lower esophageal sphincter, the strong muscular ring located at the entrance to the stomach. When this specialized muscle opens at the wrong time, stomach acid will flow back up into the esophagus, causing gastroesophageal reflux. A small, thin probe, or electrode, that measures the pH (acidity) level within the esophagus is affixed at the end of flexible nasal catheter tubing. The catheter is inserted through the nose down to the target area in the esophagus, usually determined by manometry, and connected to a data recorder. The probe records the pH level within the esophagus. Neutral pH is 7. The lower the number, the more acidic the environment. The stomach has a normal pH around 2. The pH recording may be done over the course of a day. The catheter/tubing is taped behind the ear and out of the way under clothing, and connected to a small data recorder that is worn around the waist. This code includes the analysis and interpretation of the recorded results.

Relative Value Units/Medicare Edits

Non-Facility RVU	Work	PE	MP	Total
91034	0.97	4.82	0.06	5.85
Facility RVU	Work	PE	MP	Total
91034	0.97	4.82	0.06	5.85

91035

91035 Esophagus, gastroesophageal reflux test; with mucosal attached telemetry pH electrode placement, recording, analysis and interpretation

Explanation

The physician performs a gastroesophageal reflux test using mucosal attached telemetry pH electrode placement and recording. A small capsule containing a radiotelemetry pH sensor is inserted endoscopically in the esophagus and temporarily attached to the esophageal wall. The capsule monitors esophageal pH levels over a 48-hour period. This information is transmitted to an external pager-sized receiver worn by the patient that records pH levels. After the 48-hour testing period, the data is downloaded from the receiver to a computer that contains software for analyzing pH levels. The physician provides a written interpretation of the computer analysis. The capsule does not need to be removed as it spontaneously detaches within seven to 10 days and passes through the digestive tract.

● New   ▲ Revised   + Add On   ★ Telemedicine   [Resequenced]

Coding Companion for General Surgery/Gastroenterology

Appendix

Relative Value Units/Medicare Edits

Non-Facility RVU	Work	PE	MP	Total
91035	1.59	13.1	0.12	14.81
Facility RVU	**Work**	**PE**	**MP**	**Total**
91035	1.59	13.1	0.12	14.81

91037-91038

91037 Esophageal function test, gastroesophageal reflux test with nasal catheter intraluminal impedance electrode(s) placement, recording, analysis and interpretation;

91038 prolonged (greater than 1 hour, up to 24 hours)

Explanation

The physician performs an esophageal function test with gastroesophageal reflux testing using nasal catheter intraluminal impedance electrode placement and recording. The patient fasts for a minimum of six hours. An impedance probe affixed to flexible nasal catheter tubing is inserted through the nose down to the lower esophageal sphincter following location of the lower sphincter by manometry. The impedance probe contains several electrodes that make up multiple measuring segments each 2 cm in length. The measuring segments are located at intervals above the proximal border of the lower esophageal sphincter. The patient is given a liquid or solid bolus to swallow. As the bolus passes through the esophagus, the average electrical resistance between two adjacent electrodes (impedance) is measured. The electrodes detect esophageal contraction and expansion and movement of the bolus through the esophagus in real time, as well as any gastroesophageal reflux. Esophageal function is evaluated by calculating the bolus transport time (BTT), which is the time it takes the bolus to pass from the proximal measuring segment and exit through the distal measuring segment. Contraction wave velocity (CWV), which is the speed of the contraction wave from the proximal measuring segment to the distal measuring segment, is also evaluated. This test is also referred to as multichannel intraluminal impedance testing or MII. Report 91037 for a recording of one hour or less. Report 91038 for prolonged recording of greater than one hour, up to 24 hours.

Relative Value Units/Medicare Edits

Non-Facility RVU	Work	PE	MP	Total
91037	0.97	4.1	0.05	5.12
91038	1.1	12.08	0.05	13.23
Facility RVU	**Work**	**PE**	**MP**	**Total**
91037	0.97	4.1	0.05	5.12
91038	1.1	12.08	0.05	13.23

91040

91040 Esophageal balloon distension study, diagnostic, with provocation when performed

Explanation

The physician performs a diagnostic esophageal balloon distension study, including provocation, when performed, to evaluate chest pain of undetermined etiology that is suspected to be noncardiac in origin. The patient fasts for a minimum of six hours. A local anesthetic is sprayed into the patient's throat. With the patient in an upright position, a probe is passed through the mouth into the esophagus. The subject is placed supine with the head of the exam table elevated approximately 30 degrees. Manometric pressure recordings are obtained to identify the upper and lower esophageal sphincters. The probe is removed and the physician inserts a balloon into the esophagus. The balloon is moved along the esophagus and inflated multiple times to increasing diameters at selected sites in the esophagus in an attempt to provoke chest pain in the patient. Pain is measured by conscious perception or objective responses to the stimuli. Perception of moderate to severe chest pain with low levels of balloon distension is considered to be positive for noncardiac chest pain.

Relative Value Units/Medicare Edits

Non-Facility RVU	Work	PE	MP	Total
91040	0.97	15.08	0.06	16.11
Facility RVU	**Work**	**PE**	**MP**	**Total**
91040	0.97	15.08	0.06	16.11

92950

92950 Cardiopulmonary resuscitation (eg, in cardiac arrest)

Explanation

Cardiopulmonary arrest occurs when the patient's heart and lungs suddenly stop. In a clinical setting, cardiopulmonary resuscitation, the attempt at restarting the heart and lungs, is usually directed by a physician or another health care provider who is certified in Advanced Cardiac Life Support (ACLS). The patient's lungs are ventilated by mouth-to-mouth breathing or by a bag and mask. The patient's circulation is assisted using external chest compression. An electronic defibrillator may be used to shock the heart into restarting. Medications used to restart the heart include epinephrine and lidocaine.

Relative Value Units/Medicare Edits

Non-Facility RVU	Work	PE	MP	Total
92950	4.0	5.33	0.39	9.72
Facility RVU	**Work**	**PE**	**MP**	**Total**
92950	4.0	0.98	0.39	5.37

93000-93010

93000 Electrocardiogram, routine ECG with at least 12 leads; with interpretation and report

93005 tracing only, without interpretation and report

93010 interpretation and report only

Explanation

Multiple electrodes are placed on a patient's chest to record the electrical activity of the heart. A physician interprets the findings. Report 93000 for the combined technical and professional components of an ECG; 93005 for the technical component only; and 93010 for the professional component only.

Relative Value Units/Medicare Edits

Non-Facility RVU	Work	PE	MP	Total
93000	0.17	0.24	0.02	0.43
93005	0.0	0.18	0.01	0.19
93010	0.17	0.06	0.01	0.24
Facility RVU	**Work**	**PE**	**MP**	**Total**
93000	0.17	0.24	0.02	0.43
93005	0.0	0.18	0.01	0.19
93010	0.17	0.06	0.01	0.24

93040

93040 Rhythm ECG, 1-3 leads; with interpretation and report

Explanation

One to three electrodes placed on a patient's chest are used to record electrical activity of the heart. The physician interprets the report.

Appendix

Relative Value Units/Medicare Edits

Non-Facility RVU	Work	PE	MP	Total
93040	0.15	0.2	0.02	0.37
Facility RVU	**Work**	**PE**	**MP**	**Total**
93040	0.15	0.2	0.02	0.37

93041

93041 Rhythm ECG, 1-3 leads; tracing only without interpretation and report

Explanation

An assistant records the electrical activity of the heart by placing one to three electrodes on a patient's chest in a predetermined pattern. This code describes the tracing only.

Relative Value Units/Medicare Edits

Non-Facility RVU	Work	PE	MP	Total
93041	0.0	0.16	0.01	0.17
Facility RVU	**Work**	**PE**	**MP**	**Total**
93041	0.0	0.16	0.01	0.17

93042

93042 Rhythm ECG, 1-3 leads; interpretation and report only

Explanation

A physician interprets a recording of electrical activities of a patient's heart acquired by placing one to three electrodes on the patient's chest.

Relative Value Units/Medicare Edits

Non-Facility RVU	Work	PE	MP	Total
93042	0.15	0.04	0.01	0.2
Facility RVU	**Work**	**PE**	**MP**	**Total**
93042	0.15	0.04	0.01	0.2

93503

93503 Insertion and placement of flow directed catheter (eg, Swan-Ganz) for monitoring purposes

Explanation

The physician threads a catheter to the right heart through a central intravenous line often inserted up the femoral vein to take blood samples, pressure and electrical recordings, and/or other tests. This code applies to the insertion of a flow directed catheter, such as the Swan-Ganz device, used for measuring pressure and related parameters.

Relative Value Units/Medicare Edits

Non-Facility RVU	Work	PE	MP	Total
93503	2.0	0.38	0.17	2.55
Facility RVU	**Work**	**PE**	**MP**	**Total**
93503	2.0	0.38	0.17	2.55

94002-94004

94002 Ventilation assist and management, initiation of pressure or volume preset ventilators for assisted or controlled breathing; hospital inpatient/observation, initial day

94003 Ventilation assist and management, initiation of pressure or volume preset ventilators for assisted or controlled breathing; hospital inpatient/observation, each subsequent day

94004 nursing facility, per day

Explanation

A mechanical ventilator is applied with a mask over the nose and mouth or through a tube placed into the trachea for patients requiring help breathing due to a lung disorder. Intermittent positive pressure breathing uses positive pressure during the inspiration phase of breathing. Code 94002 applies to ventilation assistance using adjustments in volume and pressure on the initial day of treatment in a hospital to an inpatient or observation patient and 94003 is reported for ventilation assistance to a hospital inpatient or observation patient provided on subsequent days. Ventilation assistance and management provided to a nursing facility patient is reported with 94004 on a per day basis.

Relative Value Units/Medicare Edits

Non-Facility RVU	Work	PE	MP	Total
94002	1.99	0.52	0.15	2.66
94003	1.37	0.42	0.11	1.9
94004	1.0	0.34	0.06	1.4
Facility RVU	**Work**	**PE**	**MP**	**Total**
94002	1.99	0.52	0.15	2.66
94003	1.37	0.42	0.11	1.9
94004	1.0	0.34	0.06	1.4

94005

94005 Home ventilator management care plan oversight of a patient (patient not present) in home, domiciliary or rest home (eg, assisted living) requiring review of status, review of laboratories and other studies and revision of orders and respiratory care plan (as appropriate), within a calendar month, 30 minutes or more

Explanation

A mechanical ventilator is applied with a mask over the nose and mouth or through a tube placed into the trachea for patients requiring help breathing due to a lung disorder. Intermittent positive pressure breathing uses positive pressure during the inspiration phase of breathing. Code 94005 reports at least 30 minutes of care plan oversight for ventilation assist and management occurring within a calendar month for a patient at home or in assisted living (domiciliary or rest home). The physician reviews lab work and other studies and orders revisions in the care plan as appropriate.

Relative Value Units/Medicare Edits

Non-Facility RVU	Work	PE	MP	Total
94005	1.5	1.04	0.13	2.67
Facility RVU	**Work**	**PE**	**MP**	**Total**
94005	1.5	1.04	0.13	2.67

94662

94662 Continuous negative pressure ventilation (CNP), initiation and management

Coding Companion for General Surgery/Gastroenterology

Explanation

A mechanical ventilator is applied with a mask over the nose and mouth or through a tube placed into the trachea for patients requiring help breathing due to a lung disorder. Intermittent negative pressure breathing uses negative pressure during the inspiration phase of breathing. This code applies to subsequent evaluation or application of continuous negative airway pressure for ventilation assistance with negative pressure during inspiration and exhalation.

Relative Value Units/Medicare Edits

Non-Facility RVU	Work	PE	MP	Total
94662	0.76	0.22	0.05	1.03
Facility RVU	Work	PE	MP	Total
94662	0.76	0.22	0.05	1.03

94760

94760   Noninvasive ear or pulse oximetry for oxygen saturation; single determination

Explanation

A sensor is placed on the ear lobe or finger to measure oxygen levels in the blood for a pulse oximetry. A light shines through the capillary bed for the measurement. This code applies to a single measurement.

Relative Value Units/Medicare Edits

Non-Facility RVU	Work	PE	MP	Total
94760	0.0	0.06	0.01	0.07
Facility RVU	Work	PE	MP	Total
94760	0.0	0.06	0.01	0.07

94761

94761   Noninvasive ear or pulse oximetry for oxygen saturation; multiple determinations (eg, during exercise)

Explanation

A sensor is placed on the ear lobe or finger to measure oxygen levels in the blood for a pulse oximetry. A light shines through the capillary bed for the measurement. This code applies to multiple measurements.

Relative Value Units/Medicare Edits

Non-Facility RVU	Work	PE	MP	Total
94761	0.0	0.1	0.01	0.11
Facility RVU	Work	PE	MP	Total
94761	0.0	0.1	0.01	0.11

96360-96361

  96360   Intravenous infusion, hydration; initial, 31 minutes to 1 hour
+ 96361   each additional hour (List separately in addition to code for primary procedure)

Explanation

A physician or an assistant under direct physician supervision infuses a hydration solution (prepackaged fluid and electrolytes) for 31 minutes to one hour through an intravenous catheter inserted by needle into a patient's vein or by infusion through an existing indwelling intravascular access catheter or port. Report 96361 for each additional hour beyond the first hour. Intravenous infusion for hydration lasting 30 minutes or less is not reported.

Relative Value Units/Medicare Edits

Non-Facility RVU	Work	PE	MP	Total
96360	0.17	0.85	0.02	1.04
96361	0.09	0.3	0.01	0.4
Facility RVU	Work	PE	MP	Total
96360	0.17	0.85	0.02	1.04
96361	0.09	0.3	0.01	0.4

96369-96371

  96369   Subcutaneous infusion for therapy or prophylaxis (specify substance or drug); initial, up to 1 hour, including pump set-up and establishment of subcutaneous infusion site(s)
+ 96370   each additional hour (List separately in addition to code for primary procedure)
+ 96371   additional pump set-up with establishment of new subcutaneous infusion site(s) (List separately in addition to code for primary procedure)

Explanation

A physician or an assistant under direct physician supervision infuses a therapeutic or prophylactic (preventive) medication other than chemotherapy or other highly complex drug or biologic agent via a subcutaneous route. Indications for subcutaneous infusion may include coma, dysphagia, nausea/vomiting, intestinal obstruction, malabsorption, or extreme weakness. Infusions are administered through a needle inserted beneath the skin; common infusion sites include the upper arm, shoulder, abdomen, and thigh. Report 96369 for infusions lasting longer than 15 minutes and up to one hour. This code includes pump set-up and the establishment of subcutaneous infusion sites. Report 96370 for each additional hour and 96371 for an additional pump set-up with the establishment of new subcutaneous infusion sites. Codes 96369 and 96371 should be reported only once per encounter.

Relative Value Units/Medicare Edits

Non-Facility RVU	Work	PE	MP	Total
96369	0.21	4.32	0.02	4.55
96370	0.18	0.25	0.01	0.44
96371	0.0	1.89	0.0	1.89
Facility RVU	Work	PE	MP	Total
96369	0.21	4.32	0.02	4.55
96370	0.18	0.25	0.01	0.44
96371	0.0	1.89	0.0	1.89

96372-96376

  96372   Therapeutic, prophylactic, or diagnostic injection (specify substance or drug); subcutaneous or intramuscular
  96373   intra-arterial
  96374   intravenous push, single or initial substance/drug
+ 96375   each additional sequential intravenous push of a new substance/drug (List separately in addition to code for primary procedure)
+ 96376   Therapeutic, prophylactic, or diagnostic injection (specify substance or drug); each additional sequential intravenous push of the same substance/drug provided in a facility (List separately in addition to code for primary procedure)

Explanation

The physician or an assistant under direct physician supervision administers a therapeutic, prophylactic, or diagnostic substance by subcutaneous or intramuscular injection (96372), intra-arterial injection (96373), or by push into an intravenous catheter or intravascular access device (96374 for a single or initial substance, 96375 for each additional sequential IV push of a new substance, and 96376 for each additional sequential IV push of the same substance after 30 minutes have elapsed). The push technique involves an infusion of less than 15 minutes. Code 96376 may be reported only by facilities.

Relative Value Units/Medicare Edits

Non-Facility RVU	Work	PE	MP	Total
96372	0.17	0.23	0.01	0.41
96373	0.17	0.35	0.01	0.53
96374	0.18	1.0	0.02	1.2
96375	0.1	0.38	0.01	0.49
96376	0.0	0.0	0.0	0.0
Facility RVU	Work	PE	MP	Total
96372	0.17	0.23	0.01	0.41
96373	0.17	0.35	0.01	0.53
96374	0.18	1.0	0.02	1.2
96375	0.1	0.38	0.01	0.49
96376	0.0	0.0	0.0	0.0

96377

96377   Application of on-body injector (includes cannula insertion) for timed subcutaneous injection

Explanation

An on-body injector is applied by a qualified health care provider in order to deliver drug therapy at and for a specified time. The provider pierces the skin and inserts a cannula for drug delivery. The cannula is connected to the device adhered to the outside of the patient's body, typically the abdomen or arm. The device is filled with the appropriate amount of medication and programmed for dose delivery.

Relative Value Units/Medicare Edits

Non-Facility RVU	Work	PE	MP	Total
96377	0.17	0.4	0.01	0.58
Facility RVU	Work	PE	MP	Total
96377	0.17	0.4	0.01	0.58

97602

97602   Removal of devitalized tissue from wound(s), non-selective debridement, without anesthesia (eg, wet-to-moist dressings, enzymatic, abrasion, larval therapy), including topical application(s), wound assessment, and instruction(s) for ongoing care, per session

Explanation

A health care provider performs wound care management to promote healing using non-selective debridement techniques to remove devitalized tissue. Non-selective debridement techniques are those in which necrotic and healthy tissue are removed. Non-selective techniques, sometimes referred to as mechanical debridement, include wet-to-moist dressings, enzymatic chemicals, autolytic debridement, abrasion, and larval therapy. Wet-to-moist debridement involves allowing a dressing to proceed from wet to moist and manually removing the dressing, which removes the necrotic and healthy tissue. Chemical enzymes are fast acting products that produce slough of necrotic tissue. Autolytic debridement is accomplished using occlusive or semi-occlusive dressings that keep wound fluid in contact with the necrotic tissue. Types of dressing applications used in autolytic debridement include hydrocolloids, hydrogels, and transparent films. Abrasion involves scraping the wound surface with a tongue blade or similar blunt instrument. Larval treatment may include larvae placement on the wound, which in turn feed off the dead tissue and/or application of the larvae digestive excretions allowing for debridement of dead tissue with no damage to viable tissue.

Relative Value Units/Medicare Edits

Non-Facility RVU	Work	PE	MP	Total
97602	0.0	0.0	0.0	0.0
Facility RVU	Work	PE	MP	Total
97602	0.0	0.0	0.0	0.0

97610

97610   Low frequency, non-contact, non-thermal ultrasound, including topical application(s), when performed, wound assessment, and instruction(s) for ongoing care, per day

Explanation

The physician performs wound treatment utilizing a device that produces low-frequency, ultrasound-generated mist. This noncontact, nonthermal modality promotes wound healing through cellular stimulation. Indicated for acute, chronic, and colonized wounds, as well as burns and ulcers, it provides wound cleansing, bacteria removal, and maintenance debridement of fibrin and tissue exudates. The device uses ultrasound technology to atomize saline, delivering a continuous mist to the treatment site. Multiple passes over the wound are made with the treatment head of the device for a predetermined treatment session. This code includes assessment of the wound, topical applications when performed, and ongoing care instructions. Report this code once per day for the duration of treatment.

Relative Value Units/Medicare Edits

Non-Facility RVU	Work	PE	MP	Total
97610	0.4	11.52	0.01	11.93
Facility RVU	Work	PE	MP	Total
97610	0.4	0.12	0.01	0.53

97810-97811

97810   Acupuncture, 1 or more needles; without electrical stimulation, initial 15 minutes of personal one-on-one contact with the patient

+ 97811   without electrical stimulation, each additional 15 minutes of personal one-on-one contact with the patient, with re-insertion of needle(s) (List separately in addition to code for primary procedure)

Explanation

The health care provider applies acupuncture therapy by inserting one or more fine needles into the patient as dictated by acupuncture meridians for the relief of pain. The needles are twirled or manipulated by hand to generate therapeutic stimulation. No electrical stimulation is employed with this procedure. Report 97810 for the initial 15 minutes of personal one-on-one contact with the patient and 97811 for each additional 15 minutes of personal one-on-one contact with the patient, with re-insertion of the needle.

Appendix

Relative Value Units/Medicare Edits

Non-Facility RVU	Work	PE	MP	Total
97810	0.6	0.41	0.05	1.06
97811	0.5	0.26	0.04	0.8
Facility RVU	**Work**	**PE**	**MP**	**Total**
97810	0.6	0.23	0.05	0.88
97811	0.5	0.19	0.04	0.73

97813-97814

97813　Acupuncture, 1 or more needles; with electrical stimulation, initial 15 minutes of personal one-on-one contact with the patient

+ 97814　with electrical stimulation, each additional 15 minutes of personal one-on-one contact with the patient, with re-insertion of needle(s) (List separately in addition to code for primary procedure)

Explanation

The health care provider applies acupuncture therapy by inserting one or more fine needles into the patient as dictated by acupuncture meridians for the relief of pain. The needles are energized by employing a micro-current for electrical stimulation. Report 97813 for the initial 15 minutes of personal one-on-one contact with the patient and 97814 for each additional 15 minutes of personal one-on-one contact with the patient, with reinsertion of the needle.

Relative Value Units/Medicare Edits

Non-Facility RVU	Work	PE	MP	Total
97813	0.65	0.51	0.05	1.21
97814	0.55	0.4	0.05	1.0
Facility RVU	**Work**	**PE**	**MP**	**Total**
97813	0.65	0.25	0.05	0.95
97814	0.55	0.21	0.05	0.81

98970-98972

98970　Qualified nonphysician health care professional online digital assessment and management, for an established patient, for up to 7 days, cumulative time during the 7 days; 5-10 minutes

98971　　11-20 minutes

98972　　21 or more minutes

Explanation

Online digital evaluation and management services are non-face-to-face encounters originating from the established patient to a qualified nonphysician health care professional for evaluation or management of a problem utilizing internet resources. The service includes all communication, prescription, and laboratory orders with permanent storage in the patient's medical record. The service may include more than one provider responding to the same patient and is only reportable once during seven days for the same encounter. Do not report this code if the online patient request is related to an E/M service that occurred within the previous seven days or within the global period following a procedure. Report 98970 if the cumulative time during the seven-day period is five to 10 minutes; 98971 for 11 to 20 minutes; and 98972 for 21 or more minutes.

Relative Value Units/Medicare Edits

Non-Facility RVU	Work	PE	MP	Total
98970	0.25	0.08	0.01	0.34
98971	0.44	0.14	0.02	0.6
98972	0.69	0.21	0.04	0.94
Facility RVU	**Work**	**PE**	**MP**	**Total**
98970	0.25	0.07	0.01	0.33
98971	0.44	0.13	0.02	0.59
98972	0.69	0.21	0.04	0.94

99000

99000　Handling and/or conveyance of specimen for transfer from the office to a laboratory

Explanation

This code is adjunct to basic services rendered. This code is reported for the handling and/or conveyance of a specimen from the provider's office to a laboratory.

Relative Value Units/Medicare Edits

Non-Facility RVU	Work	PE	MP	Total
99000	0.0	0.0	0.0	0.0
Facility RVU	**Work**	**PE**	**MP**	**Total**
99000	0.0	0.0	0.0	0.0

99001

99001　Handling and/or conveyance of specimen for transfer from the patient in other than an office to a laboratory (distance may be indicated)

Explanation

This code is adjunct to basic services rendered. This code is reported for the handling and/or conveyance of a specimen from the patient in a location other than the provider's office to the laboratory.

Relative Value Units/Medicare Edits

Non-Facility RVU	Work	PE	MP	Total
99001	0.0	0.0	0.0	0.0
Facility RVU	**Work**	**PE**	**MP**	**Total**
99001	0.0	0.0	0.0	0.0

99002

99002　Handling, conveyance, and/or any other service in connection with the implementation of an order involving devices (eg, designing, fitting, packaging, handling, delivery or mailing) when devices such as orthotics, protectives, prosthetics are fabricated by an outside laboratory or shop but which items have been designed, and are to be fitted and adjusted by the attending physician or other qualified health care professional

Explanation

This code is adjunct to basic services rendered. The qualified provider reports this code for the handling, conveyance, and/or any other service in connection with the implementation of an order involving devices such as orthotics, protectives, and prosthetics fabricated by an outside laboratory and fitted by the provider.

Appendix

Relative Value Units/Medicare Edits

Non-Facility RVU	Work	PE	MP	Total
99002	0.0	0.0	0.0	0.0
Facility RVU	**Work**	**PE**	**MP**	**Total**
99002	0.0	0.0	0.0	0.0

99024

99024 Postoperative follow-up visit, normally included in the surgical package, to indicate that an evaluation and management service was performed during a postoperative period for a reason(s) related to the original procedure

Explanation

The physician reports this code to indicate a postoperative follow-up visit, normally included in the surgical package when the physician performs an evaluation and management service for reason(s) that are related to the original procedure.

Relative Value Units/Medicare Edits

Non-Facility RVU	Work	PE	MP	Total
99024	0.0	0.0	0.0	0.0
Facility RVU	**Work**	**PE**	**MP**	**Total**
99024	0.0	0.0	0.0	0.0

99026-99027

99026 Hospital mandated on call service; in-hospital, each hour
99027 out-of-hospital, each hour

Explanation

The code reports the time for hospital mandated on call service provided by the physician. This code does not include prolonged physician attendance time for standby services or the time spent performing other reportable procedures or services. Report 99026 for each hour of hospital mandated on call service spent in the hospital and 99027 for each hour of hospital mandated on call service spent outside the hospital.

Relative Value Units/Medicare Edits

Non-Facility RVU	Work	PE	MP	Total
99026	0.0	0.0	0.0	0.0
99027	0.0	0.0	0.0	0.0
Facility RVU	**Work**	**PE**	**MP**	**Total**
99026	0.0	0.0	0.0	0.0
99027	0.0	0.0	0.0	0.0

99050

99050 Services provided in the office at times other than regularly scheduled office hours, or days when the office is normally closed (eg, holidays, Saturday or Sunday), in addition to basic service

Explanation

This code is adjunct to basic services rendered. The physician reports this code to indicate services after posted office hours in addition to basic services.

Relative Value Units/Medicare Edits

Non-Facility RVU	Work	PE	MP	Total
99050	0.0	0.0	0.0	0.0
Facility RVU	**Work**	**PE**	**MP**	**Total**
99050	0.0	0.0	0.0	0.0

99056

99056 Service(s) typically provided in the office, provided out of the office at request of patient, in addition to basic service

Explanation

This code is adjunct to basic services rendered. The physician reports this code to indicate services typically provided in the office that are provided in a different location at the request of a patient.

Relative Value Units/Medicare Edits

Non-Facility RVU	Work	PE	MP	Total
99056	0.0	0.0	0.0	0.0
Facility RVU	**Work**	**PE**	**MP**	**Total**
99056	0.0	0.0	0.0	0.0

99058

99058 Service(s) provided on an emergency basis in the office, which disrupts other scheduled office services, in addition to basic service

Explanation

This code is adjunct to basic services rendered. The physician reports this code to indicate services provided in the office on an emergency basis that disrupt other scheduled office services.

Relative Value Units/Medicare Edits

Non-Facility RVU	Work	PE	MP	Total
99058	0.0	0.0	0.0	0.0
Facility RVU	**Work**	**PE**	**MP**	**Total**
99058	0.0	0.0	0.0	0.0

99070, 99072

99070 Supplies and materials (except spectacles), provided by the physician or other qualified health care professional over and above those usually included with the office visit or other services rendered (list drugs, trays, supplies, or materials provided)
99072 Additional supplies, materials, and clinical staff time over and above those usually included in an office visit or other nonfacility service(s), when performed during a Public Health Emergency, as defined by law, due to respiratory-transmitted infectious disease

Explanation

Code 99070 is adjunct to basic services rendered. The physician or other qualified provider reports this code to indicate supplies and materials provided over and above those usually included with an office visit or services rendered. This code does not include eyeglasses; report the appropriate supply code if eyeglasses are provided. List drugs, trays, supplies, and other materials provided when using this code. Code 99072 reports additional supplies, materials, and clinical staff time necessary to perform safety protocols during a public health emergency (PHE) due to respiratory-transmitted infectious disease. Extra precautions, over and above those usually included in an office visit or other non-facility services, are taken to ensure the safety of patients and health care professionals during in-person interactions while allowing for the provision of evaluation, treatment, or procedural services. Use of this code does not depend on a specific patient diagnosis.

Relative Value Units/Medicare Edits

Non-Facility RVU	Work	PE	MP	Total
99070	0.0	0.0	0.0	0.0
99072	0.0	0.0	0.0	0.0
Facility RVU	**Work**	**PE**	**MP**	**Total**
99070	0.0	0.0	0.0	0.0
99072	0.0	0.0	0.0	0.0

99071

99071   Educational supplies, such as books, tapes, and pamphlets, for the patient's education at cost to physician or other qualified health care professional

Explanation

This code is adjunct to basic services rendered. The physician or other qualified health care provider reports this code to indicate educational supplies provided at the cost of the provider for the patient's education.

Relative Value Units/Medicare Edits

Non-Facility RVU	Work	PE	MP	Total
99071	0.0	0.0	0.0	0.0
Facility RVU	**Work**	**PE**	**MP**	**Total**
99071	0.0	0.0	0.0	0.0

99078

99078   Physician or other qualified health care professional qualified by education, training, licensure/regulation (when applicable) educational services rendered to patients in a group setting (eg, prenatal, obesity, or diabetic instructions)

Explanation

The physician or other qualified health care professional provides educational services to patients in a group setting. The topics vary according to the group but may be related to prenatal care, diet, diabetic instruction, and smoking cessation.

Relative Value Units/Medicare Edits

Non-Facility RVU	Work	PE	MP	Total
99078	0.0	0.0	0.0	0.0
Facility RVU	**Work**	**PE**	**MP**	**Total**
99078	0.0	0.0	0.0	0.0

99080

99080   Special reports such as insurance forms, more than the information conveyed in the usual medical communications or standard reporting form

Explanation

This code is adjunct to basic services rendered. The physician reports this code to indicate reports such as insurance forms, require more than the information in standard communications methods or forms.

Relative Value Units/Medicare Edits

Non-Facility RVU	Work	PE	MP	Total
99080	0.0	0.0	0.0	0.0
Facility RVU	**Work**	**PE**	**MP**	**Total**
99080	0.0	0.0	0.0	0.0

99082

99082   Unusual travel (eg, transportation and escort of patient)

Explanation

This code is adjunct to basic services rendered. The physician reports this code to indicate unusual travel for the purpose of transportation or accompanying the patient.

Relative Value Units/Medicare Edits

Non-Facility RVU	Work	PE	MP	Total
99082	0.0	0.0	0.0	0.0
Facility RVU	**Work**	**PE**	**MP**	**Total**
99082	0.0	0.0	0.0	0.0

99151-99153

99151   Moderate sedation services provided by the same physician or other qualified health care professional performing the diagnostic or therapeutic service that the sedation supports, requiring the presence of an independent trained observer to assist in the monitoring of the patient's level of consciousness and physiological status; initial 15 minutes of intraservice time, patient younger than 5 years of age

99152   initial 15 minutes of intraservice time, patient age 5 years or older

+ 99153   each additional 15 minutes intraservice time (List separately in addition to code for primary service)

Explanation

A physician or other qualified health care provider administers medication that allows a decreased level of consciousness but does not put the patient completely asleep inducing a state called moderate (conscious) sedation. This allows the patient to breathe without assistance and respond to commands. This type of sedation is used for less invasive procedures and/or as a second medication for pain. These codes report sedation services provided by the same provider performing the primary procedure with the assistance of an independently trained health care professional to assist in monitoring the patient. Report 99151 for the first 15 minutes of intraservice time for sedation services rendered to a patient younger than 5 years of age. Report 99152 for the first 15 minutes of intraservice time for sedation services rendered to a patient age 5 years or older. Report 99153 for each additional 15 minutes of intraservice time.

Relative Value Units/Medicare Edits

Non-Facility RVU	Work	PE	MP	Total
99151	0.5	1.99	0.05	2.54
99152	0.25	1.24	0.02	1.51
99153	0.0	0.3	0.01	0.31
Facility RVU	**Work**	**PE**	**MP**	**Total**
99151	0.5	0.18	0.05	0.73
99152	0.25	0.09	0.02	0.36
99153	0.0	0.3	0.01	0.31

99195

99195   Phlebotomy, therapeutic (separate procedure)

Explanation

The health care provider draws blood from the patient to right dramatically imbalanced blood levels (i.e., hemoglobin, potassium salts). The procedure is similar to drawing blood from a donor, but a number of pints may be taken to reduce the imbalance. Blood removal is performed under a physician's direction.

Relative Value Units/Medicare Edits

Non-Facility RVU	Work	PE	MP	Total
99195	0.0	3.05	0.06	3.11
Facility RVU	Work	PE	MP	Total
99195	0.0	3.05	0.06	3.11

99505

99505   Home visit for stoma care and maintenance including colostomy and cystostomy

Explanation

The home health care provider measures vital signs, inspects incisions, assesses mobility and appetite, and determines if there are problems or situations that could require a surgeon's intervention. The provider checks the stoma site and the stoma's function. The home health provider teaches and answers questions the patient may have about the care and maintenance of the colostomy and/or cystostomy. The home health provider also administers medications or draws blood so that the surgeon can continue to monitor the patient's condition. Most patients who have had a colostomy or cystostomy will be seen by a home health provider one or more times after discharge.

Relative Value Units/Medicare Edits

Non-Facility RVU	Work	PE	MP	Total
99505	0.0	0.0	0.0	0.0
Facility RVU	Work	PE	MP	Total
99505	0.0	0.0	0.0	0.0

99506

99506   Home visit for intramuscular injections

Explanation

The home health provider visits a patient's home to perform an intermuscular injection of medication per a physician's or another valid order. The home health provider brings supplies and medications that are necessary to accomplish the injection to the patient's home, including a syringe, needle, liquid disinfectant, cotton ball, and adhesive tape. The procedure involves inserting the needle, aspiration and slow injection, and at the end of the procedure a cotton ball is placed over the injection site. Adhesive tape is applied over the cotton ball.

Relative Value Units/Medicare Edits

Non-Facility RVU	Work	PE	MP	Total
99506	0.0	0.0	0.0	0.0
Facility RVU	Work	PE	MP	Total
99506	0.0	0.0	0.0	0.0

99511

99511   Home visit for fecal impaction management and enema administration

Explanation

A home health visit includes assistance with dietary management and bowel management/retraining (i.e., use of prescribed medication as well as establishing a habit regimen to treat constipation). The home health caregiver may manually remove the impaction or administer an enema. The amount of fluid administered depends on the age and size of the person receiving the enema. If necessary, a specimen is collected for diagnostic evaluation.

Relative Value Units/Medicare Edits

Non-Facility RVU	Work	PE	MP	Total
99511	0.0	0.0	0.0	0.0
Facility RVU	Work	PE	MP	Total
99511	0.0	0.0	0.0	0.0

0184T

0184T   Excision of rectal tumor, transanal endoscopic microsurgical approach (ie, TEMS), including muscularis propria (ie, full thickness)

Explanation

The physician excises a rectal tumor using the transanal endoscopic microsurgical (TEMS) approach. Following administration of appropriate anesthesia, the patient is placed in a lithotomy position. Dilation of the rectum is achieved and maintained with constant-flow carbon dioxide insufflation. Using specially designed instruments inserted via a resectoscope, full-thickness excision (including the muscularis propria) of the tumor is achieved. Dissection and suturing are performed within the rectal cavity.

0234T-0238T

0234T   Transluminal peripheral atherectomy, open or percutaneous, including radiological supervision and interpretation; renal artery
0235T   visceral artery (except renal), each vessel
0236T   abdominal aorta
0237T   brachiocephalic trunk and branches, each vessel
0238T   iliac artery, each vessel

Explanation

The physician treats a stenosed artery percutaneously or via open surgical incision to relieve a blockage. In the percutaneous approach, a needle punctures the skin at the access site and is followed by a guidewire and an introducer sheath to protect and enclose the opening. A series of catheters and guidewires are inserted until the stenosed area has been traversed. An atherectomy catheter is manipulated to the study area and activated to cut or drill a channel through the plaque lesion and reopen the artery. Contrast medium is injected to fluoroscopically visualize the degree of luminal opening. The process may be repeated with a larger diameter catheter if necessary. In the open surgical approach, the physician creates a femoral cutdown incision to expose one of the femoral arteries. The physician punctures the femoral artery with a large needle and passes a guidewire via the needle into the artery. The physician removes the needle while leaving the guidewire in place, enlarges the arterial opening slightly with a blade, and slides an introducer sheath over the guidewire into the arterial lumen. The physician slides a guidewire through the atherectomy catheter or device and inserts the guidewire/atherectomy catheter combination through the introducer sheath into the stenosed vessel. The atherectomy device is fluoroscopically positioned at the area of stenosis and then activated to remove the stenotic tissue. The physician rechecks the diameter of the lesion by angiography. Several passes with the atherectomy device may be required. The physician removes the atherectomy catheter, guidewire, and introducer sheath, closing the femoral arteriotomy with suture. Report 0234T when the blockage occurs in the renal artery; 0235T in a visceral artery; 0236T in the abdominal aorta; 0237T in the brachiocephalic trunk and branches; and 0238T in the iliac artery.

Coding Companion for General Surgery/Gastroenterology

Appendix

0312T-0317T

0312T Vagus nerve blocking therapy (morbid obesity); laparoscopic implantation of neurostimulator electrode array, anterior and posterior vagal trunks adjacent to esophagogastric junction (EGJ), with implantation of pulse generator, includes programming

0313T laparoscopic revision or replacement of vagal trunk neurostimulator electrode array, including connection to existing pulse generator

0314T laparoscopic removal of vagal trunk neurostimulator electrode array and pulse generator

0315T removal of pulse generator

0316T replacement of pulse generator

0317T neurostimulator pulse generator electronic analysis, includes reprogramming when performed

Explanation

Vagus nerve blocking therapy, also known as vagal blocking for obesity control or VBLOC, is used to treat morbid obesity while leaving digestive organs intact. A neuroregulator is inserted via laparoscope in the patient's subcutaneous tissue. Continuing with the laparoscope, an electrode is attached to the trunk of each vagal nerve at the gastroesophageal junction and the distal ends attached to the neuroregulator. Low voltage, high frequency energy waves are sent to the vagus nerves to block the signals of hunger from the nerve to the brain. The device is programmed and recharged noninvasively using an external mobile charger, transmit coil, and clinician programmer. Report 0312T for laparoscopic insertion of the entire system. Report 0313T for a laparoscopic revision or replacement of an electrode, including attachment to the neuroregulator. Report 0314T when the entire system is removed via a laparoscope. Report 0315T when only the neuroregulator is removed laparoscopically. Report 0316T for the replacement of the neuroregulator. If only analysis with or without reprogramming is performed, report 0317T.

0358T

0358T Bioelectrical impedance analysis whole body composition assessment, with interpretation and report

Explanation

Bioelectrical impedance analysis (BIA) is a relatively simple, quick, and noninvasive technique to measure body composition, the measurement of body fat in relation to lean body mass. The provider places electrodes to various parts of the body; often this may be two electrodes on the patient's right hand and right foot. Low level, imperceptible, and painless electrical current is passed through the body. Bioelectrical impedance analysis is a practical method of measuring the degree of resistance to the current as it moves through the water found in muscles and fat tissue. Muscles contain more water than fat; the more water the body has, the easier it is for the current to pass through it. Subsequently, the more fat a patient has, the more difficult it is for the current to pass through. Measurements are taken to determine how much resistance the current meets based on the various types of tissue. BIA provides an estimate of how much body water is present in order to calculate body fat. An interpretation and report are generated after the analysis has been performed.

0397T

+ 0397T Endoscopic retrograde cholangiopancreatography (ERCP), with optical endomicroscopy (List separately in addition to code for primary procedure)

Explanation

Endoscopic retrograde cholangiopancreatography (ERCP) is a diagnostic test performed via a long flexible viewing instrument (duodenoscope) that can be moved and directed around the turns of the stomach and duodenum. The duodenoscope has a thin fiberoptic bundle at the tip that transmits light, as well as a microscopic camera that can project digital video images onto a television screen. The endoscope is designed with an open channel for other instruments to be passed through for biopsies or to insert plastic or metal tubing (stents) to relieve strictures or other obstructions caused by cancer or scarring, as well as to make incisions via electrocautery. Contrast material is injected and x-rays of the bile ducts and the pancreatic duct are taken. Optical endomicroscopy (confocal laser endomicroscopy) involves a very small but strong microscope attached to the end of the scope that allows the physician to see all of the internal structures in precise detail and is frequently used as a tool to diagnose patients with Barrett's esophagus for esophageal cancer much earlier, often without a biopsy due to the high-resolution and detailed imagery, thereby increasing the likelihood of a cure. The procedure is similar in manner to an upper endoscopy. The patient is administered anesthesia, as appropriate, and is placed in the left lateral position. The physician inserts the scope through the mouth and pharynx and into the esophagus with the images being displayed on the screen in real-time with the physician reviewing the images.

0437T

+ 0437T Implantation of non-biologic or synthetic implant (eg, polypropylene) for fascial reinforcement of the abdominal wall (List separately in addition to code for primary procedure)

Explanation

Biosynthetic implants are a fairly recent tool available to surgeons for assisting in ventral hernia repairs in a possible contaminated field, as well as with patients with a significant abdominal wall fascial defect. In these cases, non-biologic or synthetic implants are often preferable to obtaining a tension-free abdominal wall closure. Prosthetic mesh is associated with a higher risk of complications such as infection, fistula, and skin erosion. The concern with these complications has led to the development of alternative materials to attain a tension-free repair in a single operative session even in cases where the patient has a highly contaminated field. Biosynthetic grafts appear to show promise in solving some of these concerns. Essentially a matrix scaffold comprised of collagen and other extracellular components contain fibroblasts that make angiogenesis, which is the natural process in the body of developing new capillary blood vessels for the purposes of healing and reproducing healthy tissue. By their very nature, these implants are more resistant to infections. A number of biosynthetic implants are available and are categorized according to a number of factors, including, but not limited to, species of origin (allogenic, xenogeneic); the specific decellularization process; whether there is cross-linking; the type of collagen used, such as dermis, pericardium, etc.; how the implant is stored; and whether or not it requires rehydration.

0546T

0546T Radiofrequency spectroscopy, real time, intraoperative margin assessment, at the time of partial mastectomy, with report

Explanation

Radiofrequency (RF) spectroscopy is a technology that pinpoints minute electromagnetic differences between normal cells and cancerous cells in real-time. One proprietary system employs RF electromagnetic fields to identify residual cancerous tissue during a partial mastectomy (lumpectomy) procedure. Differences in the tissue sample can be detected in as little as three to five minutes, allowing the surgeon to make an immediate determination of how much more breast tissue to remove during the procedure and reducing the likelihood of more surgery for the patient. This technology has been successfully used during lumpectomy procedures for ductal carcinoma in situ (DCIS) and invasive breast cancers.

0559T-0560T

0559T Anatomic model 3D-printed from image data set(s); first individually prepared and processed component of an anatomic structure

+ 0560T each additional individually prepared and processed component of an anatomic structure (List separately in addition to code for primary procedure)

Explanation

These codes describe the creation of three-dimensional (3D) printed models of individually prepared and processed elements of anatomic structures, such as bones, arteries, veins, nerves, ureters, muscles, tendons, ligaments, joints, visceral organs, and the brain. Models may be comprised of one or more distinct parts and incorporate various colors and materials. Uses of 3D-printed anatomic models are continuing to increase for a number of applications including, but not limited to, surgery planning, preparing and practicing for the procedure, training and education of health care professionals, and for patient education.

0561T-0562T

0561T Anatomic guide 3D-printed and designed from image data set(s); first anatomic guide

+ 0562T each additional anatomic guide (List separately in addition to code for primary procedure)

Explanation

Three-dimensional (3D) printed cutting or drilling guides are patient-specific surgery guides combining individualized imaging information that is used by the surgeon to navigate a procedure. Each guide is a sole, distinctive tool created to be an exact fit to the patient's natural anatomy customized to precisely match every intervention aspect, such as position and angles that mirror the actual surgery. The use of guides saves considerable time and resources; the predictability permitted by the guides allows for greater confidence in the operation room, which subsequently improves patient outcomes. In some cases, the surgery may require the use of a 3D-printed model and cutting or drilling guide for the same patient.

0581T

0581T Ablation, malignant breast tumor(s), percutaneous, cryotherapy, including imaging guidance when performed, unilateral

Explanation

The physician destroys a malignant breast tumor using percutaneous cryoablation. The patient's skin is cleansed and the ablation site is anesthetized. Imaging guidance may be used to locate the tumor. A small cryoprobe is inserted through a small incision and placed into the tumor. The device initiates ice ball formation by emitting liquid nitrogen, which freezes and destroys the cancerous tissue. Two freezing cycles are undertaken in order to achieve higher cell death. This code reports treatment of one breast.

0584T-0586T

0584T Islet cell transplant, includes portal vein catheterization and infusion, including all imaging, including guidance, and radiological supervision and interpretation, when performed; percutaneous

0585T laparoscopic

0586T open

Explanation

The physician performs an islet cell transplant in patients with type 1 diabetes, following administration of appropriate anesthesia and sedation. In 0584T, the physician inserts a catheter through a small incision in the patient's abdomen, guides it into the portal vein of the liver under ultrasound guidance, and a solution containing the islet cells is infused into the liver. Report 0585T if the

procedure is performed using a laparoscopic approach and 0586T for an open approach. Following transplantation, the beta cells in the islets begin producing and releasing insulin into the patient's bloodstream.

0598T-0599T

0598T Noncontact real-time fluorescence wound imaging, for bacterial presence, location, and load, per session; first anatomic site (eg, lower extremity)

+ 0599T each additional anatomic site (eg, upper extremity) (List separately in addition to code for primary procedure)

Explanation

The physician uses a proprietary point-of-care handheld portable imaging device to identify the presence, location, and amount of bacteria in a wound. A positive result (104 colony-forming units per gram) can indicate infection. The device produces a safe violet light that causes the bacteria, blood, and tissue in wounds to fluoresce different colors; red fluorescence is indicative of gram negative and gram-positive species, aerobes, and anaerobes including *E. coli*, *Klebsiella*, and *Staphylococcus*, while cyan fluorescence indicates *Pseudomonas aeruginosa*. The device detects *Acinetobacter*, the *Enterobacteriaceae* family, and *Pseudomonas*, which are considered by the World Health Organization to be "priority pathogens of concern" due to their multi-drug resistance. The physician can also obtain highly accurate wound area measurements, create a digital record of all images, and export the images to electronic health records. A built-in sensor detects optimal lighting conditions. When room lights cannot be turned off and required ambient lighting conditions cannot be met, the device may be used in conjunction with a compatible one-time use polyethylene drape. Report 0598T per session for the first anatomic site and 0599T for each additional anatomic site imaged during the same session.

0651T

● **0651T** Magnetically controlled capsule endoscopy, esophagus through stomach, including intraprocedural positioning of capsule, with interpretation and report

Explanation

The patient undergoes a minimally invasive diagnostic visualization of the esophagus and stomach using a robotically controlled capsule endoscopy system. The proprietary system, which does not require sedation, incorporates a miniaturized wireless endoscope within a single-use capsule that is remotely controlled during the procedure by the physician using magnetic guidance hardware. System components include a controller, which consists of a rotation platform, examination bed, and magnetic head, and a patient console, which consists of the control panel, computer, and software. The physician or nurse activates the capsule locator prior to ingestion. The patient then swallows the ingestible capsule with water prior to beginning the examination. The video camera that is contained within has its own light source and takes pictures of the patient's stomach. A data recorder, which is worn over the clothes during the examination, receives the images captured by the capsule during the procedure, and the component software displays the actual anatomical view and recently captured images. Interpretation and report are included in the procedure.

0652T-0654T

● **0652T** Esophagogastroduodenoscopy, flexible, transnasal; diagnostic, including collection of specimen(s) by brushing or washing, when performed (separate procedure)

● **0653T** with biopsy, single or multiple

● **0654T** with insertion of intraluminal tube or catheter

Explanation

The physician examines the upper gastrointestinal (GI) tract for diagnostic purposes using a transnasal approach as an alternative to conventional transoral esophagogastroduodenoscopy (EGD). Following application of a local anesthetic, the physician examines the esophagus, stomach, and duodenum via an ultra-thin flexible endoscope inserted through one of the patient's nasal passages. In 0652T, a collection of specimen cells may be obtained by brushing or washing. In 0653T, biopsy forceps are used through the endoscope to obtain one or more samples from the upper GI tract. In 0654T, the physician places a tube or catheter through the endoscope. The endoscope is removed and the patient observed.

0673T

- **0673T** Ablation, benign thyroid nodule(s), percutaneous, laser, including imaging guidance

Explanation

The physician performs percutaneous laser ablation of one or more benign thyroid nodules. With the patient under conscious sedation, a local anesthetic is injected into the subcutaneous tissue and subcapsular region of the thyroid gland. Using ultrasound guidance, the physician inserts one or more 21G spinal needles into the thyroid nodule and positions the laser fiber through the needle so that the tip is in direct contact with the nodule tissue. Laser treatment is administered with a fixed power protocol (typically 3W to 4W). Total energy delivered for each fiber is frequently in the 1200-2000 J range. In some cases, the laser fibers are retracted one or more times (pull-back technique) and additional energy is administered to address the entire volume of the nodule. Following the procedure, patients may receive a betamethasone injection intramuscularly and are then observed prior to discharge.

0686T

- **0686T** Histotripsy (ie, non-thermal ablation via acoustic energy delivery) of malignant hepatocellular tissue, including image guidance

Explanation

The physician performs a nonthermal, noninvasive ablation of liver tissue to destroy primary and metastatic tumors. The procedure, known as histotripsy, uses automated external beam therapy that delivers acoustic energy to destroy the tissue. One proprietary platform uses pulsed sound waves to generate "microbubbles" from gases that are naturally present in the targeted liver tissue. The physician plans the treatment by reviewing current MRI and CT data sets to determine the targeted tissue. Using the integrated ultrasound imaging, the physician centers the histotripsy treatment contours onto the target and creates an appropriate treatment volume. The physician then enables the platform to deliver the correct dose of energy to create a "bubble cloud" at distinct points inside the target and creates a personalized treatment plan for each target by setting the energy levels and calculating the time it will take to complete each treatment. In the treatment phase, histotripsy is delivered by the platform to the previously targeted tissue. Using short ultrasound bursts that last for microseconds, acoustic cavitation is generated from the force of the microbubbles and tissue is liquified and destroyed on a subcellular level. Ultrasound imaging is used to guide and monitor the histotripsy procedure in real-time.

Appendix

Correct Coding Initiative Update 27.3

0184T 00731-00732, 00811-00813, 0213T, 0216T, 0596T-0597T, 11000-11006, 11042-11047, 36000, 36410, 36591-36592, 44701, 45900-45990, 46040, 46080, 46220, 46600-46601, 46604-46615, 46940-46942, 51701-51703, 61650, 62324-62327, 64415-64417, 64450, 64454, 64486-64490, 64493, 69990, 94760-94761, 96360, 96365, 96372, 96374-96377, 96523, 97597-97598, 97602, 99151, 99152, 99153, 99446-99449, 99451-99452, G0471, G0500

0234T 01924-01926, 0213T, 0216T, 0596T-0597T, 11000-11006, 11042-11047, 34713-34716, 34812, 34820, 34833-34834, 35201-35206, 35226-35236, 35256-35266, 35286, 36000, 36002-36005, 36400-36410, 36420-36430, 36440, 36500, 36591-36592, 36600-36640, 37184, 43752, 49000-49002, 51701-51703, 61645-61650, 62320-62327, 64400, 64405-64408, 64415-64435, 64445-64454, 64461, 64463, 64479, 64483, 64486-64490, 64493, 64505, 64510-64530, 69990, 75893, 76000, 76942, 76998, 77002, 93000-93010, 93040-93042, 93050, 93318, 93355, 94002, 94200, 94680-94690, 95812-95816, 95819, 95822, 95829, 95955, 96360, 96365, 96372, 96374-96377, 96523, 97597-97598, 97602, 99155, 99156, 99157, 99446-99449, 99451-99452, G0471

0235T 01924-01926, 0213T, 0216T, 0596T-0597T, 11000-11006, 11042-11047, 34713-34716, 34812, 34820, 34833-34834, 35201-35206, 35226-35236, 35256-35266, 35286, 36000, 36002-36005, 36400-36410, 36420-36430, 36440, 36500, 36591-36592, 36600-36640, 37184, 43752, 49000-49002, 51701-51703, 61645-61650, 62320-62327, 64400, 64405-64408, 64415-64435, 64445-64454, 64461, 64463, 64479, 64483, 64486-64490, 64493, 64505, 64510-64530, 69990, 75726, 75736, 75774, 75893, 76000, 76942, 76998, 77002, 93000-93010, 93040-93042, 93050, 93318, 93355, 94002, 94200, 94680-94690, 95812-95816, 95819, 95822, 95829, 95955, 96360, 96365, 96372, 96374-96377, 96523, 97597-97598, 97602, 99155, 99156, 99157, 99446-99449, 99451-99452, G0471

0236T 01924-01926, 0213T, 0216T, 0596T-0597T, 11000-11006, 11042-11047, 32551, 32556-32557, 34713-34716, 34812, 34820, 34833-34834, 35201-35206, 35226-35236, 35256-35266, 35286, 36000, 36002-36005, 36400-36410, 36420-36430, 36440, 36500, 36591-36592, 36600-36640, 37184, 43752, 49000-49002, 51701-51703, 61645-61650, 62320-62327, 64400, 64405-64408, 64415-64435, 64445-64454, 64461, 64463, 64479, 64483, 64486-64490, 64493, 64505, 64510-64530, 69990, 75600, 75605, 75625, 75630, 75635, 75893, 76000, 76942, 76998, 77002, 93000-93010, 93040-93042, 93050, 93318, 93355, 94002, 94200, 94680-94690, 95812-95816, 95819, 95822, 95829, 95955, 96360, 96365, 96372, 96374-96377, 96523, 97597-97598, 97602, 99155, 99156, 99157, 99446-99449, 99451-99452, G0471

0237T 01924-01926, 0213T, 0216T, 0596T-0597T, 11000-11006, 11042-11047, 34715-34716, 34834, 35201-35206, 35226-35236, 35256-35266, 35286, 36000, 36002-36005, 36400-36410, 36420-36430, 36440, 36500, 36591-36592, 36600-36640, 37184, 43752, 51701-51703, 61645-61650, 62320-62327, 64400, 64405-64408, 64415-64435, 64445-64454, 64461, 64463, 64479, 64483, 64486-64490, 64493, 64505, 64510-64530, 69990, 75605, 75710, 75716, 75893, 76000, 76942, 76998, 77002, 93000-93010, 93040-93042, 93050, 93318, 93355, 94002, 94200, 94680-94690, 95812-95816, 95819, 95822, 95829, 95955, 96360, 96365, 96372, 96374-96377, 96523, 97597-97598, 97602, 99155, 99156, 99157, 99446-99449, 99451-99452, G0471

0238T 01924, 0596T-0597T, 11000-11006, 11042-11047, 35201-35206, 35226-35236, 35256-35266, 35286, 36000, 36002-36005, 36400-36410, 36420-36430, 36440, 36500, 36591-36592, 36600-36640, 43752,

51701-51703, 61650, 62320-62327, 64400, 64405-64408, 64415-64435, 64445-64454, 64461, 64463, 64479, 64483, 64486-64490, 64493, 64505, 64510-64530, 69990, 75630, 75635, 75710, 75716, 75736, 75774, 75893, 76000, 76942, 76998, 77002, 93000-93010, 93040-93042, 93050, 93318, 93355, 94002, 94200, 94680-94690, 95812-95816, 95819, 95822, 95829, 95955, 96360, 96365, 96372, 96374-96377, 96523, 97597-97598, 97602, 99155, 99156, 99157, 99446-99449, 99451-99452, G0471

0312T 0313T-0317T, 0466T-0468T❖, 0589T-0590T, 0596T-0597T, 12001-12007, 12011-12057, 13100-13133, 13151-13153, 36000, 36400-36410, 36420-36430, 36440, 36591-36592, 36600, 36640, 43653, 43752, 44005, 44180, 44970, 49082-49084, 49320, 50715, 51701-51703, 58660, 61650, 61885-61888, 62320-62327, 64400, 64405-64408, 64415-64435, 64445-64454, 64461, 64463, 64479, 64483, 64486-64490, 64493, 64505, 64510-64530, 64568-64570❖, 69990, 93000-93010, 93040-93042, 93318, 93355, 94002, 94200, 94680-94690, 95812-95816, 95819, 95822, 95829, 95955, 95970, 95976-95977, 96360, 96365, 96372, 96374-96377, 96523, 99155, 99156, 99157, 99446-99449, 99451-99452, G0471

0313T 0314T❖, 0466T-0468T❖, 0589T-0590T, 0596T-0597T, 11000-11006, 11042-11047, 12001-12007, 12011-12057, 13100-13133, 13151-13153, 36000, 36400-36410, 36420-36430, 36440, 36591-36592, 36600, 36640, 43653, 43752, 44005, 44180, 44970, 49082-49084, 49320, 50715, 51701-51703, 58660, 61650, 61885-61888, 62320-62327, 64400, 64405-64408, 64415-64435, 64445-64454, 64461, 64463, 64479, 64483, 64486-64490, 64493, 64505, 64510-64530, 64568-64570❖, 69990, 93000-93010, 93040-93042, 93318, 93355, 94002, 94200, 94680-94690, 95812-95816, 95819, 95822, 95829, 95955, 95970, 96360, 96365, 96372, 96374-96377, 96523, 97597-97598, 97602, 99155, 99156, 99157, 99446-99449, 99451-99452, G0471

0314T 0315T-0316T❖, 0466T-0468T❖, 0596T-0597T, 11000-11006, 11042-11047, 12001-12007, 12011-12057, 13100-13133, 13151-13153, 36000, 36400-36410, 36420-36430, 36440, 36591-36592, 36600, 36640, 43653, 43752, 44005, 44180, 44970, 49082-49084, 49320, 50715, 51701-51703, 58660, 61650, 61885-61888, 62320-62327, 64400, 64405-64408, 64415-64435, 64445-64454, 64461, 64463, 64479, 64483, 64486-64490, 64493, 64505, 64510-64530, 64568-64570❖, 69990, 93000-93010, 93040-93042, 93318, 93355, 94002, 94200, 94680-94690, 95812-95816, 95819, 95822, 95829, 95955, 96360, 96365, 96372, 96374-96377, 96523, 97597-97598, 97602, 99155, 99156, 99157, 99446-99449, 99451-99452, G0471

0315T 0596T-0597T, 11000-11006, 11042-11047, 12001-12007, 12011-12057, 13100-13133, 13151-13153, 36000, 36400-36410, 36420-36430, 36440, 36591-36592, 36600, 36640, 43752, 51701-51703, 61650, 62320-62327, 64400, 64405-64408, 64415-64435, 64445-64454, 64461, 64463, 64479, 64483, 64486-64490, 64493, 64505, 64510-64530, 69990, 93000-93010, 93040-93042, 93318, 93355, 94002, 94200, 94680-94690, 95812-95816, 95819, 95822, 95829, 95955, 96360, 96365, 96372, 96374-96377, 96523, 97597-97598, 97602, 99155, 99156, 99157, 99446-99449, 99451-99452, G0471

0316T 0315T, 0589T-0590T, 0596T-0597T, 11000-11006, 11042-11047, 12001-12007, 12011-12057, 13100-13133, 13151-13153, 36000, 36400-36410, 36420-36430, 36440, 36591-36592, 36600, 36640, 43752, 51701-51703, 61650, 62320-62327, 64400, 64405-64408, 64415-64435, 64445-64454, 64461, 64463, 64479, 64483, 64486-64490, 64493, 64505, 64510-64530, 69990, 93000-93010, 93040-93042, 93318, 93355, 94002, 94200, 94680-94690, 95812-95816, 95819, 95822, 95829,

95955, 95970, 95976-95977, 96360, 96365, 96372, 96374-96377, 96523, 97597-97598, 97602, 99155, 99156, 99157, 99446-99449, 99451-99452, G0471

0317T 36591-36592, 96523, 99446-99449, 99451-99452

0358T 36591-36592, 96523

0397T 00520, 00731-00732, 00811-00813, 0213T, 0216T, 0596T-0597T, 0632T, 12001-12007, 12011-12057, 13100-13133, 13151-13153, 31505, 31525, 31575, 36000, 36005-36015, 36400-36410, 36420-36430, 36440, 36591-36592, 36600, 36640, 43191, 43193, 43197-43200, 43202, 43210, 43235, 43239, 43752, 51701-51703, 62320-62327, 64400, 64405-64408, 64415-64435, 64445-64454, 64461, 64463, 64479, 64483, 64486-64490, 64493, 64505, 64510-64530, 69705-69706, 69990, 76000, 76942, 76975, 76998, 77001-77002, 88375, 92012-92014, 92511, 93000-93010, 93040-93042, 93318, 93355, 94002, 94200, 94680-94690, 94760-94761, 95812-95816, 95819, 95822, 95829, 95955, 96360, 96365, 96372, 96374-96377, 96523, 99155, 99156, 99157, 99211-99223, 99231-99255, 99291-99292, 99304-99310, 99315-99316, 99334-99337, 99347-99350, 99374-99375, 99377-99378, 99446-99449, 99451-99452, 99495-99496, G0463, G0471

0437T 0213T, 0216T, 0596T-0597T, 12001-12007, 12011-12057, 13100-13133, 13151-13153, 36000, 36400-36410, 36420-36430, 36440, 36591-36592, 36600, 36640, 43752, 51701-51703, 62320-62327, 64400, 64405-64408, 64415-64435, 64445-64454, 64461-64463, 64479-64483, 64486-64505, 64510-64530, 69990, 92012-92014, 93000-93010, 93040-93042, 93318, 94002, 94200, 94680-94690, 95812-95816, 95819, 95822, 95829, 95955, 96360-96368, 96372, 96374-96377, 96523, 99155, 99156, 99157, 99211-99223, 99231-99255, 99291-99292, 99304-99310, 99315-99316, 99334-99337, 99347-99350, 99374-99375, 99377-99378

0546T 11000-11006, 11042-11047, 97597-97598, 97602

0559T 76376-76377

0560T 76376-76377

0561T 76376-76377

0562T 76376-76377

0581T 0213T, 0216T, 36591-36592, 64450, 77022, 93318, 93355, 96376, 96523, 99446-99449, 99451-99452, 99495-99496, G0463, G0471, J0670, J2001

0584T 0213T, 0216T, 0585T-0586T, 0596T-0597T, 12001-12007, 12011-12057, 13100-13133, 13151-13153, 36000, 36400-36410, 36420-36430, 36440, 36481, 36591-36592, 36600, 36640, 43752, 48554❖, 51701-51703, 62320-62327, 64400, 64405-64408, 64415-64435, 64445-64450, 64461-64463, 64479-64505, 64510-64530, 76998, 77001, 92012-92014, 93000-93010, 93040-93042, 93318, 93355, 94002, 94200, 94680-94690, 95812-95816, 95819, 95822, 95829, 95955, 96360-96368, 96372, 96374-96377, 96523, 99155, 99156, 99157, 99211-99223, 99231-99255, 99291-99292, 99304-99310, 99315-99316, 99334-99337, 99347-99350, 99374-99375, 99377-99378, 99446-99449, 99451-99452, 99495-99496, G0463, G0471, J0670, J1642-J1644, J2001

0585T 0213T, 0216T, 0586T, 0596T-0597T, 12001-12007, 12011-12057, 13100-13133, 13151-13153, 36000, 36400-36410, 36420-36430, 36440, 36481, 36591-36592, 36600, 36640, 43752, 44180, 44602-44605, 48554❖, 49320, 49400, 51701-51703, 62320-62327, 64400, 64405-64408, 64415-64435, 64445-64450, 64461-64463, 64479-64505, 64510-64530, 76998, 77001, 92012-92014, 93000-93010, 93040-93042, 93318, 93355, 94002, 94200, 94680-94690, 95812-95816, 95819, 95822, 95829, 95955, 96360-96368, 96372, 96374-96377, 96523, 99155, 99156, 99157, 99211-99223, 99231-99255, 99291-99292,

99304-99310, 99315-99316, 99334-99337, 99347-99350, 99374-99375, 99377-99378, 99446-99449, 99451-99452, 99495-99496, G0463, G0471

0586T 0213T, 0216T, 0596T-0597T, 11000-11006, 11042-11047, 12001-12007, 12011-12057, 13100-13133, 13151-13153, 36000, 36400-36410, 36420-36430, 36440, 36481, 36591-36592, 36600, 36640, 43752, 44005, 44180, 44602-44605, 44820-44850, 44950, 44970, 48554❖, 49000-49010, 49255, 49320, 49570, 51701-51703, 62320-62327, 64400, 64405-64408, 64415-64435, 64445-64450, 64461-64463, 64479-64505, 64510-64530, 76998, 77001, 92012-92014, 93000-93010, 93040-93042, 93318, 93355, 94002, 94200, 94680-94690, 95812-95816, 95819, 95822, 95829, 95955, 96360-96368, 96372, 96374-96377, 96523, 97597-97598, 97602, 99155, 99156, 99157, 99211-99223, 99231-99255, 99291-99292, 99304-99310, 99315-99316, 99334-99337, 99347-99350, 99374-99375, 99377-99378, 99446-99449, 99451-99452, 99495-99496, G0463, G0471

0598T 36591-36592, 96523

0599T 36591-36592, 96523

0651T No CCI edits apply to this code.

0652T No CCI edits apply to this code.

0653T No CCI edits apply to this code.

0654T No CCI edits apply to this code.

0673T No CCI edits apply to this code.

0686T No CCI edits apply to this code.

10004 0213T, 0216T, 10012, 10035, 19281, 19283, 19285, 19287, 36000, 36410, 36591-36592, 61650, 62324-62327, 64415-64417, 64450, 64454, 64486-64490, 64493, 76000, 76380❖, 76942, 76998, 77001-77002, 77012, 77021, 96360, 96365, 96372, 96374-96377, 96523, J2001

10005 0213T, 0216T, 10004, 10008, 10010-10012, 10021, 10035, 11102-11107, 19281, 19283, 19285, 19287, 36000, 36410, 36591-36592, 61650, 62324-62327, 64415-64417, 64450, 64454, 64486-64490, 64493, 76000, 76380❖, 76942, 76998, 77001-77002, 77012, 77021, 96360, 96365, 96372, 96374-96377, 96523, J2001

10006 0213T, 0216T, 10004, 10035, 19281, 19283, 19285, 19287, 36000, 36410, 36591-36592, 61650, 62324-62327, 64415-64417, 64450, 64454, 64486-64490, 64493, 76000, 76380❖, 76942, 76998, 77001-77002, 77012, 77021, 96360, 96365, 96372, 96374-96377, 96523, J2001

10007 0213T, 0216T, 10004-10006, 10010-10012, 10021, 10035, 11102-11107, 19281, 19283, 19285, 19287, 36000, 36410, 36591-36592, 61650, 62324-62327, 64415-64417, 64450, 64454, 64486-64490, 64493, 76000, 76380❖, 76942, 76998, 77001-77002, 77012, 77021, 96360, 96365, 96372, 96374-96377, 96523, J2001

10008 0213T, 0216T, 10004, 10021, 10035, 19281, 19283, 19285, 19287, 36000, 36410, 36591-36592, 61650, 62324-62327, 64415-64417, 64450, 64454, 64486-64490, 64493, 76000, 76380❖, 76942, 76998, 77001-77002, 77012, 77021, 96360, 96365, 96372, 96374-96377, 96523, J2001

10009 0213T, 0216T, 10004-10008, 10011-10012, 10021, 10035, 11102-11106, 19281, 19283, 19285, 19287, 36000, 36410, 36591-36592, 61650, 62324-62327, 64415-64417, 64450, 64454, 64486-64490, 64493, 76000, 76380❖, 76942, 76998, 77001-77002, 77012, 77021, 96360, 96365, 96372, 96374-96377, 96523, J2001

10010 0213T, 0216T, 10004, 10021, 10035, 19281, 19283, 19285, 19287, 36000, 36410, 36591-36592, 61650, 62324-62327, 64415-64417, 64450, 64454, 64486-64490, 64493, 76000, 76380❖, 76942, 76998, 77001-77002, 77012, 77021, 96360, 96365, 96372, 96374-96377, 96523, J2001

10011 0213T, 0216T, 10004, 10006, 10008, 10010, 10035, 19281, 19283, 19285, 19287, 36000, 36410, 36591-36592, 61650, 62324-62327, 64415-64417, 64450, 64454, 64486-64490, 64493, 76000, 76380♦, 76942, 76998, 77001-77002, 77012, 77021, 96360, 96365, 96372, 96374-96377, 96523, J2001

10012 0213T, 0216T, 10035, 19281, 19283, 19285, 19287, 36000, 36410, 36591-36592, 61650, 62324-62327, 64415-64417, 64450, 64454, 64486-64490, 64493, 76000, 76380♦, 76942, 76998, 77001-77002, 77012, 77021, 96360, 96365, 96372, 96374-96377, 96523, J2001

10021 0213T, 0216T, 10006, 10011-10012, 10035, 11102-11105, 11107, 19281, 19283, 19285, 19287, 36000, 36410, 36591-36592, 61650, 62324-62327, 64415-64417, 64450, 64454, 64486-64490, 64493, 76000, 76380♦, 76942, 76998, 77001-77002, 77012, 77021, 96360, 96365, 96372, 96374-96377, 96523, J2001

10030 0213T, 0216T, 0596T-0597T, 10060-10061♦, 10080-10081♦, 10140♦, 10160♦, 11055-11057, 11401-11406♦, 11421-11426♦, 11441-11471♦, 11600-11606♦, 11620-11646♦, 11719-11721, 11765, 12001-12007, 12011-12057, 13100-13133, 13151-13153, 20500, 29580-29581, 36000, 36400-36410, 36420-36430, 36440, 36591-36592, 36600, 36640, 43752, 51701-51703, 61650, 62320-62327, 64400, 64405-64408, 64415-64435, 64445-64454, 64461-64463, 64479-64505, 64510-64530, 69990, 75989, 76000, 76380, 76942, 76998, 77002-77003, 77012, 77021, 92012-92014, 93000-93010, 93040-93042, 93318, 93355, 94002, 94200, 94680-94690, 95812-95816, 95819, 95822, 95829, 95955, 96360-96368, 96372, 96374-96377, 96523, 97597-97598, 97602-97608, 99155, 99156, 99157, 99211-99223, 99231-99255, 99291-99292, 99304-99310, 99315-99316, 99334-99337, 99347-99350, 99374-99375, 99377-99378, 99446-99449, 99451-99452, G0127, G0463, G0471, J0670, J2001

10035 00400, 0213T, 0216T, 0596T-0597T, 12001-12007, 12011-12057, 13100-13133, 13151-13153, 19281-19286♦, 36000, 36400-36410, 36420-36430, 36440, 36591-36592, 36600, 36640, 36680♦, 43752, 49412♦, 51701-51703, 62320-62327, 64400, 64405-64408, 64415-64435, 64445-64454, 64461-64463, 64479-64505, 64510-64530, 69990, 76000, 76380, 76942, 76998, 77002, 77011-77012, 77021, 92012-92014, 93000-93010, 93040-93042, 93318, 93355, 94002, 94200, 94680-94690, 95812-95816, 95819, 95822, 95829, 95955, 96360-96368, 96372, 96374-96377, 96523, 99155, 99156, 99157, 99211-99223, 99231-99255, 99291-99292, 99304-99310, 99315-99316, 99334-99337, 99347-99350, 99374-99375, 99377-99378, 99446-99449, 99451-99452, G0463, G0471, J0670, J2001

10036 00400, 0213T, 0216T, 0596T-0597T, 12001-12007, 12011-12057, 13100-13133, 13151-13153, 19281-19284♦, 19286♦, 36000, 36400-36410, 36420-36430, 36440, 36591-36592, 36600, 36640, 36680♦, 43752, 51701-51703, 62320-62327, 64400, 64405-64408, 64415-64435, 64445-64454, 64461, 64463, 64479, 64483, 64486-64490, 64493, 64505, 64510-64530, 69990, 76000, 76380, 76942, 76998, 77002, 77011-77012, 77021, 92012-92014, 93000-93010, 93040-93042, 93318, 93355, 94002, 94200, 94680-94690, 95812-95816, 95819, 95822, 95829, 95955, 96360, 96365, 96372, 96374-96377, 96523, 99155, 99156, 99157, 99211-99223, 99231-99255, 99291-99292, 99304-99310, 99315-99316, 99334-99337, 99347-99350, 99374-99375, 99377-99378, 99446-99449, 99451-99452, G0463, G0471, J0670, J2001

10060 0213T, 0216T, 0596T-0597T, 11055-11057, 11401-11406♦, 11421-11426♦, 11441-11471♦, 11600-11606♦, 11620-11646♦, 11719-11730, 11740, 11765, 12001-12007, 12011-12057, 13100-13133, 13151-13153, 20500, 29580-29581, 30000♦, 36000, 36400-36410, 36420-36430, 36440, 36591-36592, 36600, 36640, 43752, 51701-51703, 62320-62327, 64400, 64405-64408, 64415-64435, 64445-64454, 64461-64463, 64479-64505, 64510-64530, 69990, 92012-92014,

93000-93010, 93040-93042, 93318, 93355, 94002, 94200, 94680-94690, 95812-95816, 95819, 95822, 95829, 95955, 96360-96368, 96372, 96374-96377, 96523, 97597-97598, 97602-97608, 99155, 99156, 99157, 99211-99223, 99231-99255, 99291-99292, 99304-99310, 99315-99316, 99334-99337, 99347-99350, 99374-99375, 99377-99378, 99446-99449, 99451-99452, 99495-99496, G0127, G0463, G0471, J0670, J2001

10061 0213T, 0216T, 0596T-0597T, 10060, 11055-11057, 11406♦, 11424-11440♦, 11444-11451♦, 11463-11471♦, 11604-11606♦, 11623-11626♦, 11643-11646♦, 11719-11730, 11740-11750, 11760, 11765, 12001-12007, 12011-12057, 13100-13133, 13151-13153, 20500, 29580-29581, 36000, 36400-36410, 36420-36430, 36440, 36591-36592, 36600, 36640, 43752, 51701-51703, 62320-62327, 64400, 64405-64408, 64415-64435, 64445-64454, 64461-64463, 64479-64505, 64510-64530, 69990, 92012-92014, 93000-93010, 93040-93042, 93318, 93355, 94002, 94200, 94680-94690, 95812-95816, 95819, 95822, 95829, 95955, 96360-96368, 96372, 96374-96377, 96523, 97597-97598, 97602-97608, 99155, 99156, 99157, 99211-99223, 99231-99255, 99291-99292, 99304-99310, 99315-99316, 99334-99337, 99347-99350, 99374-99375, 99377-99378, 99446-99449, 99451-99452, 99495-99496, G0127, G0463, G0471, J0670, J2001

10080 0213T, 0216T, 0596T-0597T, 12001-12007, 12011-12057, 13100-13133, 13151-13153, 20500, 36000, 36400-36410, 36420-36430, 36440, 36591-36592, 36600, 36640, 43752, 51701-51703, 62320-62327, 64400, 64405-64408, 64415-64435, 64445-64454, 64461-64463, 64479-64505, 64510-64530, 69990, 92012-92014, 93000-93010, 93040-93042, 93318, 93355, 94002, 94200, 94680-94690, 95812-95816, 95819, 95822, 95829, 95955, 96360-96368, 96372, 96374-96377, 96523, 99155, 99156, 99157, 99211-99223, 99231-99255, 99291-99292, 99304-99310, 99315-99316, 99334-99337, 99347-99350, 99374-99375, 99377-99378, 99446-99449, 99451-99452, 99495-99496, G0463, G0471, J0670, J2001

10081 0213T, 0216T, 0596T-0597T, 10080, 12001-12007, 12011-12057, 13100-13133, 13151-13153, 20500, 36000, 36400-36410, 36420-36430, 36440, 36591-36592, 36600, 36640, 43752, 51701-51703, 62320-62327, 64400, 64405-64408, 64415-64435, 64445-64454, 64461-64463, 64479-64505, 64510-64530, 69990, 92012-92014, 93000-93010, 93040-93042, 93318, 93355, 94002, 94200, 94680-94690, 95812-95816, 95819, 95822, 95829, 95955, 96360-96368, 96372, 96374-96377, 96523, 99155, 99156, 99157, 99211-99223, 99231-99255, 99291-99292, 99304-99310, 99315-99316, 99334-99337, 99347-99350, 99374-99375, 99377-99378, 99446-99449, 99451-99452, 99495-99496, G0463, G0471, J0670, J2001

10120 0213T, 0216T, 0596T-0597T, 11000-11006, 11042-11047, 11055-11057, 11719-11721, 12001-12007, 12011-12057, 13100-13133, 13151-13153, 36000, 36400-36410, 36420-36430, 36440, 36591-36592, 36600, 36640, 43752, 51701-51703, 62320-62327, 64400, 64405-64408, 64415-64435, 64445-64454, 64461-64463, 64479-64505, 64510-64530, 69990, 92012-92014, 93000-93010, 93040-93042, 93318, 93355, 94002, 94200, 94680-94690, 95812-95816, 95819, 95822, 95829, 95955, 96360-96368, 96372, 96374-96377, 96523, 97597-97598, 97602, 99155, 99156, 99157, 99211-99223, 99231-99255, 99291-99292, 99304-99310, 99315-99316, 99334-99337, 99347-99350, 99374-99375, 99377-99378, 99446-99449, 99451-99452, 99495-99496, G0127, G0463, G0471, J0670, J2001

10121 0213T, 0216T, 0596T-0597T, 10120, 11000-11006, 11042-11047, 11720-11721, 12001-12007, 12011-12057, 13100-13133, 13151-13153, 36000, 36400-36410, 36420-36430, 36440, 36591-36592, 36600, 36640, 43752, 51701-51703, 62320-62327, 64400, 64405-64408, 64415-64435, 64445-64454, 64461-64463, 64479-64505, 64510-64530, 69990, 92012-92014, 93000-93010, 93040-93042, 93318, 93355, 94002, 94200,

94680-94690, 95812-95816, 95819, 95822, 95829, 95955, 96360-96368, 96372, 96374-96377, 96523, 97597-97598, 97602, 99155, 99156, 99157, 99211-99223, 99231-99255, 99291-99292, 99304-99310, 99315-99316, 99334-99337, 99347-99350, 99374-99375, 99377-99378, 99446-99449, 99451-99452, 99495-99496, G0463, G0471, J0670, J2001

10140 0213T, 0216T, 0596T-0597T, 11055-11057, 11719-11721, 12001-12007, 12011-12057, 13100-13133, 13151-13153, 29580-29581, 36000, 36400-36410, 36420-36430, 36440, 36591-36592, 36600, 36640, 43752, 51701-51703, 62320-62327, 64400, 64405-64408, 64415-64435, 64445-64454, 64461-64463, 64479-64505, 64510-64530, 69990, 76000, 76942, 76998, 77002, 77012, 77021, 92012-92014, 93000-93010, 93040-93042, 93318, 93355, 94002, 94200, 94680-94690, 95812-95816, 95819, 95822, 95829, 95955, 96360-96368, 96372, 96374-96377, 96523, 99155, 99156, 99157, 99211-99223, 99231-99255, 99291-99292, 99304-99310, 99315-99316, 99334-99337, 99347-99350, 99374-99375, 99377-99378, 99446-99449, 99451-99452, 99495-99496, G0127, G0463, G0471, J0670, J2001

10160 0213T, 0216T, 0596T-0597T, 10061✧, 10140✧, 11055-11057, 11719-11721, 12001-12007, 12011-12057, 13100-13133, 13151-13153, 29580-29581, 36000, 36400-36410, 36420-36430, 36440, 36591-36592, 36600, 36640, 43752, 51701-51703, 62320-62327, 64400, 64405-64408, 64415-64435, 64445-64454, 64461-64463, 64479-64505, 64510-64530, 69990, 92012-92014, 93000-93010, 93040-93042, 93318, 93355, 94002, 94200, 94680-94690, 95812-95816, 95819, 95822, 95829, 95955, 96360-96368, 96372, 96374-96377, 96523, 99155, 99156, 99157, 99211-99223, 99231-99255, 99291-99292, 99304-99310, 99315-99316, 99334-99337, 99347-99350, 99374-99375, 99377-99378, 99446-99449, 99451-99452, 99495-99496, G0127, G0463, G0471, J0670, J2001

10180 0213T, 0216T, 0596T-0597T, 11720-11721, 12001-12007, 12011-12057, 13100-13133, 13151-13153, 20500, 36000, 36400-36410, 36420-36430, 36440, 36591-36592, 36600, 36640, 43752, 51701-51703, 62320-62327, 64400, 64405-64408, 64415-64435, 64445-64454, 64461-64463, 64479-64505, 64510-64530, 69990, 92012-92014, 93000-93010, 93040-93042, 93318, 93355, 94002, 94200, 94680-94690, 95812-95816, 95819, 95822, 95829, 95955, 96360-96368, 96372, 96374-96377, 96523, 99155, 99156, 99157, 99211-99223, 99231-99255, 99291-99292, 99304-99310, 99315-99316, 99334-99337, 99347-99350, 99374-99375, 99377-99378, 99446-99449, 99451-99452, 99495-99496, G0463, G0471, J0670, J2001

11004 0213T, 0216T, 0437T, 0552T, 10030, 10060-10061, 11000, 11010-11012, 11042-11044, 11102-11107, 12001-12007, 12011-12018, 12021-12057, 13100-13133, 13151-13153, 15769, 15777, 20552-20553, 20560-20561, 20700-20701, 36000, 36400-36410, 36420-36430, 36440, 36591-36592, 36600, 36640, 43752, 57267, 62320-62327, 64400, 64405-64408, 64415-64435, 64445-64454, 64461-64463, 64479-64505, 64510-64530, 66987-66988, 69990, 92012-92014, 93000-93010, 93040-93042, 93318, 93355, 94002, 94200, 94680-94690, 95812-95816, 95819, 95822, 95829, 95955, 96360-96368, 96372, 96374-96377, 96523, 97597-97598, 97610, 99155, 99156, 99157, 99211-99223, 99231-99255, 99291-99292, 99304-99310, 99315-99316, 99334-99337, 99347-99350, 99374-99375, 99377-99378, 99446-99449, 99451-99452, 99495-99496, G0463, G0471

11005 0213T, 0216T, 0437T, 0552T, 10030, 10060-10061, 11000, 11004, 11010-11012, 11042-11044, 11102-11107, 12001-12007, 12011-12018, 12021-12057, 13100-13133, 13151-13153, 15769, 15777, 20552-20553, 20560-20561, 20700-20701, 36000, 36400-36410, 36420-36430, 36440, 36591-36592, 36600, 36640, 43752, 57267, 62320-62327, 64400, 64405-64408, 64415-64435, 64445-64454, 64461-64463, 64479-64505, 64510-64530, 66987-66988, 69990, 92012-92014, 93000-93010, 93040-93042, 93318, 93355, 94002, 94200, 94680-94690, 95812-95816,

11006 0213T, 0216T, 0437T, 0552T, 10030, 10060-10061, 11000, 11004-11005, 11010-11012, 11042-11044, 11102-11107, 12001-12007, 12011-12018, 12021-12057, 13100-13133, 13151-13153, 15769, 15777, 20552-20553, 20560-20561, 20700-20701, 36000, 36400-36410, 36420-36430, 36440, 36591-36592, 36600, 36640, 43752, 57267, 62320-62327, 64400, 64405-64408, 64415-64435, 64445-64454, 64461-64463, 64479-64505, 64510-64530, 66987-66988, 69990, 92012-92014, 93000-93010, 93040-93042, 93318, 93355, 94002, 94200, 94680-94690, 95812-95816, 95819, 95822, 95829, 95955, 96360-96368, 96372, 96374-96377, 96523, 97597-97598, 97610, 99155, 99156, 99157, 99211-99223, 99231-99255, 99291-99292, 99304-99310, 99315-99316, 99334-99337, 99347-99350, 99374-99375, 99377-99378, 99446-99449, 99451-99452, 99495-99496, G0463, G0471

11008 36591-36592, 96523

11042 0213T, 0216T, 0552T, 10030, 10060, 11000, 11008, 11010-11011✧, 11719-11721, 12007, 12014, 12016-12018, 12036-12041, 12044, 12046-12047, 12053, 12055-12057, 13102, 13122, 13133, 13153, 15852, 17000, 17250, 20526, 20552-20553, 20560-20561, 24300, 25259, 26340, 29000-29015, 29035-29200, 29240-29450, 29505-29581, 29584, 29730, 35702-35703, 36000, 36400-36410, 36420-36430, 36440, 36591-36592, 36600, 36640, 43752, 62320-62327, 64400, 64405-64408, 64415-64435, 64445-64454, 64461-64463, 64479-64505, 64510-64530, 64553, 66987-66988, 69990, 72295, 76000, 77001-77002, 92012-92014, 93000-93010, 93040-93042, 93318, 93355, 94002, 94200, 94680-94690, 95812-95816, 95819, 95822, 95829, 95955, 96360-96368, 96372, 96374-96377, 96523, 97022, 97597-97598, 97602, 97610, 99155, 99156, 99157, 99211-99223, 99231-99255, 99291-99292, 99304-99310, 99315-99316, 99334-99337, 99347-99350, 99374-99375, 99377-99378, 99446-99449, 99451-99452, 99495-99496, G0463, G0471

11043 0213T, 0216T, 0552T, 10030, 10060-10061, 11000, 11008, 11010-11012✧, 11042, 11719-11721, 12001-12004, 12007, 12011-12018, 12021-12031, 12041-12042, 12045, 12047-12057, 13102, 13122, 13133, 13153, 15852, 17250, 20552-20553, 20560-20561, 24300, 25001✧, 29000-29015, 29035-29200, 29240-29450, 29505-29581, 29584, 35702-35703, 36000, 36400-36410, 36420-36430, 36440, 36591-36592, 36600, 36640, 43752, 62320-62327, 64400, 64405-64408, 64415-64435, 64445-64454, 64461-64463, 64479-64505, 64510-64530, 66987-66988, 69990, 75710, 75820, 76000, 77001-77002, 92012-92014, 93000-93010, 93040-93042, 93318, 93355, 94002, 94200, 94680-94690, 95812-95816, 95819, 95822, 95829, 95955, 96360-96368, 96372, 96374-96377, 96523, 97597-97598, 97602, 97610, 99155, 99156, 99157, 99211-99223, 99231-99255, 99291-99292, 99304-99310, 99315-99316, 99334-99337, 99347-99350, 99374-99375, 99377-99378, 99446-99449, 99451-99452, 99495-99496, G0127, G0463, G0471, J0670, J2001

11044 0213T, 0216T, 0552T, 10030, 10060-10061, 11000, 11008, 11010-11012✧, 11042-11043, 11719-11721, 12001-12007, 12011-12018, 12021-12034, 12036, 12041-12042, 12045, 12047-12057, 13102, 13122, 13133, 13153, 15852, 17250, 20552-20553, 20560-20561, 24300, 25001✧, 29000-29015, 29035-29200, 29240-29450, 29505-29581, 29584, 35702-35703, 36000, 36400-36410, 36420-36430, 36440, 36591-36592, 36600, 36640, 43752, 62320-62327, 64400, 64405-64408, 64415-64435, 64445-64454, 64461-64463, 64479-64505, 64510-64530, 66987-66988, 69990, 75710, 75716,

Coding Companion for General Surgery/Gastroenterology

92012-92014, 93000-93010, 93040-93042, 93318, 93355, 94002, 94200, 94680-94690, 95812-95816, 95819, 95822, 95829, 95955, 96360-96368, 96372, 96374-96377, 96523, 97597-97598, 97602, 97610, 99155, 99156, 99157, 99211-99223, 99231-99255, 99291-99292, 99304-99310, 99315-99316, 99334-99337, 99347-99350, 99374-99375, 99377-99378, 99446-99449, 99451-99452, 99495-99496, G0463, G0471, J0670, J2001

11045 20560-20561, 29000-29015, 29035-29200, 29240-29450, 29505-29581, 29584, 36591-36592, 66987-66988, 96523, 97597-97598, 97602

11046 20560-20561, 29000-29015, 29035-29200, 29240-29450, 29505-29581, 29584, 36591-36592, 66987-66988, 96523, 97597-97598, 97602, J0670, J2001

11047 20560-20561, 29000-29015, 29035-29200, 29240-29450, 29505-29581, 29584, 36591-36592, 66987-66988, 96523, 97597-97598, 97602, J0670, J2001

11102 00170, 0213T, 0216T, 0470T-0471T, 0596T-0597T, 10011, 11000-11001, 11042-11047, 11055-11057, 11200, 11300, 11719, 12001-12007, 12011-12057, 13100-13133, 13151-13153, 15824-15829, 16000, 16020, 17000, 17250-17260, 36000, 36400-36410, 36420-36430, 36440, 36591-36592, 36600, 36640, 43752, 51701-51703, 62320-62327, 64400, 64405-64408, 64415-64435, 64445-64454, 64461-64463, 64479-64505, 64510-64530, 69990, 92012-92014, 93000-93010, 93040-93042, 93318, 93355, 94002, 94200, 94680-94690, 95812-95816, 95819, 95822, 95829, 95955, 96360-96368, 96372, 96374-96377, 96523, 96931-96936, 97597-97598, 97602, 99155, 99156, 99157, 99211-99223, 99231-99255, 99291-99292, 99304-99310, 99315-99316, 99334-99337, 99347-99350, 99374-99375, 99377-99378, 99446-99449, 99451, 99495-99496, G0127, G0168, G0463, G0471, J0670, J2001

11103 00170, 0213T, 0216T, 0470T-0471T, 0596T-0597T, 10011, 11000-11001, 11042-11047, 11719, 12001-12007, 12011-12057, 13100-13133, 13151-13153, 36000, 36400-36410, 36420-36430, 36440, 36591-36592, 36600, 36640, 43752, 51701-51703, 62320-62327, 64400, 64405-64408, 64415-64435, 64445-64454, 64461-64463, 64479-64505, 64510-64530, 69990, 92012-92014, 93000-93010, 93040-93042, 93318, 93355, 94002, 94200, 94680-94690, 95812-95816, 95819, 95822, 95829, 95955, 96360-96368, 96372, 96374-96377, 96523, 96931-96936, 97597-97598, 97602, 99155, 99156, 99157, 99211-99223, 99231-99255, 99291-99292, 99304-99310, 99315-99316, 99334-99337, 99347-99350, 99374-99375, 99377-99378, 99446-99449, 99451, 99495-99496, G0127, G0168, G0463, G0471, J0670, J2001

11104 00170, 0213T, 0216T, 0470T-0471T, 0596T-0597T, 10011, 11000-11001, 11042-11047, 11055-11057, 11102, 11200, 11300-11301, 11305-11306, 11310, 11719, 12001-12007, 12011-12057, 13100-13133, 13151-13153, 15824-15829, 16000, 16020, 17000, 17110, 17250-17260, 36000, 36400-36410, 36420-36430, 36440, 36591-36592, 36600, 36640, 43752, 51701-51703, 62320-62327, 64400, 64405-64408, 64415-64435, 64445-64454, 64461-64463, 64479-64505, 64510-64530, 69100✦, 69990, 92012-92014, 93000-93010, 93040-93042, 93318, 93355, 94002, 94200, 94680-94690, 95812-95816, 95819, 95822, 95829, 95955, 96360-96368, 96372, 96374-96377, 96523, 96931-96936, 97597-97598, 97602, 99155, 99156, 99157, 99211-99223, 99231-99255, 99291-99292, 99304-99310, 99315-99316, 99334-99337, 99347-99350, 99374-99375, 99377-99378, 99446-99449, 99451, 99495-99496, G0127, G0168, G0463, G0471, J0670, J2001

11105 00170, 0213T, 0216T, 0470T-0471T, 0596T-0597T, 10011, 11000-11001, 11042-11047, 11719, 12001-12007, 12011-12057, 13100-13133, 13151-13153, 36000, 36400-36410, 36420-36430, 36440, 36591-36592, 36600, 36640, 43752, 51701-51703, 62320-62327, 64400, 64405-64408, 64415-64435, 64445-64454, 64461-64463, 64479-64505, 64510-64530, 69990, 92012-92014, 93000-93010, 93040-93042, 93318, 93355, 94002,

94200, 94680-94690, 95812-95816, 95819, 95822, 95829, 95955, 96360-96368, 96372, 96374-96377, 96523, 96931-96936, 97597-97598, 97602, 99155, 99156, 99157, 99211-99223, 99231-99255, 99291-99292, 99304-99310, 99315-99316, 99334-99337, 99347-99350, 99374-99375, 99377-99378, 99446-99449, 99451, 99495-99496, G0127, G0168, G0463, G0471, J0670, J2001

11106 00170, 0213T, 0216T, 0470T-0471T, 0596T-0597T, 10011, 10021, 11000-11001, 11042-11047, 11055-11057, 11102, 11104, 11200, 11300-11301, 11305-11306, 11310-11311, 11400, 11440, 11719, 11755, 12001-12007, 12011-12057, 13100-13133, 13151-13153, 15824-15829, 16000, 16020, 17000, 17110-17111, 17250-17261, 17280, 36000, 36400-36410, 36420-36430, 36440, 36591-36592, 36600, 36640, 43752, 51701-51703, 62320-62327, 64400, 64405-64408, 64415-64435, 64445-64454, 64461-64463, 64479-64505, 64510-64530, 69100✦, 69990, 92012-92014, 93000-93010, 93040-93042, 93318, 93355, 94002, 94200, 94680-94690, 95812-95816, 95819, 95822, 95829, 95955, 96360-96368, 96372, 96374-96377, 96523, 96931-96936, 97597-97598, 97602, 99155, 99156, 99157, 99211-99223, 99231-99255, 99291-99292, 99304-99310, 99315-99316, 99334-99337, 99347-99350, 99374-99375, 99377-99378, 99446-99449, 99451, 99495-99496, G0127, G0168, G0463, G0471, J0670, J2001

11107 00170, 0213T, 0216T, 0470T-0471T, 0596T-0597T, 10011, 11000-11001, 11042-11047, 11719, 12001-12007, 12011-12057, 13100-13133, 13151-13153, 36000, 36400-36410, 36420-36430, 36440, 36591-36592, 36600, 36640, 43752, 51701-51703, 62320-62327, 64400, 64405-64408, 64415-64435, 64445-64454, 64461-64463, 64479-64505, 64510-64530, 69990, 92012-92014, 93000-93010, 93040-93042, 93318, 93355, 94002, 94200, 94680-94690, 95812-95816, 95819, 95822, 95829, 95955, 96360-96368, 96372, 96374-96377, 96523, 96931-96936, 97597-97598, 97602, 99155, 99156, 99157, 99211-99223, 99231-99255, 99291-99292, 99304-99310, 99315-99316, 99334-99337, 99347-99350, 99374-99375, 99377-99378, 99446-99449, 99451, 99495-99496, G0127, G0168, G0463, G0471, J0670, J2001

11400 00400, 0213T, 0216T, 0470T-0471T, 0596T-0597T, 10030✦, 10060-10061✦, 11000-11006, 11042-11047, 11102, 11104, 11900-11901, 12001-12007, 12011-12057, 13100-13133, 13151-13153, 17000✦, 17250, 36000, 36400-36410, 36420-36430, 36440, 36591-36592, 36600, 36640, 43752, 51701-51703, 62320-62327, 64400, 64405-64408, 64415-64435, 64445-64454, 64461-64463, 64479-64505, 64510-64530, 69990, 92012-92014, 93000-93010, 93040-93042, 93318, 93355, 94002, 94200, 94680-94690, 95812-95816, 95819, 95822, 95829, 95955, 96360-96368, 96372, 96374-96377, 96405-96406, 96523, 96931-96936, 97597-97598, 97602, 99155, 99156, 99157, 99211-99223, 99231-99255, 99291-99292, 99304-99310, 99315-99316, 99334-99337, 99347-99350, 99374-99375, 99377-99378, 99446-99449, 99451-99452, 99495-99496, G0168, G0463, G0471, J0670, J2001

11401 00400, 0213T, 0216T, 0470T-0471T, 0596T-0597T, 10061✦, 11000-11006, 11042-11047, 11102, 11104, 11106, 11900-11901, 12001-12007, 12011-12018, 17000✦, 17004✦, 17250, 19120✦, 36000, 36400-36410, 36420-36430, 36440, 36591-36592, 36600, 36640, 43752, 51701-51703, 62320-62327, 64400, 64405-64408, 64415-64435, 64445-64454, 64461-64463, 64479-64505, 64510-64530, 69990, 92012-92014, 93000-93010, 93040-93042, 93318, 93355, 94002, 94200, 94680-94690, 95812-95816, 95819, 95822, 95829, 95955, 96360-96368, 96372, 96374-96377, 96405-96406, 96523, 96931-96936, 97597-97598, 97602, 99155, 99156, 99157, 99211-99223, 99231-99255, 99291-99292, 99304-99310, 99315-99316, 99334-99337, 99347-99350, 99374-99375, 99377-99378, 99446-99449, 99451-99452, 99495-99496, G0168, G0463, G0471, J0670, J2001

11402 00400, 0213T, 0216T, 0470T-0471T, 0596T-0597T, 10061✦, 11000-11006, 11042-11047, 11102, 11104, 11106, 11900-11901, 12001-12007, 12011-12018, 17000✦, 17004✦, 17250, 19120✦, 36000, 36400-36410, 36420-36430, 36440, 36591-36592, 36600, 36640, 43752, 51701-51703, 62320-62327, 64400, 64405-64408, 64415-64435, 64445-64454, 64461-64463, 64479-64505, 64510-64530, 69990, 92012-92014, 93000-93010, 93040-93042, 93318, 93355, 94002, 94200, 94680-94690, 95812-95816, 95819, 95822, 95829, 95955, 96360-96368, 96372, 96374-96377, 96405-96406, 96523, 96931-96936, 97597-97598, 97602, 99155, 99156, 99157, 99211-99223, 99231-99255, 99291-99292, 99304-99310, 99315-99316, 99334-99337, 99347-99350, 99374-99375, 99377-99378, 99446-99449, 99451-99452, 99495-99496, G0168, G0463, G0471, J0670, J2001

11403 00400, 0213T, 0216T, 0419T-0420T✦, 0470T-0471T, 0596T-0597T, 10061✦, 11000-11006, 11042-11047, 11102, 11104, 11106, 11900-11901, 12001-12007, 12011-12018, 17000✦, 17004✦, 17250, 19120✦, 36000, 36400-36410, 36420-36430, 36440, 36591-36592, 36600, 36640, 43752, 51701-51703, 62320-62327, 64400, 64405-64408, 64415-64435, 64445-64454, 64461-64463, 64479-64505, 64510-64530, 69990, 92012-92014, 93000-93010, 93040-93042, 93318, 93355, 94002, 94200, 94680-94690, 95812-95816, 95819, 95822, 95829, 95955, 96360-96368, 96372, 96374-96377, 96405-96406, 96523, 96931-96936, 97597-97598, 97602, 99155, 99156, 99157, 99211-99223, 99231-99255, 99291-99292, 99304-99310, 99315-99316, 99334-99337, 99347-99350, 99374-99375, 99377-99378, 99446-99449, 99451-99452, 99495-99496, G0168, G0463, G0471, J0670, J2001

11404 00400, 0213T, 0216T, 0470T-0471T, 0596T-0597T, 10061✦, 11000-11006, 11042-11047, 11102, 11104, 11106, 11900-11901, 12001-12007, 12011-12018, 17000✦, 17004✦, 17250, 19120✦, 36000, 36400-36410, 36420-36430, 36440, 36591-36592, 36600, 36640, 43752, 51701-51703, 62320-62327, 64400, 64405-64408, 64415-64435, 64445-64454, 64461-64463, 64479-64505, 64510-64530, 69990, 92012-92014, 93000-93010, 93040-93042, 93318, 93355, 94002, 94200, 94680-94690, 95812-95816, 95819, 95822, 95829, 95955, 96360-96368, 96372, 96374-96377, 96405-96406, 96523, 96931-96936, 97597-97598, 97602, 99155, 99156, 99157, 99211-99223, 99231-99255, 99291-99292, 99304-99310, 99315-99316, 99334-99337, 99347-99350, 99374-99375, 99377-99378, 99446-99449, 99451-99452, 99495-99496, G0168, G0463, G0471, J0670, J2001

11406 00400, 0213T, 0216T, 0470T-0471T, 0596T-0597T, 11000-11006, 11042-11047, 11102, 11104, 11106, 11900-11901, 12001-12007, 12011-12018, 17000✦, 17004✦, 17250, 19120✦, 36000, 36400-36410, 36420-36430, 36440, 36591-36592, 36600, 36640, 43752, 51701-51703, 62320-62327, 64400, 64405-64408, 64415-64435, 64445-64454, 64461-64463, 64479-64505, 64510-64530, 69990, 92012-92014, 93000-93010, 93040-93042, 93318, 93355, 94002, 94200, 94680-94690, 95812-95816, 95819, 95822, 95829, 95955, 96360-96368, 96372, 96374-96377, 96405-96406, 96523, 96931-96936, 97597-97598, 97602, 99155, 99156, 99157, 99211-99223, 99231-99255, 99291-99292, 99304-99310, 99315-99316, 99334-99337, 99347-99350, 99374-99375, 99377-99378, 99446-99449, 99451-99452, 99495-99496, G0168, G0463, G0471, J0670, J2001

11420 00400, 0213T, 0216T, 0470T-0471T, 0596T-0597T, 10030✦, 10060-10061✦, 11000-11006, 11042-11047, 11102, 11104, 11106, 11719, 11900-11901, 12001-12007, 12011-12057, 13100-13133, 13151-13153, 17000✦, 17250, 36000, 36400-36410, 36420-36430, 36440, 36591-36592, 36600, 36640, 43752, 51701-51703, 62320-62327, 64400, 64405-64408, 64415-64435, 64445-64454, 64461-64463, 64479-64505, 64510-64530, 69990, 92012-92014, 93000-93010, 93040-93042, 93318, 93355, 94002, 94200, 94680-94690, 95812-95816,

95819, 95822, 95829, 95955, 96360-96368, 96372, 96374-96377, 96405-96406, 96523, 96931-96936, 97597-97598, 97602, 99155, 99156, 99157, 99211-99223, 99231-99255, 99291-99292, 99304-99310, 99315-99316, 99334-99337, 99347-99350, 99374-99375, 99377-99378, 99446-99449, 99451-99452, 99495-99496, G0168, G0463, G0471, J0670, J2001

11421 00400, 0213T, 0216T, 0470T-0471T, 0596T-0597T, 10061✦, 11000-11006, 11042-11047, 11102, 11104, 11106, 11719, 11900-11901, 12001-12007, 12011-12018, 17000✦, 17004✦, 17250, 36000, 36400-36410, 36420-36430, 36440, 36591-36592, 36600, 36640, 43752, 51701-51703, 62320-62327, 64400, 64405-64408, 64415-64435, 64445-64454, 64461-64463, 64479-64505, 64510-64530, 69990, 92012-92014, 93000-93010, 93040-93042, 93318, 93355, 94002, 94200, 94680-94690, 95812-95816, 95819, 95822, 95829, 95955, 96360-96368, 96372, 96374-96377, 96405-96406, 96523, 96931-96936, 97597-97598, 97602, 99155, 99156, 99157, 99211-99223, 99231-99255, 99291-99292, 99304-99310, 99315-99316, 99334-99337, 99347-99350, 99374-99375, 99377-99378, 99446-99449, 99451-99452, 99495-99496, G0168, G0463, G0471, J0670, J2001

11422 00400, 0213T, 0216T, 0470T-0471T, 0596T-0597T, 10061✦, 11000-11006, 11042-11047, 11102, 11104, 11106, 11900-11901, 12001-12007, 12011-12018, 17000✦, 17004✦, 17250, 36000, 36400-36410, 36420-36430, 36440, 36591-36592, 36600, 36640, 43752, 51701-51703, 62320-62327, 64400, 64405-64408, 64415-64435, 64445-64454, 64461-64463, 64479-64505, 64510-64530, 69990, 92012-92014, 93000-93010, 93040-93042, 93318, 93355, 94002, 94200, 94680-94690, 95812-95816, 95819, 95822, 95829, 95955, 96360-96368, 96372, 96374-96377, 96405-96406, 96523, 96931-96936, 97597-97598, 97602, 99155, 99156, 99157, 99211-99223, 99231-99255, 99291-99292, 99304-99310, 99315-99316, 99334-99337, 99347-99350, 99374-99375, 99377-99378, 99446-99449, 99451-99452, 99495-99496, G0168, G0463, G0471, J0670, J2001

11423 00400, 0213T, 0216T, 0470T-0471T, 0596T-0597T, 10061✦, 11000-11006, 11042-11047, 11102, 11104, 11106, 11900-11901, 12001-12007, 12011-12018, 17000✦, 17004✦, 17250, 36000, 36400-36410, 36420-36430, 36440, 36591-36592, 36600, 36640, 43752, 51701-51703, 62320-62327, 64400, 64405-64408, 64415-64435, 64445-64454, 64461-64463, 64479-64505, 64510-64530, 69990, 92012-92014, 93000-93010, 93040-93042, 93318, 93355, 94002, 94200, 94680-94690, 95812-95816, 95819, 95822, 95829, 95955, 96360-96368, 96372, 96374-96377, 96405-96406, 96523, 96931-96936, 97597-97598, 97602, 99155, 99156, 99157, 99211-99223, 99231-99255, 99291-99292, 99304-99310, 99315-99316, 99334-99337, 99347-99350, 99374-99375, 99377-99378, 99446-99449, 99451-99452, 99495-99496, G0168, G0463, G0471, J0670, J2001

11424 00400, 0213T, 0216T, 0470T-0471T, 0596T-0597T, 11000-11006, 11042-11047, 11102, 11104, 11106, 11900-11901, 12001-12007, 12011-12018, 17000✦, 17004✦, 17250, 36000, 36400-36410, 36420-36430, 36440, 36591-36592, 36600, 36640, 43752, 51701-51703, 62320-62327, 64400, 64405-64408, 64415-64435, 64445-64454, 64461-64463, 64479-64505, 64510-64530, 69990, 92012-92014, 93000-93010, 93040-93042, 93318, 93355, 94002, 94200, 94680-94690, 95812-95816, 95819, 95822, 95829, 95955, 96360-96368, 96372, 96374-96377, 96405-96406, 96523, 96931-96936, 97597-97598, 97602, 99155, 99156, 99157, 99211-99223, 99231-99255, 99291-99292, 99304-99310, 99315-99316, 99334-99337, 99347-99350, 99374-99375, 99377-99378, 99446-99449, 99451-99452, 99495-99496, G0168, G0463, G0471, J0670, J2001

Coding Companion for General Surgery/Gastroenterology

11426 00400, 0213T, 0216T, 0470T-0471T, 0596T-0597T, 11000-11006, 11042-11047, 11102, 11104, 11106, 11900-11901, 12001-12007, 12011-12018, 17000✦, 17004✦, 17250, 36000, 36400-36410, 36420-36430, 36440, 36591-36592, 36600, 36640, 43752, 51701-51703, 62320-62327, 64400, 64405-64408, 64415-64435, 64445-64454, 64461-64463, 64479-64505, 64510-64530, 69990, 92012-92014, 93000-93010, 93040-93042, 93318, 93355, 94002, 94200, 94680-94690, 95812-95816, 95819, 95822, 95829, 95955, 96360-96368, 96372, 96374-96377, 96405-96406, 96523, 96931-96936, 97597-97598, 97602, 99155, 99156, 99157, 99211-99223, 99231-99255, 99291-99292, 99304-99310, 99315-99316, 99334-99337, 99347-99350, 99374-99375, 99377-99378, 99446-99449, 99451-99452, 99495-99496, G0168, G0463, G0471, J0670, J2001

11440 00170, 0213T, 0216T, 0419T-0420T✦, 0470T-0471T, 0596T-0597T, 10030✦, 10060✦, 11000-11006, 11042-11047, 11102, 11104, 11900-11901, 12001-12007, 12011-12057, 13100-13133, 13151-13153, 17000✦, 17250, 36000, 36400-36410, 36420-36430, 36440, 36591-36592, 36600, 36640, 41825-41827✦, 42104-42107✦, 43752, 51701-51703, 62320-62327, 64400, 64405-64408, 64415-64435, 64445-64454, 64461-64463, 64479-64505, 64510-64530, 67810, 69990, 92012-92014, 93000-93010, 93040-93042, 93318, 93355, 94002, 94200, 94680-94690, 95812-95816, 95819, 95822, 95829, 95955, 96360-96368, 96372, 96374-96377, 96405-96406, 96523, 96931-96936, 97597-97598, 97602, 99155, 99156, 99157, 99211-99223, 99231-99255, 99291-99292, 99304-99310, 99315-99316, 99334-99337, 99347-99350, 99374-99375, 99377-99378, 99446-99449, 99451-99452, 99495-99496, G0168, G0463, G0471, J0670, J2001

11441 00170, 0213T, 0216T, 0419T-0420T✦, 0470T-0471T, 0596T-0597T, 10061✦, 11000-11006, 11042-11047, 11102, 11104, 11106, 11900-11901, 12001-12007, 12011-12018, 17000✦, 17004✦, 17250, 36000, 36400-36410, 36420-36430, 36440, 36591-36592, 36600, 36640, 41826-41827✦, 42104-42107✦, 43752, 51701-51703, 62320-62327, 64400, 64405-64408, 64415-64435, 64445-64454, 64461-64463, 64479-64505, 64510-64530, 67810, 69990, 92012-92014, 93000-93010, 93040-93042, 93318, 93355, 94002, 94200, 94680-94690, 95812-95816, 95819, 95822, 95829, 95955, 96360-96368, 96372, 96374-96377, 96405-96406, 96523, 96931-96936, 97597-97598, 97602, 99155, 99156, 99157, 99211-99223, 99231-99255, 99291-99292, 99304-99310, 99315-99316, 99334-99337, 99347-99350, 99374-99375, 99377-99378, 99446-99449, 99451-99452, 99495-99496, G0168, G0463, G0471, J0670, J2001

11442 00170, 0213T, 0216T, 0470T-0471T, 0596T-0597T, 10061✦, 11000-11006, 11042-11047, 11102, 11104, 11106, 11900-11901, 12001-12007, 12011-12018, 17000✦, 17004✦, 17250, 36000, 36400-36410, 36420-36430, 36440, 36591-36592, 36600, 36640, 41826-41827✦, 42106-42107✦, 43752, 51701-51703, 62320-62327, 64400, 64405-64408, 64415-64435, 64445-64454, 64461-64463, 64479-64505, 64510-64530, 67810, 69990, 92012-92014, 93000-93010, 93040-93042, 93318, 93355, 94002, 94200, 94680-94690, 95812-95816, 95819, 95822, 95829, 95955, 96360-96368, 96372, 96374-96377, 96405-96406, 96523, 96931-96936, 97597-97598, 97602, 99155, 99156, 99157, 99211-99223, 99231-99255, 99291-99292, 99304-99310, 99315-99316, 99334-99337, 99347-99350, 99374-99375, 99377-99378, 99446-99449, 99451-99452, 99495-99496, G0168, G0463, G0471, J0670, J2001

11443 00170, 0213T, 0216T, 0470T-0471T, 0596T-0597T, 10061✦, 11000-11006, 11042-11047, 11102, 11104, 11106, 11900-11901, 12001-12007, 12011-12018, 17000✦, 17004✦, 17250, 36000, 36400-36410, 36420-36430, 36440, 36591-36592, 36600, 36640, 42106-42107✦, 43752, 51701-51703, 62320-62327, 64400,

64405-64408, 64415-64435, 64445-64454, 64461-64463, 64479-64505, 64510-64530, 67810, 69990, 92012-92014, 93000-93010, 93040-93042, 93318, 93355, 94002, 94200, 94680-94690, 95812-95816, 95819, 95822, 95829, 95955, 96360-96368, 96372, 96374-96377, 96405-96406, 96523, 96931-96936, 97597-97598, 97602, 99155, 99156, 99157, 99211-99223, 99231-99255, 99291-99292, 99304-99310, 99315-99316, 99334-99337, 99347-99350, 99374-99375, 99377-99378, 99446-99449, 99451-99452, 99495-99496, G0168, G0463, G0471, J0670, J2001

11444 00170, 0213T, 0216T, 0470T-0471T, 0596T-0597T, 11000-11006, 11042-11047, 11102, 11104, 11106, 11900-11901, 12001-12007, 12011-12018, 17000✦, 17004✦, 17250, 36000, 36400-36410, 36420-36430, 36440, 36591-36592, 36600, 36640, 42107✦, 43752, 51701-51703, 62320-62327, 64400, 64405-64408, 64415-64435, 64445-64454, 64461-64463, 64479-64505, 64510-64530, 67810, 69990, 92012-92014, 93000-93010, 93040-93042, 93318, 93355, 94002, 94200, 94680-94690, 95812-95816, 95819, 95822, 95829, 95955, 96360-96368, 96372, 96374-96377, 96405-96406, 96523, 96931-96936, 97597-97598, 97602, 99155, 99156, 99157, 99211-99223, 99231-99255, 99291-99292, 99304-99310, 99315-99316, 99334-99337, 99347-99350, 99374-99375, 99377-99378, 99446-99449, 99451-99452, 99495-99496, G0168, G0463, G0471, J0670, J2001

11446 00170, 0213T, 0216T, 0470T-0471T, 0596T-0597T, 11000-11006, 11042-11047, 11102, 11104, 11106, 11900-11901, 12001-12007, 12011-12018, 15002✦, 17000✦, 17004✦, 17250, 36000, 36400-36410, 36420-36430, 36440, 36591-36592, 36600, 36640, 43752, 51701-51703, 62320-62327, 64400, 64405-64408, 64415-64435, 64445-64454, 64461-64463, 64479-64505, 64510-64530, 67810, 69990, 92012-92014, 93000-93010, 93040-93042, 93318, 93355, 94002, 94200, 94680-94690, 95812-95816, 95819, 95822, 95829, 95955, 96360-96368, 96372, 96374-96377, 96405-96406, 96523, 96931-96936, 97597-97598, 97602, 99155, 99156, 99157, 99211-99223, 99231-99255, 99291-99292, 99304-99310, 99315-99316, 99334-99337, 99347-99350, 99374-99375, 99377-99378, 99446-99449, 99451-99452, 99495-99496, G0168, G0463, G0471, J0670, J2001

11450 0213T, 0216T, 0470T-0471T, 0596T-0597T, 11000-11006, 11042-11047, 11102, 11104, 11106, 11900-11901, 12001-12007, 12011-12057, 17000✦, 17004✦, 17250, 36000, 36400-36410, 36420-36430, 36440, 36591-36592, 36600, 36640, 43752, 51701-51703, 62320-62327, 64400, 64405-64408, 64415-64435, 64445-64454, 64461-64463, 64479-64505, 64510-64530, 69990, 92012-92014, 93000-93010, 93040-93042, 93318, 93355, 94002, 94200, 94680-94690, 95812-95816, 95819, 95822, 95829, 95955, 96360-96368, 96372, 96374-96377, 96405-96406, 96523, 96931-96936, 97597-97598, 97602, 99155, 99156, 99157, 99211-99223, 99231-99255, 99291-99292, 99304-99310, 99315-99316, 99334-99337, 99347-99350, 99374-99375, 99377-99378, 99446-99449, 99451-99452, 99495-99496, G0168, G0463, G0471, J0670, J2001

11451 0213T, 0216T, 0470T-0471T, 0596T-0597T, 11000-11006, 11042-11047, 11102, 11104, 11106, 11900-11901, 12001-12007, 12011-12057, 13100-13133, 13151-13152, 13160, 15002✦, 15004✦, 17000✦, 17004✦, 17250, 36000, 36400-36410, 36420-36430, 36440, 36591-36592, 36600, 36640, 43752, 51701-51703, 62320-62327, 64400, 64405-64408, 64415-64435, 64445-64454, 64461-64463, 64479-64505, 64510-64530, 69990, 92012-92014, 93000-93010, 93040-93042, 93318, 93355, 94002, 94200, 94680-94690, 95812-95816, 95819, 95822, 95829, 95955, 96360-96368, 96372, 96374-96377, 96405-96406, 96523, 96931-96936, 97597-97598, 97602, 99155, 99156, 99157, 99211-99223, 99231-99255, 99291-99292, 99304-99310, 99315-99316, 99334-99337, 99347-99350, 99374-99375, 99377-99378, 99446-99449, 99451-99452, 99495-99496, G0168, G0463, G0471, J0670, J2001

11462 0213T, 0216T, 0470T-0471T, 0596T-0597T, 10061✦, 11000-11006, 11042-11047, 11102, 11104, 11106, 11900-11901, 12001-12007, 12011-12057, 15002✦, 17000✦, 17004✦, 17250, 36000, 36400-36410, 36420-36430, 36440, 36591-36592, 36600, 36640, 43752, 51701-51703, 62320-62327, 64400, 64405-64408, 64415-64435, 64445-64454, 64461-64463, 64479-64505, 64510-64530, 69990, 92012-92014, 93000-93010, 93040-93042, 93318, 93355, 94002, 94200, 94680-94690, 95812-95816, 95819, 95822, 95829, 95955, 96360-96368, 96372, 96374-96377, 96405-96406, 96523, 96931-96936, 97597-97598, 97602, 99155, 99156, 99157, 99211-99223, 99231-99255, 99291-99292, 99304-99310, 99315-99316, 99334-99337, 99347-99350, 99374-99375, 99377-99378, 99446-99449, 99451-99452, 99495-99496, G0168, G0463, G0471, J0670, J2001

11463 0213T, 0216T, 0470T-0471T, 0596T-0597T, 11000-11006, 11042-11047, 11102, 11104, 11106, 11900-11901, 12001-12007, 12011-12057, 13100-13132, 13151-13152, 13160, 15002✦, 15004✦, 17000✦, 17004✦, 17250, 36000, 36400-36410, 36420-36430, 36440, 36591-36592, 36600, 36640, 43752, 51701-51703, 62320-62327, 64400, 64405-64408, 64415-64435, 64445-64454, 64461-64463, 64479-64505, 64510-64530, 69990, 92012-92014, 93000-93010, 93040-93042, 93318, 93355, 94002, 94200, 94680-94690, 95812-95816, 95819, 95822, 95829, 95955, 96360-96368, 96372, 96374-96377, 96405-96406, 96523, 96931-96936, 97597-97598, 97602, 99155, 99156, 99157, 99211-99223, 99231-99255, 99291-99292, 99304-99310, 99315-99316, 99334-99337, 99347-99350, 99374-99375, 99377-99378, 99446-99449, 99451-99452, 99495-99496, G0168, G0463, G0471, J0670, J2001

11470 0213T, 0216T, 0470T-0471T, 0596T-0597T, 11000-11006, 11042-11047, 11102, 11104, 11106, 11900-11901, 12001-12007, 12011-12057, 15002✦, 17000✦, 17004✦, 17250, 36000, 36400-36410, 36420-36430, 36440, 36591-36592, 36600, 36640, 43752, 51701-51703, 62320-62327, 64400, 64405-64408, 64415-64435, 64445-64454, 64461-64463, 64479-64505, 64510-64530, 69990, 92012-92014, 93000-93010, 93040-93042, 93318, 93355, 94002, 94200, 94680-94690, 95812-95816, 95819, 95822, 95829, 95955, 96360-96368, 96372, 96374-96377, 96405-96406, 96523, 96931-96936, 97597-97598, 97602, 99155, 99156, 99157, 99211-99223, 99231-99255, 99291-99292, 99304-99310, 99315-99316, 99334-99337, 99347-99350, 99374-99375, 99377-99378, 99446-99449, 99451-99452, 99495-99496, G0168, G0463, G0471, J0670, J2001

11471 0213T, 0216T, 0470T-0471T, 0596T-0597T, 11000-11006, 11010, 11042-11047, 11102, 11104, 11106, 11900-11901, 12001-12007, 12011-12057, 13100-13121, 13131-13133, 13151-13152, 13160, 15002✦, 15004✦, 17000✦, 17004✦, 17250, 36000, 36400-36410, 36420-36430, 36440, 36591-36592, 36600, 36640, 43752, 51701-51703, 62320-62327, 64400, 64405-64408, 64415-64435, 64445-64454, 64461-64463, 64479-64505, 64510-64530, 69990, 92012-92014, 93000-93010, 93040-93042, 93318, 93355, 94002, 94200, 94680-94690, 95812-95816, 95819, 95822, 95829, 95955, 96360-96368, 96372, 96374-96377, 96405-96406, 96523, 96931-96936, 97597-97598, 97602, 99155, 99156, 99157, 99211-99223, 99231-99255, 99291-99292, 99304-99310, 99315-99316, 99334-99337, 99347-99350, 99374-99375, 99377-99378, 99446-99449, 99451-99452, 99495-99496, G0168, G0463, G0471, J0670, J2001

11600 00400, 0213T, 0216T, 0596T-0597T, 10061✦, 11000-11006, 11042-11047, 11102, 11104, 11106, 11900-11901, 12001-12007, 12011-12018, 17000✦, 17004✦, 17250, 17262-17266✦, 17271-17276✦, 17281-17286✦, 19120✦, 36000, 36400-36410, 36420-36430, 36440, 36591-36592, 36600, 36640, 43752, 51701-51703, 62320-62327, 64400, 64405-64408, 64415-64435, 64445-64454, 64461-64463, 64479-64505, 64510-64530, 69990, 92012-92014, 93000-93010, 93040-93042, 93318,

93355, 94002, 94200, 94680-94690, 95812-95816, 95819, 95822, 95829, 95955, 96360-96368, 96372, 96374-96377, 96523, 97597-97598, 97602, 99155, 99156, 99157, 99211-99223, 99231-99255, 99291-99292, 99304-99310, 99315-99316, 99334-99337, 99347-99350, 99374-99375, 99377-99378, 99446-99449, 99451-99452, 99495-99496, G0168, G0463, G0471, J0670, J2001

11601 00400, 0213T, 0216T, 0419T-0420T✦, 0596T-0597T, 10061✦, 11000-11006, 11042-11047, 11102, 11104, 11106, 11900-11901, 12001-12007, 12011-12018, 17000✦, 17004✦, 17250, 17264-17266✦, 17273-17276✦, 17282-17286✦, 19120✦, 36000, 36400-36410, 36420-36430, 36440, 36591-36592, 36600, 36640, 43752, 51701-51703, 62320-62327, 64400, 64405-64408, 64415-64435, 64445-64454, 64461-64463, 64479-64505, 64510-64530, 69990, 92012-92014, 93000-93010, 93040-93042, 93318, 93355, 94002, 94200, 94680-94690, 95812-95816, 95819, 95822, 95829, 95955, 96360-96368, 96372, 96374-96377, 96523, 97597-97598, 97602, 99155, 99156, 99157, 99211-99223, 99231-99255, 99291-99292, 99304-99310, 99315-99316, 99334-99337, 99347-99350, 99374-99375, 99377-99378, 99446-99449, 99451-99452, 99495-99496, G0168, G0463, G0471, J0670, J2001

11602 00400, 0213T, 0216T, 0596T-0597T, 10061✦, 11000-11006, 11042-11047, 11102, 11104, 11106, 11900-11901, 12001-12007, 12011-12018, 17000✦, 17004✦, 17250, 17266✦, 17274-17276✦, 17283-17286✦, 19120✦, 36000, 36400-36410, 36420-36430, 36440, 36591-36592, 36600, 36640, 43752, 51701-51703, 62320-62327, 64400, 64405-64408, 64415-64435, 64445-64454, 64461-64463, 64479-64505, 64510-64530, 69990, 92012-92014, 93000-93010, 93040-93042, 93318, 93355, 94002, 94200, 94680-94690, 95812-95816, 95819, 95822, 95829, 95955, 96360-96368, 96372, 96374-96377, 96523, 97597-97598, 97602, 99155, 99156, 99157, 99211-99223, 99231-99255, 99291-99292, 99304-99310, 99315-99316, 99334-99337, 99347-99350, 99374-99375, 99377-99378, 99446-99449, 99451-99452, 99495-99496, G0168, G0463, G0471, J0670, J2001

11603 00400, 0213T, 0216T, 0596T-0597T, 10061✦, 11000-11006, 11042-11047, 11102, 11104, 11106, 11900-11901, 12001-12007, 12011-12018, 17000✦, 17004✦, 17250, 17274-17276✦, 17283-17286✦, 19120✦, 36000, 36400-36410, 36420-36430, 36440, 36591-36592, 36600, 36640, 43752, 51701-51703, 62320-62327, 64400, 64405-64408, 64415-64435, 64445-64454, 64461-64463, 64479-64505, 64510-64530, 69990, 92012-92014, 93000-93010, 93040-93042, 93318, 93355, 94002, 94200, 94680-94690, 95812-95816, 95819, 95822, 95829, 95955, 96360-96368, 96372, 96374-96377, 96523, 97597-97598, 97602, 99155, 99156, 99157, 99211-99223, 99231-99255, 99291-99292, 99304-99310, 99315-99316, 99334-99337, 99347-99350, 99374-99375, 99377-99378, 99446-99449, 99451-99452, 99495-99496, G0168, G0463, G0471, J0670, J2001

11604 00400, 0213T, 0216T, 0596T-0597T, 11000-11006, 11042-11047, 11102, 11104, 11106, 11900-11901, 12001-12007, 12011-12018, 17000✦, 17004✦, 17250, 17274-17276✦, 17283-17286✦, 19120✦, 36000, 36400-36410, 36420-36430, 36440, 36591-36592, 36600, 36640, 43752, 51701-51703, 62320-62327, 64400, 64405-64408, 64415-64435, 64445-64454, 64461-64463, 64479-64505, 64510-64530, 69990, 92012-92014, 93000-93010, 93040-93042, 93318, 93355, 94002, 94200, 94680-94690, 95812-95816, 95819, 95822, 95829, 95955, 96360-96368, 96372, 96374-96377, 96523, 97597-97598, 97602, 99155, 99156, 99157, 99211-99223, 99231-99255, 99291-99292, 99304-99310, 99315-99316, 99334-99337, 99347-99350, 99374-99375, 99377-99378, 99446-99449, 99451-99452, 99495-99496, G0168, G0463, G0471, J0670, J2001

Coding Companion for General Surgery/Gastroenterology

11606 00400, 0213T, 0216T, 0596T-0597T, 11000-11006, 11042-11047, 11102, 11104, 11106, 11900-11901, 12001-12007, 12011-12018, 15002✦, 15004✦, 17000✦, 17004✦, 17250, 17286✦, 19120✦, 36000, 36400-36410, 36420-36430, 36440, 36591-36592, 36600, 36640, 43752, 51701-51703, 62320-62327, 64400, 64405-64408, 64415-64435, 64445-64454, 64461-64463, 64479-64505, 64510-64530, 69990, 92012-92014, 93000-93010, 93040-93042, 93318, 93355, 94002, 94200, 94680-94690, 95812-95816, 95819, 95822, 95829, 95955, 96360-96368, 96372, 96374-96377, 96523, 97597-97598, 97602, 99155, 99156, 99157, 99211-99223, 99231-99255, 99291-99292, 99304-99310, 99315-99316, 99334-99337, 99347-99350, 99374-99375, 99377-99378, 99446-99449, 99451-99452, 99495-99496, G0168, G0463, G0471, J0670, J2001

11620 00400, 0213T, 0216T, 0596T-0597T, 10061✦, 11000-11006, 11042-11047, 11102, 11104, 11106, 11900-11901, 12001-12007, 12011-12018, 17000✦, 17004✦, 17250, 17262-17266✦, 17271-17276✦, 17281-17286✦, 36000, 36400-36410, 36420-36430, 36440, 36591-36592, 36600, 36640, 43752, 51701-51703, 62320-62327, 64400, 64405-64408, 64415-64435, 64445-64454, 64461-64463, 64479-64505, 64510-64530, 69990, 92012-92014, 93000-93010, 93040-93042, 93318, 93355, 94002, 94200, 94680-94690, 95812-95816, 95819, 95822, 95829, 95955, 96360-96368, 96372, 96374-96377, 96523, 97597-97598, 97602, 99155, 99156, 99157, 99211-99223, 99231-99255, 99291-99292, 99304-99310, 99315-99316, 99334-99337, 99347-99350, 99374-99375, 99377-99378, 99446-99449, 99451-99452, 99495-99496, G0168, G0463, G0471, J0670, J2001

11621 00400, 0213T, 0216T, 0596T-0597T, 10061✦, 11000-11006, 11042-11047, 11102, 11104, 11106, 11900-11901, 12001-12007, 12011-12018, 17000✦, 17004✦, 17250, 17266✦, 17273-17276✦, 17282-17286✦, 36000, 36400-36410, 36420-36430, 36440, 36591-36592, 36600, 36640, 43752, 51701-51703, 62320-62327, 64400, 64405-64408, 64415-64435, 64445-64454, 64461-64463, 64479-64505, 64510-64530, 69990, 92012-92014, 93000-93010, 93040-93042, 93318, 93355, 94002, 94200, 94680-94690, 95812-95816, 95819, 95822, 95829, 95955, 96360-96368, 96372, 96374-96377, 96523, 97597-97598, 97602, 99155, 99156, 99157, 99211-99223, 99231-99255, 99291-99292, 99304-99310, 99315-99316, 99334-99337, 99347-99350, 99374-99375, 99377-99378, 99446-99449, 99451-99452, 99495-99496, G0168, G0463, G0471, J0670, J2001

11622 00400, 0213T, 0216T, 0596T-0597T, 10061✦, 11000-11006, 11042-11047, 11102, 11104, 11106, 11900-11901, 12001-12007, 12011-12018, 17000✦, 17004✦, 17250, 17274-17276✦, 17283-17286✦, 36000, 36400-36410, 36420-36430, 36440, 36591-36592, 36600, 36640, 43752, 51701-51703, 62320-62327, 64400, 64405-64408, 64415-64435, 64445-64454, 64461-64463, 64479-64505, 64510-64530, 69990, 92012-92014, 93000-93010, 93040-93042, 93318, 93355, 94002, 94200, 94680-94690, 95812-95816, 95819, 95822, 95829, 95955, 96360-96368, 96372, 96374-96377, 96523, 97597-97598, 97602, 99155, 99156, 99157, 99211-99223, 99231-99255, 99291-99292, 99304-99310, 99315-99316, 99334-99337, 99347-99350, 99374-99375, 99377-99378, 99446-99449, 99451-99452, 99495-99496, G0168, G0463, G0471, J0670, J2001

11623 00400, 0213T, 0216T, 0596T-0597T, 11000-11006, 11042-11047, 11102, 11104, 11106, 11900-11901, 12001-12007, 12011-12018, 17000✦, 17004✦, 17250, 17276✦, 17284-17286✦, 36000, 36400-36410, 36420-36430, 36440, 36591-36592, 36600, 36640, 43752, 51701-51703, 62320-62327, 64400, 64405-64408, 64415-64435, 64445-64454, 64461-64463, 64479-64505, 64510-64530, 69990, 92012-92014, 93000-93010, 93040-93042, 93318, 93355, 94002, 94200, 94680-94690, 95812-95816, 95819, 95822, 95829, 95955, 96360-96368, 96372, 96374-96377, 96523, 97597-97598, 97602, 99155, 99156, 99157,

11624 99211-99223, 99231-99255, 99291-99292, 99304-99310, 99315-99316, 99334-99337, 99347-99350, 99374-99375, 99377-99378, 99446-99449, 99451-99452, 99495-99496, G0168, G0463, G0471, J0670, J2001

11624 00400, 0213T, 0216T, 0596T-0597T, 11000-11006, 11042-11047, 11102, 11104, 11106, 11900-11901, 12001-12007, 12011-12018, 17000✦, 17004✦, 17250, 17286✦, 36000, 36400-36410, 36420-36430, 36440, 36591-36592, 36600, 36640, 43752, 51701-51703, 62320-62327, 64400, 64405-64408, 64415-64435, 64445-64454, 64461-64463, 64479-64505, 64510-64530, 69990, 92012-92014, 93000-93010, 93040-93042, 93318, 93355, 94002, 94200, 94680-94690, 95812-95816, 95819, 95822, 95829, 95955, 96360-96368, 96372, 96374-96377, 96523, 97597-97598, 97602, 99155, 99156, 99157, 99211-99223, 99231-99255, 99291-99292, 99304-99310, 99315-99316, 99334-99337, 99347-99350, 99374-99375, 99377-99378, 99446-99449, 99451-99452, 99495-99496, G0168, G0463, G0471, J0670, J2001

11626 00400, 0213T, 0216T, 0596T-0597T, 11000-11006, 11042-11047, 11102, 11104, 11106, 11900-11901, 12001-12007, 12011-12018, 15002✦, 17000✦, 17004✦, 17250, 17286✦, 36000, 36400-36410, 36420-36430, 36440, 36591-36592, 36600, 36640, 43752, 51701-51703, 62320-62327, 64400, 64405-64408, 64415-64435, 64445-64454, 64461-64463, 64479-64505, 64510-64530, 69990, 92012-92014, 93000-93010, 93040-93042, 93318, 93355, 94002, 94200, 94680-94690, 95812-95816, 95819, 95822, 95829, 95955, 96360-96368, 96372, 96374-96377, 96523, 97597-97598, 97602, 99155, 99156, 99157, 99211-99223, 99231-99255, 99291-99292, 99304-99310, 99315-99316, 99334-99337, 99347-99350, 99374-99375, 99377-99378, 99446-99449, 99451-99452, 99495-99496, G0168, G0463, G0471, J0670, J2001

11640 00170, 0213T, 0216T, 0596T-0597T, 10061, 11000-11006, 11042-11047, 11102, 11104, 11106, 11900-11901, 12001-12007, 12011-12018, 17000✦, 17004✦, 17250, 17262-17266✦, 17272-17276✦, 17281-17286✦, 36000, 36400-36410, 36420-36430, 36440, 36591-36592, 36600, 36640, 41826-41827✦, 42107✦, 43752, 51701-51703, 62320-62327, 64400, 64405-64408, 64415-64435, 64445-64454, 64461-64463, 64479-64505, 64510-64530, 67810, 69990, 92012-92014, 93000-93010, 93040-93042, 93318, 93355, 94002, 94200, 94680-94690, 95812-95816, 95819, 95822, 95829, 95955, 96360-96368, 96372, 96374-96377, 96523, 97597-97598, 97602, 99155, 99156, 99157, 99211-99223, 99231-99255, 99291-99292, 99304-99310, 99315-99316, 99334-99337, 99347-99350, 99374-99375, 99377-99378, 99446-99449, 99451-99452, 99495-99496, G0168, G0463, G0471, J0670, J2001

11641 00170, 0213T, 0216T, 0596T-0597T, 10061, 11000-11006, 11042-11047, 11102, 11104, 11106, 11900-11901, 12001-12007, 12011-12018, 17000✦, 17004✦, 17250, 17274-17276✦, 17283-17286✦, 36000, 36400-36410, 36420-36430, 36440, 36591-36592, 36600, 36640, 41827✦, 42107✦, 43752, 51701-51703, 62320-62327, 64400, 64405-64408, 64415-64435, 64445-64454, 64461-64463, 64479-64505, 64510-64530, 67810, 69990, 92012-92014, 93000-93010, 93040-93042, 93318, 93355, 94002, 94200, 94680-94690, 95812-95816, 95819, 95822, 95829, 95955, 96360-96368, 96372, 96374-96377, 96523, 97597-97598, 97602, 99155, 99156, 99157, 99211-99223, 99231-99255, 99291-99292, 99304-99310, 99315-99316, 99334-99337, 99347-99350, 99374-99375, 99377-99378, 99446-99449, 99451-99452, 99495-99496, G0168, G0463, G0471, J0670, J2001

11642 00170, 0213T, 0216T, 0596T-0597T, 10061, 11000-11006, 11042-11047, 11102, 11104, 11106, 11900-11901, 12001-12007, 12011-12018, 17000✦, 17004✦, 17250, 17276✦, 17284-17286✦, 36000, 36400-36410, 36420-36430, 36440, 36591-36592, 36600, 36640, 41827✦, 42107✦, 43752, 51701-51703, 62320-62327, 64400, 64405-64408, 64415-64435, 64445-64454, 64461-64463, 64479-64505, 64510-64530, 67810, 69990,

92012-92014, 93000-93010, 93040-93042, 93318, 93355, 94002, 94200, 94680-94690, 95812-95816, 95819, 95822, 95829, 95955, 96360-96368, 96372, 96374-96377, 96523, 97597-97598, 97602, 99155, 99156, 99157, 99211-99223, 99231-99255, 99291-99292, 99304-99310, 99315-99316, 99334-99337, 99347-99350, 99374-99375, 99377-99378, 99446-99449, 99451-99452, 99495-99496, G0168, G0463, G0471, J0670, J2001

11643 00170, 0213T, 0216T, 0596T-0597T, 11000-11006, 11042-11047, 11102, 11104, 11106, 11900-11901, 12001-12007, 12011-12018, 17000✦, 17004✦, 17250, 17286✦, 36000, 36400-36410, 36420-36430, 36440, 36591-36592, 36600, 36640, 42107✦, 43752, 51701-51703, 62320-62327, 64400, 64405-64408, 64415-64435, 64445-64454, 64461-64463, 64479-64505, 64510-64530, 67810, 69990, 92012-92014, 93000-93010, 93040-93042, 93318, 93355, 94002, 94200, 94680-94690, 95812-95816, 95819, 95822, 95829, 95955, 96360-96368, 96372, 96374-96377, 96523, 97597-97598, 97602, 99155, 99156, 99157, 99211-99223, 99231-99255, 99291-99292, 99304-99310, 99315-99316, 99334-99337, 99347-99350, 99374-99375, 99377-99378, 99446-99449, 99451-99452, 99495-99496, G0168, G0463, G0471, J0670, J2001

11644 00170, 0213T, 0216T, 0596T-0597T, 11000-11006, 11042-11047, 11102, 11104, 11106, 11900-11901, 12001-12007, 12011-12018, 15002✦, 17000✦, 17004✦, 17250, 36000, 36400-36410, 36420-36430, 36440, 36591-36592, 36600, 36640, 43752, 51701-51703, 62320-62327, 64400, 64405-64408, 64415-64435, 64445-64454, 64461-64463, 64479-64505, 64510-64530, 67810, 69990, 92012-92014, 93000-93010, 93040-93042, 93318, 93355, 94002, 94200, 94680-94690, 95812-95816, 95819, 95822, 95829, 95955, 96360-96368, 96372, 96374-96377, 96523, 97597-97598, 97602, 99155, 99156, 99157, 99211-99223, 99231-99255, 99291-99292, 99304-99310, 99315-99316, 99334-99337, 99347-99350, 99374-99375, 99377-99378, 99446-99449, 99451-99452, 99495-99496, G0168, G0463, G0471, J0670, J2001

11646 00170, 0213T, 0216T, 0596T-0597T, 11000-11006, 11042-11047, 11102, 11104, 11106, 11900-11901, 12001-12007, 12011-12018, 15002✦, 15004✦, 17000✦, 17004✦, 17250, 36000, 36400-36410, 36420-36430, 36440, 36591-36592, 36600, 36640, 43752, 51701-51703, 62320-62327, 64400, 64405-64408, 64415-64435, 64445-64454, 64461-64463, 64479-64505, 64510-64530, 67810, 69990, 92012-92014, 93000-93010, 93040-93042, 93318, 93355, 94002, 94200, 94680-94690, 95812-95816, 95819, 95822, 95829, 95955, 96360-96368, 96372, 96374-96377, 96523, 97597-97598, 97602, 99155, 99156, 99157, 99211-99223, 99231-99255, 99291-99292, 99304-99310, 99315-99316, 99334-99337, 99347-99350, 99374-99375, 99377-99378, 99446-99449, 99451-99452, 99495-99496, G0168, G0463, G0471, J0670, J2001

11770 0213T, 0216T, 0596T-0597T, 10080-10081, 11000-11006, 11042-11047, 11900-11901, 12001-12007, 12011-12057, 13100-13133, 13151-13153, 17250, 20500, 36000, 36400-36410, 36420-36430, 36440, 36591-36592, 36600, 36640, 43752, 51701-51703, 62320-62327, 64400, 64405-64408, 64415-64435, 64445-64454, 64461-64463, 64479-64505, 64510-64530, 69990, 92012-92014, 93000-93010, 93040-93042, 93318, 93355, 94002, 94200, 94680-94690, 95812-95816, 95819, 95822, 95829, 95955, 96360-96368, 96372, 96374-96377, 96405-96406, 96523, 97597-97598, 97602, 99155, 99156, 99157, 99211-99223, 99231-99255, 99291-99292, 99304-99310, 99315-99316, 99334-99337, 99347-99350, 99374-99375, 99377-99378, 99446-99449, 99451-99452, 99495-99496, G0463, G0471, J0670, J2001

11771 0213T, 0216T, 0596T-0597T, 10080-10081, 11000-11006, 11042-11047, 11770, 11900-11901, 12001-12007, 12011-12057, 13100-13133, 13151-13153, 17250, 20500, 36000, 36400-36410, 36420-36430, 36440, 36591-36592, 36600, 36640, 43752, 51701-51703, 62320-62327, 64400,

64405-64408, 64415-64435, 64445-64454, 64461-64463, 64479-64505, 64510-64530, 69990, 92012-92014, 93000-93010, 93040-93042, 93318, 93355, 94002, 94200, 94680-94690, 95812-95816, 95819, 95822, 95829, 95955, 96360-96368, 96372, 96374-96377, 96405-96406, 96523, 97597-97598, 97602, 99155, 99156, 99157, 99211-99223, 99231-99255, 99291-99292, 99304-99310, 99315-99316, 99334-99337, 99347-99350, 99374-99375, 99377-99378, 99446-99449, 99451-99452, 99495-99496, G0463, G0471, J0670, J2001

11772 0213T, 0216T, 0596T-0597T, 10080-10081, 11000-11006, 11042-11047, 11770-11771, 11900-11901, 12001-12007, 12011-12057, 13100-13133, 13151-13153, 17250, 17313✦, 36000, 36400-36410, 36420-36430, 36440, 36591-36592, 36600, 36640, 43752, 51701-51703, 62320-62327, 64400, 64405-64408, 64415-64435, 64445-64454, 64461-64463, 64479-64505, 64510-64530, 69990, 92012-92014, 93000-93010, 93040-93042, 93318, 93355, 94002, 94200, 94680-94690, 95812-95816, 95819, 95822, 95829, 95955, 96360-96368, 96372, 96374-96377, 96405-96406, 96523, 97597-97598, 97602, 99155, 99156, 99157, 99211-99223, 99231-99255, 99291-99292, 99304-99310, 99315-99316, 99334-99337, 99347-99350, 99374-99375, 99377-99378, 99446-99449, 99451-99452, 99495-99496, G0463, G0471, J0670, J2001

11960 0213T, 0216T, 0596T-0597T, 11000-11006, 11042-11047, 11970✦, 12001-12007, 12011-12057, 13100-13133, 13151-13160, 29848, 36000, 36400-36410, 36420-36430, 36440, 36591-36592, 36600, 36640, 43752, 51701-51703, 62320-62327, 64400, 64405-64408, 64415-64435, 64445-64454, 64461-64463, 64479-64505, 64510-64530, 69990, 92012-92014, 93000-93010, 93040-93042, 93318, 93355, 94002, 94200, 94680-94690, 95812-95816, 95819, 95822, 95829, 95955, 96360-96368, 96372, 96374-96377, 96523, 97597-97598, 97602, 99155, 99156, 99157, 99211-99223, 99231-99255, 99291-99292, 99304-99310, 99315-99316, 99334-99337, 99347-99350, 99374-99375, 99377-99378, 99446-99449, 99451-99452, 99495-99496, G0463, G0471

11970 0213T, 0216T, 0596T-0597T, 11000-11006, 11042-11047, 12001-12007, 12011-12057, 13100-13133, 13151-13153, 36000, 36400-36410, 36420-36430, 36440, 36591-36592, 36600, 36640, 43752, 51701-51703, 62320-62327, 64400, 64405-64408, 64415-64435, 64445-64454, 64461-64463, 64479-64505, 64510-64530, 69990, 92012-92014, 93000-93010, 93040-93042, 93318, 93355, 94002, 94200, 94680-94690, 95812-95816, 95819, 95822, 95829, 95955, 96360-96368, 96372, 96374-96377, 96523, 97597-97598, 97602, 99155, 99156, 99157, 99211-99223, 99231-99255, 99291-99292, 99304-99310, 99315-99316, 99334-99337, 99347-99350, 99374-99375, 99377-99378, 99446-99449, 99451-99452, 99495-99496, G0463, G0471

11971 0213T, 0216T, 0596T-0597T, 11000-11006, 11042-11047, 11960-11970✦, 12001-12007, 12011-12057, 13100-13133, 13151-13153, 36000, 36400-36410, 36420-36430, 36440, 36591-36592, 36600, 36640, 43752, 51701-51703, 62320-62327, 64400, 64405-64408, 64415-64435, 64445-64454, 64461-64463, 64479-64505, 64510-64530, 69990, 92012-92014, 93000-93010, 93040-93042, 93318, 93355, 94002, 94200, 94680-94690, 95812-95816, 95819, 95822, 95829, 95955, 96360-96368, 96372, 96374-96377, 96523, 97597-97598, 97602, 99155, 99156, 99157, 99211-99223, 99231-99255, 99291-99292, 99304-99310, 99315-99316, 99334-99337, 99347-99350, 99374-99375, 99377-99378, 99446-99449, 99451-99452, 99495-99496, G0463, G0471, J0670, J2001

11981 0213T, 0216T, 11000-11006, 11042-11047, 11982✦, 36000, 36410, 36591-36592, 61650, 62324-62327, 64415-64417, 64450, 64454, 64486-64490, 64493, 96360, 96365, 96372, 96374-96377, 96523, 97597-97598, 97602, G0516-G0517✦, J0670, J2001

11982 0213T, 0216T, 11000-11006, 11042-11047, 11976✦, 20701, 36000, 36410, 36591-36592, 61650, 62324-62327, 64415-64417, 64450, 64454,

Coding Companion for General Surgery/Gastroenterology

64486-64490, 64493, 96360, 96365, 96372, 96374-96377, 96523, 97597-97598, 97602, G0517✦, J0670, J2001

11983 0213T, 0216T, 11000-11006, 11042-11047, 11976, 11981-11982, 36000, 36410, 36591-36592, 61650, 62324-62327, 64415-64417, 64450, 64454, 64486-64490, 64493, 96360, 96365, 96372, 96374-96377, 96523, 97597-97598, 97602, G0516-G0518✦, J0670, J2001

12001 0213T, 0216T, 0543T-0544T, 0545T, 0567T-0574T, 0580T, 0581T, 0582T, 11042, 11055-11056, 11719, 11740-11750, 11900-11901, 20560-20561, 36000, 36400-36410, 36420-36430, 36440, 36591-36592, 36600, 36640, 43752, 51701-51703, 64400, 64405-64408, 64415-64435, 64445-64450, 64479-64484, 64490-64505, 64510-64530, 66987-66988, 69990, 92012-92014, 93000-93010, 93040-93042, 93318, 93355, 94002, 94200, 94680-94690, 95812-95816, 95819, 95822, 95829, 95955, 96360-96368, 96372, 96374-96377, 96523, 97597-97598, 97602-97608, 99155, 99156, 99157, 99211-99223, 99231-99255, 99291-99292, 99304-99310, 99315-99316, 99334-99337, 99347-99350, 99374-99375, 99377-99378, 99446-99449, 99451-99452, 99495-99496, G0168, G0463, G0471, J0670, J2001

12002 0213T, 0216T, 0543T-0544T, 0545T, 0567T-0574T, 0580T, 0581T, 0582T, 11042, 11740, 11900-11901, 12001, 12013-12014✦, 20560-20561, 20701, 36000, 36400-36410, 36420-36430, 36440, 36591-36592, 36600, 36640, 43752, 51701-51703, 64400, 64405-64408, 64415-64435, 64445-64450, 64479-64484, 64490-64505, 64510-64530, 66987-66988, 69990, 92012-92014, 93000-93010, 93040-93042, 93318, 93355, 94002, 94200, 94680-94690, 95812-95816, 95819, 95822, 95829, 95955, 96360-96368, 96372, 96374-96377, 96523, 97597-97598, 97602-97608, 99155, 99156, 99157, 99211-99223, 99231-99255, 99291-99292, 99304-99310, 99315-99316, 99334-99337, 99347-99350, 99374-99375, 99377-99378, 99446-99449, 99451-99452, 99495-99496, G0168, G0463, G0471, J0670, J2001

12004 0213T, 0216T, 0543T-0544T, 0545T, 0567T-0574T, 0580T, 0581T, 0582T, 11042, 11900-11901, 12001-12002, 12015✦, 20560-20561, 20701, 36000, 36400-36410, 36420-36430, 36440, 36591-36592, 36600, 36640, 43752, 51701-51703, 64400, 64405-64408, 64415-64435, 64445-64450, 64479-64484, 64490-64505, 64510-64530, 66987-66988, 69990, 92012-92014, 93000-93010, 93040-93042, 93318, 93355, 94002, 94200, 94680-94690, 95812-95816, 95819, 95822, 95829, 95955, 96360-96368, 96372, 96374-96377, 96523, 97597-97598, 97602-97608, 99155, 99156, 99157, 99211-99223, 99231-99255, 99291-99292, 99304-99310, 99315-99316, 99334-99337, 99347-99350, 99374-99375, 99377-99378, 99446-99449, 99451-99452, 99495-99496, G0168, G0463, G0471, J0670, J2001

12005 0213T, 0216T, 0543T-0544T, 0545T, 0567T-0574T, 0580T, 0581T, 0582T, 11042-11043, 11900-11901, 12001-12004, 12016✦, 20560-20561, 20700-20701, 36000, 36400-36410, 36420-36430, 36440, 36591-36592, 36600, 36640, 43752, 51701-51703, 64400, 64405-64408, 64415-64435, 64445-64451, 64479-64484, 64490-64505, 64510-64530, 66987-66988, 69990, 92012-92014, 93000-93010, 93040-93042, 93318, 93355, 94002, 94200, 94680-94690, 95812-95816, 95819, 95822, 95829, 95955, 96360-96368, 96372, 96374-96377, 96523, 97597-97598, 97602-97608, 99155, 99156, 99157, 99211-99223, 99231-99255, 99291-99292, 99304-99310, 99315-99316, 99334-99337, 99347-99350, 99374-99375, 99377-99378, 99446-99449, 99451-99452, 99495-99496, G0168, G0463, G0471, J0670, J2001

12006 0213T, 0216T, 0543T-0544T, 0545T, 0567T-0574T, 0580T, 0581T, 0582T, 11042-11043, 11900-11901, 12001-12005, 12017✦, 20560-20561, 20700-20701, 36000, 36400-36410, 36420-36430, 36440, 36591-36592, 36600, 36640, 43752, 51701-51703, 64400, 64405-64408, 64415-64435, 64445-64451, 64479-64484, 64490-64505, 64510-64530, 66987-66988,

69990, 92012-92014, 93000-93010, 93040-93042, 93318, 93355, 94002, 94200, 94680-94690, 95812-95816, 95819, 95822, 95829, 95955, 96360-96368, 96372, 96374-96377, 96523, 97597-97598, 97602-97608, 99155, 99156, 99157, 99211-99223, 99231-99255, 99291-99292, 99304-99310, 99315-99316, 99334-99337, 99347-99350, 99374-99375, 99377-99378, 99446-99449, 99451-99452, 99495-99496, G0168, G0463, G0471, J0670, J2001

12007 0213T, 0216T, 0543T-0544T, 0545T, 0567T-0574T, 0580T, 0581T, 0582T, 11900-11901, 12001-12006, 12018✦, 15772, 15774, 20560-20561, 20700-20701, 36000, 36400-36410, 36420-36430, 36440, 36591-36592, 36600, 36640, 43752, 51701-51703, 64400, 64405-64408, 64415-64435, 64445-64451, 64479-64484, 64490-64505, 64510-64530, 66987-66988, 69990, 92012-92014, 93000-93010, 93040-93042, 93318, 93355, 94002, 94200, 94680-94690, 95812-95816, 95819, 95822, 95829, 95955, 96360-96368, 96372, 96374-96377, 96523, 97597-97598, 97602-97608, 99155, 99156, 99157, 99211-99223, 99231-99255, 99291-99292, 99304-99310, 99315-99316, 99334-99337, 99347-99350, 99374-99375, 99377-99378, 99446-99449, 99451-99452, 99495-99496, G0168, G0463, G0471, J0670, J2001

12011 0213T, 0216T, 0567T-0574T, 0580T, 0581T, 0582T, 11042, 11900-11901, 12001, 20560-20561, 36000, 36400-36410, 36420-36430, 36440, 36591-36592, 36600, 36640, 43752, 51701-51703, 64400, 64405-64408, 64415-64435, 64445-64450, 64479-64484, 64490-64505, 64510-64530, 66987-66988, 69990, 92012-92014, 93000-93010, 93040-93042, 93318, 93355, 94002, 94200, 94680-94690, 95812-95816, 95819, 95822, 95829, 95955, 96360-96368, 96372, 96374-96377, 96523, 97597-97598, 97602-97608, 99155, 99156, 99157, 99211-99223, 99231-99255, 99291-99292, 99304-99310, 99315-99316, 99334-99337, 99347-99350, 99374-99375, 99377-99378, 99446-99449, 99451-99452, 99495-99496, G0168, G0463, G0471, J0670, J2001

12013 0213T, 0216T, 0567T-0574T, 0580T, 0581T, 0582T, 11042, 11900-11901, 12011, 20560-20561, 20701, 36000, 36400-36410, 36420-36430, 36440, 36591-36592, 36600, 36640, 43752, 51701-51703, 64400, 64405-64408, 64415-64435, 64445-64450, 64479-64484, 64490-64505, 64510-64530, 66987-66988, 69990, 92012-92014, 93000-93010, 93040-93042, 93318, 93355, 94002, 94200, 94680-94690, 95812-95816, 95819, 95822, 95829, 95955, 96360-96368, 96372, 96374-96377, 96523, 97597-97598, 97602-97608, 99155, 99156, 99157, 99211-99223, 99231-99255, 99291-99292, 99304-99310, 99315-99316, 99334-99337, 99347-99350, 99374-99375, 99377-99378, 99446-99449, 99451-99452, 99495-99496, G0168, G0463, G0471, J0670, J2001

12014 0213T, 0216T, 0567T-0574T, 0580T, 0581T, 0582T, 11900-11901, 12011-12013, 20560-20561, 20700-20701, 36000, 36400-36410, 36420-36430, 36440, 36591-36592, 36600, 36640, 43752, 51701-51703, 64400, 64405-64408, 64415-64435, 64445-64451, 64479-64484, 64490-64505, 64510-64530, 66987-66988, 69990, 92012-92014, 93000-93010, 93040-93042, 93318, 93355, 94002, 94200, 94680-94690, 95812-95816, 95819, 95822, 95829, 95955, 96360-96368, 96372, 96374-96377, 96523, 97597-97598, 97602-97608, 99155, 99156, 99157, 99211-99223, 99231-99255, 99291-99292, 99304-99310, 99315-99316, 99334-99337, 99347-99350, 99374-99375, 99377-99378, 99446-99449, 99451-99452, 99495-99496, G0168, G0463, G0471, J0670, J2001

12015 0213T, 0216T, 0567T-0574T, 0580T, 0581T, 0582T, 11042, 11900-11901, 12011-12014, 20560-20561, 20700-20701, 36000, 36400-36410, 36420-36430, 36440, 36591-36592, 36600, 36640, 43752, 51701-51703, 64400, 64405-64408, 64415-64435, 64445-64451, 64479-64484, 64490-64505, 64510-64530, 66987-66988, 69990, 92012-92014, 93000-93010, 93040-93042, 93318, 93355, 94002, 94200, 94680-94690, 95812-95816, 95819, 95822, 95829, 95955, 96360-96368, 96372,

96374-96377, 96523, 97597-97598, 97602-97608, 99155, 99156, 99157, 99211-99223, 99231-99255, 99291-99292, 99304-99310, 99315-99316, 99334-99337, 99347-99350, 99374-99375, 99377-99378, 99446-99449, 99451-99452, 99495-99496, G0168, G0463, G0471, J0670, J2001

12016 0213T, 0216T, 0567T-0574T, 0580T, 0581T, 0582T, 11900-11901, 12011-12015, 15772, 15774, 20560-20561, 20700-20701, 36000, 36400-36410, 36420-36430, 36440, 36591-36592, 36600, 36640, 43752, 51701-51703, 64400, 64405-64408, 64415-64435, 64445-64451, 64479-64484, 64490-64505, 64510-64530, 66987-66988, 69990, 92012-92014, 93000-93010, 93040-93042, 93318, 93355, 94002, 94200, 94680-94690, 95812-95816, 95819, 95822, 95829, 95955, 96360-96368, 96372, 96374-96377, 96523, 97597-97598, 97602-97608, 99155, 99156, 99157, 99211-99223, 99231-99255, 99291-99292, 99304-99310, 99315-99316, 99334-99337, 99347-99350, 99374-99375, 99377-99378, 99446-99449, 99451-99452, 99495-99496, G0168, G0463, G0471, J0670, J2001

12017 0213T, 0216T, 0567T-0574T, 0580T, 0581T, 0582T, 11010, 11900-11901, 12011-12016, 15772, 15774, 20560-20561, 20700-20701, 36000, 36400-36410, 36420-36430, 36440, 36591-36592, 36600, 36640, 43752, 51701-51703, 64400, 64405-64408, 64415-64435, 64445-64451, 64479-64484, 64490-64505, 64510-64530, 66987-66988, 69990, 92012-92014, 93000-93010, 93040-93042, 93318, 93355, 94002, 94200, 94680-94690, 95812-95816, 95819, 95822, 95829, 95955, 96360-96368, 96372, 96374-96377, 96523, 97597-97598, 97602-97608, 99155, 99156, 99157, 99211-99223, 99231-99255, 99291-99292, 99304-99310, 99315-99316, 99334-99337, 99347-99350, 99374-99375, 99377-99378, 99446-99449, 99451-99452, 99495-99496, G0168, G0463, G0471

12018 0213T, 0216T, 0567T-0574T, 0580T, 0581T, 0582T, 11010, 11900-11901, 12011-12017, 15772, 15774, 20560-20561, 20700-20701, 36000, 36400-36410, 36420-36430, 36440, 36591-36592, 36600, 36640, 43752, 51701-51703, 64400, 64405-64408, 64415-64435, 64445-64451, 64479-64484, 64490-64505, 64510-64530, 64625, 66987-66988, 69990, 92012-92014, 93000-93010, 93040-93042, 93318, 93355, 94002, 94200, 94680-94690, 95812-95816, 95819, 95822, 95829, 95955, 96360-96368, 96372, 96374-96377, 96523, 97597-97598, 97602-97608, 99155, 99156, 99157, 99211-99223, 99231-99255, 99291-99292, 99304-99310, 99315-99316, 99334-99337, 99347-99350, 99374-99375, 99377-99378, 99446-99449, 99451-99452, 99495-99496, G0168, G0463, G0471

12020 0213T, 0216T, 0543T-0544T, 0545T, 0567T-0574T, 0580T, 0581T, 0582T, 11000-11006, 11042-11047, 11900-11901, 12021, 15772, 15774, 20560-20561, 20700-20701, 36000, 36400-36410, 36420-36430, 36440, 36591-36592, 36600, 36640, 43752, 51701-51703, 64400, 64405-64408, 64415-64435, 64445-64451, 64479-64484, 64490-64505, 64510-64530, 66987-66988, 69990, 92012-92014, 93000-93010, 93040-93042, 93318, 93355, 94002, 94200, 94680-94690, 95812-95816, 95819, 95822, 95829, 95955, 96360-96368, 96372, 96374-96377, 96523, 97597-97598, 97602-97608, 99155, 99156, 99157, 99211-99223, 99231-99255, 99291-99292, 99304-99310, 99315-99316, 99334-99337, 99347-99350, 99374-99375, 99377-99378, 99446-99449, 99451-99452, 99495-99496, G0168, G0463, G0471, J0670, J2001

12021 0213T, 0216T, 0543T-0544T, 0567T-0574T, 0580T, 0581T, 0582T, 11042, 11900-11901, 20560-20561, 20700-20701, 36000, 36400-36410, 36420-36430, 36440, 36591-36592, 36600, 36640, 43752, 51701-51703, 64400, 64405-64408, 64415-64435, 64445-64451, 64479-64484, 64490-64505, 64510-64530, 66987-66988, 69990, 92012-92014, 93000-93010, 93040-93042, 93318, 93355, 94002, 94200, 94680-94690, 95812-95816, 95819, 95822, 95829, 95955, 96360-96368, 96372, 96374-96377, 96523, 97597-97598, 97602-97608, 99155, 99156, 99157, 99211-99223, 99231-99255, 99291-99292, 99304-99310, 99315-99316,

99334-99337, 99347-99350, 99374-99375, 99377-99378, 99446-99449, 99451-99452, 99495-99496, G0168, G0463, G0471, J2001

12031 0213T, 0216T, 0543T-0544T, 0567T-0574T, 0580T, 0581T, 0582T, 11042, 11055-11056, 11900-11901, 12051❖, 20560-20561, 20700-20701, 36000, 36400-36410, 36420-36430, 36440, 36591-36592, 36600, 36640, 43752, 51701-51703, 64400, 64405-64408, 64415-64435, 64445-64451, 64479-64484, 64490-64505, 64510-64530, 66987-66988, 69990, 92012-92014, 93000-93010, 93040-93042, 93318, 93355, 94002, 94200, 94680-94690, 95812-95816, 95819, 95822, 95829, 95955, 96360-96368, 96372, 96374-96377, 96523, 97597-97598, 97602-97608, 99155, 99156, 99157, 99211-99223, 99231-99255, 99291-99292, 99304-99310, 99315-99316, 99334-99337, 99347-99350, 99374-99375, 99377-99378, 99446-99449, 99451-99452, 99495-99496, G0168, G0463, G0471, J0670, J2001

12032 0213T, 0216T, 0543T-0544T, 0567T-0574T, 0580T, 0581T, 0582T, 11042-11043, 11900-11901, 12031, 12042❖, 12052-12053❖, 15772, 15774, 20560-20561, 20700-20701, 36000, 36400-36410, 36420-36430, 36440, 36591-36592, 36600, 36640, 43752, 51701-51703, 64400, 64405-64408, 64415-64435, 64445-64451, 64479-64484, 64490-64505, 64510-64530, 66987-66988, 69990, 92012-92014, 93000-93010, 93040-93042, 93318, 93355, 94002, 94200, 94680-94690, 95812-95816, 95819, 95822, 95829, 95955, 96360-96368, 96372, 96374-96377, 96523, 97597-97598, 97602-97608, 99155, 99156, 99157, 99211-99223, 99231-99255, 99291-99292, 99304-99310, 99315-99316, 99334-99337, 99347-99350, 99374-99375, 99377-99378, 99446-99449, 99451-99452, 99495-99496, G0168, G0463, G0471, J0670, J2001

12034 0213T, 0216T, 0543T-0544T, 0567T-0574T, 0580T, 0581T, 0582T, 11042-11043, 11900-11901, 12031-12032, 12044❖, 12054❖, 15772, 15774, 20560-20561, 20700-20701, 36000, 36400-36410, 36420-36430, 36440, 36591-36592, 36600, 36640, 43752, 51701-51703, 64400, 64405-64408, 64415-64435, 64445-64451, 64479-64484, 64490-64505, 64510-64530, 66987-66988, 69990, 92012-92014, 93000-93010, 93040-93042, 93318, 93355, 94002, 94200, 94680-94690, 95812-95816, 95819, 95822, 95829, 95955, 96360-96368, 96372, 96374-96377, 96523, 97597-97598, 97602-97608, 99155, 99156, 99157, 99211-99223, 99231-99255, 99291-99292, 99304-99310, 99315-99316, 99334-99337, 99347-99350, 99374-99375, 99377-99378, 99446-99449, 99451-99452, 99495-99496, G0168, G0463, G0471, J0670, J2001

12035 0213T, 0216T, 0543T-0544T, 0567T-0574T, 0580T, 0581T, 0582T, 11042-11044, 11900-11901, 12031-12034, 12045❖, 12055❖, 15772, 15774, 20560-20561, 20700-20701, 36000, 36400-36410, 36420-36430, 36440, 36591-36592, 36600, 36640, 43752, 51701-51703, 64400, 64405-64408, 64415-64435, 64445-64451, 64479-64484, 64490-64505, 64510-64530, 64625, 66987-66988, 69990, 92012-92014, 93000-93010, 93040-93042, 93318, 93355, 94002, 94200, 94680-94690, 95812-95816, 95819, 95822, 95829, 95955, 96360-96368, 96372, 96374-96377, 96523, 97597-97598, 97602-97608, 99155, 99156, 99157, 99211-99223, 99231-99255, 99291-99292, 99304-99310, 99315-99316, 99334-99337, 99347-99350, 99374-99375, 99377-99378, 99446-99449, 99451-99452, 99495-99496, G0168, G0463, G0471, J0670, J2001

12036 0213T, 0216T, 0543T-0544T, 0567T-0574T, 0580T, 0581T, 0582T, 11043, 11900-11901, 12031-12035, 12046❖, 12056❖, 15772, 15774, 20560-20561, 20700-20701, 36000, 36400-36410, 36420-36430, 36440, 36591-36592, 36600, 36640, 43752, 51701-51703, 64400, 64405-64408, 64415-64435, 64445-64451, 64479-64484, 64490-64505, 64510-64530, 64625, 66987-66988, 69990, 92012-92014, 93000-93010, 93040-93042, 93318, 93355, 94002, 94200, 94680-94690, 95812-95816, 95819, 95822, 95829, 95955, 96360-96368, 96372, 96374-96377, 96523, 97597-97598, 97602-97608, 99155, 99156, 99157, 99211-99223,

99231-99255, 99291-99292, 99304-99310, 99315-99316, 99334-99337, 99347-99350, 99374-99375, 99377-99378, 99446-99449, 99451-99452, 99495-99496, G0168, G0463, G0471, J0670, J2001

12037 0213T, 0216T, 0543T-0544T, 0567T-0574T, 0580T, 0581T, 0582T, 11043-11044, 11900-11901, 12031-12036, 12057♣, 15772, 15774, 20560-20561, 20700-20701, 36000, 36400-36410, 36420-36430, 36440, 36591-36592, 36600, 36640, 43752, 51701-51703, 64400, 64405-64408, 64415-64435, 64445-64451, 64479-64484, 64490-64505, 64510-64530, 64625, 66987-66988, 69990, 92012-92014, 93000-93010, 93040-93042, 93318, 93355, 94002, 94200, 94680-94690, 95812-95816, 95819, 95822, 95829, 95955, 96360-96368, 96372, 96374-96377, 96523, 97597-97598, 97602-97608, 99155, 99156, 99157, 99211-99223, 99231-99255, 99291-99292, 99304-99310, 99315-99316, 99334-99337, 99347-99350, 99374-99375, 99377-99378, 99446-99449, 99451-99452, 99495-99496, G0168, G0463, G0471, J0670, J2001

12041 0213T, 0216T, 0543T-0544T, 0567T-0574T, 0580T, 0581T, 0582T, 11055-11056, 11740, 11900-11901, 12031, 20560-20561, 20700-20701, 36000, 36400-36410, 36420-36430, 36440, 36591-36592, 36600, 36640, 43752, 51701-51703, 64400, 64405-64408, 64415-64435, 64445-64451, 64479-64484, 64490-64505, 64510-64530, 66987-66988, 69990, 92012-92014, 93000-93010, 93040-93042, 93318, 93355, 94002, 94200, 94680-94690, 95812-95816, 95819, 95822, 95829, 95955, 96360-96368, 96372, 96374-96377, 96523, 97597-97598, 97602-97608, 99155, 99156, 99157, 99211-99223, 99231-99255, 99291-99292, 99304-99310, 99315-99316, 99334-99337, 99347-99350, 99374-99375, 99377-99378, 99446-99449, 99451-99452, 99495-99496, G0168, G0463, G0471, J0670, J2001

12042 0213T, 0216T, 0567T-0574T, 0580T, 0581T, 0582T, 11042, 11740, 11900-11901, 12041, 15772, 15774, 20560-20561, 20700-20701, 36000, 36400-36410, 36420-36430, 36440, 36591-36592, 36600, 36640, 43752, 51701-51703, 64400, 64405-64408, 64415-64435, 64445-64451, 64479-64484, 64490-64505, 64510-64530, 66987-66988, 69990, 92012-92014, 93000-93010, 93040-93042, 93318, 93355, 94002, 94200, 94680-94690, 95812-95816, 95819, 95822, 95829, 95955, 96360-96368, 96372, 96374-96377, 96523, 97597-97598, 97602-97608, 99155, 99156, 99157, 99211-99223, 99231-99255, 99291-99292, 99304-99310, 99315-99316, 99334-99337, 99347-99350, 99374-99375, 99377-99378, 99446-99449, 99451-99452, 99495-99496, G0168, G0463, G0471, J0670, J2001

12044 0213T, 0216T, 0567T-0574T, 0580T, 0581T, 0582T, 11043-11044, 11900-11901, 12041-12042, 12054♣, 15772, 15774, 20560-20561, 20700-20701, 36000, 36400-36410, 36420-36430, 36440, 36591-36592, 36600, 36640, 43752, 51701-51703, 64400, 64405-64408, 64415-64435, 64445-64451, 64479-64484, 64490-64505, 64510-64530, 66987-66988, 69990, 92012-92014, 93000-93010, 93040-93042, 93318, 93355, 94002, 94200, 94680-94690, 95812-95816, 95819, 95822, 95829, 95955, 96360-96368, 96372, 96374-96377, 96523, 97597-97598, 97602-97608, 99155, 99156, 99157, 99211-99223, 99231-99255, 99291-99292, 99304-99310, 99315-99316, 99334-99337, 99347-99350, 99374-99375, 99377-99378, 99446-99449, 99451-99452, 99495-99496, G0168, G0463, G0471, J0670, J2001

12045 0213T, 0216T, 0567T-0574T, 0580T, 0581T, 0582T, 11042, 11900-11901, 12041-12044, 12055♣, 15772, 15774, 20560-20561, 20700-20701, 36000, 36400-36410, 36420-36430, 36440, 36591-36592, 36600, 36640, 43752, 51701-51703, 64400, 64405-64408, 64415-64435, 64445-64451, 64479-64484, 64490-64505, 64510-64530, 64625, 66987-66988, 69990, 92012-92014, 93000-93010, 93040-93042, 93318, 93355, 94002, 94200, 94680-94690, 95812-95816, 95819, 95822, 95829, 95955, 96360-96368, 96372, 96374-96377, 96523, 97597-97598, 97602-97608, 99155, 99156,

99157, 99211-99223, 99231-99255, 99291-99292, 99304-99310, 99315-99316, 99334-99337, 99347-99350, 99374-99375, 99377-99378, 99446-99449, 99451-99452, 99495-99496, G0168, G0463, G0471, J0670, J2001

12046 0213T, 0216T, 0567T-0574T, 0580T, 0581T, 0582T, 11043-11044, 11900-11901, 12041-12045, 12056♣, 15772, 15774, 20560-20561, 20700-20701, 36000, 36400-36410, 36420-36430, 36440, 36591-36592, 36600, 36640, 43752, 51701-51703, 64400, 64405-64408, 64415-64435, 64445-64451, 64479-64484, 64490-64505, 64510-64530, 64625, 66987-66988, 69990, 92012-92014, 93000-93010, 93040-93042, 93318, 93355, 94002, 94200, 94680-94690, 95812-95816, 95819, 95822, 95829, 95955, 96360-96368, 96372, 96374-96377, 96523, 97597-97598, 97602-97608, 99155, 99156, 99157, 99211-99223, 99231-99255, 99291-99292, 99304-99310, 99315-99316, 99334-99337, 99347-99350, 99374-99375, 99377-99378, 99446-99449, 99451-99452, 99495-99496, G0168, G0463, G0471, J0670, J2001

12047 0213T, 0216T, 0567T-0574T, 0580T, 0581T, 0582T, 11900-11901, 12037-12046, 12057♣, 15772, 15774, 20560-20561, 20700-20701, 36000, 36400-36410, 36420-36430, 36440, 36591-36592, 36600, 36640, 43752, 51701-51703, 64400, 64405-64408, 64415-64435, 64445-64451, 64479-64484, 64490-64505, 64510-64530, 64625, 66987-66988, 69990, 92012-92014, 93000-93010, 93040-93042, 93318, 93355, 94002, 94200, 94680-94690, 95812-95816, 95819, 95822, 95829, 95955, 96360-96368, 96372, 96374-96377, 96523, 97597-97598, 97602-97608, 99155, 99156, 99157, 99211-99223, 99231-99255, 99291-99292, 99304-99310, 99315-99316, 99334-99337, 99347-99350, 99374-99375, 99377-99378, 99446-99449, 99451-99452, 99495-99496, G0168, G0463, G0471, J0670, J2001

12051 0213T, 0216T, 0567T-0574T, 0580T, 0581T, 0582T, 11042, 11055, 11900-11901, 12041, 20560-20561, 20700-20701, 36000, 36400-36410, 36420-36430, 36440, 36591-36592, 36600, 36640, 43752, 51701-51703, 64400, 64405-64408, 64415-64435, 64445-64451, 64479-64484, 64490-64505, 64510-64530, 66987-66988, 69990, 92012-92014, 93000-93010, 93040-93042, 93318, 93355, 94002, 94200, 94680-94690, 95812-95816, 95819, 95822, 95829, 95955, 96360-96368, 96372, 96374-96377, 96523, 97597-97598, 97602-97608, 99155, 99156, 99157, 99211-99223, 99231-99255, 99291-99292, 99304-99310, 99315-99316, 99334-99337, 99347-99350, 99374-99375, 99377-99378, 99446-99449, 99451-99452, 99495-99496, G0168, G0463, G0471, J0670, J2001

12052 0213T, 0216T, 0567T-0574T, 0580T, 0581T, 0582T, 11042, 11900-11901, 12051, 15772, 20560-20561, 20700-20701, 36000, 36400-36410, 36420-36430, 36440, 36591-36592, 36600, 36640, 43752, 51701-51703, 64400, 64405-64408, 64415-64435, 64445-64451, 64479-64484, 64490-64505, 64510-64530, 66987-66988, 69990, 92012-92014, 93000-93010, 93040-93042, 93318, 93355, 94002, 94200, 94680-94690, 95812-95816, 95819, 95822, 95829, 95955, 96360-96368, 96372, 96374-96377, 96523, 97597-97598, 97602-97608, 99155, 99156, 99157, 99211-99223, 99231-99255, 99291-99292, 99304-99310, 99315-99316, 99334-99337, 99347-99350, 99374-99375, 99377-99378, 99446-99449, 99451-99452, 99495-99496, G0168, G0463, G0471, J0670, J2001

12053 0213T, 0216T, 0567T-0574T, 0580T, 0581T, 0582T, 11900-11901, 12051-12052, 15772, 15774, 20560-20561, 20700-20701, 36000, 36400-36410, 36420-36430, 36440, 36591-36592, 36600, 36640, 43752, 51701-51703, 64400, 64405-64408, 64415-64435, 64445-64451, 64479-64484, 64490-64505, 64510-64530, 66987-66988, 69990, 92012-92014, 93000-93010, 93040-93042, 93318, 93355, 94002, 94200, 94680-94690, 95812-95816, 95819, 95822, 95829, 95955, 96360-96368, 96372, 96374-96377, 96523, 97597-97598, 97602-97608, 99155, 99156, 99157, 99211-99223, 99231-99255, 99291-99292, 99304-99310,

CCI Edits

99315-99316, 99334-99337, 99347-99350, 99374-99375, 99377-99378, 99446-99449, 99451-99452, 99495-99496, G0168, G0463, G0471, J0670, J2001

12054 0213T, 0216T, 0567T-0574T, 0580T, 0581T, 0582T, 11042, 11900-11901, 12051-12053, 15772, 15774, 20560-20561, 20700-20701, 36000, 36400-36410, 36420-36430, 36440, 36591-36592, 36600, 36640, 43752, 51701-51703, 64400, 64405-64408, 64415-64435, 64445-64451, 64479-64484, 64490-64505, 64510-64530, 64625, 66987-66988, 69990, 92012-92014, 93000-93010, 93040-93042, 93318, 93355, 94002, 94200, 94680-94690, 95812-95816, 95819, 95822, 95829, 95955, 96360-96368, 96372, 96374-96377, 96523, 97597-97598, 97602-97608, 99155, 99156, 99157, 99211-99223, 99231-99255, 99291-99292, 99304-99310, 99315-99316, 99334-99337, 99347-99350, 99374-99375, 99377-99378, 99446-99449, 99451-99452, 99495-99496, G0168, G0463, G0471, J0670, J2001

12055 0213T, 0216T, 0567T-0574T, 0580T, 0581T, 0582T, 11900-11901, 12051-12054, 15772, 15774, 20560-20561, 20700-20701, 36000, 36400-36410, 36420-36430, 36440, 36591-36592, 36600, 36640, 43752, 51701-51703, 64400, 64405-64408, 64415-64435, 64445-64451, 64479-64484, 64490-64505, 64510-64530, 64625, 66987-66988, 69990, 92012-92014, 93000-93010, 93040-93042, 93318, 93355, 94002, 94200, 94680-94690, 95812-95816, 95819, 95822, 95829, 95955, 96360-96368, 96372, 96374-96377, 96523, 97597-97598, 97602-97608, 99155, 99156, 99157, 99211-99223, 99231-99255, 99291-99292, 99304-99310, 99315-99316, 99334-99337, 99347-99350, 99374-99375, 99377-99378, 99446-99449, 99451-99452, 99495-99496, G0168, G0463, G0471, J0670, J2001

12056 0213T, 0216T, 0567T-0574T, 0580T, 0581T, 0582T, 11900-11901, 12051-12055, 15772, 15774, 20560-20561, 20700-20701, 36000, 36400-36410, 36420-36430, 36440, 36591-36592, 36600, 36640, 43752, 51701-51703, 64400, 64405-64408, 64415-64435, 64445-64451, 64479-64484, 64490-64505, 64510-64530, 64625, 66987-66988, 69990, 92012-92014, 93000-93010, 93040-93042, 93318, 93355, 94002, 94200, 94680-94690, 95812-95816, 95819, 95822, 95829, 95955, 96360-96368, 96372, 96374-96377, 96523, 97597-97598, 97602-97608, 99155, 99156, 99157, 99211-99223, 99231-99255, 99291-99292, 99304-99310, 99315-99316, 99334-99337, 99347-99350, 99374-99375, 99377-99378, 99446-99449, 99451-99452, 99495-99496, G0168, G0463, G0471, J0670, J2001

12057 0213T, 0216T, 0548T, 0567T-0574T, 0580T, 0581T, 0582T, 11900-11901, 12051-12056, 15772, 15774, 20560-20561, 20700-20701, 36000, 36400-36410, 36420-36430, 36440, 36591-36592, 36600, 36640, 43752, 51701-51703, 64400, 64405-64408, 64415-64435, 64445-64451, 64479-64484, 64490-64505, 64510-64530, 64625, 66987-66988, 69990, 92012-92014, 93000-93010, 93040-93042, 93318, 93355, 94002, 94200, 94680-94690, 95812-95816, 95819, 95822, 95829, 95955, 96360-96368, 96372, 96374-96377, 96523, 97597-97598, 97602-97608, 99155, 99156, 99157, 99211-99223, 99231-99255, 99291-99292, 99304-99310, 99315-99316, 99334-99337, 99347-99350, 99374-99375, 99377-99378, 99446-99449, 99451-99452, 99495-99496, G0168, G0463, G0471, J0670, J2001

13100 0213T, 0216T, 0543T-0544T, 0548T, 0567T-0574T, 0580T, 0581T, 0582T, 11000, 11010-11012, 11042-11044, 11900-11901, 13102, 13160◆, 15772, 15774, 20560-20561, 20700-20701, 36000, 36400-36410, 36420-36430, 36440, 36591-36592, 36600, 36640, 43752, 51701-51703, 64400, 64405-64408, 64415-64435, 64445-64451, 64479-64484, 64490-64505, 64510-64530, 66987-66988, 69990, 92012-92014, 93000-93010, 93040-93042, 93318, 93355, 94002, 94200, 94680-94690, 95812-95816, 95819, 95822, 95829, 95955, 96360-96368, 96372,

96374-96377, 96523, 97597-97598, 97602-97608, 99155, 99156, 99157, 99211-99223, 99231-99255, 99291-99292, 99304-99310, 99315-99316, 99334-99337, 99347-99350, 99374-99375, 99377-99378, 99446-99449, 99451-99452, 99495-99496, G0168, G0463, G0471, J0670, J2001

13101 0213T, 0216T, 0543T-0544T, 0548T, 0567T-0574T, 0580T, 0581T, 0582T, 11000, 11010-11012, 11042-11044, 11900-11901, 13100, 13160◆, 15772, 15774, 20560-20561, 20700-20701, 36000, 36400-36410, 36420-36430, 36440, 36591-36592, 36600, 36640, 43752, 51701-51703, 64400, 64405-64408, 64415-64435, 64445-64451, 64479-64484, 64490-64505, 64510-64530, 64625, 66987-66988, 69990, 92012-92014, 93000-93010, 93040-93042, 93318, 93355, 94002, 94200, 94680-94690, 95812-95816, 95819, 95822, 95829, 95955, 96360-96368, 96372, 96374-96377, 96523, 97597-97598, 97602-97608, 99155, 99156, 99157, 99211-99223, 99231-99255, 99291-99292, 99304-99310, 99315-99316, 99334-99337, 99347-99350, 99374-99375, 99377-99378, 99446-99449, 99451-99452, 99495-99496, G0168, G0463, G0471, J0670, J2001

13102 0543T-0544T, 0548T, 0567T-0574T, 0580T, 0581T, 0582T, 11900-11901, 13160◆, 20560-20561, 20701, 36591-36592, 66987-66988, 69990, 96523, J0670, J2001

13120 0213T, 0216T, 0543T-0544T, 0548T, 0567T-0574T, 0580T, 0581T, 0582T, 11000, 11010-11012, 11042-11044, 11900-11901, 13122, 13160◆, 15772, 15774, 20560-20561, 20700-20701, 36000, 36400-36410, 36420-36430, 36440, 36591-36592, 36600, 36640, 43752, 51701-51703, 64400, 64405-64408, 64415-64435, 64445-64451, 64479-64484, 64490-64505, 64510-64530, 66987-66988, 69990, 92012-92014, 93000-93010, 93040-93042, 93318, 93355, 94002, 94200, 94680-94690, 95812-95816, 95819, 95822, 95829, 95955, 96360-96368, 96372, 96374-96377, 96523, 97597-97598, 97602-97608, 99155, 99156, 99157, 99211-99223, 99231-99255, 99291-99292, 99304-99310, 99315-99316, 99334-99337, 99347-99350, 99374-99375, 99377-99378, 99446-99449, 99451-99452, 99495-99496, G0168, G0463, G0471, J0670, J2001

13121 0213T, 0216T, 0543T-0544T, 0548T, 0567T-0574T, 0580T, 0581T, 0582T, 11000, 11010-11012, 11042-11044, 11900-11901, 13120, 13160◆, 15772, 15774, 20560-20561, 20700-20701, 36000, 36400-36410, 36420-36430, 36440, 36591-36592, 36600, 36640, 43752, 51701-51703, 64400, 64405-64408, 64415-64435, 64445-64451, 64479-64484, 64490-64505, 64510-64530, 64625, 66987-66988, 69990, 92012-92014, 93000-93010, 93040-93042, 93318, 93355, 94002, 94200, 94680-94690, 95812-95816, 95819, 95822, 95829, 95955, 96360-96368, 96372, 96374-96377, 96523, 97597-97598, 97602-97608, 99155, 99156, 99157, 99211-99223, 99231-99255, 99291-99292, 99304-99310, 99315-99316, 99334-99337, 99347-99350, 99374-99375, 99377-99378, 99446-99449, 99451-99452, 99495-99496, G0168, G0463, G0471, J0670, J2001

13122 0543T-0544T, 0548T, 0567T-0574T, 0580T, 0581T, 0582T, 11900-11901, 13160◆, 20560-20561, 20701, 36591-36592, 66987-66988, 69990, 96523, J0670, J2001

13131 0213T, 0216T, 0548T, 0567T-0574T, 0580T, 0581T, 0582T, 11000, 11010-11012, 11042-11044, 11900-11901, 13133, 13160◆, 15772, 15774, 20560-20561, 20700-20701, 36000, 36400-36410, 36420-36430, 36440, 36591-36592, 36600, 36640, 43752, 51701-51703, 64400, 64405-64408, 64415-64435, 64445-64451, 64479-64484, 64490-64505, 64510-64530, 64625, 66987-66988, 69990, 92012-92014, 93000-93010, 93040-93042, 93318, 93355, 94002, 94200, 94680-94690, 95812-95816, 95819, 95822, 95829, 95955, 96360-96368, 96372, 96374-96377, 96523, 97597-97598, 97602-97608, 99155, 99156, 99157, 99211-99223, 99231-99255, 99291-99292, 99304-99310, 99315-99316, 99334-99337, 99347-99350, 99374-99375, 99377-99378, 99446-99449, 99451-99452, 99495-99496, G0168, G0463, G0471, J0670, J2001

13132 0213T, 0216T, 0548T, 0567T-0574T, 0580T, 0581T, 0582T, 11000, 11010-11012, 11042-11044, 11056, 11900-11901, 13131, 13160◆, 15772, 15774, 20560-20561, 20700-20701, 36000, 36400-36410, 36420-36430, 36440, 36591-36592, 36600, 36640, 43752, 51701-51703, 64400, 64405-64408, 64415-64435, 64445-64451, 64479-64484, 64490-64505, 64510-64530, 64625, 66987-66988, 69990, 92012-92014, 93000-93010, 93040-93042, 93318, 93355, 94002, 94200, 94680-94690, 95812-95816, 95819, 95822, 95829, 95955, 96360-96368, 96372, 96374-96377, 96523, 97597-97598, 97602-97608, 99155, 99156, 99157, 99211-99223, 99231-99255, 99291-99292, 99304-99310, 99315-99316, 99334-99337, 99347-99350, 99374-99375, 99377-99378, 99446-99449, 99451-99452, 99495-99496, G0168, G0463, G0471, J0670, J2001

13133 0548T, 0567T-0574T, 0580T, 0581T, 0582T, 11900-11901, 13160◆, 20560-20561, 20700-20701, 36591-36592, 64451, 66987-66988, 69990, 96523, J0670, J2001

13151 0213T, 0216T, 0548T, 0567T-0574T, 0580T, 0581T, 0582T, 11000, 11010-11012, 11042-11044, 11056, 11900-11901, 13153-13160◆, 15772, 15774, 20560-20561, 20700-20701, 36000, 36400-36410, 36420-36430, 36440, 36591-36592, 36600, 36640, 40654◆, 43752, 51701-51703, 64400, 64405-64408, 64415-64435, 64445-64451, 64479-64484, 64490-64505, 64510-64530, 64625, 66987-66988, 69990, 92012-92014, 93000-93010, 93040-93042, 93318, 93355, 94002, 94200, 94680-94690, 95812-95816, 95819, 95822, 95829, 95955, 96360-96368, 96372, 96374-96377, 96523, 97597-97598, 97602-97608, 99155, 99156, 99157, 99211-99223, 99231-99255, 99291-99292, 99304-99310, 99315-99316, 99334-99337, 99347-99350, 99374-99375, 99377-99378, 99446-99449, 99451-99452, 99495-99496, G0168, G0463, G0471, J0670, J2001

13152 0213T, 0216T, 0548T, 0567T-0574T, 0580T, 0581T, 0582T, 11000, 11010-11012, 11042-11044, 11900-11901, 13151, 13160◆, 15772, 15774, 20560-20561, 20700-20701, 36000, 36400-36410, 36420-36430, 36440, 36591-36592, 36600, 36640, 43752, 51701-51703, 64400, 64405-64408, 64415-64435, 64445-64451, 64479-64484, 64490-64505, 64510-64530, 64625, 66987-66988, 69990, 92012-92014, 93000-93010, 93040-93042, 93318, 93355, 94002, 94200, 94680-94690, 95812-95816, 95819, 95822, 95829, 95955, 96360-96368, 96372, 96374-96377, 96523, 97597-97598, 97602-97608, 99155, 99156, 99157, 99211-99223, 99231-99255, 99291-99292, 99304-99310, 99315-99316, 99334-99337, 99347-99350, 99374-99375, 99377-99378, 99446-99449, 99451-99452, 99495-99496, G0168, G0463, G0471, J0670, J2001

13153 0548T, 0567T-0574T, 0580T, 0581T, 0582T, 11900-11901, 13160◆, 20560-20561, 20700-20701, 36591-36592, 64451, 66987-66988, 69990, 96523, J0670, J2001

13160 0213T, 0216T, 0596T-0597T, 10180, 11000-11006, 11010-11012, 11042-11047, 11102, 11104, 11106, 11900-11901, 12001-12007, 12011-12057, 36000, 36400-36410, 36420-36430, 36440, 36591-36592, 36600, 36640, 43752, 51701-51703, 62320-62327, 64400, 64405-64408, 64415-64435, 64445-64454, 64461-64463, 64479-64505, 64510-64530, 69990, 92012-92014, 93000-93010, 93040-93042, 93318, 93355, 94002, 94200, 94680-94690, 95812-95816, 95819, 95822, 95829, 95955, 96360-96368, 96372, 96374-96377, 96523, 97597-97598, 97602-97608, 99155, 99156, 99157, 99211-99223, 99231-99255, 99291-99292, 99304-99310, 99315-99316, 99334-99337, 99347-99350, 99374-99375, 99377-99378, 99446-99449, 99451-99452, 99495-99496, G0168, G0463, G0471

15002 01951-01952, 0213T, 0216T, 0596T-0597T, 11000-11006, 11042-11047, 11102, 11104, 11106, 11400-11421◆, 11423-11444◆, 11450◆, 11600-11604◆, 11620-11624◆, 11640-11643◆, 12001-12007, 12011-12057, 13100-13133, 13151-13153, 36000, 36400-36410,

36420-36430, 36440, 36591-36592, 36600, 36640, 43752, 51701-51703, 62320-62327, 64400, 64405-64408, 64415-64435, 64445-64454, 64461-64463, 64479-64505, 64510-64530, 69990, 92012-92014, 93000-93010, 93040-93042, 93318, 93355, 94002, 94200, 94680-94690, 95812-95816, 95819, 95822, 95829, 95955, 96360-96368, 96372, 96374-96377, 96523, 97597-97598, 97602, 99155, 99156, 99157, 99211-99223, 99231-99255, 99291-99292, 99304-99310, 99315-99316, 99334-99337, 99347-99350, 99374-99375, 99377-99378, 99446-99449, 99451-99452, 99495-99496, G0168, G0463, G0471, J0670, J2001

15003 11000-11006, 11042-11047, 36591-36592, 96523, 97597-97598, 97602, J0670, J2001

15004 01951-01952, 0213T, 0216T, 0596T-0597T, 11000-11006, 11042-11047, 11102, 11104, 11106, 11400-11421◆, 11423-11450◆, 11462◆, 11470◆, 11600-11604◆, 11620-11644◆, 12001-12007, 12011-12057, 13100-13133, 13151-13153, 36000, 36400-36410, 36420-36430, 36440, 36591-36592, 36600, 36640, 51701-51703, 62320-62327, 64400, 64405-64408, 64415-64435, 64445-64454, 64461-64463, 64479-64505, 64510-64530, 69990, 92012-92014, 93000-93010, 93040-93042, 93318, 93355, 94002, 94200, 94680-94690, 95812-95816, 95819, 95822, 95829, 95955, 96360-96368, 96372, 96374-96377, 96523, 97597-97598, 97602, 99155, 99156, 99157, 99211-99223, 99231-99255, 99291-99292, 99304-99310, 99315-99316, 99334-99337, 99347-99350, 99374-99375, 99377-99378, 99446-99449, 99451-99452, 99495-99496, G0168, G0463, G0471, J0670, J2001

15005 11000-11006, 11042-11047, 36591-36592, 96523, 97597-97598, 97602, J0670, J2001

15100 01951-01952, 0213T, 0216T, 0596T-0597T, 11000-11006, 11042-11047, 11102, 11104, 11106, 12001-12007, 12011, 12014-12041, 12044-12057, 13100-13133, 13151-13153, 15050, 15852, 16020-16030, 29000-29015, 29035-29085, 29105-29200, 29240-29450, 29505-29581, 29584, 36000, 36400-36410, 36420-36430, 36440, 36591-36592, 36600, 36640, 43752, 51701-51703, 62320-62327, 64400, 64405-64408, 64415-64435, 64445-64454, 64461-64463, 64479-64505, 64510-64530, 69990, 92012-92014, 93000-93010, 93040-93042, 93318, 93355, 94002, 94200, 94680-94690, 95812-95816, 95819, 95822, 95829, 95955, 96360-96368, 96372, 96374-96377, 96523, 97597-97598, 97602-97608, 99155, 99156, 99157, 99211-99223, 99231-99255, 99291-99292, 99304-99310, 99315-99316, 99334-99337, 99347-99350, 99374-99375, 99377-99378, 99446-99449, 99451-99452, 99495-99496, G0168, G0463, G0471, J0670, J2001

15101 11000-11006, 11042-11047, 36591-36592, 96523, 97597-97598, 97602, J0670, J2001

15120 01951-01952, 0213T, 0216T, 0490T, 0596T-0597T, 11000-11006, 11042-11047, 11102, 11104, 11106, 12001-12007, 12011-12057, 13100-13133, 13151-13153, 15050, 15852, 16020-16030, 20526-20553, 20560-20561, 25259, 26340, 29000-29015, 29035-29200, 29240-29450, 29505-29581, 29584, 36000, 36400-36410, 36420-36430, 36440, 36591-36592, 36600, 36640, 43752, 51701-51703, 62320-62327, 64400, 64405-64408, 64415-64435, 64445-64454, 64461-64463, 64479-64505, 64510-64530, 69990, 92012-92014, 93000-93010, 93040-93042, 93318, 93355, 94002, 94200, 94680-94690, 95812-95816, 95819, 95822, 95829, 95955, 96360-96368, 96372, 96374-96377, 96523, 97597-97598, 97602-97608, 99155, 99156, 99157, 99211-99223, 99231-99255, 99291-99292, 99304-99310, 99315-99316, 99334-99337, 99347-99350, 99374-99375, 99377-99378, 99446-99449, 99451-99452, 99495-99496, G0168, G0463, G0471, J0670, J2001

15121 11000-11006, 11042-11047, 36591-36592, 96523, 97597-97598, 97602, J0670, J2001

15200 01951-01952, 0213T, 0216T, 0490T, 0596T-0597T, 11000-11006, 11042-11047, 11102, 11104, 11106, 12001-12007, 12011-12057, 13100-13133, 13151-13153, 15852, 16020-16030, 20527-20553, 20560-20561, 29000-29015, 29035-29200, 29240-29450, 29505-29581, 29584, 36000, 36400-36410, 36420-36430, 36440, 36591-36592, 36600, 36640, 43752, 51701-51703, 62320-62327, 64400, 64405-64408, 64415-64435, 64445-64454, 64461-64463, 64479-64505, 64510-64530, 69990, 92012-92014, 93000-93010, 93040-93042, 93318, 93355, 94002, 94200, 94680-94690, 95812-95816, 95819, 95822, 95829, 95955, 96360-96368, 96372, 96374-96377, 96523, 97597-97598, 97602-97608, 99155, 99156, 99157, 99211-99223, 99231-99255, 99291-99292, 99304-99310, 99315-99316, 99334-99337, 99347-99350, 99374-99375, 99377-99378, 99446-99449, 99451-99452, 99495-99496, G0168, G0463, G0471, J0670, J2001

15201 11000-11006, 11042-11047, 36591-36592, 96523, 97597-97598, 97602, J0670, J2001

15220 01951-01952, 0213T, 0216T, 0490T, 0596T-0597T, 11000-11006, 11042-11047, 11102, 11104, 11106, 12001-12007, 12011-12057, 13100-13133, 13151-13153, 15852, 16020-16030, 20527-20553, 20560-20561, 29000-29015, 29035-29200, 29240-29450, 29505-29581, 29584, 36000, 36400-36410, 36420-36430, 36440, 36591-36592, 36600, 36640, 43752, 51701-51703, 62320-62327, 64400, 64405-64408, 64415-64435, 64445-64454, 64461-64463, 64479-64505, 64510-64530, 69990, 92012-92014, 93000-93010, 93040-93042, 93318, 93355, 94002, 94200, 94680-94690, 95812-95816, 95819, 95822, 95829, 95955, 96360-96368, 96372, 96374-96377, 96523, 97597-97598, 97602-97608, 99155, 99156, 99157, 99211-99223, 99231-99255, 99291-99292, 99304-99310, 99315-99316, 99334-99337, 99347-99350, 99374-99375, 99377-99378, 99446-99449, 99451-99452, 99495-99496, G0168, G0463, G0471, J0670, J2001

15221 11000-11006, 11042-11047, 36591-36592, 96523, 97597-97598, 97602, J0670, J2001

15240 01951-01952, 0213T, 0216T, 0596T-0597T, 11000-11006, 11042-11047, 11102, 11104, 11106, 12001-12007, 12011-12057, 13100-13133, 13151-13153, 15852, 16020-16030, 20526, 20551-20553, 20560-20561, 25259, 26340, 29000-29015, 29035-29200, 29240-29450, 29505-29581, 29584, 36000, 36400-36410, 36420-36430, 36440, 36591-36592, 36600, 36640, 43752, 51701-51703, 62320-62327, 64400, 64405-64408, 64415-64435, 64445-64454, 64461-64463, 64479-64505, 64510-64530, 69990, 92012-92014, 93000-93010, 93040-93042, 93318, 93355, 94002, 94200, 94680-94690, 95812-95816, 95819, 95822, 95829, 95955, 96360-96368, 96372, 96374-96377, 96523, 97597-97598, 97602-97608, 99155, 99156, 99157, 99211-99223, 99231-99255, 99291-99292, 99304-99310, 99315-99316, 99334-99337, 99347-99350, 99374-99375, 99377-99378, 99446-99449, 99451-99452, 99495-99496, G0168, G0463, G0471, J0670, J2001

15241 11000-11006, 11042-11047, 36591-36592, 96523, 97597-97598, 97602, J0670, J2001

15260 01951-01952, 0213T, 0216T, 0596T-0597T, 11000-11006, 11042-11047, 11102, 11104, 11106, 12001-12007, 12011-12057, 13100-13133, 13151-13153, 15852, 16020-16030, 29000-29015, 29035-29200, 29240-29450, 29505-29581, 29584, 36000, 36400-36410, 36420-36430, 36440, 36591-36592, 36600, 36640, 43752, 51701-51703, 62320-62327, 64400, 64405-64408, 64415-64435, 64445-64454, 64461-64463, 64479-64505, 64510-64530, 69990, 92012-92014, 93000-93010, 93040-93042, 93318, 93355, 94002, 94200, 94680-94690, 95812-95816, 95819, 95822, 95829, 95955, 96360-96368, 96372, 96374-96377, 96523, 97597-97598, 97602-97608, 99155, 99156, 99157, 99211-99223, 99231-99255, 99291-99292, 99304-99310, 99315-99316, 99334-99337,

99347-99350, 99374-99375, 99377-99378, 99446-99449, 99451-99452, 99495-99496, G0168, G0463, G0471, J0670, J2001

15261 11000-11006, 11042-11047, 36591-36592, 96523, 97597-97598, 97602, J0670, J2001

15850 11000-11006, 11042-11047, 36591-36592, 96523, 97597-97598, 97602, J0670, J2001

15851 0213T, 0216T, 0596T-0597T, 11000-11006, 11042-11047, 12001-12007, 12011-12057, 13100-13133, 13151-13153, 36000, 36400-36410, 36420-36430, 36440, 36591-36592, 36600, 36640, 43752, 51701-51703, 62320-62327, 64400, 64405-64408, 64415-64435, 64445-64454, 64461-64463, 64479-64505, 64510-64530, 69990, 92012-92014, 93000-93010, 93040-93042, 93318, 93355, 94002, 94200, 94680-94690, 95812-95816, 95819, 95822, 95829, 95955, 96360-96368, 96372, 96374-96377, 96523, 97597-97598, 97602-97608, 99155, 99156, 99157, 99211-99223, 99231-99255, 99291-99292, 99304-99310, 99315-99316, 99334-99337, 99347-99350, 99374-99375, 99377-99378, 99446-99449, 99451-99452, 99495-99496, G0463, G0471, J0670, J2001

15852 0213T, 0216T, 0596T-0597T, 12001-12007, 12011-12057, 13100-13133, 13151-13153, 36000, 36400-36410, 36420-36430, 36440, 36591-36592, 36600, 36640, 43752, 51701-51703, 62320-62327, 64400, 64405-64408, 64415-64435, 64445-64454, 64461-64463, 64479-64505, 64510-64530, 69990, 92012-92014, 93000-93010, 93040-93042, 93318, 93355, 94002, 94200, 94680-94690, 95812-95816, 95819, 95822, 95829, 95955, 96360-96368, 96372, 96374-96377, 96523, 97597-97598, 97602-97608, 99155, 99156, 99157, 99211-99223, 99231-99255, 99291-99292, 99304-99310, 99315-99316, 99334-99337, 99347-99350, 99374-99375, 99377-99378, 99446-99449, 99451-99452, 99495-99496, G0463, G0471, J2001

15920 0213T, 0216T, 0596T-0597T, 11000-11006, 11010-11012, 11042-11047, 11102, 11104, 11106, 12001-12007, 12011-12057, 13100-13133, 13151-13153, 15757✢, 36000, 36400-36410, 36420-36430, 36440, 36591-36592, 36600, 36640, 43752, 51701-51703, 62320-62327, 64400, 64405-64408, 64415-64435, 64445-64454, 64461-64463, 64479-64505, 64510-64530, 69990, 92012-92014, 93000-93010, 93040-93042, 93318, 93355, 94002, 94200, 94680-94690, 95812-95816, 95819, 95822, 95829, 95955, 96360-96368, 96372, 96374-96377, 96523, 97597-97598, 97602, 99155, 99156, 99157, 99211-99223, 99231-99255, 99291-99292, 99304-99310, 99315-99316, 99334-99337, 99347-99350, 99374-99375, 99377-99378, 99446-99449, 99451-99452, 99495-99496, G0463, G0471

15922 0213T, 0216T, 0596T-0597T, 11000-11006, 11010-11012, 11042-11047, 12001-12007, 12011-12057, 13100-13133, 13151-13153, 15756-15757✢, 15920, 36000, 36400-36410, 36420-36430, 36440, 36591-36592, 36600, 36640, 43752, 51701-51703, 62320-62327, 64400, 64405-64408, 64415-64435, 64445-64454, 64461-64463, 64479-64505, 64510-64530, 69990, 92012-92014, 93000-93010, 93040-93042, 93318, 93355, 94002, 94200, 94680-94690, 95812-95816, 95819, 95822, 95829, 95955, 96360-96368, 96372, 96374-96377, 96523, 97597-97598, 97602, 99155, 99156, 99157, 99211-99223, 99231-99255, 99291-99292, 99304-99310, 99315-99316, 99334-99337, 99347-99350, 99374-99375, 99377-99378, 99446-99449, 99451-99452, 99495-99496, G0463, G0471

15931 0213T, 0216T, 0596T-0597T, 11000-11006, 11010-11012, 11042-11047, 11102, 11104, 11106, 12001-12007, 12011-12057, 13100-13133, 13151-13153, 15756-15757✢, 15936-15937✢, 36000, 36400-36410, 36420-36430, 36440, 36591-36592, 36600, 36640, 43752, 51701-51703, 62320-62327, 64400, 64405-64408, 64415-64435, 64445-64454, 64461-64463, 64479-64505, 64510-64530, 69990, 92012-92014, 93000-93010, 93040-93042, 93318, 93355, 94002, 94200, 94680-94690, 95812-95816, 95819, 95822, 95829, 95955, 96360-96368, 96372, 96374-96377, 96523, 97597-97598, 97602, 99155, 99156, 99157,

99211-99223, 99231-99255, 99291-99292, 99304-99310, 99315-99316, 99334-99337, 99347-99350, 99374-99375, 99377-99378, 99446-99449, 99451-99452, 99495-99496, G0463, G0471

15933 0213T, 0216T, 0596T-0597T, 11000-11006, 11010-11012, 11042-11047, 11102, 11104, 11106, 12001-12007, 12011-12057, 13100-13133, 13151-13153, 15756-15757✧, 15931, 15936-15937✧, 36000, 36400-36410, 36420-36430, 36440, 36591-36592, 36600, 36640, 43752, 51701-51703, 62320-62327, 64400, 64405-64408, 64415-64435, 64445-64454, 64461-64463, 64479-64505, 64510-64530, 69990, 92012-92014, 93000-93010, 93040-93042, 93318, 93355, 94002, 94200, 94680-94690, 95812-95816, 95819, 95822, 95829, 95955, 96360-96368, 96372, 96374-96377, 96523, 97597-97598, 97602, 99155, 99156, 99157, 99211-99223, 99231-99255, 99291-99292, 99304-99310, 99315-99316, 99334-99337, 99347-99350, 99374-99375, 99377-99378, 99446-99449, 99451-99452, 99495-99496, G0463, G0471

15934 0213T, 0216T, 0596T-0597T, 11000-11006, 11010-11012, 11042-11047, 11102, 11104, 11106, 12001-12007, 12011-12057, 13100-13133, 13151-13153, 15756-15757✧, 15937✧, 36000, 36400-36410, 36420-36430, 36440, 36591-36592, 36600, 36640, 43752, 51701-51703, 62320-62327, 64400, 64405-64408, 64415-64435, 64445-64454, 64461-64463, 64479-64505, 64510-64530, 69990, 92012-92014, 93000-93010, 93040-93042, 93318, 93355, 94002, 94200, 94680-94690, 95812-95816, 95819, 95822, 95829, 95955, 96360-96368, 96372, 96374-96377, 96523, 97597-97598, 97602, 99155, 99156, 99157, 99211-99223, 99231-99255, 99291-99292, 99304-99310, 99315-99316, 99334-99337, 99347-99350, 99374-99375, 99377-99378, 99446-99449, 99451-99452, 99495-99496, G0463, G0471

15935 0213T, 0216T, 0596T-0597T, 11000-11006, 11010-11012, 11042-11047, 11102, 11104, 11106, 12001-12007, 12011-12057, 13100-13133, 13151-13153, 15756-15757✧, 15934, 36000, 36400-36410, 36420-36430, 36440, 36591-36592, 36600, 36640, 43752, 51701-51703, 62320-62327, 64400, 64405-64408, 64415-64435, 64445-64454, 64461-64463, 64479-64505, 64510-64530, 69990, 92012-92014, 93000-93010, 93040-93042, 93318, 93355, 94002, 94200, 94680-94690, 95812-95816, 95819, 95822, 95829, 95955, 96360-96368, 96372, 96374-96377, 96523, 97597-97598, 97602, 99155, 99156, 99157, 99211-99223, 99231-99255, 99291-99292, 99304-99310, 99315-99316, 99334-99337, 99347-99350, 99374-99375, 99377-99378, 99446-99449, 99451-99452, 99495-99496, G0463, G0471

15940 0213T, 0216T, 0596T-0597T, 11000-11006, 11010-11012, 11042-11047, 11102, 11104, 11106, 12001-12007, 12011-12057, 13100-13133, 13151-13153, 15756-15757✧, 36000, 36400-36410, 36420-36430, 36440, 36591-36592, 36600, 36640, 43752, 51701-51703, 62320-62327, 64400, 64405-64408, 64415-64435, 64445-64454, 64461-64463, 64479-64505, 64510-64530, 69990, 92012-92014, 93000-93010, 93040-93042, 93318, 93355, 94002, 94200, 94680-94690, 95812-95816, 95819, 95822, 95829, 95955, 96360-96368, 96372, 96374-96377, 96523, 97597-97598, 97602, 99155, 99156, 99157, 99211-99223, 99231-99255, 99291-99292, 99304-99310, 99315-99316, 99334-99337, 99347-99350, 99374-99375, 99377-99378, 99446-99449, 99451-99452, 99495-99496, G0463, G0471

15941 0213T, 0216T, 0596T-0597T, 11000-11006, 11010-11012, 11042-11047, 11102, 11104, 11106, 12001-12007, 12011-12057, 13100-13133, 13151-13153, 15756-15757✧, 15940, 36000, 36400-36410, 36420-36430, 36440, 36591-36592, 36600, 36640, 43752, 51701-51703, 62320-62327, 64400, 64405-64408, 64415-64435, 64445-64454, 64461-64463, 64479-64505, 64510-64530, 69990, 92012-92014, 93000-93010, 93040-93042, 93318, 93355, 94002, 94200, 94680-94690, 95812-95816, 95819, 95822, 95829, 95955, 96360-96368, 96372,

96374-96377, 96523, 97597-97598, 97602, 99155, 99156, 99157, 99211-99223, 99231-99255, 99291-99292, 99304-99310, 99315-99316, 99334-99337, 99347-99350, 99374-99375, 99377-99378, 99446-99449, 99451-99452, 99495-99496, G0463, G0471

15944 0213T, 0216T, 0596T-0597T, 11000-11006, 11010-11012, 11042-11047, 11102, 11104, 11106, 12001-12007, 12011-12057, 13100-13133, 13151-13153, 15756-15757✧, 36000, 36400-36410, 36420-36430, 36440, 36591-36592, 36600, 36640, 43752, 51701-51703, 62320-62327, 64400, 64405-64408, 64415-64435, 64445-64454, 64461-64463, 64479-64505, 64510-64530, 69990, 92012-92014, 93000-93010, 93040-93042, 93318, 93355, 94002, 94200, 94680-94690, 95812-95816, 95819, 95822, 95829, 95955, 96360-96368, 96372, 96374-96377, 96523, 97597-97598, 97602, 99155, 99156, 99157, 99211-99223, 99231-99255, 99291-99292, 99304-99310, 99315-99316, 99334-99337, 99347-99350, 99374-99375, 99377-99378, 99446-99449, 99451-99452, 99495-99496, G0463, G0471

15945 0213T, 0216T, 0596T-0597T, 11000-11006, 11010-11012, 11042-11047, 11102, 11104, 11106, 12001-12007, 12011-12057, 13100-13133, 13151-13153, 15756-15757✧, 15944, 36000, 36400-36410, 36420-36430, 36440, 36591-36592, 36600, 36640, 43752, 51701-51703, 62320-62327, 64400, 64405-64408, 64415-64435, 64445-64454, 64461-64463, 64479-64505, 64510-64530, 69990, 92012-92014, 93000-93010, 93040-93042, 93318, 93355, 94002, 94200, 94680-94690, 95812-95816, 95819, 95822, 95829, 95955, 96360-96368, 96372, 96374-96377, 96523, 97597-97598, 97602, 99155, 99156, 99157, 99211-99223, 99231-99255, 99291-99292, 99304-99310, 99315-99316, 99334-99337, 99347-99350, 99374-99375, 99377-99378, 99446-99449, 99451-99452, 99495-99496, G0463, G0471

15946 0213T, 0216T, 0596T-0597T, 11000-11006, 11010-11012, 11042-11047, 11102, 11104, 11106, 12001-12007, 12011-12057, 13100-13133, 13151-13153, 36000, 36400-36410, 36420-36430, 36440, 36591-36592, 36600, 36640, 43752, 51701-51703, 62320-62327, 64400, 64405-64408, 64415-64435, 64445-64454, 64461-64463, 64479-64505, 64510-64530, 69990, 92012-92014, 93000-93010, 93040-93042, 93318, 93355, 94002, 94200, 94680-94690, 95812-95816, 95819, 95822, 95829, 95955, 96360-96368, 96372, 96374-96377, 96523, 97597-97598, 97602, 99155, 99156, 99157, 99211-99223, 99231-99255, 99291-99292, 99304-99310, 99315-99316, 99334-99337, 99347-99350, 99374-99375, 99377-99378, 99446-99449, 99451-99452, 99495-99496, G0463, G0471

15950 0213T, 0216T, 0596T-0597T, 11000-11006, 11010-11011, 11042-11047, 11102, 11104, 11106, 12001-12007, 12011-12057, 13100-13133, 13151-13153, 36000, 36400-36410, 36420-36430, 36440, 36591-36592, 36600, 36640, 43752, 51701-51703, 62320-62327, 64400, 64405-64408, 64415-64435, 64445-64454, 64461-64463, 64479-64505, 64510-64530, 69990, 92012-92014, 93000-93010, 93040-93042, 93318, 93355, 94002, 94200, 94680-94690, 95812-95816, 95819, 95822, 95829, 95955, 96360-96368, 96372, 96374-96377, 96523, 97597-97598, 97602, 99155, 99156, 99157, 99211-99223, 99231-99255, 99291-99292, 99304-99310, 99315-99316, 99334-99337, 99347-99350, 99374-99375, 99377-99378, 99446-99449, 99451-99452, 99495-99496, G0463, G0471

15951 0213T, 0216T, 0596T-0597T, 11000-11006, 11010-11012, 11042-11047, 11102, 11104, 11106, 12001-12007, 12011-12057, 13100-13133, 13151-13153, 15950, 36000, 36400-36410, 36420-36430, 36440, 36591-36592, 36600, 36640, 43752, 51701-51703, 62320-62327, 64400, 64405-64408, 64415-64435, 64445-64454, 64461-64463, 64479-64505, 64510-64530, 69990, 92012-92014, 93000-93010, 93040-93042, 93318, 93355, 94002, 94200, 94680-94690, 95812-95816, 95819, 95822, 95829, 95955, 96360-96368, 96372, 96374-96377, 96523, 97597-97598, 97602, 99155, 99156, 99157, 99211-99223, 99231-99255, 99291-99292,

99304-99310, 99315-99316, 99334-99337, 99347-99350, 99374-99375, 99377-99378, 99446-99449, 99451-99452, 99495-99496, G0463, G0471

15952 0213T, 0216T, 0596T-0597T, 11000-11006, 11010-11012, 11042-11047, 11102, 11104, 11106, 12001-12007, 12011-12057, 13100-13133, 13151-13153, 36000, 36400-36410, 36420-36430, 36440, 36591-36592, 36600, 36640, 43752, 51701-51703, 62320-62327, 64400, 64405-64408, 64415-64435, 64445-64454, 64461-64463, 64479-64505, 64510-64530, 69990, 92012-92014, 93000-93010, 93040-93042, 93318, 93355, 94002, 94200, 94680-94690, 95812-95816, 95819, 95822, 95829, 95955, 96360-96368, 96372, 96374-96377, 96523, 97597-97598, 97602, 99155, 99156, 99157, 99211-99223, 99231-99255, 99291-99292, 99304-99310, 99315-99316, 99334-99337, 99347-99350, 99374-99375, 99377-99378, 99446-99449, 99451-99452, 99495-99496, G0463, G0471

15953 0213T, 0216T, 0596T-0597T, 11000-11006, 11010-11012, 11042-11047, 11102, 11104, 11106, 12001-12007, 12011-12057, 13100-13133, 13151-13153, 15952, 36000, 36400-36410, 36420-36430, 36440, 36591-36592, 36600, 36640, 43752, 51701-51703, 62320-62327, 64400, 64405-64408, 64415-64435, 64445-64454, 64461-64463, 64479-64505, 64510-64530, 69990, 92012-92014, 93000-93010, 93040-93042, 93318, 93355, 94002, 94200, 94680-94690, 95812-95816, 95819, 95822, 95829, 95955, 96360-96368, 96372, 96374-96377, 96523, 97597-97598, 97602, 99155, 99156, 99157, 99211-99223, 99231-99255, 99291-99292, 99304-99310, 99315-99316, 99334-99337, 99347-99350, 99374-99375, 99377-99378, 99446-99449, 99451-99452, 99495-99496, G0463, G0471

15956 0213T, 0216T, 0596T-0597T, 11000-11006, 11010-11012, 11042-11047, 11102, 11104, 11106, 12001-12007, 12011-12057, 13100-13133, 13151-13153, 36000, 36400-36410, 36420-36430, 36440, 36591-36592, 36600, 36640, 43752, 51701-51703, 62320-62327, 64400, 64405-64408, 64415-64435, 64445-64454, 64461-64463, 64479-64505, 64510-64530, 69990, 92012-92014, 93000-93010, 93040-93042, 93318, 93355, 94002, 94200, 94680-94690, 95812-95816, 95819, 95822, 95829, 95955, 96360-96368, 96372, 96374-96377, 96523, 97597-97598, 97602, 99155, 99156, 99157, 99211-99223, 99231-99255, 99291-99292, 99304-99310, 99315-99316, 99334-99337, 99347-99350, 99374-99375, 99377-99378, 99446-99449, 99451-99452, 99495-99496, G0463, G0471

15958 0213T, 0216T, 0596T-0597T, 11000-11006, 11010-11012, 11042-11047, 11102, 11104, 11106, 12001-12007, 12011-12057, 13100-13133, 13151-13153, 15956, 36000, 36400-36410, 36420-36430, 36440, 36591-36592, 36600, 36640, 43752, 51701-51703, 62320-62327, 64400, 64405-64408, 64415-64435, 64445-64454, 64461-64463, 64479-64505, 64510-64530, 69990, 92012-92014, 93000-93010, 93040-93042, 93318, 93355, 94002, 94200, 94680-94690, 95812-95816, 95819, 95822, 95829, 95955, 96360-96368, 96372, 96374-96377, 96523, 97597-97598, 97602, 99155, 99156, 99157, 99211-99223, 99231-99255, 99291-99292, 99304-99310, 99315-99316, 99334-99337, 99347-99350, 99374-99375, 99377-99378, 99446-99449, 99451-99452, 99495-99496, G0463, G0471

16020 01951-01952, 0213T, 0216T, 0596T-0597T, 11000, 11719, 12001-12007, 12011-12057, 13100-13133, 13151-13153, 16000✦, 36000, 36400-36410, 36420-36430, 36440, 36591-36592, 36600, 36640, 43752, 51701-51703, 62320-62327, 64400, 64405-64408, 64415-64435, 64445-64454, 64461-64463, 64479-64505, 64510-64530, 69990, 92012-92014, 93000-93010, 93040-93042, 93318, 93355, 94002, 94200, 94680-94690, 95812-95816, 95819, 95822, 95829, 95955, 96360-96368, 96372, 96374-96377, 96523, 97022, 97597-97598✦, 97602-97608✦, 99155, 99156, 99157, 99211-99223, 99231-99255, 99291-99292, 99304-99310, 99315-99316, 99334-99337, 99347-99350, 99374-99375, 99377-99378, 99446-99449, 99451-99452, 99495-99496, G0463, G0471, J0670, J2001

16025 01951-01952, 0213T, 0216T, 0596T-0597T, 11000, 11102, 11104, 11106, 12001-12007, 12011-12057, 13100-13133, 13151-13153, 16020✦, 36000, 36400-36410, 36420-36430, 36440, 36591-36592, 36600, 36640, 43752, 51701-51703, 62320-62327, 64400, 64405-64408, 64415-64435, 64445-64454, 64461-64463, 64479-64505, 64510-64530, 69990, 92012-92014, 93000-93010, 93040-93042, 93318, 93355, 94002, 94200, 94680-94690, 95812-95816, 95819, 95822, 95829, 95955, 96360-96368, 96372, 96374-96377, 96523, 97022, 97597-97598✦, 97602-97608✦, 99155, 99156, 99157, 99211-99223, 99231-99255, 99291-99292, 99304-99310, 99315-99316, 99334-99337, 99347-99350, 99374-99375, 99377-99378, 99446-99449, 99451-99452, 99495-99496, G0463, G0471, J0670, J2001

16030 01951-01952, 0213T, 0216T, 0596T-0597T, 11000, 11102, 11104, 11106, 12001-12007, 12011-12057, 13100-13133, 13151-13153, 16020-16025✦, 36000, 36400-36410, 36420-36430, 36440, 36591-36592, 36600, 36640, 43752, 51701-51703, 62320-62327, 64400, 64405-64408, 64415-64435, 64445-64454, 64461-64463, 64479-64505, 64510-64530, 69990, 92012-92014, 93000-93010, 93040-93042, 93318, 93355, 94002, 94200, 94680-94690, 95812-95816, 95819, 95822, 95829, 95955, 96360-96368, 96372, 96374-96377, 96523, 97022, 97597-97598✦, 97602-97608✦, 99155, 99156, 99157, 99211-99223, 99231-99255, 99291-99292, 99304-99310, 99315-99316, 99334-99337, 99347-99350, 99374-99375, 99377-99378, 99446-99449, 99451-99452, 99495-99496, G0463, G0471, J0670, J2001

16035 01951-01952, 0213T, 0216T, 0479T✦, 0491T✦, 0596T-0597T, 11000-11006, 11010, 11042-11047, 11102, 11104, 11106, 12001-12007, 12011-12057, 13100-13133, 13151-13153, 36000, 36400-36410, 36420-36430, 36440, 36591-36592, 36600, 36640, 43752, 51701-51703, 62320-62327, 64400, 64405-64408, 64415-64435, 64445-64454, 64461-64463, 64479-64505, 64510-64530, 69990, 92012-92014, 93000-93010, 93040-93042, 93318, 93355, 94002, 94200, 94680-94690, 95812-95816, 95819, 95822, 95829, 95955, 96360-96368, 96372, 96374-96377, 96523, 97597-97598, 97602-97608✦, 99155, 99156, 99157, 99211-99223, 99231-99255, 99291-99292, 99304-99310, 99315-99316, 99334-99337, 99347-99350, 99374-99375, 99377-99378, 99446-99449, 99451-99452, 99495-99496, G0463, G0471

16036 11000-11006, 11042-11047, 36591-36592, 96523, 97597-97598, 97602

17311 0213T, 0216T, 0596T-0597T, 11000-11006, 11010-11012, 11042-11047, 11102, 11104, 11106, 11420-11446✦, 11470-11471✦, 11600-11606, 11620-11646, 11750✦, 11765✦, 15837-15838, 15920, 17260-17286✦, 30120✦, 36000, 36400-36410, 36420-36430, 36440, 36591-36592, 36600, 36640, 40510✦, 40520-40527, 42810✦, 43752, 51701-51703, 62320-62327, 64400, 64405-64408, 64415-64435, 64445-64454, 64461-64463, 64479-64505, 64510-64530, 67840✦, 67961-67966✦, 69110✦, 69990, 88300-88314, 88331-88332, 88342, 88344, 92012-92014, 93000-93010, 93040-93042, 93318, 93355, 94002, 94200, 94680-94690, 95812-95816, 95819, 95822, 95829, 95955, 96360-96368, 96372, 96374-96377, 96523, 97597-97598, 97602, 99155, 99156, 99157, 99211-99223, 99231-99255, 99291-99292, 99304-99310, 99315-99316, 99334-99337, 99347-99350, 99374-99375, 99377-99378, 99446-99449, 99451-99452, 99495-99496, G0416, G0463, G0471, J0670, J2001

17312 11000-11006, 11042-11047, 36591-36592, 88302-88309, 88314, 96523, 97597-97598, 97602, J0670, J2001

17313 0213T, 0216T, 0596T-0597T, 11000-11006, 11010-11012, 11042-11047, 11102, 11104, 11106, 11400-11406✦, 11450-11471✦, 11600-11606, 11620-11646, 11770-11771✦, 15830, 15832-15837, 15920, 17260-17286✦, 26596, 36000, 36400-36410, 36420-36430, 36440, 36591-36592, 36600, 36640, 43752, 51701-51703, 54060✦,

62320-62327, 64400, 64405-64408, 64415-64435, 64445-64454, 64461-64463, 64479-64505, 64510-64530, 69990, 88300-88314, 88331-88332, 88342, 88344, 92012-92014, 93000-93010, 93040-93042, 93318, 93355, 94002, 94200, 94680-94690, 95812-95816, 95819, 95822, 95829, 95955, 96360-96368, 96372, 96374-96377, 96523, 97597-97598, 97602, 99155, 99156, 99157, 99211-99223, 99231-99255, 99291-99292, 99304-99310, 99315-99316, 99334-99337, 99347-99350, 99374-99375, 99377-99378, 99446-99449, 99451-99452, 99495-99496, G0416, G0463, G0471, J0670, J2001

17314 11000-11006, 11042-11047, 36591-36592, 88314, 96523, 97597-97598, 97602, J0670, J2001

17315 11000-11006, 11042-11047, 36591-36592, 88302-88309, 88314, 96523, 97597-97598, 97602

19000 00400, 0213T, 0216T, 0596T-0597T, 12001-12007, 12011-12057, 13100-13133, 13151-13153, 36000, 36400-36410, 36420-36430, 36440, 36591-36592, 36600, 36640, 43752, 51701-51703, 62320-62327, 64400, 64405-64408, 64415-64435, 64445-64454, 64461-64463, 64479-64505, 64510-64530, 69990, 92012-92014, 93000-93010, 93040-93042, 93318, 93355, 94002, 94200, 94680-94690, 95812-95816, 95819, 95822, 95829, 95955, 96360-96368, 96372, 96374-96377, 96523, 99155, 99156, 99157, 99211-99223, 99231-99255, 99291-99292, 99304-99310, 99315-99316, 99334-99337, 99347-99350, 99374-99375, 99377-99378, 99446-99449, 99451-99452, 99495-99496, G0463, G0471, J0670, J2001

19001 36591-36592, 96523, J2001

19020 00400, 0213T, 0216T, 0596T-0597T, 11000-11006, 11042-11047, 12001-12007, 12011-12057, 13100-13133, 13151-13153, 20500, 36000, 36400-36410, 36420-36430, 36440, 36591-36592, 36600, 36640, 43752, 51701-51703, 62320-62327, 64400, 64405-64408, 64415-64435, 64445-64454, 64461-64463, 64479-64505, 64510-64530, 69990, 92012-92014, 93000-93010, 93040-93042, 93318, 93355, 94002, 94200, 94680-94690, 95812-95816, 95819, 95822, 95829, 95955, 96360-96368, 96372, 96374-96377, 96523, 97597-97598, 97602, 99155, 99156, 99157, 99211-99223, 99231-99255, 99291-99292, 99304-99310, 99315-99316, 99334-99337, 99347-99350, 99374-99375, 99377-99378, 99446-99449, 99451-99452, 99495-99496, G0463, G0471, J0670, J2001

19081 00400, 0213T, 0216T, 0596T-0597T, 10005, 10007, 10009, 10011, 10021, 10035-10036, 12001-12007, 12011-12057, 13100-13133, 13151-13153, 19100-19101, 19281-19288, 36000, 36400-36410, 36420-36430, 36440, 36591-36592, 36600, 36640, 43752, 51701-51703, 62320-62327, 64400, 64405-64408, 64415-64435, 64445-64454, 64461-64463, 64479-64505, 64510-64530, 69990, 76000, 76098, 76380, 76942, 76998, 77002, 77011-77012, 77021, 88172, 92012-92014, 93000-93010, 93040-93042, 93318, 93355, 94002, 94200, 94680-94690, 95812-95816, 95819, 95822, 95829, 95955, 96360-96368, 96372, 96374-96377, 96523, 99155, 99156, 99157, 99211-99223, 99231-99255, 99291-99292, 99304-99310, 99315-99316, 99334-99337, 99347-99350, 99374-99375, 99377-99378, 99446-99449, 99451-99452, G0463, G0471, J0670, J2001

19082 00400, 0213T, 0216T, 0596T-0597T, 10005, 10007, 10009, 10011, 10021, 10035-10036, 12001-12007, 12011-12057, 13100-13133, 13151-13153, 19100-19101✦, 19281-19288, 36000, 36400-36410, 36420-36430, 36440, 36591-36592, 36600, 36640, 43752, 51701-51703, 61650, 62320-62327, 64400, 64405-64408, 64415-64435, 64445-64454, 64461, 64463, 64479, 64483, 64486-64490, 64493, 64505, 64510-64530, 69990, 76000, 76098, 76380, 76942, 76998, 77002, 77011-77012, 77021, 88172, 93000-93010, 93040-93042, 93318, 93355, 94002, 94200, 94680-94690, 95812-95816, 95819, 95822, 95829, 95955, 96360, 96365, 96372, 96374-96377, 96523, 99155, 99156, 99157, 99211-99223, 99231-99255, 99291-99292, 99304-99310,

19083 00400, 0213T, 0216T, 0596T-0597T, 10005, 10007, 10009, 10011, 10021, 10035-10036, 12001-12007, 12011-12057, 13100-13133, 13151-13153, 19100-19101, 19281-19288, 36000, 36400-36410, 36420-36430, 36440, 36591-36592, 36600, 36640, 43752, 51701-51703, 62320-62327, 64400, 64405-64408, 64415-64435, 64445-64454, 64461-64463, 64479-64505, 64510-64530, 69990, 76000, 76098, 76380, 76942, 76998, 77002, 77011-77012, 77021, 88172, 92012-92014, 93000-93010, 93040-93042, 93318, 93355, 94002, 94200, 94680-94690, 95812-95816, 95819, 95822, 95829, 95955, 96360-96368, 96372, 96374-96377, 96523, 99155, 99156, 99157, 99211-99223, 99231-99255, 99291-99292, 99304-99310, 99315-99316, 99334-99337, 99347-99350, 99374-99375, 99377-99378, 99446-99449, 99451-99452, G0463, G0471, J0670, J2001

19084 00400, 0213T, 0216T, 0596T-0597T, 10005, 10007, 10009, 10011, 10021, 10035-10036, 12001-12007, 12011-12057, 13100-13133, 13151-13153, 19100-19101✦, 19281-19288, 36000, 36400-36410, 36420-36430, 36440, 36591-36592, 36600, 36640, 43752, 51701-51703, 61650, 62320-62327, 64400, 64405-64408, 64415-64435, 64445-64454, 64461, 64463, 64479, 64483, 64486-64490, 64493, 64505, 64510-64530, 69990, 76000, 76098, 76380, 76942, 76998, 77002, 77011-77012, 77021, 88172, 93000-93010, 93040-93042, 93318, 93355, 94002, 94200, 94680-94690, 95812-95816, 95819, 95822, 95829, 95955, 96360, 96365, 96372, 96374-96377, 96523, 99155, 99156, 99157, 99211-99223, 99231-99255, 99291-99292, 99304-99310, 99315-99316, 99334-99337, 99347-99350, 99374-99375, 99377-99378, 99446-99449, 99451-99452, G0463, G0471, J0670, J2001

19085 00400, 0213T, 0216T, 0596T-0597T, 10005, 10007, 10009, 10011, 10021, 10035-10036, 12001-12007, 12011-12057, 13100-13133, 13151-13153, 19100-19101, 19281-19288, 36000, 36400-36410, 36420-36430, 36440, 36591-36592, 36600, 36640, 43752, 51701-51703, 62320-62327, 64400, 64405-64408, 64415-64435, 64445-64454, 64461-64463, 64479-64505, 64510-64530, 69990, 76000, 76098, 76380, 76942, 76998, 77002, 77011-77012, 77021, 88172, 92012-92014, 93000-93010, 93040-93042, 93318, 93355, 94002, 94200, 94680-94690, 95812-95816, 95819, 95822, 95829, 95955, 96360-96368, 96372, 96374-96377, 96523, 99155, 99156, 99157, 99211-99223, 99231-99255, 99291-99292, 99304-99310, 99315-99316, 99334-99337, 99347-99350, 99374-99375, 99377-99378, 99446-99449, 99451-99452, G0463, G0471, J0670, J2001

19086 00400, 0213T, 0216T, 0596T-0597T, 10005, 10007, 10009, 10011, 10021, 10035-10036, 12001-12007, 12011-12057, 13100-13133, 13151-13153, 19100-19101✦, 19281-19288, 36000, 36400-36410, 36420-36430, 36440, 36591-36592, 36600, 36640, 43752, 51701-51703, 61650, 62320-62327, 64400, 64405-64408, 64415-64435, 64445-64454, 64461, 64463, 64479, 64483, 64486-64490, 64493, 64505, 64510-64530, 69990, 76000, 76098, 76380, 76942, 76998, 77002, 77011-77012, 77021, 88172, 93000-93010, 93040-93042, 93318, 93355, 94002, 94200, 94680-94690, 95812-95816, 95819, 95822, 95829, 95955, 96360, 96365, 96372, 96374-96377, 96523, 99155, 99156, 99157, 99211-99223, 99231-99255, 99291-99292, 99304-99310, 99315-99316, 99334-99337, 99347-99350, 99374-99375, 99377-99378, 99446-99449, 99451-99452, G0463, G0471, J0670, J2001

19100 00400, 0213T, 0216T, 0596T-0597T, 10005, 10007, 10009, 10011, 10021, 10035, 12001-12007, 12011-12057, 13100-13133, 13151-13153, 19281, 19283, 19285, 19287, 36000, 36400-36410, 36420-36430, 36440, 36591-36592, 36600, 36640, 43752, 51701-51703, 62320-62327, 64400, 64405-64408, 64415-64435, 64445-64454, 64461-64463,

64479-64505, 64510-64530, 69990, 76380, 76942, 76998, 77012, 77021, 92012-92014, 93000-93010, 93040-93042, 93318, 93355, 94002, 94200, 94680-94690, 95812-95816, 95819, 95822, 95829, 95955, 96360-96368, 96372, 96374-96377, 96523, 99155, 99156, 99157, 99211-99223, 99231-99255, 99291-99292, 99304-99310, 99315-99316, 99334-99337, 99347-99350, 99374-99375, 99377-99378, 99446-99449, 99451-99452, 99495-99496, G0463, G0471, J0670, J2001

19101 00400, 0213T, 0216T, 0596T-0597T, 10005, 10007, 10009, 10011, 10021, 10035, 12001-12007, 12011-12057, 13100-13133, 13151-13153, 19100, 36000, 36400-36410, 36420-36430, 36440, 36591-36592, 36600, 36640, 43752, 51701-51703, 62320-62327, 64400, 64405-64408, 64415-64435, 64445-64454, 64461-64463, 64479-64505, 64510-64530, 69990, 76380, 76942, 76998, 77012, 77021, 88172, 92012-92014, 93000-93010, 93040-93042, 93318, 93355, 94002, 94200, 94680-94690, 95812-95816, 95819, 95822, 95829, 95955, 96360-96368, 96372, 96374-96377, 96523, 99155, 99156, 99157, 99211-99223, 99231-99255, 99291-99292, 99304-99310, 99315-99316, 99334-99337, 99347-99350, 99374-99375, 99377-99378, 99446-99449, 99451-99452, 99495-99496, G0463, G0471, J0670, J2001

19105 0213T, 0216T, 0581T✣, 0596T-0597T, 12001-12007, 12011-12057, 13100-13133, 13151-13153, 36000, 36400-36410, 36420-36430, 36440, 36591-36592, 36600, 36640, 43752, 51701-51703, 62320-62327, 64400, 64405-64408, 64415-64435, 64445-64454, 64461-64463, 64479-64505, 64510-64530, 69990, 76940, 76942, 76998, 92012-92014, 93000-93010, 93040-93042, 93318, 93355, 94002, 94200, 94680-94690, 95812-95816, 95819, 95822, 95829, 95955, 96360-96368, 96372, 96374-96377, 96523, 99155, 99156, 99157, 99211-99223, 99231-99255, 99291-99292, 99304-99310, 99315-99316, 99334-99337, 99347-99350, 99374-99375, 99377-99378, 99446-99449, 99451-99452, 99495-99496, G0463, G0471, J0670, J2001

19110 00400, 0213T, 0216T, 0596T-0597T, 10005, 10007, 10009, 10011, 10021, 10035, 11000-11006, 11042-11047, 12001-12007, 12011-12057, 13100-13133, 13151-13153, 19081, 19083, 19085, 19100, 19112, 36000, 36400-36410, 36420-36430, 36440, 36591-36592, 36600, 36640, 43752, 51701-51703, 62320-62327, 64400, 64405-64408, 64415-64435, 64445-64454, 64461-64463, 64479-64505, 64510-64530, 69990, 76942, 76998, 92012-92014, 93000-93010, 93040-93042, 93318, 93355, 94002, 94200, 94680-94690, 95812-95816, 95819, 95822, 95829, 95955, 96360-96368, 96372, 96374-96377, 96523, 97597-97598, 97602, 99155,

64445-64454, 64461-64463, 64479-64505, 64510-64530, 69990, 76942, 76998, 92012-92014, 93000-93010, 93040-93042, 93318, 93355, 94002, 94200, 94680-94690, 95812-95816, 95819, 95822, 95829, 95955, 96360-96368, 96372, 96374-96377, 96523, 97597-97598, 97602, 99155, 99156, 99157, 99211-99223, 99231-99255, 99291-99292, 99304-99310, 99315-99316, 99334-99337, 99347-99350, 99374-99375, 99377-99378, 99446-99449, 99451-99452, 99495-99496, G0463, G0471, J0670, J2001

19125 00400, 0213T, 0216T, 0596T-0597T, 10005, 10007, 10009, 10011, 10021, 11000-11006, 11042-11047, 12001-12007, 12011-12057, 13100-13133, 13151-13153, 19081, 19083, 19085, 19100-19101, 19110-19120, 36000, 36400-36410, 36420-36430, 36440, 36591-36592, 36600, 36640, 43752, 51701-51703, 62320-62327, 64400, 64405-64408, 64415-64435, 64445-64454, 64461-64463, 64479-64505, 64510-64530, 69990, 92012-92014, 93000-93010, 93040-93042, 93318, 93355, 94002, 94200, 94680-94690, 95812-95816, 95819, 95822, 95829, 95955, 96360-96368, 96372, 96374-96377, 96523, 97597-97598, 97602, 99155, 99156, 99157, 99211-99223, 99231-99255, 99291-99292, 99304-99310, 99315-99316, 99334-99337, 99347-99350, 99374-99375, 99377-99378, 99446-99449, 99451-99452, 99495-99496, G0463, G0471, J0670, J2001

19126 11000-11006, 11042-11047, 19081, 19083, 19085, 36591-36592, 96523, 97597-97598, 97602

19294 0213T, 0216T, 0596T-0597T, 11000-11006, 11042-11047, 12001-12007, 12011-12057, 13100-13133, 13151-13153, 36000, 36400-36410, 36420-36430, 36440, 36591-36592, 36600, 36640, 43752, 51701-51703, 62320-62327, 64400, 64405-64408, 64415-64435, 64445-64454, 64461-64463, 64479-64505, 64510-64530, 69990, 92012-92014, 93000-93010, 93040-93042, 93318, 94002, 94200, 94680-94690, 95812-95816, 95819, 95822, 95829, 95955, 96360-96368, 96372, 96374-96377, 96523, 97597-97598, 97602, 99155, 99156, 99157, 99211-99223, 99231-99255, 99291-99292, 99304-99310, 99315-99316, 99334-99337, 99347-99350, 99374-99375, 99377-99378

19296 0213T, 0216T, 0596T-0597T, 11000-11006, 11042-11047, 12001-12007, 12011-12057, 13100-13133, 13151-13153, 19297✣, 36000, 36400-36410, 36420-36430, 36440, 36591-36592, 36600, 36640, 43752, 51701-51703, 62320-62327, 64400, 64405-64408, 64415-64435, 64445-64454, 64461-64463, 64479-64505, 64510-64530, 69990, 76000, 76380, 76942, 76965, 76998, 77001-77002, 77012, 77021, 92012-92014, 93000-93010, 93040-93042, 93318, 93355, 94002, 94200, 94680-94690, 95812-95816, 95819, 95822, 95829, 95955, 96360-96368,

---

IMPORTANT

Note: The following URL and password will provide you with access to download and view the complete list of CCI edits:

https://www.optum360coding.com/productupdates

2022 password: **CODING22**

Please note that you should log in each quarter to ensure you receive the most current updates. An email reminder will also be sent to you when the updates are available.

CPT Index

A

ABBI Biopsy, 19081-19086
Abdomen, Abdominal
  Abscess, 49020-49040
    Incision and Drainage
      Skin and Subcutaneous Tissue, 10060-10061
    Open, 49040
      Peritoneal, 49020
      Peritonitis, Localized, 49020
      Retroperitoneal, 49060
      Subdiaphragmatic, 49040
      Subphrenic, 49040
  Biopsy
    Incisional, 11106-11107
    Open, 49000
    Percutaneous, 49180
    Punch, 11104-11105
    Skin, Tangential, 11102-11103
  Cannula/Catheter
    Insertion, 49419-49421
    Removal, 49422
  Catheter
    Removal, 49422
  Celiotomy, 49000
  Cyst
    Destruction/Excision, 49203-49205
    Sclerotherapy, 49185
  Delivery
    Peritoneal Abscess
      Open, 49020
      Peritonitis, Localized, 49020
  Drainage, 49020-49040
    Fluid, 49082-49083
    Retroperitoneal
      Open, 49060
    Skin and Subcutaneous Tissue, 10060-10061
    Subdiaphragmatic
      Open, 49040
    Subphrenic
      Open, 49040
  Endometrioma, 49203-49205
    Destruction/Excision, 49203-49205
  Excision
    Tumor, Abdominal Wall, 22900
  Exploration, 49000-49084
    Blood Vessel, 35840
  Hernia Repair, 49491-49590, 49650-49657
  Incision, 49000-49084
  Incision and Drainage
    Pancreatitis, 48000
  Injection
    Air, 49400
    Contrast Material, 49400
  Insertion
    Catheter, 49324, 49418-49421
    Venous Shunt, 49425
  Intraperitoneal
    Catheter Exit Site, 49436
    Catheter Insertion, 49324, 49418-49421, 49425, 49435
    Catheter Removal, 49422
    Catheter Revision, 49325
    Shunt
      Insertion, 49425
      Ligation, 49428
      Removal, 49429
      Revision, 49426
  Laparoscopy, 49320-49327
  Laparotomy
    Exploration, 47015, 49000-49002
    Hemorrhage Control, 49002
    Reopening, 49002
    with Biopsy, 49000
  Needle Biopsy
    Mass, 49180
  Pancreatitis, 48000
  Paracentesis, 49082-49083
  Peritoneal Abscess, 49020
  Peritoneal Lavage, 49084

Abdomen, Abdominal — *continued*
  Placement Guidance Devices, 49411-49412
  Repair
    Hernia, 49491-49590, 49650-49657
    Suture, 49900
  Revision
    Venous Shunt, 49426
  Suture, 49900
  Tumor
    Destruction/Excision, 49203-49205
  Wall
    Debridement
      Infected, 11005-11006
    Implant
      Fascial Reinforcement, 0437T
    Reconstruction, 49905
    Removal
      Mesh, 11008
      Prosthesis, 11008
    Repair
      Hernia, 49491-49590
        by Laparoscopy, 49650-49651
    Tumor
      Excision, 22900-22905
  Wound Exploration
    Penetrating, 20102
Abdominal Plane Block
  Bilateral, 64488-64489
  Unilateral, 64486-64487
Ablation
  Anus, 46615
  Breast Tumor, 0581T
  Colon, [44401, 45346]
  Cryosurgical
    Breast Tumor, 0581T
    Fibroadenoma, 19105
    Liver Tumor(s), 47381, 47383
  Endoscopic
    Duodenum/Jejunum, [43270]
    Esophagus, 43229 [43270]
    Hepatobiliary System, [43278]
    Stomach, [43270]
  Endovenous, 36473-36479
  Liver
    Tumor, 47370-47371, 47380-47383
      Cryoablation, 47381, 47383
      Laparoscopic, 47370-47371
      Microwave, 47370
      Open, 47380-47381
      Percutaneous, 47382
      Radiofrequency, 47370, 47380, 47382
  Radiofrequency
    Liver Tumor(s), 47382
  Rectum, [45346]
  Thyroid
    Percutaneous, 0673T
  Vein
    Endovenous, 36473-36479
Abscess
  Abdomen, 49020-49040
    Peritoneal, 49020
    Peritonitis, Localized, 49020
    Retroperitoneal, 49060
    Skin and Subcutaneous Tissue, 10060-10061
    Subdiaphragmatic, 49040
    Subphrenic, 49040
  Anal, 46045-46050
  Appendix, 44900
  Arm
    Upper, 23930
  Bartholin's Gland
    Puncture Aspiration, 10160
  Bladder, 49406
  Breast, 19020
  Elbow, 23930
  Hip, 26990
  Kidney
    Percutaneous, 49405
  Leg
    Lower, 27603

Abscess — *continued*
  Liver
    Injection, 47015
    Marsupialization, 47300
    Open, 47010
    Percutaneous, 49405
  Lung
    Percutaneous, 49405
  Lymph Node, 38300-38305
  Lymphocele, 49062
  Neck, 21501-21502
  Olecranon Process, 23930
  Pelvis, 26990
    Transrectal, 45000, 49407
  Perirenal or Renal
    Percutaneous, 49405
  Peritoneal, 49020, 49406-49407
  Posterior Spine, 22010-22015
  Rectum, 45005-45020, 46040, 46060
  Retroperitoneal, 49060
  Skin, 10060-10061
    Puncture Aspiration, 10160
  Soft Tissue Catheter Drainage, 10030
  Spine, 22010-22015
  Spleen, 49405
  Subdiaphragmatic, 49040
  Subphrenic, 49040
    Percutaneous, 49406
  Thoracostomy, 32551
  Thorax, 21501-21502
  Visceral, 49405
Access
  Small Bowel via Biliary Tree, Percutaneous, 47541
Acetabulum
  Tumor
    Excision, 27076
Acid
  Perfusion Test
    Esophagus, 91013, 91030
  Reflux Test, 91034-91038
Acromioclavicular Joint
  Arthrocentesis, 20605-20606
Acupuncture
  One or More Needles
    with Electrical Stimulation, 97813-97814
    without Electrical Stimulation, 97810-97811
  Trigger Point, [20560, 20561]
Adenoma
  Pancreas
    Excision, 48120
  Thyroid Gland
    Excision, 60200
Adhesion, Adhesions
  Intestinal
    Enterolysis, 44005
      Laparoscopic, 44180
Administration
  Injection
    Intramuscular Antibiotic, 96372
    Therapeutic, Diagnostic, Prophylactic
      Intra–arterial, 96373
      Intramuscular, 96372
      Intravenous, 96374-96376
      Subcutaneous, 96372
Adrenal Gland
  Biopsy, 60540-60545
  Excision
    Laparoscopy, 60650
    Retroperitoneal, 60545
  Exploration, 60540-60545
Adrenalectomy, 60540
  Laparoscopic, 60650
  with Excision Retroperitoneal Tumor, 60545
After Hours Medical Services, 99050, 99056-99058
Albumin
  Serum Plasma, 82040
  Whole Blood, 82040

Allogeneic Donor
  Backbench Preparation
    Intestine, 44715-44721
    Liver, 47143-47147
    Pancreas, 48551-48552
Allogeneic Transplantation
  Backbench Preparation, 44715-44721
    Intestine, 44715-44721
    Liver, 47143-47147
    Pancreas, 48551-48552
Allograft Preparation
  Intestines, 44715-44721
  Liver, 47143-47147
  Pancreas, 48551-48552
Alloplastic Dressing
  Burns, 15002, 15004-15005
Allotransplantation
  Intestines, 44135-44136
Almen Test
  Blood, Feces, 82270
Altemeier Procedure
  Rectum Prolapse, Excision, 45130-45135
Amussat's Operation, 44025
Amylase
  Blood, 82150
  Urine, 82150
Anal
  Abscess, 46045
  Bleeding, 46614
  Fissurectomy, 46200, 46261
  Fistula, 46262-46288, 46706-46707, 46715-46716
  Fistulectomy, 46270-46285
  Fistulotomy, 46270-46280
  Polyp, 46615
  Sphincter
    Dilation, 45905
    Incision, 46080
  Tumor, 46615
  Ulceration, 46200, 46261
Analgesia, 99151-99153
Analysis
  Electronic
    Pulse Generator, 95980-95982
  Physiologic Data, Remote, [99091, 99457]
Anastomosis
  Arteriovenous Fistula
    Direct, 36821
    Revision, 36832-36833
      with Thrombectomy, 36833
      without Thrombectomy, 36832
    with Graft, 36825-36830, 36832
    with Thrombectomy, 36831
  Bile Duct
    to Bile Duct, 47800
    to Intestines, 47760, 47780
  Bile Duct to Gastrointestinal, 47760, 47780-47785
  Caval to Mesenteric, 37160
  Colorectal, 44620, 44626
  Gallbladder to Intestine, 47720-47740
  Hepatic Duct to Intestine, 47765, 47802
  Ileo–Anal, 45113
  Intestine to Intestine, 44130
  Intestines
    Colo–anal, 45119
    Enterostomy, 44620-44626
    Ileoanal, 44157-44158
    Resection
      Laparoscopic, 44202-44205
  Intrahepatic Portosystemic, 37182-37183
  Jejunum, 43820-43825
  Microvascular
    Free Transfer Jejunum, 43496
  Pancreas to Intestines, 48520-48540, 48548
  Portocaval, 37140
  Renoportal, 37145
  Splenorenal, 37180-37181
  Stomach, 43825
    to Duodenum, 43810
    to Jejunum, 43820-43825, 43860-43865
  Vein to Vein, 37140-37183

Battle's Operation, 44950, 44960
Bed
  Sore/Pressure Ulcer/Decubitus
    Excision, 15920-15935, 15940-15958
Belsey IV Procedure, 43280, 43327-43328
Benzidine Test
  Blood, Feces, 82270
Bernstein Test, 91030
Bile Duct
  Anastomosis
    with Intestines, 47760, 47780-47785
  Biopsy
    Endoscopy, 43261, 47553
    Percutaneous, 47543
  Catheterization
    Drainage, 47533-47537
  Cyst
    Excision, 47715
  Destruction
    Calculi (Stone), 43265
  Dilation
    Endoscopic, 47555-47556 [43277]
    Percutaneous, 47542
  Drainage
    Catheter Insertion, 47533-47534
    Change Biliary Catheter, 47535-47536
    Removal, 47537
  Endoscopy
    Biopsy, 47553
    Cannulation, 43273
    Destruction
      Calculi (Stone), 43265
      Tumor, [43278]
    Dilation, 47555-47556 [43277]
    Exploration, 47552
    Intraoperative, 47550
    Placement
      Stent, [43274]
    Removal
      Calculi, 43264, 47554
      Foreign Body, [43275]
      Stent, [43275, 43276]
    Specimen Collection, 43260
    Sphincter Pressure, 43263
    Sphincterotomy, 43262 [43274,
      43276, 43277]
  Exploration
    Atresia, 47700
    Endoscopy, 47552
  Incision
    Sphincter, 43262, 47460
  Incision and Drainage, 47420-47425
  Insertion
    Catheter, 47533-47534
      Revision, 47535-47536
    Stent, 47538-47540, 47801
  Placement
    Percutaneous, 47538-47540
    Stent, [43274]
  Reconstruction
    Anastomosis, 47800
  Removal
    Calculi (Stone), 43264, 47420-47425
      Percutaneous, 47544
    Foreign Body, [43275]
    Stent, [43275, 43276]
  Repair
    Gastrointestinal Tract, 47785
    with Intestines, 47760, 47780
  Tumor
    Ablation, [43278]
    Destruction, [43278]
    Excision, 47711-47712
Bilirubin
  Blood, 82247-82248
  Total
    Direct, 82247-82248
    Total Blood, 82247-82248
Billroth I or II, 43631-43634
Bioelectrical Impedance Whole Body Analysis,
  0358T
Bioimpedance
  Whole Body Analysis, 0358T
Biopsy
  ABBI, 19081-19086
  Abdomen, 49000, 49321

Biopsy — *continued*
  Abdomen — *continued*
    Mass, 49180
  Adrenal Gland, 60540-60545
    Laparoscopic, 60650
    Open, 60540-60545
  Anal
    Endoscopy, 46606-46607
  Arm, Lower, 25065-25066
  Arm, Upper, 24065-24066
  Back/Flank, 21920-21925
  Bile Duct
    Endoscopic, 47553
    Percutaneous, 47543
  Breast, 19081-19101
    ABBI, 19081-19086
    Localization Clip Placement, 19081-
      19086
      with Magnetic Resonance Guid-
        ance, 19085-19086
      with Stereotactic Guidance,
        19081-19082
      with Ultrasound Guidance,
        19083-19084
    with Magnetic Resonance Imaging,
      19085-19086
    with Stereotactic Guidance, 19081-
      19082
    with Ultrasound Guidance, 19083-
      19084
  Colon, 44025, 44100
    Endoscopic, 44389, 45380, 45391-
      45392
    Multiple
      with Colostomy, Cecostomy,
        44322
  Colon–Sigmoid
    Endoscopic, 45305, 45331
  Duodenum, 44010
  Elbow, 24065-24066
  Esophagus
    Endoscopic, 43193, 43198, 43202,
      43238-43239, 43242
  Fallopian Tube, 49321
  Forearm, Soft Tissue, 25065-25066
  Gallbladder
    Endoscopic, 43261
  Gastrointestinal, Upper
    Endoscopic, 43239
  Ileum
    Endoscopic, 44382
  Intestines, Small, 44010, 44020, 44100
    Endoscopic, 44361, 44377, 44382,
      44386
  Leg
    Lower, 27613-27614
    Upper, 27323-27324
  Liver, 47000-47001, 47100, 47700
  Lymph Nodes, 38500-38530, 38570
    Injection Procedure
      Identification of Sentinel Node,
        38792
      Radioactive Tracer, 38792
    Laparoscopic, 38570-38572
    Needle, 38505
    Open, 38500, 38510-38530
    Superficial, 38500
  Muscle, 20200-20206
  Neck, 21550
  Needle
    Abdomen
      Mass, 49180
  Omentum, 49321
  Ovary, 49321
  Pancreas, 43261, 48100-48102
  Pelvis, 27040-27041
  Peritoneum
    Laparoscopic, 49321
  Rectum, 45100, 45305, 45331
  Retroperitoneal Area, 49010, 49180
  Skin Lesion, 11102-11107
  Stomach, 43605
  Thigh, 27323-27324
  Thorax, 21550
  Thyroid
    Percutaneous Needle Core, 60100

Bladder
  Repair
    Fistula, 44660-44661, 45800-45805
  Suture
    Fistula, 44660-44661, 45800-45805
Bleeding Time, 85002
Blood Vessel(s)
  Exploration
    Abdomen, 35840
  Repair
    Graft Defect, 35870
  Shunt Creation
    Direct, 36821
    Thomas Shunt, 36835
    with Graft, 36825-36830
    with Transposition, 36818-36819
  Shunt Revision
    with Graft, 36832
Blood
  Bleeding Time, 85002
  Cell
    Sedimentation Rate
      Manual, 85651
  Cell Count
    Blood Smear, 85007-85008
    Differential WBC Count, 85004-85007
    Hematocrit, 85014
    Hemoglobin, 85018
    Microhematocrit, 85013
  Feces, 82270
    by Hemoglobin Immunoassay, 82274
  Gases
    by Pulse Oximetry, 94760
  Occult, 82270
  Platelet
    Count, 85008
  Smear
    Microscopic Examination, 85007-
      85008
  Test(s)
    Panels
      Electrolyte, 80051
      Lipid Panel, 80061
  Urea Nitrogen, 84525
Bone
  Debridement, 11044, 11047
Brachytherapy
  Placement of Device
    Breast, 19296-19298
    Genitalia, 55920
    Pelvis, 55920
Brain
  Neurostimulation
    Analysis, 95980-95982
Breast
  Ablation
    Cryosurgery, 19105
    Fibroadenoma, 19105
  Abscess
    Incision and Drainage, 19020
  Biopsy, 19100-19101
    ABBI, 19081-19086
    with Localization Device Placement,
      19081-19086
      MRI Guided, 19085-19086
      Stereotactic Guided, 19081-
        19082
      Ultrasound Guided, 19083-19084
      with Specimen Imaging, 19085-19086
  Catheter Placement
    for Interstitial Radioelement Applica-
      tion, 19296-19298, 20555
  Catheter Placement for Application Intersti-
    tial Radioelement, 19296-19298
  Cryosurgical Ablation, 19105
  Cyst
    Excision, 19120
    Puncture Aspiration, 19000-19001
  Excision
    Biopsy, 19100-19101
    Chest Wall Tumor, 21601-21603
    Cyst, 19120
    Lactiferous Duct Fistula, 19112
    Lesion, 19120-19126
      Needle Localization, 19125-
        19126

Breast — *continued*
  Excision — *continued*
    Mastectomy, 19300-19307
    Nipple Exploration, 19110
    Tumors, 19120, 21601-21603
  Exploration
    Abscess, 19020
    Nipple, 19110
  Mastectomy
    Complete, 19303
    Gynecomastia, 19300
    Modified Radical, 19307
    Partial, 19301-19302
    Radical, 19303-19306
  Needle Biopsy, 19100
  Removal
    Modified Radical, 19307
    Partial, 19300-19302
    Radical, 19305-19306
    Simple, Complete, 19303
  Stereotactic Localization, 19081
  Tumor
    Excision
      Benign, 19120
      Chest Wall, 21601-21603
      Malignant, 19120
      with Ribs, 21601-21603
Breath Test
  Hydrogen, 91065
  Methane, 91065
Brisement Injection, 20550-20551
Bulla
  Incision and Drainage
    Puncture Aspiration, 10160
BUN, 84525
Burhenne Procedure, 43500
  Bile Duct, Removal of Calculus, 43264,
    47420-47425, 47554
Burns
  Debridement, 15002-15005, 16020-16030
  Dressing, 16020-16030
  Escharotomy, 15002-15005, 16035-16036
  Excision, 15002, 15004-15005
  Tissue Culture Skin Grafts, 15100-15101,
    15120-15121
Bursa
  Ankle, 27604
    Aspiration or Injection, 20605-20606
  Arm
    Lower
      Aspiration or Injection, 20605-
        20606
    Upper, 23931
      Aspiration or Injection, 20610-
        20611
  Elbow, 23931
    Aspiration or Injection, 20605-20606
  Finger, 20600-20604
  Hip
    Aspiration or Injection, 20610-20611
  Injection, 20600-20611
  Joint, 20600-20611
  Knee
    Aspiration or Injection, 20610-20611
  Leg
    Lower, 27604
      Aspiration or Injection, 20605-
        20606
    Upper
      Aspiration or Injection, 20610-
        20611
  Shoulder
    Aspiration or Injection, 20610-20611
  Toe, 20600-20604
  Wrist
    Aspiration or Injection, 20605-20606
Bypass Graft
  Excision
    Abdomen, 35907
  Repair
    Abdomen, 35907
  Secondary Repair, 35870
  Thrombectomy, 37184-37186

C

Calcium
  Deposits
    Removal, Calculi–Stone
      Bile Duct, 43264, 47420-47425,
        47554
      Gallbladder, 47480
      Hepatic Duct, 47400
      Pancreas, 48020
      Pancreatic Duct, 43264
Calculus
  Destruction
    Bile Duct, 43265
    Pancreatic Duct, 43265
  Removal
    Bile Duct, 43264, 47554
    Biliary Tract, 47400-47425, 47480
    Liver, 47400
    Pancreatic Duct, 43264, 48020
Cannulation
  Arterial, 36620-36625
  Arteriovenous, 36810-36815
  Endoscopic
    Common Bile Duct, 43273
    Pancreatic Duct, 43273
    Papilla, 43273
  Vein to Vein, 36800
Cannulization
  Arteriovenous (AV), 36810-36815, 36901-
    36903
  Declotting, 36593, 36860-36861
  Dialysis Circuit, 36901-36903
  External
    Declotting, 36860-36861
  Vein to Vein, 36800
Capsule
  Biopsy of Intestine, 44100
  Endoscopy, 91110-91111 [91113]
    Magnetically Controlled, 0651T
Carbuncle
  Incision and Drainage, 10060-10061
Cardiac Catheterization
  Flow Directed, 93503
  Insertion Swan-Ganz, 93503
Cardiology
  Diagnostic
    Electrocardiogram
      Evaluation, 93000, 93010
      Recording, 93000-93005
      Rhythm, 93040-93042
      Tracing, 93005
  Therapeutic
    Cardiopulmonary Resuscitation,
      92950
Cardioplasty, 43320
Cardiopulmonary Resuscitation, 92950
Carotid Artery
  Excision, 60605
Carotid Body
  Lesion
    Carotid Artery, 60605
    Excision, 60600
Carpal Bone
  Ligament Release, 29848
Carpal Tunnel Syndrome
  Decompression, 64721
    Arthroscopy, 29848
  Median Nerve Neuroplasty, 64721
Case Management Services
  Online, 99446-99449, 98970-98972
  Referral, [99451, 99452]
  Team Conferences, 99366-99368
  Telephone Calls
    Consult Physician, 99446-99449
    Physician, 99441-99443
Catheter
  Blood Specimen Collection, 36592
  Breast
    for Interstitial Radioelement Applica-
      tion, 19296-19298
  Central Venous
    Repair, 36575
    Replacement, 36580-36581, 36584
    Repositioning, 36597
    Declotting, 36593, 36861

Catheter — *continued*
  Drainage
    Biliary, 47533-47537
    Peritoneal, 49406-49407
    Pleural, 32556-32557
    Retroperitoneal, 49406-49407
  Embolization
    Peritoneal, 49423
  Enteral Alimentation, 44015
  Exchange
    Drainage, 49423
    Peritoneal, 49423
  Flow Directed, 93503
  Intracatheter
    Obstruction Clearance, 36596
  Intraperitoneal
    Tunneled
      Laparoscopic, 49324
      Open, 49421
      Percutaneous, 49418-49419
  Pericatheter
    Obstruction Clearance, 36595
  Placement
    Breast
      for Interstitial Radioelement
        Placement, 19296-19298,
        20555
    Muscle and/or Soft Tissue, 20555
  Removal
    Central Venous, 36589
    Obstruction, 36595-36596
    Peritoneum, 49422
  Repair
    Central Venous, 36575
    Intraperitoneal, 49325
  Replacement
    Central Venous, 36580-36581, 36584
  Repositioning, 36597
  Transcatheter Therapy, 36640
Catheterization
  Abdomen, 49324, 49418-49421
  Arterial
    Arteriovenous Shunt
      Dialysis Circuit, 36901-36903
      Cutdown, 36625
      Percutaneous, 36620
  Arteriovenous Shunt
    Dialysis Circuit, 36901-36903
  Bile Duct
    Change, 47535-47536
    Percutaneous, 47533-47534
    Removal, 47537
  Cardiac
    Flow Directed, 93503
    Insertion Swan-Ganz, 93503
  Central, 36555-36563, 36578-36583
  Dialysis, 49418-49421
  Dialysis Circuit, 36901-36903
  Gastrointestinal, 43241
  Hepatic Vein, 37182-37183
  Interstitial Radioelement Application
    Breast, 19296-19298
    Genitalia, 55920
    Muscle, 20555
    Pelvic Organs, 55920
    Soft Tissue, 20555
  Intraperitoneal Tunneled, 49324, 49421
  Jejunum
    for Enteral Therapy, 44015
  Peripheral, 36568-36571, 36584 [36572,
    36573]
  Pleural Cavity, 32550-32551
  Portal Vein, 37182-37183
  Removal
    Obstructive Material
      Intracatheter, 36596
      Pericatheter, 36595
  Venous
    Central–Line, 36555-36563, 36578-
      36583
    Peripheral, 36568-36571, 36584-
      36585 [36572, 36573]
    with Cholecystostomy, 47490
Cauterization
  Anus
    Bleeding Control, 46614

Cauterization — *continued*
  Anus — *continued*
    Destruction of Hemorrhoid(s), 46930
    Fissure, 46940-46942
    Removal
      Polyp
        Multiple, 46612
        Single, 46610
      Tumor
        Multiple, 46612
        Single, 46610
  Colon
    Bleeding Control, 45334, 45382
    Removal Tumor, 45333, 45384
  Esophagus
    Removal Tumor, 43216, 43250
  Lower Esophageal Sphincter
    Thermal via Endoscopy, 43257
  Rectum
    Bleeding Control, 45317
    Removal Polyp
      Multiple, 45315
      Single, 45308
    Removal Tumor, 45308
      Multiple, 45315
      Single, 45308
  Small Intestine
    Bleeding Control, 44366, 44378,
      44391
    Removal Polyp(s), 44366, 44392
    Removal Tumor(s), 44365-44366,
      44392
Cecostomy
  Contrast, 49465
  Laparoscopic, 44188
  Obstructive Material Removal, 49460
  Radiological Evaluation, 49465
  Skin Level, 44320
  Tube Imaging, 49465
  Tube Insertion
    Open, 44300
    Percutaneous, 49442
  Tube Replacement, 49450
  with Colectomy, 44141
Celestin Procedure, 43510
Celiotomy, 49000
Cell
  Count
    Bacterial Colony, 87086
Central Venous Catheter (CVC)
  Insertion
    Central, 36555-36563, 36578-36583
    Non-tunneled, 36555-36556
    Peripheral, 36568-36569, 36584-
      36585 [36572, 36573]
      with Port, 36570-36571
    Tunneled
      with Port, 36560-36561
      with Pump, 36563
      without Port or Pump, 36557-
        36558
  Removal, 36589
  Repair, 36575-36576
  Replacement, 36580-36585
    Catheter Only, 36578
  Repositioning, 36597
Central Venous Catheter Removal, 36589-
  36590
Cervical Lymphadenectomy, 38720-38724
Cervicectomy
  Pelvic Exenteration, 45126
Change
  Stent
    (Endoscopic), Bile or Pancreatic Duct,
      [43275, 43276]
  Tube
    Gastrostomy, 43762-43763
Cheek
  Wound Repair, 13131-13133
Chemistry Tests
  Organ or Disease Oriented Panel
    Electrolyte, 80051
    Lipid Panel, 80061
Chemodenervation
  Anal Sphincter, 46505
  Internal Anal Sphincter, 46505

Chemodenervation — *continued*
  Muscle
    Trunk, 64646-64647
    Trunk Muscle, 64646-64647
Chemosurgery
  Mohs Technique, 17311-17315
Chemotherapy
  Intra–arterial
    Catheterization, 36640
  Peritoneal Cavity
    Catheterization, 49418
Chest Wall
  Debridement, 11044, 11047
  Reconstruction, 49904
    Lung Tumor Resection, 32504
  Resection, 32503
  Tumor
    Excision, 21601-21603
Chest
  Exploration
    Penetrating Wound, 20101
  Tube, 32551
  Wound Exploration
    Penetrating, 20101
Child Procedure, 48146
Chin
  Wound Repair, 13131-13133
Chloride
  Panels
    Electrolyte, 80051
CHOL, 82465, 83718-83722
Cholangiography
  Injection, 47531-47533
  Repair
    with Bile Duct Exploration, 47700
    with Cholecystectomy, 47620
    with Cholecystectomy, 47563, 47605
Cholangiopancreatography
  Destruction of Calculus, 43264-43265
  Diagnostic, 43260
  Exchange Stent, [43276]
  Papillotomy, 43262
  Pressure Measurement Sphincter of Oddi,
    43263
  Removal
    Calculus, 43264-43265
    Foreign Body, [43275, 43276]
    Stent, [43275, 43276]
  Specimen Collection, 43260
  Sphincterotomy, 43262 [43274, 43276,
    43277]
  Stent Placement, [43274]
  with Ablation, [43278]
  with Biopsy, 43261
  with Optical Endomicroscopy, 0397T
  with Surgery, 43262-43265 [43274, 43275,
    43276]
Cholecystectomy
  Donor Liver Preparation, 47143
  Laparoscopic, 47562-47570
    with Cholangiography, 47563
    with Exploration Common Duct,
      47564
  Open Approach, 47600-47620
    with Cholangiography, 47605, 47620
    with Choledochoenterostomy, 47612
    with Exploration Common Duct,
      47610
Cholecystoenterostomy
  Direct, 47720
  Laparoscopic, 47570
  Roux-en-Y, 47740-47741
  with Gastroenterostomy, 47721, 47741
Cholecystostomy
  Open, 47480
  Percutaneous, 47490
  with Placement Peripancreatic Drains,
    48000
Cholecystotomy
  Open, 47480
  Percutaneous, 47490
  with Choledochostomy, 47420
  with Choledochotomy, 47420
Choledochoscopy, 47550
Choledochostomy, 47420-47425
Choledochotomy, 47420-47425

Cholesterol
Lipid Panel, 80061
Measurement
HDL, 83718
LDL, 83721-83722
VLDL, 83719
Serum, 82465
Testing, 83718-83722
Cimino Type Procedure, 36821
Clavicle
Arthrocentesis, 20605
Closure
Anal Fistula, 46288
Enterostomy, 44620-44626
Laparoscopic, 44227
Esophagostomy, 43420-43425
Fistula
Anal, 46288, 46706
Anorectal, 46707
Enterovesical, 44660-44661
Ileoanal Pouch, 46710-46712
Tracheoesophageal, 43305, 43312, 43314
Gastrostomy, 43870
Skin
Abdomen
Complex, 13100-13102
Intermediate, 12031-12037
Layered, 12031-12037
Simple, 12001-12007
Superficial, 12001-12007
Arm, Arms
Complex, 13120-13122
Intermediate, 12031-12037
Layered, 12031-12037
Simple, 12001-12007
Superficial, 12001-12007
Axilla, Axillae
Complex, 13131-13133
Intermediate, 12031-12037
Layered, 12031-12037
Simple, 12001-12007
Superficial, 12001-12007
Back
Complex, 13100-13102
Intermediate, 12031-12037
Layered, 12031-12037
Simple, 12001-12007
Superficial, 12001-12007
Breast
Complex, 13100-13102
Intermediate, 12031-12037
Layered, 12031-12037
Simple, 12001-12007
Superficial, 12001-12007
Buttock
Complex, 13100-13102
Intermediate, 12031-12037
Layered, 12031-12037
Simple, 12001-12007
Superficial, 12001-12007
Chest
Complex, 13100-13102
Intermediate, 12031-12037
Layered, 12031-12037
Simple, 12001-12007
Superficial, 12001-12007
Extremity, Extremities
Intermediate, 12031-12037
Layered, 12031-12037
Simple, 12001-12007
Superficial, 12001-12007
Forearm, Forearms
Complex, 13120-13122
Intermediate, 12031-12037
Layered, 12031-12037
Simple, 12001-12007
Superficial, 12001-12007
Leg, Legs
Complex, 13120-13122
Intermediate, 12031-12037
Layered, 12031-12037
Simple, 12001-12007
Superficial, 12001-12007

Closure — continued
Skin — continued
Lower
Arm, Arms
Complex, 13120-13122
Intermediate, 12031-12037
Layered, 12031-12037
Simple, 12001-12007
Superficial, 12001-12007
Extremity, Extremities
Intermediate, 12031-12037
Layered, 12031-12037
Simple, 12001-12007
Superficial, 12001-12007
Leg, Legs
Complex, 13120-13122
Intermediate, 12031-12037
Layered, 12031-12037
Simple, 12001-12007
Superficial, 12001-12007
Neck
Complex, 13131-13133
Intermediate, 12041-12047
Layered, 12041-12047
Simple, 12001-12007
Superficial, 12001-12007
Scalp
Complex, 13120-13122
Intermediate, 12031-12037
Layered, 12031-12037
Simple, 12001-12007
Superficial, 12001-12007
Trunk
Complex, 13100-13102
Intermediate, 12031-12037
Layered, 12031-12037
Simple, 12001-12007
Superficial, 12001-12007
Upper
Arm, Arms
Complex, 13120-13122
Intermediate, 12031-12037
Layered, 12031-12037
Simple, 12001-12007
Superficial, 12001-12007
Extremity
Intermediate, 12031-12037
Layered, 12031-12037
Simple, 12001-12007
Superficial, 12001-12007
Leg, Legs
Complex, 13120-13122
Intermediate, 12031-12037
Layered, 12031-12037
Simple, 12001-12007
Superficial, 12001-12007
CNP, 94662
CNPB (Continuous Negative Pressure Breathing), 94662
Coccygectomy, 15920-15922
Coccyx
Pressure Ulcer, 15920-15922
Tumor
Excision, 49215
Colectomy
Miles', 44155
Partial, 44140
Transanal Approach, 44147
with
Anastomosis, 44140
Laparoscopic, 44213
Coloproctostomy, 44145-44146
Colostomy, 44141-44144
Laparoscopic, 44205
Ileocolostomy, Laparoscopic, 44205
Ileostomy, 44144
Mobilization Splenic Flexure, 44139
Laparoscopic, 44213
Removal Ileum, 44160
Total
Laparoscopic
with
Ileoproctostomy, 44210
Ileostomy, 44210-44212

Colectomy — continued
Total — continued
Laparoscopic — continued
with — continued
Proctectomy, 44211-44212
Proctectomy and Ileoanal Anastomosis, 44211
Proctectomy and Ileostomy, 44212
Rectal Mucosectomy, 44211
without Proctectomy, 44210
Open
with
Complete Proctectomy, 45121
Ileal Reservoir, 44158
Ileoanal Anastomosis, 44157
Ileoproctostomy, 44150
Ileostomy, 44150-44151
Proctectomy, 44155-44158
Collection and Processing
Brushings
Abdomen, 49320
Anus, 46600-46601
Biliary Tract, 47552
Colon, 44388, 45300, 45330, 45378
Duodenum, 43235, 44360, 44376
Esophagus, 43197, 43200, 43235
Hepatobiliary System, 43260
Ileum, 44376, 44380
Jejunum, 43235
Omentum, 49320
Peritoneum, 49320
Rectum, 45300, 45330
Small Intestine, 44385
Stomach, 43235
Specimen
Duodenum, 43756-43757
Hematoma, 10140
Implantable Venous Access Device, 36591
Stomach, 43754
Venous Access Device, 36591
Venous Blood, 36591-36592
Venous Catheter, 36592
Washings
Abdomen, 49320
Anus, 46600-46601
Biliary, 47552
Colon, 44388, 45300, 45330, 45378
Duodenum, 43235, 44360, 44376
ERCP, 43260
Esophageal, 43197, 43200, 43235
Hepatobiliary System, 43260
Ileum, 44376, 44380
Jejunum, 43235
Omentum, 49320
Peritoneum, 49320
Small Intestine, 44360, 44376, 44380, 44385
Stomach, 43235
Upper GI, 43235
Collis Procedure, 43338
Colon–Sigmoid
Biopsy
Endoscopy, 45331
Decompression, 45378
Volvulus, 45337
Dilation, 45340
Endoscopy
Ablation
Polyp, [45346]
Tumor, [45346]
Biopsy, 45331
Dilation, 45340
Exploration, 45330, 45335
Hemorrhage, 45334
Needle Biopsy, 45342
Placement
Stent, 45327, 45347
Removal
Foreign Body, 45332
Polyp, 45333, 45338

Colon–Sigmoid — continued
Endoscopy — continued
Removal — continued
Tumor, 45333, 45338
Ultrasound, 45341-45342
Volvulus, 45337
Exploration
Endoscopy, 45330, 45335
Hemorrhage
Endoscopy, 45334
Needle Biopsy
Endoscopy, 45342
Removal
Foreign Body, 45332
Repair
Volvulus
Endoscopy, 45337
Ultrasound
Endoscopy, 45341-45342
Colon
Biopsy, 44025, 44100, 44322
by Colonoscopy, 45378
Endoscopic, 44389, 45380, 45392
Capsule Endoscopy, [91113]
Colostomy, 44320-44322
Revision, 44340-44346
Colotomy, 44322
Colostomy, 44322
Destruction
Lesion, [44401, 45388]
Tumor, [44401, 45388]
Endoscopy
Band Ligation, [45398]
Biopsy, 44389, 44407, 45380, 45392
Collection of Specimen, 44388, 45378
Decompression, 44408, 45393
Destruction
Lesion, [44401, 45388]
Tumor, [44401, 45388]
Dilation, 44405, 45386
Exploration, 44388, 45378
Hemorrhage, 44391, 45382
Injection, Submucosal, 44404, 45381
Mucosal Resection, 44403, 45349 [45390]
Placement
Stent, 44402, 45389
Removal
Foreign Body, 44390, 45379
Polyp, 44392, 44394, 45384-45385
Tumor, 44392, 44394, 45384-45385
Ultrasound, 44406-44407, 45391-45392
via Stoma, 44388-44394, 44402-44408 [44401]
Excision
Partial, 44140-44147, 44160
Laparoscopic, 44204-44208
Total, 44150-44158
Laparoscopic, 44210-44212
Exclusion, 44700
Exploration, 44025
Endoscopic, 44388, 45378, 45381, 45386
Hemorrhage
Endoscopic Control, 44391, 45382
Hernia, 44050
Incision
Creation
Stoma, 44320-44322
Exploration, 44025
Revision
Stoma, 44340-44346
Intraluminal Imaging, [91113]
Lavage
Intraoperative, 44701
Lesion
Destruction, [44401, 45388]
Excision, 44110-44111
Lysis
Adhesions, 44005
Motility Study, 91117
Obstruction, 44025-44050

Destruction — continued
Lesion
Anus, 46900-46917, 46924
Colon, [44401, 45388]
Gastrointestinal, Upper, [43270]
Intestines
Large, [44401, 45388]
Small, 44369
Rectum, 45320
Molluscum Contagiosum, 46900-46924
Muscle Endplate
Trunk, 64646-64647
Nerve, 64646-64647
Polyp
Rectum, 45320
Tumor
Abdomen, 49203-49205
Bile Duct, [43278]
Chemosurgery, 17311-17315
Colon, [44401, 45388]
Intestines
Large, [44401, 45388]
Small, 44369
Mesentery, 49203-49205
Pancreatic Duct, [43278]
Peritoneum, 49203-49205
Rectum, 45190, 45320
Retroperitoneal, 49203-49205
Tumor or Polyp
Rectum, 45320
Device
Adjustable Gastric Restrictive Device, 43770-43774
Drug Delivery, 20700-20701
Handling, 99002
Subcutaneous Port
for Gastric Restrictive Device, 43770, 43774, 43886-43888
Venous Access
Collection of Blood Specimen, 36591-36592
Implanted, 36591
Venous Catheter, 36592
Fluoroscopic Guidance, 77001
Insertion
Catheter, 36578
Central, 36560-36563
Obstruction Clearance, 36595-36596
Peripheral, 36570-36571
Removal, 36590
Repair, 36576
Replacement, 36582-36583, 36585
Obstruction Clearance, 36595-36596
Removal, 36590
Repair, 36576
Replacement, 36582-36583, 36585
Catheter, 36578
Dialysis
Arteriovenous Fistula
Revision
without Thrombectomy, 36832
Thrombectomy, 36831
Arteriovenous Shunt, 36901-36909
Revision
with Thrombectomy, 36833
Thrombectomy, 36831
Dialysis Circuit, 36901-36909
Peritoneal
Catheter Insertion, 49418-49421
Catheter Removal, 49422
Diaphragm
Imbrication for Eventration, 39545
Repair
Esophageal Hiatal, 43280-43282, 43325
for Eventration, 39545
Hernia, 39503-39541
Neonatal, 39503
Laceration, 39501
Resection, 39560-39561
Differential Count
White Blood Cell Count, 85007

Digit(s)
Skin Graft
Split, 15120-15121
Dilation
Anal
Endoscopic, 46604
Sphincter, 45905, 46940
Bile Duct
Endoscopic, 47555-47556 [43277]
Colon
Endoscopy, 45386
Colon–Sigmoid
Endoscopy, 45340
Esophagus, 43450-43453
Endoscopic Balloon, 43195, 43220, 43249 [43213, 43214, 43233]
Endoscopy, 43195-43196, 43220-43226, 43248-43249 [43213, 43214, 43233]
Surgical, 43510
Gastric/Duodenal Stricture, 43245
Open, 43510
Intestines, Small
Endoscopy, 44370
Open, 44615
Stent Placement, 44379
Pancreatic Duct
Endoscopy, [43277]
Rectum
Endoscopy, 45303
Sphincter, 45910
Discharge Services
Observation Care, 99217, 99234-99236
Dissection
Donor Organs
Liver, 47143
Pancreas, 48551
Hygroma, Cystic
Axillary, 38550-38555
Cervical, 38550-38555
Lymph Nodes, 38542
Mediastinal, 60521-60522
Neurovascular, 32503
Diverticulectomy, 44800
Esophagus, 43130-43135
Diverticulum
Meckel's
Excision, 44800
Repair
Large Intestine, 44604-44605
Small Intestine, 44602-44603
Division
Anal Sphincter, 46080
Rectal Stricture, 45150
Saphenous Vein, 37700-37735
Donor Procedures
Backbench Preparation Prior to Transplan-
tation
Intestine, 44715-44721
Liver, 47143-47147
Pancreas, 48551-48552
Intestine, 44132-44133
Liver, 47140-47142
Preparation Fecal Microbiota, 44705
Drainage
Abdomen
Abdominal Fluid, 49082-49083
Paracentesis, 49082-49083
Peritoneal, 49020
Peritoneal Lavage, 49084
Peritonitis, Localized, 49020
Retroperitoneal, 49060
Subdiaphragmatic, 49040
Subphrenic, 49040
Wall
Skin and Subcutaneous Tissue, 10060-10061
Complicated, 10061
Multiple, 10061
Simple, 10060
Single, 10060
Abscess
Abdomen, 49040
Peritoneal
Open, 49020
Peritonitis, localized, 49020

Drainage — continued
Abscess — continued
Abdomen — continued
Retroperitoneal
Open, 49060
Skin and Subcutaneous Tissue
Complicated, 10061
Multiple, 10061
Simple, 10060
Single, 10060
Subdiaphragmatic, 49040
Subphrenic, 49040
Anal
Incision and Drainage, 46045-46060
Ankle
Incision and Drainage, 27603
Appendix
Incision and Drainage, 44900
Arm, Upper
Incision and Drainage, 23930-23931
Bartholin's Gland
Puncture Aspiration, 10160
Biliary Tract, 47400-47425, 47480, 47533-47536
Breast
Incision and Drainage, 19020
Elbow
Incision and Drainage, 23930-23931
Ganglion Cyst, 20600-20605
Hematoma
Incision and Drainage, 27603
Hip
Incision and Drainage, 26990
Leg, Lower, 27603
Incision and Drainage, 27603
Liver
Incision and Drainage
Open, 47010
Injection, 47015
Repair, 47300
Lymph Node, 38300-38305
Lymphocele, 49062, 49185
Neck
Incision and Drainage, 21501-21502
Pelvic
Percutaneous, 49406
Supralevator, 45020
Transrectal, 49407
Transvaginal, 49407
Pelvis, 26990
Incision and Drainage, 26990, 45000
Peritoneum
Open, 49020
Rectum
Incision and Drainage, 45005-45020, 46040, 46060
Retroperitoneal
Laparoscopic, 49323
Open, 49060
Skin
Incision and Drainage
Complicated, 10061
Multiple, 10061
Simple, 10060
Single, 10060
Puncture Aspiration, 10160
Soft Tissue
Image-Guided by Catheter, 10030
Percutaneous, 10030
Subfascial, 22010-22015
Spine, Subfascial, 22010-22015
Subdiaphragmatic
Incision and Drainage, 49040
Subphrenic, 49040
Thoracostomy, 32551
Thorax
Incision and Drainage, 21501-21502
Visceral, 49405

Drainage — continued
Bile Duct
Transhepatic, 47533-47534
Bursa
Arm, Upper, 23931
Arthrocentesis, 20600-20612
Elbow, 23931
Leg, 27604
Cyst
Breast, 19000-19001
Ganglion, 20612
Liver, 47010
Pilonidal, 10080-10081
Elbow, 23930
Extraperitoneal Lymphocele
Laparoscopic, 49323
Open, 49062
Percutaneous, Sclerotherapy, 49185
Fluid
Abdominal, 49082-49083
Peritoneal
Percutaneous, 49406
Transrectal, 49407
Transvaginal, 49407
Retroperitoneal
Percutaneous, 49406
Transrectal, 49407
Transvaginal, 49407
Visceral, 49405
Ganglion Cyst, 20612
Hematoma
Ankle, 27603
Joint, 20600-20610
Superficial, 10140
Joint
Hip, 26990
Pelvis, 26990
Liver
Abscess or Cyst, 47010
Lymph Node, 38300-38305
Lymphocele, 49062
Laparoscopic, 49323
Percutaneous, Sclerotherapy, 49185
Pancreas
Pseudocyst, 48510
Peritonitis, 49020
Pleura, 32556-32557
Postoperative Wound Infection, 10180
Pseudocyst
Gastrointestinal, Upper
Transmural Endoscopic, 43240
Pancreas
Open, 48510
Rectum Injury, 45562
Seroma, 10140, 49185
Skin, 10060-10180
Via Tube Thoracostomy, 32551
Dressings
Burns, 16020-16030
Change Under Anesthesia, 15852
Drug Delivery Implant
Insertion, 11981
Removal, 11982-11983
with Reinsertion, 11983
Drug
Delivery Device, 20700-20701
Infusion, 96369-96371
Dry Needle Insertion, [20560, 20561]
Duhamel Procedure, 45120
Duodenectomy
Near Total, 48153-48154
Total, 48150-48152
Duodenostomy
Injection, 49465
Insertion, 49441
Obstructive Material Removal, 49460
Replacement, 49451
Duodenotomy, 44010
Duodenum
Biopsy, 44010
Contrast Injection, 49465
Correction Malrotation, 44055
Endoscopy, 43235-43259 [43233, 43266, 43270]
Diagnostic, 43235
Dilation, 43245

Duodenum — *continued*
  Endoscopy — *continued*
    Placement Catheter or Tube, 43241
    Ultrasound, 43242, 43253, 43259
  Excision, 48150-48154
  Exclusion, 48547
  Exploration, 44010
  Incision, 44010
  Intubation, 43756-43757
  Motility Study, 91022
  Removal Foreign Body, 44010
  Repositioning Feeding Tube, 43761

E

Ear
  External
    Repair
      Complex, 13151-13153
      Intermediate, 12051-12057
      Simple, 12011-12018
      Superficial, 12011-12018
    Removal Skin Lesions
      Excision
        Benign, 11440-11446
        Malignant, 11640-11646
ECG, 93000-93010, 93040-93042
Education, 99078
  Services (group), 99078
  Supplies, 99071
EGD, 43235-43259 [43233, 43266, 43270]
EKG, 93000-93010
  Rhythm Strips, 93040-93042
  Routine, 93000-93010
Elastography
  Ultrasound, Parenchyma, 76981-76983
Elbow
  Abscess
    Incision and Drainage, 23930
  Arthrocentesis, 20605-20606
  Biopsy, 24065-24066
  Excision
    Tumor
      Soft Tissue, 24077-24079
      Subcutaneous, 24075
      [24071]
      Subfascial, 24076 [24073]
  Exploration, 24065-24066, 24075-24079
    [24071, 24073]
  Hematoma
    Incision and Drainage, 23930
  Incision and Drainage
    Abscess, Deep, 23930
    Bursa, 23931
    Hematoma, 23930
  Radical Resection
    Soft Tissue Tumor, 24077-24079
  Tumor
    Excision, 24076 [24071]
    Radical Resection, 24077-24079
Electrical Stimulation
  Acupuncture, 97813-97814
Electrocardiogram, 93000-93010
  Rhythm Strips, 93040-93042
    Interpretation and Report Only, 93042
    Tracing Only Without Interpretation
      and Report, 93041
    with Interpretation and Report, 93040
  Routine 12-Lead, 93000-93010
Electrocardiography
  12-Lead ECG, 93000
  Evaluation, 93000, 93010
  Rhythm, 93040
    1-3 Leads, 93040
    Evaluation, 93042
    Interpretation and Report Only, 93042
    Tracing and Evaluation, 93040
    Tracing Only without Interpretation
      and Report, 93005, 93041
  Routine; at Least 12 Leads, 93000-93010
    Interpretation and Report Only, 93010
    Tracing Only, without Interpretation
      and Report, 93005
    with Interpretation and Report, 93000
  Tracing, 93005
Electrogastrography, 91132-91133

Electronic Analysis
  Neurostimulator Pulse Generator, 95980-95982
  Pulse Generator, 95980-95982
    Gastric Neurostimulator, 95980-95982
Electrosurgery
  Anal, 46924
  Rectal Tumor, 45190
Empyema
  Thoracostomy, 32551
Endometrioma
  Abdomen
    Destruction, 49203-49205
    Excision, 49203-49205
  Mesenteric
    Destruction, 49203-49205
    Excision, 49203-49205
  Peritoneal
    Destruction, 49203-49205
    Excision, 49203-49205
  Retroperitoneal
    Destruction, 49203-49205
    Excision, 49203-49205
Endorectal Pull-Through
  Proctectomy, Total, 45110, 45112, 45120-45121
Endoscopic Retrograde Cholangiopancreatography
  Ablation Lesion/Polyp/Tumor, [43278]
  Balloon Dilation, [43277]
  Destruction of Calculi, 43265
  Diagnostic, 43260
  Measure Pressure Sphincter of Oddi, 43263
  Placement
    Stent, [43274]
      with Removal and Replacement, [43276]
  Removal
    Calculi or Debris, 43264
    Foreign Body, [43275]
    Stent, [43275]
      with Stent Exchange, [43276]
  Removal Calculi or Debris, 43264
  with Optical Endomicroscopy, 0397T
Endoscopy
  Adrenal Gland
    Biopsy, 60650
    Excision, 60650
  Anal
    Ablation
      Polyp, 46615
      Tumor, 46615
    Biopsy, 46606-46607
    Collection of Specimen, 46600-46601
    Diagnostic, 46600-46601
    Dilation, 46604
    Exploration, 46600
    Hemorrhage, 46614
    High Resolution, 46601, 46607
    Removal
      Foreign Body, 46608
      Polyp, 46610, 46612
      Tumor, 46610, 46612
  Bile Duct
    Biopsy, 47553
    Cannulation, 43273
    Destruction
      Calculi (Stone), 43265
      Tumor, [43278]
    Diagnostic, 47552
    Dilation, 47555-47556 [43277]
    Exchange
      Stent, [43276]
    Exploration, 47552
    Intraoperative, 47550
    Percutaneous, 47552-47556
    Removal
      Calculi (Stone), 43264, 47554
      Foreign Body, [43275]
      Stent, [43275]
    Specimen Collection, 43260
    Sphincter Pressure, 43263
    Sphincterotomy, 43262 [43274]
    Stent Placement, [43274]
  Cannulization
    Papilla, 43273

Endoscopy — *continued*
  Capsule, 91110-91111 [91113]
    Magnetically Controlled, 0651T
  Colon
    Ablation, [44401, 45388]
    Band Ligation, [45398]
    Biopsy, 44389, 44407, 45380, 45392
    Collection of Specimen, 44388, 45378
    Decompression, 44408, 45393
    Destruction
      Lesion, [44401, 45388]
      Tumor, [44401, 45388]
    Dilation, 44405, 45386
    Exploration, 44388, 45378
    Hemorrhage, 44391, 45382
    Injection, Submucosal, 44404, 45381
    Placement
      Stent, 44402, 45389
    Removal
      Foreign Body, 44390, 45379
      Polyp, 44392, 44394, 45384-45385
      Tumor, 44392, 44394, 45384-45385
    Ultrasound, 44406-44407, 45391-45392
    via Stoma (Colostomy), 44388-44394, 44402-44408 [44401]
  Colon-Sigmoid
    Ablation
      Polyp, [45346]
      Tumor, [45346]
    Biopsy, 45331
    Dilation, 45340
    Exploration, 45330
      Specimen Collection, 45331
    Hemorrhage, 45334
    Injection, 45335
    Needle Biopsy, 45342
    Placement
      Stent, 45327, 45347
    Removal
      Foreign Body, 45332
      Polyp, 45333, 45338
      Tumor, 45333, 45338
    Specimen Collection, 45330
    Ultrasound, 45341-45342
    Volvulus, 45321, 45337
  Duodenum Ultrasound, 43253
  Endomicroscopy
    Esophageal, 43206
    Gastrointestinal, 43252
  Esophagus
    Biopsy, 43193, 43198, 43202
    Dilation, 43195-43226, 43229, 43248-43249 [43212, 43213, 43214, 43233]
    Exploration, 43191, 43197, 43200
    Hemorrhage, 43227
    Injection, 43192, 43201, 43204
      Varices, 43243
    Insertion Stent, [43212]
    Mucosal Resection, [43211]
    Needle Biopsy, 43232
    Removal
      Foreign Body, 43194, 43215
      Polyp, 43216-43217, 43229
      Tumor, 43216-43217, 43229
    Specimen Collection, 43197, 43200
    Ultrasound, 43231-43232, 43237-43238, 43242, 43253
    Vein Ligation, 43205
    with Optical Endomicroscopy, 43206
  Gastrointestinal
    Ablation
      Lesion, [43270]
      Polyp, [43270]
      Tumor, [43270]
    Capsule, 91110-91111 [91113]
      Magnetically Controlled, 0651T
    Upper
      Biopsy, 43239
      Catheterization, 43241
      Destruction of Lesion, [43270]
      Dilation, 43245, 43248-43249 [43233]

Endoscopy — *continued*
  Gastrointestinal — *continued*
    Upper — *continued*
      Drainage of Pseudocyst, 43240
      Exploration, 43235, 43252
      Foreign Body, 43247
      Gastric Bypass, 43644-43645
      Gastroenterostomy, 43644-43645
      Hemorrhage, 43255
      Inject Varices, 43243
      Injection, 43236, 43253
      Mucosal Resection, 43254
      Needle Biopsy, 43232, 43238, 43242
      Removal, 43247, 43250-43251
      Roux-En-Y, 43644
      Stent Placement, [43266]
      Thermal Radiation, 43257
      Tube Placement, 43246
      Ultrasound, 43237-43242, 43253, 43259
      Vein Ligation, 43244
      with Optical Endomicroscopy, 43252
  Ileum
    Biopsy, 44382
    Stent Insertion, 44384
    via Stoma, 44384
  Intestines, Small
    Ablation
      Polyp, 44369
      Tumor, 44369
    Biopsy, 44361, 44377
    Destruction
      Lesion, 44369
      Tumor, 44369
    Diagnostic, 44376
    Exploration, 44360
    Hemorrhage, 44366, 44378
    Insertion
      Stent, 44370, 44379
      Tube, 44379
    Pelvic Pouch, 44385-44386
    Placement
      Stent, 44370, 44379
      Tube, 44372-44373, 44379
    Removal
      Foreign Body, 44363
      Lesion, 44365
      Polyp, 44364-44365
      Tumor, 44364-44365
    Tube Placement, 44372
    Tube Revision, 44373
    via Stoma, 44380, 44382-44384 [44381]
      Tumor, 44364-44365
  Jejunum, 43253
  Pancreatic Duct
    Cannulation, 43273
    Destruction
      Calculi (Stone), 43265
      Tumor, [43278]
    Dilation, [43277]
    Removal
      Calculi (Stone), 43264
      Foreign Body, [43275]
      Stent, [43275, 43276]
    Specimen Collection, 43260
    Sphincter Pressure, 43263
    Sphincterotomy, 43262 [43274]
    Stent Placement, [43274]
  Rectum
    Ablation
      Polyp, 45320
      Tumor, 45320
    Biopsy, 45305
    Destruction
      Tumor, 45320
    Dilation, 45303
    Exploration, 45300
    Hemorrhage, 45317
    Removal
      Foreign Body, 45307
      Polyp, 45308-45315
      Tumor, 45308-45315

● New   ▲ Revised   + Add On   AMA: CPT Assist [Resequenced]

Endoscopy — continued
Rectum — continued
Volvulus, 45321
Sleep
Drug-induced, 42975
Spleen
Removal, 38120
Stomach, Ultrasound Examination, 43253
Endotracheal Tube
Intubation, 31500
Endovascular
Therapy
Ablation
Vein, 36473-36479
Endovenous Catheter Ablation, 36473-36479
Enema
Home Visit for Fecal Impaction, 99511
Enterectomy, 44126-44128, 44137
Donor, 44132-44133
for Congenital Atresia, 44126-44128
Laparoscopic, 44202-44203
Partial, 44133
Resection, 44120-44121
Transplanted Allograft, 44137
with Enterostomy, 44125
Enteroenterostomy, 44130
Enterolysis, 44005
Laparoscopic, 44180
Enterorrhaphy, 44602-44603, 44615
Enteroscopy
Intestines, Small
Biopsy, 44361, 44377
Control of Bleeding, 44378
Destruction
Lesion, 44369
Tumor, 44369
Diagnostic, 44376
Exploration, 44360
Hemorrhage, 44366
Pelvic Pouch, 44385-44386
Removal
Foreign Body, 44363
Lesion, 44364-44365
Polyp, 44364-44365
Tumor, 44364-44365
Tube Placement, 44372
Tube Revision, 44373
via Stoma, 44380, 44382-44384
[44381]
Tumor, 44364-44365
Enterostomy
Closure, 44227, 44620-44626
Tube Placement, 44300
with Enterectomy
Intestine, Small, 44125
with Enteroenterostomy, 44130
with Proctectomy, 45119, 45397
Enterotomy
Biopsy, 44020
Decompression, 44021
Excision of Lesion, 44110-44111
Exploration, 44020
Foreign Body Removal, 44020
Intestinal Stricturoplasty, 44615
Epigastric
Hernia Repair, 49570-49572
Laparoscopic, 49652
Epiploectomy, 49255
ERCP (Cholangiopancreatography), 43260-
43265 [43274, 43275, 43276, 43277,
43278]
Escharotomy
Burns, 16035-16036
Graft Site, 15002-15005
Esophageal Acid Infusion Test, 91030
Esophageal Myotomy
Lower Esophageal, 43497
Esophageal Varices
Decompression, 37181
Injection Sclerosis, 43204, 43243
Ligation, 43205, 43244
Esophagectomy
McKeown, 43112
Partial, 43116-43124
Total, 43107-43113, 43124, 43286-43288
Tri-incisional, [43211]

Esophagoenterostomy
with Total Gastrectomy, 43260
Esophagogastroduodenoscopy
Ablation Lesions/Polyps/Tumors, [43270]
Band Ligation of Varices, 43244
Biopsy (Single or Multiple), 43239, 0653T
Collection of Specimen, 43235
Control of Bleeding, 43255
Delivery of Thermal Energy, 43257
Diagnostic, 43235, 0652T
Dilation, 43245, 43248-43249 [43233]
Directed Submucosal Injection(s), 43236
Drainage of Pseudocyst, 43240
Endoscopic Ultrasound Examination, 43237,
43259
Fine Needle Aspiration/Biopsy(s), 43238,
43242
Guide Wire Insertion, 43248
Injection
Anesthetic Agent, 43253
Diagnostic Substance(s), 43253
Fiducial Marker(s), 43253
Neurolytic Agent, 43253
Sclerosis Agent, 43243
Submucosal, 43236
Therapeutic Substance(s), 43253
Injection Varices, 43243
Insertion Intraluminal Tube or Catheter,
43241, 0654T
Mucosal Resection, 43254
Optical Endomicroscopy, 43252
Placement
Endoscopic Stent, [43266]
Gastrostomy Tube, 43246
Removal
Foreign Body, 43247
Lesion/Polyp/Tumor, 43250-43251
Transnasal, 0652T-0654T
Ultrasound Guided, 43237-43238, 43253,
43259
Esophagogastrostomy, 43112, 43320
Esophagojejunostomy, 43340-43341
Esophagomyotomy, 43330-43331
Abdominal, 43330
Heller Type, 43279, 43330
Laparoscopic, 43279
Thoracic Approach, 43331
With Fundoplasty, 43279
Esophagoplasty, 43300-43312
Congenital Defect, 43313-43314
Esophagoscopy
Dilation Over Guidewire, 43196
Transnasal
Biopsy, 43198
Collection of Specimen, 43197
Transoral
Ablation of Lesion, 43229
Collection of Specimen, 43191, 43200
Dilation, 43195-43226, 43229 [43212,
43213, 43214]
Exploration, 43200
Guide Wire Insertion, 43196, 43226,
43229 [43212]
Hemorrhage, 43227
Injection, 43192, 43201, 43204
Ligation of Varices, 43205
Mucosal Resection, [43211]
Needle Biopsy, 43232
Removal
Foreign Body, 43194, 43215
Polyp, 43216-43217, 43229
Tumor, 43216-43217, 43229
Stent Placement, [43212]
With Diverticulectomy, 43180
With Optical Endomicroscopy, 43206
With Ultrasound Examination, 43231-
43232
Ultrasound, 43231-43232
Vein Ligation, 43205
With Optical Endomicroscopy, 43206
Esophagostomy
Closure, 43420-43425
External Fistulization, 43351-43352
With Esophagectomy, 43124
Esophagotomy, 43020

Esophagus
Ablation
Lesion, 43229
Polyp, 43229
Tumor, 43229
Acid Perfusion Test, 91030
Acid Reflux Tests, 91034-91038
Balloon Distension, 43249 [43233]
Provocation Study, 91040
Biopsy
Endoscopy, 43198, 43202
Dilation, 43450-43453
Endoscopic, 43195-43226, 43229,
43248-43249 [43212, 43213,
43214, 43233]
Strictures
Duodenal, 43245
Gastric, 43245
Surgical, 43510
Endoscopy
Biopsy, 43193, 43198, 43202
Diagnostic, 43191, 43197, 43200
Dilation
Balloon, 43195 [43214, 43233]
Dilator Over Guide Wire, 43196,
43226, 43248
Retrograde by Balloon or Dilator,
[43213]
Transendoscopic with Balloon,
43220, 43249
Exploration, 43200
Hemorrhage, 43227
Injection, 43192, 43201, 43204, 43243,
43253
Insertion Stent, [43212]
Mucosal Resection, [43211]
Needle Biopsy, 43232
Removal
Foreign Body, 43194, 43215
Polyp, 43216-43217
Tumor, 43216-43217
Specimen Collection, 43191, 43197,
43200
Ultrasound, 43231-43232
Vein Ligation, 43205
Excision
Diverticula, 43130-43135
Partial, 43116-43124
Total, 43107-43113, 43124
Exploration
Endoscopy, 43200
Hemorrhage, 43227
Incision, 43020
Injection
Sclerosis Agent, 43204
Submucosal, 43192, 43201
Insertion
Sengstaken Tamponade, 43460
Stent, [43212]
Tamponade, 43460
Tube, 43510
Intraluminal Imaging, 91110-91111
Intubation with Specimen Collection,
43753-43755
Lengthening, 43283, 43338
Lesion
Excision, 43100-43101
Ligation, 43405
Motility Study, 91010-91013
Mucosal Resection, [43211]
Myotomy
Lower Esophageal, 43497
Needle Biopsy
Endoscopy, 43232
Reconstruction, 43300, 43310, 43313
Creation
Stoma, 43351-43352
Esophagostomy, 43351-43352
Fistula, 43305, 43312, 43314
Gastrointestinal, 43360-43361
Removal
Foreign Bodies, 43020, 43194, 43215
Lesion, 43216-43217
Polyp, 43216-43217
Repair, 43300, 43310, 43313

Esophagus — continued
Repair — continued
Esophagogastric Fundoplasty, 43325-
43328
Laparoscopic, 43280
Esophagogastrostomy, 43112, 43320
Esophagojejunostomy, 43340-43341
Esophagomyotomy, 43279
Esophagoplasty, 43300-43312
Fistula, 43305, 43312, 43314, 43420-
43425
Muscle, 43330-43331
Nissan Procedure, 43280
Paraesophageal Hernia
Laparoscopic, 43281-43282
Laparotomy, 43332-43333
Thoracoabdominal Incision,
43336-43337
Thoracotomy, 43334-43335
Pre-existing Perforation, 43405
Thal-Nissen Procedure, 43325
Toupet Procedure, 43280
Wound, 43410-43415
Stapling Gastroesophageal Junction, 43405
Suture
Gastroesophageal Junction, 43405
Wound, 43410-43415
Ultrasound, 43231-43232
Vein
Ligation, 43205
ESR, 85651
Established Patient
Critical Care, 99291-99292
Hospital Inpatient Services, 99221-99223,
99231-99236
Hospital Observation Services, 99217-
99220, 99234-99236 [99224, 99225,
99226]
Initial Inpatient Consultation, 99251-99255
Office and/or Other Outpatient Consulta-
tions, 99241-99245
Office Visit, 99211-99215
Online Evaluation and Management Ser-
vices
Nonphysician, 98970-98972
Physician, [99421, 99422, 99423]
Outpatient Visit, 99211-99215
Prolonged Services, 99354-99359 [99415,
99416, 99417]
with Patient Contact, 99354-99357
without Patient Contact, 99358-99359
Telephone Services, 99441-99443
Evacuation
Stomach, 43753
Evaluation and Management
Case Management Services, 99366-99368
Consultation, 99241-99255
Critical Care, 99291-99292
Hospital, 99221-99223, 99231-99233
Hospital Services
Initial, 99221-99223, 99231-99233
Observation Care, 99217-99220
Subsequent, 99231
Internet Communication
Consult Physician, 99446-99449
[99451]
Nonphysician, 98970-98972
Physician, [99421, 99422, 99423]
Referral, [99452]
Medical
Team Conference, 99366-99368
Observation Care, 99217-99220
Office and Other Outpatient, 99202-99215
Online Assessment
Consult Physician, 99446-99449
[99451]
Nonphysician, 98970-98972
Physician, [99421, 99422, 99423]
Referral, [99452]
Online Evaluation
Consult Physician, 99446-99449
[99451]
Nonphysician, 98970-98972
Physician, [99421, 99422, 99423]
Referral, [99452]
Physician Standby Services, 99360

Exploration — *continued*
  Rectum
    Endoscopic, 45300
    Injury, 45562-45563
  Retroperitoneal Area, 49010
  Stomach, 43500
Extremity
  Penetrating Wound, 20103
  Wound Exploration, 20103

F

Fenestration Procedure
  Tracheostomy, 31610
Fibroadenoma
  Ablation
    Cryosurgical, 19105
  Excision, 19120-19126
Fibula
  Tumor
    Radical Resection, 27615-27616
Fine Needle Aspiration, 10021 [10004, 10005,
  10006, 10007, 10008, 10009, 10010, 10011,
  10012]
  Evaluation
    Abdominal Mass, 49180
    Breast, 19081-19086
    General, 10021 [10004, 10005, 10006,
      10007, 10008, 10009, 10010,
      10011, 10012]
    Muscle, 20206
    Pancreas, 48102
    Retroperitoneal Mass, 49180
    Soft Tissue Drainage, 10030
    Thyroid, 60100
    Transendoscopic
      Colon, 45392
      Esophagogastroduodenoscopy,
        43238, 43242
      Esophagus, 43238
      Surgically Altered Stomach,
        43242
Finger
  Tumor
    Excision, 26115-26116 [26111, 26113]
    Radical Resection, 26117-26118
Fissurectomy, 46200, 46261-46262
Fistula
  Anal
    Repair, 46262-46288, 46706
  Anorectal
    Repair, 46707
  Arteriovenous, 36831-36833
    Injection, 36901-36903
    Revision
      with Thrombectomy, 36831
      without Thrombectomy, 36832
      Thrombectomy without revision,
        36831
    Autogenous Graft, 36825
  Enterovesical
    Closure, 44660-44661
  Ileoanal Pouch
    Repair, 46710-46712
  Tracheoesophageal
    Repair, 43305, 43312, 43314
Fistulectomy
  Anal, 46060, 46262-46285
Fistulization
  Esophagus, 43351-43352
  Intestines, 44300-44346
    Laparoscopic, 44187-44188
    Mucofistula, 44144
Fistulotomy
  Anal, 46270-46280
Flap
  Free
    Microvascular Transfer, 49906
    Omental, 49906
  Omentum
    Free
      with Microvascular Anastomosis,
        49906
Fluid Collection
  Incision and Drainage
    Skin, 10140

Fluid Drainage
  Abdomen, 49082-49084
Fluorescence Wound Imaging
  Noncontact, 0598T-0599T
Fluoroscopy
  Nasogastric, 43752
  Needle Biopsy, 77002
  Orogastric, 43752
  Venous Access Device, 36598, 77001
FNA (Fine Needle Aspiration), 10021 [10004,
  10005, 10006, 10007, 10008, 10009, 10010,
  10011, 10012]
FOBT (Fecal Occult Blood Test), 82270, 82274
Follow–up Services
  Post-op, 99024
Foreign Body
  Removal
    Anal, 46608
    Bile Duct, [43275]
    Colon, 44025, 44390, 45379
    Colon–Sigmoid, 45332
    Duodenum, 44010
    Esophagus, 43020, 43194, 43215
    Gastrointestinal, Upper, 43247
    Intestines, Small, 44020, 44363
    Muscle, 20520-20525
    Pancreatic Duct, [43275]
    Peritoneum, 49402
    Rectum, 45307, 45915
    Skin
      Stomach, 43500
    Subcutaneous, 10120-10121
    Tendon Sheath, 20520-20525
Fredet–Ramstedt Procedure, 43520
Frickman Operation, 45550
Fructose Intolerance Breath Test, 91065
FTG, 15200-15261
FTSG, 15200-15261
Full Thickness Graft, 15200-15261
Fundoplasty
  Esophagogastric
    Endoscopic, [43210]
    Laparoscopic, 43279-43280, 43283
    Laparotomy, 43327
    Thoracotomy, 43328
    with Gastroplasty, 43842-43843
  Esophagomyotomy
    Laparoscopic, 43279
  with Fundic Patch, 43325
  with Paraesophageal Hernia
    Laparoscopic, 43281-43282
    with Fundoplication
      Laparotomy, 43332-43333
      Thoracoabdominal Incisional,
        43336-43337
      Thoracotomy, 43334-43335
Furuncle
  Incision and Drainage, 10060-10061

G

Gallbladder
  Anastomosis
    with Intestines, 47720-47741
  Cholecystectomy, 47600
    Laparoscopic, 47562
      with Cholangiogram, 47564
    Open, 47600
      with Cholangiogram, 47605
      with Choledochoenterostomy,
        47612
      with Exploration Common Duct,
        47610
      with Transduodenal Sphinctero-
        tomy or Sphincteroplasty,
        47620
  Cholecystostomy
    for Drainage, 47480
    for Exploration, 47480
    for Removal of Stone, 47480
    Percutaneous, 47490
  Excision, 47562-47564, 47600-47620
  Exploration, 47480
  Incision, 47490
  Incision and Drainage, 47480
  Removal Calculi, 47480

Gallbladder — *continued*
  Repair
    with Gastroenterostomy, 47741
    with Intestines, 47720-47740
Ganglion
  Cyst
    Aspiration/Injection, 20612
    Drainage, 20612
  Wrist
    Excision, 25111-25112
Gastrectomy
  Longitudinal, 43775
  Partial, 43631
    Distal with Vagotomy, 43635
    with Gastroduodenostomy, 43631
      with Roux–en–Y Reconstruction,
        43633
    with Gastrojejunostomy, 43632
      with Intestinal Pouch, 43634
  Sleeve, 43775
  Total, 43621-43622
    with Esophagoenterostomy, 43620
    with Intestinal Pouch, 43622
Gastric
  Analysis Test, 43755-43757
  Electrodes
    Neurostimulator
      Implantation
        Laparoscopic, 43647
        Open, 43881
      Removal
        Laparoscopic, 43648
        Open, 43882
      Replacement
        Laparoscopic, 43647
        Open, 43881
      Revision
        Laparoscopic, 43648
        Open, 43882
  Intubation, 43753-43755
    Diagnostic, 43754-43757
    Therapeutic, 43753
  Lavage
    Therapeutic, 43753
  Restrictive Procedure
    Laparoscopy, 43770-43774
    Open, 43886-43888
  Tests
    Manometry, 91020
Gastroduodenostomy, 43810
  with Gastrectomy, 43631-43632
Gastroenterology, Diagnostic
  Breath Hydrogen Test, 91065
  Colon Motility Study, 91117
  Duodenal Intubation and Aspiration, 43756-
    43757
  Esophagus Tests
    Acid Perfusion, 91030
    Acid Reflux Test, 91034-91038
    Balloon Distension Provocation Study,
      91040
    Intubation with Specimen Collection,
      43754-43755
    Manometry, 91020
    Motility Study, 91010-91013
  Gastric Tests
    Manometry, 91020
  Gastroesophageal Reflux Test
    See Acid Reflux, 91034-91038
  Manometry, 91020
  Rectum
    Manometry, 91122
    Sensation, Tone, and Compliance Test,
      91120
  Stomach
    Intubation with Specimen Collection,
      43754-43755
    Manometry, 91020
    Stimulation of Secretion, 43755
Gastroenterostomy
  for Obesity, 43644-43645, 43842-43848
Gastroesophageal Reflux Test, 91034-91038
Gastrointestinal Tract
  Imaging Intraluminal
    Colon, [91113]
    Distal Ileum, [91113]

Gastrointestinal Tract — *continued*
  Imaging Intraluminal — *continued*
    Esophagus, 91111
    Esophagus Through Ileum, 91110
    Reconstruction, 43360-43361
    Transit and Pressure Measurements, 91112
    Upper
      Dilation, 43249
    X–ray
      Guide Intubation, 49440
Gastrointestinal, Upper
  Biopsy
    Endoscopy, 43239
  Dilation
    Endoscopy, 43245
    Esophagus, 43248
  Endoscopy
    Catheterization, 43241
    Destruction
      Lesion, [43270]
    Dilation, 43245
    Drainage
      Pseudocyst, 43240
    Exploration, 43235
    Hemorrhage, 43255
    Inject Varices, 43243
    Needle Biopsy, 43238, 43242
    Removal
      Foreign Body, 43247
      Lesion, 43250-43251
      Polyp, 43250-43251
      Tumor, 43250-43251
    Resection, Mucosa, 43254
    Stent Placement, [43266]
    Thermal Radiation, 43257
    Tube Placement, 43246
    Ultrasound, 43237-43238, 43242,
      43253
  Exploration
    Endoscopy, 43235
  Hemorrhage
    Endoscopic Control, 43255
  Injection
    Submucosal, 43236
    Varices, 43243
  Lesion
    Destruction, [43270]
  Ligation of Vein, 43244
  Needle Biopsy
    Endoscopy, 43238, 43242
  Removal
    Foreign Body, 43247
    Lesion, 43250-43251
    Polyp, 43250-43251
    Tumor, 43250-43251
  Stent Placement, [43266]
  Tube Placement
    Endoscopy, 43237-43238, 43246
  Ultrasound
    Endoscopy, 43237-43238, 43242,
      43259
Gastrojejunostomy, 43860-43865
  Contrast Injection, 49465
  Conversion from Gastrostomy Tube, 49446
  Removal
    Obstructive Material, 49460
  Replacement
    Tube, 49452
  Revision, 43860
    with Vagotomy, 43865
  with Duodenal Exclusion, 48547
  with Partial Gastrectomy, 43632
  with Vagotomy, 43825
  without Vagotomy, 43820
Gastroplasty
  Collis, 43283, 43338
  Esophageal Lengthening Procedure, 43283,
    43338
  Laparoscopic, 43283, 43644-43645
  Restrictive for Morbid Obesity, 43842-43848
    Other Than Vertical Banded, 43843
  Wedge, 43283, 43338
Gastrorrhaphy, 43840
Gastroschisis, 49605-49606
Gastrostomy
  Closure, 43870

CPT Index

CPT Index

Gastrostomy — *continued*
Laparoscopic
 Permanent, 43832
 Temporary, 43653
 Temporary, 43830
 Laparoscopic, 43653
 Neonatal, 43831
Tube
 Change of, 43762-43763
 Conversion to Gastro-jejunostomy Tube, 49446
 Directed Placement
  Endoscopic, 43246
  Percutaneous, 49440
 Insertion
  Endoscopic, 43246
  Percutaneous, 49440
 Percutaneous, 49440
 Removal
  Obstructive Material, 49460
 Replacement, 49450
 Repositioning, 43761
with Pancreatic Drain, 48001
with Pyloroplasty, 43640
with Vagotomy, 43640
Gastrotomy, 43500-43501, 43510
Globulin
Immune, 90389
Glucose
Blood Test, 82948
Graft
Anal, 46753
Skin
 Full Thickness, Free
  Axillae, 15240-15241
  Extremities (Excluding Hands/Feet), 15240-15241
  Mouth, Neck, 15240-15241
  Scalp, 15220-15221
  Trunk, 15200-15201
 Preparation Recipient Site, 15002, 15004-15005
 Split Graft, 15100-15101, 15120-15121
Groin Area
Repair
 Hernia, 49550-49557
Gross Type Procedure, 49610-49611
Group Health Education, 99078
Guaiac Test
Blood in Feces, 82270
Guide
3D Printed, Anatomic, 0561T-0562T

H

Halsted Mastectomy, 19305
Halsted Repair
Hernia, 49495
Hand
Tumor
 Excision, 26115 [26111]
 Radical Resection, 26116-26118 [26113]
Handling
Device, 99002
Specimen, 99000-99001
Hartmann Procedure, 44143
Closure of, 44227, 44626
Laparoscopy
 Partial Colectomy with Colostomy, 44206
Open, 44143
Harvesting
Intestines, 44132-44133
Liver, 47140-47142
Hct, 85013-85014
HDL (High Density Lipoprotein), 83718
Heart
Catheterization
 Flow–Directed, 93503
Resuscitation, 92950
Heller Procedure, 43279, 43330-43331
Hematochezia, 82270, 82274
Hematoma
Arm, Upper
 Incision and Drainage, 23930

Hematoma — *continued*
Incision and Drainage
 Neck, 21501-21502
 Skin, 10140
 Thorax, 21501-21502
Leg, Lower, 27603
Pelvis, 26990
Puncture Aspiration, 10160
Skin
 Incision and Drainage, 10140
 Puncture Aspiration, 10160
Hemoglobin
Antibody
 Fecal, 82274
Hemogram
Manual, 85014-85018
Hemorrhage
Abdomen, 49002
Anal
 Endoscopic Control, 46614
Colon
 Endoscopic Control, 44391, 45382
Colon–Sigmoid
 Endoscopic Control, 45334
Esophagus
 Endoscopic Control, 43227
Gastrointestinal, Upper
 Endoscopic Control, 43255
Intestines, Small
 Endoscopic Control, 44366, 44378
Liver
 Control, 47350
Rectum
 Endoscopic Control, 45317
Hemorrhoidectomy
External, 46250 [46320]
Internal and External, 46255-46262
Ligation, 46221 [46945, 46946]
Whitehead, 46260
Hemorrhoidopexy, [46947]
Hemorrhoids
Destruction, 46930
Excision, 46250-46262 [46320]
Incision, 46083
Injection
 Sclerosing Solution, 46500
Ligation, 45350, 46221 [45398, 46945, 46946]
Stapling, [46947]
Hemothorax
Thoracostomy, 32551
Hepatectomy
Extensive, 47122
Left Lobe, 47125
Partial
 Donor, 47140-47142
 Lobe, 47120
Right Lobe, 47130
Hepatic Duct
Anastomosis
 with Intestines, 47765, 47802
Exploration, 47400
Incision and Drainage, 47400
Removal
 Calculi (Stone), 47400
Repair
 with Intestines, 47765, 47802
Hepaticoenterostomy, 47802
Hepaticostomy, 47400
Hepaticotomy, 47400
Hepatotomy
Abscess, 47010
Cyst, 47010
Hernia
Repair
 Abdominal, 49560, 49565, 49590
  Incisional, 49560
  Recurrent, 49565
 Diaphragmatic, 39503-39541
  Chronic, 39541
  Neonatal, 39503
 Epigastric, 49570
  Incarcerated, 49572
 Femoral, 49550
  Incarcerated, 49553
  Recurrent, 49555

Hernia — *continued*
Repair — *continued*
 Femoral — *continued*
  Recurrent Incarcerated, 49557
  Reducible, 49550
 Incisional, 49561, 49566
  Incarcerated, 49561
 Inguinal, 49491, 49495-49500, 49505
  Incarcerated, 49492, 49496, 49501, 49507, 49521
  Infant, Incarcerated Strangulated, 49496, 49501
  Infant, Reducible, 49495, 49500
  Laparoscopic, 49650-49651
  Pediatric, Reducible, 49500, 49505
  Recurrent, Incarcerated Strangulated, 49521
  Recurrent, Reducible, 49520
  Sliding, 49525
  Strangulated, 49492
 Lumbar, 49540
 Mayo, 49585
 Recurrent Incisional
  Incarcerated, 49566
 Umbilicus, 49580, 49585
  Incarcerated, 49582, 49587
 Spigelian, 49590
Hgb, 85018
Hidradenitis
Excision, 11450-11471
Suppurative
 Incision and Drainage, 10060-10061
High Density Lipoprotein, 83718
Hill Procedure, 43842-43843
Histotripsy
Hepatocellular Tissue
 Malignant, 0686T
Hofmeister Operation, 43632
Home Services
Enema Administration, 99511
Intramuscular Injections, 99506
Stoma Care, 99505
Hospital Services
Inpatient Services
 Initial Care New or Established Patient, 99221-99223
 Initial Hospital Care, 99221-99223
 Prolonged Services, 99356-99357
 Subsequent Hospital Care, 99231-99233
Observation
 Discharge Services, 99234-99236
 Initial Care, 99218-99220
 New or Established Patient, 99218-99220
Same Day Admission
 Discharge Services, 99234-99236
Humerus
Excision, 24077-24079
Radical Resection, 24077-24079
Tumor
 Excision, 24075-24079 [24071, 24073]
Hydration, 96360-96361
Hydrocelectomy, 49491-49501
Hygroma, Cystic
Axillary or Cervical Excision, 38550-38555
HyperTED, 90389
Hypopharynx
Diverticulectomy, 43130, 43180

I

Identification
Sentinel Node, 38792, 38900
Ileocolostomy, 44160
Ileoproctostomy, 44150
Ileoscopy
via Stoma, 44380, 44382-44384 [44381]
Ileostomy, 44310, 45136
Continent (Kock Pouch), 44316
Laparoscopic, 44186-44187
Nontube, 44187
Revision, 44312-44314
IM Injection
Diagnostic, Prophylactic, Therapeutic, 96372

Image-Guided Fluid Collection Drainage, Percutaneous, 10030
Imaging, Fluorescence
Noncontact, Wound, 0598T-0599T
Imbrication
Diaphragm, 39545
Immune Globulin Administration, 96372, 96374-96375
Immune Globulins
Tetanus, 90389
Immunization
Passive
 Hyperimmune Serum Globulin, 90389
Immunoassay
Infectious Agent, 86318
Implant
Abdominal Wall
 Fascial Reinforcement, 0437T
Breast
 Removal
  Tissue Expander, 11971
 Replacement
  Tissue Expander, 11970
Drug Delivery Device, 11981, 11983
Electrode
 Gastric Implantation
  Laparoscopic
   Neurostimulator, 43647
  Open
   Neurostimulator, 43881
Fascial Reinforcement
 Abdominal Wall, 0437T
Mesh
 Closure of Necrotizing Soft Tissue Infection, 49568
 Hernia Repair, 49568, 49652-49657
Neurostimulator
 Gastric, 43647, 43881, 64590
Receiver
 Nerve, 64590
Reservoir Vascular Access Device
 Declotting, 36593
Incision and Drainage
Abdomen
 Fluid, 49082-49083
 Pancreatitis, 48000
Abscess
 Abdomen, Abdominal
  Open, 49040
  Pancreatitis, 48000
  Peritoneal, 49020
  Peritonitis, Localized, 49020
  Retroperitoneal, 49060
  Skin and Subcutaneous Tissue
   Complicated, 10061
   Multiple, 10061
   Simple, 10060
   Single, 10060
  Subdiaphragmatic, 49040
  Subphrenic, 49040
 Anal, 46045-46050
 Appendix
  Open, 44900
 Arm, Upper, 23930-23931
 Breast, 19020
 Leg, Lower, 27603
 Liver
  Open, 47010
 Lymph Node, 38300-38305
 Neck, 21501-21502
 Pelvis, 26990, 45000
 Peritoneum
  Open, 49020
 Rectum, 45005-45020, 46040, 46050-46060
 Retroperitoneal
  Open, 49060
 Skin, 10060-10061
 Spine, 22010-22015
 Subdiaphragmatic
  Open, 49040
 Subphrenic
  Open, 49040
 Thorax, 21501-21502
 Bile Duct, 47420-47425

● New   ▲ Revised   + Add On   AMA: CPT Assist [Resequenced]

Coding Companion for General Surgery/Gastroenterology

Intestine(s) — continued
Transplantation — continued
Removal of Allograft, 44137
Intestines, Small
Anastomosis, 43845, 44130
Biopsy, 44020, 44100
Endoscopy, 44361
Catheterization
Jejunum, 44015
Closure
Stoma, 44620-44625
Decompression, 44021
Destruction
Lesion, 44369
Tumor, 44369
Endoscopy, 44360
Biopsy, 44361, 44377
Control of Bleeding, 44366, 44378
via Stoma, 44382
Destruction
Lesion, 44369
Tumor, 44369
Diagnostic, 44376
Exploration, 44360
Hemorrhage, 44366
Insertion
Stent, 44370, 44379
Tube, 44379
Pelvic Pouch, 44385-44386
Place Tube, 44372
Removal
Foreign Body, 44363
Lesion, 44365
Polyp, 44364-44365
Tumor, 44364-44365
Tube Placement, 44372
Tube Revision, 44373
via Stoma, 44380, 44382-44384
[44381]
Enterostomy, 44620-44626
Tube Placement, 44300
Excision, 44120-44128
Partial with Anastomosis, 44140
Exclusion, 44700
Exploration, 44020
Gastrostomy Tube, 44373
Hemorrhage, 44378
Hemorrhage Control, 44366
Ileostomy, 44310-44316, 45136
Continent, 44316
Incision, 44010, 44020
Creation
Pouch, 44316
Stoma, 44300-44310
Decompression, 44021
Exploration, 44020
Revision
Stoma, 44312
Stoma Closure, 44620-44626
Insertion
Catheter, 44015
Duodenostomy Tube, 49441
Jejunostomy Tube, 44015, 44372
Jejunostomy, 44310
Laparoscopic, 44186
Lesion
Excision, 44110-44111
Lysis
Adhesions, 44005
Removal
Foreign Body, 44020, 44363
Repair
Diverticula, 44602-44603
Fistula, 44640-44661
Hernia, 44050
Malrotation, 44055
Obstruction, 44050, 44615
Ulcer, 44602-44603, 44605
Volvulus, 44050
Wound, 44602-44603, 44605
Revision
Jejunostomy Tube, 44373, 49451-49452
Specimen Collection, 43756-43757
Suture
Diverticula, 44602-44603, 44605

Intestines, Small — continued
Suture — continued
Fistula, 44640-44661
Plication, 44680
Stoma, 44620-44625
Ulcer, 44602-44603, 44605
Wound, 44602-44603, 44605
Intramuscular Injection, 96372, 99506
Intraoperative
Radiation Therapy Applicator, 19294
Intravenous Therapy, 96360-96361, 96374-96377
Introduction
Breast
Localization Device
with Biopsy, 19081-19086
Contraceptive Capsules
Implantable, 11981
Drug Delivery Implant, 11981, 11983
Gastrointestinal Tube, 44500
Needle or Catheter
AV Shunt
Dialysis Circuit, 36901-36903
Tissue Expanders, Skin, 11960-11971
Intubation
Duodenal, 43756-43757
Endotracheal Tube, 31500
Gastric, 43753-43755
Intussusception
Reduction
Laparotomy, 44050
Ischial
Excision
Tumor, 27078
Ischiectomy, 15941
Ischium
Pressure Ulcer, 15940-15946
Islet Cell
Transplant, 0584T-0586T
Isthmusectomy
Thyroid Gland, 60210-60225
IV Infusion Therapy
Hydration, 96360-96361
IV Injection, 96374-96376
IV, 96374-96376
Hydration, 96360-96361
Ivor Lewis, 43117
Ivy Bleeding Time, 85002

J

Jaboulay Operation
Gastroduodenostomy, 43810
Janeway Procedure, 43832
Jejunostomy
Catheterization, 44015
Insertion
Catheter, 44015
Laparoscopic, 44186
Non–tube, 44310
with Pancreatic Drain, 48001
Jejunum
Transfer with Microvascular Anastomosis, Free, 43496
Joint
Drainage
Hip, 26990
Pelvis, 26990

K

K+, 84132
Kader Operation
Incision, Stomach, Creation of Stoma, 43830-43832
Kocher Pylorectomy
Gastrectomy, Partial, 43631
Kock Pouch, 44316
Kock Procedure, 44316
Kraske Procedure, 45116

L

Lactase Deficiency Breath Test, 91065
Lactiferous Duct
Excision, 19112
Exploration, 19110

Ladd Procedure, 44055
Lane's Operation, 44150
Laparoscopy
Abdominal, 49320-49327
Surgical, 49321-49326
Adrenal Gland
Biopsy, 60650
Excision, 60650
Adrenalectomy, 60650
Appendectomy, 44970
Aspiration, 49322
Biopsy, 49321
Lymph Nodes, 38570
Ovary, 49321
Cecostomy, 44188
Cholecystectomy, 47562-47564
Cholecystoenterostomy, 47570
Closure
Enterostomy, 44227
Colectomy
Partial, 44204-44208, 44213
Total, 44210-44212
Colostomy, 44188
Diagnostic, 49320
Drainage
Extraperitoneal Lymphocele, 49323
Electrode
Implantation
Gastric
Antrum, 43647
Removal
Gastric, 43648
Replacement
Gastric, 43647
Revision
Gastric, 43648
Enterectomy, 44202
Enterolysis, 44180
Enterostomy
Closure, 44227
Esophageal Lengthening, 43283
Esophagogastric Fundoplasty, 43280
Esophagomyotomy, 43279
Esophagus
Esophageal Lengthening, 43283
Esophagogastric Fundoplasty, 43280
Esophagomyotomy, 43279
Gastric Restrictive Procedures, 43644-43645, 43770-43774
Gastrostomy
Temporary, 43653
Hernia Repair
Epigastric, 49652
Incarcerated or Strangulated, 49653
Incisional, 49654
Incarcerated or Strangulated, 49655
Recurrent, 49656
Incarcerated or Strangulated, 49657
Initial, 49650
Recurrent, 49651
Spigelian, 49652
Incarcerated or Strangulated, 49653
Umbilical, 49652
Incarcerated or Strangulated, 49653
Ventral, 49652
Incarcerated or Strangulated, 49653
Ileostomy, 44187
Jejunostomy, 44186-44187
Liver
Ablation
Tumor, 47370-47371
Lymphadenectomy, 38571-38573
Lymphatic, 38570-38573
Lysis of Intestinal Adhesions, 44180
Mobilization
Splenic Flexure, 44213
Omentopexy, 49326
Ovary
Biopsy, 49321
Pelvis, 49320

Laparoscopy — continued
Placement Interstitial Device, 49327
Proctectomy, 45395-45397
Complete, 45395
with Creation of Colonic Reservoir, 45397
Proctopexy, 45400-45402
Rectum
Resection, 45395-45397
Removal
Spleen, 38120
Resection
Intestines
with Anastomosis, 44202-44203
Rectum, 45395-45397
Splenectomy, 38120
Splenic Flexure
Mobilization, 44213
Stomach, 43651-43653
Gastric Bypass, 43644-43645
Gastric Restrictive Procedures, 43770-43774, 43848, 43886-43888
Gastroenterostomy, 43644-43645
Roux–en–Y, 43644
Surgical, 38570-38572, 43651-43653, 44188-44188, 44212-44227, 44970, 45395-45397, 45400-45402, 47370-47371, 49321-49327, 49650-49651
Vagus Nerve, 0312T-0314T
Vagus Nerves Transection, 43651-43652
Laparotomy, Exploratory, 47015, 49000-49002
Laparotomy
Electrode
Gastric
Implantation, 43881
Removal, 43882
Replacement, 43881
Revision, 43882
Esophagogastric Fundoplasty, 43327
Exploration, 47015, 49000-49002
Hemorrhage Control, 49002
Hiatal Hernia, 43332-43333
Surgical, 44050
with Biopsy, 49000
Laryngoplasty
Cricotracheal Resection, 31592
Laser Surgery
Anus, 46614, 46917, 46924
Cautery
Anus, 46614
Colon, 44391, 45317, 45382
Esophagus, 43227
Hemorrhoids, 46930
Rectum, 45317, 45334
Small Intestine, 44366, 44378
Incompetent Vein, 36478-36479
Lesion
Anus, 46917, 46924
Colon, 45320
Rectum, 45320
Polyp, Colon, 45320
Tumor
Colon, 45320
Rectum, 45190
Lavage
Colon, 44701
Gastric, 43753
Peritoneal, 49084
LDL, 83721-83722
Leg
Lower
Abscess
Incision and Drainage, 27603
Biopsy, 27613-27614
Bursa
Incision and Drainage, 27604
Hematoma
Incision and Drainage, 27603
Skin Graft
Full Thickness, 15220-15221
Split, 15100-15101
Tumor, 27615-27619 [27632, 27634]
Upper
Biopsy, 27323-27324
Pressure Ulcer, 15950-15958

Leg — *continued*
Upper — *continued*
Tumor
Excision, 27327-27364 [27329, 27337, 27339]
Wound Exploration
Penetrating, 20103
Lengthening
Esophageal, 43338
Lesion
Anal
Destruction, 46900-46917, 46924
Excision, 45108, 46922
Breast
Excision, 19120-19126
Carotid Body
Excision, 60600-60605
Colon
Excision, 44110-44111
Esophagus
Ablation, 43229
Excision, 43100-43101
Removal, 43216
Intestines
Excision, 44110
Intestines, Small
Destruction, 44369
Excision, 44111
Lymph Node
Incision and Drainage, 38300-38305
Mesentery
Excision, 44820
Pancreas
Excision, 48120
Rectum
Excision, 45108
Skin
Biopsy, 11102-11107
Excision
Benign, 11400-11471
Malignant, 11600-11646
Stomach
Excision, 43611
LeVeen Shunt
Insertion, 49425
Revision, 49426
Ligament
Injection, 20550
Release
Transverse Carpal, 29848
Transverse Carpal Release, 29848
Wrist
Release, 29848
Ligation
Esophageal Varices, 43204
Gastroesophageal, 43405
Hemorrhoids, 45350, 46221 [45398, 46945, 46946, 46948]
Shunt
Peritoneal
Venous, 49428
Thoracic Duct, 38380
Abdominal Approach, 38382
Thoracic Approach, 38381
Vein
Clusters, 37785
Esophagus, 43205, 43244
Gastric, 43244
Saphenous, 37700-37735
Limited Neck Dissection
with Thyroidectomy, 60252
Lipoprotein
Blood, 83718-83721
LDL, 83721-83722
Lithotripsy
Bile Duct Calculi (Stone)
Endoscopic, 43265
Pancreatic Duct Calculi (Stone)
Endoscopic, 43265
Liver
Ablation
Tumor, 47370-47371, 47380-47383
Cryoablation, 47381, 47383
Laparoscopic, 47370-47371
Microwave, 47370
Open, 47380-47381

Liver — *continued*
Ablation — *continued*
Tumor — *continued*
Percutaneous, 47382
Radiofrequency, 47370, 47380, 47382
Abscess
Aspiration, 47015
Incision and Drainage
Open, 47010
Injection, 47015
Aspiration, 47015
Biopsy, 47100
Cholangiography Injection
Existing Access, 47531
New Access, 47532
Cyst
Aspiration, 47015
Incision and Drainage
Open, 47010
Excision
Extensive, 47122
Partial, 47120, 47125-47130, 47140-47142
Injection, 47015
Cholangiography
Existing Access, 47531
New Access, 47532
Lobectomy, 47125-47130
Partial, 47120
Needle Biopsy, 47000-47001
Repair
Abscess, 47300
Cyst, 47300
Wound, 47350-47362
Suture
Wound, 47350-47362
Transplantation
Allograft preparation, 47143-47147
Trisegmentectomy, 47122
Lobectomy
Contralateral Subtotal
Thyroid Gland, 60212, 60225
Liver, 47120-47130
Thyroid Gland
Partial, 60210-60212
Total, 60220-60225
Localization
Nodule Radiographic, Breast
with Biopsy, 19081-19086
Longmire Operation, 47765
Lord Procedure
Anal Sphincter, Dilation, 45905
Low Frequency Ultrasound, 97610
Lumpectomy, 19301-19302
Lung
Excision
Tumor, 32503-32504
Tumor
Removal, 32503-32504
Lymph Duct
Injection, 38790
Lymph Node(s)
Abscess
Incision and Drainage, 38300-38305
Biopsy, 38500, 38510-38530, 38570
Needle, 38505
Dissection, 38542
Excision, 38500, 38510-38530
Abdominal, 38747
Inguinofemoral, 38760-38765
Laparoscopic, 38571-38573
Limited, for Staging
Para–Aortic, 38562
Pelvic, 38562
Retroperitoneal, 38564
Pelvic, 38770
Radical
Axillary, 38740-38745
Cervical, 38720-38724
Suprahyoid, 38720-38724
Retroperitoneal Transabdominal, 38780
Thoracic, 38746
Exploration, 38542

Lymph Node(s) — *continued*
Hygroma, Cystic
Axillary
Cervical
Excision, 38550-38555
Removal
Abdominal, 38747
Inguinofemoral, 38760-38765
Pelvic, 38747, 38770
Retroperitoneal Transabdominal, 38780
Thoracic, 38746
Lymph Vessels
Incision, 38308
Lymphadenectomy
Abdominal, 38747
Bilateral Pelvic
Total, 38571-38573
Gastric, 38747
Inguinofemoral, 38760-38765
Injection
Sentinel Node, 38792
Limited, for Staging
Para–Aortic, 38562
Pelvic, 38562
Retroperitoneal, 38564
Peripancreatic, 38747
Portal, 38747
Radical
Axillary, 38740-38745
Cervical, 38720-38724
Groin Area, 38760-38765
Suprahyoid, 38700
Retroperitoneal Transabdominal, 38780
Thoracic, 38746
Lymphadenitis
Incision and Drainage, 38300-38305
Lymphangiography
Injection, 38790
Lymphangiotomy, 38308
Lymphatic Channels
Incision, 38308
Lymphatic Cyst
Drainage
Laparoscopic, 49323
Open, 49062
Lymphocele
Drainage
Laparoscopic, 49323
Extraperitoneal
Open Drainage, 49062
Lysis
Adhesions
Intestinal, 44005

M

MacEwen Operation
Hernia Repair, Inguinal, 49495-49500, 49505
Incarcerated, 49496, 49501, 49507, 49521
Laparoscopic, 49650-49651
Recurrent, 49520
Sliding, 49525
Mallory–Weiss Procedure, 43502
Mammary Abscess, 19020
Mandated Services
Hospital, On Call, 99026-99027
Manometric Studies
Rectum
Anus, 91122
Manometry
Esophagogastric, 91020
Mapping
Sentinel Lymph Node, 38900
Marsupialization
Liver
Cyst or Abscess, 47300
Pancreatic Cyst, 48500
Mastectomy
Gynecomastia, 19300
Modified Radical, 19307
Partial, 19301-19302
Radical, 19305-19306
Simple, Complete, 19303
Subcutaneous, 19300

Mastotomy, 19020
Maydl Operation, 45563
Mayo Hernia Repair, 49580-49587
Mayo Operation
Varicose Vein Removal, 37700-37735, 37785
McBurney Operation
Hernia Repair, Inguinal, 49495-49500, 49505
Incarcerated, 49496, 49501, 49507, 49521
Recurrent, 49520
Sliding, 49525
McKeown Esophagectomy, 43112
McVay Operation
Hernia Repair, Inguinal, 49495-49500, 49505
Incarcerated, 49496, 49501, 49507, 49521
Laparoscopic, 49650-49651
Recurrent, 49520
Sliding, 49525
Meckel's Diverticulum
Excision, 44800
Median Nerve Compression
Decompression, 64721
Endoscopy, 29848
Median Nerve
Decompression, 64721
Neuroplasty, 64721
Release, 64721
Transposition, 64721
Medical Team Conference, 99366-99368
Mesentery
Lesion
Excision, 44820
Repair, 44850
Suture, 44850
Mesh
Implantation
Hernia, 49568
Removal
Abdominal Infected, 11008
Microbiology, 87086-87088
Micrographic Surgery
Mohs Technique, 17311-17315
Mile Operation, 44155-44156
Miller–Abbott Intubation, 44500
Mobilization
Splenic Flexure, 44139
Laparoscopic, 44213
Model
3D Printed, Anatomic, 0559T-0560T
Moderate Sedation, 99151-99153
Modified Radical Mastectomy, 19307
Mohs Micrographic Surgery, 17311-17315
Molluscum Contagiosum Destruction
Anus, 46900-46924
Monitoring
Prolonged, with Physician Attendance, 99354-99360 [99415, 99416, 99417]
Moschcowitz Operation
Repair, Hernia, Femoral, 49550-49557
Mosenthal Test, 81002
Motility Study
Colon, 91117
Duodenal, 91022
Esophagus, 91010-91013
Mousseaux–Barbin Procedure, 43510
Mucosa
Excision of Lesion
via Esophagoscopy, 43229
via Small Intestinal Endoscopy, 44369
via Upper GI Endoscopy, [43270]
Mucosectomy
Rectal, 45113
Mucous Membrane
See Mouth, Mucosa
Rectum
Proctoplasty for Prolapse, 45505
Muscle(s)
Biopsy, 20200-20206
Chemodenervation
Trunk, 64646-64647
Debridement
Infected, 11004-11006

Muscle(s) — *continued*
Removal
Foreign Body, 20520-20525
Myomectomy
Anorectal, 45108
Myotomy
Esophagus
Lower Esophageal, 43497
Peroral Endoscopic, 43497
Myxoid Cyst
Aspiration/Injection, 20612
Drainage, 20612
Wrist
Excision, 25111-25112

N

Nails
Drainage, 10060-10061
Nasogastric Tube
Placement, 43752
Neck
Biopsy, 21550
Exploration
Lymph Nodes, 38542
Incision and Drainage
Abscess, 21501-21502
Hematoma, 21501-21502
Skin Graft
Full Thickness, 15240-15241
Split, 15120-15121
Tumor, 21555-21558 [21552, 21554]
Wound Exploration
Penetrating, 20100
Needle Biopsy
Abdomen Mass, 49180
Breast, 19100
Colon
Endoscopy, 45392
Colon Sigmoid
Endoscopy, 45342
Esophagus
Endoscopy, 43232, 43238
Fluoroscopic Guidance, 77002
Gastrointestinal, Upper
Endoscopy, 43238, 43242
Liver, 47000-47001
Lymph Node, 38505
Muscle, 20206
Pancreas, 48102
Retroperitoneal Mass, 49180
Thyroid Gland, 60100
Needle Insertion, Dry, [20560, 20561]
Needle Localization
Breast
with Biopsy, 19081-19086
with Lesion Excision, 19125-19126
Nerves
Avulsion, 64755-64760
Decompression, 64719-64721
Destruction, 64646-64647
Incision, 43640-43641, 64755-64760
Injection
Anesthetic or Steroid, 64486-64489
Neurolytic Agent, 64646-64647
Neuroplasty, 64719-64721
Transection, 43640-43641, 64755-64760
Transposition, 64719-64721
Neuroplasty
Peripheral Nerve, 64719-64721
Neurostimulator
Analysis, 0317T
Gastric Nerve
Electronic Analysis, 95980-95982
Implantation/Replacement, 43647, 43881, 64590
Revision/Removal, 43648, 43882, 64595
Vagus Nerve
Electronic Analysis/Programming, 0317T
Implantation, 0312T
Removal, 0314T-0315T
Replacement, 0313T, 0316T
Revision, 0313T, 0316T

New Patient
Hospital Inpatient Services, 99221-99223, 99231-99236
Hospital Observation Services, 99217-99220
Initial Inpatient Consultations, 99251-99255
Initial Office Visit, 99202-99205
Office and/or Other Outpatient Consultations, 99241-99245
Outpatient Visit, 99211-99215
Newborn Care
Standby for C–Section, 99360
Nitrate Reduction Test
Urinalysis, 81000-81003, 81007
Noble Procedure, 44680
Node Dissection, Lymph, 38542
Non–office Medical Services, 99056

O

O2 Saturation, 94760-94761
Observation
Discharge, 99217
Initial, 99218-99220
Same Date Admit/Discharge, 99234-99236
Subsequent, [99224, 99225, 99226]
Obstruction Clearance
Venous Access Device, 36595-36596
Obstruction Colon, 44025-44050
Obstructive Material Removal
Gastrostomy, Duodenostomy, Jejunostomy, Gastro-jejunostomy, or Cecostomy Tube, 49460
Occult Blood, 82270
by Hemoglobin Immunoassay, 82274
Oddi Sphincter
Pressure Measurement, 43263
Oesophageal Neoplasm
Endoscopic Removal
Ablation, 43229
Bipolar Cautery, 43216
Hot Biopsy Forceps, 43216
Snare, 43217
Excision, Open, 43100-43101
Oesophageal Varices
Injection Sclerosis, 43204, 43243
Ligation, 43205, 43244
Office and/or Other Outpatient Visits
Consultation, 99241-99245
Established Patient, 99211-99215
New Patient, 99202-99205
Office Visit
Established Patient, 99211-99215
New Patient, 99202-99205
Prolonged Service, 99354-99355 [99415, 99416, 99417]
Outpatient Visit
Established Patient, 99211-99215
New Patient, 99202-99205
Prolonged Service, 99354-99355 [99415, 99416, 99417]
Office Medical Services
After Hours, 99050
Emergency Care, 99058
Office or Other Outpatient Consultations, 99241-99245, 99354-99355
Omentectomy, 49255
Omentum
Excision, 49255
Flap, 49904-49905
Free
with Microvascular Anastomosis, 49906
Omphalocele
Repair, 49600-49611
Omphalomesenteric Duct, Persistent
Excision, 44800
Omphalomesenteric Duct
Excision, 44800
Online Internet Assessment/Management
Nonphysician, 98970-98972
Physician, [99421, 99422, 99423]
Online Medical Evaluation
Nonphysician, 98970-98972
Physician, [99421, 99422, 99423]
Open Biopsy, Adrenal Gland, 60540-60545
Operation/Procedure
Collis, 43283, 43338

Operation/Procedure — *continued*
Fredet-Ramstedt, 43520
Heller, 43330-43331
Jaboulay Gastroduodenostomy, 43810
Nissen, 43280
Ramstedt, 43520
Schlatter Total Gastrectomy, 43620-43622
Stamm, 43830
Laparoscopic, 43653
Toupet, 43280
Winiwarter Cholecystoenterostomy, 47720-47740
Optical Endomicroscopic Images, 88375
Optical Endomicroscopy, 43206, 43252, 0397T
Orbits
Skin Graft
Split, 15120-15121
Organ or Disease Oriented Panel
Electrolyte, 80051
Lipid Panel, 80061
Orogastric Tube
Placement, 43752
Ostectomy
Pressure Ulcer
Ischial, 15941, 15945
Sacral, 15933, 15935
Trochanteric, 15951, 15953, 15958
Other Nonoperative Measurements and Examinations
Acid Perfusion
Esophagus, 91013, 91030
Acid Reflux
Esophagus, 91034-91038
Bernstein Test, 91030
Breath Hydrogen, 91065
Gastric Motility (Manometric) Studies, 91020
Manometry
Anorectal, 91122
Esophageal, 91010
Outpatient Visit, 99202-99215
Oximetry (Noninvasive)
Blood O^2 Saturation
Ear or Pulse, 94760-94761
Oxygen Saturation
Ear Oximetry, 94760-94761
Pulse Oximetry, 94760-94761

P

Pain Management
Intravenous Therapy, 96360-96361, 96374-96376
Pancoast Tumor Resection, 32503-32504
Pancreas, Endocrine Only
Islet Cell
Transplantation, 48160, 0584T-0586T
Pancreas
Anastomosis
with Intestines, 48520-48540, 48548
Biopsy, 48100
Needle Biopsy, 48102
Cyst
Anastomosis, 48520-48540
Repair, 48500
Debridement
Peripancreatic Tissue, 48105
Excision
Ampulla of Vater, 48148
Duct, 48148
Partial, 48140-48146, 48150-48154, 48160
Peripancreatic Tissue, 48105
Total, 48155-48160
Lesion
Excision, 48120
Needle Biopsy, 48102
Placement
Drains, 48000-48001
Pseudocyst
Drainage
Open, 48510
Removal
Calculi (Stone), 48020
Repair
Cyst, 48500

Pancreas — *continued*
Resection, 48105
Suture, 48545
Transplantation, 48160
Allograft Preparation, 48551-48552
X–ray with Contrast
Injection Procedure, 48400
Pancreatectomy
Partial, 48140-48146, 48150-48154, 48160
Total, 48155-48160
with Transplantation, 48160
Pancreatic Duct
Destruction
Calculi (Stone), 43265
Tumor, [43278]
Dilation
Endoscopy, [43277]
Endoscopy
Collection
Specimen, 43260
Destruction
Calculi (Stone), 43265
Tumor, [43278]
Dilation, [43277]
Removal
Calculi (Stone), 43264
Foreign Body, [43275]
Stent, [43275, 43276]
Sphincter Pressure, 43263
Sphincterotomy, 43262
Incision
Sphincter, 43262
Placement
Stent, [43274]
Removal
Calculi (Stone), 43264
Foreign Body, [43275]
Stent, [43275, 43276]
Tumor
Destruction, [43278]
Pancreaticojejunostomy, 48548
Pancreatitis
Incision and Drainage, 48000
Pancreatography
Injection Procedure, 48400
Pancreatorrhaphy, 48545
Pancreatotomy
Sphincter, 43262
Papilla Excision, 46230 [46220]
Papilloma
Destruction
Anus, 46900-46924
Papillotomy, 43262
Destruction
Anus, 46900-46924
Paracentesis
Abdomen, 49082-49083
Parathyroid Gland
Excision, 60500-60502
Exploration, 60500-60505
Parathyroidectomy, 60500-60505
Parietal Cell Vagotomies, 43641
Park Posterior Anal Repair, 46761
Paronychia
Incision and Drainage, 10060-10061
Partial Colectomy, 44140-44147, 44160, 44204-44208, 44213
Partial Esophagectomy, 43116-43124
Partial Gastrectomy, 43631-43635, 43845
Partial Hepatectomy, 47120, 47125-47130, 47140-47142
Partial Mastectomies, 19301-19302
Partial Pancreatectomy, 48140-48146, 48150, 48153-48154, 48160
Partial Splenectomy, 38101, 38120
Patey's Operation
Mastectomy, Modified Radical, 19307
Patterson's Test
Blood Urea Nitrogen, 84525
PEG, 43246
Pelvic Bone
Drainage, 26990
Pelvic Exenteration
for Colorectal Malignancy, 45126
Pelvic Lymphadenectomy, 38562, 38765
Laparoscopic, 38571-38573

Pelvis
Abscess
Incision and Drainage, 26990, 45000
Biopsy, 27040-27041
Exclusion
Small Intestine, 44700
Exenteration
for Colorectal Malignancy, 45126
Hematoma
Incision and Drainage, 26990
Tumor, 27047-27049, 27075-27078 [27043, 27045]
Pentagastrin Test, 43755-43757
Percutaneous
Access, Biliary, 47541
Aspiration
Bartholin's Gland, 10160
Atherectomies, 0234T-0238T
Biopsy, Gallbladder/Bile Ducts, 47553
Perineum
Debridement
Infected, 11004, 11006
Peritoneal Free Air, 49400
Peritoneal Lavage, 49084
Peritoneoscopy
Biopsy, 49321
Exploration, 49320
Peritoneum
Abscess
Incision and Drainage, 49020
Exchange
Drainage Catheter, 49423
Laparoscopic
Drainage
Lymphocele, 49323
Ligation
Shunt, 49428
Removal
Cannula
Catheter, 49422
Foreign Body, 49402
Shunt, 49429
Venous Shunt, 49427
Persistent, Omphalomesenteric Duct
Excision, 44800
PFG (Percutaneous Fluoroscopic Gastrostomy), 49440
PFT (Pulmonary Function Test), 94662, 94760-94761
Phlebectasia
Ablation, 36473-36479
Removal, 37718-37735, 37765-37766, 37785
with Tissue Excision, 37735
Phlebectomy
Stab, 37765-37766
Phlebotomy
Therapeutic, 99195
Physical Examination
Office and/or Other Outpatient Services, 99202-99215
Physician Services
Case Management Services, 99366-99368
Online, [99421, 99422, 99423]
Prolonged, [99417]
with Direct Patient Contact, 99354-99357
Outpatient Office, 99354-99355
with Direct Patient Services
Inpatient, 99356-99357
without Direct Patient Contact, 99358-99359
Standby, 99360
Team Conference, 99367
Telephone, 99441-99443
PICC Line Insertion, 36568-36569, 36584 [36572, 36573]
Pilonidal Cyst
Excision, 11770-11772
Incision and Drainage, 10080-10081
Placement
Adjustable Gastric Restrictive Device, 43770
Catheter
Bile Duct, 47533-47540

Placement — *continued*
Catheter — *continued*
for Interstitial Radioelement Application
Breast, 19296-19298
Genitalia, 55920
Muscle, 20555
Pelvic Organs, 55920
Soft Tissue, 20555
Pleural, 32550
Catheter, Cardiac, 93503
Cecostomy Tube, 44300, 49442
Colonic Stent, 45327, 45347, 45389
Drainage
Pancreas, 48001
Duodenostomy Tube, 49441
Enterostomy Tube, 44300
Fiducial Markers
Duodenum/Jejunum, 43253
Esophagus, 43253
Intra-abdominal, 49411
Intrapelvic, 49411
Retroperitoneum, 49411
Stomach, 43253
Gastrostomy Tube, 43246, 49440
Interstitial Device
Intra-abdominal, 49327, 49411-49412
Intrapelvic, 49411
Retroperitoneum, 49411
Jejunostomy Tube
Endoscopic, 44372
Percutaneous, 49441
Nasogastric Tube, 43752
Needle
for Interstitial Radioelement Application
Genitalia, 55920
Muscle, 20555
Pelvic Organs, 55920
Soft Tissue, 20555
Muscle or Soft Tissue
for Radioelement Application, 20555
Pelvic Organs and/or Genitalia, 55920
Orogastric Tube, 43752
Radiation Delivery Device
Therapy Applicator for IORT, 19294
Seton
Anal, 46020
Pleural Cavity
Catheterization, 32550
Incision
Pneumothorax, 32551
Puncture and Drainage, 32554-32557
Pleuritis, Purulent, 21501-21502
Pneumoperitoneum, 49400
Polya Anastomosis, 43632
Polya Gastrectomy, 43632
Polyp
Esophagus
Ablation, 43229
Port-A-Cath
Insertion, 36560-36563, 36568-36571 [36572, 36573]
Removal, 36589-36590
Replacement, 36575-36585
Port
Peripheral
Insertion, 36569-36571 [36572, 36573]
Removal, 36590
Replacement, 36578, 36585
Venous Access
Insertion, 36560-36561
Removal, 36590
Repair, 36576
Replacement, 36578, 36582-36583
Portoenterostomy, Hepatic, 47802
Post–op Visit, 99024
Postoperative Wound Infection
Incision and Drainage, 10180
Potassium
Serum, 84132
Preparation
for Transplantation
Intestines, 44715-44721

Preparation — *continued*
for Transplantation — *continued*
Liver, 47143-47147
Pancreas, 48551-48552
Tumor Cavity
Intraoperative Radiation Therapy (IORT), 19294
Pressure Breathing
Negative
Continuous (CNP), 94662
Pressure Measurement of Sphincter of Oddi, 43263
Pressure Ulcer (Decubitus)
Excision, 15920-15935, 15940-15958
Coccygeal, 15920-15922
Ischial, 15940-15946
Sacral, 15931-15935
Trochanter, 15950-15958
Procidentia
Rectal
Excision, 45130-45135
Repair, 45900
Proctectomy
Laparoscopic, 45395-45397
with Colectomy/Ileostomy, 44211-44212
Open Approach, 45110-45123
with Colectomy, 45121
with Colectomy/Ileostomy, 44155-44158
Proctopexy, 45400-45402, 45540-45550
with Sigmoid Excision, 45550
Proctoplasty, 45500-45505
Proctorrhaphy
Fistula, 45800-45825
Prolapse, 45540-45541
Proctosigmoidoscopy
Ablation
Polyp or Lesion, 45320
Biopsy, 45305
Destruction
Tumor, 45320
Dilation, 45303
Exploration, 45300
Hemorrhage Control, 45317
Placement
Stent, 45327
Removal
Foreign Body, 45307
Polyp, 45308-45315
Tumor, 45315
Volvulus Repair, 45321
Proctotomy, 45160
Prolapse
Anus, 46750-46751
Proctopexy, 45400-45402, 45540-45550
Proctoplasty, 45505-45520
Rectum, 45130-45135, 45900, 46753
Prolonged Services, [99417]
Before or After Direct Patient Contact, 99358-99359
Inpatient or Observation, 99356-99357
Physician Standby Services, 99360
with Direct Patient Contact, 99354-99355
Prosthesis
Hernia
Mesh, 49568
Intestines, 44700
Protein
Urine
by Dipstick, 81000-81003
Pseudocyst, Pancreas
Drainage
Open, 48510
PTA, 36902-36903, 36905-36906
PTE (Prolonged Tissue Expansion), 11960
Puestow Procedure, 48548
Pulmonology
Diagnostic
Oximetry
Ear or Pulse, 94760-94761
Therapeutic
Pressure Ventilation
Negative CNPB, 94662
Ventilation Assist, 94002-94005

Pulse Generator
Electronic Analysis, 95980-95982
Pump Stomach for Poison, 43753
Puncture Aspiration
Abscess
Skin, 10160
Bulla, 10160
Cyst
Breast, 19000-19001
Skin, 10160
Hematoma, 10160
Puncture
Chest
with Imaging Guidance, 32555, 32557
without Imaging Guidance, 32554, 32556
Pleural Cavity
Drainage, 32556-32557
Pyloric Sphincter
Incision, 43520
Reconstruction, 43800
Pyloromyotomy, 43520
Pyloroplasty, 43800
with Vagotomy, 43640
Pyothorax
Incision and Drainage, 21501-21502

Q

Quadrantectomy, 19301-19302

R

Radiation Therapy
Intraoperative, 19294
Radical Excision of Lymph Nodes
Axillary, 38740-38745
Cervical, 38720-38724
Suprahyoid, 38700
Radical Mastectomies, Modified, 19307
Radical Neck Dissection
with Thyroidectomy, 60254
Radioelement Substance
Catheter Placement
Breast, 19296-19298
Muscle and/or Soft Tissue, 20555
Pelvic Organs or Genitalia, 55920
Needle Placement
Muscle and/or Soft Tissue, 20555
Pelvic Organs and Genitalia, 55920
Radiofrequency Spectroscopy
Partial Mastectomy, 0546T
Radiological Marker
Preoperative Placement
Excision of Breast Lesion, 19125-19126
Radiotherapy
Afterloading
Catheter Insertion, 19296-19298
Ramstedt Operation
Pyloromyotomy, 43520
RBC, 85007, 85014, 85651
RBL (Rubber Band Ligation)
Hemorrhoids, 46221
Reconstruction
Abdominal Wall
Omental Flap, 49905
Anal
Congenital Absence, 46730-46740
Fistula, 46742
Graft, 46753
Sphincter, 46750-46751, 46760-46761
Bile Duct
Anastomosis, 47800
Chest Wall
Omental Flap, 49905
Esophagus, 43300, 43310, 43313
Creation
Stoma, 43351-43352
Esophagostomy, 43351-43352
Fistula, 43305, 43312, 43314
Gastrointestinal, 43360-43361
Intestines, Small
Anastomosis, 44130
Pyloric Sphincter, 43800

Reconstruction — *continued*
　Stomach
　　for Obesity, 43644-43645, 43845-43848
　　Gastric Bypass, 43644-43653, 43752-43846
　　Roux–en–Y, 43644, 43846
　　with Duodenum, 43810, 43860-43865
　　with Jejunum, 43820-43825, 43860-43865
　　Wound Repair, 13100-13160
Rectal Bleeding
　Endoscopic Control, 45317
Rectal Prolapse
　Excision, 45130-45135
　Repair, 45900
Rectal Sphincter
　Dilation, 45910
Rectocele
　Repair, 45560
Rectopexy
　Laparoscopic, 45400-45402
　Open, 45540-45550
Rectoplasty, 45500-45505
Rectorrhaphy, 45540-45541, 45800-45825
Rectum
　Abscess
　　Incision and Drainage, 45005-45020, 46040, 46060
　Biopsy, 45100
　Dilation
　　Endoscopy, 45303
　Endoscopy
　　Destruction
　　　Tumor, 45320
　　Dilation, 45303
　　Exploration, 45300
　　Hemorrhage, 45317
　　Removal
　　　Foreign Body, 45307
　　　Polyp, 45308-45315
　　　Tumor, 45308-45315
　　Volvulus, 45321
　Excision
　　Partial, 45111, 45113-45116, 45123
　　Total, 45110, 45112, 45119-45120
　　with Colon, 45121
　Exploration
　　Endoscopic, 45300
　　Surgical, 45990
　Hemorrhage
　　Endoscopic, 45317
　Injection
　　Sclerosing Solution, 45520
　Lesion
　　Excision, 45108
　Manometry, 91122
　Prolapse
　　Excision, 45130-45135
　Removal
　　Fecal Impaction, 45915
　　Foreign Body, 45307, 45915
　Repair
　　Fistula, 45800-45825, 46706-46707
　　Injury, 45562-45563
　　Prolapse, 45505-45541, 45900
　　Rectocele, 45560
　　Stenosis, 45500
　　with Sigmoid Excision, 45550
　Sensation, Tone, and Compliance Test, 91120
　Stricture
　　Excision, 45150
　Suture
　　Fistula, 45800-45825
　　Prolapse, 45540-45541
　Tumor
　　Destruction, 45190, 45320
　　Excision, 45160-45172
Rectus Sheath Block
　Bilateral, 64488-64489
　Unilateral, 64486-64487
Red Blood Cell (RBC)
　Hematocrit, 85014
　Morphology, 85007
　Platelet Estimation, 85007

Red Blood Cell (RBC) — *continued*
　Sedimentation Rate
　　Automated
　　　Manual, 85651
Reflux Study
　Gastroesophageal, 91034-91038
Rehydration, 96360-96361
Reinsertion
　Drug Delivery Implant, 11983
Release
　Carpal Tunnel, 64721
　Ligament
　　Transverse Carpal, 29848
　Nerve, 64719-64721
　　Carpal Tunnel, 64721
　Scar
　　Colostomy, 44340
　　Ileostomy, 44312
　　Skin, 11042 [11045]
Remote Monitoring Physiologic Data, [99091, 99457]
Removal
　Adrenal Gland, 60650
　Allograft
　　Intestinal, 44137
　Breast
　　Modified Radical, 19307
　　Partial, 19301-19302
　　Radical, 19305-19306
　　Simple, Complete, 19303
　　Subcutaneous, 19300
　Calculi (Stone)
　　Bile Duct, 43264, 47420-47425
　　　Percutaneous, 47554
　　Gallbladder, 47480
　　Hepatic Duct, 47400
　　Pancreas, 48020
　　Pancreatic Duct, 43264
　Catheter
　　Central Venous, 36589
　　Peritoneum, 49422
　Drug Delivery Implant, 11982-11983
　Electrode
　　Stomach, 43648, 43882
　Fecal Impaction
　　Rectum, 45915
　Foreign Bodies
　　Anal, 46608
　　Bile Duct, [43275]
　　Colon, 44025, 44390, 45379
　　Colon–Sigmoid, 45332
　　Duodenum, 44010
　　Esophagus, 43020, 43194, 43215
　　Gastrointestinal, Upper, 43247
　　Intestines, Small, 44020, 44363
　　Muscle, 20520-20525
　　Pancreatic Duct, [43275]
　　Peritoneum, 49402
　　Rectum, 45307, 45915
　　Stomach, 43500
　　Subcutaneous, 10120-10121
　　Tendon Sheath, 20520-20525
　Infusion Pump
　　Intravenous, 36590
　Lung
　　Apical Tumor, 32503-32504
　Lymph Nodes
　　Abdominal, 38747
　　Inguinofemoral, 38760-38765
　　Pelvic, 38770
　　Retroperitoneal Transabdominal, 38780
　　Thoracic, 38746
　Mesh
　　Abdominal Wall, 11008
　Neurostimulator
　　Pulse Generator, 64595
　　Receiver, 64595
　Obstructive Material
　　Gastrostomy, Duodenostomy, Jejunostomy, Gastro-jejunostomy, or Cecostomy Tube, 49460
　Polyp
　　Anal, 46610, 46612
　　Colon, 44392, 45385
　　Colon–Sigmoid, 45333

Removal — *continued*
　Polyp — *continued*
　　Endoscopy, 44364-44365, 44394
　　Esophagus, 43217, 43250
　　Gastrointestinal, Upper, 43250-43251
　　Rectum, 45315
　Prosthesis
　　Abdomen, 49606
　　Abdominal Wall, 11008
　Pulse Generator
　　Vagus Nerve Blocking Therapy, 0314T-0315T
　Seton
　　Anal, 46030
　Shunt
　　Peritoneum, 49429
　Stent
　　Bile Duct, [43275, 43276]
　　Pancreatic Duct, [43275, 43276]
　Stone (Calculi)
　　Bile Duct, 43264, 47420-47425
　　　Percutaneous, 47554
　　Gallbladder, 47480
　　Hepatic Duct, 47400
　　Pancreas, 48020
　　Pancreatic Duct, 43264
　Subcutaneous Port for Gastric Restrictive Procedure, 43887-43888
　Suture
　　Anal, 46754
　　Anesthesia, 15850-15851
　Tissue Expanders, 11971
　Transplant Intestines, 44137
　Vein
　　Clusters, 37785
　　Saphenous, 37718-37735
　　Secondary, 37785
　　Varicose, 37765-37766
　Wire
　　Anal, 46754
Renal Arteries
　Atherectomy, 0234T
Renal Disease Services
　Arteriovenous Fistula
　　Revision, 36832-36833
　　Thrombectomy, 36831
　Arteriovenous Shunt
　　Revision, 36832-36833
　　Thrombectomy, 36831
Rendezvous Procedure
　Biliary Tree Access, 47541
Repair
　Abdomen, 49900
　　Hernia, 49491-49525, 49565, 49570, 49582-49590
　　Omphalocele, 49600-49611
　　Suture, 49900
　Anal
　　Anomaly, 46744-46748
　　Fistula, 46288, 46706-46716
　　High Imperforate, 46730-46742
　　Low Imperforate, 46715-46716
　　Park Posterior, 46761
　　Stricture, 46700-46705
　Aneurysm
　　Arteriovenous, 36832
　Arteriovenous Aneurysm, 36832
　Artery
　　Angioplasty, 36902-36903, 36905-36908
　　Dialysis Circuit, 36902-36903, 36905-36908
　Bile Duct
　　with Intestines, 47760, 47780-47785
　　Wound, 47900
　Bladder
　　Fistula, 44660-44661, 45800-45805
　Blood Vessel(s)
　　Graft Defect, 35870
　Bypass Graft, 35907
　　Fistula, 35870
　Cannula, 36860-36861
　Central Venous Catheter, 36575-36576
　Cloacal Anomaly, 46744-46748
　Colon
　　Fistula, 44650-44661

Repair — *continued*
　Colon — *continued*
　　Hernia, 44050
　　Malrotation, 44055
　　Obstruction, 44050
　Cyst
　　Liver, 47300
　Diaphragm
　　for Eventration, 39545
　　Hernia, 39503-39541
　　Lacerations, 39501
　Esophagus, 43300, 43310-43314
　　Esophagogastrostomy, 43112, 43320
　　Esophagojejunostomy, 43340-43341
　　Fistula, 43305, 43312, 43314, 43420-43425
　　Fundoplasty, 43325-43328
　　Hiatal Hernia, 43332-43337
　　Muscle, 43330-43331
　　Preexisting Perforation, 43405
　　Wound, 43410-43415
　Fistula
　　Anal, 46706
　　Anoperineal, 46715-46716
　　Anorectal, 46707
　　Graft-Enteric Fistula, 35870
　　Ileoanal Pouch, 46710-46712
　　Rectourethral, 46740-46742
　　Rectovaginal, 46740-46742
　Gallbladder
　　with Gastroenterostomy, 47741
　　with Intestines, 47720-47740
　Hepatic Duct
　　with Intestines, 47765, 47802
　Hernia
　　Abdomen, 49565, 49590
　　　Incisional or Ventral, 49560
　　Diaphragmatic, 39503-39541
　　Epigastric
　　　Incarcerated, 49572
　　　Reducible, 49570
　　Femoral, 49550
　　　Incarcerated, 49553
　　　Initial
　　　　Incarcerated, 49553
　　　　Reducible, 49550
　　　Recurrent, 49555
　　　Recurrent Incarcerated, 49557
　　　Reducible Recurrent, 49555
　　Hiatus, 43332-43337
　　Incisional
　　　Initial
　　　　Incarcerated, 49566
　　　　Reducible, 49560
　　　Recurrent
　　　　Reducible, 49565
　　Inguinal
　　　Initial
　　　　by Laparoscopy, 49650
　　　　Incarcerated, 49496, 49501, 49507
　　　　Reducible, 49491, 49495, 49500, 49505
　　　　Strangulated, 49492, 49496, 49501, 49507
　　　Laparoscopy, 49650-49651
　　　Older Than 50 Weeks, Younger Than 6 Months, 49496
　　　Preterm Older Than 50 Weeks and Younger Than 6 Months, Full Term Infant Younger Than 6 Months, 49495-49496
　　　Preterm Up to 50 Weeks, 49491-49492
　　　Recurrent
　　　　by Laparoscopy, 49651
　　　　Incarcerated, 49521
　　　　Reducible, 49520
　　　　Strangulated, 49521
　　　Sliding, 49525
　　Intestinal, 44025-44050
　　Lumbar, 49540
　　Paracolostomy, 44346

Revision — *continued*
  Gastric Restrictive Procedure — *continued*
    Subcutaneous Port Component, 43886
  Gastrostomy Tube, 44373
  Ileostomy, 44312-44314
  Infusion Pump
    Intravenous, 36576-36578, 36582-36583
  Jejunostomy Tube, 44373
  Shunt
    Intrahepatic Portosystemic, 37183
  Stomach
    for Obesity, 43848
  Subcutaneous Port for Gastric Restrictive Procedure, 43886
  Venous Access Device, 36576-36578, 36582-36583, 36585
Rib
  Excision, 21601-21603
  Resection, 21601-21603
Ripstein Operation
  Laparoscopic, 45400
    with Sigmoid Resection, 45402
  Open, 45540-45541
    with Sigmoid Excision, 45550
Roux–en–Y Procedures
  Biliary Tract, 47740-47741, 47780-47785
  Pancreas, 48540
  Stomach, 43621, 43633, 43644, 43846
    Laparoscopic, 43644
Rubber Band Ligation
  Hemorrhoids, 46221

S

Sacrum
  Pressure Ulcer, 15931-15935
  Tumor
    Excision, 49215
Saundby Test, 82270
Schlatter Operation, 43620
Sclerotherapy
  Percutaneous (Cyst, Lymphocele, Seroma), 49185
Scribner Cannulization, 36810
Sedation
  Moderate
    with Independent Observation, 99151-99153
Sedimentation Rate
  Blood Cell
    Manual, 85651
Segmentectomy
  Breast, 19301-19302
Sengstaken Tamponade
  Esophagus, 43460
Sentinel Node
  Injection Procedure, 38792
Seroma
  Incision and Drainage
    Skin, 10140
  Sclerotherapy, Percutaneous, 49185
Serum
  Albumin, 82040
SG, 93503
Shock Wave (Extracorporeal) Therapy, 43265
Shunt(s)
  Arteriovenous Shunt
    Dialysis Circuit, 36901-36909
  Creation
    Arteriovenous
      Direct, 36821
      Thomas Shunt, 36835
      Transposition, 36818
      with Graft, 36825-36830
  LeVeen
    Insertion, 49425
    Ligation, 49428
    Removal, 49429
    Revision, 49426
  Peritoneal
    Venous
      Injection, 49427
      Ligation, 49428
      Removal, 49429

Shunt(s) — *continued*
  Revision
    Arteriovenous, 36832
    Transvenous Intrahepatic Portosystemic, 37182-37183
Sigmoidoscopy
  Ablation
    Polyp, [45346]
    Tumor, [45346]
  Biopsy, 45331
  Collection
    Specimen, 45331
  Exploration, 45330
  Hemorrhage Control, 45334
  Injection
    Submucosal, 45335
  Mucosal Resection, 45349
  Needle Biopsy, 45342
  Placement
    Stent, 45347
  Removal
    Foreign Body, 45332
    Polyp, 45333, 45338
    Tumor, 45333, 45338
  Repair
    Volvulus, 45337
  Ultrasound, 45341-45342
Sinus
  Pilonidal
    Excision, 11770-11772
    Incision and Drainage, 10080-10081
Sistrunk Operation
  Cyst, Thyroid Gland, Excision, 60200
Skin Graft and Flap
  Autograft
    Split-Thickness, 15100-15101, 15120-15121
  Free
    Full Thickness Skin Graft, 15200-15261
    Recipient Site Preparation, 15002-15005
    Split Graft, 15100-15101, 15120-15121
Skin
  Abscess
    Incision and Drainage, 10060-10061
    Puncture Aspiration, 10160
  Biopsy, 11102-11107
  Cyst
    Puncture Aspiration, 10160
  Debridement, 11004-11006, 11042-11044, 11047 [11045, 11046]
    Infected, 11004-11006
    Subcutaneous Tissue, 11042-11044, 11047 [11045, 11046]
    Infected, 11004-11006
  Decubitus Ulcer(s)
    Excision, 15920-15935, 15940-15958
  Excision
    Debridement, 11004-11006, 11042-11044 [11045, 11046]
    Hemangioma, 11400-11446
    Lesion
      Benign, 11400-11446
      Malignant, 11600-11646
  Grafts
    Free, 15200-15261
  Incision and Drainage, 10060-10180
  Wound Repair
    Abdomen
      Complex, 13100-13102
      Intermediate, 12031-12037
      Layered, 12031-12037
      Simple, 12001-12007
      Superficial, 12001-12007
    Arm, Arms
      Complex, 13120-13122
      Intermediate, 12031-12037
      Layered, 12031-12037
      Simple, 12001-12007
      Superficial, 12001-12007
    Axilla, Axillae
      Complex, 13131-13133
      Intermediate, 12031-12037
      Layered, 12031-12037
      Simple, 12001-12007
      Superficial, 12001-12007

Skin — *continued*
  Wound Repair — *continued*
    Back
      Complex, 13100-13102
      Intermediate, 12031-12037
      Layered, 12031-12037
      Simple, 12001-12007
      Superficial, 12001-12007
    Breast
      Complex, 13100-13102
      Intermediate, 12031-12037
      Layered, 12031-12037
      Simple, 12001-12007
      Superficial, 12001-12007
    Buttock
      Complex, 13100-13102
      Intermediate, 12031-12037
      Layered, 12031-12037
      Simple, 12001-12007
      Superficial, 12001-12007
    Chest
      Complex, 13100-13102
      Intermediate, 12031-12037
      Layered, 12031-12037
      Simple, 12001-12007
      Superficial, 12001-12007
    Extremity, Extremities
      Complex/Intermediate, 12031-12037
      Layered, 12031-12037
      Simple, 12001-12007
      Superficial, 12001-12007
    Forearm, Forearms
      Complex, 13120-13122
      Intermediate, 12031-12037
      Layered, 12031-12037
      Simple, 12001-12007
      Superficial, 12001-12007
    Leg, Legs
      Complex, 13120-13122
      Intermediate, 12031-12037
      Layered, 12031-12037
      Simple, 12001-12007
      Superficial, 12001-12007
    Lower
      Arm, Arms
        Complex, 13120-13122
        Intermediate, 12031-12037
        Layered, 12031-12037
        Simple, 12001-12007
        Superficial, 12001-12007
      Extremity, Extremities
        Complex, 13120-13122
        Intermediate, 12031-12037
        Layered, 12031-12037
        Simple, 12001-12007
        Superficial, 12001-12007
      Leg, Legs
        Complex, 13120-13122
        Intermediate, 12031-12037
        Layered, 12031-12037
        Simple, 12001-12007
        Superficial, 12001-12007
    Neck
      Complex, 13131-13133
      Intermediate, 12041-12047
      Layered, 12041-12047
      Simple, 12001-12007
      Superficial, 12001-12007
    Trunk
      Complex, 13100-13102
      Intermediate, 12031-12037
      Layered, 12031-12037
      Simple, 12001-12007
      Superficial, 12001-12007
    Upper
      Arm, Arms
        Complex, 13120-13122
        Intermediate, 12031-12037
        Layered, 12031-12037
        Simple, 12001-12007
        Superficial, 12001-12007
      Extremity
        Complex, 13120-13122
        Intermediate, 12031-12037
        Layered, 12031-12037

Skin — *continued*
  Wound Repair — *continued*
    Upper — *continued*
      Extremity — *continued*
        Simple, 12001-12007
        Superficial, 12001-12007
      Leg, Legs
        Complex, 13120-13122
        Intermediate, 12031-12037
        Layered, 12031-12037
        Simple, 12001-12007
        Superficial, 12001-12007
Sleep Endoscopy
  Drug-induced, 42975
Sleeve Gastrectomy, 43775
Small Bowel
  Endoscopy, 44360-44380, 44382-44386 [44381]
    with Tumor Removal
      Ablation, 44369
      Bipolar Cautery, 44365
      Hot Biopsy Forceps, 44365
      Snare Technique, 44364
  Enterectomy, 44120-44128
    Laparoscopic, 44202-44203
  Enterotomy, 44020-44021
    for Lesion Removal, 44110-44111
Soave Procedure, 45120
Soft Tissue
  Image-Guided Drainage with Catheter, 10030
Sore, Bed
  Excision, 15920-15935, 15940-15958
Special Services
  After Hours Medical Services, 99050
  Analysis
    Remote Physiologic Data, [99091]
  Device Handling, 99002
  Emergency Care in Office, 99058
  Group Education, 99078
  Non–office Medical Services, 99056
  On Call, Hospital Mandated, 99026-99027
  Postoperative Visit, 99024
  Prolonged Attendance, 99354-99360 [99415, 99416, 99417]
  Remote Physiological Monitoring, [99091, 99457]
  Reports and Forms
    Medical, 99080
  Specimen Handling, 99000-99001
  Supply of Materials, 99070, 99072
    Educational, 99071
  Unusual Travel, 99082
Specific Gravity
  with Urinalysis, 81000-81003
Specimen Collection
  Intestines, 43756-43757
  Stomach, 43754-43755
  Venous Catheter, 36591-36592
Specimen Handling, 99000-99001
Spectroscopy
  Radiofrequency, Partial Mastectomy, 0546T
Sphincter of Oddi
  Pressure Measurement
    Endoscopy, 43263
Sphincter
  Anal
    Dilation, 45905
    Incision, 46080
  Pyloric
    Incision, 43520
    Reconstruction, 43800
Sphincteroplasty
  Anal, 46750-46751, 46760-46761
  Bile Duct, 47460, 47542
Sphincterotomy
  Anal, 46080
  Bile Duct, 47460
Spine
  Incision and Drainage
    Abscess, 22010-22015
Spleen
  Excision, 38100-38102
    Laparoscopic, 38120
  Repair, 38115

● **New** ▲ **Revised** + **Add On** **AMA: CPT Assist** **[Resequenced]**

Coding Companion for General Surgery/Gastroenterology

CPT © 2021 American Medical Association. All Rights Reserved.

● New   ▲ Revised   + Add On   AMA: CPT Assist[Resequenced]

© 2021 Optum360, LLC

Coding Companion for General Surgery/Gastroenterology

907

CPT Index

Thoracic
Duct
  Ligation, 38380
    Abdominal Approach, 38382
    Thoracic Approach, 38381
  Suture, 38380
    Abdominal Approach, 38382
    Cervical Approach, 38380
    Thoracic Approach, 38381
Empyema
  Incision and Drainage, 21501-21502

Thoracostomy
Tube, 32551

Thoracotomy
Esophagogastric Fundoplasty, 43328
Hiatal Hernia Repair, 43334-43335
Neonatal, 39503

Thorax
Biopsy, 21550
Incision
  Pneumothorax, 32551
Incision and Drainage
  Abscess, 21501-21502
  Hematoma, 21501-21502
Tumor, 21555-21558 [21552, 21554]

Thrombectomy
Arterial, Mechanical, 37184-37185
Arteriovenous Fistula
  Graft, 36904-36906
Bypass Graft
  Noncoronary/Nonintracranial, 37184-
    37186
Dialysis Circuit, 36904-36906
Dialysis Graft
  without Revision, 36831
Percutaneous
  Noncoronary, Nonintracranial, 37184-
    37186
Vein, 37187-37188
Venous, Mechanical, 37187-37188

Thrombocyte (Platelet)
Count, 85008

Thymectomy, 60520-60521
Sternal Split
  Transthoracic Approach, 60521-60522
Transcervical Approach, 60520

Thymus Gland, 60520
Excision, 60520-60521

Thyroglossal Duct
Cyst
  Excision, 60280-60281

Thyroid Gland
Ablation
  Nodule, 0673T
Cyst
  Aspiration, 60300
  Excision, 60200
  Incision and Drainage, 60000
  Injection, 60300
Excision
  for Malignancy
    Limited Neck Dissection, 60252
    Radical Neck Dissection, 60254
  Partial, 60210-60225
  Secondary, 60260
  Total, 60240, 60271
    Cervical Approach, 60271
    Removal All Thyroid Tissue,
      60260
    Sternal Split
      Transthoracic Approach,
        60270
    Transcervical Approach, 60520
Needle Biopsy, 60100
Tumor
  Excision, 60200

Thyroid Isthmus
Transection, 60200

Thyroidectomy
Partial, 60210-60225
Secondary, 60260
Total, 60240, 60271
  Cervical Approach, 60271
    for Malignancy
      Limited Neck Dissection,
        60252

Thyroidectomy — continued
Total — continued
  Cervical Approach — continued
    for Malignancy — continued
      Radical Neck Dissection,
        60254
  Removal All Thyroid Tissue, 60260
  Sternal Split
    Transthoracic Approach, 60270

Thyrolingual Cyst
Incision and Drainage, 60000

TIG (Tetanus Immune Globulin) Vaccine, 90389
TIG, 90389

Time
Bleeding, 85002

TIPS (Transvenous Intrahepatic Portosystemic Shunt) Procedure, 37182-37183

Tissue
Culture
  Skin Grafts, 15100-15101, 15120-
    15121
Expander
  Insertion
    Skin, 11960
  Removal
    Skin, 11971
  Replacement
    Skin, 11970

TMJ
Arthrocentesis, 20605-20606

Total
Bilirubin Level, 82247
Esophagectomy, 43107-43113, 43124,
  43286-43288
Gastrectomy, 43620-43622
Splenectomy, 38100, 38102

Toupet Procedure, 43280
Toxin, Botulinum
Chemodenervation
  Internal Anal Sphincter, 46505
  Trunk Muscle, 64646-64647

Trachea
Incision
  Emergency, 31603-31605
  Planned, 31600-31601
  with Flaps, 31610

Tracheal
Tube, 31500

Tracheoesophageal Fistula
Repair, 43305, 43312, 43314

Tracheostomy
Emergency, 31603-31605
Planned, 31600-31601
with Flaps, 31610

Transection
Nerve, 64755-64760
  Vagus, 43640-43641

Transfer
Jejunum
  Free, 43496

Transluminal
Angioplasty
  Arterial, 36902-36903, 36905-36906
Atherectomies, 0234T-0238T

Transnasal
Esophagogastroduodenoscopy, 0652T-
  0654T
Esophagoscopy, 43197-43198

Transplant
Islet Cell, 0584T-0586T

Transplantation
Backbench Preparation Prior to Transplan-
  tation
  Intestine, 44715-44721
  Liver, 47143-47147
  Pancreas, 48551-48552
Intestines
  Allograft Preparation, 44715-44721
  Allotransplantation, 44135-44136
  Donor Enterectomy, 44132-44133
  Removal of Allograft, 44137
Islet Cell, 0584T-0586T
Liver
  Allograft Preparation, 47143-47147
Pancreas
  Allograft Preparation, 48551-48552

Transplantation — continued
Pancreatic Islet Cell, 0584T-0586T
  with Pancreatectomy, 48160

Transposition
Nerve, 64719-64721

Transversus Abdominis Plane (TAP) Block
Bilateral, 64488-64489
Unilateral, 64486-64487

Travel, Unusual, 99082
Trendelenburg Operation, 37785
Tri-incisional Esophagectomy, 43112
Trigger Point
Acupuncture, [20560, 20561]

Trisegmentectomy, 47122
Trochanter
Pressure Ulcer, 15950-15958

Truncal Vagotomies, 43640
Truncus Brachiocephalicus
Atherectomy, 0237T

Trunk
Skin Graft
  Full Thickness, 15200
  Split, 15100-15101

Tube Change
Colonic, 49450
Duodenostomy, 49451
Gastro-Jejunostomy, 49452
Gastrostomy, 43762-43763, 49446
Jejunostomy, 49451

Tube Placement
Cecostomy, 44300, 49442
Chest, 32551
Colonic, 49442
Duodenostomy, 49441
Enterostomy, 44300
Gastrostomy, 43246, 49440
Jejunostomy, 49441
Nasogastric, 43752
Orogastric, 43752

Tubes
Chest, 32551
Endotracheal, 31500
Gastrostomy, 43246, 49440

Tudor "Rabbit Ear"
Urethra, Repair
  Fistula, 45820-45825

Tumor
Abdomen
  Destruction
    Excision, 49203-49205
Abdominal Wall, 22900-22905
Acetabulum
  Excision, 27076
Arm, Lower, 25075-25078 [25071, 25073]
Arm, Upper, 24075-24079 [24071, 24073]
Back, 21930-21936
Bile Duct
  Ablation, [43278]
  Extrahepatic, 47711
  Intrahepatic, 47712
Breast
  Cryoablation, 0581T
  Excision, 19120-19126
Chest Wall
  Excision, 21601-21603
Coccyx, 49215
Colon
  Destruction, [44401, 45388]
  Removal, 44392, 44394, 45384-45385
Destruction
  Abdomen, 49203-49205
  Chemosurgery, 17311-17315
Esophagus
  Ablation, 43229
Flank, 21930-21936
Forearm
  Radical Resection, 25077
Ilium, 27075-27076
Innominate
  Excision, 27077
Intestines, Small
  Destruction, 44369
  Removal, 44364-44365
Ischial Tuberosity, 27078
Leg, Lower, 27615-27619 [27632]

Tumor — continued
Leg, Upper
  Excision, 27327-27364 [27329, 27337,
    27339]
Liver
  Ablation, 47380-47383
Neck, 21555-21558 [21552, 21554]
Olecranon Process, 24075-24077 [24071,
  24073]
Pancreatic Duct
  Ablation, [43278]
Pelvis, 27047-27049 [27043, 27045]
Rectum, 45160-45190, 0184T
Retroperitoneal
  Destruction
    Excision, 49203-49205
Sacrum, 49215
Soft Tissue
  Forearm
    Radical Resection, 25077
Stomach
  Excision, 43610-43611
Thorax, 21555-21558 [21552, 21554]
Thyroid
  Excision, 60200

Tylectomy, 19120-19126

U

UCX (Urine Culture), 87086-87088
Ulcer
Anal
  Destruction, 46940-46942
  Excision, 46200
Pressure, 15920-15935, 15940-15958
Stomach
  Excision, 43610

Ulnar Nerve
Neuroplasty, 64719
Reconstruction, 64719
Release, 64719
Transposition, 64719

Ultrasound
Colon
  Endoscopic, 45391-45392
Colon–Sigmoid
  Endoscopic, 45341-45342
Esophagus
  Endoscopy, 43231-43232
Gastrointestinal, Upper
  Endoscopic, 43242, 43259
Guidance
  Esophagogastroduodenoscopy
    Examination, 43237, 43259
    Fine Needle Aspiration/Biopsy,
      43238, 43242
    with Drainage Pseudocyst with
      Placement
      Catheters/Stents, 43240
    with Injection Diagnostic or
      Therapeutic Substance,
      43253
  Needle Biopsy, 43232, 43242, 45342
Needle or Catheter Insertion, 20555

Umbilical
Hernia
  Repair, 49580-49587
  Omphalocele, 49600-49611

Umbilicus
Repair
  Hernia, 49580-49587
  Omphalocele, 49600-49611

Unilateral Simple Mastectomy, 19303
Upper
Gastrointestinal Bleeding
  Endoscopic Control, 43255
Gastrointestinal Endoscopy, Biopsy, 43239

Urea Nitrogen, 84525
Blood, 84525
Semiquantitative, 84525

Urethra
Repair
  Fistula, 45820-45825
Suture
  Fistula, 45820-45825

Urethroplasty, 46744-46746
Urinalysis, 81000-81003, 81007